Oxford Textbook of

Medical Education

Oxford Textbook of
Medical Education

Edited by

Kieran Walsh

Clinical Director
BMJ Learning, London, UK

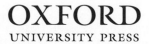

OXFORD

UNIVERSITY PRESS

OXFORD

UNIVERSITY PRESS

Great Clarendon Street, Oxford, OX2 6DP,
United Kingdom

Oxford University Press is a department of the University of Oxford.
It furthers the University's objective of excellence in research, scholarship,
and education by publishing worldwide. Oxford is a registered trade mark of
Oxford University Press in the UK and in certain other countries

© Oxford University Press 2013

Chapter 59 Adapted from The Lancet, 376, Frenk et al., 'Health professionals for a new century:
transforming education to strengthen health systems in an interdependent world', pp. 1923–1958,
© 2010, with permission from Elsevier.

The moral rights of the author have been asserted

First Edition published in 2013

Impression: 1

Published in the United States of America by Oxford University Press
198 Madison Avenue, New York, NY 10016, United States of America

British Library Cataloguing in Publication Data

Data available

Library of Congress Control Number: 2013938049

ISBN 978–0–19–965267–9

Printed and bound in China by
C&C Offset Printing Co. Ltd.

For Sarah Jane, Tommie Jack, and Catie Sue

Foreword

In the 1970s, in Sweden, Roger Saljo was interested in how people learn and why there are differences in the ways people go about learning. He asked a group of people from a variety of backgrounds the question 'what do you actually mean by learning?' (Saljo 1979). His respondents provided answers ranging from those individuals who thought learning was something to be taken for granted to those for whom learning was something that can be 'explicitly talked about and become the object of conscious planning and analysis' (Saljo 1979). Saljo categorized the responses into a hierarchy beginning with learning as simply an increase in knowledge; through learning as memorizing; to the acquisition of facts and skills of purely practical value; and onto learning as the abstraction of meaning, in which what is studied is in some way changed, and not simply reproduced. Learning is thus a constructive act with what is learned acting as the starting point for further learning. The final category identified learning as an interpretive process aimed at understanding or interpreting the world in which the learner lives. Saljo's work in Sweden with Ference Marton and then later with Noel Entwistle and others in Edinburgh, and that of John Biggs in Australia, went on to define and elaborate issues such as *surface*, *deep*, and *strategic* learners, orientations and approaches to learning, and, eventually, to ways of measuring differences in learning between people and to estimating the effects these differences have on learning outcomes.

In the 1990s, Michael Eraut in England was interested in how professional knowledge and competence developed. He classified knowledge underpinning professional practice into three types: *Propositional*, *Personal*, and *Process* knowledge. He further subdivided *Process* knowledge into five subtypes: *acquiring information*, *skilled behaviour*, *deliberative processes*, *giving information*, and *self-monitoring*. His work has gone on to make clear how professionals learn in the workplace and has shown that much of this learning is informal, commonplace, and is largely unstructured or recognized as learning. He has argued that the context of learning and the context of use of knowledge are both centrally important to effective practice (Eraut 1994).

Both David Irby in San Francisco and Scott Wright in Baltimore have been interested in the qualities of excellent teachers (Irby 1995; Wright et al. 1998). Their work has been exceptionally helpful in clarifying how faculty development programmes can be structured to help aspiring teachers achieve the best standards including understanding the importance of effective teacher-learner relationships, excellent communication skills and enthusiasm for their subject.

More recently, Tim Dornan in Manchester (and latterly in Maastricht), has been interested in the relationship between medical learner, clinical teacher, and the patient (McLachlan et al. 2012). This triadic relationship is central to medical education and yet remains largely unstudied despite the enormous number of teaching encounters engaging these three protagonists that occur each day across the world. Thinking about this triad has engaged other researchers in considering notions of power (Bleakley et al. 2011; Rees et al. 2013) of 'absence' (Bleakley et al. 2008) (when just the learner and teacher are 'present' and the patient is either simulated, considered as a paper case, or as most often happens, does not appear at all—in for example lectures or seminars about 'basic science') and of collaborative learning (Bell et al. 2009) between patient, student and doctor.

I have picked these four examples of research into teaching and, especially, into medical teaching, because not only do they demonstrate the cardinal importance of the learner, the teacher, and the patient in any teaching episode, but also because they give a flavour of the extensive range of enquiry that underpins contemporary medical education. I could have chosen any number of other examples from this range but I particularly wanted to use material that has influenced my own practice as a clinical teacher over the last thirty years.

During this time the role and importance of teaching has grown both in medical schools and in the health services, and along with this increasing professionalization has come a burgeoning appreciation of, and demand for, high quality research evidence that can be used by students and practitioners to develop and improve the study and practice of medical teaching. Specific training and qualifications in medical education are now widely available in the UK and in many other countries, and the number of textbooks and journals publishing material about medical education has increased—in both paper and in electronic formats, greatly enabling the retrieval of source materials that in earlier years could be found only after extensive reading and searching. Most recently, specific standards for medical teachers have been published by regulators and professional bodies indicating that medical education is becoming a discipline in its own right (Academy of Medical Educators 2012; Collins 2009; General Medical Council 2012).

This growth in the awareness of the power of medical education to improve the quality of care has been accompanied by the development a robust scholarly archive that provides a strong grounding for building a vigorous future.

For Calman (1999), the purpose of medical education is to produce a skilled workforce but, of course, in doing so the overarching aim is to improve the quality of care for patients, and for populations, through effective practice, leadership and clinically focused research. Brian Hodges believes that in order to bring about the paradigmatic changes that are required to produce such doctors, we need 'a corps of medical educators and clinical teachers with a strong grasp of theory, sustained by well-honed pedagogical and research skills' (Hodges 2011).

This then is the book for the modern clinical teacher. It is a comprehensive and evidence-based guide to all those who have a role or an interest in the training and education of doctors; and, unlike many other textbooks in the field, it covers the educational principles, the underpinning evidence, and the application of what is known to all aspects of medical education from curriculum design to standard setting for assessment, and from selecting students for medical school to continuing professional development of practising clinicians.

The editor, Kieran Walsh, deserves our congratulations for bringing together an outstanding international group of experienced authors who have jointly produced a text that is authoritative and comprehensive but which is also, and this is a most important quality indicator for any text, immensely readable and enjoyable.

John Bligh
Professor of Medical Education
Cardiff University
Wales , UK

References

Academy of Medical Educators (2012) *Professional Standards 2012*. London: Academy of Medical Educators

Bell, K., Boshuizen, H.P.A., Scherpbier, A., and Dornan, T. (2009) When only the real thing will do: junior medical students' learning from real patients. *Med Educ.* 43(11): 1036–1043

Bleakley, A. and Bligh, J. (2008) Students learning from patients: let's get real in medical education. *Adv Health Sci Educ.* 13(1): 89–107

Bleakley, A., Bligh, J., and Browne, J. (2011) *Medical Education for the Future: Identity, Power and Location*. London: Springer

Byrne, P.S., (1971) quoting Jean Piaget in: Byrne, P.S. 'Men Capable of Doing New Things' (The W Victor Johnson Oration). *Can Fam Physician.* 17(12): 29–35

Calman, K. (1999) Foreword. In N. Boaden, and J. Bligh, (eds) *Community Based Medical Education: towards a shared agenda for learning*. London: Hodder Arnold

Collins, J.P. (2009) An academy of surgical educators: why, how and who. *ANZ J Surg.* 79: A70

Eraut, M. (1994) *Developing Professional Knowledge and Competence*. London: Falmer Press

General Medical Council (2012) *Recognising and Approving Trainers: the implementation plan*. London: General Medical Council

Hodges, B. (2011) Foreword. In A. Bleakley, J. Bligh, and J. Browne (eds) *Medical Education for the Future: Identity, Power and Location* (p. vi). Springer: Dordrecht

Irby, D.M. (1995) Teaching and learning in ambulatory settings: a thematic review of the literature. *Acad Med.* 70: 898–931

McLachlan, E., King, N., Wenger, E., and Dornan, T. (2012) Phenomenological analysis of patient experiences of medical student teaching encounters. *Med Educ.* 46(10): 963–973

Rees, C.E., Ajjawi, R., and Monrouxe, L.V. (2013) The construction of power in family medicine bedside teaching: a video observation study. *Med Educ.* 47(2): 154–165

Saljo, R. (1979) Learning about learning. *Higher Educ.* 8: 443–451

Wright, S.M., Kern, D.E., Kolodner, K., Howard, D.M., and Brancati, F.L. (1998) Attributes of excellent attending-physician role models. *N Engl J Med.* 339: 1986–1993

Preface

All is now flux in medical education where once all was stasis.

Reproduced from *British Medical Journal*, Chris McManus, 'New pathways to medical education: learning to learn at Harvard', 311, p. 67, copyright 1995, with permission from BMJ Publishing Group Ltd

Medical education is an important business. We rely on those who are responsible for medical education to deliver newly qualified doctors who are fit to start work, junior doctors in training who are able to practice under supervision, and fully qualified specialists and general practitioners who are fit to practice independently and, perhaps more importantly, are equipped with lifelong learning skills that will keep them up to date over a 30 year career. At the same time the medical educator must ensure that curricula are designed according to best practice principles, that assessments are valid and reliable and that evaluations of education programmes are fair and useful to a range of stakeholders. When all these things go right, then doctors and other healthcare professionals have the necessary knowledge, skills and behaviours to provide the best possible care for their patients; when they go wrong, teachers, learners and patients alike suffer. But there is a great deal of complexity and some controversy and one might reasonably ask: 'where is the medical educator to find all that they need to deliver their service?'. The purpose of this book is to provide a comprehensive and evidence-based reference guide for those who have a scholarly interest in medical education. The aim of the book is to give an account of the theoretical educational principles that lay the foundations of best practice in medical education, to explain the evidence base that backs up best practice, and finally to explicitly state how to put both theory and evidence into practice for the benefit of learners and ultimately patients. As Chris McManus says 'medical education is currently in a state of flux' and the aim of this book is to capture the current state of that flux, albeit safe in the knowledge that the pace of change will continue unabated for some time to come.

In putting together the book I have been delighted and proud to work with a wide range of authors who have contributed to the content. Recruitment of authors from different backgrounds, disciplines and continents was a deliberate attempt to create a book that would be both original and international. The only factor that all contributors have in common is the achievement of excellence in their fields—something that is clearly reflected in the content of their chapters. All were given broadly the same brief—to create content that was academically sound with a strong evidence base; to create content that would answer the majority of relevant questions on the topic; and, that most difficult of tasks, to follow these rules and at the same time create content that was accessible and practical and useful to readers. My brief was to try to put it all together and create a coherent volume. If I have to any degree succeeded then it is very much down to individual authors who have given time, energy and care to their chapters. Amongst this final cohort of authors we've faced numerous challenges—but all of these authors have delivered and this book is a credit to them and their perseverance and professionalism.

The Oxford textbooks have had a long tradition in many of the major medical specialties and it has been an honour to work with staff at the Oxford University Press to help create the first Oxford textbook in this still young specialty. Particular praise must go to Chris Reid who had the vision to take the idea forward and to Fiona Richardson and Geraldine Jeffers for making that vision a reality.

My colleagues at BMJ Learning also deserve special mention and particular thanks must go to Catrin Thomas and Edward Briffa for their encouragement and support. Medical education has always been a practical specialty and it continues to be a constant source of personal learning to put the new ideas in the various chapters of this book into practice for the benefit of the users of BMJ Learning.

Lastly and most importantly this book would not have been possible without the help of my family—Sarah Jane, Tommie Jack and Catie Sue—and this book is dedicated to them. With their encouragement I have tried to examine the various ideas and concepts in medical education with an open mind and in a spirit of enquiry. I feel that the future of medical education will always belong to those with an enquiring mind—those who, like the father of modern surgery, never stop asking questions.

When I was a boy I wanted to know all about the clouds and the grasses, and why the leaves changed colour in the autumn, I watched the ants, bees, birds, tadpoles, and caddis-worms: I pestered people with questions about what nobody knew or cared anything about.

John Hunter (1728–1793) (Sampson Handley 1939 p. 313)

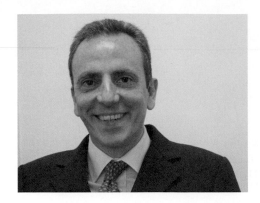

References

McManus IC. New pathways to medical education: learning to learn at
    Harvard Medical School. BMJ 1995; 311: 67
Sampson Handley W. Makers of John Hunter (1728–93). BMJ 1939; 1: 313

Dr Kieran Walsh
London, UK

Acknowledgements

Chapter 45:
We would like to acknowledge the support of the Academy for Innovation in Medical Education, University of Ottawa and its founder, the late Dr Meridith Marks (1962–2012).

Chapter 52:
I would like to thank Dr Bryan Burford, Dr Jane Margetts and Mr Paul Crampton for their helpful comments and suggestions on this chapter.

Chapter 59:
This chapter is adapted from The Lancet, 376, Frenk et al., 'Health professionals for a new century: transforming education to strengthen health systems in an interdependent world', pp. 1923–1958, Copyright 2010, with permission from Elsevier.

Contents

About the editor *xvii*

Contributors *xvii*

Abbreviations *xxv*

PART 1
Introduction *1*

1. **Introduction** *3*
   Kieran Walsh

PART 2
Curriculum *11*

2. **Curriculum design in context** *13*
   Janet Grant, Mohamed Y. H. Abdelrahmen,
   and Anand Zachariah

3. **Problem-based learning** *25*
   Mark A. Albanese and Laura C. Dast

4. **Interprofessional education: learning
   together in health and social care** *38*
   Hugh Barr and Richard Gray

5. **Student choice in the undergraduate
   curriculum: student-selected components** *50*
   Simon C. Riley and Michael J. Murphy

6. **Integrated learning** *63*
   David Prideaux, Julie Ash, and Anaise Cottrell

7. **Instructional design for medical education** *74*
   John Sweller, Jeroen J.G. van Merriënboer

8. **Using concept maps in medical education** *86*
   Dario M. Torre and Barbara J. Daley

9. **Creating the learning environment** *100*
   Rachel Isba

PART 3
Identity *111*

10. **Identities, self and medical education** *113*
    Lynn V. Monrouxe

11. **Personality and medical education** *124*
    Eva Doherty

12. **Medical education and its context in society** *136*
    Elise Paradis, Fiona Webster, and Ayelet Kuper

PART 4
Delivery *149*

13. **Small group learning** *151*
    Joy Rudland

14. **Large group teaching** *163*
    Janet Tworek, Rachel Ellaway, and Tim Dornan

15. **E-learning** *174*
    John Sandars

16. **Simulation-based medical education** *186*
    Margaret Bearman, Debra Nestel,
    and Pamela Andreatta

17. **Simulated patients in medical education** *198*
    Jennifer Cleland, Keiko Abe, and Jan-Joost Rethans

18. **Work-based learning** *209*
    Clare Morris and Martina Behrens

19. **Learning in ambulatory care** 221
John Dent

20. **The humanities in medical education** 233
John Spicer, Debbie Harrison, and Jo Winning

21. **Study skills** 244
Raja C. Bandaranayke

PART 5
Supervision 255

22. **Educational supervision** 257
Susan Kilminster and David Cottrell

23. **Mentoring** 265
Erik Driessen and Karlijn Overeem

24. **Professionalism** 275
John Goldie, Al Dowie, Phil Cotton, and Jill Morrison

25. **The resident as teacher** 288
Tzu-Chieh Yu, Susan E. Farrell, and Andrew G. Hill

26. **Students learning to teach** 300
Michael T. Ross and Terese Stenfors-Hayes

27. **Patient involvement in medical education** 311
Angela Towle and William Godolphin

PART 6
Stages 323

28. **Undergraduate medical education** 325
H. Thomas Aretz and Elizabeth G. Armstrong

29. **Postgraduate medical education** 340
Jamiu O. Busari and Ashley Duits

30. **Continuing professional development** 350
Karen V. Mann and Joan M. Sargeant

31. **Remediation** 362
David Mendel, Alex Jamieson, and Julia Whiteman

32. **Transitions in medical education** 372
Michiel Westerman and Pim W. Teunissen

PART 7
Selection 383

33. **Selection into medical education, training and practice** 385
Fiona Patterson

34. **Study dropout in medical education** 398
Gilbert Reibnegger and Simone Manhal

PART 8
Assessment 407

35. **Principles of assessment** 409
Lambert W. T. Schuwirth and Julie Ash

36. **Setting standards** 421
Danette W. McKinley and John J. Norcini

37. **Choosing instruments for assessment** 432
Sean McAleer and Madawa Chandratilake

38. **Test-enhanced learning** 443
Douglas P. Larsen and Andrew C. Butler

39. **Assessing learners' needs** 453
Casey B. White, Lou Ann Cooper,
Mary Edwards, and Jennifer Lyon

40. **Self-regulated learning in medical education** 465
Timothy J. Cleary, Steven J. Durning, Larry D. Gruppen,
Paul A. Hemmer, and Anthony R. Artino, Jr.

41. **Formative assessment** 478
Diana F. Wood

42. **Technology enhanced assessment in medical education** 489
Zubair Amin

43. **Assessing professionalism** 500
Richard Hays

44. **Assessment in the context of relicensure** 513
W. Dale Dauphinee

45. **Objective structured clinical examinations** 524
Susan Humphrey-Murto, Claire
Touchie, and Sydney Smee

46. **Workplace-based assessment** 537
Gominda Ponnamperuma

47. **Written assessment** 549
Kevin Hays

48. **Successful feedback: embedded in the culture** 564
Julian Archer and Joan M. Sargeant

PART 9
Quality 575

49. **Evaluation** 577
John Goldie and Jill Morrison

50. **Continuous quality improvement** 589
Jan Kleijnen, Diana Dolmans,
Jos Willems, and Hans van Hout

51. **Cost and value in medical education** *601*
Kieran Walsh

PART 10
Research and scholarship *613*

52. **Theoretical perspectives in medical education research** *615*
Jan Illing

53. **Quantitative research methods in medical education** *626*
Tyrone Donnon

54. **Qualitative research in medical education** *638*
Patricia McNally

55. **Publishing in medical education** *648*
Steven L. Kanter, Victoria A. Groce, and Eliza Beth Littleton

56. **Scholarship in medical education** *658*
Christie L. Palladino, Maryellen E. Gusic, Ruth-Marie E. Fincher, and Janet P. Hefler

PART 11
Global medical education *669*

57. **Medical education in developing countries** *671*
Francesca Celletti, Erich Buch, and Badara Samb

58. **Medical education in the emerging market economies** *683*
Manisha Nair and Premila Webster

PART 12
The future *695*

59. **The future of health professional education** *697*
Julio Frenk, Lincoln Chen, and Catherine Michaud

60. **Faculty development for teaching improvement: from individual to organizational change** *711*
Yvonne Steinert

61. **Educational leadership** *722*
Judy McKimm, Phil Cotton, Anne Garden, and Gillian Needham

Index *737*

About the editor

Dr Kieran Walsh is Clinical Director of BMJ Learning—the education service of the BMJ Group. He is responsible for the editorial direction of BMJ Online Learning, BMJ Masterclasses and BMJ onExamination. He has written over 200 articles for publication—mainly in the field of medical education. He has previously written two books—the first on cost and value in medical education and the second a dictionary of medical education quotations. He has worked in the past as a hospital doctor—specialising in care of the elderly medicine and neurology.

Contributors

Dr Mohamed Y. H. Abdelrahmen
Consultant Surgeon, Khartoum University Clinic, and
Director of Examinations, Evaluation and Accreditation
Sudan Medical Council
Khartoum, Sudan

Keiko Abe
Department of General Medicine
Nagoya University Graduate School of Medicine
65 Tsurumai-cho Showa-ku
Nagoya, 466-8560
Japan

Mark A. Albanese PhD
Director of Research, National Conference of Bar Examiners
302 South Bedford Street;
Departments of Population Health Sciences and Educational
Leadership and Policy Analysis School of Medicine and
Public Health
University of Wisconsin-Madison
610 Walnut Street, 1007C
Madison, Wisconsin
USA

Professor Zubair Amin
Yong Loo Lin School of Medicine
National University Hospital
Singapore

Professor Pamela Andreatta
SimPORTAL
University of Minnesota Medical School
A509 Mayo (MMC 394)
420 Delaware St SE
Minneapolis, MN 55455
USA

Dr Julian Archer
NIHR Career Development Fellow
Academic Clinical Lecturer in Medical Education
Director of the Collaboration for the Advancement of Medical
Education Research & Assessment (CAMERA)
Plymouth University Peninsula Schools of Medicine & Dentistry
C408 Portland Square
University of Plymouth Campus
Plymouth, PL4 8AA
UK

Dr H. Thomas Aretz
Vice President, Partners HealthCare International
Associate Professor of Pathology
Harvard Medical School
100 Cambridge Street, Suite 2002
Boston, MA 02114
USA

Elizabeth G. Armstrong, PhD
Clinical Professor in Pediatrics
Harvard Macy Institute
100 Cambridge Street, Suite 2002
Boston, Massachusetts 02114
USA

Dr. Anthony R. Artino, Jr
Associate Professor of Preventive Medicine and Biometrics
Uniformed Services University of the Health Sciences
4301 Jones Bridge Road
Bethesda, MD 20814
USA

Dr Julie Ash
Head, Health Professional Education
School of Medicine
Flinders University
GPO Box 2100 Adelaide, 5001
Australia

Professor Raja C. Bandaranayake
International Consultant in Medical Education and Visiting Professor
Gulf Medical University
Ajman
UAE

Professor Hugh Barr
President
CAIPE
PO Box 680
Fareham PO14 9NH
UK

Margaret Bearman PhD
Associate Professor
HealthPEER - Health Professional Education and Education Research
Monash University
Clayton Campus Victoria 3800
Australia

Dr Martina Behrens
Principal Lecturer Clinical Education and Leadership
Faculty of Health & Social Studies
University of Bedfordshire
Luton LU2 8LE
UK

Professor Eric Buch
Dean, Faculty of Health Science
University of Pretoria
Pretoria
South Africa

Professor Jamiu O. Busari
Associate Professor of Medical Education and Clinical Director, Pediatric Residency Program
Department of Paediatrics
Atrium Medical Center Parkstad, Henri Dunantstraat 5
6401CX, Heerlen
The Netherlands

Dr Andrew C. Butler
Department of Psychology & Neuroscience
Duke University
Box 90086
Durham, NC 27708
USA

Dr Francesca Celletti
Medical Officer
World Health Organization
Geneva
Switzerland

Dr Madawa Chandratilake
Centre of Medical Education
Dundee University
Dundee
UK

Dr Lincoln Chen
China Medical Board
2 Arrow St.
Cambridge MA, 02138
USA

Professor Timothy J. Cleary
Associate Professor at the Graduate School of Applied and Professional Psychology (GSAPP)
Rutgers
The State University of New Jersey
152 Frelinghuysen Road
Piscataway, NJ 08854-8085
USA

Dr Jennifer Cleland
Senior Clinical Lecturer, Lead, Medical Education Research and Clinical Communication
University of Aberdeen
DMDE/CAPC, West Wing Polwarth Building
Foresterhill
Aberdeen, AB25 2ZD
UK

Lou Ann Cooper
College of Medicine—Chapman Education Center
University of Florida
PO Box 100213
1600 S.W. Archer Rd.
Gainesville, FL 32610-0206
USA

Professor Phil Cotton
Academic Unit of General Practice and Primary Care
University of Glasgow
1 Horselethill Road
Glasgow G12 9LX
UK

Anaise Cottrell
Australian Securities and Investments Commission
Level 7 100 Pirie St
Adelaide 5000
Australia

Professor David Cottrell
Dean of Medicine
University of Leeds
Level 8, Worsley Building
Clarendon Way
Leeds LS2 9NL
UK

Barbara J. Daley, PhD
Associate Dean—Education Outreach, Professor, Adult and
Continuing Education Program
School of Education
University of Wisconsin-Milwaukee
PO Box 413, Milwaukee, WI 53201
USA

Laura C. Dast
University of Wisconsin School of Medicine and Public Health
4283 Health Science Learning Center
750 Highland Avenue
Madison, WI 53705
USA

Professor W. Dale Dauphinee
Clinical and Health Informatics Research Group
McGill University
1140 Pine Avenue West
Montreal, QC H3A 13A
Canada

Dr John Dent
AMEE International Relations Officer
Hon Reader in Medical Education and Orthopaedic Surgery
Tay Park House, 484 Perth Road
Dundee, DD1 1LR
UK

Dr Eva Doherty
Senior Lecturer and Director of Human Factors and Patient Safety
National Surgical Training Centre
Royal College of Surgeons in Ireland
Dublin
Ireland

Professor Diana Dolmans
Department of Educational Development and Research
Maastricht University
PO Box 616, 6200 MD Maastricht
The Netherlands

Tyrone Donnon
Associate Professor at the Medical Education & Research Unit
Community Health Science, Faculty of Medicine, University of
Calgary
AB T2N 1N4
Canada

Professor Tim Dornan
Department of Educational Development and Research
Maastricht University
PO Box 616, 6200 MD Maastricht
The Netherlands

Dr Al Dowie
Senior University Teacher in Medical Ethics and Law
Glasgow University Medical School
Glasgow
UK

Professor Ashley Duits
Professor of Medical Education
Institute of Medical Education
University of Groningen
Groningen
The Netherlands

Dr Erik Driessen
Department of Educational Research and Development, Faculty of
Health, Medicine and Life Sciences
Maastricht University
PO Box 616
6200MD Maastricht
The Netherlands

Professor Steven J. Durning
Professor of Medicine and Pathology
Uniformed Services University of the Health Sciences
4301 Jones Bridge Road
Bethesda MD 20814-4799
USA

Mary Edwards
Distance Education and Liaison Librarian
Health Science Center Libraries
University of Florida
PO Box 100206
1600 S.W. Archer Rd.
Gainesville, FL 32610-0206
USA

Rachel Ellaway
Assistant Dean, Informatics and Associate Professor
Northern Ontario School of Medicine

Assistant Professor Susan E. Farrell
Brigham and Women's Hospital
Department of Emergency Medicine
75 Francis Street
Boston, MA 02115
USA

Professor Ruth-Marie E. Fincher
Vice Dean for Academic Affairs
Medical College of Georgia, Georgia Health Sciences University
Augusta GA
USA

Professor Julio Frenk
Harvard School of Public Health
677 Huntington Ave
Boston MA, 02115-6018
USA

Professor Anne Garden
Head, Lancaster Medical School
Furness College
Lancaster University
Lancaster
LA1 4YB
UK

Professor William Godolphin
Department of Pathology & Laboratory Medicine
University of British Columbia
G227-2211 Wesbrook Mall
Vancouver, BC, V6T 2B5
Canada

Dr John Goldie
Academic Unit of General Practice and Primary Care
University of Glasgow
1 Horselethill Road
Glasgow G12 9LX
UK

Professor Janet Grant
Director of the Centre for Medical Education in Context
(CenMEDIC)
CenMEDIC
27 Church Street
Hampton, TW12 2EB
UK

Dr Richard Gray
CAIPE
PO Box 680
Fareham PO14 9NH
UK

Victoria A. Groce
Project Coordinator, Office of the Vice Dean
University of Pittsburgh School of Medicine
Pittsburgh, PA 15261
USA

Professor Larry D. Gruppen
University of Michigan Medical School
G1113 Towsley Center
1500 E. Medical Center Drive
Ann Arbor, MI 48109-5201
USA

Professor Maryellen E. Gusic
Vice Dean for Education
Indiana University School of Medicine
Indianapolis, IN
USA

Professor Janet P. Hafler
Assistant Dean, Educational Scholarship
Yale University School of Medicine
New Haven, CT
USA

Dr Debbie Harrison
Honorary Research Fellow
Birkbeck College
University of London
43 Gordon Square
London WC1H 0PD
UK

Professor Richard Hays
Bond University
Gold Coast
Queensland, 4229
Australia

Dr Kevin Hayes
Senior Lecturer in Obstetrics and Gynaecology and Medical
Education
St George's University of London
London
UK

Professor Paul A. Hemmer
Professor of Medicine
Uniformed Services University of the Health Sciences
4301 Jones Bridge Road
Bethesda, MD 20814
USA

Professor Andrew G. Hill
South Auckland Clinical School
Department of Surgery, University of Auckland
Middlemore Hospital
Private Bag 93 311, Otahuhu
Auckand, 1640
New Zealand

Susan Humphrey-Murto
Associate Professor, Faculty of Medicine
The Ottawa Hospital-Riverside Campus
1967 Riverside Drive, Box 37
Ottawa, Ontario
K1H 7W9 Canada

Dr Jan Illing
Medical Education Research Group
Durham University
Durham
UK

Rachel Isba
Clinical Lecturer in Medical Education
Lancaster Medical School, Furness College
Lancaster University
Lancaster, LA1 4YB
UK

Dr Alex Jamieson
London Deanery
Stewart House, 32 Russell Square
London WC1B 5DN
UK

Dr Steven L. Kanter
Vice Dean, University of Pittsburgh School of Medicine
M-240 Scaife Hall, Terrace and DeSoto Streets
Pittsburgh, PA 15261
USA

Susan Kilminster
Leeds Institute of Medical Education
Level 7, Worsley Building
Clarendon Way
Leeds LS2 9NL
UK

Dr Jan Kleijnen
Praaglaan 129
6229 HR Maastricht
The Netherlands

Professor Ayelet Kuper
Wilson Centre for Research in Education
Assistant Professor, Department of Medicine
University of Toronto Faculty of Medicine
Toronto
Canada

Professor Douglas P. Larsen
Department of Neurology
Campux Box 8111
660 S. Euclid Avenue
St. Louis, MO 63110
USA

Dr. Eliza Beth Littleton
Research Assistant Professor of Medicine
University of Pittsburgh School of Medicine
Pittsburgh, PA 15261
USA

Jennifer Lyon
Clinical Research Librarian
Health Science Center Libraries
University of Florida
PO Box 100206
1600 S.W. Archer Rd.
Gainesville, FL 32610-0206
USA

Simone Manhal
Assistant of the Vice Rector for Studies and Teaching
Rectorate Medical University of Graz Harrachgasse 21/VI
A-8010 Graz
Austria

Professor Emeritus Karen V. Mann
Division of Medical Education
Dalhousie Faculty of Medicine, Clinical Research Centre
5489 University Avenue, Halifax
Nova Scotia B3H 4R2
Canada

Dr Sean McAleer
Centre of Medical Education
Dundee University
Dundee
UK

Professor Judy McKimm
College of Medicine
Swansea University
Swansea
UK

Dr Danette McKinley
Director, Research and Data Resources
Foundation for Advancement of International Medical Education and
Research (FAIMER)
3624 Market Street, 4th Floor
Philadelphia, PA 19104
USA

Dr Patricia McNally
Assistant Dean, Medical Education, Adjunct Associate Professor,
Department of Neurology
Stritch School of Medicine
Loyola University Chicago
2160 S. First Ave., Bldg. 120, Room 320
Maywood, IL 60153
USA

Dr David Mendel
Associate Director, Continuing Professional Development Unit
London Deanery
Stewart House, 32 Russell Square
London WC1B 5DN
UK

Dr Catherine Michaud
Independent Consultant PO Box 1546
Duxbury, MA 02331
USA

Dr Lynn V. Monrouxe
Director of Medical Education Research
Institute of Medical Education, School of Medicine
Cardiff University
Cardiff, UK

Clare Morris
Head of Department
Clinical Education and Leadership University of Bedfordshire
Luton, LU2 8LE
UK

Professor Jill Morrison
Dean for Learning and Teaching
College of Medical, Veterinary and Life Sciences
University of Glasgow, 1, Horselethill Road
Glasgow, G12 9LX
UK

Dr Michael J. Murphy
Clinical Reader Centre for Undergraduate
Medicine Medical Education
Institute University of Dundee
Dundee
UK

Dr. Manisha Nair
Department of Public Health
University of Oxford
Third floor, Rosemary Rue Building, Old Road Campus
Headington, Oxford, OX3 7LF
UK

Professor Gillian Needham
Postgraduate Dean
NHS Education for Scotland
North of Scotland Deanery
Forest Grove House, Foresterhill
Aberdeen, AB25 2ZP
UK

Professor Debra Nestel
Professor of Simulation Education in Healthcare
School of Rural Health, HealthPEER
Faculty of Medicine, Nursing and Health Sciences
Monash University
Victoria
Australia

Professor John Norcini
President and Chief Executive Officer
Foundation for Advancement of International Medical
Education and Research (FAIMER)
3624 Market Street, 4th Floor
Philadelphia, PA 19104
USA

Dr Karlijn Overeem
Department of Educational Research and Development,
Faculty of Health, Medicine and Life Sciences
Maastricht University
PO Box 616
6200MD Maastricht
The Netherlands

Professor Christie L. Palladino
Educational Researcher, Education Discovery Institute
Medical College of Georgia
Georgia Health Sciences University
Augusta GA
USA

Dr Elise Paradis
Assistant Professor
Department of Social and Behavioral Sciences
University of California, San Francisco
San Francisco CA
USA

Professor Fiona Patterson
Department of Social and Developmental Psychology
University of Cambridge
Work Psychology Group
27 Brunel Parkway, Pride Park
Derby DE24 8HR
UK

Dr Gominda Ponnamperuma
Faculty of Medicine
University of Colombo
Colombo
Sri Lanka

Professor David Prideaux
Emeritus Professor of Medical Education
Health Professional Education, School of Medicine
Flinders University
GPO Box 2100, Adelaide 5001
Australia

O. Univ.-Prof. Mag. Dr. Gilbert Reibnegger
Professor of Medical Chemistry
Institute of Medical Chemistry
Medical University of Graz
Harrachgasse 21/II
A-8010 Graz
Austria

Jan-Joost Rethans
Skillslab
Maastricht University
PO Box 616
6200 MD Maastricht
The Netherlands

Dr Simon C. Riley
Centre for Medical Education University of Edinburgh
Chancellor's Building, 49 Little France Crescent
Edinburgh, EH16 2SB
UK

Dr Michael T. Ross
Programme Co-Director, MSc Clinical Education
Centre for Medical Education
The University of Edinburgh
The Chancellor's Building, 49 Little France Crescent
Edinburgh EH16 4SB
UK

Joy Rudland
Director of the Faculty Education Unit
Faculty of Medicine
University of Otago
Otago
New Zealand

Dr Badara Samb
Health Systems and Services
World Health Organization
Geneva
Switzerland

Dr John Sandars
Associate Professor
Leeds Institute of Medical Education
Level 7, Worsley Building
University of Leeds
Leeds, LS2 9LN
UK

Professor Joan M. Sargeant
Division of Medical Education, Dalhousie Faculty of Medicine
Clinical Research Centre
5489 University Avenue, P.O.Box 15000,
Halifax, Nova Scotia B3H 4R2
Canada

Professor Lambert W.T. Schuwirth
Health Professions Education, Flinders Medical Centre
Bedford Park
Adelaide
Australia

Sydney Smee
The Medical Council of Canada
2283 St-laurent Blvd, Suite 100
Ottawa, Ontario
K1G 5A2 Canada

Dr John Spicer
Head of School of General Practice
London Deanery
University of London
Stewart House, 32 Russell Square
London WC1B 5DN
UK.

Dr Terese Stenfors-Hayes
Department of Learning, Informatics, Management and Ethics
Karolinska Institutet
17177 Stockholm
Sweden

Professor Yvonne Steinert
Richard and Sylvia Cruess Chair in Medical Education
Director Centre for Medical Education, Faculty of Medicine,
McGill University
1110 Pine Avenue West Montreal, Quebec,
Canada H3A 1A3

Professor John Sweller
School of Education
University of New South Wales
Sydney NSW 2052
Australia

Dr Pim W. Teunissen
Researcher Department of Educational
Development and Research School of Health
Professions Education (SHE)
Universiteitssingel 60,
6229 ER Maastricht
The Netherlands

Professor Dario M. Torre
Director at the Department of Medicine
Drexel University College of Medicine
245 North 15th Street, 6209 New College Building
Philadelphia, PA 19102
USA

Claire Touchie
The Medical Council of Canada
2283 St-laurent Blvd, Suite 100
Ottawa, Ontario
K1G 5A2 Canada

Dr Angela Towle
Centre for Health Education Scholarship
Faculty of Medicine
University of British Columbia
Vancouver, British Columbia
Canada V5Z 1M9

Janet Tworek
Faculty of Education
University of Calgary
Calgary
Canada

Professor Doctor Hans van Hout
Flevolaan 30A
1411 KD Naarden
The Netherlands

Dr Jeroen J. G. van Merriënboer
School of Health Professions Education, Department of
Educational Development and Research
Faculty of Health, Medicine and Life Sciences
Maastricht University
Maastricht
The Netherlands

Dr Kieran Walsh
Clinical Director of BMJ Learning
BMJ Group
BMA House, Tavistock Square
London WC1H 9JR
UK

Professor Fiona Webster
Assistant Professor, Department of Family and Community Medicine
University of Toronto Faculty of Medicine
Toronto
Canada

Dr Premila Webster
Department of Public Health
University of Oxford
Third floor, Rosemary Rue Building, Old Road Campus
Headington, Oxford, OX3 7LF
UK

Dr Michiel Westerman
VU Medical Centre Institute for Medical Education
Postbus 70571007 MB
Amsterdam
The Netherlands

Casey B. White
Associate Residency Program Director and Education Specialist
Department of Anesthesiology
University of Florida College of Medicine

Dr Julia Whiteman
London Deanery
Stewart House, 32 Russell Square
London WC1B 5DN
UK

Dr Jos Willems
Chambertinlaan 26
6213 EW Maastricht
The Netherlands

Dr Jo Winning
Senior Lecturer in Literary and Cultural Studies
School of Arts, Birkbeck College
University of London
43 Gordon Square
London WC1H 0PD
UK

Dr Diana F. Wood
Director of Medical Education and Clinical Dean
University of Cambridge School of Clinical Medicine
Addenbrookes Hospital
Hills Road Cambridge CB2 0SP
UK

Dr Tzu-Chieh Yu
South Auckland Clinical School
Department of Surgery, University of Auckland
Middlemore Hospital
Private Bag 93 311, Otahuhu
Auckland, 1640
New Zealand

Dr. Anand Zachariah
Professor of Medicine, Christian Medical College
Vellore, Tamil Nadu
India

Abbreviations

16PF	Sixteen Personality Factor questionnaire
AAFP	American Association of Family Physicians
AAI	Appraisal and Assessment Instrument
AAMC	Association of American Medical Colleges
ABG	arterial blood gases
ABIM	American Board of Internal Medicine
ABMS	American Board of Medical Specialists
ACCME	Accreditation Council for CME
ACGME	Accreditation Council for Graduate Medical Education
ACTC	Ambulatory Care Teaching Centre
ADH	antidiuretic hormone
AHRQ	Agency for Healthcare Research and Quality
AI	appreciative inquiry
AIDS	acquired immune deficiency syndrome
AMEE	Association for Medical Education in Europe
AoME	Academy of Medical Educators
APA ESP	Academic Pediatric Association's Educational Scholars Program
ASEAN	Association of Southeast Asian Nations
ATEEM	Anaesthetic Theatre Educational Environment Measure
BCI	Basic Character Inventory
BDI	Beck Depression Inventory
BEME	Best Evidence Medical Education
CA	conversation analysis
CAL	computer-assisted learning
CARE	Consultation and Relational Empathy
CAS	complex adaptive system
CAT	classroom assessment technique
CAT	computer adaptive testing (
CBD	case-based discussion
CBE	competency-based education
CBL	case-based learning
CBT	cognitive-behaviour therapy
CEX	clinical evaluation exercise
CFPC	College of Family Physicians of Canada
CHAT	cultural–historical activity theory
CIPP	context, inputs, processes, and products
CL	cooperative learning
CLEI	Clinical Learning Environment Inventory
CLIC	Consortium of Longitudinal Integrated Clerkships
CME	continuing medical education
COGME	Council on Graduate Medical Education
COE	community-oriented education
CoP	communities of practice
COPC	Community-Oriented Primary Care Model
COPD	chronic obstructive pulmonary disease
CPA	creative professional activity
CPI	California Personality Inventory
CPD	continuous professional development
CQI	continuous quality improvement
CSR	chart-stimulated recall
CV	curriculum vitae
DA	discourse analysis
DDD-E	Decide, Design, Develop, and Evaluate
DI	discrimination index
DOPS	direct observation of procedural skills
D-RECT	Dutch Residency Educational Climate Test
DREEM	Dundee Ready Educational Environment Measure
DSM-5	*Diagnostic and Statistical Manual of Mental Disorders*
DSU	day surgery unit
DTC	Diagnostic and Treatment Centre
DV	dependent variable
EBL	enquiry-based learning
EBM	evidence-based medicine
EI	emotional intelligence
EMAR	Educational Management Research Model
EME	emerging market economy
EMQ	extended matching questions
EPA	entrustable professional activities
EPQ	Eysenck Personality Questionnaire
ESR	erythrocyte sedimentation rate
EUA	European University Association
FAIMER	Foundation for Advancement of International Medical Education and Research
FBC	full blood count

FGM	female genital mutilation	MOOC	massively open, online courses
GAMSAT	Graduate Australian Medical Schools Admission Test	MSCEIT	Mayer–Salovey–Caruso Emotional Intelligence Test
		MSF	multisource feedback
GEA	Group on Educational Affairs	MSLES	Medical School Learning Environment Survey
GHQ	General Health Questionnaire	MUSM	Mercer University School of Medicine
GMA	general mental ability	NACE	narcissism, aloofness, confidence, and empathy
GMC	General Medical Council	NCAS	National Clinical Assessment Service
GP	general practitioner	NCD	non-communicable disease
GPA	grade point average	NEO-PI-R	Revised NEO Personality Inventory
GROP	get rid of patients	NHS	National Health Service
GTA	Gynecology Teaching Associate	OBE	outcome-based education
HIV	human immunodeficiency virus	OSCE	objective structured clinical examination
HDS	Hogan Development Survey	OECD	Organization for Economic Cooperation and Development
HPAT	Health Professions Admission Test		
ICMJE	International Committee of Medical Journal Editors	OSATS	objective structured assessment of technical skills
		OSTE	objective structured teaching examination
IDEAL	International Database for Enhanced Assessment and Learning Consortium	PAL	peer-assisted learning
		PALS	peer-assisted learning scheme
IE	institutional ethnography	PAR	Physician Achievement Review
IFA	instructions for authors	PAR	participatory action research
IFOM	International Foundations of Medicine	PAT	peer assessment tool
IPE	interprofessional education	PBA	procedure-based assessment
IPPI	integrated procedural performance instrument	PBIT	practice-based improvement tool
ISM	Integrated Systems Model	PBL	problem-based learning
IT	information technology	PBLM	problem-based learning module
ITER	in-training evaluation report	PDCA	plan, do, check, act
ITC	item total score correlations	PDP	personal development plan
IV	independent variable	PEPFAR	President's Emergency Plan for AIDS Relief
IVIMEDs	the international virtual medical school	PESTLE	political; economic; sociodemographic; technological; legal and environmental
JCAHO	Joint Commission on Accreditation of Healthcare Organisations		
		PHEEM	Postgraduate Hospital Educational Environment Measure
JRCPTB	Joint Royal College of Physicians Training Board		
JET	joint evaluation team	PI	Patient Instructor
JMHPE	Joint Master of Health Professions Education	PI	performance improvement
KT	knowledge translation	PIM	Performance Improvement Module
KTA	knowledge-to-action	PME	postgraduate medical education
LIC	longitudinal integrated clerkships	PPIK	process, personality, interests, knowledge
LMS	learning management systems	PQA	Personal Qualities Assessment
LPP	legitimate peripheral participation	PRCC	Parallel Rural Community Curriculum
MaSP	Maastricht Assessment of Simulated Patients	PRECEDE	*Predisposing, Reinforcing and Enabling Causes in Educational Diagnosis and Evaluation Model*
MBPI	Myers–Briggs Personality Type Indicator		
MBTI	Myers–Briggs Type Indicator	PTSD	post-traumatic stress disorder
MCA	membership categorization analysis	QA	quality assurance
MCAT	Medical College Admission Test	QABME	Quality Assurance of Basic Medical Education
MCD	membership categorization devices	QI	quality improvement
MCI	Medical Council of India	RCPSC	Royal College of Physicians and Surgeons of Canada
MCQ	multiple-choice question	RCT	randomized controlled trial
MCW	Medical College of Wisconsin	RIME	reporter–interpreter–manager–educator
MDG	Millennium Development Goals	RISE	Research, Innovation, and Scholarship in Education
MEQ	modified essay question	RLO	reusable learning object
MEPI	Medical Education Partnership Initiative	SAI	Self-assessment Inventory
MESP	Medical Education Scholars Program	SAMA	South African Medical Association
MEU	Medical Education Unit	SAQ	short answer questions
MHPE	Masters in Health Professions Education	SBA	single best answer
MLCF	Medical Leadership Competency Framework	SBE	simulation-based education
MLE	managed learning environment	SC	selection centre
MMI	multiple mini-interview	SCORM	Sharable Content Object Reference Model
MMPI	Minnesota Multiphasic Personality Inventory	SCT	script concordance test
MOC	Maintenance of Certification	SDL	self-directed learning

SGPA	science grade point averages
SJT	situational judgement test
SMP	senior mentor programme
SOLO	structure of observed learning outcome
SP	simulated patient
SPAP	specialty-based practice assessment programme
SPRAT	Sheffield Peer Review Assessment Tool
SRL	self-regulated learning
SSC	student-selected components
SSM	special study module
SSRI	selective serotonin reuptake inhibitor
STEEM	Surgical Theatre Educational Environment Measure
STEPS	Simulation-based Training for Enhancement of Procedural Skills
SWOT	strengths, weaknesses, opportunities, and threats
TAB	Team Assessment of Behaviours
TAT	Thematic Apperception Test

TBL	task-based learning
TBL	team-based learning
TOSCE	team-observed structural clinical examination
TPI	Teaching Perspectives Inventory
TQM	total quality management
UCAS	Universities and Colleges Admissions Service
UGME	undergraduate medical education
uGPA	undergraduate grade point average
UKCAT	UK Clinical Aptitude Test
UMAT	Undergraduate Medical Admissions Test
VARK	visual, audio, read/write, kinetic inventory
VLE	virtual learning environment
WPBA	workplace-based assessment
WFME	World Federation of Medical Education
WHO	World Health Organization
ZPD	zone of proximal development

PART 1

Introduction

CHAPTER 1

Introduction

Kieran Walsh

In considering the usual medical curriculum of today, and asking where in it clinical science is to play its part, I would start from the statement that this curriculum is already overloaded.

Thomas Lewis

Reproduced from *British Medical Journal*, Thomas Lewis, 'The Huxley lecture on clinical science within the university', 1, p. 631, copyright 1935, with permission from BMJ Publishing Group Ltd

Curriculum

Reform in medical education has been around a long time. The above quote from Thomas Lewis sounds like it originated in the 1990s when the General Medical Council in the UK first started to look at curriculum overload seriously and so it comes as a surprise to see that Lewis was concerned about this problem some 60 years beforehand. Each generation thinks that it is the first to invent medical education reform and so sets out in its texts and papers how it will transform medical education for learners and ultimately patients. The aim of this introduction is to be more modest in its ambitions. Its aim is to set out the current state of the art in the theoretical framework, the evidence base and the practice of medical education, and to do so in the context of a rich history that reaches back over 2000 years when Hippocrates gave his famous dictum on the benefits of a practical education—'he who desires to practice surgery must go to war' (Corpus Hippocraticum 400 BC). In so doing I hope that the *Oxford Textbook of Medical Education* will stand the test of time.

Any medical education initiative will thrive or fail on the basis of its curriculum, and so this title purposefully starts off with a thorough grounding on how to design curricula and on the basics of commonly used curricular frameworks (from problem-based learning to interprofessional education). Janet Grant and colleagues lay the foundations for this section in their chapter on curriculum design (Chapter 2). One of the strongest themes to emerge from the chapter is the need for a contextual curriculum. They state that 'history and current practice suggest the need for a contextual approach to curriculum design and development, drawing on local conditions and opportunities, relying on local experience and strengths' (Chapter 2). They emphasize the importance of delivering curricula that will meet local needs and stress the importance of 'the practicing profession itself' being the driving force behind curriculum design (Chapter 2).

Albanese and Dast start their chapter by claiming that 'launching a problem-based learning (PBL) curriculum is not for the faint-hearted'

(Chapter 3). Their chapter gives a comprehensive overview of this form of learning—which has become almost ubiquitous in medical education. The chapter recommends the Integrated Systems Model as a means of 'making sense of the findings from the literature and for providing guidance when the literature is either non-existent or conflicting' (Chapter 3). The chapter continues the contextual theme commenced in the first chapter, and the authors would likely agree with Feletti (1995) when he states that 'problem-based learning is grounded in the belief that learning is most effective when students are actively involved and learn in the context in which knowledge is to be used'.

Healthcare today is sufficiently complex for it to be impossible for any single clinician to provide comprehensive care to a range of different patients. And if healthcare professionals work in teams, then surely it makes sense for them to learn in teams? The chapter on interprofessional education explains the advantages and disadvantages that this particular format confers on medical education. Here again there is the importance of context—captured well by Hutchinson when she wrote in 2006: 'moving some roles to other healthcare professionals will require review of medical students' and doctors' training'.

And how are we as educators to weave all these different formats into a coherent whole? According to John Sweller and Jeroen van Merriënboer, only through proper instructional design. Doctors and medical students at all levels have to learn vast amounts of information that is necessary for them to carry out their work. Instructional design guidelines help them to structure knowledge in a way that will enable them to access relevant knowledge quickly and easily—when and where they need to. Their example of chess as a game where expertise is 'critically dependent on long-term memory' and the ability to source this memory at will was fascinating to this enthusiastic but untalented player (Chapter 7). And I always thought it was my problem-solving skills!

Another surprise comes in Isba's chapter on the learning environment (Chapter 9). Certainly it is true that the environment in which doctors learn has immediate and long term impact on the outcomes of their education. However, Rachel Isba's thoughts on how medical students and doctors can in turn influence their own environment and that instead of their being one overall environment there may be lots of 'micro-environments' seems to turn yet another commonly held truism on its head (Chapter 9).

What all the chapters in the curriculum section have in common is how the authors outline their views in a keen and yet balanced way. In the past curriculum design has been described as a war and as John Last (1985) has said 'the war for time and students' minds is a sad, futile, self destructive activity in many medical schools'.

Here's hoping for more objective détente in the future.

Identity

Lynn Monrouxe's chapter forms the cornerstone of this section. Professional identity formation is likely to be as important in the education of healthcare professionals as the acquisition of new knowledge and skills. Despite the progress that has been made by researchers into identity formation in medical education, there is still much work to be done. As Schwartz and colleagues (2011) have said, to 'truly capture the complexity of this construct [identity], we must move beyond isolated sub-disciplines … and design innovative research studies that capture multiple components and processes of identity'.

Closely linked to identity is personality. Certain personality traits have been shown to affect the performance of medical students and doctors, and as Doherty says in Chapter 11 certain personality factors can affect how doctors cope with and even perceive stressful situations. The chapter also cites a memorable definition of the ideal prospective doctor. According to Munro et al. (2008, p. 103), such a prospective doctor should be 'steady, sane and nice'—an epithet that few would disagree with.

Delivery

Medical education has always been rich in the variety of forms of that it can be used in its delivery.

Small group learning has always existed in medical education—but in the past 20 years, there has been a movement to define small group learning and outline best practice in its application. Joy Rudland gives a thorough overview of this form of learning and also details some varieties on the core small group format—such as snowballing or goldfish bowling. According to Rudland, 'snowballing interaction takes place when subgroups combine with other groups to share their understanding—ultimately resulting in the whole class discussing the topic' (Chapter 13). Snowballing as well as goldfish bowling enables small group techniques to be used in large groups which will be an increasing necessity to extract maximum value from this form of learning in straitened economic circumstances.

And then there is large group teaching—certainly no form of medical education has received as much critical attention as the lecture. It can be difficult to find many researchers that have positive things to say about lectures—unless they are being ironic. Peter Medawar (1979) claims that 'no sleep is so deeply refreshing as that which, during lectures, Morpheus invites us so insistently to enjoy' and this quote sums up much of the poor press that lectures have received over the years. Thankfully, Tim Dornan and colleagues

take a different view. They condemn as fruitless the questioning as to whether or not 'large group teaching is or is not a good thing' and suggest that educationalists would be better off spending their time considering 'how lectures work, for whom, in what ways, with what outcomes, and how the activity, method, and system of lecturing can be improved' (Chapter 14). When we have answers to some of these questions it is likely that large group teaching will have 'a growing rather than shrinking role in contemporary medical education' (Chapter 14).

Another increasingly used mode of delivery is e-learning. This has been the 'latest advance' in medical education for some time now. In its early years, great promises were made as to its potential but today it is worth asking to what extent it has lived up to this potential. John Sandars' chapter provides a realistic portrayal of the achievements of e-learning as it has started to come of age. As with lectures the question as to whether e-learning is as good as or better than other forms of learning is likely to be too simplistic to provide useful answers. As Sandars says 'there has been increasing recognition that the effective use of e-learning depends on a structured approach for development and implementation, with a skilful alignment of the needs of the learner, the content or educational experience to be delivered, the instructional design, the available technology and the context within which the e-learning intervention is to be implemented' (Chapter 15). His chapter gives an excellent primer on how to achieve this.

Simulation is another mode of educational delivery has come into its own in the past ten years. Analogies are continually made between the roles of simulation in aviation and simulation in medicine. Some analogies are sound, others more tenuous but regardless of this there is no doubt that the airline industry was quicker out of the blocks than medicine. The Wright brothers got Wright Flyer I off the ground at Kittyhawk in 1903—by 1909 not only had aircraft simulators been invented, a commercial aircraft simulation industry had started to develop in the United States (fig. 1.1).

It says something about the innate conservatism of the medical profession that it has taken as long as it has to roll out simulation to a wide range of healthcare professionals in a wide range of specialties. The chapter by Bearman and colleagues explains the pedagogical rationale for simulation based medical education and the evidence base that it is effective and gives a comprehensive guide to setting up simulation-based medical education programmes. The authors state that 'effective educational design is about deep

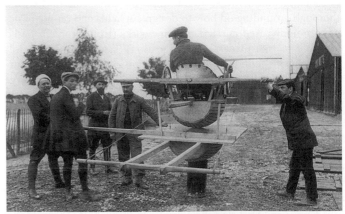

Figure 1.1 The Antoinette trainer—an early aircraft simulator.
Cour des ateliers Levavasseur à Chalons, 1910.

thought and considered decisions, not about following recipes' and they certainly give a detailed account of effective instructional design in simulation (Chapter 16).

Ultimately most medical education is delivered in the workplace and so it is vitally important that work-based learning is delivered as it should be. As Clare Morris and Martina Behrens state, 'medicine has a long tradition of recognizing the workplace as a significant site for learning; the future of medicine relies upon a revitalization of working-learning relationships throughout a medical career' (Chapter 18). The issue of work-based learning as an issue in continuous professional development is thus likely to become more important in the future. Of course work-based learning is crucially dependent on the learner's actual place or work. In modern health systems, the delivery of healthcare increasingly occurs in ambulatory settings and so learning must follow the healthcare professional and their patients to such settings. As William Hensel (1988 p. 2695) writes, 'giving students the opportunity to care for ambulatory patients allows them to learn valuable lessons absent from the inpatient experience'. And John Dent elegantly lays out the rich vein of learning opportunities now available in ambulatory care settings. If in the past, ambulatory care has meant mainly outpatients but today ambulatory care can stretch from screening clinics to clinical investigation units. We will do our learners a disservice if we do not enable them to experience these rich learning opportunities.

According to Paul McCoubrie (2004), 'the arguments for and against different methods of teaching medical students how to be a doctor has been raging for decades and will continue to run and run. A study that provides firm evidence of the superiority of one method over another will, I wager, never be done'. When thinking about delivery of education, the issues of who the learner is, what they need to learn about, why they need to learn and how they prefer to learn will always take precedence over the mode of delivery regardless of how modern or innovative it may be.

Supervision

Inadequate supervision has short- and long-term consequences for both learners and patients. In the short term it can lead to medical accidents and in the long term can result in specialists or generalists who, although they may be technically fully qualified, are not fully trained. Worse than poor supervision is no supervision at all and it is worthwhile reflecting how frequently we as trainees spent practicing under the direct guidance of our seniors or indeed how often now as seniors we spend time directly observing and feeding back to trainees about various aspects of their practice. Sue Kilminster and David Cottrell outline the 'empirical evidence that supervisory guidance is far too infrequent, and even where guidance is given, there is little or no feedback' (Chapter 22) and give direct advice on how to improve supervision at an institutional as well as at an individual level. As John Launer (2006, p. 171) says, 'supervision does not have to be solemn' but an even more fundamental rule is that supervision has to happen in the first place.

Closely related to supervision is mentoring. Effective mentoring can play a key role in enabling learners at all levels to progress with their education and their careers. Chapter 23 outlines the various roles of a mentor and types of mentoring relationships. It explains how to set up mentoring programmes and how to overcome common difficulties that are encountered in their establishment. If in

the past mentorship has been a 'fortuitous relationship that fosters the development of the adult learner', the challenge for the future is to ensure that all learners get the opportunity to benefit from this form of relationship rather than it being a matter having the good fortune to stumble upon a helpful senior (Longhurst 1994, p. 53).

If this is the role of senior healthcare professionals in medical education, what of the role of the patient? As Angela Towle and William Godolphin state 'patients have always been involved in medical education but too often in the past they have been used as convenient and passive tools for learning and practice' (Chapter 27). Their chapter looks at better ways of involving patients in medical education. It explains why it is helpful to involve patients as active partners and also examines the evidence that involving patients can improve outcomes. Many of us already involve patients in relatively simple ways—perhaps as patient educators—this chapter lays down the gauntlet by asking how we can involve patients in high-level strategic decision making at our institutions. As Linda Hutchinson (2006, p. 1502) has said 'medical education has an important role in shifting to a truly patient led culture' and so this is an example where medical education can lead the way for the health service.

Stages

In ideal circumstances medical education progresses seamlessly and inexorably from undergraduate to postgraduate education to continuous professional development (albeit not to remediation—apart from in exceptional circumstances).

Undergraduate medical education has undergone a period of major reform over the past 30 years. Aretz's chapter outlines the background to these reforms, the pedagogical principles on which they were based and the evidence base that they have made a difference. It also sets out the steps that need to be taken in setting up any undergraduate curriculum—regardless of its type—from planning to implementation to evaluation. Undergraduate education forms the foundation of all medical education and with proper thought and planning hopefully we can consign to history Michael Simpson's partly tongue-in-cheek memories of medical school: 'whoever it was who claimed to have been educated mainly during the holidays must have been an Old Boy of my medical school' (Simpson 1979, p. 94).

Following postgraduate training, healthcare professionals subsequently move onto the phase in their careers when they must undertake continuous professional development. It is vital that fully qualified doctors keep up to date throughout their careers—to do this they need to participate in continuous professional development. Despite its importance, continuous professional development is perhaps one of the less studied components of medical education. The chapter by Karen Mann and Joan Sargeant on CPD has as its theme the artificial separation between 'knowledge translation (KT), quality improvement (QI) and CPD' and the need to integrate these sometimes parallel activities. Their explicit purpose is 'to convey the significant shifts occurring in the field, particularly the change in focus from how physicians learn effectively to how they translate and apply that learning into practice, and from an emphasis on the transmission of knowledge to individuals, to a culture of lifelong learning in which individuals learn in many ways and in a variety of professional domains' (Chapter 30).

As learners progress from stage to stage, they must undergo a series of transitions. In their chapter on transitions in medical education, Pim Teunissen and Michiel Westerman emphasize the biggest steps that learners must take—from preclinical studies to clinical studies, from undergraduate study to work, and from training under supervision to independent practice. The literature on transitions traditionally looks at transitions as challenges to be overcome or perhaps avoided altogether by means of better preparation and education in the pre-transition phase. In this regard the chapter turns another truism on its head—the authors suggest that transitions be seen not just as threats but as 'opportunities for rapid personal and professional development' (Chapter 32).

Selection

Selecting for medical school is important—the more suited the student is to the practice of medicine, the better our workforce will be. However, this seemingly simple statement has a range of implications and begs a number of questions. How best should we select for medical school? Should we assess cognitive ability or aptitude or personality or emotional intelligence? How should we assess these attributes—by interviews or exam results or references or by a combination of some or all of these? At an even more basic level, as Fiona Patterson asks, should schools 'aim to select for individuals who will make successful students or, should the focus be on selecting those that will make competent clinicians'? Writing over 20 years ago Thomas McKeown (1986, p. 200) claimed that 'few medical schools would now consider seriously an applicant who had an A in biology, C in chemistry, D in physics and an intense interest in natural history and foreign travel, the credentials that Darwin, a slow starter, might have offered': we would do well to ask whether our current selection systems would do better.

Closely related to selection is dropout. Medical school dropout can have serious consequences for medical schools, tutors, society and those dropping out. A high dropout rate can certainly have professional and cost implications for institutions. And yet medical dropout is understudied. Chapter 34 gives a comprehensive outline of what factors predict medical dropout and what if anything can be done to lower dropout rates.

Assessment

When reading the medical education literature, one could be forgiven for thinking that the most important problem facing medical education today is the search for an assessment tool with near-perfect objectivity, reliability and validity and that an incremental increase in any one of these measures is worth all the time, effort and expense in its achievement. Lambert Schuwirth and Julie Ash's chapter on assessment forms the foundation of this section of this title and sets outs its stall in the first paragraph. The authors state that they 'want to defend the position that assessment is based on human judgement, and that the role of the technical aspects is to support the plausibility, credibility and trustworthiness of assessment and should not be a substitute for them' (Chapter 35). They call for 'assessment *for* learning' where the results of assessment are sufficiently information rich to steer learning and at the same time produce results that we can safely rely upon in high stakes examination.

If assessment is to achieve all that we expect of it, then it must be based on sound standards. In Chapter 36, John Norcini and Danette McKinley describe standard setting as 'the process of translating a description of the characteristics denoting the desired level performance into a number that applies to a particular test'. As they state there is no single best way of setting standards, rather the 'selection of a standard setting method is dependent on the goals and stakes associated with the assessment' (Chapter 36). Similarly to Lambert Schuwirth and Julie Ash in the previous chapter, the authors stress that standard setting is inevitably based on human judgement even though such judgement should come from experts; should follow due process; and should fit with the goals of assessment.

According to Brian Jolly (2008), 'there are no quick and easy assessment tools—they all require time and effort' and the authors of Chapter 37 on choosing instruments for assessment would surely agree. As Sean McAleer and Madawa Chandratilake outline, there are no intrinsically 'good' or 'bad' forms of assessment—rather different assessment instruments are likely to be helpful in different circumstances. Different instruments will have different levels of validity, reliability and feasibility when used in different contexts—so it is vital that assessment instruments are chosen carefully and for the correct purpose. This chapter outlines the steps that those involved in assessing learners must take when choosing an assessment instrument. It explains the evidence base that underlies each step and gives practical advice and tips on how to overcome potential pitfalls in choosing assessment instruments.

Tests undoubtedly enhance learning—the question is how we can use testing to have the best possible impact on our learners. Although doctors need much more than just knowledge to practice effectively, there is a growing evidence base that expertise is founded on knowledge that doctors can rapidly recall and put into practice. The chapter by Doug Larsen and colleagues explains the role of test-enhanced learning in medical education. It outlines different forms of test-enhanced learning and their relative effectiveness. As Doug Larsen and Andrew Butler state 'tests that require the production of information rather than the recognition of information generate greater retrieval effort and therefore have a greater mnemonic benefit' (Chapter 38). David Smyth (1978 p.1082) captured the frustration that many doctors have felt about their undergraduate education when he stated that 'the objection I have to much of my medical education is not that I memorized things, but that I memorized the wrong things'—with more relevant curricula and more effective assessments there should be few excuses for this recurring in the future.

Assessment drives learning and nowhere is this truer than in assessing professionalism. If we want newly qualified doctors who behave in a professional manner, then the absolute minimum that we must do is assess professionalism and ideally carry out a valid and reliable assessment that will have a positive impact on doctors' behaviours. The chapter by Richard Hays (Chapter 43) explains the educational rationale for assessing professionalism, the research base for this practice and also gives a thorough account of how best to assess professionalism in practical settings. Richard Hays' take home messages are reassuringly simple on the assessment of professionalism: he advises that we assess early and often—using multiple methods and approaching the issue from multiple perspectives.

One method that can be used to assess professionalism as well as a range of other attributes is the objective structured clinical examination (OSCE). Setting up an OSCE is a complex logistical task. There is a lot to prepare and make ready to ensure that those undergoing the exam receive a fair, valid, and reliable assessment. The chapter by Susan Humphrey-Murto and colleagues give a comprehensive account of this now common form of assessment. Once again the context of the assessment is as important as the format. For example the answer to the age old question about whether to use rating scales or checklists depends on the context. As the authors state studies comparing checklists and rating scales 'demonstrate checklists as being more appropriate for assessing structured tasks and junior trainees, and rating scales as better for distinguishing novices from experts' (Chapter 45). A debate that has been almost as contentious in the past is the one about what method of standard setting to use in OSCEs. The authors cite the borderline group method as certainly the most 'easily implemented and widely used approach' (Chapter 45).

In 1979 Hilliard Jason wrote that 'we in the health professions have only begun to emerge from the strikingly arrogant posture of asserting that our licences are awarded for life and that we can be fully entrusted to pursue whatever continuing learning we choose, without the need for external monitoring' (Jason 1979, p. 277) Thirty years later we are still just emerging from that posture. Dale Dauphinee has been a long time champion of recertification and here gives a practical account of how to implement recertification programmes that are fair, valid and reliable and that promote good behaviours amongst doctors whilst at the same time ensuring the safety of patients and the public. Recertification is a high-stakes assessment and like all assessments its validity 'must be established with each use and in each setting'. As Dale Dauphinee reminds us, 'validity does not lie in the test, but in each use and its interpretation'. Like Karen Mann and Joan Sargeant in the chapter on continuous professional development, Dauphinee urges that recertification builds on the framework of the quality improvement cycle and becomes for the vast majority of doctors a process whereby they can improve their practice for the benefit of the patients and community that they serve.

Regardless of the format of the assessment, feedback is likely to be a vital factor in ensuring its maximum impact. Chapter 48 by Julian Archer and Joan Sargeant explains how to give feedback in a wide range of circumstances. The authors run through the features that make for good feedback—they suggest that feedback content should be 'clear, mutually understood, specific and relevant' and that 'the feedback process should be timely, interactive, non-judgemental and accompanied by explanation' (Chapter 48). However this is only a small part of their theme. They suggest that to get maximum value from feedback, both teachers and learners should see feedback not as something to be delivered but rather as part of a wider two-way conversational process whereby information is shared amongst all relevant parties.

What all the assessment chapters have in common is that the authors realize the importance of assessment in medical education and in their various ways strive to reach a point where they will have a clear and true view of a candidates' ability. The authors search not an existential truth but a practical and useful one. Alan Bennett claims that 'truth is no more at issue in an examination than thirst at a wine-tasting or fashion at a striptease', but these chapters make me think that Bennett (2004) exaggerates and that we are getting closer to forms of assessment that will bring us closer to the truth.

Quality

In putting together the quality section, I was fortunate in being able to recruit some of the leading lights in evaluation and quality assurance.

John Goldie and Jill Morrison start the section off with a comprehensive account of evaluation in medical education. Without sound evaluation, we won't be able to assess the quality of medical education programmes and then measure the effectiveness of our quality improvement initiatives. As the authors say, 'evaluation should be planned during the setting up of educational programmes' and not left until the end (Chapter 49). Even though different evaluation models have clear underlying theoretical constructs, evaluation is ultimately a practical matter with the amount of funding available determining its scope and the 'political milieu' in which the evaluators operate having an important influence on the process.

Quality assurance is of course more than simple evaluation. It encompasses measurement of the quality of medical education, delving into the causes of possible variations in quality and introducing systems to assure high-quality education. Chapter 50 explains how to measure quality, how to analyse the results of measurements and how to use all of this to 'create a culture of continuous quality improvement'. The authors unequivocally call for quality management that 'is not too complex but a feasible part of the day-to-day practice of all staff' (Chapter 50).

This section ends with my own contribution on cost and value in medical education. I was keen to contribute myself so that at least I could look all authors in the eye and say yes I have given of 10 000 words and 100 references also (!) but more importantly as I feel that this is still a much neglected subject. Writing over 100 years ago, Arthur Hawkyard (1910, p. 1095) complained that the 'cost of medical education has also increased a good deal these last few years, thus affecting those who are putting their sons into the profession'.

Today there continues to be concerns that the cost of medical education remains a barrier to entry to young people from poorer sections of society; that medical student debt can drive graduates towards specialities that will enable them to become high earners rather than the healthcare professionals that a community needs; and that developing countries still cannot afford to produce the number of healthcare professionals that they require (and that even when they do, such health professionals often migrate to other countries where they feel they will have better career and life opportunities). Will we have to wait another 100 years before delivering healthcare professionals at an affordable cost or indeed ensuring that we get sufficient value out of the funding that we do spend on medical education? Former Secretary of State for Health, Iain MacLeod will be remembered for a number of reasons: for chain-smoking through the press conference when Richard Doll's study on smoking and lung cancer was released; for being one of first to disassociate mainstream conservatism from Enoch Powell's 'Rivers of Blood' speech; but for me he will always be the person who flipped an age old aphorism to come up with his own: 'money is the root of all progress' (Nairne 1988, p. 1518). More and more I think he was right.

Research and scholarship

In the last 30 years medical educational research has helped to lead the many reforms that were necessary in undergraduate and postgraduate medical education. Jan Illing's chapter introduces the various theoretical frameworks and perspectives that exist in medical education research. As Stewart Petersen (1999, p. 1223) has said 'some debates in medical education can appear to the outsider to have an almost religious fervour to them, which may be off putting'—in contrast Chapter 52 outlines the various theories that underlie research in an impartial yet enthusiastic fashion.

Jan Illing captures the cause of much misunderstanding when she states that 'researchers new to medical education who have medical training arrive in medical education research having been exposed to the scientific method and its *positivist* stance in relation to knowledge creation, and with little awareness of other theoretical perspectives' (Chapter 52).

Continuing on this vein in Chapter 54, Patty McNally explains how the majority of health professionals feel more comfortable with quantitative research methods—as these methods are most commonly used in clinical research. Writing over 50 years ago Leslie Witts (1960) claimed that 'in a world into which fifty million children are born each year we ought to have better guides to education than the speculations of Plato and Dewey' and since then there has been a flowering of different research methods—many of them qualitative—that have been used in medical education research and published in a growing number of medical education research journals.

Regardless of the research method used, we need to write up our findings and ideally in a way that is accessible to editors of journals and their readers. All too often medical education research is not written up or is written up in a way that perplexes rather than enlightens the readers. William Bean, writing about writing in 1952, complained that the 'so-called medical literature is stuffed to bursting with junk, written in a hopscotch style characterised by a Brownian movement of uncontrolled parts of speech which seethe in restless unintelligibility' (Bean 1952, p. 3). We would do well to ask whether our own specialty of medical education has sometimes contributed to this sea of restless unintelligibility. If medical education is to flourish as a discipline, then it is vital that those involved in medical education have the knowledge and skills and confidence to write papers with a clear message and to submit them to academic journals. It has been a pleasure to invite fellow editor Steve Kanter to give a comprehensive guide to writing and getting published in medical education. His chapter gives an overview of writing and publishing skills that are important regardless of the discipline but also explains specifically what will help the reader get published in medical education. The chapter also gives an account of different types of papers and explains the types of articles most likely to be accepted by the main medical education journals. Kanter emphasizes planning ahead 'not just because it is better to think ahead than to discover a significant error after submitting a manuscript to a journal but rather because planning ahead *is* the thinking that concludes with a substantive contribution to the field' (Chapter 55). Proper planning will lead to publication and dissemination of findings and build on the current state of scholarship in medical education. As Jennifer Leaning (1997) has written 'Hippocrates and Maimonides still abide, but the vast changes in situation and circumstance since they spoke create the need for other canons'—it is only through publication that such new canons come to renew or indeed replace the old.

Publication is of course just one component of scholarship and the authors of Chapter 56 give a scholarly account of the other components. In the past all that one needed to be a medical teacher was to have content expertise in that which was being taught. But in recent years this has changed as educators and learners alike have realized that more than just content expertise is necessary to become a competent educator. Chapter 56 defines scholarship in medical education and sets out ways in which those responsible for educational programmes can start to professionalize medical education. In 1961 William Bean complained about teaching institutes—'reports of teaching institutes, the kind of thing that the linguistically destitute cheerfully call workshops, often are about as inspiring as a workshop'. The authors of Chapter 56 adopt a more enlightened approach and outline the many and varied ways in which educators can develop their expertise. The chapter also explains the importance of academic standards in medical education and ways to help teachers reach those standards and reward them when they have done so.

Global medical education

Medical education in the developing world faces many challenges. There is inadequate funding, inadequate numbers of staff and inadequate infrastructure. In many countries, there is a continuous drain on the graduates that medical education produces who are tempted to leave their home country in search of work in the Western world. Medical education in the developing world needs to be cost effective and needs to produce doctors who can deliver the sort of healthcare that is needed by patients and communities in developing countries. The chapter by Badara Samb and colleagues outlines what form such medical education should take. Here the authors are frank—they state that an 'insufficient collaboration between the health and education sectors creates a crippling mismatch between medical education and the realities of health service delivery' and that the 'challenge of medical education in low- and middle-income countries relates to the quantity of doctors graduating from medical schools: the quality of medical education; and its relevance to population health needs and expectations' (Chapter 57). Too often in the past medical education curricula from Western countries have been parachuted into developing countries without sufficient thought given to the appropriateness of these curricula in their new context. We should also be wary of thinking that the sharing of educational expertise should be unidirectional and that there is nothing that we in the West can learn from developing countries (Walsh 2012). On cost grounds alone there may be unexpected sharing of expertise—medical schools in Africa can produce graduates at one tenth of the cost of North American schools. At times of cost constraint perhaps it is Western countries that need to import rather than export curricula.

The emerging market economies are currently restructuring their healthcare systems. As their population becomes healthier and grows older, the type of healthcare that the population needs will change. And the healthcare providers within these economies will need to change too. Chapter 58 by Manisha Nair and Premila Webster looks at how medical education in the emerging economies has evolved over the past number of years and examines how education will likely change in the future. Like in developing countries, the future will ideally lie in alignment—alignment of undergraduate and postgraduate training, of educational delivery and population needs, and of the skill mix of graduates and the outcomes required in the healthcare system.

The future

It is just over one hundred years since the publication of Abraham Flexner's report on the state of medical education in the USA. The report set in train a series of reforms which have led to our current system of medical education. One hundred years later, is it time for another great revolutionary change? Medicine and medical education are under enormous pressures, not least of which is the need to deliver cost-effective healthcare in a patient-centred way. In reflecting on questions of the future it is worth reflecting to what degree Flexner's report was revolutionary in the first place rather than evolutionary. According to Nicholas Christakis (1995, p. 706):

> reforms such as increasing generalist training, increasing ambulatory care exposure, providing social science courses, teaching lifelong and self-learning skills, rewarding teaching, clarifying the school mission, and centralizing curriculum control have appeared almost continuously since 1910

and it is a sobering and salutary thought that many of these ideas constitute the themes of some of the chapters of this book. Do we really need revolution—or should we just be putting into practice the evidence that we have developed over the past 100 years of what is effective medical education? If ideas have been around a long time then certainly the pace of change has been slow. In 1956 George Pickering commented wryly that 'no country has produced so many excellent analyses of the present defects of medical education as has Britain, and no country has done less to implement them'.

Perhaps the future might lie in incremental implementation of what we do know about medical education. In Chapter 59 Frenk and colleagues call for further 'instructional reforms (competency-driven, interprofessional, and transprofessional education; IT-empowered, local-global educational resources; and a new professionalism), and institutional reforms (joint planning; global networks; and a culture of critical inquiry)'. Perhaps it is this alignment of these two types of reforms that will finally enable the system to change.

And who will be the leaders that will guide us towards this bright future? Back to William Bean for the last time. According to Bean (1965):

> somewhere betwixt and between the extremes of the dynamic power seeker who triples his efforts as he loses sight of his goals and the ineffectual one driven about by every casual breeze, we find good deans of good medical schools who produce the inspiration and leadership as well as exert the firm hand of the helmsman in just the right combination.

That is undoubtedly the type of leader that we want—but how will we develop such leaders? Chapter 61 by Judy McKimm and colleagues outlines a number of different models of leadership and theoretical frameworks that underpin them. Interestingly the authors go some way to exploding the myth that leadership and management are completely separate spheres of activity. According to the authors the two concepts are inextricably linked—a leader cannot lead if they do not know some of the details of perhaps the change management process that an institution may have to undergo and equally all managers must show some degree of leadership. Perhaps it is distributed leadership that will be the way of the future.

My own view is that to reach a future that we want we should learn from the lessons of the past and yet stop short of romanticizing it. The rose-tinted glasses perspective is caught well by this quote from Ezekiel Emanuel (2006):

> at the end of their careers, physicians tend to wax poetic about the art of medicine and how it is being lost. (The same art seems to be lost every generation.)

When we look critically at the current state of medical education, we should remember that the past was often about passive undergraduate education, unsupervised postgraduate education, and optional and sometimes non-existent continuing medical education—all the while interspersed with largely intermittent, invalid and irreproducible assessments in programmes that were never evaluated. We have made progress, we are doing better and we must build on the progress that we have made. We should also perhaps stop searching for holy grails and rather look for the best format of medical education that will work in the particular context in which we are working—be it a contextualized curriculum or assessment or evaluation (Chapter 2).

There are no doubt more lessons but it is impossible to touch on them all or even on all chapters in this short introduction. Even though an introduction is not a lecture, I am wary of imposing to heavily on attention spans. If Chevalier Jackson was right and the primary purpose of medical education is to keep the medical student awake, then now is probably a good time for me to stop, and allow you dear reader to start.

References

Bean W. (1952) A testament of duty; some structures on moral responsibilities in clinical research. *J Lab Clin Med.* 39: 3

Bean WB. (1961) Report of the First Institute on Clinical Teaching: Report of the 6th AAMC Teaching Institute. *Arch Intern Med.* 107(3): 465

Bean WB. (1965) Fundamentals of medical education. *Arch Intern Med.* 115 (4):500

Bennett A. (2004) *The History Boys.* London: Faber and Faber

Christakis NA. (1995) The similarity and frequency of proposals to reform US medical education: constant concerns. *JAMA.*274(9): 706–711

Emanuel EJ. (2006) Changing premed requirements and the medical curriculum. *JAMA* 296(9): 1128

Feletti G. (1995) The disaster simulation: a problem-based learning or assessment experience for primary care professionals. *Med Teach.* 17(1): 39–45

Hawkyard A. (1910) Contract practice and the medical profession. *BMJ.* 2: 1095

Hensel WA. (1988) Graduate medical education confronted. *JAMA.* 259(18): 2695

Hippocrates. Corpus Hippocraticum 400 BCHutchinson L. (2006) Medical education: Challenges of training doctors in the new English NHS. *BMJ.* 332: 1502

Jason H. (1979) Continuing education—where does it begin? *Med Teach.* 1(6): 277

Jolly BC. (2008) The long case is mortal. BMJ. http://www.bmj.com/content/336/7655/1250/reply#bmj_el_196478?sid=90b7a8a2-7af4-4018-b137-261049bb6944 Accessed 5 October 2011

Last JM. (1985) Personal view. *BMJ.* 290:1900

Launer J. (2006) Reflective practice and clinical supervision: emotion and interpretation in supervision. *Work Based Learning in Primary Care.* 4(2): 171

Leaning J. (1997) Human rights and medical education: Why every medical student should learn the Universal Declaration of Human Rights. *BMJ.* 315: 1390

Lewis T. The Huxley lecture on clinical science within the university. *BMJ* 1935; 1: 631

Longhurst MF. (1994) The mentoring experience. *Med Teach.* 16(1): 53

McCoubrie P. (2004) The PBL debate is a distraction. *BMJ* (Published 21 July 2004) http://www.bmj.com/content/329/7457/92/reply#bmj_el_67922?sid=3f545f3a-8b62-4679-979a-2c0b244a4cd7 (accessed 15 October 2011)

McKeown T. (1986) Personal view. *BMJ.* 293:200

Medawar, P. B. (1979) *Advice to a Young Scientist.* New York: HarperCollins

Munro, D., Bore, M. and Powis, D. (2008). Personality determinants of success in medical school and beyond. 'Steady, Sane and Nice'. In S. Boag, (ed.).*Personality Down Under: Perspectives from Australia* (pp. 103–111). New York: Nova Science Publisher

Nairne P. (1988) Green College Lectures: The National Health Service: reflections on a changing service. *BMJ.* 296: 1518

Petersen S. (1999) Time for evidence based medical education: Tomorrow's doctors need informed educators not amateur tutors. *BMJ.* 318: 1223

Pickering G. (1956). The purpose of medical education. *BMJ.* 2(4985): 113–116

Schwartz, S. J, Vignoles, V. L., and Luyckx, K. (2011). Epilogue: What's next for identity theory and research? In: S. J. Schwartz, K. Luyckx, and V. L. Vignoles (eds) *Handbook of Identity Theory and Research (Volumes 1 & 2)* (pp. 933–938). New York, NY: Springer Science + Business Media

Simpson MA. (1979) A study in irrelevancy. *Med Teach.* 1(2): 94

Smyth DH. (1978) Personal view. *BMJ.* 2:1082

Walsh K. (2012) Medical education: what the West could learn from Africa. *Med Educ.* 46 (3): 336

Witts LJ. (1960) Traditional tutorial wisdom. *BMJ.* 1: 1550

PART 2

Curriculum

CHAPTER 2

Curriculum design in context

Janet Grant, Mohamed Y. H. Abdelrahmen,
and Anand Zachariah

The only task which 'educational theory' can legitimately
pursue … is to develop theories of educational practice that are
intrinsically related to practitioners' own accounts of what they
are doing, that will improve the quality of their involvement in
these practices and thereby allow them to practise better.

Wilfred Carr

Context and diversity

History and current practice suggest the need for a contextual
approach to curriculum design and development, drawing on
local conditions and opportunities, relying on local experience
and strengths. The relevant community of practice for curriculum
designers will be the constituency whom they consciously serve.

This implies that diversity in curriculum design is essential.
Where some schools will opt for orientation towards the community, or towards primary care, others will wish to produce the academics, scientists and researchers who will generate new knowledge
to support clinical work, or the tertiary specialists who may also be
required. Both approaches are important and need to interact with
each other. Medicine has a rich ecology. Medical schools must populate all corners of that environment to train the best health professionals and provide high quality and effective healthcare. And
each medical school must do so in the manner best suited to their
purpose, constituency and context.

What is curriculum?

According to Grant (2012), 'educators and philosophers have
addressed the question of what to teach and how to teach it at least
since Plato wrote *The Republic* in about 360 BCE. It might seem surprising then, that it is only relatively recently, perhaps in the last 40 to
50 years, that curriculum design has become a topic of debate in its
own right…'.

The power and role of curriculum are well recognized. The
debate about what a curriculum should be has advanced accordingly, with a consequent terminological confusion and no single
definition. To illustrate, table 2.1 characterizes the range, using
some commonly cited authors from within and outside medical
education.

Curriculum can be conceptualized in many ways differing in the balance of social, societal, educational, and instrumental focus. But all agree
that a curriculum should transmit and develop knowledge, skills, and
attitudes. It is not the student's concept, but the teacher's or institution's,
perhaps informed by other authorities. This profoundly challenges ideas
of learner centredness, suggesting that this is simply another approach
to delivering outcomes that are not the learner's own, as limitations on
extracurricular choices might suggest (Nikkar-Esfahani et al. 2012). But
where a subject is to be mastered, it cannot be otherwise.

Curriculum theory

Curriculum theorists, addressing the design and enactment of
curriculum, tend to approach this in one or a combination of four
ways, articulating the curriculum as:

- a body of knowledge (syllabus) to be transmitted

- a mechanism to achieve predefined endpoints which can be
  stated, for example, as objectives, competences or outcomes
  (Grant 1999, 2012)

- a process or 'proposal for action' which sets out essential features
  of the educational encounter (Smith 1996, 2000)

- praxis or informed committed actions which shape and change
  the world.

Curriculum has social and societal dimensions as the basis of
planned induction into the next stage. The philosopher and social
reformer, John Dewey argued that education and learning are social
and interactive processes, the school itself being a social institution
through which social reform should take place. And simultaneously, the curriculum must derive from, reflect and facilitate a set
of academic, social or professional values, being neither a neutral
nor value-free document.

Table 2.1 What is curriculum?

Author	Definition
Bobbit (1918)	Things which learners must do and experience to develop the abilities to do the things well and that make up the affairs of adult life.
Taba (1962)	A statement of aims and of specific objectives; indicating selection and organisation of content; implying certain patterns of learning and teaching, whether because the objectives demand them or the content organization requires them. It includes a programme of evaluation of the outcomes.
Bell (1971)	The socially valued knowledge, skills, and attitudes made available to students through a variety of arrangements during the time they are in education.
Stenhouse (1976)[2]	An attempt to communicate the essential principles and features of an educational proposal in a form that is open to critical scrutiny and capable of effective translation into practice.
Oliver (1977)	'The educational programme of the school' divided into four basic elements: (1) studies, (2) experiences, (3) service, and (4) hidden curriculum.
Tanner and Tanner (1980)	The planned and guided learning experiences and intended outcomes, formulated through the school's systematic reconstruction of knowledge and experiences, for the learners' continuous growth in personal social competence.
Hass (1987)	All of the experiences that individual learners have in a programme of education whose purpose is to achieve broad goals and related specific objectives, planned in terms of a framework of theory and research or professional practice.
Schubert (1987)	The contents of a subject, concepts and tasks to be acquired, planned activities, the desired learning outcomes and experiences, product of culture and an agenda to reform society.
Grundy (1987)	A programme of activities designed so that pupils will attain certain educational and other schooling ends or objectives.
Armstrong (1989)	A master plan for selecting content and organizing learning experiences to change and develop learners' behaviours and insights.
Oliva (1989)	The programme, a plan, content, and learning experiences.
Goodlad and Su (1992)	A plan covering learning opportunities for a specific time frame and place, to facilitate behaviour changes in students through planned learning experiences received by students with the guidance of the school.
Prideaux (2003)	The expression of educational ideas in practice . . . .All the planned learning experiences of an educational institution.
Fish and Coles (2005)	All the activities, experiences and learning opportunities for which an institution or a teacher takes responsibility—*either deliberately or by default*. This includes the formal and the informal, the overt and the covert, the recognised and the overlooked, the intentional and the unintentional.
Kern, Thomas and Hughes (2009)	A planned breadth of educational experiences, from one or more sessions on a special subject to a year-long course, from a clinical rotation or clerkship to an entire training programme.

The limits of curriculum

A curriculum is an aspirational statement; not a predictor of reality but a reflection of values, beliefs, intentions and hopes. It is the basis of management, administration and the assessment system. Nonetheless, translation into practice will be limited by a variety of factors.

The curriculum stated and experienced

Hafferty (1998) points out that the curriculum is limited by 'at least three interrelated spheres of influence'. These include the formal curriculum, the informal curriculum and the hidden curriculum. The idea of the hidden curriculum was first posited by Dewey (1916) and explored by others including Paulo Freire (2006) and Haralambos et al. (1991) who suggested that 'the hidden curriculum consists of those things pupils learn through the experience of attending school rather than the stated educational objectives of such institutions'.

Given that medicine is learned in the context of the healthcare service, and that role models transmit such fundamental values as

professionalism (Barret 2012; Skiles 2005) this statement is important. If the health service or teachers' behaviour are in contradiction with curriculum aspirations, those aspirations will be limited. A task of curriculum implementation, then, is to support faculty and their work context.

As Boelen and Woollard (2009) assert 'social accountability entails a duty to venture into a field over which the institution has no formal authority, namely, the functioning of the healthcare system'. So the curriculum must describe induction into the profession, through which learners acquire the knowledge, skills, attitudes and expertise to be an independent practitioner through increasing exposure to the healthcare system in which they will serve. This context of practice will present important lessons that are sometimes difficult to characterize or predict and so are often not mentioned in the objectified curriculum but are extraordinarily powerful learning experiences.

Contrary to this, Eisner (1994) put forward the idea of the 'null curriculum', suggesting that what is not taught will be regarded as unimportant and ignored by students. So as curriculum choices are made, dismissing certain content can have serious repercussions. Fish and Coles (2005) echo this: 'the curriculum, then, is determined as much by what is not offered, what is omitted, and what has been rejected, as it is by positive decisions'. These omissions are powerful messages in their own right. If basic science, primary care or community experiences, for example, are omitted, then the message will be clear.

But perhaps Eisner's observation only applies to the written curriculum, if it applies at all. It is too easy to think of curriculum as just the written document that allows a school to manage its resources, guide its teachers, inform its students and determine its assessments. In reality, the curriculum that shapes the learner is determined by other forces.

The curriculum and practice

The context of practice is just such a force. Stenhouse (1976) recognizes that a curriculum is limited by its contextual ability to be translated into practice. For example, a new, approved specialty curriculum for surgery could not inhibit a decline in achieved surgical skill which was a function of reduced working hours and operating opportunities (Parsons et al. 2010).

A curriculum within this professional induction process becomes increasingly problematic as the student, then trainee, then qualified independent practitioner progresses through the stages of a medical career. At each stage of this 'situated learning' (Lave and Wenger 1991), the unpredictability and richness of the service, the individual qualities of patients and their problems, and the increasingly specific, individual and sometimes flexible roles of doctors, cause increasing individuality of the trainee's knowledge and experience (Gale and Marsden 1983; Grant and Marsden 1987). This, in turn, makes a specific curriculum appropriate to all learners, increasingly difficult to define. Whereas a curriculum is relatively manageable in medical school, it becomes more challenging for specialty training where the service becomes more important as the basis of learning. For the practising clinician, learning needs will often derive from practice and so a shared curriculum for continuing professional development becomes less relevant to individual practice (Grant 2011). Thus, moving through the training and career stages of medicine presents an increasing limiting force on curriculum.

The power of a written curriculum, however, is unlimited if it aligns all aspects of the context of study and professional induction. As Fish and Coles (2005) assert 'a curriculum for practice must take "practice" as its starting point, and this means basing such a curriculum on and in ... the lived experience of practitioners ... '.

For the curriculum designer wishing to identify content, outcomes, processes and assessment systems, that is either a challenging limiting factor or a liberating force.

The contradictions of curriculum

Far from liberation, it has been argued that a curriculum which sets out clear, often competence-based outcomes instigates a teach-to-test paradigm (Schwartz and Sharpe 2010) which disempowers and de-professionalizes teachers, denying their ability to respond to students, find the teachable moment and exercise professional discretion. Where teach-to-test is dominant, students become instrumental in their learning. Carl Rogers' (1969) view of education as a process of liberating students to learn has perhaps been entirely overturned by curricula linked closely to high-stakes testing.

And yet the medical education rhetoric is contradictory, speaking often of a learner-centredness within a highly controlled curriculum (Ludmerer 1999; McLean and Gibbs 2009). However, a safe doctor must have a certain obligatory knowledge base and skill-set, and experience in applying these. A curriculum could be seen as an insurance policy against unsafe practice, with necessary strict limits on negotiation with the learner.

There is a tension between a learner-centred declared philosophy and the reality that in medicine, the school must ensure mastery; curriculum is at the centre of these opposing forces.

Curriculum ideology

Some key authors (Kelly 2009; Schiro 2008), addressing ideology and theory, decline to define curricula, having shown that a curriculum can have various ideological identities, for example:

- social utility (Bobbitt 1918)
- transmission of professional culture (Stenhouse 1976)
- social reconstruction (Kliebard 2004)
- description and prescription (Tyler 1949)
- scholar academic ideology (Schiro 2008)
- learner-centred ideology focusing on individual learner needs (Schiro 2008)
- the 'performative' curriculum to produce a product for the workforce (Barnett et al. 2010).

Such ideologies are reflections of differing social values about education.

The most influential educational thinker in the past century is almost dismissive of curriculum as central to the educational development of the young: according to Bruner (1996):

> ... education is not just about conventional school matters like curriculum or standards or testing. What we resolve to do in school only makes sense when considered in the broader context of what the society intends to accomplish through its educational investment in the young. How one conceives of education ... is a function of how one conceives of culture and its aims, professed and otherwise.
>
> Bruner 1996)

So understanding curriculum theory and ideology is essential. We do this with Crawford's (2009) caveats in mind:

> to regard universal knowledge as the whole of knowledge is to take no account of ... those features of actual thinkers who are always in particular *situations* ... We do not usually encounter things in a disinterested way ... '.

So, knowledge is based in practice.

The curriculum and the knowledge base

Curriculum theory adopts a neutral stance towards the knowledge base, assuming that the curriculum development process will identify this. This is an important function, because medical knowledge emerges in a particular social and political context, which shapes the form of that knowledge. An example will highlight the importance of this design stage—see box 2.1.

So politics, ideology and social context are determining influences not just on curriculum and education models, but on medical knowledge itself. It is therefore important for curriculum to be cognisant of the context of practice, and adopt a critical perspective on the knowledge base it offers.

Box 2.1 The curriculum and knowledge

Where healthcare is provided as a human right through welfare medicine, as in the UK (see Timmins 2001), medicine enters the scale of macroeconomics and governments spend a substantial portion of their budget on health (Foucault 1978, 2003). This fuels the growth of scientific research, large hospitals and the pharmaceutical and equipment industries. Western medicine has its growth in this ecological niche, with government investment in healthcare for problems of western countries, and at a cost that their health systems can afford (Zachariah et al. 2010).

When such knowledge is universalized, as has happened over the last half century, it results in mismatches between the setting of origin (the West, for example) and the settings where it is applied (the non-West, for example), creating problems of relevance, appropriateness and cost. So this raises questions: should we think not just of one universal knowledge base for medicine, but of multiple knowledge bases and local knowledge systems appropriate for the local setting, anywhere in the world? If the answer is in the affirmative (as we think it should be), then there are challenges for current curriculum theory.

What are the translations that are required to reinterpret and apply the received knowledge to the setting of practice? This applies not only to the knowledge component but equally to the teaching and learning processes promulgated since these are also culture bound and socially determined rather than absolute (Shiraev and Levy 2007). There is little robust evidence to suggest that any one educational approach is superior to another, so the decision about these too, must derive from context. For curricula to serve their societies they have not only to understand the educational process in context, and the context of practice and the healthcare system; they must also reinterpret the body of knowledge and the practice of medicine for the local situation.

In this, there is tension between absolutist views of knowledge (Peters 1966) and Dewey's (1916) pragmatic view whereby value is a quality situated in events, so no part of knowledge has a natural 'right' to be in the curriculum but must enjoy acceptance by the relevant community. Michael Young's (1971) seminal work on the sociology of education argued that knowledge, whether scientific or otherwise, is socially constructed and best understood through a study of the social contexts and conditions in which it is generated.

Influences on curriculum design

Curriculum development and design are based on implicit or explicit ideas, theories and purposes. There are three main sources of such influence: politics, paradigms of learning and professional and social theories.

Politics and the curriculum

Kelly (2009) points out that '... all of education is essentially a political activity ... the education system is a device by which an advanced society prepares its young for adult life in the society. In countries having a socialized healthcare system, this is even more

the case, where governments take an interest in the medical school curriculum, as is the case, for example, in the United Kingdom where the Foundation curriculum was derived from government, not professional imperative and reviews of medical education are often government driven. Health is a key political concern. So the curriculum that produces the healthcare workers will also be of political import.

Paradigms of learning

Just as education is a socially constructed process, likewise learning theories change according to dominant social ideas. Eventually, the original often reappears under a new guise: such as defining outcomes as competences rather than behavioural objectives which are, essentially the same entity (Grant 1999).

Table 2.2 presents the main paradigms of learning that have informed curriculum design in the current era. There are numerous specific theories within each. The relative prominence of each paradigm reflects its contemporary dominant social and economic values.

Ideas about adult learning from the 1970s (Houle 1972; Knowles1973; Kidd 1978) are not included as a paradigm, being only assumptions, models, aspirations or prescriptions for behaviour rather than a theory (Brookfield 1994) with little evidence base (Merriam and Caffarella 1998). Recent work suggests that there is no 'correct' model of adult learning, just as there is no parallel correct way for children to learn, but rather that such learning is influenced by the particular features of culture, context and practices (Tusting and Barton 2003).

It is clear that no one theory is sufficient to explain or determine actual learning. No single theory can describe the entire educational process. Different stages and topics require different types of learning. Education and training, particularly in a complex profession such as medicine, is a rich process with multifaceted outcomes, hence a wide variety of teaching and learning experiences of all these types, from lectures to free forms, is required.

Learning theories will not show how best to construct a curriculum. They simply offer ways of thinking, describing and conceptualizing.

Professional and social theories

Professional and social theories are less well described than the learning theories we have considered. Nonetheless, they are influential.

Prominent among professional theories are the frameworks that underpin the approaches of regulators who often define similar core areas of competence that apply to medical students, junior doctors in postgraduate training, and practising physicians. The three frameworks in table 2.3 inform almost all others used worldwide and have influenced the construction of curricula and the organization of defined outcomes. So they have credibility as an instrument, if not the status of a theory.

That professional and social theories are shared, reflecting current social and cultural imperatives, is demonstrated by Skochelak (2010) who analysed 15 US reports calling for change in medical education published in the previous 10 years. She found 'remarkable congruence' in their recommendations around eight themes:

Table 2.2 Paradigms of learning

Paradigm	Characteristics	Effect on curriculum design
Behaviourism (Skinner 1974)	Ignores internal mental processes. Focus on external stimuli, for reward and punishment, to control behaviour. Teacher transmits learning by breaking subject matter into small chunks (behavioural objectives or competences) which are rehearsed repeatedly until mastery.	Attainment of behavioural objectives is the priority. Little concern with learning processes.
Cognitive theories (Ausubel 1968; Gagné, 1985)	Replaced behaviourism. Suggested that people are not simply to be trained, but are rational so we should understand thinking, memory, knowing and problem-solving processes. Cognitive structure is central to success in learning allowing new knowledge to be coherently assimilated and, in turn, to allow those structures to adapt to new information.	Less rigorous approach to the definition of learning outcomes. More interest in teaching and learning processes and the learning environment. Greater focus towards the individual learner. Emphasis on acquiring a solid knowledge base from which new learning can benefit by assimilation and adaptation.
Constructivism (Piaget 1970, Vygotsky 1934/1986, Bruner 1973)	Further development of cognitive theory. Learners seen as actively constructing new ideas and concepts based on their existing knowledge. Robust cognitive structures (the knowledge base, or mental models, called 'mental sets' or 'schemata' by Piaget) are fundamental to the ability to 'go beyond the information given'. Constructivism assumes that the student's ability to construct their own understanding is independent of the teaching method. A scaffold of knowledge is important.	Curricula designed around teaching and learning processes. Bruner introduced the spiral *curriculum* organized so that the student continually builds on what they have already learned. Led to ideas such as enquiry and discovery learning.
Social learning theory (Bandura, 1977; Lave and Wenger 1991; Vygotsky 1978; perhaps Kolb 1984)	People learn through observation and considered experience. Internal mental states are important in how this occurs. Learning for Vygotsky (1978) best occurs in the *zone of proximal development* (the distance between assisted and independent action). The modelling process involves successful attention, retention, reproduction and motivation to imitate (Bandura 1977) Learning is situated in practice, starting with peripheral participation under supervision, and ending with full participation with full responsibility (Lave and Wenger 1991).	Introduction of live (role) models, verbal instructional models (descriptions and explanations of behaviour), and symbolic models (books or films). Curricula constructed towards independence through stages of being taught and being supervised.
Humanism (Maslow 1943; Rogers 1969)	Learning seen as the process of fulfilling personal potential. Learner seen as having cognitive and affective needs. Emphasis placed on human freedom and dignity through learning. Assumes learners act with intentionality and values (Huitt 2001).	Learning seen as student-centred and personal. Teacher is facilitator of individual student's learning and personal fulfilment (self-actualization) in a co-operative, supportive environment.

◆ integrating the educational continuum

◆ the need for evaluation and research

◆ the need for new methods of financing

◆ the importance of leadership

◆ the need for social accountability

◆ the need for new technology in education and practice

◆ the need to align education with changing healthcare delivery systems

◆ the need to align education with future workforce patterns.

These themes derive from social and economic development, and politics. They seem reactive, pragmatic and instrumental, viewing medical education largely as a production line for future medical employment and deployment. Although understandable, if the profession's own theories of practice are outweighed by economic, and even social, imperatives, there is danger in the venture. When instrumentalist authorities suggest that '… medical schools need to adapt their *product* [our italics] …' (Farry and Williamson 2004) we might be alarmed. Barnett et al. (2010) worry about the growing domination of the principle of 'performativity', in higher education, which merely relates universities to the labour market: 'it implies doing, rather than knowing, and performance rather than understanding. In the performative society, there is a mistrust of all things that cannot easily be quantified and measured'.

This antiprofessional view affects curricula as they strive towards an instrumental and measurable outcome, perhaps perversely limiting the ultimate power of the independent graduate to operate to society's greater benefit.

Table 2.3 Professional frameworks

Framework	Characteristics
US Accreditation Council for Graduate Medical Education	◆ Patient care ◆ Practice-based learning and improvement ◆ Medical knowledge ◆ Interpersonal and communication skills ◆ Professionalism ◆ Systems-based practice
UK General Medical Council	The doctor as: 1. A scholar and a scientist 2. A practitioner 3. A professional
Royal College of Physicians and Surgeons of Canada: CanMEDS	Medical expert, made up of: ◆ Communicator ◆ Collaborator ◆ Manager ◆ Health advocate ◆ Scholar ◆ Professional

Table 2.4 Types of curricula

A curriculum may be	
◆ Task-based	◆ Community based
◆ Spiral	◆ Horizontally integrated
◆ Problem-based	◆ Vertically integrated
◆ Case-based	◆ Traditional
◆ Modular	◆ Discipline based
◆ Community orientated	◆ Theme based
	◆ Core and options

The current dominant social concept is that of the social accountability of medical schools:

> the obligation of medical schools to direct education, research and service activities towards addressing the priority health concerns of the community, region or nation that they are mandated to serve.
>
> Boelen and Heck 1995

Although it is difficult to argue against this idea, it is still a problematical one which fails to address satisfactorily the limited power of medical education in relation to healthcare provision (the ultimate employer), the role of exploratory academic scientific research, the professional knowledge and skills of medicine, the autonomy of a professional, the largely unknown causal relationship between teaching and learning processes, careers choice and outcomes.

As with learning theories, these ideas simply offer ways of thinking, describing and conceptualizing. It is still for each agency to define its own curriculum on the basis of its own values and intentions. There is no more rational and empowered approach.

Curriculum models and the design process

The literature is replete with curriculum models, each of which has its proponents and detractors. As Prideaux (2003) indicates, 'a curriculum is the result of human agency. It is underpinned by a set of values and beliefs about what students should know and how they come to know it. The curriculum of any institution is often contested and problematic'.

This leaves the choice of model fully open to each institution. The choices are bewildering, not independent and often borrowed from other areas of education (see table 2.4).

Within each of these are many variants. In curriculum design, there is no one truth, no strong evidence, no universal choice. For example, the literature is equivocal on clinical problem solving: on the one hand the traditional curriculum has been shown to produce better clinical problem-solvers (Goss et al. 2011); while on the other, more modern variants claim to do so (Norman 1988).

At a higher level, Print (1993) suggests that most curricula can be:

◆ prescriptive (obligatory) OR descriptive (reflecting complex practice)

◆ rational (objectives-based) OR dynamic (fluid and reactive).

Given that there is no consistent evidence that undergraduate medical education can securely predict later doctor performance (Norman et al. 2008), then the choice of curriculum model must be a function entirely of local vision, values, need, culture and context.

How then, is the contextual curriculum to be designed? The democratization of social processes means that there are much wider considerations than the views of content experts alone. However, some components seem to be held in common (Grant 2012). These include stating the overall purpose, vision, mission and values; performing a contextual analysis; stating educational goals; deciding how the curriculum will be organized; stating specific learner objectives; deciding on the educational philosophy and values; selecting educational opportunities; deciding on the assessment; deciding on the evaluation; and setting out the administration plan (Grant 2012; Fish and Coles 2005).

Unfortunately, the literature cannot advise the curriculum developer what best to decide at each stage. So designers must make their own decisions. For example, 60 years after Tyler's (1949) seminal work, there is still no agreement about the use, effect and structure of objectives as a way of expressing intended learning outcomes. The current atavistic fashion for competence-based curricula is hotly debated as being merely a derivative of post-war behaviourism (Hyland 1993; Grant 1999) in need of recontextualizing within social, political and cultural practices (Jeris et al. 2005). It is argued that the 'reductive and formulaic' use of competences which 'seek to atomize complex forms of behaviour' (Fleming 2006) could be replaced by more process and procedural statements (Lum 2004), and in any case, competences cannot describe undertakings of a social character (Davis 2005)—such as medicine. Even at the level of the original basic claims, Kjaer et al. (2011) conclude that 'it is unlikely that a competency-based curriculum can justify a significant reduction on time spent on clinical training'. These arguments are a reprise of those aired when objectives were first mooted over 60 years ago.

The highly marketed introduction of e-learning is also now under a critical gaze, with student satisfaction and learning outcomes not delivering on earlier hopes (Kaznowska, Rogers, and Usher 2011).

The equally aggressively disseminated problem-based learning now is finding its own level as one learning method among many, rather than a full curriculum design.

There is no aspect of education or educational planning which is not subject to constant debate. Research evidence cannot and will not decide: education is too complex a phenomenon for objective or replicable analysis. Only openly articulated values and purpose will allow the local choices that must be made at each step of curriculum design.

The case for curriculum heterogeneity

A curriculum is a social, ideological, and political instrument, which must inform and guide the actions and outcomes of educational institutions, teachers, learners, and managers. Curriculum trends are not evidence-based but are social and philosophical. So each country and institution must build its own, on the basis of its own culture, context, and needs. For example, the current focus on teaching professionalism has revealed considerable regional and subregional cultural differences that require different interpretations of the term (Chandratilake et al. 2012; van der Horst and Lemmens 2012) and a determination to 'move the field beyond a Western individualist focus' (Ho et al. 2012).

But this is an issue of ephemeral ideological, not western, domination which oppresses all. It is a question of whether there is a research or philosophical base to inform educational recommendations. Clearly, national regulators must have their say, and global standards (WFME 2003) might help schools to produce a curriculum of their own. But medical education research, which is derivative of educational research as a whole, does not tell us what any curriculum should say. Only a locally owned process made on the basis of negotiation and professional judgement will lead to a relevant curriculum.

Localizing content

Simply looking at the causes of death in different countries explains why a curriculum must be based on context. Comparing causes of male adult deaths in UK and India shows that: cancer causes 17% of deaths in the UK but 9% of deaths in India; TB causes 10% of deaths in India but is a rare cause of death in the UK (Office of the Registrar General India Ministry of Home Affairs 2009). Although

the disease profile is different in developing countries, the resources for students are western textbooks.

Further, when a disease category (the basic unit of medical knowledge) emerges it is assumed that it operates in the same way across the world and that treatments are universally applicable. Let us analyse this assumption taking the example of post-traumatic stress disorder (PTSD).

PTSD emerged as a disease category in the context of Vietnam war veterans' demand for public acknowledgement of the suffering that US troops underwent. In this setting, the definition of the syndrome included feelings of guilt and the need for trauma counselling and compensation to resolve this. The entity of PTSD that emerged to address the social needs of war veterans became universalized with the same criteria and guidelines for care even if the settings did not correspond. For example, post-Bhopal, or after the Asian tsunami or communal conflict, the context of the trauma had to guide the care of survivors (Jacob 2010). In the instance of the Asian tsunami, PTSD rates were unexpectedly low and it is thought that this is due to the community support provided to the survivors (Tharyan 2005). This example emphasizes the need to understand context in relation to our knowledge of any health problem. There is a culture surrounding any disease category, related to its context of origin which, though invisible, travels with it when it is transplanted to another setting. The culture of that knowledge continues to trouble the category as it is used in other settings (Tharu 2010).

Local curricula are not just a matter of determining the common problems in a particular country or region or of training students within the context of the healthcare system. They are about developing a critical perspective to knowledge and a knowledge base appropriate to specific local circumstance. This requires careful study and research of local health problems for which there is no precedent (see fig. 2.1). It also requires appropriate learning resources.

Harmonizing curriculum and resource

Despite the lack of consistent evidence suggesting better outcomes in more resource-intensive curricula, or in modern curricula as opposed to traditional ones, the following ideas tend to dominate the discourse: skills labs, e-learning, disintegration of the science base in the name of integration, teaching and learning methods that require a more intensive student-staff ratio. Journals and conferences report curriculum innovation, while stasis does not publicize itself so well.

Consider the case study outlined in box 2.2, which is derived from a number of instances.

Although the scenario outlined in box 2.2 is from a developing country, its lessons apply to all curriculum developers everywhere. Start from the circumstances, identify the vision, use available resources and design independently—appropriate to local conditions, context and culture. Medical education curricula will be enriched by becoming homogenously heterogeneous.

The contextual curriculum

Bellack (1969) states that 'the history of curriculum thought and practice cannot be separated from the general history of American education, which, in turn, cannot be divorced from the broader stream of cultural and intellectual history'.

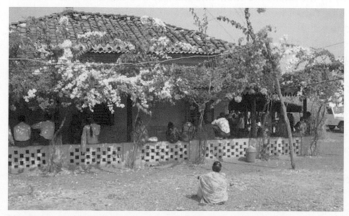

Figure 2.1 Healthcare in context—a clinic in Cuttack, Orissa, India.

This is true of any country, and calls into question the international transferability of curriculum ideas, even within the west. That does not seem to deter, however, their export and import. Bleakley et al. (2011) draw our attention to this in what they refer to as the 'post-colonial dilemma' and its neocolonial sequelae, according to which countries almost voluntarily seem to feel the need to follow (sometimes unsuccessful and often unproven) medical education practices under the uncritical guise of international benchmarking, modernization or innovation, sometimes despite current better comparative health outcomes or satisfactory quality of medical graduate resulting from the current system. They juxtapose, for example, a call for the importation of western educational ideas into Japan (Onishi and Yoshida 2004) despite better existing health outcomes in Japan at many points in the age spectrum compared with the US, suggesting, perhaps a superior medical education there (Rao 2006, 2007). Bleakley et al. (2011) note the

> apologetic stance taken by authors in the east about their slowness in adopting western methods, even though, following Khoo's (2003) observations, those methods will demand an 'intense re-socialization of learners into metropolitan Western mindsets … '.

However, there are differences in educational and assessment cultures, even within and between western countries (Segouin and Hodges 2005; Hodges et al. 2009; Jippes and Majoor 2008). The case for a contextual curriculum applies across the board.

Wong (2011) states that:

> unlike a single universal definition of medical education, a sociocultural conceptualisation of medical education recognises that many different models of effective teaching may exist in the world.

Box 2.2 Case study

A new medical school was to be opened in a developing country, with ambitions for a well-run, not-for-profit medical school to serve the community. The location and land were found.

Buildings for the school were erected, consisting of a few large lecture rooms, offices, a library, a general laboratory, a computer laboratory, and a small dissecting room. They hoped to expand in future.

The curriculum was planned to be community based, directed towards the needs of the local population, with learning objectives to be prioritized accordingly, based on evidence of community needs.

Eventually a curriculum was designed to fit the regulator's standards. It adopted a student-centred model which the local curriculum designers had heard about and had had international consultancy visits to support.

The curriculum was tailored to health system demands, involving all stakeholders: academics, the Health Ministry and community leaders, who were all concerned about the competencies of the graduates.

Lack of self-confidence and expertise meant that the curriculum model comprised parts of models existing elsewhere. They adopted 'modern methods': faculty-intensive teaching, with communication skills and clinical skills learned in the community setting.

Their building blocks consisted mainly of community residences and family visits, while the teaching was planned to be delivered by educators working in district hospitals and primary healthcare centres.

They needed administrative and teaching staff. Finding individuals to work as administrators who had experience with educational institutions was a challenge and they settled on recruiting professionals in accounting and general management. Recruiting appropriately experienced teaching staff was difficult. There was a scarcity of expert teachers. It was impossible to offer the high salary that a full-time expert would demand. So the founders were not able to bring in experts in all subjects. A part-time option was an affordable and more convenient alternative (albeit less effective for students).

After much deliberation, they decided to recruit the most needed professors as part-timers and those with fewer qualifications and experience as full-timers to monitor the students' learning process. Curriculum implementation looked challenging. They thought about inviting the diaspora and foreign students on electives but regarded this as unsustainable.

Student applications were more than expected, although it felt gratifying for the founders. Consequently they decided to accept a larger number of students than they had the capacity for, driven partly by the financial benefit and stability that this may yield even if it demanded that staff put in extra effort. They believed that, in the long run, it would benefit the school; a decision that would later prove to be daunting, given the chosen teaching and learning methods.

Tenders for equipment were studied but with large student numbers and financial constraints, the cheapest was accepted.

The school was opened and gradually it started to face different problems, most of which could be traced to limited resources in relation to a resource-intensive curriculum design. The school's budget was mainly used to pay for teaching the large number of students. The curriculum as planned could not be implemented. It was too late to plan an appropriate curriculum.

Each year, the student-staff ratio worsened. The local healthcare service was not analysed for its educational potential. There was a continuous need for supplies and materials. Information provided to the students needed constant updating, new references and evidence based information. The library could not cope.

The circumstances were alarming; the situation needed a pause so that the issues could be addressed. Goodwill was there, but time to plan, reflect, change and evaluate was limited.

There was a clear vision, goals were set, the curriculum was written, the community was the motive and the students were the asset that they wanted to invest in with their limited resources.

How could such a vision be achieved?

(continued)

Box 2.2 (Continued)

In a low resource setting, curriculum designers need the self-confidence to create their own solutions. Sadly, even the literature on health professions education in low-resource circumstances frequently recommends high-resource solutions, such as technology-based learning and teacher-intensive approaches (Wootton et al. 2011) or culturally inappropriate pedagogical ideas (Murray et al. 2011) rather than analysing the opportunities of the local context. Excellence cannot be equated with others' innovations, however, nor with elaborate resources. Open educational resources which are affordable, cost cutting and sustainable can help (Yuan et al. 2008) where they are appropriate to the context and the technology is sufficiently available. But management and prioritization of existing resources towards achievement of an appropriate curriculum vision of excellence requires new models, developed in local circumstances.

The college graduated their first batch and it was time to review the curriculum. Definite strengths and weaknesses in the curriculum were observed.

It became clear that overcoming low resources involved using community settings that would guarantee exposure for students. Clinical learning, skills training, peer education, disseminating the culture of supervision and feedback, and integration of teaching with health service needs were all situated in the available locations. When curriculum review started from context, it led to learning in that context. So the curriculum developed new models on its own terms.

Strengths were found in the committed staff who felt ownership and responsibility for curriculum implementation. The graduates excelled in communication, clinical skills and understanding their communities' health problems.

Partnership with health service providers proved beneficial and the stakeholders who supported them were willing to continue their support. An entire contextual model of their own developed.

The original staff-intensive curriculum was a weakness. Furthermore, improper deployment of staff, with university professors teaching in primary healthcare settings, resulted at times in a poor understanding of the true community health needs. Another challenge was faced when the model of integration lost the intensity of basic science subjects and students were not happy with their knowledge, feeling underprivileged when compared to their peers from other universities.

The school faculty were frustrated by their limited involvement in academic research; mainly due to limitation of funds. This is being addressed and opportunities for community-based clinical and scientific research are being sought.

The curriculum was revised. The spirit of the college and its real social commitment towards the community increased when the context became the driver. In developing countries, the role of the doctor as a healer is often over-ruled by the high expectations of the local community as a wise-man, which gives a sociocultural dimension to the way the doctor is viewed. This was fundamental in planning their contextual curriculum that produces doctors who are aware of their local health service and community needs, and can meld easily with their communities.

This leaves the onus for decision-making on the curriculum designer, using professional judgement, reflecting on the local context and vision. As Bruner (1996) states, 'you cannot understand mental activity unless you take into account the cultural setting and its resources; the very things that give mind its shape and scope. Learning, remembering, talking, and imaging: all of them are made possible by participating in a culture'.

In practice, curriculum planning, design and development tend to be shared, logical processes. However, the content and variables to be taken into consideration, and subsequent choices made, will differ depending on local contexts, and the challenge is to ensure that the medical school will produce graduates who are appropriate for the healthcare needs of the population and the healthcare system. In this, the symbiotic relationship with the healthcare service and the research activity which underpins the development of knowledge and practice, are key elements. There is no authoritative source of information or guidance about how best to proceed.

In designing a contextual curriculum, the technical aspects of curriculum design still apply. Decisions will still be required about:

◆ the vision

◆ how to express outcomes

◆ what the content will be

◆ how to organize the curriculum

◆ what teaching and learning methods will be offered and encouraged and

◆ how the assessment system will run.

However, these must be consequential, not primary, decisions. They should be made on the basis of local professional knowledge and judgement, and on context.

For many, the driving vision will be of a socially accountable institution, closely linked with the healthcare service, and with the healthcare priorities and problems that medicine and communities face. But medicine is an academic discipline, and so for others, the medical school will primarily be a seat of high learning, of academic discourse and scientific research. These goals are not in contradiction with social accountability.

A contextual curriculum demands a change of emphasis, away from a narrow focus on educational method and the unending search for the most effective methods of teaching and learning, for which there will not be a robust differentiating evidence base, and towards context and vision, for which there will be demonstrated health benefits and benefits to the scientific and cultural basis of medicine. In a contextual curriculum, the medical education decisions become secondary and no longer drive curriculum design, as shown in fig. 2.2.

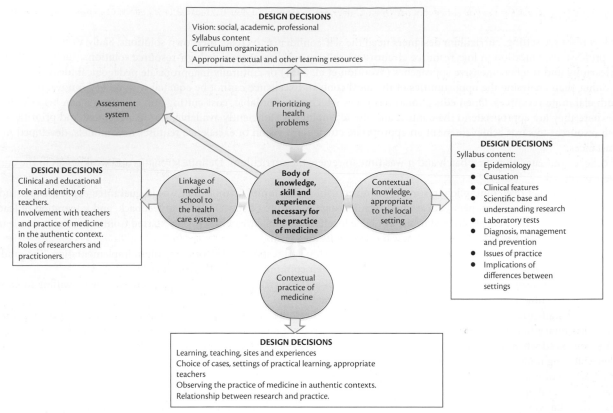

Figure 2.2 Design decisions.

What context means

In designing curricula, we might be careful about what we wish for. Aspiration to control learning, and achieve global harmonization and international benchmarking is high. In a comment on the 2011 London riots, a community-based general practitioner, Mike Fitzpatrick (2011), wrote that 'the lesson that emerges from the Hackney riots is that far from empowering individuals and communities, professional intrusion damages personal autonomy ... '

There is a parallel. Although we must ensure that our students and specialty trainees are safe and are acquiring the necessary skills and knowledge of the profession, the current drive towards a unified curriculum philosophy in professional education may possibly subvert the development of the locally relevant, culturally sensitive, responsible, creative and engaged doctor we purport to value, emerging from medical schools which are individual, fit for national and local purpose and for the development of the profession as a whole. A contextual curriculum is required.

Conclusions

◆ A curriculum is an ideological statement that must reflect relevant values deriving from the local political, cultural, professional and social context.

◆ There is pressure for increasing international homogenization of ideas at a time when heterogeneity is required to address the cultural, social, philosophical and healthcare needs of different societies and contexts.

◆ For medical education to be effective and relevant, it must derive its solutions locally, relating the educational process to locally relevant medical knowledge and practice; and to the link between medical schools and the healthcare system. A contextual curriculum is required.

◆ The practising profession itself must be the driving force for the development of curricula fully integrated with the development of the healthcare services and the knowledge and skill base of the profession appropriate to the local circumstance.

◆ In curriculum theory, there is terminological confusion; no single definition; and a deficit of evidence about process, theory, and underlying assumptions about education. In the absence of evidence, professional judgment in context must inform curriculum design.

References

Apple MW (2004) *Ideology and Curriculum*. 3rd edn. London: Routledge Falmer

Armstrong, D.G. (1989) *Developing and Documenting the Curriculum*. Boston: Allyn and Bacon

Ausubel, D. (1968) *Educational Psychology. A Cognitive View*. London; Holt, Rinehart and Winston

Bandura, A. (1977) *Social Learning Theory*. New York: General Learning Press

Barnett, R., Parry, G. and Coate, K. (2010) Conceptualising curriculum change. *Teaching in Higher Education*, 6(4): 435–449

Barret, M. (2012) Clinical experiences during preclinical training: the function of modelled behaviour and the evidence of professionalism principles. *Int J Med Educ.*, 3:37–45

Bell R (1971) *Thinking about Curriculum*. Maidenhead: Open University Press

Bellack, A.A. (1969) History of curriculum thought and practice. *Rev Educ Res.* 39(3): 283–292

Bleakley, A., Bligh, J., Browne, J. (2011) *Medical Education for the Future. Identity, Power and Location*. Springer: London

Bobbitt F. (1918) *The Curriculum*. Boston: Houghton Mifflin

Boelen, C. and Heck, J.E. (1995) *Defining and Measuring the Social Accountability of Medical Schools*. Geneva: World Health Organization.

Boelen, C. and Woollard, B. (2009) Social accountability and accreditation: a new frontier for educational institutions. *Med Educ.* 43(9): 887–894

Brookfield, S.D. (1994) Adult learning. An overview. In A. Tuijnman (ed.) (1994) *International Encyclopedia of Education*. Oxford: Pergamon Press

Bruner, J. (1973) *Going Beyond the Information Given*. New York: Norton

Bruner J. (1996) *The Culture of Education*. Harvard University Press: Cambridge, MA

Carr, W. (1995) *For Education. Towards Critical Educational Inquiry*. Open University Press: Buckingham, UK

Cavenagh, P., Leinster, S.J., and Miles, S. (eds) *The Changing Face of Medical Education*. Oxford: Radcliffe Publishing Company

Chandratilake, M., McAleer, S. and Gibson, J. (2012) Cultural similarities and differences in medical professionalism: A multi-region study. *Med Educ.* 46(3): 257–266

Clarkson, J. (2009) What is comparative education? In W. Bignold and L. Gayton (eds) Sharp, J (series ed) (2009) *Global Issues and Comparative Education* (pp. 4–17). Exeter: Learning Matters

Crawford, M. (2009) *The Case for Working with Your Hands or Why Office Work is Bad for Us and Fixing Things Feel Good*. London: Viking

Davis, A. (2005) Social externalism and the ontology of competence. *Philosophical Explorations*. 8(3): 295–306.

Dewey J (1916) *Democracy and education. An introduction to the philosophy of education*. New York: The MacMillan Company. http://www.ilt.columbia.edu/Publications/dewey.html Accessed 15 February 2013

Eisner, E.W. (1994) *The Educational Imagination: On Design and Evaluation of School Programs*. 3rd. edn. New York: Macmillan

Farry, P. and Williamson, M. (2004) Aligning medical education with the healthcare needs of the population. *N Zealand Med J.*, 117: 1204 http://www.nzma.org.nz/journal/117-1204/1114. Accessed 16 March 2012

Fish, D. and Coles, C. (2005) *Medical Education. Developing a Curriculum for Practice*. Maidenhead: Open University Press

Fitzpatrick, M. (2011) Reflections on the riots in Hackney. *Br J Gen Pract*. 61: 591–634

Fleming, M. (2006) The use and misuse of competence frameworks and statements with particular attention to describing achievements in literature. Report of an international conference organised jointly by the Council of Europe, Language Policy Division, and the Jagiellonian University. Retrieved from www.coe.int/t/dg4/linguistic/source/krakow%20abstracts.pdf Accessed 15 February 2013

Foucault, M. (1978) The crises of medicine or the crises of anti-medicine. In *Foucault Studies*, No. 1, December 2004 (talk originally delivered in 1978), 5–19. Translated by E.C Knowlton Jr., W.J. King and C. O'Farrel

Foucault, M. (2003) *The Essential Foucault: Selections from the Essential Works*, 1954–1984. Eds P. Rabinow, and N. Rose. New York and London: The New Press

Freire, P. (2006) *Pedagogy of the Oppressed*, 30th Anniversary ed. New York: Continuum

Gagné, R. (1985). *The Conditions of Learning* (4th edn). New York: Holt, Rinehart & Winston

Gale, J. and Marsden, P. (1983) *Medical Diagnosis. From Student to Clinician*. Oxford: Oxford University Press

Goodlad, J. and Su Z. (1992) Organization of the curriculum. In P. Jackson (ed.) *Handbook of Research on Curriculum*, New York: MacMillan, pp. 327–344

Goss, B., Reid, K., Dodds, A. and McColl, G. (2011) Comparison of medical students' diagnostic reasoning skills in a traditional and a problem based learning curriculum. *Int J Med Educ*. 2: 87–93

Grant, J. (1999) The incapacitating effects of competence: A critique. *J Health Sci Educ*. 4(3): 271–277

Grant, J. (2011) *The Good CPD Guide*. Oxford: Radcliffe.

Grant, J. (2012) Principles of curriculum design. In T. Swanwick (ed.) *Understanding medical Education. Evidence, Theory and Practice*. pp. 1–15. Chichester: John Wiley & Sons

Grant, J. and Marsden, P. (1987) The structure of memorised knowledge in students and clinicians: an explanation for diagnostic expertise. *Med Educ*. 21: 92–98

Grundy, S. (1987) *Curriculum: Product or praxis*. Lewes: Falmer Press

Hafferty FW (1998) Beyond curriculum reform: Confronting medicine's hidden curriculum. *Acad Med*. 73: 403–407

Haralambos, M, Heald, R.M, Holborn M (1991) *Sociology: Themes and Perspectives*. Bishopsbriggs: Collins Educational

Hass G (1987) *Curriculum Planning. A New Approach*. Boston: Allyn and Bacon

Ho, M-J., Lin, C-W., Lingard, L. and Ginsburg, S. (2012) A cross-cultural study of students' approaches to professional dilemmas: Sticks or ripples. *Med Educ*. 46(3): 245–256

Hodges, BD., Maniate, J.M., Martimianakis, M.A., Alsuwadan, M., Segouin, C. (2009) Cracks and crevices: globalisation discourse and medical education. *Med Teach*. 31(10): 910–917

Houle, C.O. (1972) *The Design of Education*. San Francisco: Jossey-Bass

Huitt, W. (2001) *Humanism and open education. Educational Psychology Interactive*. Valdosta: Valdosta Statge University. http://www.edpsycinteractive.org/topics/affect/humed.html Accessed 15 February 2013

Hyland, T. (1993) Competence, knowledge and education. *J Philosophy Educ*. 27(1): 57–68.

Jackson, N. (2002) Pressures for curriculum change. LTSN Generic Centre. http://78.158.56.101/archive/palatine/files/1049.pdf Accessed 17 February 2013

Jacob, K.S. (2010) TSD, DSM and India: A critique In A. Zachariah, R. Srivatsan, and S. Tharu (eds) *Towards a Critical Medical Practice. Reflections on the Dilemmas of Medical Culture Today* (pp. 57–68) Hyderabad: Orient BlackSwan

Jeris, L., Johnson, K., Isopahkala, U., Winterton, J. and Anthony, K. (2005) The politics of competence. Views from around the globe. *Human Resource Development Journal*. 8(3): 379–384

Jippes, M. and Majoor, G.D.(2008) Influence of national culture on the adoption of integrated and problem-based curricula in Europe. *Med Educ*.;42(3): 279–285

Kaznowska, E., Rogers, J., and Usher, A. (2011) The State of E-Learning in Canadian Universities, 2011: If Students Are Digital Natives, Why Don't They Like E-Learning? Toronto: Higher Education Strategy Associates

Kelly, A.V. (2009) *The Curriculum. Theory and Practice*. 6th edn. London: Sage

Kern DE, Thomas PA, Hughes MT (2009) *Curriculum development for medical education: A six-step approach*. Baltimore: The Johns Hopkins University Press

Khoo, H.E. (2003) Implementation of problem-based learning in Asian medical schools and students' perceptions of their experience. *Med Educ*. 37(5): 401–409

Kidd, J.R. (1978) *How Adults Learn*. Englewood Cliffs: Prentice-Hall

Kjaer, N.K., Kodal, T., Shaughnessy, A.F. and Qvesel, D. (2011) Introducing competency-based postgraduate medical training: Gains and losses. *Int J Med Educ*. 2: 110–115

Kliebard, H. (2004) *The Struggle for the American Curriculum, 1893–1958*. New York: Routledge Falmer

Kolb, D.A. (1984) *Experiential Learning. Experience as the Source of Learning and Development*. Englewood Cliffs: Prentice-Hall

Knowles, M. (1973) *The Adult Learner. A Neglected Species*. Houston: Gulf Publishing Company

Knowles, M. (1980). *The Modern Practice of Adult Education: From Pedagogy to Andragogy*. Wilton, Connecticut: Association Press

Lave, J. and Wenger, E. (1991) *Situated learning. Legitimate peripheral participation*. Cambridge: Cambridge University Press

Ludmerer, K.M. (1999) *Time to Heal: American Medical Education from the Turn of the Century to the Era of Managed Care*. Oxford, England: Oxford University Press

Lum, G. (2004) On the non-discursive nature of competence. *Educational Philosophy and Theory*. 36(5): 485–496

Maslow, A.H. (1943) A theory of human motivation. *Psychol Rev*. 50 (4): 370–396

McLean, M., and Gibbs, TJ. (2009) Learner-centred medical education: Improved learning or increased stress? *Education for Health*, 22: 3. http://www.educationforhealth.net/. Accessed 19 March 2012

Merriam, S.B. and Caffarella, R.S. (1998) *Learning in Adulthood. A Comprehensive Guide*. 2nd edn. New York: Jossey-Bass

Murray, J.P., Wenger, A.F.Z., Downes, E.A. and Terrazas, S.B. (2011) *Educating Health Professionals in Low-Resource Countries*. New York: Springer

Nikkar-Esfahani. A., Jamjoom, A.A.B., Fitzgerald, E.F. (2012) Extracurricular participation in research and audit by medical students. *Med Teach*. e1–e8, Early Online, http://informahealthcare.com/doi/pdf/10.3109/01 42159X.2012.670324. Accessed April 2012

Norman, G.R. (1988) Problem-solving skills, solving problems and problem-based learning. *Med Educ*. 22(4): 279–286

Norman, G.R., Wenghofer, E. and Klass, D. (2008) Predicting doctor performance outcomes of curriculum interventions: Problem-based learning and continuing competence. *Med Educ*. 42: 794–799

Office of the Registrar General India Ministry of Home Affairs (2009) Report on Causes of Death in India 2001–2003. http://nrhm-mis.nic.in/Publications.aspx Accessed 19 February 2013

Oliva, P.F. (1989) *Supervision for today's schools*. New York: Longman

Oliver, A.I. (1977) *Curriculum Improvement : A Guide to Problems, Principles, and Process*. New York: Harper & Row

Onishi, H. and Yoshida, I. (2004) Rapid change in Japanese medical education. *Med Teach*. 26(5): 403–408

Parsons, B.A., Blencowe, N.S., Hollowood, A.D. and Grant, J.R. (2010) Surgical training: the impact of changes in curriculum and experience. *J Surg Educ*. 68(1): 44–51

Peters, R.S. (1966) *Ethics and Education*. London: Allen and Unwin

Piaget, J. (1970) *The Science of Education and the Psychology of the Child*. London: Longman

Prideaux, D. (2003) Curriculum design. *BMJ*. 326: 268–270

Print, M. (1993) *Curriculum development and design*. 2nd edn. Crows Nest NSW: Allen and Unwin

Rao, K.H. and Rao, R.H. (2007) Reflections on the state of medical education in Japan. *Keio Journal of Medicine*. 55: 41–51

Rao, R.H. (2006) Perspectives in medical education. 1. Implementing a more integrated, interactive and interesting curriculum to improve Japanese medical education. *Keio J Med*. 56: 75–84

Rogers C.R. (1969). *Freedom to Learn: A View of What Education Might Become*. Columbus: Charles E. Merrill

Schiro, M.S. (2008) *Curriculum theory. Conflicting visions and enduring concerns*. Los Angeles: Sage

Schubert, W.H. (1987) Curriculum history and the dilemma of social control. *Rev Educ*.13(2): 131–136

Schwartz, B. and Sharpe, K. (2010) *Practical Wisdom*. New York: Riverhead Books

Segouin, C. and Hodges, B. (2005) Educating physicians in France and Canada: are the differences based on evidence or history? *Med. Educ*. 39: 1205–1212

Shiraev, E. and Levy, D. (2007) *Cross-Cultural Psychology. Critical Thinking and Contemporary Applications*. 3rd ed. Boston: Pearson

Skiles, J. (2005) Teaching professionalism. A medical student's opinion. *The Clinical Teacher*. 2: 66–71

Skinner, B.F. (1974) *About Behaviourism*. New York: Random House

Skochelak, S.E. (2010) A decade of reports calling for change in medical education: What do they say? *Acad Med*. 85(9): S26–S33

Smith, M.K. (1996, 2000) Curriculum theory and practice. *The Encyclopaedia of Informal Education*. www.infed.org/biblio/b-curric.htm. Accessed 18 February 2012

Stenhouse L (1976) *An introduction to Curriculum Research and Development*. London: Heinemann

Taba H (1962) *Curriculum Development: Theory and Practice*. New York; John Wiley & Sons, Inc.

Tanner, D., Tanner, L. (1980) *Curriculum Development*. New York: Macmillan

Tharu, S. (2010) Medicine and government: Histories of the present. In: A. Zachariah, R. Srivatsan, and S. Tharu (eds) *Towards a Critical Medical Practice. Reflections on the Dilemmas of Medical Culture Today* (pp. 69–92). Hyderabad: Orient BlackSwan

Tharyan, P. (2005). Traumatic bereavement and the Asian Tsunami: Perspectives from Tamil Nadu, India. *Bereavement Care*. 24(2): 23–25

Timmins, N. (2001) *The Five Giants. A Biography of the Welfare State*. 2nd edn. London: HarperCollins

Tusting, K. and Barnet, D. (2003) *Models of Adult Learning: A literature Review*. Leicester: National Institute of Adult Continuing Education

Tyler R.W. (1949) *Basic Principles of Curriculum and Instruction*. Chicago: University of Chicago Press

van der Horst, F. and Lemmens, P. (2012) Medical education and professionalism across different cultures. *Med Educ*. 46(3): 238–244

Vygotsky, L. (1934/1986) *Thought and language*. Cambridge, MA: MIT Press

Vygotsky, L. (1978) Interaction between learning and development. In *Mind in Society*. (Trans. M. Cole). (pp. 79–91). Cambridge, MA: Harvard University Press

Wong, A.K. (2011) Culture in medical education: Comparing a Thai and a Canadian residency programme. *Med Educ*. 45(12): 1209–1219

Wootton, R., Vladzymyrskyy, A., Zolfo, M. and Bonnardot, L. (2011) Experience with low-cost telemedicine in three different settings. Recommendations based on a proposed framework for network performance evaluation. *Global Health Action*. 4: 7214

WFME (World Federation for Medical Education) (2003) Standards for basic medical education postgraduate medical education and continuing professional development. http://www.wfme.org/standards/ Accessed April 2012

Young, M.F.D (ed) (1971) *Knowledge and Control*. London: Collier-Macmillan

Yuan, L., MacNeil, S. and Kraan, W. (2008). *Open Educational Resources—Opportunities and Challenges for Higher Education*. http://wiki.cetis.ac.uk/images/0/0b/OER_Briefing_Paper.pdf Accessed 15 February 2013

Zachariah, A. (2010) Development of the cardiovascular epidemic in India and inappropriate tertiary care treatment guidelines. In A. Zachariah, R. Srivatsan, and S. Tharu (eds) *Towards a Critical Medical Practice. Reflections on the Dilemmas of Medical Culture Today* (pp. 187–200). Hyderabad: Orient BlackSwan

Zachariah, A., Srivatsan, R., Tharu, S. (2010) The dilemmas of medical culture today. In A. Zachariah, R. Srivatsan, and S. Tharu (eds) *Towards a Critical Medical Practice. Reflections on the Dilemmas of Medical Culture Today* (pp. 1–34). Hyderabad: Orient BlackSwan

CHAPTER 3

Problem-based learning

Mark A. Albanese and Laura C. Dast

Discussion clarifies thinking.
John McMichael

Reproduced from *British Medical Journal*, John McMichael, 2, pp. 510, copyright 1955, with permission from BMJ Publishing Group Ltd.

Introduction

From its beginnings as a unique curriculum at an emerging medical school (McMaster University) in the late 1960s, problem-based learning (PBL) has become one of the most common curriculum elements in medical education. It may even be one of the major curriculum approaches instead of just a new innovation. It has supplanted the traditional lecture-based learning model in many schools and has expanded around the world and into a host of other disciplines beyond medical education.

What is PBL?

PBL began with the opening of McMaster University in 1969. The originators borrowed heavily from different disciplines, including case studies from business (Neville and Norman 2007). As PBL grew, it mutated. To clarify what constituted PBL, Barrows published a taxonomy of PBL (Barrows 1986). The taxonomy was anchored at one end by case-based learning where a fully digested patient case is presented by an instructor and at the other end by reiterative PBL, where patient case material unfolds as students prod and probe with minimal guidance by the facilitator. The reiterative part involves students reflecting on their actions as they solved the case.

PBL uses patient problems as a context for students to acquire knowledge about the basic and clinical sciences. Barrows (1985) described the PBL process as: encountering the problem first; problem-solving with clinical reasoning skills and identifying learning needs in an interactive process; self-study; applying newly gained knowledge to the problem; and summarizing what has been learned. In the reiterative form, the process concludes with students' evaluating the information resources they used and how they might have better managed the problem. In recent years, other methods have been developed. The Maastricht 7 Step method has become popular. (Wood 2003) has become popular as more of a 'how to' list of instructions to the tutor and student participants in a PBL session.

1. The process begins with a patient problem. Resources accompanying the problem include detailed objectives, print materials, audiovisual resources, multiple choice self-assessment exercises and resource faculty.

2. Students work in small groups; 6–8 students per group is recommended.

3. The small groups are moderated by one or more facilitators.

4. Students determine their own learning needs to address the problem, give assignments to each other to obtain needed information and then return to report what they have learned and continue with the problem. This happens repeatedly as students secure more information and keep probing deeper.

5. Students return for a final debriefing and analyse the approach they took after getting feedback on their case report.

6. Student evaluation occurs in a small group session and is derived from input from self, peer and facilitator.

The Maastricht 7 Step method (Wood 2003) is more of a 'how to' list of instructions to the tutor and student participants in a PBL session:

Step 1 Identify and clarify unfamiliar terms presented in the scenario; scribe lists those that remain unexplained.

Step 2 Define the problem or problems to be discussed; students may have different views on the issues, but all should be considered; scribe records a list of agreed problems.

Step 3 'Brainstorming' session to discuss the problem(s), suggesting explanations on the basis of prior knowledge; students draw on each other's knowledge and identify areas of incomplete knowledge; scribe records all discussion.

Step 4 Review steps 2 and 3 and arrange explanations into tentative solutions; scribe organizes the explanations and restructures if necessary.

Step 5 Formulate learning objectives; group reaches consensus on the objectives; tutor ensures objectives are focused, achievable, comprehensive, and appropriate.

Step 6 Private study (students gather information related to each objective).

Step 7 Group shares results of private study; tutor checks learning and may assess the group.

There are many derivatives of these two approaches. While the 'McMaster Philosophy' had three key features: self-directed learning; PBL; and small group learning; the only characteristic that cuts across all of what has passed as PBL is that learning is based upon a patient problem. Because such variations on PBL can be considered corruptions of basic PBL, we will adhere to reiterative PBL as the base and discuss departures from the base model as evidence exists to support them.

Theories underlying PBL

There have been a number of theories explaining why PBL should be superior to other forms of instruction. Some theories focus on the learning process, while others consider motivation and human needs. We will review three theories that focus on the learning process and then introduce the Integrated Systems Model, which we believe provides a framework for considering the processes underlying learning in PBL.

Contextual learning

Contextual learning was one of the first and probably most referenced principle used to support PBL. The premise is that when we learn material in the context of how it will be used, it promotes learning and the ability to use information. In PBL, the problem is usually portrayed in the real-life context of a patient coming to visit a doctor. Colliver (2000, p. 259) criticized the contextual learning argument on the grounds that it was drawn from a weak research base and that almost all of clinical education occurs in the contextually relevant process of patient care.

Information-processing theory

Some have argued that information-processing theory underlies PBL (Schmidt 1983). This theory involves: prior knowledge activation, encoding specificity and elaboration of knowledge. Prior knowledge activation refers to students using knowledge they already possess to understand and structure new information. Encoding specificity refers to transfer of learning being more likely to occur as the situation in which something is learned more closely resembles the situation in which it will be applied. Elaboration of knowledge refers to information being better understood and remembered if there is opportunity for elaboration (discussion, answering questions). These elements are commonly part of PBL. That encoding specificity incorporates most of the salient features of contextual learning theory, suggests that information processing theory provides a more comprehensive basis of theoretical support for PBL.

Cooperative learning

Cooperative learning (CL) is another concept that supports PBL. CL situations are those where individuals perceive that they can reach their goals if and only if other group members also do so. The small groups used in PBL fit this definition. Qin, Johnson, and Johnson (1995) conducted a meta-analysis of studies assessing the effect of cooperative versus competitive learning on problem-solving. Cooperation was defined by the presence of joint goals, mutual rewards, shared resources, and complementary roles among members of a group. CL situations were those where individuals perceived that they can reach their goals if and only if the other participants can attain their goals. Competition was defined by the presence of a goal or reward that only one or a few group members could achieve by outperforming the others. The authors concluded that overall, 'cooperation resulted in higher-quality problem solving than did competition'. One possible reason for the success of CL is that it enables material to better mesh with students' level of cognitive development. In cooperative efforts, learners exchanged ideas and corrected each other's errors more frequently and effectively than did individuals competing with each other. Students who are struggling to understand material may be more able to identify the sources of other students' misunderstandings than is an expert.

There are a number of other potentially relevant theories—amongst these are Self-determination Theory (Williams et al. 1999) and Control Theory (Glasser 1986).

Thus, while PBL began with no particular theory undergirding its design, over the intervening years, numerous theories have been advanced in its support. Albanese and colleagues (2009a, b) proposed the Integrated Systems Model (ISM) as an overarching model to explain behaviour in the relatively chaotic healthcare learning environment. The value of the ISM is its ability to incorporate a number of different models and theories into a cohesive unit.

The ISM student world

The general structure of the ISM has six major parts:

1. Superstructure

2. Change/adaptation

3. Feedback/regeneration

4. Environment/context and resources

5. Functional interactions

6. All parts of the system behave as a complex adaptive system (CAS).

In applying the ISM to medical students, the learner is represented as a form of CAS (Plsek 2001). The CAS is built of interacting microsystems in which alignment of new material to be learned with the student's existing cognitive structure (also called scaffolding) is critical for learning to occur. Within ISM, students are characterized as learning workers. Their mission is to learn the knowledge, skills, abilities and professional attributes that will prepare them for practice. The superstructure of the ISM is built upon Stufflebeam's Context, Inputs, Processes and Products (CIPP) (Stufflebeam 1966, 1971, 2000, 2003) evaluation model and augmented by several models from human factors engineering (Carayon et al. 2006; Karsh 2006) The student is the sum of the Inputs, Processes and Products and an upper change loop. The upper change loop is critical to adapting to the world and enabling the learner to adapt to the demands of medical education. The context envelops the student and provides the environment in which the student operates—the educational institution and larger community. The inputs for a student are what they bring with them to their latest learning job, including the sum of their genetics, education, life experiences, social supports and reserve capacity. The process is the means by which the student learns.

The reserve is the region that sits atop the inputs into which resources are sequestered for needs beyond the norm. The reserve powers the change loop which enables the learner to do what it takes to succeed. The change loop is there to 'plug gaps'. The degree of alignment of new material with the existing cognitive structure and processes will determine the degree of energy needed to learn.

If the student's cognitive framework has a gap that leaves no way to absorb new material, the new material must be reduced to a level that the gap can be filled and then the new material absorbed. Even if the cognitive structure has a fit for the new material and can absorb it, repetition is necessary to ensure that the fit endures.

Breaking sophisticated material down to a more basic level to fill a gap requires the expenditure of substantial time and energy. This engages the change loop and draws on reserves. Even if the instructor does the task of breaking the material down, the learners must fill the gap before they can absorb the material that is expected, essentially a double load. In terms of time, it is even more. The brain must be able to re-structure in response to the new material. This requires down-time when the learner is focusing on other things, such as sleeping, exercising or socializing. Without re-structuring, there comes a point where to absorb new material, material that has already been absorbed needs to be expelled. This is counter-productive and learning starts to shut down no matter how hard the learner tries. A learner cannot afford to have too much of their reserves devoted to filling gaps or they will fall behind.

Unlike previous applications of ISM, where change was different from the norm, students are learning workers (Albanese 1999). Their primary mission is to learn and evolve to become a more skilled individual who can assume professional roles and perform more complex tasks. For a learning-worker, learning itself generates resource return as well as the reinforcement received from the system, such as positive feedback from other group members, or grades, or promotion. These things build back the reserves needed to keep the learner at work.

The ISM and PBL

The ISM is a radical departure from models that typically describe undergraduate medical education in the literature because of: (1) the characterization of students and teachers as CASs; (2) the concept of resource reserves needed for learning; (3) the need to align content complexity and structure of instruction with the existing level of cognitive development; and (4) the need for alignment of the instructional operations with the research and service operations of the institution. Additionally, the integration of different models in one organism represents a clarification of the different types of change models and how they relate to one another. Despite its unique characteristics, ISM melds well with findings from PBL research.

Practical matters

Characteristics of problems

From an ISM perspective, problems (also called cases) need to fulfil the criteria outlined in Box 3.1.

Hays (2002) states that an appropriate problem should: (1) present a common problem that graduates would be expected to be able to handle, and be prototypical of that problem; (2) be serious or potentially serious—where appropriate management might affect the outcome; (3) have implications for prevention; (4) provide interdisciplinary input and cover a broad area; (5) lead to an encounter of faculty members' objectives; (6) present a concrete task; and (7) have a degree of complexity appropriate for the students' prior knowledge.

Problem formats can range from brief paragraphs describing a symptom or symptoms to elaborate simulations or even simulated

> **Box 3.1** Characteristics of Problem Selection
>
> Problems should
>
> - Be targeted to the level of the learner's cognitive development
> - Help students achieve the needed objectives for the curriculum
> - Challenge students to reach beyond their comfort zone
> - Support working as a group in a cooperative manner and
> - Be easily identified as mission critical.

patients. Barrows (1986) suggests that a relatively unorganized, unsynthesized, and open-ended form promotes the application of clinical reasoning skills, structuring of knowledge in useful contexts, and the development of self-directed learning. ISM recommends starting with more structure for students early in the curriculum and gradually becoming less structured as the students' cognitive structures become more sophisticated and better able to integrate unstructured information.

The problem-based learning modules (PBLM) were developed at Southern Illinois University and are aligned with Barrows unstructured PBL form. PBLMs provide specialized written simulations—with sufficient flexibility to enable students to pursue almost unlimited types of inquiry.

The Focal Problem developed at Michigan State University is a more structured form. They start with a written narrative of a clinical problem as it unfolds. After descriptions of significant developments occur, 'stop and think' questions are inserted. This problem design helps students focus on the steps in the decision-making process when problems have more than one solution (Jones et al. 1984; Wales and Stager 1972; Pawlak et al. 1989).

Sources of problems

PBL cases can be obtained from a number of sources. The AAMC has developed MedEdPORTAL (http://services.aamc.org/jsp/mededportal/) as a repository of peer-reviewed materials for medical education. Cases in this system are all evaluated by peers for their quality.

The PBLMs mentioned earlier are patient cases in a book format permitting free inquiry. The patient can be asked any question in any sequence. Similarly, any component of the physical examination can be performed and any diagnostic test can be ordered in any sequence. The results are provided as they would be in a real clinical situation.

Problem selection issues

Problems are the central feature of a PBL curriculum. The ISM considers it essential that they provide a developmentally appropriate sequence that addresses skills and abilities that lead students to develop competence. However, care needs to be exercised in problem selection. Hays (2002) warns of biases in PBL problems toward more acute problems in younger people in urban settings. He further elaborates that many problems that have objectives pertaining to rural health describe poor healthcare in a rural setting and patients having to be rescued by clinicians in large teaching hospitals. In addition, objectives addressing the healthcare of indigenous peoples often illustrate dominant culture stereotypes.

Besides the biases that can creep into the cases themselves, it is challenging to ensure that all student groups achieve the objectives of the problems. Coulson and Osbourne (1984) analysed learning issues identified by students in PBL groups. They found that groups identified an average of 61% of the learning objectives that faculty deemed essential. Dolmans et al. (1992) found that 62% of faculty-generated objectives were definitely identified. Thus, PBL groups may typically only achieve about 60% of the learning objectives. Unless cases are 'spiralled' in which the objectives are present in multiple cases with each presentation addressing them at a deeper level, PBL can leave gaps. Further, it is important that each sequential presentation not be too much deeper or students will have to expend their reserve filling the gaps so they can meaningfully interact with the case.

Using PBL in the clinical years raises some important questions. One would expect that a real patient would be the ultimate PBL problem. PBL would then seem like a natural partner to patient care in that it can provide some structured exposure to clinical content that is difficult to orchestrate with real patients. However, PBL has not always integrated well into the clinical setting. Dornan and colleagues (2005) interviewed 14 general physicians after the University of Manchester extended PBL into the clinical years. They describe the loss of student excitement in clinical discovery because of preoccupation with PBL cases.

The ISM offers some warnings about PBL use in the clinical years. Systems will use whatever they can to build reserves and particularly to survive in a hostile environment. PBL can be used by healthcare systems to offset the inefficiencies inherent in student teaching. Comments about teaching on the wards made by clinicians in Dornan's study (2005, p. 167) included mention of constraints resulting from 'falling numbers of beds, shorter lengths of stay, changing work patterns, pressure on staff and a narrower range of "material."'. Outpatients fared little better, with comments that dealt with space constraints, work pressure, productivity targets, patient expectations, and the time-cost of teaching. As the clinical environment appears to be increasingly hostile to teaching, PBL may become the fallback to maintain clinical education at a reasonable level of quality. This may be especially true if medical education continues to progress toward competency-based education (Irby et al. 2010); students will need to demonstrate core skills that may not be reliably obtained during the course of clinical encounters. PBL could become the surrogate for such experience.

Facilitators

The ISM has much to say about facilitators and support system needed for PBL.

Role definition and expectations

The role of the facilitator and expectations for their availability must be established before facilitators are recruited. The amount of time that facilitators need to be available to students should be determined. This includes the number of times per week groups are scheduled to meet and how much of the rest of the time facilitators need to be available (including expectations for how long a response should take to email).

Facilitating in PBL is a complex task. Facilitators need a working knowledge of the language and terms used in the case as well as of the case content. They need to be able to manage group dynamics without interfering with initiative. Facilitators must apply the student grading system in a fair and unbiased manner. Facilitators must also be sensitive to boundaries and need to maintain a minimum level of social distance from students. Personal relationships with students compromise a facilitator's ability to function and can be as disruptive to group dynamics as problems among students.

Selection of facilitators

Being a facilitator for PBL groups means being there whenever the group formally meets. Competing demands on faculty time need to be addressed. Medical faculty have the misfortune of being central to the three different missions of teaching, research and service. However, the model of faculty being 'triple threats' in teaching, research and service is giving way to more specialization. There are now research faculty and clinical faculty titles that bring promotion with more focus. These faculties either free up the other faculty for their scheduled teaching activities or teach themselves.

A second concern is providing backups in the event of sickness or other unavoidable absence. There should be a backup for each facilitator or a backup pool of faculty. How many backups are needed in a pool can start at 10% and be adjusted as experience is gained and absence rates and backup faculty availability rates can be better estimated. Specific individual faculty as backup for each facilitator has merits in allowing more specific planning for the role they will need to assume. The availability of backup faculty on any given date might be slim, requiring a search and some prodding. Sometimes, schools might encourage new faculty who must commit time toward their tenure work to enter the backup pool and transition into full teaching roles when their research or practice has become established.

A third concern is whether faculty need content expertise to be effective facilitators. ISM recommends that facilitators have operational knowledge of the content and principles of the case as well as understanding where students are likely to have difficulties. Facilitators also need to be able to help the group maintain positive dynamics and constructive working relationships. From a content expertise perspective, the facilitator does not necessarily need to be an expert in the discipline from which a case is drawn. For example, a facilitator for a case about nosocomial infection with *Clostridium difficile* does not have to be either an infectious disease specialist or a microbiologist. What the facilitator does need is to be expert in the case-specific elements, particularly those that students may unearth related to the case. So a rheumatologist could serve effectively as a facilitator for the case if they have acquired an understanding of *Clostridium difficile* infections expected of a generalist in the context of the specific case. The facilitator's role is not to be an expert source, but to be able to guide students in their search for relevant information. Physicians would have a natural advantage in this regard. Their knowledge of the basic sciences underlying a case is likely to be better developed from a clinical perspective, but not so far removed from students' understanding. Basic scientists provide a strong biological conceptual basis for reviewing the case, but generally have a limited clinical perspective. ISM would give a nod to physicians serving as facilitators, particularly generalists. It would even argue that higher level residents might be ideally placed to serve as facilitators. They would be not so far removed from the level of the student in their understanding of the biological sciences of a case, yet they would be more advanced in their clinical expertise and skills at seeking information.

The research on facilitator expertise is not definitive. In the original McMaster PBL curriculum, tutors were not required to have any particular content expertise (Neville and Norman 2007). Curriculum developers believed that content experts could not resist the temptation to lecture which would short circuit the students' learning. Miflin (2004) argues that given the norms when PBL originated, tutors were expected to be physicians and that tutors having general medical expertise was an unstated assumption. In subsequent research, several studies found better learning outcomes if the facilitator had content expertise (Eagle et al. 1992; Davis et al. 1992). Zeitz and Paul (1993) argue that these two studies were experiments in PBL in a larger traditional curriculum and that the learners were novices regarding PBL. In their experience, the outcomes are better for novices if the faculty facilitators are content experts. However, after one to two months, students in a PBL curriculum are so skilled in student-centred, self-directed learning that they no longer depend on expert facilitators. They further argue that it is not feasible to have facilitators be content experts for all problems that they will facilitate. They have found that facilitators develop 'case expertness' by facilitating the case from three to five times.

What may be as important as content knowledge are group management skills. The ISM warns that the facilitator provides a level of motivation for participation that can be good or bad. Students may posture for the facilitator hoping for a good assessment or even a recommendation. This can lead to subtle jockeying for dominant roles. The facilitator needs to be aware of this type of behaviour and discourage it in a constructive manner. These are fairly sophisticated interpersonal skills that may not be mastered by all faculty. Training should be geared toward sensitivity to these types of dynamics and strategies for addressing them.

Training facilitators

The ISM argues that effective organization and appropriately targeting cases are key elements. Faculty and student time is precious; both must be used to maximum advantage. Facilitators need to be given specific guidelines for how they are to interact with students. Moving from content expert to facilitator is not necessarily a natural act—so having them practice the role during training will be helpful. 'Standardized' students, individuals who are trained to act like students, can help.

Facilitators should also be given all information about the case and any associated materials that students receive plus materials that will allow them to guide students in their search for knowledge. This includes the 'next steps' that students are expected to take. Anything that can help facilitators to more quickly reach case expertness is useful (Zeitz and Paul 1993).

Facilitators also need to be prepared for students to have a negative reaction to the experience, particularly in the early period. Students are generally unused to having faculty facilitating learning instead of delivering instruction. Over time, students become more self-reliant, but early on it can be a difficult adjustment.

PBL may be susceptible to the regressive and task-avoiding behaviours seen in clinical psychology groups (Bowman and Hughes 2005). PBL shares four characteristics that can promote these problems: extended contact time (often >6 hours per week), the non-directive tutor role that facilitates uncertainty, the unpredictable nature of group processes and the potential intimacy of PBL. These characteristics may induce undesirable behaviour in

students and facilitators. To avoid facilitator problems (wanting to be 'one of the gang', liked by students and in control; subverting the primary task with a new agenda; having a relationship with a student), they argue that training and follow up should provide: clear statements of the primary task of PBL tutors, clear boundaries on the staff role and availability, ongoing review and monitoring of tutor work, and social activities that are friendly but not intimate. They also recommend monthly supervision, peer observation and mentoring for all PBL tutors.

A final facilitator training issue is in assessing student contributions to the group. If this is one of the role expectations, they need to be carefully trained to do it properly.

How many facilitators per group or groups per facilitator

How many facilitators for how many groups has not been studied in a systematic manner. The ISM gives some guidance and there have been studies that provide additional suggestions. ISM directs that there be a sufficient number of facilitators so that the role of the facilitator can be fulfilled. This may seem obvious, but it forces one to define the exact role of the facilitator and then assess whether it can be achieved by having one or more facilitators per group; or maybe having one facilitator who circulates among multiple groups. Suppose the primary role of the facilitator is to ensure that students stay on track. One could have either one facilitator per group who meets with their group during scheduled time; or, one could have one facilitator for several groups who signs off student work plans before they break up and begin their assignments. If the students are headed on a wild goose chase, rather than just signing off, the facilitator could give them some guidance that will help them get back on track. The facilitator would then review a revised plan and sign off if appropriate. If the role of the facilitator is also to assess each student's contributions to the group deliberations, then this would take one facilitator per group to get a complete perspective and maybe two if one wanted to ensure that rater bias did not affect scores. If the assessment is to consider the longitudinal contributions of each student over the entire case, then the rater(s) would need to be there for all the meetings. Clearly, the expected role of the facilitator has a major influence on the number of facilitators needed per group.

There have been studies that examined the impact of having one facilitator for more than one group. Farrell and colleagues (1999) studied whether a single facilitator could effectively tutor four groups, each of which had three or four second-year students. They found improvements in learning that were comparable to those made by students who had a more traditional experience. In a study that undoubtedly stretches the definition of PBL to the extreme, Khaliq (2005) reported substantial increases in student satisfaction ratings after introducing problem-solving exercises into lectures.

Small groups

Optimal size

Recommendations for optimal group size tend to have little empirical support and are generally anecdotal. The ISM recommends that group size be sufficient for the PBL groups to meet their goals. There is more to this recommendation than first appears. It forces one to examine what the exact role of the group is in the PBL process and to choose a group size and composition that will best facilitate

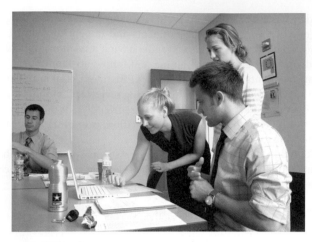

Figure 3.1 PBL in action.

students achieving the purpose of having a group. ISM makes the further caution that groups need to be large enough that assignments will not deplete the reserves of any member. A rough guideline is that each person should have enough 'air time' to talk for at least 10 minutes in any structured session. It would be a rare group where air time is equal among all participants, but there must be sufficient opportunity for all members to make a verbal contribution. The expectation should also be there that each group member will make a verbal contribution at each meeting. At the least, each group member should present the results of their assignment from the previous meeting and contribute meaningfully to the discussion of the implications of the results of their investigations and then contribute to the creation of the new assignments (fig. 3.1).

In studies of PBL that define group size, often there are six to seven students per group (Lohman and Finkelstein 2002; Trappler 2006) although some elements of PBL have been used in much larger groups of even 100 plus students (Woods 1996). Recommendations for optimal group size tend to be anecdotal. 'Groups should contain no more than seven members and no less than five. More than seven results in too many opportunities for reluctant members to hide. Fewer than five puts the spotlight on members permanently and removes much of the opportunity for "think" time'. (Matheson 2007).

Composition

Groups should be composed of students—but what varieties? ISM recommends randomization but stratification according to gender and academic ability. There is some evidence that men and women function differently in a group environment, so balance is needed to avoid any style from superseding. Also, students who are 'couples', especially if married, should be assigned to different groups. Personal relationships within a small group have potential for disrupting group dynamics. Perhaps of greatest importance is diversity in academic ability, particularly if there is a desire for students to teach students. If a cooperative model is used, the stronger students are expected to bring along the weaker students. The cooperative model drives this by having the group assessed by a presentation of their results, and all members being equally likely to be called upon to present results. Thus, it is in the best interest of the group for each member to be equally prepared. Even if a cooperative model is not used, ISM would recommend stratifying by academic ability.

Too many low ability students in the same group would not be desirable (Hojat et al. 1997).

ISM cautions that there are limits on the degree of academic diversity desired. If the low ability student(s) are so far below the rest of the group in their academic preparation, student efforts to break the material down into more digestible sizes can become frustrating. The further down they have to drill in order to reach the level of cognitive scaffolding of the lowest level learner, the more likely that the effort spent drilling will start to deplete the reserves of the advanced learners. Additionally, the fast-track building back up of the cognitive structures of a learner who is far below the level of their peers can be even more painful.

Schools may want to consider in advance under what circumstances students could join different groups. Groups may take differing amount of times to 'gel' but there should be a 'way out' for a group that is truly dysfunctional.

Structure (role assignments)

In the ISM students behave as CASs. Throw them together in a group and lay out expectations that impact upon their survival and they will succeed in achieving both. However, it might not be pretty and there may be blood.

To help make small group operations civilized and efficient, recommendations for role assignments have been made. Barrows (1985) recommends that students assume three separate administrative roles to make the process work smoothly: PBL Module reader, Action Master List Handler, and Recorder. In the context Barrows was describing, students were working through what they call PBL Modules. They were also instructed to formulate action lists. So, he recommends having one student in the role of module reader, another handling the list of actions that need to be taken and a third who is general recorder of activities.

There have also been recommendations for group member behaviour. Matheson (2007) recommends that attendance at PBL sessions be mandatory to avoid erosion and to underline the seriousness of the enterprise. He further recommends that groups need to set rules and standards of acceptable behaviour that consider such things as when interruption is permitted, the attitudes towards latecomers, whether eating is allowed during a session, what to do if the tasks for the day were completed before time was up and so on.

Technology is also becoming a problem for small group management and may interfere with problem-solving. Davis (2007) provides detailed recommendations.

Time management

Baker (2007, personal communication) observed that when students identify learning issues they state them in general terms. This can lead to inefficiencies and the follow-up discussion can be lengthy and unfocused. PBL adherents may not consider this to be bad, but simply the stage that students need to go through to become effective problem-solvers. It may be alright to let the group flounder a bit in the interest of developing problem-solving skills, but they should make progress in becoming more efficient over time. If this does not happen, and particularly if there is backsliding, the facilitator should take the initiative in pointing out the elements that are unclear before allowing students to go off in their independent assignments.

Time is an important issue and if the students are not managing it well, the facilitator should assist by noting the time and pointing out how much progress still needs to be made. As students become more skilled in working in PBL small groups, they will generally improve their time management (Sungur and Tekkaya 2006). However, at the start there is value in having a formally appointed time-keeper in addition to the roles described earlier, especially if the group continually runs over the allotted time.

Resources

Space

It is desirable for rooms to be dedicated to PBL and used only by an individual group. 'This helps create a sense of group cohesion and gives the group a place to call "home."' (Matheson 2007, personal communnication) However, dedicated space in today's crowded centres can be hard to come by. While dedicated space is nice, it is not clear if the lack of dedicated space will have detrimental effects on learning.

Instructional/IT resources

A well-stocked library is an important resource. After a PBL course on neurobiology was introduced Nolte et al. (1988) reported library book use increased 20-fold. With the more recent advent of on-line references, having good internet access is essential. Having general web-searching capability with search engines such as Google Scholar will be useful for looking for non-library references such as policy statements and current events. However, there needs to be guidelines for internet usage to avoid having the problem-solving process subverted by web searches (Kerfoot et al. 2005). ISM would signal this as being especially problematic early in the curriculum when students have relatively primitive cognitive structures. Without having much cognitive scaffolding to draw upon in determining what information they need to address a problem, their searches can be scattered and chaotic; wasting much time in the process. Providing training in advanced searching by academic librarians can be helpful.

Also beneficial are white-boards and blackboards. Some schools have adopted electronic blackboards that enable electronic capturing of the material written on the board. With evolving technology such as tablet devices, technology will continue to become more powerful and easier to use. Anything available in the clinical environment should be made available to students as they mature in their professional roles. Access to confidential information, however, must be limited to appropriate situations and with full compliance with any regulations that exist.

Lectures can also be an instructional resource, but they should be limited. Barrows (1985) recommends limiting lecture to 1–1.5 hours per day. Barrows also recommends that basic science research faculty should be a resource available to meet with students for 4–6 hours per week.

Creature comforts

The instructional environment in the small group should be informal and as low stress as possible. Lighting should be sufficient to see all the types of educational resources that will be shared. The environment should be comfortable, but not so comfortable as to make it difficult for students to stay awake. Students should be able to bring food and drink into the meeting room.

Standardized patients

As early as 1973 Barrows and Tamblyn (1976) report using standardized patients for both teaching and assessing students in PBL groups. When learning communication skills and physical exam skills, it can be especially useful to have standardized patients who can meet with groups. Depending on the goals of the session, there may be times when teaching patients should be employed. These individuals are skilled in playing the part of a patient with a particular condition as well as in the art of teaching and in the components of the examination that are being learned. In cases where the goal is simply to give students an opportunity to work through the history and physical examination with a 'real' person, there may not be the need for such extensive training. Generally speaking, standardized patients are expensive to deploy. Their use should be carefully considered for benefits derived.

Administration and governance

Barrows (1985) believes PBL is most compatible with an organ-based curriculum, in which courses are aligned with different organs of the body. Thus, a course on the cardiovascular system would have anatomy, physiology and biochemistry integrated together. ISM would also support having the curriculum organized by organ system because it tends to align better with patient care than does the traditional discipline-based course structure. The caveat ISM would add is that there still needs to be theory addressed for students to be able to adequately develop their cognitive structures. New information will be better absorbed if cognitive structures are built that have a superstructure with logical places for knowledge to fit and be recalled when learned.

However, ISM offers some cautions about organ-system based teaching when a medical school is organized around discipline-based departments. Interdisciplinary collaboration can be difficult to sustain in a disciplinary-based school because it cuts across the organizational structure of the school, thereby requiring extra resources to sustain. Thus, once the 'newness' of a PBL curriculum wears off, and resources devoted to make the change are redirected to other purposes, you are still left with the underlying structure of the school. If it does not align with PBL, it will be a constant drag on resources that will draw on the system reserves. Long term, this can undermine the PBL curriculum and may be one of the reasons that many PBL curricula have migrated toward hybrids.

Some newer schools in the US have (or are) organizing themselves differently than has been traditionally the case. For example, Florida State University, a recently opened school with a PBL curriculum, has organized itself around five interdisciplinary departments: Biomedical Sciences, Medical Humanities and Social Sciences, Clinical Sciences, Geriatrics, and Family Medicine and Rural Health. The University of New Mexico School of Medicine, another school with a PBL curriculum, has grouped its biological sciences into five departments: Biochemistry and Molecular Biology, Cell Biology and Physiology, Molecular Genetics/Microbiology, Neurosciences, and Pathology. Organ-based curricula and PBL require interdisciplinary collaboration to be most effective. The interdisciplinary structures of these departments are more likely to sustain an organ-system and PBL curriculum in the face of administrative changes and budget reductions because they require less resources to maintain than in a school with discipline-based departments.

In hybrid curricula, care needs to be exercised to avoid 'curriculum creep', where the activities outside the PBL envelope expand to choke off time available for students to adequately engage with the PBL process. Medical school is notorious for expanding beyond the bounds of human endurance. Barnes and colleagues (1977) analysed the reading speed of second year medical students for clinical texts and used it to evaluate how much time it would take students to complete assignments in a second year Introduction to Clinical Medicine Course. They concluded it would take students 47 hours per week. Klatt and Klatt (2011) conducted a student survey to address similar concerns. They concluded that students would have to spend 28 to 41 hours per week to complete a single reading without factoring in study time.

It is not just PBL being in competition with other types of learning in the curriculum that should be of concern. Because medical school resides in a larger complex medical system, constant vigilance is needed to ensure that the educational mission is not corrupted by the needs of some other part of the system.

Evaluation

ISM recommends having both formative and summative evaluation in place. Formative evaluation is timed to identify and resolve small problems before they become big problems, thereby improving the education while making more efficient use of resources. Summative evaluations are designed to assess how effective the total learning experience has been.

For formative evaluation purposes, Barrows (1985) recommends that the course coordinator meet weekly with groups. Modern technology enables students to report issues as they occur in real time through email, texting or posting to a website. Students should be encouraged to report issues that are detracting from their learning experience as early as possible. Confidentiality should be assured for them because the PBL process is such a personal one that any criticisms can be misinterpreted or taken personally. This becomes especially problematic with formative evaluation because it occurs while the PBL process is still in progress.

Summative evaluation relies on information that is generally collected after the completion of the learning experience. The goal is to determine the effectiveness of the experience. Student ratings are the most commonly used summative evaluation data. Success in achieving programme goals and objectives by students can also be a source of information. For PBL curricula in the preclinical years, preceptor ratings of students have been useful. For entire curricula, the ratings of graduates and the residency supervisors of the graduates have also been useful (Hojat et al. 1997). Performance on objective examinations, especially external ones, can also serve as summative evidence, however, they have been criticized as being not sensitive to the types of skills that PBL is attempting to develop. Generally, one is better off using a range of different types of data to evaluate a programme. Each type of data one collects generally has its own weaknesses, but in aggregate the weaknesses average out. Longitudinal databases can be especially valuable for summative evaluation.

Grading systems

Grading students in PBL offers challenges because of the desire for students to help other students learn. If the grading system is not properly designed, it can obstruct this goal. In particular, competitive grading with a fixed quota for the highest grades can leave students unwilling to help others for fear they would disadvantage themselves. There is also the component of PBL that has students working in groups and producing reports based on group work. Distinguishing individual performance in this type of activity is difficult and imprecise. A pass/fail grading system is most compatible with these elements of PBL. However, many faculty and students alike believe that a pass/fail system does not provide the motivation for achieving excellence. To recognize excellence, an honors grade is sometimes added. The other concern is that assessors appear to be loath to award failing grades. A marginal or low pass grade is sometimes used as a buffer between fail and pass. Which system to use depends upon the goals of the school and the proclivities of its faculty. Including narrative feedback in addition to letter grades, which is more common in clerkship education, can be another mechanism of rewarding excellence. This also can contribute to the longitudinal database where areas of improvement may be evident over longer spans of time than one course would capture.

Student assessment

Assessing student performance is challenging. The following is a brief overview. For more details see Nendaz and Tekian (1999). Figure 3.2 shows the different forms of assessment that can be used.

Multiple choice exams

The use of multiple choice examinations is common because of the breadth of testing and ease of scoring. Whether multiple-choice question (MCQs) can assess the content at the level of problem solving that PBL is designed to promote is an open question. Some believe that well-written MCQs are capable of assessing these problem-solving skills but others do not. Certainly writing sophisticated questions is a complex skill, one that is unlikely to be prevalent among all faculty.

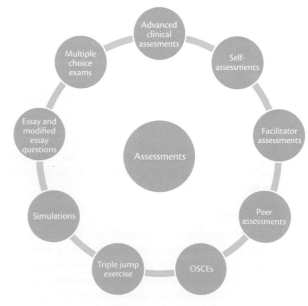

Figure 3.2 Assessments.

Case and Swanson (2001) recommend using 'case clusters', in which several multiple-choice questions are drawn from the same patient presentation. A potential problem with these types of items is that they tend to have higher correlations with one another than they do with questions drawn from different patient presentations. This will tend to inflate the internal consistency reliability estimate for these items over what it would be if each MCQ was drawn from a different patient presentation. While this may not be a critical concern in low stakes exams, in some extreme cases, reliabilities have been found to increase from 0.56 to 0.80 (Albanese and Sabers 1988). Another issue is that over the entire test, there needs to be at least 11 or more different patient presentations to obtain a result that has acceptable generalizability (Petrusa et al. 1991). The most important consideration, however, is whether the entire mix of MCQs meets the overall test design (often referred to as the table of specifications)—a critical factor in ensuring the content validity of the examination.

A form of multiple choice examination called the progress test has been used widely in PBL A progress test reflects the end objectives of the curriculum and samples knowledge across all disciplines and content areas relevant for the medical degree. The Maastricht exam was composed of 250 true–false questions while the McMaster exam contained 180 MCQs. At Maastricht the progress test is administered four times per year to all students while McMaster administers theirs three times per year. The Maastricht progress test has been found to have a high correlation with a test on clinical reasoning ($r = 0.93$). (Boshuizen et al. 1997) The McMaster version was submitted to an extensive psychometric analysis and showed test-retest reliabilities over successive administrations ranging from 0.53 to 0.64; predictive validity of the cumulative score was approximately 0.60 (Blake et al. 1996).

The main problem with progress tests is that they can be inefficient. Neophyte examinees can spend much time attempting questions they can only hope to guess upon and advanced examinees spend time answering questions that are trivial for them. Measurement specialists prefer to administer tests that are appropriate for the level of learner since these items provide the most information about a learner's ability. However, if the progress test is the only major knowledge evaluation taking up students' time in the curriculum, some inefficiency is probably acceptable. The most critical issue is that every item should discriminate at some point in the curriculum. Easy items should discriminate among students early in the curriculum and the most difficult questions should discriminate among advanced students. A question that does not discriminate between students at any level should be eliminated.

Essay and modified essay questions

Essay questions provide the least structure and have the potential to offer insight into the thought processes underlying choices when confronted with a patient problem. However, a student who is not skilled at writing essays could appear to be less accomplished than they are—simply because they do not write well.

A form of essay called the modified essay question has been used to assess PBL. It consists of a standardized series of open questions about a problem in which the information on the case is ordered sequentially. Students receive new information only after answering a certain question (Verwijnen et al. 1982). A variation described by Saunders et al (1990) covered nine areas of internal medicine

content. The advantage of the essay-type questions is in their relative ease of construction. The disadvantage is in complexity of scoring and the large amount of time needed to do it. Achieving reliable scores among graders is difficult.

Simulations

Simulations in medical education were first described by McGuire and Babbott (1967). Simulations can be used in assessment—some simulations end with the diagnosis, others with management of the patient.

Triple jump exercise

The primary goal of a triple jump exercise is to assess clinical problem-solving and self-directed learning skills (Painvin et al. 1979). In a triple jump exercise, students discuss a written clinical scenario and identify the related learning goals, review the learning materials individually, and return to present their conclusions and judge their own performances. Students sometimes have 3 hours to complete their exercise, sometimes a week. This type of assessment is often used for formative evaluation purposes. It is less used for grading purposes because it is time consuming, limiting the number of scenarios that can be assessed.

Objective structured clinical exams (OSCEs)

OSCEs have achieved widespread adoption in recent years, undoubtedly spurred on by the adoption of the United States Medical Licensing Examination Step 2 Clinical Skills, a short-type OSCE consisting of 12 stations that was implemented in 2004. The strengths of the OSCE are its face validity and standardized clinical experience for all examinees. There are few other ways of assessing complex skills and abilities such as communication skills with the same degree of standardization and reliability. The primary limitation of the OSCE is its cost. It requires substantial infrastructure to administer: personnel to recruit, train and manage standardized patients and facilities, at least 11 places to put the stations, usually examination rooms, and money to pay the standardized patients. Increasingly, schools are setting up assessment centres that include examining rooms that can be used for teaching and then assessing using the OSCE format.

Peer assessments

Peer evaluations have a certain appeal because clinicians do it informally on a daily basis as they make decisions about which peers they feel comfortable making referrals. The ISM would issue a cautionary note in using peer assessments for students. Because students are still learning what it means to be a professional, they do not have a solid basis for making peer judgements of knowledge. Also, students may be competing with one another, making peer evaluations contain at least some level of conflict of interest. Complicating matters further, if a cooperative learning model is being used, students are expected to teach their peers. If they are expected to teach and assess their peers, the two activities can be antagonistic. And, if after peer assessments, students are expected to come back and continue to work in their small groups, group dynamics can be disrupted. If peer assessments are used for grading students, care should be exercised. ISM would be more supportive of peer assessments of teaching contributions to colleagues than it would of learning accomplishment and group contributions.

Facilitator assessments

There is increasing interest in having what has been termed tutorial-based assessments, with the primary assessor being the facilitator (or tutor). Several tools have been proposed to assess facilitator or tutor perceptions of student performance, but they vary markedly in their length and the frequency with which they are to be used. Hebert and Bravo (1996) propose use of what they call Tutotest, an exhaustive 44 item instrument. Ladouceur et al. (2004) propose use of a somewhat shorter instrument composed of 31 items, but this is still a formidable burden for facilitators. Several investigators have explored use of forms with five or fewer items (Eva et al. 2007; Chaves et al. 2006; Sim et al. 2006). The longer forms have been recommended for use at the end of a unit, while the shorter forms have been recommended for use at the end of each session. Thus, an instrument completed at the end of each unit will have one assessment completed every 2–6 weeks, while one completed at the end of each session will have from 4 to 18 assessments completed by the end of a unit. The latter approach has been found to improve the psychometric properties of the resulting scores.

Self-assessment

One of the goals of PBL is to develop self-directed learning skills. A key component of achieving this is the ability to accurately assess one's strengths and weaknesses and identify ways to address weaknesses. Self-assessment is a key to achieving self-directed learning skills. It is not clear, however, if anyone is really good at doing this. At the least, if there is anything at stake from self-assessments, there is obvious conflict of interest.

Studies comparing self-assessment to actual performance have found tendencies for poor performers to overestimate their performance and high performers to underestimate their performance (Kruger and Dunning 1999; Ward et al. 2002). This pattern is pervasive across skills. As a consequence, using self-assessments in grading may penalize the high performers and give undeserved increases in grades to the poorest performers. While self-assessment is a good activity for students to experience, it should be used with care in assigning grades.

Advanced clinical assessments

For more advanced students, there are assessments of clinical competence that can be employed such as the Mini-CEX (Norcini et al. 2003), script Concordance tests (Brailovsky et al. 2001) and oral examinations (Anastakis et al. 1991).

Effectiveness of PBL

The question that has dogged PBL since its inception has been to what degree it produces the types of changes in learners that it was designed to produce. These include whether they are self-directed learners who have a deeper knowledge of their discipline and who are better prepared to apply the science of medicine to patient care. Demonstrating these changes has been a challenge. There have been hundreds of studies designed to test these differences and at least 13 major reviews since 1990.

The attempts to do systematic reviews have either resorted to a small set of controlled studies (Vernon and Blake 1993; Colliver 2000; Newman 2003) or adopted a thematic approach (Berkson 1993) or what might be called a 'best evidence approach' that used effect sizes when possible and a thematic approach when not (Albanese and

Mitchell 1993). For those who are certain that PBL is excellent, these reviews have been disappointing. Vernon and Blake (1993) concluded that results generally support the superiority of the PBL approach over more traditional academic methods. Albanese and Mitchell (1993) while acknowledging the weaknesses of the research literature concluded that PBL was more nurturing and enjoyable and that PBL graduates performed as well and sometimes better on clinical examinations and faculty assessments. However, they also concluded that PBL graduates showed potentially important gaps in their cognitive knowledge base, did not demonstrate expert reasoning patterns, and that PBL was costly. Berkson (1993) was unequivocal in her conclusion that the graduate of PBL is not distinguishable from their traditional counterpart. She further argued that the experience of PBL can be stressful for the student and faculty and implementation may be unrealistically costly. Dochy and colleagues (2003) concluded that PBL had a positive robust effect on the skills of students but a negative non-robust effect on knowledge. Smits and colleagues (2002) concluded that there was:

> no consistent evidence that problem-based learning in continuing medical education was superior to other educational strategies in improving doctors' knowledge and performance. (p. 155).

Newman's review was no more encouraging. Only for the outcome 'accumulation of knowledge' was there more than 3 studies that met the inclusion criteria. For this outcome, of 39 effect sizes computed, 16 favoured the PBL group, and 23 the control. Generally, the state of the literature was not sufficient to make much out of it in his review. Dochy and colleagues (2003) performed a meta-analysis of 43 studies, concluding that PBL had a negative effect on the knowledge base of students (effect size = −0.776) but a positive effect on their application of that knowledge (effect size = +0.658). Gijbels and colleagues (2005) reported another meta-analysis of 40 studies in which they analysed the effects of PBL as a function of the type of cognitive skill assessed in the outcome: Concepts, Principles and Application. They found a slight negative effect size for concepts (−0.042) and positive effect sizes for principles and application (0.748 and 0.401, respectively).

However, the analysis of PBL must make a distinction between those studies conducted before 1993 and those conducted since. The three reviews that came out that year apparently moved curricula toward what might be called hybrids—a combination of structured activities directed at giving students the disciplinary conceptual frameworks (usually via lecture) combined with substantial time devoted to PBL. At the risk of cherry-picking only the studies that have shown positive results, we will highlight what have been some of the findings of interest in that time.

Hoffman and colleagues (2006) present results for the USMLE Steps 1 and 2, and residency director perceptions of their graduates versus all other graduates for the period one year before implementation of PBL (1996 graduating year) and post implementation (1997–2006 graduating years). Medical College Admission Test (MCAT) scores of the classes were also presented to show how USMLE performance compared to entry-level academic status.

MCAT effect sizes (using class means in comparison to the national mean and standard deviations) would be expected to be comparable to Step 1 and Step 2 effect sizes unless the curriculum disproportionately affected student ability. In the pre-PBL year, the Step 1 effect size was almost identical to the MCAT effect size, which was approximately one quarter of a standard deviation below the national mean. The Step 2 effect size was even more negative, approximately one half standard deviation below the national mean. There was a significant improvement in the transitional year that continued for the 8–9 years since PBL was introduced. In that period, the MCAT effect sizes rose from –0.23 to an average of –0.06, a +0.29 rise; but the changes in Step 1 and Step 2 were larger. Step 1 increased from –0.25 to an average of +0.30. Step 2 increased from –0.50 to an average of 0.38. Thus, during the PBL period, Step 1 and Step 2 performance exceeded that which would have been predicted from MCAT scores by over one quarter and one half standard deviation, respectively. The type of PBL used in their curriculum would probably be termed hybrid. They have about 10 hours of lectures concurrent with an equal amount of time spent in PBL. This exceeds the limit on lectures that Barrows (1985) recommended (1.5 hours/day—7.5 hours per week). One other point is that concurrent with implementing PBL, they reduced the class size from 112 to 96 students.

Schmidt and colleagues (2006) obtained self-ratings of professional competence from a survey of 820/2081 (39%) of graduates of a PBL school and 621/3268 (19%) of graduates of a traditional school in the Netherlands. For interpersonal competencies such as working in a team, interpersonal skills and skills required for running meetings, the PBL graduates rated themselves more skilled by an effect size of 1.30. For PBL-related competencies such as self-directed learning, problem solving and information gathering, the PBL graduates rated themselves as more skilled by an effect size of 0.78. For general academic competencies and task-supporting competencies, the differences were 0.14 and 0.31 respectively, small but yet more positive for PBL graduates.

Schafer and colleagues (2006) reported a randomized trial of PBL versus traditional curricula regarding basic science and clinical knowledge. Students who had applied for the PBL track but due to limits were randomly assigned to the PBL track ($N = 122$) or to the traditional track ($N = 129$) and the remaining students in the traditional track ($N = 617$) were compared at three time points (beginning of first, third and fifth semester) using a 200-item progress test (1/3 basic science, 2/3 clinical). The results showed comparable gains by all groups on the basic science portion of the exam but by the third administration, performance on the clinical section by the PBL students exceeded that of the other two groups by effect sizes greater than 1.17.

Albanese and colleagues (2006) examined the relationship of undergraduate science grade point averages (SGPA) to Step 1 failure rate for students in a PBL track and traditional track at one medical school and those at three other traditional medical schools. While the overall failure rates for the three different groups were not different by a great margin (2%), the pattern by which the three groups reached the overall failure rate was different for the PBL track. The traditional track and the three traditional medical schools had a relatively linear relationship between SGPA and Step 1 failure rate. The PBL school, however, had almost no failures among those with SGPA values below 3.0. For SGPA values between 3.0 and 3.4, the PBL students had a much higher rate of failure that merged with the other two groups for SGPA values beyond 3.4.

These results raise the spectre that PBL may be better for some students, particularly those who have had relatively poor grades in prior course work (SGPA < 3.0), and worse for students who did relatively well in prior course work (SGPA: 3.0–3.4). These results need to be confirmed with other schools, but it may explain why the results from studies of PBL have been so variable. If some students do better and others do worse, effects will be difficult to find as they will cancel each other out. Another factor that may affect studies of PBL is that Schmidt et al. (2009) found the attrition rates of PBL schools in the Netherlands to be substantially below that of the conventional schools. Assuming academic problems are the main reason for attrition, the higher rate of elimination of poorer-performing students in the conventional schools may inflate their outcomes, masking the overall poorer performance of students in the conventional curricula (Albanese 2009).

Conclusions

- PBL provides important positive features, including patient problems that motivate learning, early exposure to clinical thinking and a nurturing learning environment.

- Systems that recognize and duly reward faculty for facilitator teaching and provide mechanisms for relief from the pressures of clinical service and research will be most likely to sustain a PBL curriculum.

- If one is open to broadly defining PBL, its various strains have been found to fit almost any budget and any physical layout.

- While studies of the efficacy of PBL are not conclusive, there is some evidence of improved clinical knowledge and skills in PBL-trained students and it has been consistently found that students and faculty enjoy PBL, potentially reducing student attrition in some cases.

References

Albanese, M.A. (1999) Students are not customers: a new model for medical education, *Acad Med.* 74(11): 1172–1184

Albanese M.A. (2009) Life is tough for curriculum researchers. *Med Educ.* 43: 199–201

Albanese M.A., Colliver J., and Dottl S.L. (2006) Effects of tutors with case expertise on problem-based learning issues Proceedings of the Annual Meeting of the Association for Medical Education in Europe. 14–18 September 2006. Cotone Congressi, Genoa, Italy, Abstract 10H1, p. 208

Albanese M.A., Mejicano G.C., Xakellis G., and Kokotailo P., (2009a) Physician practice change I: a critical review and description of an integrated systems model, *Acad Med.* 8(84): 1043–1055

Albanese M.A., Mejicano G.C., Xakellis G., and Kokotailo P. (2009b) Physician practice change II: implications for the future of continuing medical education. *Acad Med.* 8(84), 1056–1065.

Albanese M.A. and Mitchell S. (1993) Problem-based learning: a review of literature on its outcomes and implementation issues. *Acad Med.* 68: 52–81

Albanese M.A. and Sabers D.L. (1988) Multiple true-false items: a study of interitem correlations, scoring alternatives and reliability estimation. *J Educ Meas.* 25(2): 111–123

Anastakis D.J., Cohen R., and Reznick R.K. (1991) The structured oral examination as a method for assessing surgical residents. *Am J Surg.* 162(1): 67–70

Barnes, H.V., Albanese, M., and Schroeder, J. (1977) An approach to realistic reading assignments in an Introduction to Clinical Medicine Course (ICMC). In P. Stillman (ed.) *Update: Introduction to Clinical Medicine*. Monograph published by the Group on Medical Education, Association of American Medical Colleges.

Barrows, H.S. (1985) *How to Design a Problem-based Curriculum for the Preclinical Years*. New York: Springer Publishing Company

Barrows, H.S. (1986) A taxonomy of problem-based learning methods. *Med Educ.* 20: 481–486

Barrows, H.S. and Tamblyn, R.M. (1976) An evaluation of problem-based learning in small groups utilizing a simulated patient. *J Med Educ.* 51: 52–54

Berkson, L. (1993) Problem-based learning: have the expectations been met? *Acad Med.* 68(10): S79–S88

Blake, J.M., Norman, G.R., Keane, D.R., Mueller, C.B., Cunnington, J., and Didyk, N. (1996) Introducing progress testing in McMaster University's problem-based medical curriculum: psychometric properties and effect on learning. *Acad Med.* 71: 1002–1007

Boshuizen, H.P., van der Vleuten, C.P., Schmidt, H.G., and Machiels-Bongaerts, M. (1997) Measuring knowledge and clinical reasoning skills in a problem-based curriculum. *Med Educ.* 31: 115–121

Bowman, D. and Hughes, P. (2005) Emotional responses of tutors and students in problem-based learning: lessons for staff development. *Med Educ.* 39(2): 145–153

Brailovsky, C., Charlin, B., Beausoleil, S., Côté S., and van der Vleuten, C. (2001) Measurement of clinical reflective capacity early in training as a predictor of clinical reasoning performance at the end of residency: an experimental study on the script concordance test. *Med Educ.* 35: 430–436

Carayon, P., Schoofs Hundt, A., Karsh B.T., et al. (2006) Work system design for patient safety: The SEIPS model. *Qual Saf Health Care.* 15: i50–i58

Case, S.M. and Swanson, D.B. (2001) Constructing written test questions for the basic and clinical sciences. 3rd edn. Philadelphia, PA: National Board of Medical Examiners

Chaves, J.F., Baker, C.M., Chaves, J.A., and Fisher, M.L. (2006) Self, peer and tutor assessments of MSN competencies using the PBL-evaluator. *J. Nursing Educ.* 45(1): 25–31

Colliver, J.A. (2000) Effectiveness of problem-based learning curricula: Research and theory. *Acad Med.* 75(3): 259–268

Coulson, R.L. and Osborne, C.E. (1984) Insuring curricular content in a student-directed problem-based learning program. In H.G. Schmidt and ML. de Volder, eds., *Tutorials in Problem-based Learning*, pp. 225–229. Maastricht, The Netherlands: Van Gorcum, Assen

Davis S. (2007) Establishing small group ground rules. http://www.oucom.ohiou.edu/fd/group_ground_rules.htm, accessed 18 February 2013

Davis, W.K., Nairn, R., Paine, M.E., Anderson, R.M., and Oh, M.S. (1992) Effects of expert and non-expert facilitators on the small-group process and on student performance. *Acad Med.* 67: 470–474

Dochy, F., Segers, M., Van den Bossche, P., and Gijbels, D. (2003) Effects of problem-based learning: a meta-analysis. *Learning and Instruction*, 13, 533–568.

Dolmans, D.H.J.M., De Grave, W., Wolfhagen, I.H.A.P., and van der Vleuten, C.P.M. (2005) Problem-based learning: future challenges for educational practice and research. *Med Educ.* 39: 732–741

Dolmans, D.H.J.M., Gijselaers, W.H., and Schmidt, H.G. (1992) Do students learn what their teachers intend they learn? Guiding processes in problem-based learning. Paper presented at the Annual Meeting of the American Educational Research Association, San Francisco, California, April 1992

Dornan, T., Scherpbier, A., King, N., and Boshuizen, H. (2005) Clinical teachers and problem-based learning: a phenomenological study. *Med Educ.* 39: 163–170

Eagle, C.J., Harasym, P.H., and Mandin, H. (1992) Effects of tutors with case expertise on problem-based learning issues. *Acad Med.* 67: 465–469

Eva, K.W., Solomon, P., Neville, A.J., et al. (2007) Using a sampling strategy to address psychometric challenges in tutorial-based assessments. *Adv Health Sciences Educ.* 12(1): 19–33

Farrell, T., Albanese, M.A., and Pomrehn, P. (1999) Problem-based learning in ophthalmology: A pilot program for curricular renewal, *Arch Ophthalmol.* 117: 1223–1226

Gijbels, D., Dochy, F., Van den Bossche, P., and Segers, M. (2005) Effects of problem-based learning: a meta-analysis from the angle of assessment. *Rev Educ Res.* 75: 27–61

Glasser, W. (1986) *Control Theory in the Classroom*. New York, NY: Harper and Row.

Hays, R. (2002) Problems with problems in problem-based curricula, *Med Educ.* 36: 790

Hebert, R. and Bravo, G. (1996) Development and validation of an evaluation instrument for medical students in tutorials. *Acad Med.* 71(5): 488–494

Hoffman, K., Hosokawa, M., Blake, R., Headrick, L., and Johnson, G. (2006) Problem-based learning outcomes: Ten years of experience at the University of Missouri-Columbia School of Medicine. *Acad Med.* 81(7): 17–25

Hojat, M., Gonnella, J., Erdmann, J., and Veloske, J. (1997). The fate of medical students with different levels of knowledge: are the basic medical sciences relevant to physician competence? *Adv Health Sciences Educ.* 1: 179–196

Irby, D.M., Cooke, M., and O'Brien, B.C. (2010) Calls for reform of medical education by the Carnegie Foundation for the Advancement of Teaching: 1910 and 2010. *Acad Med.* 85(2): 220–227

Jones, J.W., Bieber, L.L., Echt, R., Scheifley, V., and Ways, P.O. (1984). A problem-based curriculum—ten years of experience. In: H.G. Schmidt and M.L. de Volder, (eds) *Tutorials in Problem-based Learning* (pp. 181–198). Assen, The Netherlands: Van Gorcum

Karsh, B.T., Holden, R.J., Alper, S.J., and Or, C.K. (2006) A human factors engineering paradigm for patient safety: designing to support the performance of the healthcare professional. *Qual Saf Health Care.* 15: 59–65

Kerfoot, B.P., Masser, B.A., and Hafler, J.P. (2005) Influence of new educational technology on problem-based learning at Harvard Medical School. *Med Educ.* 39(4): 380–387

Khaliq, F. (2005). Introduction of problem-solving activities during conventional lectures. *Med Educ.* 5(39): 1146–1147

Klatt, E.C. and Klatt, C.A. (2011) How much is too much reading for medical students? Assigned reading and reading rates at one medical school. *Acad Med.* 87(9): 1079–1083

Kruger, J. and Dunning, D. (1999) Unskilled and unaware of it: how difficulties in recognizing one's own incompetence lead to inflated self-assessments. *J Personality and Social Psychology.* 77(6): 1121–1134

Ladouceur, M.G., Rideout, D.M., Black, M.E., Crooks, D.L., O'Mara, L.M., and Schmuck, M.L. (2004) Development of an instrument to assess individual student performance in small group tutorials. *J. Nursing Educ.* 43(10): 447–455

Lohman, M.C. and Finkelstein, M. (2002) Designing cases in problem-based learning to foster problem-solving skill. *Eur J Dent Educ.* 6(3): 121–127

McGuire, C.H. and Babbott, D. (1967) Simulation technique in the measurement of problem-solving skills. *J Educ Meas.* 4(1): 1–10

McMichael, J. (1955) Adult education: for the academic clinical teacher. *BMJ.* 2: 510

Miflin, B. (2004) Problem-based learning: the confusion continues. *Med Educ.* 38: 921–926

Nendaz, M.R. and Tekian, A. (1999) Assessment in problem-based learning medical schools: a literature review. *Teach andLearn Med.* 11(4): 232–243

Neville, A.J. and Norman, G.R. (2007) PBL in the undergraduate MD program at McMaster University: three iterations in three decades. *Acad Med.* 82(4): 370–374

Newman, M. (2003) A pilot systematic review and meta-analysis on the effectiveness of problem based learning. On behalf of the Campbell Collaboration Systematic Review Group on the effectiveness of problem based learning. Newcastle, UK: University of Newcastle, Learning and Teaching Support Network

Nolte, J, Eller, P., and Ringel, S.P. (1988) Shifting toward problem-based learning in a medical school neurobiology course. In: *Research in Medical Education*, Proceedings of the Twenty-Seventh Annual Conference, pp. 66–71. Washington, DC: Association of American Medical Colleges

Norcini, J.J., Blank, L.L., Duffy, F.D., and Fortna, G.S. (2003). The Mini-CEX: A Method for Assessing Clinical Skills. *Ann Intern Med.* 138(6): 476–481

Painvin, C., Neufeld, V., Norman, G., Walker, I., and Whelan G. (1979) The 'triple jump' exercise—a structured measure of problem solving and self directed learning. *Annual Conf Res in Med Educ.* 18: 73–77

Pawlak, S.M., Popovich, N.G., Blank, J.W., and Russell, J.D. (1989) Development and validation of guided design scenarios for problem-solving instruction. *Am J Pharm Educ.* 53: 7–16

Petrusa, E.R., Blackwell, T., Carline, J., et al. (1991) A multi-institutional trial of an objective structured clinical examination. *Teach andLearn Med.* 3: 86–94

Plsek, P. (2001) Redesigning health care with insights from the science of complex adaptive systems. In: Committee on Quality of Health Care in America. Institute of Medicine. Crossing the Quality Chasm: A New Health System for the 21st Century (pp. 309–323). Washington, DC: The National Academies Press,. http://www.nap.edu/openbook.php?record_id=10027andpage=309 Accessed 18 February 2013

Qin, Z., Johnson, D.W., and Johnson, R.T. (1995) Cooperative versus competitive efforts and problem solving. *Rev Educ Res.* 65(2): 129–143

Saunders, N.A., McIntosh, J., McPherson, J., and Engel, C.E. (1990) A comparison between University of Newcastle and University of Sydney final-year students: knowledge and competence. In: Z.M. Nooman, H.G. Schmidt, and E.S. Ezzat (eds) *Innovation in Medical Education: An Evaluation of Its Present Status* (pp. 50–63). New York: Springer Publishing Company

Schafer, T., Huenges, B., Burger, A., and Rusche, H. (2006) A randomized controlled study on the progress in knowledge in a traditional versus problem-based curriculum. Proceedings of the 2006 Annual Meeting of the Association for Medical Education in Europe. 14–18 September 2006. Cotone Congressi, Genoa, Italy, Abstract 10H2, p. 208

Schmidt, H.G. (1983) Problem-based learning: rationale and description. *Med Educ.* 17: 11–16

Schmidt, H.G., Cohen-Schotanus, J., and Arends, L.R. (2009) Impact of problem-based, active learning on graduation rates for 10 generations of Dutch medical students. *Med Educ.* 43: 211–218

Schmidt, H.G., Vermeulen, L., and van der Molen, H.T. (2006) Longterm effects of problem-based learning on the attitudes of undergraduate health care students. *Med Educ.* 40(6): 562–567

Sim, S.M., Azila, N.M., Lian, L., Tan, C.P., and Tan, N.H. (2006) A simple instrument for the assessment of student performance in problem-based learning tutorials. *Ann Acad Med Singapore.* 35(9): 634–641

Smits, P., Verbeek, J., and De Buisonje, C. (2002) Problem based learning in continuing medical education: a review of controlled evaluation studies. *BMJ.* 324: 153–156

Stufflebeam, D.L. (1966) A depth study of the evaluation requirement. *Theory Pract.* 5: 121–133

Stufflebeam, D.L. (1971) The relevance of the CIPP evaluation model for educational accountability. Presented at the annual meeting of the American Association of School Administrators, Atlantic City, NJ, 24 February 1971. http://www.eric.ed.gov/PDFS/ED062385.pdf Accessed 19 March 2013

Stufflebeam, D.L. (2000). The CIPP model for evaluation. In: D.L. Stufflebeam, G. F. Madaus andand T. Kellaghan (eds) *Evaluation Models* (Chapter 16, pp. 279–317). 2nd edn. Boston: Kluwer Academic Publishers.

Stufflebeam, D.L., (2003) The *CIPP Model for Evaluation: An update, a review of the model's development, a checklist to guide implementation* Presented at the *2003* Annual *Conference of the Oregon Program Evaluators Network (OPEN), Portland, Oregon.*

Sungur, S. and Tekkaya, C. (2006) Effects of problem-based learning and traditional instruction on self-regulated learning. *J Educ Res.* 99(5): 307–320

Trappler, B. (2006) Integrated problem-based learning in the neuroscience curriculum—the SUNY Downstate experience. *BMC Med Educ.* (6: 47

van der Vleuten, C.P.M., Verwijnen, G.M., and Wijnen, W.H.F.W. (1996) Fifteen years of experience with Progress Testing in a problem-based learning curriculum. *Med Teach.* 18: 103–109

Vernon, D.T.A., and Blake, R.L. (1993) Does problem-based learning work? A meta-analysis of evaluative research. *Acad Med.* 68: 550–563.

Verwijnen, M., Imbos, T., Snellen, H., Stalenhoef, B., Sprooten, Y., and van der Vleuten C. (1982) The evaluation system at the medical school of Maastricht. In: H.G. Schmidt, M. Vries, and E.S. Ezzat (eds) *Innovation in Medical Education: An evaluation of its present status* (pp. 41–49). New York: Springer

Wales, C.E. and Stager, R. (1972) Design of an educational system. *Eng Educ.* 62: 456–459

Ward, M., Gruppen, L., and Regehr, G. (2002) Measuring self-assessment: current state of the art. *Adv Health Sciences Educ.* 7: 63–80

Williams, G.C., Saizow, R.B., and Ryan, R.M. (1999) The importance of self-determination theory for medical education. *Acad Med.* 74(9): 992–995

and Wood, D.F. (2003) ABC of learning and teaching in medicine: problem based learning. *BMJ.* 326: 328–330

Woods, D.R. (1996) Instructor's Guide for '*Problem-based Learning: how to gain the most from PBL*' 3rd edn. Hamilton. W. L. Griffin Printing, Ontario

Zeitz, H.J. and Paul, H. (1993) Facilitator expertise and problem-based learning in PBL and traditional curricula. *Acad Med.* 68(3): 203–204

CHAPTER 4

Interprofessional education: learning together in health and social care

Hugh Barr and Richard Gray

After almost 50 years of inquiry, there is now sufficient evidence to indicate that interprofessional education enables effective collaborative practice which in turn optimizes health-services, strengthens health systems and improves health outcomes.

WHO, 2010

Framework for Action in Interprofessional Education and Collaborative Practice. Geneva: WHO, 2010. Available at: http://www.who.int/hrh/resources/ framework_action/en. Accessed 10th May 2013.

Introduction

Advances made in medical and health care would have been inconceivable had it not been for the strength of the professional institutions established and the lead which they have given, albeit at a price. Professions proliferate and specialities within them, driven by medical and technological progress, making collaboration more complex, more costly, more protracted and more problematic. Patients benefit, but care fragments (General Medical Council 2011).

Nor is that all: doctors, along with other professionals, are working with a more damaged, more dependent and more demanding clientele than in the past, evident in wealthier countries by the number of older people living longer with chronic, complex and multiple problems (Department of Health 2010) and in poorer countries by the number of families at the mercy of infant mortality, malnutrition, the killer childhood diseases and the human immunodeficiency virus (HIV) pandemic (Crisp 2010). Confronted by problems beyond their roles and responsibilities, doctors have three choices: to set aside those problems for which they have neither authorization nor training; to go beyond their role at risk of stress and overload for themselves and less than adequate care for their patients; or to work in partnership with other professions to spread the load and respond more fully to the range of needs.

It does not take long for the perceptive doctor to recognize how poverty, unemployment, family breakdown, homelessness, or migration may be compounding the medical problem presented. It takes longer to mobilize the resources needed to respond. Bridges must be built across organizational, professional and attitudinal divides before medicine can reach out not only to the other health professions, but also

to social work and, with its help, to community, education, housing, income maintenance, legal, police, social care, and youth services.

Beyond organizational solutions

What then is to be done? Policy makers invariably turn first to organizational 'solutions'—joint planning, joint finance, coordinating machinery and service integration. Outcomes often disappoint. The integration of some services distances them from others (Leutz 2009) while the implications for the workforce are often overlooked. The structural fallacy has long since been exposed where policymakers rely on organizational solutions without heeding the human factor (Carrier and Kendall 1995).

Efforts are redoubled as one round of reorganization follows another in the confident (or overconfident) expectation that this time the projected improvements will result. Reorganization destabilizes working relations as boundaries are redrawn, power redistributed, roles redefined, posts jettisoned and new ones sometimes substituted. Recurrent reorganization demoralizes and debilitates, generating stress and prompting defensive behaviour between professions and between organizations (Hinshelwood and Skogstad 2000; Obholzer 1994) at the very time when collaboration may be most critical to implement change in a spirit of give and take.

Towards reconciling workforce and interprofessional agendas

Hard lessons have been learned; policy makers today appreciate better than did their forebears the need to take workforce planning into account. Proposals to remodel services are more often complemented by those to remodel the workforce and professional education as an agent of change (Frenk et al. 2010). Policy makers call for core curricula across pre-licensure programmes to instill common values, knowledge and skills in the belief that these changes will transcend barriers between the professions and free up the deployment of personnel, in response to the exigencies of the services, and career progression, in response to the aspirations of the workers.

Reforms follow in professional education paving the way for interprofessional education (IPE), but often stop short. Common studies are not enough to further collaborative practice unless and until they are complemented by interactive learning between the professions. Profession-specific studies must be safeguarded to observe regulations, to respect the identity and integrity of each profession and, above all, to ensure that it retains and reinforces its distinctive expertise within the interprofessional team.

Pre-licensure IPE proposals, however, invariably call for common studies to be refined and extended during an ongoing process of negotiation, accommodation and mutual consent between the professions and with other stakeholders. They also introduce interactive studies in small groups so that students from the participant professions can 'deal in differences' as they exchange experience, expertise and insights, and explore ways to work more closely and more effectively together in practice.

That goes to the heart of IPE where members of the participant professions learn with, from and about each other to promote collaboration and to improve quality of care and health outcomes (CAIPE 2002; WHO 2010). The collaboration includes flexible working, for example between members of an interprofessional team as they grow to trust each other and boundaries between roles become permeable and modified by mutual consent within the constraints of law and patient safety. Conversely, workforce strategies can further collaborative practice insofar as the associated educational reforms build on IPE expertise, experience and evidence and engage the professions as partners (Box 4.1).

The interprofessional learning process

IPE enshrines and extends the principles of adult learning. Responsibility for managing the learning rests not only on the student but also on the group—an interprofessional group with differing perceptions and expectations on how to progress its learning—which may be an early test of collaborative practice. Members negotiate how, within the objectives as given, each of them can contribute to a process of cooperative, collaborative, reflective and socially constructed learning (Clark 2006, 2009), coping with conflict out of which insight, understanding and skills may come (Kolb 1984). Learners become a community of practice, negotiating the meaning of phenomena and problems as they engage in a process which relies for its success upon the willingness and ability of the learners to enter into new experiences, reflect on them from different perspectives, create concepts that integrate their observations into logical theories and use them to make decisions and solve problems (Lave and Wenger 1991; Wenger 1998). During 'situated learning' they call on a shared repertoire of communal learning resources facilitating change where the meaning of the activities that occur is a constantly negotiated and renegotiated interpretation of those held by all

---

Box 4.1 A case study

Medical and social work teachers wrote, developed and implemented an interprofessional 5-day module entitled 'Looking after the vulnerable—who cares?' The students were third-year medical students, for whom this was a voluntary student-selected module (SSC), and second-year social work students on a Masters programme, for whom this module was an integral part of their course. The latter group tended to be older with more practical caring experience and had spent more time with clients in practice during their courses.

The module focused on client groups who were deemed to have particular health and social care needs including young people who were care leavers, the homeless, asylum seekers or refugees, and victims of domestic abuse. The purpose of the module was to highlight the importance of integrated interprofessional responses to the needs of the client groups.

Each day was co-facilitated by a medical and a social work teacher. During the first day student perception and stereotypes were explored focusing on both the client groups and each other. Although the teachers anticipated that this would not be an easy session, neither of them was prepared for the degree of anger that emerged, particularly from some social work students towards medical students. This appeared to be related to their previous experiences with paediatricians who were perceived as being cold and uncaring. In contrast, the medical students did not demonstrate anger towards the social work students.

As the anger appeared to be disrupting learning, additional time was spent during the day discussing with the students what was happening. As a satisfactory resolution was not achieved, it was decided to continue with the programme to achieve the planned outcomes for the day. By the end of the first day both teachers felt dissatisfied that they had neither addressed the disruption satisfactorily nor effectively completed the planned timetable. The problems encountered were outside their usual teaching experience. Both teachers felt confused.

---

the participants. The learning process accommodates complexity. Rational deduction is no longer enough; linearity no longer holds where multiple remedies may be more effective than troubleshooting and quick fixes (Plsek and Greenhalgh 2001). The learning takes place in 'the zone of complexity' between familiar and unfamiliar tasks, and familiar and unfamiliar environments (Fraser and Greenhalgh 2001).

Participants reflect as they evaluate their beliefs, assumptions and hypotheses while recognizing and accepting the uncertainty generated (Dewey 1933, 1938). Problematic practice turns into learning opportunities as participants individually, in pairs or in groups grow and develop (Jarvis 1992). Learning is cyclical (Kolb 1984), heightening understanding and self-awareness, bridging theory and practice, evaluating and cultivating identity (Tate 2004), empowering and transformative, if sometimes disorienting as it interprets new experiences (Mezirow 1981).

Interprofessional learning entails more than reflection-in-action (immediately based on practice know-how); it entails reflection-on-action (later taking into account guiding principles for practice)

(Schön 1983, and1987). It goes beyond first order reflection limited by participants' own personal and professional views to second order reflection where interprofessional learning becomes transformative as participants step back to become aware of their frames of reference; 'meta-cognition' where they 'decentre' their learning taking into account points of view other than their own (Dahlgren 2009; Wackerhausen 2009).

Psychodynamic insights cultivate critical awareness of behaviour in groups, as groups and between groups exemplified in IPE by approaches originating from experiential learning developed by the London-based Tavistock Institute of Human Relations (Bion 1961). Interprofessional learning utilizes and develops the skills of independent learning in a state of educational sensitivity where cognitive dissonance, often at the point of consciousness, is recognized as discomfort and used as a focus for further learning and development (Eraut 1996). The process reveals implicit behaviours and motives that affect attitudes and interprofessional relationships (Jaques 1994). Students reflect constantly, assisted by feedback on experience which carries over into further learning throughout their professional lives.

Perspectives from social psychology are also illuminating. According to the contact hypothesis (Allport1954), interprofessional learning needs to satisfy specified conditions before it is likely to modify reciprocal attitudes and perceptions, counter prejudice and negative stereotyping and improve group and inter-group relations. The learning must be interactive and cooperative between the participant groups; it must be characterized by positive expectations and enjoy the backing of the host institution (McMichael and Gilloran 1984; Carpenter 1995; Carpenter and Hewstone 1996; Dickinson and Carpenter 2005).

General systems theory (von Bertalanffy 1971 cited by Loxley 1997) provides an antidote in IPE to the limitations of specialist disciplines in addressing complex problems. It treats wholes as more than the sum of their parts, interactions between parties as purposeful, boundaries between them as permeable, and cause and effect as interdependent not linear. Many interprofessional teachers find the biopsychosocial model (Engel 1977) especially helpful in developing interprofessional learning as a means to counter reductionism in the definition of the problems to be addressed and the specialties to respond while accommodating both. Systems theory offers a unifying and dynamic framework within which the professions may variously relate their work in response to the needs of individuals, families, communities, and the environment—beyond health and social care as commonly understood.

Choosing from a repertoire of learning methods

Experienced teachers introduce a repertoire of learning methods during IPE (Barr 2002). These are some of them.

Ice breaking

Ice breaking is especially important in IPE if students from different professions exhibit diverse needs and are reluctant to engage with each other. One example involves interprofessional groups of students on their first day at university in competing in a treasure hunt around the city tracking down its many health and social care agencies. Another is 'the balloon game'. Each of a number of students is assigned a profession—accountant, doctor, journalist, priest and so on—as they climb into the basket ready for take-off. All goes well until the gas supply begins to run low without warning. Saving the majority of the passengers depends upon one being sacrificed. Which profession should it be? Following a vote, the unfortunate profession holder elects to be thrown overboard. The gas runs lower. Which profession should be the next to go? And so the process is repeated as one by one the professions are deemed less valuable to society than those that remain until just one is left to return safely to earth. Games help IPE to be fun. Debates can also be helpful where students propose and oppose motions as they expose attitudes, perceptions and sometimes prejudices to challenge.

Case-based learning

Case-based learning is perhaps the most common method in IPE where teachers devise and select cases relevant to practice which contain multiple and progressively more complex problems for their interprofessional student groups to assess as they develop a more rounded or holistic understanding of needs beyond those which any one profession may identify alone. The way is then open to explore how each profession can best exercise its role and deploy its expertise to complement that of the others within the team (Higgs and Jones 2000).

Observation-based learning

Observation-based learning was introduced into IPE from the training of child psychotherapists and, in its most sophisticated applications, follows much the same process of critical reflection. It applies also where groups of students from different professions follow the patient throughout their treatment experience, (D'Avray 2007), or make joint visits by invitation to patients in their homes, viewing their lives from different perspectives (Lennox and Anderson 2007). Each profession, in both examples, sees the patient through its lens. Differences in perception become apparent later and are facilitated by the teacher. Shadowing is yet another example of observation based learning where students, typically on part-time continuing IPE courses, spend time with each other at each other's place of work.

Experiential learning

Experiential learning may be said to occur in any of these examples. It refers in IPE more precisely to situations where learning is contrived between students from different professions in group settings designed to engender interpersonal and interprofessional interaction and to mirror working relationships in practice as discussed above from a psychodynamic perspective.

Appreciative inquiry

Appreciative inquiry (AI) is a process originated by Cooperrider grounded in the belief that all organizations have positive experiences on which to build (Cooperrider and Whitney 2005). Participants exchange their experiences of good practice in pairs and small groups leading to the identification of best practice and ways to disseminate it. AI has been introduced into work-based IPE to generate change in practice. It can reverse the downward spiral where learning has become preoccupied with negative relationships and problematic practice.

Problem-based learning

Problem-based learning (PBL) has been introduced into IPE via progressive models of medical education pioneered at McMaster University in Canada (Barrows 1996) as student-centred, self-directed, facilitated small group learning focusing on the resolution of problems. It was transposed into IPE in the first instance at Linkoping University in Sweden (Willhelmsson et al. 2009) and adapted for IPE by other universities worldwide as commended by the WHO (1988). Although PBL can be a useful alternative approach to traditional medical teaching, it uses a rigid framework that is based on medical diagnostic principles and may not be appropriate or acceptable to other professional groups who may express negativity towards the process. Enquiry-based learning (EBL) addresses these issues by using questions rather than problems to stimulate learning. In addition, learning and teaching styles can be varied allowing for flexible implementation.

Continuous quality improvement

Continuous quality improvement (CQI) merits critical comparison with PBL but is applied more often in work based interprofessional learning and practice. Its roots lie in the work of W. Edward Deming (Walton, 1988) in Japan and the United States in total quality management as a grassroots response by practising professionals to improve systems and services from the bottom up. It applies Deming's cyclical process—plan, do, check and act (PDCA)—to analyse problematic situations in the work and to effect small-scale change as a concerted response by the professions directly involved. Interprofessional learning is a byproduct that benefits ongoing teamwork between the participants and carries over into subsequent quality improvement endeavours.

Collaborative inquiry

Collaborative inquiry was developed by Reason (1994) based on the work of Heron (1971) as a process to involve all the interested parties as co-participants in an investigation (Heron and Reason 2008). It was introduced into work-based IPE in the UK as means to review and improve health services before CQI was imported from the United States. Like CQI, its application in IPE is post-licensure and work based where the learning is generated in the doing.

Simulation-based learning

Simulation-based learning in IPE is another ambiguous term. It has referred for many years to exercises such as role play where students are variously assigned parts—perhaps patient, carer or one of several professions—as they enact scenarios that simulate collaborative practice. However, it refers also to the creation of virtual learning environments (e.g. at St George's University of London <www.elu.sgul.ac.uk>—accessed 1 March 2012 and Cumbria University—Walsh and van Soeren 2012) and increasingly to the extension of laboratory-based simulated learning on manikins, notably from medical education, into IPE where students from, for example, medicine, nursing and physiotherapy practice their respective interventions as members of an interprofessional team observed by their fellows and followed by debriefing (Freeth et al. 2006, Mikkelsen Krykjebo et al. 2006).

Didactic teaching

Didactic teaching is used sparingly in IPE. Given the uncertainty and discomfort which teachers can experience in responding spontaneously as they facilitate IPE sessions, they may retreat into the comfort of more familiar didactic teaching. This should be resisted. IPE teachers need to learn to live with uncertainty as a normal part of the teaching process.

Evidence-based practice is one sphere of learning which is arguably handled more effectively and more expeditiously in didactic teaching than in group discussion (though exponents of PBL may beg to differ). Impact on practice—especially collaborative practice—nevertheless needs to be explored between the interested professions, teasing out implications for their roles and responsibilities and demarcations and overlaps between them.

E-enhanced learning

E-learning can be mistakenly seen as another learning method. It is better treated as a medium—more precisely several media—for the learning methods in Table 4.1. That explains our preference for the term 'e-enhanced learning'.

E-enhanced interprofessional learning is increasing rapidly employing one or more of the following technologies:

* access to information through the internet
* virtual learning environments and tools to enhance reflective learning such as e-portfolios
* use of e-communication tools to enable synchronous discussion
* electronic simulation
* 'Web 2.0' technologies and social networking.

(Barr, Helme and D'Avray 2011; Bromage et al. 2010)

In IPE it can obviate logistical problems by freeing students from the constraints of timetabling, room availability and practice

Table 4.1 Some interprofessional learning methods

Methods	Projected outcome
Ice breaking	Loosening up, opening up
Case-based learning	Understanding – needs from multiple perspectives – professional responses, roles and relationships
Observational learning	Heightening awareness of people and situations from different professional perspectives
Experiential learning	Enhancing awareness of the behaviour of self and others in groups
Appreciative inquiry	Enhancing motivation to collaborate for positive change
Problem-based learning	Enhancing collaborative and analytic competence
Continuous quality improvement	Enhanced collaborative and analytic competence
Collaborative inquiry	Enhanced collaborative and analytic competence
Lab-based simulation	Enhanced collaborative and analytic competence

placements patterns. It can enable both collaborative and personal learning. Students may either use materials collaboratively as a group or access them individually in their own place and at their own pace.

It may be tempting to substitute e-enhanced learning for face-to-face learning in cost-conscious times, but to do so would detract from the interpersonal interactions behind the interprofessional ones. On-line and face-to-face learning are better blended.

Practice-based learning

Similarly, practice-based learning is the context in which many if not all of methods discussed above may be introduced into IPE.

Opportunities for interprofessional learning during uniprofessional placements may be serendipitous (accidental or incidental), opportunist (responsive to chance encounters including those with students from other professions), or planned in advance between the student and the clinical supervisor. Some practice teachers collaborate across professions to generate interprofessional learning opportunities. An interprofessional practice teacher may be designated to work with an ad hoc interprofessional student group concurrently in the same placement setting in parallel with their uniprofessional practice teachers (Barr and Brewer 2012).

Meetings may also be arranged between students on placement in the same organization or community to get acquainted, compare their experiences, discuss cases and engage in joint activities (Jaques and Higgins 1986). Others may be placed in an interprofessional team where they work alongside members from other professions and observe team process, behaviour and decision-making (Reeves et al. 2010). Yet others may be lucky enough to be part of an interprofessional student team, for example on an interprofessional training ward (Fallsberg and Hammer 2000; Jacobsen et al. 2009; Ponzer et al. 2004; Reeves and Freeth 2002).

Mixing and matching learning methods

Teachers 'import' these and other learning methods into IPE from their respective fields of professional education. Medical teachers, for example, often bring with them PBL, drawing on experience gained from its adoption in medical curricula, and lab-based simulated learning.

To opt for any one method alone would be to miss the opportunity to respond to the range and diversity of students' needs and learning styles. Experienced teachers 'mix and match' the methods and ring the changes to hold the interest of their students.

Tension can, however, arise between learning approaches. Switching between the constructivist learning and the didactic teaching in IPE, or during concurrent interprofessional and professional sequences, may not come easily. Students' learning styles are influenced by the prevalent learning approaches in their respective professional courses and during their earlier schooling. The teacher, as facilitator, needs to be sensitive and responsive if and when students find the transition difficult. Unfamiliar approaches may need to be justified, explained and tested.

The range of learning methods being introduced into IPE exemplifies the 'new pedagogy' grounded in expository, interactive, conversational and experiential practice-based methods where the learners actively construct knowledge for themselves from an array

of experiences rather than focusing on knowledge-based subject matter transferred from the teacher to the taught (Barr et al. 2011 citing Bruner 1966).

Preparing teachers as facilitators

University and practice teachers often feel underprepared and undervalued for their interprofessional role. They find it daunting to be confronted by students from diverse backgrounds with different perspectives, expectations, assumptions and styles of learning. Some are anxious about working with students and teachers from other professions whose discourses differ from their own. They may worry about how to field questions, handle prejudice or mediate conflict between the professional groups (as the case study in Box 4.1 illustrates). They may need opportunities to develop insight into ways in which their own interprofessional experiences impact for better or worse on their relationships with their students and their fellow teachers (Barr 2009).

Some may be accustomed to facilitating uniprofessional learning, atuned to the dynamics of small groups; others may be wedded to didactic teaching and ill-at-ease as facilitators of socially constructed learning. Initial preparation is essential with ongoing support (Anderson, Cox and Thorpe 2009; Barr and Coyle 2012; Freeman, Wright and Lindquist 2010; Gray 2009; Rees and Johnson 2007,).

Demystifying facilitation

Facilitating interprofessional learning requires insights and skills additional to those in facilitating professional learning. It enables students from different professions to enhance each other's learning; sensitive to each other's differing perspectives and perceptions, as they translate problems into learning opportunities. It optimizes learning by calling on resources within and beyond the interprofessional group. The facilitator may encourage the student group to view its learning experience as a microcosm of working life, a test bed under safe and controlled conditions to develop collaborative capabilities.

The facilitators remain sensitive to the perspectives, perceptions and particular needs of each individual and profession, aware of ways in which their own attitudes and behaviour can intrude positively or negatively on students' experience. They understand how students behave in interprofessional groups, the roles which each may play in leading or obstructing its work, assisting or impeding the learning of others, and the conflicts and rivalries which may intrude, overlain by power and status differentials. They are ready to extend extra support where students are less accustomed to learning in small groups. They resist pressure to assume the teaching role unless and until the group has exhausted its own learning capacity (Barr et al. 2011; Barr and Low 2012; Howkins and Bray 2008).

Building on experience

IPE gains much from the experience that teachers bring from recent and concurrent education (as students, clinical supervisors or teachers) and from practice to enhance the relevance of their teaching. Some may well have IPE and/or collaborative practice experience. If so, that will be a bonus. Past encounters with other professions may, however, have been more or less positive, colouring attitudes towards students and fellow teachers from those professions. Teachers moving into IPE need time to reflect on such experiences and their implication for their newfound role.

Each profession brings distinctive experience and expertise to IPE to be compared and combined during an ongoing process of accommodation and development within the teaching team. Doctors bring in-depth knowledge and understanding of health conditions from which students and teachers from other professions may gain much. In Japan, for example, medical teachers write IPE case materials for use in seven universities (Endoh, Magara, and Nagai 2012). Doctors are well placed to relate teaching and learning about patient safety to the care and treatment of patients with particular conditions and risks.

Acquiring additional identities

Making the transition from practice to professional teaching and then interprofessional teaching entails not only transferring and augmenting skills, but also the acquisition of additional identities along a developmental pathway with milestones to be achieved. It is not the loss of an identity that can cause difficulty during transition but the associated loss of clarity and certainty which is replaced by the emergence of confusion and uncertainty as the transition progresses towards the new identity. It is this transition that needs to be managed effectively to enable interprofessional teacher development to occur (Gray 2009). Doctors who become teachers remain doctors whether or not they continue in practice. That affirms their commitment to practice driven professional and interprofessional education and the distinctive and indispensable contribution which medicine makes to IPE and collaborative practice (Box 4.2).

Boundaries and identities

Professional boundaries provide a structure during pre-licensure education, which is important in cultivating students' professional identity, but can also produce feelings of tribalism that block IPE. If professional boundaries are challenged and perceived as being breached, then confrontation can occur between professionals, with associated anxiety and stress. A transition period then occurs whilst individuals struggle to make sense out of the confusion of an open interprofessional culture as they endeavour to form a larger tribe with different interprofessional boundaries and different interprofessional identities (Atkins 1998). Boundaries around undergraduate professional learning can be made more flexible to minimize the effect of tribalism during IPE by incorporating integrated and appropriate interprofessional learning focused on areas that overlap artificial discipline-specific topics and are of direct relevance to future professional work (Anderson, Smith, and Thorpe 2010; Kinnair, Anderson, and Thorpe 2012). This is exemplified by Anderson, Ford, and Thorpe (2011) who evaluated a workshop for interprofessional student groups that effectively enhanced their communication using the power of story telling by disabled people and their carers.

A further insight into ways of addressing tribalism is provided by Brown and Williams (1984) who distinguished between different models of social identity theory. The Decategorization model plays down the differences between professionals and the Common Group In-group identity model focuses on the

---

Box 4.2 Implications for the case study

Considering the discussion in Box 4.1, it was not at all surprising that anger emerged during the first day of the module, especially from the social work students. As second-year Masters' students, this group tended to be older, with many having had previous experience as social care professionals. They had the opportunity of considering many options but decided at this later stage that they wished to become social workers. Consequently, many would have developed particularly strong professional identities and at the time of the module may not have been ready to relinquish resultant professional ties to enable them to embark upon the second transition to develop interprofessional identities. The module being a compulsory part of their programme may have intensified this anger.

In contrast, for the medical students this was a voluntary student-selected module. Hence members of this group self-selected the module already being receptive to IPE and having an interest in interprofessional issues. It is likely that this group having achieved professional identities were already working towards an interprofessional identity.

When considering the above issues it is surprising that more anger, negativity and suspicion was not expressed on this first day. If the teachers had anticipated this and understood the reasons, sufficient protected time would have been offered to reflect on past assumptions leading to conflict. An initial effective ice breaker may have helped participants to start to engage in an interactive process. Much of the conflict appeared to be based on assumptions developed from past experiences and this situation may be considered a microcosm of practice. Second order reflection could have been facilitated using dissonance created from the conflict as a focus for learning. Feelings could have been discussed, reasons acknowledged and ways of helping students work through the situation explored.

---

formation of a new larger group which all previous different professional groups can join. Both these models again explain the need for developing an IPE curriculum that overlaps artificial discipline-specific topics.

When professionals from different backgrounds come together to learn, it is necessary to implement a number of conditions including the group agreeing and focusing on a common purpose (Allport 1954) with positive and successful expectations (Hewstone and Brown 1986). Again this need can be addressed by encouraging interprofessional learners to focus on patient care and to understand the perspective of patients.

Patient involvement

Involving patients in IPE can provide a meaningful platform that addresses these needs (Anderson, Ford, and Thorpe 2011). Quality of patient care is integral to the IPE process and to the collaborative practice for which it prepares (CAIPE 2002). The involvement of patients and/or their families and carers provides a natural and clear focus that transcends artificial professional boundaries and ensures relevance grounded in practice (Figure 4.1).

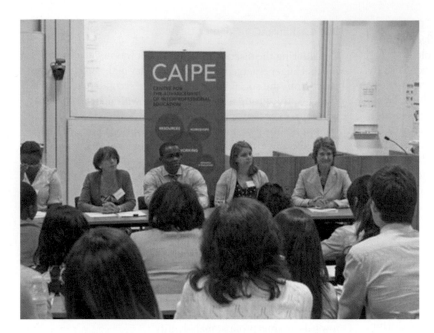

Figure 4.1 Centre for the Advancement of Interprofessional Education

How then can patient involvement best be incorporated into professional and interprofessional education? The content of the modern undergraduate medical curriculum integrates learning based on systems of the body with clinical problems presented by patients (Brighton and Sussex Medical School [BSMS] 2009). Bernstein (1971) described this as an integrated code curriculum. Both patient contact and IPE can occur from the beginning of the course with an emphasis on communication skills. This process theoretically allows medical students to develop flexible attitudes and creative thinking that can cross both subject and professional boundaries with a constant focus on the patient/client. This not only allows opportunities for students to develop their professional identities (Stephenson, Higgs, and Sugarman 2001), but also provides opportunities for IPE to occur (Martin 2005).

In what ways then can patients be involved in IPE?

- Patients used in a passive role to be examined
- Patients used in a partially active role, e.g. taking a case history
- Patient acting as an expert resource in group, facilitated by other
- Patient specifically invited to a session to teach, facilitate or lecture
- Patient an equal member of teaching team with full involvement in planning and assessment.

As one descends through the list so the patient becomes more actively involved in the process of teaching and is more empowered. However, it should be emphasized that no role should be considered superior or inferior to any other. It is a matter of involving the patient in the most relevant way at the most appropriate time in order to demonstrate that patients are valued and involved as part of the interprofessional team.

Outcomes

Attempts to frame competency based outcomes for IPE have been taking shape for some years. Barr distinguished between:

- Common competencies held by all (or a number) the professions
- Complementary competencies that distinguished one profession and complemented those which distinguished other professions
- Collaborative competencies which every profession needed to collaborate within its own ranks, with other professions, with non-professionals, within organizations, between organizations, with patients and their carers, volunteers and with community groups (Barr 1998).

Barr saw collaborative competencies as being the ability to:

- Recognize and respect the roles, responsibilities and competences of other professions in relation to one's own, knowing when, where and how to involve those others through agreed channels
- Work with other professions to review services, effect change, improve standards, solve problems, and resolve conflict in the provision of care and treatment
- Work with other professions to assess, plan, provide, and review care for individual patients and support carers
- Tolerate differences, misunderstandings, ambiguities, shortcomings, and unilateral change in another profession
- Enter into interdependent relationships, teaching and sustaining other professions
- Learn from, and be sustained by, those other professions
- Facilitate interprofessional case conferences, meetings, team working, and networking (Barr 1998, 2002).

Major strides have since been made in framing interprofessional competencies in terms which have come to enjoy wide currency: in the UK led by Sheffield Hallam and Sheffield Universities (Combined Universities Interprofessional Learning Unit 2010);

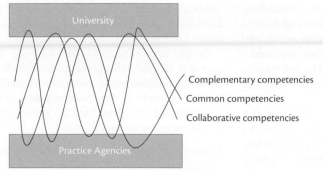

Figure 4.2 The pre-licensure professional learning process

in Canada led by the University of British Columbia (Canadian Interprofessional Collaborative 2010); and in the United States (US) by a broad based interprofessional collaborative (Interprofessional Education Collaborative 2011).

The last of these three competency statements from the US is, in our view, the best grounded, most comprehensive and likely to have the most impact. It defines and distinguishes between professional and interprofessional competencies, calling on international sources and formulations by a range of US professional bodies including the Association of American Medical Colleges (2008) and the Accredited Colleges for Graduate Medical Education (2011).

It divides the competencies into four domains:

◆ *Values and ethics for interprofessional practice*, i.e. the values that should underpin relationships among the professions

◆ *Roles and responsibilities* grounded in mutual appreciation of diversity and difference

◆ *Interprofessional communication*—beyond basic communication skills

◆ *Teams and teamwork*—learning to be a good team player.

Core competencies are needed to:

◆ Embed essential content in all health professions education curricula

◆ Guide curricular development and assessment strategies to achieve productive outcomes

◆ Provide the foundation for an interprofessional learning continuum

◆ Inform the evaluation of interprofessional programmes

◆ Prompt dialogue between education and practice

◆ Inform accreditation and licensing criteria.

It is too soon (at the time of writing) to gauge the impact of the US statement against these expectations. In Canada, however, participants during a Delphi study have been invited to contribute towards agreeing performance indicators which will break down competency statements into assessment criteria for students (<www.CIHC/cihc-2012-01 January.html>—accessed 30 January 2012). In Australia, Curtin University has prepared a user-friendly digest from the Sheffield and Canadian statements to inform the assessment of its students and the evaluation of its programmes (Brewer 2011). In the Philippines, the University of Manila has adapted and tested the Curtin digest (Paterno 2011).

Pulling the strands together

Figure 4.2 is a visual presentation of uniprofessional, multiprofessional, and interprofessional education as three interwoven strands throughout pre-licensure programmes iterating between learning in the university and in practice settings leading respectively to complementary, common and collaborative competencies.

Assembling the evidence

Pressure to assemble evidence to support claims made for IPE built up during the late 1990s at a time of mounting concern to establish the evidence-base, not only for professional practice, but also for professional education (Hargreaves 1996). The first of six international conferences in the *All Together Better Health* series held in London in 1997 seemed an ideal opportunity to focus on the effectiveness of interprofessional practice and IPE as a means to promote it.

Two propositions were put:

◆ that IPE improves collaborative practice

◆ that interprofessional practice improves the quality of care.

Distinguished scholars were invited from both sides of the Atlantic to address these propositions. Outcomes fell short of expectations which, with benefit of hindsight, were naïve although some progress was made in reframing questions and mapping territory. The answers, it became painfully clear, were going to be more complex than the propositions. There would be no quick fix.

Tracking down isolated evaluations was not enough. Sustained and systematic searches were needed to collate evaluations that would provide a baseline for future policy, pointers for future evaluations and verify or vitiate claims being made for IPE. Systematic reviews were beginning in healthcare practice, notably under the auspices of the Cochrane Collaboration, which prompted a team of UK researchers to explore the application of its methodology to determine the efficacy of IPE under its Effective Practice and Organisation of Care Group (EPOC). Criteria for the review that followed focused narrowly on direct benefit to patients attributable to an IPE intervention evaluated by a randomized, controlled trial, a controlled before and after study, or an interrupted time series study. None were found despite an exhaustive search of over a thousand abstracts from electronic databases and scrutiny of 89 papers (Zwarenstein et al. 2001). The group faced an unenviable choice: abandon its search; renew it after an interval in accordance with its obligation to the Cochrane Collaboration; or try another approach. The review has been updated twice so far in accordance with the researchers' obligation to Cochrane, searching the same and some additional sources. The first of these updates found six studies which met the same inclusion criteria as before, of which four reported a range of positive outcomes (Reeves et al. 2008). The second also found six such studies, four of which reported a range of positive outcomes (Reeves et al. 2010)

Prepared though the group was to replicate the review in this way, most of its members were doubtful about the translation of a methodology derived from experimental research in medicine into the evaluation of education where quasi-experimental methods were more common and, in the opinion of the group, more realistic. There was a need too to include qualitative paradigms especially to evaluate the learning process. Studies, they had discovered, which reported before and after changes attributed to the IPE left a 'black hole' which qualitative evaluation of the learning process could have filled.

The group, known from then on as the interprofessional joint evaluation team (JET), determined to conduct a less restrictive but no less rigorous and systematic review which would take into account a continuum of outcomes and a range of research methodologies. Its report (Barr et al. 2005) was based on the 107 robust evaluations found, which met quality checks for presentation and rigour. A third of the studies came from the UK and over half from the United States with the remainder widely spread. Evenly divided between community and hospital based care, two thirds related to chronic conditions. Four fifths were post qualification and typically work-based workshops. Almost all had been published since 1991.

Reported outcomes were classified modifying Kirkpatrick's (1967) categories and collated as follows (with multiple coding):

- Reactions to the interprofessional learning 45 (42%)
- Changes in attitudes/perceptions 21 (20%)
- Acquisition of knowledge/skills 38 (36%)
- Changes in behaviour 21 (20%)
- Changes in organizational practice 37 (35%)
- Benefit to patients 20 (19%).

The first three outcomes spanned pre- and post-licensure IPE; the last three referred invariably to work-based continuing interprofessional education where service improvement was an explicit objective.

The inference was clear, albeit derived from only a few studies. Pre-licensure IPE could lay foundations for collaborative practice by effecting attitudinal change and enhancing knowledge and skills; work-based post-licensure IPE was needed to build on those foundations before impact on practice and patient care would be apparent. It remained to be seen whether subsequent pre-licensure IPE interventions would develop the capacity to meet the higher order outcomes or whether the constraints, for example the immaturity of the student group and the time for interprofessional studies in crowded professional curricula, would render such expectations unrealistic.

The group did conduct a further study (Hammick et al. 2007) applying a higher threshold for inclusion criteria to the same data generating a subsample of 21 studies. These were analysed by precept, process and product (Biggs 1993; Dunkin and Biddle 1974).

Findings confirmed that IPE was generally well received, enabling knowledge and skills necessary for collaborative practice to be learnt.

Cooper and colleagues (2001) had also conducted a systematic review of IPE for undergraduate students in the health professions including qualitative and quantitative paradigms. They found more 'evaluative literature' than 'research data'. Half of 141 studies which they included were from the UK. Thirty (21%) met one or more of the following inclusion criteria:

- Increasing interprofessional understanding and cooperation
- Promoting competent teamwork
- Making effective/efficient use of resources
- Promoting high quality, comprehensive patient care.

Students, Cooper and her colleagues concluded, had benefitted from their interprofessional learning regarding changes in knowledge, skills, attitudes and beliefs.

In the absence of another broader-based review to follow up that by JET, publication of the reports from the two further Cochrane reviews has had the inadvertent effect of reinstating the Cochrane methodology as the one for systematic reviews of IPE and of renewing the belief that progress in securing the evidence base for IPE remains minimal. That is not corroborated by reference to the literature of recent years, notably the quality and quantity of IPE evaluations being published in the *Journal of Interprofessional Care* (<www.informaworld.com/jic>) along with other peer reviewed journals, assisted by the publication of guides to inform the evaluation of IPE (Freeth et al. 2005a, b).

Verification would depend on conducting another broad-based review replicating the methodology devised and tested by JET (Barr et al. 2005). JET has, however, been disbanded. We know of no other group ready to take on the task. Nor does assembling further evidence seem to be high on the agenda for interprofessional activists. Priority is being given instead to the production of reports which drive prospectively the promotion and development of IPE rather than review it retrospectively. We refer, as examples, to the report of the WHO study group (WHO 2010), the Frenk report (Frenk et al., 2011), the Australian review (L-TIPP 2009), the CAIPE guide (Barr and Low 2012) and, not least, the outcome statements cited above (Canadian Interprofessional Health Collaborative 2010; Combined Universities Interprofessional Learning Unit 2010; Interprofessional Education Collaborative 2011). Different though these papers are in form and purpose, they are all grounded in critical reviews of experience by interprofessional researchers and teachers.

In the absence of an inclusive and up-to-date systematic review, we end instead with working assumptions derived from the sources that we have cited, our wider reading, our experience and that of others with whom it is our privilege to work.

Pre-licensure IPE has progressed beyond the stage when it focused on the modification of reciprocal attitudes, the improvement of relationships and the acquisition of shared knowledge. Important though those objectives remain, they have been overtaken by the drive towards competency-based outcomes, which now enjoy currency in the UK and North America and are taking hold more widely. Criteria are being deduced for student assessment though not yet, to our knowledge, for programme evaluation where dated before and after measures of attitudinal change continue to be used extensively (Parsell and Bligh 1999). Time is needed for tools for student assessment and for programme evaluation to catch up with the dramatic progress made in formulating and agreeing outcomes.

Efforts are being redoubled in the leading IPE countries—Australasia, Canada, Japan, the United Kingdom and the United States—to invoke learning technology and to strengthen interprofessional practice learning to meet the outcomes set. These and other developments promise to improve the efficiency and effectiveness of pre-licensure IPE. Constraints can be eased but will remain for reasons that we gave above. Pre-licensure IPE should be regarded as the first stage in interprofessional learning carried forward throughout continuing professional development (Barr 2009).

Nor is that enough: IPE, however assiduously it may be developed, cannot stand alone. Its effectiveness depends (like that of the professional education of which it forms part) upon building it into strategies for service development within a culture of mutual learning and support.

Another broad-based up-to-date systemic review is overdue. A more pressing need, in our view, is to commission an independent, international and comparative evaluation of pre-licensure IPE in a number of locations based on a synthesis of process and outcomes derived by mutual consent from the most authoritative sources.

Conclusions

♦ IPE is extending into more fields of practice encompassing more professions in more countries and employing a widening range of learning methods.

♦ The evidence base being assembled indicates that pre-licensure IPE, when systematically planned and delivered, can modify attitudes and perceptions between professions, and heighten awareness of the need to improve practice through closer collaboration grounded in shared values, commitments and knowledge bases.

♦ Definitions of competency-based outcomes are challenging teachers and students to raise their game beyond aspirations and attitudinal change to generate the collaborative workforce which policy and practice now demands.

♦ Allowance must nevertheless be made for students' capacity for interprofessional development during the formative stages of their professional journeys.

♦ Much depends on creating ongoing interprofessional learning opportunities woven into continuing professional development. That is the next challenge.

References

Allport, G. (1954) *The nature of prejudice* (25th edn) Cambridge MA: Perseus Books Publishing LLC.

Accredited Colleges for Graduate Medical Education (2011) *Common Program Requirements*. Chicago: ACGME

Anderson, E., Cox, D., and Thorpe, L. (2009) Preparation of educators involved in interprofessional education. *J Interprofessional Care.* 23(1): 81–94

Anderson, E., Ford, J., and Thorpe, L. (2011) Learning to listen: Improving students' communication with disabled people. *Med Teach.* 33: 44–52

Anderson, E., Smith, R., and Thorpe, L. (2010) Learning from lives together: medical and social work students' experiences of learning from people with disabilities in the community. *Health and Social Care in the Community.* 18(3): 229–240

Association of American Medical Colleges (2008) *Learn, Serve, Lead.* Washington DC: AAMC

Atkins, J. (1998) Tribalism, loss and grief: issues for multiprofessional education. *J Interprofessional Care.* 12 (3): 303–307

Barr, H. (1998) Competent to collaborate: Towards a competency-based model for interprofessional education. *J Interprofessional Care.* 12(2): 181–188

Barr, H. (2002) *Interprofessional Education: Today, Yesterday and Tomorrow.* London: LTSN Health Sciences and Practice

Barr, H. (2009) An anatomy of continuing interprofessional education. *J Continuing Education in the Health Professions* 29(3): 147–150

Barr, H. (2009) Interprofessional education. In: J. Dent and R. Harden (eds) *A Practical Guide for Medical Teachers.* 3rd edn (pp. 187–192). Edinburgh: Churchill Livingstone

Barr, H. and Brewer, M. (2012) Interprofessional practice based education In: J. Higgs, R. Barnett, S. Billett, M. Hutchings, and F. Trede (eds) Rotterdam: Sense Publishers

Barr, H. and Coyle, J. (2012) Facilitating interprofessional learning. In: S. Loftus et al. (eds) *Educating Health Professionals: Becoming a University Teacher.* Rotterdam: Sense Publishing

Barr, H., Helme, M., and D'Avray, L. (2011) Developing interprofessional education in health and social care courses in the United Kingdom. Paper 12. The Higher Education Academy: Health Sciences and Practice www.health.heacademy.ac.uk

Barr, H., Koppel, I., Reeves, S., Hammick, M., and Freeth, D. (2005) *Effective Interprofessional Education: Argument, Assumption and Evidence.* Oxford: Blackwell with CAIPE

Barr, H. and Low, H. for CAIPE (2012) *Developing interprofessional learning in pre-registration education programmes.* London: CAIPE www.caipe.org.uk

Barrows, H.S. (1996) Problem-based learning in medicine and beyond: A brief overview. In: L. Wilkerson and W. H. Gijselaers (eds) *New Directions for Teaching and Learning.* San Francisco: Jossey-Bass

Bernstein, B. (1971). *Class, Codes and Control.* London: Routledge and Kegan Paul.

Bertalanffy, L. von (1971) *General systems theory.* London: Allen Lane. The Penguin Press

Biggs, J. (1993) From theory to practice: A cognitive systems approach. *Higher Educ Res and Devel.* 12: 73–85

Bion, W. R. (1961) *Experiences in Groups and Other Papers.* London: Tavistock Publications.

Brewer, M. (2011) *Interprofessional Capability Framework.* Perth: Curtin University Faculty of Health Sciences

Brighton and Sussex Medical School (2009). Undergraduate Prospectus 2010.

Bromage, A., Clouder, L., Thistlethwaite, J., and Gordon, F. (2010) *Interprofessional e-learning and Collaborative Work: Practices and technologies.* IGI Global

Brown, R., and Williams, J. (1984). Group identification: the same thing to all people? *Human Relations.* 37: 547–564

Bruner, J. (1966) *Towards a Theory of Instruction.* Harvard: Harvard University Press

CAIPE (2002) Interprofessional education—a definition. www.caipe.org.uk

Canadian Interprofessional Health Collaborative. A national competency framework for interprofessional collaboration. www.cihc.ca/files/CIHC_IPCompetencies_Feb1210.pdf Accessed 18 February 2013

Carpenter, J. (1995) Interprofessional education for medical and nursing students: evaluation of a programme, *Med Educ.* 29(4): 265–272

Carpenter, J. and Hewstone, M. (1996) Shared learning for doctors and social workers: evaluation of a programme. *Br J Social Work.* 26: 239–257

Carrier, J. and Kendall, I. (1995) Professionalism and interprofessionalism in health and community care: Some theoretical issues. In: P. Owens, J.

Carrier and J. Horder (eds) *Interprofessional Issues in Community and Health Care* (pp. 9–36). Basingstoke: MacMillan.

Clark, P. (2006). What would a theory of interprofessional education look like? Some suggestions for developing a theoretical framework for teamwork training. *J Interprofessional Care*. 20: 577–589

Clark, P. (2009) Reflecting on reflection in interprofessional education: Implications for theory and practice. *JInterprofessional Care*. 23(3): 213–223

Colyer, H., Helme, M., and Jones, I. (2005) *The Theory–Practice Relationship in Interprofessional Education*. London: Higher Education Academy: Health Sciences and Practice. http://www.health.heacadamy.ac.uk/publication/occasionalpaper

Combined Universities Interprofessional Learning Unit (2010) *Interprofessional Capability Framework 2010 Mini-Guide*. London: Higher Education Academy Subject Centre for Health Sciences and Practice

Cooper, H., Carlisle, C., Gibbs, T., and Watkins, C. (2001) Developing an evidence based for interdisciplinary learning: A systematic review. *J Adv Nursing*. 26(2): 228–237

Cooperrider, D.L. and Whitney, D. (2005) *Appreciate Inquiry: A Positive Revolution in Change*. San Francisco: Berret-Koehler Publishers

Crisp, N. (2010) *Turning the World Upside Down: The Search for Global Health in the 21st Century*. London: RSM Press

Dahlgren, L. (2009) Interprofessional learning—some remarks from a learning perspective. *J Interprofessional Care*. 23(5): 448–454

D'Avray, L. (2007) Interprofessional learning in practice in South East London. In: H. Barr (ed.) *Piloting Interprofessional Education: Four English Case Studies*. Higher Education Academy: Health Sciences and Practice. Paper 830–42. http://www.health.heacadamy.ac.uk/publication/occasionalpaper

Department of Health (2010) *Healthy Lives, Healthy People: Our Strategy for Public Health in England*. London: HMSO

Dewey, J. (1910) *How we think: a Restatement of the Relation of Reflective Thinking to the Educative Process*. Boston Mass: Heath

Dewey, J. (1938) *Logic: The Theory of Inquiry*. Troy MO: Holt, Rinehart & Winston

Dickinson, C. and Carpenter, J. (2005) Contact is not enough: An inter-group perspective on stereotypes and stereotype change in interprofessional education. In: H. Colyer, M. Helme and I. Jones (eds). *The Theory-Practice Relationship in Interprofessional Education*. (pp. 23–30). London: Higher Education Academy, Health Sciences and Practice. "http://www.health.heacademy.ac.uk"www.health.heacademy.ac.uk/publication/occasionalpaper

Dunkin, M. and Biddle, B. (1974) The study of teaching. New York: Holt Reinhart & Winston

Endoh, K., Magara, A. and Nagai, Y. (eds) (2012) *CIPES-21: End of Project Report*. Niigata: Niigata University of Health and Welfare

Engel, G. (1977), The need for a new medical model: a challenge for biomedicine. *Science*. 196(4286): 129–136

Eraut, M. (1996). *Developing Professional Knowledge and Competence*. London: Falmer Press

Fallsberg, M.B. and Hammer, M. (2000) Strategies and focus at an integrated interprofessional training ward. *J Interprofessional Care*. 14(4): 337–350

Fraser, S.W. and Greenhalgh, T. (2001) Coping with complexity: education for capability. *BMJ*. 323: 799–803

Freeman, S., Wright, A., and Lindqvist, S. (2010) Facilitator training for educators involved in interprofessional learning. *J Interprofessional Care*. 24(4): 375–385

Freeth, D., Hammick, M., Reeves, S., Koppel, I. and Barr, H. (2005a) *Effective Interprofessional Education: Development, Delivery and Evaluation*. Oxford: Blackwell with CAIPE

Freeth, D., Reeves, S., Koppel I., Hammick, M and Barr, H. (2005b) *Evaluating Interprofessional Education: A Self-Help Guide*. London: Higher Education Academy, Health Sciences and Practice www.health.heacademy.ac.uk

Freeth, D., Ayida, G., Berridge, E., Sadler, C., and Strachen, A. (2006) MOSES: Multidisciplinary Obstetric Simulated Emergency Scenarios. *J Interprofessional Care*. 20(5): 552–554

Frenk, J., Chen, L., Bhutta, Z A., et al. (2010) Health professionals for a new century: transforming education to strengthen health systems in an interdependent world. A Global Independent Commission. *The Lancet*. 4 December 377(9773):p.1235.

General Medical Council (2011) *The State of Medical Education and Practice in the UK*. London: GMC

Gray, R. (2009) *The preparation and support required for teachers involved with interprofessional education (IPE)*. University of Brighton: EdD thesis.

Hammick, M., Freeth, D., Reeves, S., and Barr, H. (2007) A Best Evidence Systematic Review Of Interprofessional Education. Dundee: Best Evidence Medical Education Guide no. 9. *Med Teach*. 29: 735–751

Hargreaves, D. (1996) *Teaching as a Research Based Profession: Possibilities and Prospects*. 1996. London: Teacher Training Agency

Heron, J. (1971) *Cooperative Inquiry: Research into the Human Condition*. Unpublished: University of Surrey

Heron, J. and Reason, P. (2008) Extending epistemology in cooperative inquiry. In: P. Reason and H. Bradbury (eds) *Handbook of Action Research*. 2nd edn. London: Sage

Hewstone, B., and Brown, R. (1986). Contact is not enough; an intergroup perspective on the 'contact hypothesis'. In: M. Hewstone and R. Brown (eds) *Contact and Conflict in Intergroup Encounters*. Oxford: Blackwell.

Higgs, J. and Jones, M.A. (2000) Clinical reasoning in health professions. In J. Higgs and M.A. Jones (eds) *Clinical Reasoning in Health Professions* (pp. 3–14). London: Butterworth Heinemann Medical

Hinshelwood, R.D. and Skogstad, W. (eds) (2000) *Observing Organisations: Anxiety, defence and Culture in Health Care*. London: Routledge

Horder, J. (2004) Interprofessional collaboration and interprofessional education. *Br J Gen Pract*. v 54 (501): 243

Howkins, E. and Bray, J. (2008) *Preparing for Interprofessional Teaching: Theory and Practice*. Oxford: Radcliffe Publishing

Interprofessional Education Collaborative Expert Panel (2011) *Core competencies for interprofessional collaborative practice: report of an expert panel*. Washington DC: Interprofessional collaborative

Jacobsen, F., Fink, A.M., Marcussen, V., Larsen, K., and Hansen, T.B. (2009) Interprofessional undergraduate clinical learning: Results from a three year project in a Danish interprofessional training unit. *J Interprofessional Care*. 23: 30–40

Jaques, D. (1994). *Learning in Groups*. London: Kogan Page

Jaques, D. and Higgins, P (1986) *Training for Teamwork: The Report of the Thamesmead Interdisciplinary Project*. Oxford: Oxford Polytechnic

Jarvis, P. (1992) Reflective practice and nursing. *Nurse Education Today*. 12: 174–181

Kinnair, J., Anderson, E., and Thorpe, N. (2012) Development of interprofessional education in mental health practice: Adapting the Leicester Model. *J Interprofessional Care*. 26 (3): 189-197 Early Online: 1–9.

Kirkpatrick, D. L. (1967) Evaluation of training. In: R. Craig and L. Bittel (eds) *Training and Development Handbook* (pp. 87–112). New York: McGraw-Hill

Kolb, D. A. (1984) *Experiential Learning: Experience as the Source of Learning and Development*. New Jersey: Prentice Hall

Lave, J. and Wenger, E. (1991) *Situated Learning: Legitimate Peripheral Participation*. Cambridge. Cambridge University Press

Lennox, A. and Anderson, E. (2007). *The Leicester model of interprofessional education: A practical guide for implementation in health and social care*. Special report 9. Newcastle: Higher Education Academy: Medicine, Dentistry and Veterinary Medicine

Leutz, W. (2009) Partnership working: Key concepts and approaches. In: J. Glasby and H. Dickinson (eds) *International Perspectives on Health and Social Care: Partnership Working in Action* (pp. 42–55). Oxford: Wiley-Blackwell with CAIPE

Loxley, A. (1997) *Collaboration is Health and Social Welfare: Working with Difference*. London: Jessica Kingsley Publishers

L-TIPP (2009) Interprofessional health education in Australia: The way forward. Sydney: Learning and Teaching for Interprofessional Practice, Australia with the University of Sydney, the University of Technology Sydney and the Australian Learning and Teaching Council

Martin, J. (2005). Inter-professional Education reframed by social practice theory. In H. Colyer, M. Helme, and I. Jones (eds) *The Theory–Practice Relationship in Interprofessional Education. Occasional Paper No 7.* London: Higher Education Academy 49–58

McMichael, P. and Gilloran, A. (1984) *Exchanging Views: Courses in Collaboration.* Edinburgh: Moray House College of Education

Meads, G. and Ashcroft, J., with Barr, H., Scott, R., and Wild, A. (2005) *The Case for Interprofessional Collaboration in Health and Social Care.* Oxford: Blackwell with CAIPE

Mezirow, J. (1981) A critical theory of adult learning and education. *Adult Educ.* 32(1): 3–24

Mikkelsen Kyrkjebo, J., Brattebo, G., and Smith-Strom, H. (2006) Improving patient safety by using interprofessional training in health professional education. *J Interprofessional Care.* 20(5): 507–516

Obholzer, A. (1994) Managing social anxieties in public sector organisations. In: A Obolzer and V Zagier Roberts (eds) *The Unconscious at Work: Individual and Organisational Stress in Human Services* (pp. 169–178). London: Routledge

Parsell, G. and Bligh, J. (1999) The development of a questionnaire to assess the readiness of health care students for interprofessional learning (RIPLS). *Med Educ.*33: 95–100

Paterno, E. (2011) *Applicability of Curtin University's interprofessional evaluation tools at the University of the Philippines Manila.* Poster presentation. The Network Towards Unity for Health Annual Conference, Graz, Austria 17–21 September 2011

Plsek, P.E. and Greenhalgh, T. (2001) The challenge of complexity in health care. *BMJ.* 323: 625–628

Ponzer, S., Hylin, U., Kusoffsky, A., et al. (2004) Interprofessional training in the context of clinical practice: goals and students' perceptions on clinical education wards. *Med Educ.* 38: 727–736

Reason, P. (1994) *Participation in Human Inquiry.* London: Sage

Rees, D. and Johnson, R. (2007) All together now? Staff views and experiences of a pre-qualifying interprofessional curriculum. *J Interprofessional Care.* 21(5): 543–555

Reeves, S. and Freeth, D. (2002) The London training ward: An innovative interprofessional learning initiative. *J Interprofessional Care.* 16(1): 41–52

Reeves, S., Lewin, S., Espin, S., and Zwarenstein, M. (2010) *Interprofessional Teamwork for Health and Social Care.* Oxford: Wiley-Blackwell

Reeves, S., Zwarenstein, M., Goldman, J., Barr, H., Freeth, D., Hammick, M., and Koppel, I. (2008) *Interprofessional Education: Effects on Professional Practice and Health Care Outcomes.* Cochrane Database of Systematic Review, Issue 1. Art No: CD002213

Reeves, S., Zwarenstein, M., Goldman, J., Barr, H., Freeth, D., Hammick, M., and Koppel, I. (2010) The effectiveness of professional practice; Key findings from a new systematic review. *J Interprofessional Care.* 24(3): 230–241

Reeves, S., Zwarenstein, M., Goldman, J., Barr, H., Freeth, D., Hammick, M., and Koppel, I. (2011) Interprofessional education: effects on professional practice and health care outcomes. *The Cochrane Database of Systematic Review* 72 (10) 1595–1602

Schön, D. (1983) *The Reflective Practitioner.* New York: Basic Books

Schön, D. (1987) *Educating the Reflective Practitioner: Toward a New Design for Teaching and Learning in the Professions.* San Francisco. Jossey-Bass

Stephenson, A., Higgs, R., and Sugarman, J. (2001). Teaching professional development in medical schools. *The Lancet.* 357: 867–870

Tate, S. (2004) Using critical reflection as a teaching tool. In S. Tate and M. Sills (eds) *The development of critical reflection in the health professions.* London: LTSN Health Sciences and Practice. "http://www.heacademyhealth.ac.uk"www.heacademyhealth.ac.uk/publication/occasionalpaper 8–17

Wackerhausen, S. (2009) Collaboration, professional identity and reflection across boundaries. *J Interprofessional Care.* 23(5): 455–473

Walsh, M. and van Soeren, M. (2012) Interprofessional learning and virtual communities: An opportunity for the future. *J Interprofessional Care.* 26(1): 43–48

Walton, M. (1988) *The Deming Management Method.* New York: Putnam Publishing Group

Wenger, E. (1998) *Communities of Practice: Learning, Meaning and Identity.* Cambridge MA: Cambridge University Press.

WHO (1988) *Learning Together to Work Together for Health.* Geneva: World Health Organization

WHO (2010) *Framework for Action on Interprofessional Education and Collaborative Practice.* Geneva: World Health Organization

Willhelmsson, M., Pelling, S., Ludvigsson, J., Hammar, M., Dahlgren, L.-O., and Faresjo, T. (2009) Twenty years experience of interprofessional education in Linkoping—ground-breaking and sustainable. *J Interprofessional Care.* 23(2): 121–133

Zwarenstein, M., Reeves, S., Barr, H., Hammick, M., Koppel, I., and Atkins, J. (2001) *Interprofessional Education: Effects on Professional Practice and Health Care Outcomes.* (Cochrane Review) http//www2.Cochrane.org/reviews/en/ab000072.html Accessed 18 February 2013

CHAPTER 5

Student choice in the undergraduate curriculum: student-selected components

Simon C. Riley and Michael J. Murphy

> The burden we place on a medical student is far too heavy
> . . . a system of medical education that is actually calculated
> to obstruct the acquisition of sound knowledge and to
> heavily favour the crammer and grinder is a disgrace.
>
> Thomas Huxley
>
> Huxley, T. H. (1876) Lecture delivered at the opening of
> Johns Hopkins University, Baltimore.

Introduction

In December 1993, the Education Committee of the UK General Medical Council (GMC) issued a set of recommendations on undergraduate medical education. The publication of *Tomorrow's Doctors* (GMC 1993) represented an attempt to revitalize undergraduate medical education. The lengthy introduction took a self-consciously historical sweep through the subject, noting previous concerns expressed by the GMC as far back as 1869 about overcrowding of undergraduate curricula, and examining the reasons why exhortations to reform had gone largely unheeded. The authors echoed these concerns, and bemoaned the failure of existing curricula to 'provide components of the course that are truly inspirational, that pertain to the proper function of a university and that are the hallmark of scholarship' (para 11, p. 5, GMC 1993). They saw *Tomorrow's Doctors* as establishing a facilitatory framework, enabling reforms which would aim to equip graduates with 'the capacity and incentive to acquire new knowledge' and, more specifically, with 'the necessary knowledge, skills and attitudes to enable them to enter the pre-registration period of training with confidence and enthusiasm' (para 19, p. 6, GMC 1993).

A key element of this envisaged framework was to be a part of the course:

> which goes beyond the limits of the core, that allows students to study in depth areas of particular interest to them, that provides them with insights into scientific method and the discipline of research, and that engenders an approach to medicine that is constantly questioning and self-critical.
>
> para 24, p. 7, GMC 1993.

The distinction from core may mislead those who have not studied *Tomorrow's Doctors* in detail, insofar as what is 'core' may be perceived as more important, and what is not, as less important. If anything, this part of the curriculum was seen as the principal vehicle for those changes that would express most fully the overarching philosophy of promoting a substantially new approach and perspective to undergraduate learning. Specifically, the provision of opportunities for students to express their individuality and to explore areas of particular interest to them was seen as a crucial way to harness their engagement with the process of reform. Existing opportunities for students to express choice, such as intercalated degree courses and electives, were seen as insufficient on their own to provide the degree of student choice envisaged, which should be 'a thread running throughout the course rather than confined to a discrete period'. (para 29, p. 9, GMC 1993). In any case, in many medical schools intercalated degrees are undertaken by a small proportion of students. For more extensive student choice to become a reality, student-chosen modules would have to be embedded throughout the entire curriculum. The term used initially for these was 'special study modules'. This was replaced in the next edition of *Tomorrow's Doctors* (GMC 2003) by the term that remains in use today: student-selected components (SSCs).

Definition and characteristics of student-selected components

SSCs have been defined as follows:

> Student-Selected Components (SSCs) are an integral part of the undergraduate medical curriculum contributing to the overall curricular learning outcomes and providing students with choice in studying, in depth, areas of particular interest. The principal learning outcome is the progressive development of skills in research, critical

appraisal, and synthesis of evidence for maintaining good medical practice. SSCs contribute to the development of a broad range of personal and professional skills, such as team-working, communication, time and resource management and self-directed learning. They also provide opportunities to explore career options

The Scottish Doctor 2007; Riley et al. 2008.

The quintessential feature of a SSC is the exercise of at least some degree of student choice. Many of the 'special study modules' envisaged by the original *Tomorrow's Doctors* are indeed modular, but the replacement of the term was a de facto acknowledgment that many SSCs are instead longitudinal elements in the curriculum performed in parallel with other curricular tasks. Many medical schools use both formats throughout the curriculum.

Although SSCs vary in time and size, most are comparatively small, and many of their perceived benefits relate to this. Exposure to working individually or in small groups facilitates acquisition of generic skills in, for example, self-directed learning and teamwork. Moreover, the provision of detailed staff feedback on the performance of individual students allows the true formative value of these curriculum components to be realized.

In some medical schools, students are permitted, within defined curricular boundaries, to design their own SSCs, with the advice and support of staff, providing the fullest possible expression of student choice. Much more frequently, students are presented with a 'menu' of staff-designed options from which to choose. Even when students are allocated to their preferred choice, student input into the design and purpose of staff-designed modules is much more limited, or even minimal. Furthermore, it is not always possible to allocate students to their preferred modules, for which reason they are often asked to rank their preferences. Thus the student experience of choice is not uniform, rather it is a spectrum. At one extreme of the spectrum are SSCs designed by the students themselves, while at the other are allocated SSCs in which they have expressed varying levels of interest (and potentially minimal interest). Medical schools have to strive to ensure that there are few, if any, in the latter category, recognizing the need to do so if student choice is to be meaningful. Such varied student experience may help to explain the mixed student view of SSCs, which ranges from supportive (Bidwai 2000; Mohammed 2001; Cross 2003; QABME reports, GMC) to critical (Payne et al. 2000; Leung 2002; QABME reports, GMC).

Implementation of student-selected components

Since 1993, schools throughout the United Kingdom have implemented the reforms in undergraduate medical education in various ways. There is a limited literature and no systematic overview of this process, either in general or specifically as it pertains to SSCs. However, the GMC has, under the auspices of its Quality Assurance of Basic Medical Education (QABME) framework, inspected every medical school at least once, and in most cases more than once. The reports of these inspections collectively hold a mirror up to the reforms as they have been implemented in practice. Along with the second and third editions of *Tomorrow's Doctors* (GMC 2003, 2009), they also provide the basis for evaluating the GMC's own view of, and response to, the implementation of the reforms.

What can be gleaned from these documents about the realization of the vision of SSCs articulated in the original *Tomorrow's Doctors*? The clearest message to emerge from the reports is that many schools have encountered substantial difficulties in trying to ensure that genuine choice is available to all students throughout the entire undergraduate curriculum (Christopher et al. 2002; QABME reports, GMC). This should not be surprising, given the scale of the task, either for existing medical schools struggling to radically overhaul their historically over-burdened curricula, or for new schools trying to establish entire curricula de novo (another key development in the UK since 1993 has been the creation of a tranche of new medical schools, often based over two or more geographically distinct teaching bases). It is reflected in repeated exhortations in GMC QABME reports to increase the range of SSCs, and the time to be devoted to them, as well as concerns relating to the percentage of students receiving their preferred (i.e. first-choice) allocations. Over-reliance on particular modes of delivery, for instance library- or classroom-based SSCs, difficulties in engaging particular groups of teaching staff, 'badging' of curriculum elements as student-selected where student choice is in reality severely constrained, all likewise attest to the practical barriers that must be overcome if genuine student choice is to be provided.

Ensuring consistency of assessment of SSCs is another recurring concern. SSCs were conceived from the outset as a broad range of educational opportunities that would inevitably reflect 'the interests, resources and individual enthusiasms of medical school staff and … the wider range of opportunities within their universities' (GMC, 1993). It was therefore entirely predictable that the implementation of heterogeneous programmes, assessed by staff of varying backgrounds and experience, would be associated with the twin coexisting problems of comparing modules that vary in educational aims and content, and in the standards applied to assessment. Generic assessment criteria represent an attempt to deal with the former, although standardisation and reliability of assessment is harder to address, and is discussed in detail later.

Finally, confusion over what is core and what is non-core, or perhaps more specifically, how core learning outcomes may be or should be delivered, has characterized some programmes of SSCs (QABME reports, GMC). The core is 'a distillate of essential knowledge and skills from all fields of medicine' (GMC 1993, para 30, p. 10), the satisfactory completion of which is mandatory for all. Clearly SSCs build on this 'distillate', reinforcing core learning outcomes. Nevertheless, with depth of knowledge and insight now recognised in the latest version of *Tomorrow's Doctors* (2009) as important generic educational outcomes, these can clearly be achieved with good curriculum design and largely irrespective of the topic or field of study (fig. 5.1). However, there must be a clear distinction between the educational remit of those parts of the curriculum completed by every student, and those completed only by some, and the purpose of SSCs—so that these core learning outcomes are achieved by all students (Murdoch-Eaton et al. 2004; Riley et al. 2009).

In the 2003 and 2009 editions of *Tomorrow's Doctors*, the GMC has progressively reduced the amount of curriculum time that must be devoted to SSCs. Currently, it stands at more than 10%, compared with one third as originally stated in the 1993 version. This represents a substantial slimming-down of the student-selected 'thread'. In effect it acknowledges the scale of the difficulty in establishing programmes of modules as extensive as originally envisaged, and that perhaps the balance between core and choice components needed to be modified. It also presumably represents an attempt to replace quantity with quality, replacing a thicker 'thread' in which genuine student choice was compromised with a

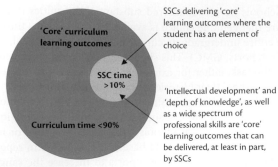

Figure 5.1 Full integration of learning outcomes into core and SSC timetable

thinner one in which it achieves fuller expression. However, given the primacy of the student-selected part of the curriculum in delivering the desired radical 're-booting' of undergraduate medical education, it remains to be seen if this scaling-back will achieve its intended effect.

A global perspective on student choice in undergraduate medical education

Other countries have also recognized the need for medical curricula reform (Christakis 1995), although they have not embraced student choice (and specifically SSCs as a curriculum theme) as enthusiastically as the UK. Governance, accreditation, and organizational issues relating to the regulation of undergraduate medical education may act as barriers to the practical implementation of student choice. These and other differences have been highlighted by the Bologna and Tuning processes to align tertiary education, including medical education, across Europe (Cumming 2010). For example, some countries consider that the acquisition of research competencies should be reserved for postgraduate training. In others, including the UK, research skills are seen as sufficiently important that they should be inculcated at undergraduate level, where they are commonly taught in SSCs. As a result of failure to reach a clear consensus about this, research has not been fully adopted as a standard competency or requirement within curriculum design in the pan-European Tuning process. Nevertheless, the Medical Education in Europe network (MEDINE2 2013) has shown that the establishment of evidence-based medicine is influencing the acceptance of developing broader research skills throughout European medical curricula.

Alternatively, the advantages of providing student choice within the curriculum may simply not be perceived to be sufficiently well-established to justify the considerable organizational change involved (Davis and Harden 2003). Other contributory factors include the absence of an evidence base, lack of resources (Ali and Baig 2012), or cultural issues (Bleakley et al. 2008) which establish delays, while British medical schools are used as a proving ground for student choice.

More widely, student choice is seen as a vehicle for delivering the 'global minimum essential requirements' for a physician (Schwarz and Wojtczak 2002), including critical thinking and research, professional values, attitudes, behaviour and ethics, communication skills, management of information, the scientific foundation of medicine, population health and health systems, and clinical skills.

The international recognition of basic medical education (World Federation for Medical Education) includes acceptance that student choice has a role to play in medical curricula (WFME 2003; WHO-WFME 2005; Karle 2006, 2008). It is a consideration also in training doctors for the transformational change of healthcare delivery in low and middle income countries (Celletti et al. 2011).

Existing models of student choice in medical curricula

Prior to 1993, student choice in British medical schools existed largely, although not exclusively, in two distinct forms. First, student electives were undertaken by most if not all students, typically at the end of their penultimate year or embedded in their final year before graduation. These were often in far-flung geographical locations, and the learning experience could be inconsistent. Second, intercalated science degrees were undertaken by varying proportions of students approximately half-way through the undergraduate curriculum, with selection usually dependent upon prior academic performance. *Tomorrow's Doctors* (GMC 2009) acknowledged these and supported their continuation as vehicles for the expression of student choice, and in the case of intercalated degrees, excellent opportunities to explore areas of particular interest. Nevertheless, they were viewed as insufficient on their own to adequately and consistently deliver to all students the concepts underlying the student-selected choice part of the curriculum. Each of these historical models of student choice has continued alongside the reforms of the last couple of decades, and will be discussed in more detail later.

SSCs: the wider context

Curriculum design has, in many contemporary schools, moved beyond the long-standing Flexner preclinical/clinical model (Cooke et al. 2006). In particular, students gain clinical experience and training at a much earlier stage than previously. The challenges posed by this restructuring of the undergraduate curriculum mean that it is important to determine, define, map, and blueprint what students should achieve, as well as how and when, and to implement the appropriate assessments to ensure this (Harden 2001; Robley et al. 2005; Willett 2008). The UK GMC describes the curriculum in terms of a core set of learning outcomes and competencies (GMC 2009), and the implementation of SSCs has occurred in the context of this framework. The sections of this chapter which address the practical implementation of SSCs will therefore focus on this curriculum model. The reader should be aware however that there is a wider debate about competency-based medical education (Lurie 2012), and curricula defined by learning outcomes (Harden 2007; Frank et al. 2010), although this debate is beyond the scope of this chapter.

Learning outcomes and competencies: the role of SSCs

An important question is: how can SSCs deliver learning outcomes and competencies? All learning outcome frameworks include competencies (e.g. how to investigate and manage a patient), generic skills (e.g. information retrieval), and professional attributes (e.g.

ability to reflect). The most widely used framework currently is the one provided in the 2009 edition of *Tomorrow's Doctors*. Many learning outcomes and competencies are generic, and can be delivered in virtually any clinical or medical environment. Selected examples are shown in box 5.1.

Delivery of SSCs: curriculum issues

Significant issues that arise when considering how to develop and deliver SSCs into a curriculum include:

◆ Curriculum mapping: Detailed mapping of competencies and learning outcomes is required if SSCs are to be integrated into the curriculum, in order to ensure that all students broadly achieve the same learning outcomes at the same time. In addition, these must be identified and defined in a form which students can decode and respond to (Murdoch-Eaton and Whittle 2012). Certainly in the UK, the GMC requires SSCs to be fully integrated into the curriculum, which includes assessment, although there remains a tension about whether students learn what is expected (Hafferty 1998; Murphy et al. 2008).

◆ Assessment: Assessment of student acquisition of learning outcomes and competencies must be appropriate and robust. Competencies can be viewed as assessable key tasks, which have been well defined by Stark et al. (2005). Opportunities have arisen with more recent development and increased acceptance of new assessments in medical education, highlighting work-based and professionalism methodologies.

Box 5.1 Generic learning outcomes and competencies

◆ Clinical skills: Generic competencies, relating to for instance prescribing or patient safety, can be delivered across a wide range of specialties. Others may be specialty-specific.

◆ Communication skills: These can be delivered in a host of ways, including student–tutor interaction, case report, poster of project, project report, formal or semi-formal oral presentation, patient communication from developing an information leaflet.

◆ Team-working skills: These may encompass work within a peer group, or with multiprofessional colleagues.

◆ Critical appraisal skills: A grounding in evidence-based medicine equips students to evaluate the medical literature in a broad sense—including clinical guidelines, protocols, meta-analyses, and clinical audits.

◆ A more in-depth understanding of a chosen field of core medicine, or of a specialist field of medicine that may potentially be regarded as a postgraduate specialism beyond the core curriculum.

◆ An awareness of issues pertaining to medical ethics and governance, cultural competencies and social accountability.

◆ Professional awareness and enhancement, including developing a maturity to learning and effective reflective skills, together with career exploration.

◆ Prior learning: This has a major effect on how a student interacts with a series of tasks and skills of increasing complexity. A student's learning has to be sequential and ordered for competencies to be successfully and fully achieved. For instance, students performing a medical literature review on a topic early in their studies can build on these skills later, and would be unlikely to achieve a much more complex integrated task, for example performing a systematic review, without an initial, perhaps naïve skill base. In a wider context, students on a graduate programme can respond differently to undergraduates (Shehmar et al. 2010).

◆ Provision of choice: We have already alluded to the fact that genuine choice varies within and between schools. In most medical schools, provision of the teaching capacity required to ensure genuine student choice is a perennial problem for curriculum planners (Payne et al. 2000). One approach to this is to deal with the problem at the level of the individual student. For example, allocations can be coordinated longitudinally to ensure that a student who fares badly one year receives their preferred allocation in a subsequent year. A more convincing way of addressing this problem is to allow students to design their own modules ('self-propose'). Giving students autonomy at an early stage in the curriculum represents an important learning outcome in itself (Murphy et al. 2009a).

◆ Breadth versus depth: Students vary in the clarity and focus of their choices. Some are single-minded and will, if permitted, choose modules and projects in the same specialty or field. This allows them to acquire increasing depth of experience and may provide the basis for pursuing a career in the specialty. In many ways this is in tune with GMC advice. Portfolio considerations provide a counter-balancing tension—should students be required to gain experience across a range of specialties in order to ensure a broader base of experience? Furthermore, less confident or motivated, or weaker students may want to stay within their comfort zone or perform projects they perceive as easier. In whatever circumstances, students need good advice and then need to act upon it.

◆ Creating real opportunities and challenges: The implementation of outcome- and competency-based curricula has been associated with a perceived loss of 'scholarship'—opportunities for students to be ambitious, experimental or to undertake otherwise challenging tasks. Students may acquire competencies in a 'tick-box' manner that is inimical to genuine immersion in a field or topic. SSCs provide ideal vehicles to counteract this. Indeed, this was their explicit purpose as articulated in the original *Tomorrow's Doctors* (GMC 1993). In the event that the project is comparatively unsuccessful, learning outcomes can and should be defined as skills and competencies (and aligned with the assessment scheme) so that the student is not unfairly penalized. Indeed, students can gain as much, or more, from the need to address problems, as long as they receive effective supervision and formative feedback, and assessment is focused on the educational process and student development.

◆ Learner-centred versus teacher-centred curriculum: This is a tension in modern curriculum design (Ludmerer 2004; McLean and Gibbs 2010). By enabling active experiential engagement with their learning, SSCs provide an opportunity for students to become the focus of the teaching experience and to gain autonomy (Graffam 2007), rather than being passive passengers in a traditional content-based curriculum. This applies across SSCs and especially to modules self-proposed by students. Through the process of developing generic skills in SSCs, students are initiated as lifelong learners to ensure their continued professional development throughout their careers (Murdoch-Eaton and Whittle 2012).

• Curriculum change: Making profound changes to medical curricula, with SSCs being one of the more contentious issues, should be recognized as an enormous challenge. To be successful they require careful planning and management, and commitment from both faculty and students (Lowry 1992; Bland et al. 2000), but the rewards are enormous (Hirsch et al. 2007).

Different types of SSCs

This section describes a range of different types of SSCs that have been developed by different schools, together with the specific literature associated with them. Two of the most widely used models will be covered in detail—clinical attachments and research projects.

Clinical attachment

The clinical attachment is a near-universal model for delivering clinical training. As a result there is a danger that this type of SSC can be delivered, and experienced by the student, in a way that is no different from a non-student-selected attachment. Clinical attachment SSCs should offer more time to undertake greater depth of study beyond core, either in a topic or area that is core, or that has limited or no coverage in the core curriculum. Alternatively, students may choose to spend time gaining experience in specialties that lack clear exposure within the curriculum, although they permeate a wide spectrum of medicine. These may include laboratory-based disciplines like pathology and histopathology, clinical biochemistry and microbiology, or radiology. Other specialties may have a similarly limited profile in undergraduate teaching, for instance dermatology, medical genetics, occupational medicine (Fletcher and Agius 1995), ophthalmology, otolaryngology (Newbegin et al. 2007), plastic surgery, psychiatry, and forensic science.

SSCs of this kind permit the attainment of more specialized clinical skills, or involvement in the care of patients with more complex problems, and can involve performing some type of case report, or a small audit project. Students also get an opportunity for career exploration and their supervisor may subsequently become a personal referee, or future senior colleague. In this environment, assessments can be more wide-ranging, testing depth of knowledge and clinical skills, but also appraising a broader range of professional skills using multisource feedback and reflective appraisals. In this regard, these types of SSC are popular (Vieira et al. 2004) and motivation would be expected to be greater in a student who has chosen their module and field of study.

Performing a research project

This type of project work may encompass clinical audit, clinical research, laboratory-based research, review of the literature, perhaps even a systematic review, with a meta-analysis potentially feasible with appropriate support. The definition of 'research' is taken here in its broadest sense, and not as a narrow view of a hypothesis-led study design for the acquisition of new findings. In most medical schools there are many opportunities to perform different types of projects, on different topics, whether in groups or as individuals. The SSC may be an in-depth clinical experience combined with a project in a specialty, and this model allows students to attain a broad range of research and professional skills (McLean and Howarth 2008; Murdoch-Eaton et al. 2010). It is important that the project is carefully designed; is feasible in what will be a relatively short timeframe; and is adequately resourced. Students also need support from their tutor and potentially from a wider team (Riley et al. 2008; Riley 2009).

This kind of teaching–research nexus provides an ideal educational environment. Allowing students to develop research skills and awareness at such an early stage in their careers has long-term benefits (Jenkins et al. 2007; Laidlaw et al. 2009). Students gain critical appraisal skills and applied insight into evidence-based medicine, often viewing the literature through the prism of analysis of their own data. This learning experience and the project output can be optimized if the student is well integrated into the academic community for the particular specialty (MacDougall and Riley 2010). Students with this kind of experience are then in a position to apply these skills as doctors throughout their careers (Dyrbye et al. 2007; West et al. 2011).

Assessment of research-type SSCs raises a range of issues (Riley et al. 2008, 2010). Research projects are often reliant upon a wider team in the ward, clinic or laboratory. Students may be working alongside or following on from others in their project—perhaps to collect a more substantial dataset or following up on an earlier study. A full acknowledgement of materials and existing datasets and particularly of contributions from other members of the team is essential, and may become a learning outcome in itself, by allowing the student's own contribution to be established, as well as their ability to work in a team. In addition, a project may start out as a good idea, and be well planned, but (particularly for more speculative or challenging projects), can rapidly plunge into difficulty. Often in such circumstances the student is not at fault.

In these types of SSC, faculty have a good opportunity to get to know the students well, potentially much better than in short, core modules. The value of this faculty insight into individual students should be recognized, and assessment of performance and professionalism using a range of methods including workplace assessments and multisource feedback may be appropriate to build into assignments. The assessments should have a degree of flexibility and focus more on gaining skills in the research process, to be able to compensate for the sometimes lack of results.

Through this type of project, students can also explore the spectrum of academic and clinical research paths for their future careers (Ahn et al. 2007; Dyrbye et al. 2007; Fancher et al. 2009; Kanna et al. 2006; Laskowitz et al. 2010). There are concerns that have been expressed worldwide regarding recruitment and development of the next generation of academic faculty (Schor et al. 2005; Collins et al. 2010; Funston and Young 2012). This format of SSC provides students with essential elements for the exploration of academic medicine. It allows a choice of field and topic across the spectrum of clinical and laboratory research; an opportunity to perform a project and develop research skills; and perhaps most importantly develops insight and even establishes professional relationships and mentors within the particular sphere of academic interest. Some student research projects are published in peer-reviewed scientific journals (Dyrbye et al. 2008; Griffin and Hindocha 2011; van Eyk et al. 2010), which will further develop student's enthusiasm for and insight into research and academic medicine, as well as benefiting their curriculum vitae (Riley 2009).

Other types of SSC associated with specific competencies

Selected examples of other types of SSC are listed in table 5.1, according to the skills or knowledge acquired.

Wider opportunities

Tomorrow's Doctors (GMC 1993) suggested that substantial amounts of time might be spent on topics outside medicine. Although opportunities to study such topics are widely available (Murdoch-Eaton and Jolly 2000; QABME reports, GMC), the time actually dedicated to them is usually limited in any given curriculum. These topics can be outside the conventional core of medicine, and in some cases may be unrelated to medicine. SSCs in complementary and alternative medicine, acupuncture, Chinese medicine, spirituality and medicine (Neely and Minford 2008; Bell et al. 2010), sports medicine, healthcare for the homeless, the history of medicine (Metcalfe and Brown 2011), museum object handling as a patient enrichment activity (Chatterjee and Noble 2009), or literature pertaining to medicine (Charon et al. 1995) have all been delivered (QABME reports, GMC).

Other SSCs are medical in the most tangential way. Many institutions run SSCs in humanities (Hodgson and Smart 1998), languages, literature (Charon et al. 1995; Kuper, 2006), creative writing (Thomas 2006), arts (Lazarus and Rosslyn, 2003), journalism (Gibson, 2006), and performing arts (GMC QABME reports). These modules allow students to develop core professional skills, engage with a wider academic community or social group, as well as to take a break to reflect, reassess and re-motivate themselves in an intense medical curriculum and timetable. This is an important and explicit recognition that maintaining or developing other interests and an appropriate professional work-life balance is essential to prevent burn-out.

Electives

Medical student electives represent a model of student choice that shares characteristics with SSCs, but that is nevertheless distinct. As the term elective indicates, they offer substantial student ownership over the educational content of the module, the setting and location. They provide excellent opportunities for self-directed and opportunistic learning. They are often considered formally to be part of the student-selected strand of the curriculum, or, if not, they fall under the same administrative aegis. However, there are several important differences. Some of these relate to the historical timing of electives immediately prior to or during the final year. First, by this point in their undergraduate training, students should have acquired many of the practical and other skills they will require as doctors. Some of the terminologies applied to these modules (e.g. clerkships or externships) are telling, indicating as they do the responsibility placed on students (although, crucially, not the degree of responsibility). Second, many students undertake placements overseas, and the choice of geographic location is influenced not only by professional considerations. This has led to the coining of the term 'medical tourism', as part of a sharper focus on the ethical issues surrounding students undertaking electives abroad (Dowell and Merrylees 2009). Issues raised include the potential harm incurred by visiting students undertaking roles that exceed their capabilities, as well as the failure of elective modules to address the needs of the host local communities in a sustainable way (Murdoch-Eaton and Green 2011; Petrosoniak et al. 2010; Shah and Wu 2008). Third, the educational content of many of these modules is poorly defined, although, the 2009 edition of *Tomorrow's Doctors* requires SSC learning outcomes to be mapped to curricula.

The model for student electives described above is shifting, partly in response to wider changes in undergraduate medical training. Increasingly, students undertake additional elective summer placements earlier in their training, when their clinical experience will be more limited. Some students undertake these electives with an explicit career agenda, for instance to seek future employment as a resident (Mueller et al. 2010). Many schools are taking more care to ensure that students are thoroughly prepared for proposed elective placements, especially from educational, ethical (Shah and Wu 2008, Elit et al. 2011), pastoral, personal safety and health standpoints (Sharafeldin et al. 2010). Balandin et al (2007) offer anecdotal evidence that short attachments are useful. As a specific example, in student clinical exchanges between Japan and England, professionalism and cultural competency developed through reflection

Table 5.1 Other types of SSC associated with specific competencies

Teaching skills	Students may gain experience teaching their peers or near-peers (Ross and Cameron 2007), for instance their classmates. Alternatively, this may be as some sort of outreach into the wider community, for instance in primary (Brown 2005) and secondary schools (Furmedge 2008; GMC QABME Reports). This may take the form of delivering information on a medical or health topic or providing a service, including community health or sex education (Jobanputra et al. 1999), which exposes students to challenging environments (Faulder et al. 2004). These initiatives also give school pupils insight into tertiary education in general, and health-related disciplines in particular.
Medical ethics	Ethical principles can be learned by their application to a topic of interest to the student, linked in with faculty who can explore a range of scenarios and quandaries (Mills and Bryden 2010). Such modules are favoured by North American schools (Charon et al. 1995; Charon 2001).
Social accountability	From a more local or specific view that may incorporate multicultural aspects of medicine and disabilities (GMC QABME Reports) through to a global view of health issues, social accountability is important in translating educational outcomes to promote transformative change and to begin to address some of the crises in delivering healthcare (GCSA; RCP 2005; Murdoch-Eaton et al. 2011)

(Nishigori et al. 2009). International partnerships may be an effective approach that helps to ensure that travelling students are well prepared and that both participating institutions are clearly aware of expectations and requirements (Balandin et al. 2007), although this does impact on freedom of choice.

Intercalated degrees

The role of intercalated degrees in enhancing 'the intellectual development of the student by studying in depth a subject of their choice' is undeniable (GMC 1993). Possession of an intercalated degree enhances career prospects. In the UK, science degrees are formally recognized in scoring schemes for medical recruitment, and are perceived as being particularly important for academic track training posts. However, not every student on a programme undertakes an intercalated degree. Hence, generic skills learning outcomes will not be achieved by all. Although the teaching capacity of host (science) departments has historically limited medical student numbers, globalization of third-level education has ensured that many departments and institutions are adapting rapidly to meet increasing demand.

There are good reasons to welcome the expansion in numbers undertaking these degrees and in the range of subjects which may be studied. These include the acquisition of a wide range of professional competencies that are key to understanding, handling and effectively utilising both generic and specific skills and knowledge in the increasingly complex clinical workplace. Students with an intercalated degree perform better in subsequent assessments. However, the effects are slight (Howman and Jones 2011; Mahesan et al 2011), and indeed graduate entry students perform similarly to direct entry students (Shehmar et al. 2010). An intercalated degree also gives insight into the opportunities presented by research and academic medicine (Hunter et al. 2007; Collins et al. 2010).

SSCs: practical aspects

There is a range of pragmatic issues that must be covered by a faculty SSC course or programme lead. All require planning and careful management (fig. 5.2) and some of these are detailed next.

Advice to students

It is important to ensure that students receive appropriate and timely advice to enable them to make the most of what are usually limited SSC opportunities within the curriculum (Riley et al. 2009). They need guidance on how to engage fully and strategically with the opportunities provided. Making the most appropriate choice is obviously important, and should encompass professional and personal strategic aims, but it can be difficult for students to look further than short-term aims, to see the benefits of SSCs in developing their educational and professional skills in the longer term (Richardson 2009). At the time that students are making choices, they should also be advised on the importance of proper preparation and planning. Tasks may include participating in preparatory meetings with faculty, revisiting prior learning, reading preliminary material, gaining ethical approval, developing and piloting a questionnaire, or requesting notes from medical records (Riley et al. 2008, 2009). Students need to be made aware that much more self-directed learning is expected during SSCs, and that they will be expected to take the initiative in trying to solve problems themselves, but also knowing when to seek help.

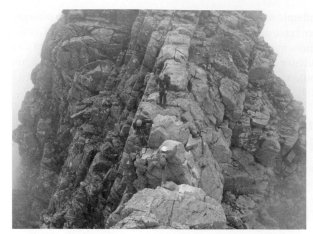

Figure 5.2 SSCs, like this activity, require planning, careful management, development of an appropriate set of skills, a good team—and commitment
Reproduced with permission from Grahame Nicoll.

Student support

Faculty tutors should be approachable and should set clear limits on their student's autonomy. They have an important role as mentors and role models (Cruess et al. 2008). SSC programme information should be readily accessible and detailed, as SSC students are likely to be spread across multiple sites, and working to different timetables. Virtual learning environments (VLEs) represent a major advance in effective programme delivery (Ellaway and Masters 2008; Masters and Ellaway 2008; McGee and Kanter 2011). SSCs are often used as pioneering vehicles to advance the utility of medical education technology. The VLE may deliver course materials including online lectures, workbooks or resources, or online workspaces such as blogs and wikis (Sandars 2006).

Administrative and financial support

SSC programmes are administratively complex and require administrative support, as well as help to develop the VLE, portfolio, feedback and assessment tools. Infrastructure support and advice must also be available for:

+ literature searches
+ ethical and governance problems (Robinson et al. 2007)
+ database management
+ applied medical statistics (MacDougall 2008).

UK medical schools have developed different strategies to address financial and cost issues (GMC QABME reports). Costs may be for faculty time or for recruitment of facilitators. Research project costs can also be substantial and may rely on students being supported by existing research grant funding, or students and faculty applying for additional funding (Barroso and Sebastiao 2012). One imaginative student-centred solution has been for each SSC to have a tariff based on real costs. Students are provided with their own fixed SSC budget. The choices they make then have to be balanced against their personal budget, which they have to manage through the duration of their programme (GMC QABME reports).

Staff engagement

With increasing demands upon time, and more detailed clinical contracts, recruitment and retention of staff as tutors, facilitators, supervisors and teachers is a challenge. A clear strategy needs to be established to ensure sufficient tutors are available for effective course delivery that is sustainable in the long term (McLean and Van Wyk 2006; Riley et al. 2008). There are encouraging signs that in many schools, recruitment of motivated and enthusiastic faculty for SSCs is satisfactory (GMC QABME reports). SSCs deliver medical teaching in a way that offers a different experience that is interesting and rewarding (Dahlstrom et al. 2005). Students who have chosen the specialty are more motivated and keen to impress a potential future mentor. The dynamic is therefore different from teaching on a core rotation, where student numbers are greater and their motivation is variable, the teaching is repetitive and it is be difficult to get to know the students as individuals.

Excellent communication between the SSC programme faculty and administrators, and individual faculty course leaders, supervisors and tutors is essential. Faculty engagement with the VLE is vital in enabling this.

Assessment of SSCs

We have already highlighted the two perennial difficulties posed by assessment of SSCs: comparing modules that vary in educational aims and content, and ensuring consistency in the standards applied to assessment. It should perhaps be stated at the outset that, short of standard-setting the assessment of individual modules across a programme of SSCs, it is impossible to achieve the same level of consistency that is expected in other summative assessments. It is possible to identify 'hawks' and 'doves' within programmes of SSCs—assessors that consistently award grades that differ significantly from the average (Murphy et al. 2009a)—although there are methodological issues that limit the application of this kind of analysis. Interestingly, the study by Murphy et al. (2009) showed it was possible to influence the marking behaviour of assessors—but not in the intended way. Feedback letters were sent to assessors, comparing the grades they awarded with the average grades awarded in the entire SSC programme, in the hope that, if there were 'hawks' and 'doves' among the outliers, they might thus be influenced to apply a different standard of assessment, closer to the average). In the event, the grades awarded across the entire programme were higher after the introduction of feedback letters. The most commonly used approach to improve reliability has been to moderate assessments by a second marker, either within the same department as the first marker, or centrally by a member of the teaching organization. This approach has been used to balance out a 'halo' effect in the marking behaviour of supervisors assessing both students and project work that they have supervised (MacDougall et al. 2008).

The GMC, in its supplement on Assessment in Undergraduate Medical Education (GMC 2011) acknowledges the particular difficulties posed by SSCs. It provides some guidance on, for example, the provision of clear marking criteria for presentation, analysis of findings, formulation of hypotheses and the outcomes of tested hypotheses. Its advice on second marking also implicitly acknowledges the issues surrounding halo and leniency effects, as noted above.

Developments in SSC assessment

The assessable key tasks in SSCs have been described (Stark et al. 2005), although these should not be taken as fully inclusive. Since their publication there has been an increased diversity in types of SSCs that students perform, together with major developments in methods to assess professionalism (Hilton and Southgate 2007; Parker 2006; Cruess and Cruess 2006, 2008) and performance (Pulito et al. 2007), together with improvements to optimize the effectiveness of assessment in context (West and Shanafelt 2007). It is important to continue to look beyond medical education for these developments. The following methodologies have been utilised in the SSC domain to assess generic professional skills and competencies:

◆ Learning portfolios: These are important in the postgraduate domain (Hrisos et al. 2008), and for continuing professional development; training in their use at an undergraduate level is important (van Tartwijk and Driessen 2009). Students need to recognize the value of their portfolio and its management (Davis et al. 2009).

◆ Reflection, responding to feedback and self-assessment: The ability to respond appropriately to feedback is an essential skill (Hounsell et al. 2008). Feedback needs to be clearly defined, and then delivered appropriately by faculty (Nicol and McFarlane-Dick 2006; Van de Ridder et al. 2008). The ability to reflect is an important skill to develop in the transition to becoming a professional (Korszun et al. 2006; Stern and Papadakis 2006), although evidence for the effectiveness of reflection is limited (Colthart et al. 2008).

◆ Workplace and multisource feedback and assessment: These methodologies can be used effectively in SSCs (Davies et al. 2008; Rees and Shepherd 2005), particularly when used longitudinally throughout the programme (Violato et al. 2008).

◆ Peer feedback: Giving and receiving feedback is an important professional skill that can be developed through peer feedback in SSCs (Cottrell et al. 2006; Dannefer et al. 2005). Issues that should be considered in the implementation of peer feedback include: whether it is used in a formative or summative way; whether it is presented anonymously or by named peers; and what to do when major problems come to light. Students usually require high levels of support, certainly in early years (Schonrock-Adema et al. 2007).

Plagiarism

Most work submitted by students is provided electronically. Use of software to detect duplication—and possible plagiarism—has become widespread in recent years. Plagiarism is considered a problem across the entire higher education sector, and different institutions deal with it in different ways. In 2004 Baroness Deech, the Independent Adjudicator for Higher Education, highlighted the level of inconsistency in the application of penalties for student plagiarism (OIAHE 2004). This prompted the Benchmark Plagiarism Tariff to examine the penalties applied for student plagiarism in higher education (Tennant and Rowell 2009), and confirmed wide variation in the penalties applied. While it is feasible to give students controlled access to the software (Whittle and Murdoch-Eaton 2008), this is controversial, with concerns that students might manipulate their writing in order to reduce similarity indices. Student work that is flagged up by the software must undergo a preliminary screen—making judgements about poor scholarship and plagiarism solely on such indices is inappropriate. There needs to be a clear process to establish whether and to what extent plagiarism has occurred, and how to deal with it, at an institutional level. Plagiarism seems to be infrequent (Riley et al. 2010), although when detected, it often raises deeper underlying problems with individual students, which then need to be considered and addressed. Plagiarism also represents a spectrum of academic misconduct that exhibits significant cultural differences worldwide. For example, in some cultures, extensive quotation of colleagues is perceived as being complimentary rather than intellectually lazy. It is important to educate students about plagiarism, particularly international students entering into a new academic environment.

SSC assessment: final thoughts

Much of the focus above and elsewhere has been on the summative assessment of SSCs. Whilst the concerns expressed are valid and the difficulties posed substantial, it is important also to highlight the considerable value of the formative aspects of SSC assessment. In many SSCs, the academic and professional dynamic established between faculty and student is different to the norm, because of the specific interest the student has expressed in the specialty and field of study (MacDougall and Riley 2010). This often encourages more detailed and helpful feedback than is normally provided. The importance of this feedback cannot be over-emphasized; it can be hugely helpful in guiding students, especially in the early years of undergraduate medical training. Moves to centralize the assessment of SSCs into a smaller panel of experienced assessors (GMC 2011) may achieve the intended aim of improving consistency of marking, but there is a risk by doing so of jeopardizing the detail and value of formative feedback if individual supervisors lose ownership of the assessment of students.

Problems can also lie at the other end of the spectrum with students who perform poorly in their SSCs. In core attachments of short duration, there can be a reluctance to fail students (Cleland et al. 2008). In this different environment and dynamic, students should be performing at their optimum, having chosen the topic or field of study, and potentially aiming to impress for career advancement purposes. When appropriate, clear notice should be taken if a student is assessed as performing poorly—considering the deeper insight the supervisor will have into their professional performance. Procedures should be in place to identify and offer remedial action and support for these students, and to manage this burden on faculty resources (Frellsen et al. 2008). These students' problems often prove to be complex (Ford et al. 2008).

Final considerations

When Henry Kissinger, the US Secretary of State, visited China in 1971, he is reported to have asked his counterpart, Zhou Enlai, for his assessment of the 1789 French Revolution. The oft-quoted reply—'It is too early to say'—may be apocryphal, but seems apposite here. The GMC's advocacy of student choice in the undergraduate medical curriculum in 1993 was fundamentally an experiment that is still in progress. There was no evidence base for student choice per se, although the logic behind the recommendation was

inescapable. Two decades later, an appraisal of this innovation is timely, but cannot be conclusive.

The implementation of SSCs has coincided with major changes in the globalization of higher education. These developments may seem unrelated, but the need to cater for students of differing backgrounds and needs would have necessitated changes to the undergraduate curriculum in any case, and this underlines one of the major advantages of SSC programmes—the flexibility they bring to curriculum planning and delivery, to respond to both educational issues and the rapidly evolving environment surrounding delivery of medical care. SSC programmes are in a constant state of turnover and renewal, with existing modules being replaced by new ones. This allows for the commissioning of modules that address particular imperatives, whether due to an influx of overseas students, or a desire to widen access or promote interprofessional learning. Indeed, many novel approaches to curriculum development and delivery have been piloted and tested in SSCs: delivering learner-centred education, formative and summative feedback, reflective writing, portfolios, together with assessment modalities including varied forms of peer assessment and multisource feedback. Some of these innovative assessments are well-established in other disciplines, for instance the humanities (Kuper et al. 2006). The innovation lies in their application to medicine.

The explicit requirement for more active student ownership of learning has acted as a driver to change attitudes on the part of faculty and students alike. Medical educators tasked with designing, developing and delivering SSC programmes and individual modules, and also the students themselves, have real opportunities to push the boundaries of what is permissible and feasible. In particular, the concept of allowing students to design their own modules has fundamentally changed the dynamic between faculty and students, allowing for a more equal partnership in learning. Students highly value the opportunities presented (GMC QABME reports). Feedback on SSCs, from faculty and students is usually very good—often more positive than for other parts of the curriculum.

How important is the absence of compelling evidence that student choice as represented in SSCs improves important outcomes like academic performance? The problems associated with SSCs are not trivial: perennial difficulties include finding the appropriate administrative support for complex programmes; providing teaching capacity; and dealing with inconsistency in assessment. If these are to be endured there should be evidence that SSCs are 'worth the trouble'. The evidence of the long-term benefits of SSCs in preparing students so they are fit for purpose as clinical trainees remains limited, and the evidence base for SSCs generally remains likewise slender (Murphy et al. 2013). This partly reflects the challenges with performing the required type of educational research (Gill and Griffin 2009; Ringsted et al. 2012). SSCs are being implemented within a complex and continuously changing environment, and are integral to the major upheaval and reorganization of whole curricula. In addition, some of the perceived benefits of SSCs are shared with problem-based learning (PBL). Both are student-centred, involve small group work, and require self-directed learning. It becomes difficult or impossible to control for the wide range of confounding factors that may affect benefits, or detriments, to student educational outcomes.

It is not possible therefore to provide at this point a definitive assessment of student choice as delivered in SSCs. Indeed their future role is uncertain. The GMC has over the past two decades progressively and substantially slimmed down the student-selected thread in the curriculum. As highlighted previously, this may simply be an acknowledgement of the difficulty in establishing programmes of modules as extensive as originally envisaged, rather than a reflection of second thoughts about the role of student choice. Even if that is the case, it may be asking a lot of an SSC thread that occupies as little as 10% of curriculum time, to deliver the ambitious revitalization of undergraduate medical education envisioned in *Tomorrow's Doctors*. Nevertheless, the changes brought about by SSCs, particularly in the relationship between students and faculty, have been profound, and it will require a major shift in educational priorities if these are to be reversed.

Conclusions

If SSCs are to be delivered effectively in a medical curriculum, the following are key considerations:

- Learning outcomes must be clearly defined and fully embedded within the whole curriculum, so that all outcomes are successfully attained by every student.

- The provision of student choice facilitates the development of a student-centred learning approach and student autonomy.

- Programme sustainability must be carefully considered. This includes creating an environment so that student choice curriculum elements are viewed as clear opportunities by both students and faculty.

- There must be full integration of the formative and summative assessment of SSCs with the core curriculum, complementing and adding value beyond the core assessment paradigms to facilitate student development.

- SSCs must be continually developed and revitalized with innovative new courses, utilizing advances in curriculum design, technology and assessment methodologies to reflect rapid developments across the fields of medical education and medicine.

References

Ahn, J., Watt, C.D., Man, L.X., Greeley, S.A., and Shea, J.A. (2007) Educating future leaders of medical research: Analysis of student opinions and goals from the MD-PhD SAGE (Students' Attitudes, Goals, and Education) survey. *Acad Med.* 82: 633–645

Ali, S.K. and Baig, L.A. (2012) Problems and issues in implementing innovative curriculum in the developing countries: the Pakistani experience. *BMC Med Educ.* 12: 31

Balandin, S., Lincoln, M., Sen, R., Wilkins, D.P., and Trembath, D. (2007) Twelve tips for effective international clinical placements. *Med Teach.* 29: 872–877

Barroso, S. and Sebastiao, A.M. (2012) Research possibilities for pre-graduate students. In: M.A.R.B. Castanho and G. Güner-Akdogan (eds) *The Researching, Teaching and Learning Triangle* (pp. 17–25). Mentoring in Academia and Industry, volume 10 New York: Springer

Bell, D., Harbinson, M., Toman, G., Crawford, V., and Cunningham, H. (2010) Wholeness of healing: An innovative student-selected component introducing United Kingdom medical students to the spiritual dimension of healthcare. *South Med J.*103: 1204–1209

Bidwai, A. (2000) SSMs are my saviour. *Student BMJ.* 8: 339–340

Bland, C.J., Starnaman, S., Wersal, L., Moorhead-Rosenberg, L., Zonia, S., and Henry, R. (2000) Curricular change in medical schools: How to succeed. *Acad Med.* 75: 575–594

Bleakley, A., Brice, J., and Bligh, J. (2008) Thinking the post-colonial in medical education. *Med Educ.* 42: 266–270

Brown, W.S. (2005) Medics to teach in primary schools. *Student BMJ.* 13: 93

Celletti, F., Reynold, T.A., Wright, A., Stoertz, A., and Dayrit, M. (2011) Educating a new generation of doctors to improve the health of populations in low- and middle-income countries. *PLoS Medicine.* 8: 1001–1108

Charon, R. (2001) Narrative medicine: A model for empathy, reflection, profession and trust. *JAMA.* 286: 1897–1902

Charon, R., Banks, J.T., Connelly, J.E., et al. (1995) Literature and medicine: contributions to clinical practice. *Ann Intern Med.* 122: 599–606

Chatterjee, H.J. and Noble, N. (2009) Object therapy: A student-selected component exploring the potential of museum object handling as an enrichment activity for patients in hospital. *Global J Health Sci.* 1: 42–49

Christakis, N.A. (1995) The similarity and frequency of proposals to reform US medical education: constant concerns. *JAMA.* 274: 706–711

Christopher, D.F., Harte, K., and George, C.F. (2002) The implementation of Tomorrow's Doctors. *Med Educ.* 36: 282–288

Cleland, J.A., Knight, L.V., Rees, C.E., Tracey, S., and Bond, C.M. (2008) Is it me or is it them? Factors that influence the passing of underperforming students. *Med Educ.* 42: 800–809

Collins, J.P., Farish, S., McCalman, J.S., and McColl, G.J. (2010) A mandatory intercalated degree programme: revitalising and enhancing academic and evidence-based medicine. *Med Educ.* 32: 541–546

Colthart, I., Bagnall, G., Evans, A., et al. (2008) A systematic review of the literature on the effectiveness of self-assessment on the identification of learner needs, learner activity and impact on clinical practice; BEME guide no. 10. *Med Teach.* 30: 124–145

Cooke, M., Irby, D.M., Sullivan, W., and Ludmerer, K.M. (2006) American Medical Education 100 years after the Flexner report. *N Engl J Med.* 355: 1339–1344

Cottrell, S., Diaz, S., Cather, A., and Shumway, J. (2006) Assessing medical student professionalism: An analysis of a peer assessment. *Med Educ Online.* 11: 8

Cross, P. (2003) Getting the most out of SSMs. Student BMJ. 11: 336–337

Cruess, R.L. and Cruess, S.R. (2006). Teaching professionalism: general principles. *Med Teach.* 28: 205–208

Cruess, R.L. and Cruess, S.R. (2008) Understanding medical professionalism: a plea for an inclusive and integrated approach. *Med Educ.* 42: 755–757

Cruess, S.R., Cruess, R.L., and Steinert, Y. (2008) Role modelling—making the most of a powerful teaching strategy. *BMJ.* 336: 718–721

Cumming, A. (2010) The Bologna process, medical education and integrated learning. *Med. Teach.* 32: 316–318

Dahlstrom, J., Dorai-Raj, A., McGill, D., Owen, C., Tymms, K., and Watson, D.A.R. (2005) What motivates senior clinicians to teach medical students? *BMC Med Educ.* 5: 27–37

Dannefer, E.F., Henson, L.C., Bierer, S.B. et al. (2005) Peer assessment of professional competence. *Med Educ.* 39: 713–722

Davies, H., Archer, J., Bateman, A. et al. (2008) Specialty-specific multi-source feedback: assuring validity, informing training. *Med Educ.* 42: 1014–1020

Davis, M.H. and Harden, R.M. (2003) Planning and implementing an undergraduate medical curriculum: the lessons learned. *Med Teach.* 25: 596–608

Davis, M.H., Ponnamperuma, G.G., and Ker, J.S. (2009) Student perceptions of a portfolio assessment process. *Med Educ.* 43: 89–98

Dowell, J. and Merrylees, N. (2009) Electives: isn't it time for a change? *Med Educ.* 43: 121–126

Dyrbye, L., Thomas, M.R., Natt, N., and Rohren, C.H. (2007) Prolonged delays for research training in medical school are associated with poorer subsequent clinical knowledge. *J Gen Intern Med.* 22: 1101–1106

Dyrbye, L.N., Davidson, L.W., and Cook, D.A. (2008) Publications and presentations resulting from required research by students at Mayo Medical School, 1976–2003. *Acad Med.* 83: 604–610

Elit, L., Hunt, M., Redwood-Campbell, L., Ranford, J., Adelson, N., and Schwartz, L. (2011) Ethical issues encountered by medical students during international health electives. *Med Educ.* 45: 704–711

Ellaway, R. and Masters, K. (2008) AMEE Guide 32: e-learning in medical education Part 1; Learning, teaching and assessment. *Med. Teach.* 30: 455–473

Fancher, T.L., Wun, T., Hotz, C.S., and Henderson, M.C. (2009) Jumpstarting academic careers with a novel intern research rotation: the AIMS rotation. *Am J Med.* 122: 1061–1066

Faulder, G.S., Riley, S.C., Stone, N., and Glasier, A. (2004) Teaching sex education improves medical students' confidence in dealing with sexual health issues. *Contraception.* 70: 135–139

Fletcher, G. and Agius, R.M. (1995) The Special Study Module: a novel approach to undergraduate teaching in occupational medicine. *Occupational Medicine.* 45: 326–328

Ford, M., Masterton, G., Cameron, H., and Kristmundsdottir, F. (2008) Supporting struggling medical students. *Clin Teach.* 5: 1–7

Frank, J.R., Snell, L.S., Cate, O.T. et al. (2010) Competency-based medical education: theory to practice. *Med Teach.* 32: 638–645

Frellsen, S.L., Baker, E.A., Papp, K.K., and Durning, S.J. (2008) Medical school policies regarding struggling medical students during the internal medicine clerkships: results of a national survey. *Acade Med.* 83: 876–881

Funston, G.M. and Young, A.M.H. (2012) Action is required to safeguard the future of academic medicine in the UK. *Nat Med.* 18: 194

Furmedge, D.S. (2008) Teaching skills: a school-based special study module. *Med Educ.* 42: 1140

General Medical Council (1993, revised in 2003, revised 2009) *Tomorrow's Doctors: Recommendations on Undergraduate Medical Education.* London: GMC

General Medical Council (2011) Assessment in undergraduate medical education: Advice supplementary to *Tomorrow's Doctors* (2009). London: GMC

General Medical Council. UK Medical Schools—Quality Assurance of Basic Medical Education (QABME) reports. London, GMC http://www.gmc-uk.org/education/undergraduate/undergraduate_qa.asp Accessed 1 Aprll 2012

Gibson, E. (2006) Media medicine. *Student BMJ.* 14: 212–213

Gill, D. and Griffin, A.E. (2009) Reframing medical education research: let's make the publishable meaningful and the meaningful publishable. *Med Educ.* 43: 933–935

Global Consensus Group for Social Accountability of Medical Schools (GCSA) www.healthsocialaccountability.org Accessed 1 February 2011

Graffam, B. (2007) Active learning in medical education: strategies for beginning implementation. *Med Teach.* 29: 38–42

Griffin, M.F. and Hindocha, S. (2011) Publication practices of medical students at British medical schools: Experience, attitudes and barriers to publish. *Med Teach.* 33: e1–e8

Hafferty, F.W. (1998) Beyond curriculum reform: Confronting medicine's hidden curriculum. *Acad Med.* 73: 403–407

Harden, R.M. (2001) AMEE Guide No 21: Curriculum mapping: a tool for transparent and authentic teaching and learning. *Med Teach.* 23: 123–137

Harden, R.M. (2007) Learning outcomes as a tool to assess progression. *Med Teach.* 29: 678–682

Hilton, S. and Southgate, L. (2007) Professionalism in medical education. *Teaching and Teacher Education.* 23: 265–279

Hirsh, D.A., Ogur, B., Thibault, G.E. and Cox, M. (2007) 'Continuity' as an organizing principle for clinical education reform. *N Engl J Med.* 356: 858–866.

Hodgson, K. and Smart, N. (1998) Humanities in medical education. *Student BMJ.* e-volume 6.

Hounsell, D., McCune, V., Hounsell, J., and Litjens, J. (2008) The quality of guidance and feedback to students. *Higher Education Research & Development.* 27: 55–67

Howman, M. and Jones, M. (2011) Does undertaking an intercalated BSc influence first year clinical exam results at a London medical school? *BMC Med Educ.* 11: 6

Hrisos, S., Illing, J.C., and Burford, B.C. (2008) Portfolio learning for foundation doctors: early feedback on its use in the workplace. *Med Educ.* 42: 214–223

Hunter, A.-B., Laursen, S.L., and Seymour, E. (2007) Becoming a scientist: the role of undergraduate research in students' cognitive, personal and professional development. *Sci Educ.* 91: 36–74

Huxley, T.H. (1876) Lecture delivered at the opening of Johns Hopkins University, Baltimore

Jenkins, A., Healy, M., and Zetter, R. (2007) Linking teaching and research in disciplines and departments. York: The Higher Education Academy

Jobanputra, J., Clack, A.R., Cheeseman, G.J., Glasier, A., and Riley, S.C. (1999) A Feasibility study of adolescent sex education: medical students as peer educators in Edinburgh schools. *Br J Obs Gynaecol.* 106: 887–891

Kanna, B., Deng, C., Erickson, S.N., Valerio, J.A., Dimitrov, V., and Soni, A. (2006) The research rotation; competency-based structured and novel approach to research training of internal medicine residents. *BMC Med Educ.* 6: 52–59.

Karle, H. (2006) Global standards and accreditation in medical education: a view from the WFME. *Acad Med.* 81(Suppl): S43–S48.

Karle, H. on behalf of the Executive Council, World Federation for Medical Education (2008) International recognition of basic medical education programmes. *Med. Educ.* 42: 12–17

Korszun, A., Winterburn, P.J., Sweetland, H., Tapper-Jones, L., and Houston, H. (2006) Assessment of professional attitude and conduct in medical undergraduates. *Med Teach.* 27: 704–708

Kuper, A. (2006) Literature and medicine: A problem with assessment. *Acad Med.* 81(Suppl): S128–S137.

Laidlaw, A., Guild, S., and Struthers, J. (2009) Graduate attributes in the disciplines of Medicine, Dentistry and Veterinary Medicine: a survey of expert opinions. *BMC Med Educ.* 9: 28

Laskowitz, D.T., Drucker, R.P., Parsonnet, J., Cross, P.C., and Gesundheit, N. (2010) Engaging students in dedicated research and scholarship during medical school: The long term experiences of Duke and Stanford. *Acad Med.* 85: 419–428

Lazarus, P.A. and Rosslyn, F.M. (2003) The arts in medicine: setting up and evaluating a new special study module at Leicester Warwick Medical School. *Med Educ.* 37: 553–559

Leung, W.-C. (2002) Is there a better alternative to special study modules? *Student BMJ.* 10: 4–5

Lowry, S. (1992) Strategies for implementing curriculum change. *BMJ.* 305: 1482–1485

Ludmerer, K.M. (2004) Learner-centred medical education. *N Engl J Med.* 351: 1163–1164

Lurie, S.J. (2012) History and practice of competency-based assessment. *Med Educ.* 46: 49–57

MacDougall, M. (2008) Ten tips for promoting autonomous learning and effective engagement in the teaching of statistics to undergraduate medical students involved in short term research projects. *J Appl Quant Methods.* 3: 223–240

MacDougall, M. and Riley, S.C. (2010) Initiating undergraduate medical students into communities of research practise: what do supervisors recommend? *BMC Med Educ.* 10: 83

MacDougall, M., Riley, S.C., Cameron, H.C. and McKinstry, B. (2008) Halo and horns in the assessment of undergraduate medical students: a consistency-based approach. *J Appl Quant Methods.* 3: 116–128

Mahesan, N., Crichton, S., Sewell, H., and Howell, S. (2011) The effect of an intercalated BSc on subsequent academic performance. *BMC Med Educ.* 11: 76

Masters, K. and Ellaway, R. (2008) e-learning in medical education Guide 32: Part 2: Technology, management and design. *Med Teach.* 30: 474–489

McGee, J.B. and Kanter, S.L. (2011) How we develop and sustain innovation in medical education technology: Keys to success. *Med Teach.* 33: 279–285

McLean, M. and Gibbs, T. (2010) Twelve tips to designing and implementing a learner-centred curriculum: Prevention is better than cure. *Med Teach.* 32: 225–230

McLean, M. and Howarth, F.C. (2008) Does undergraduate research constitute scholarship? Drawing on the experiences of one medical faculty. *J Scholarship Teaching Learning.* 8: 72–87

McLean, M. and Van Wyk, J. (2006) 12 tips for recruiting and retaining facilitators in a problem based learning programme. *Med Teach.* 28: 675–679

Medical Education in Europe (2013) MEDINE2. Integrating the Research Component in Medical Education in Europe. http://medine2.com/ Accessed 14 April 2013

Metcalfe, N.H. and Brown, A.K. (2011) History of medicine student selected components at UK medicals schools: a questionnaire-based study. *J Roy Soc Med Short Reports.* 2: 77

Mills, S. and Bryden, D.C. (2010) A practical approach to teaching medical ethics. *J Med Ethics.* 36: 50–54

Mohammed, A. (2001) Special study modules are not a waste of time. *Student BMJ.* 9: 34.

Mueller, P.S., McConahey, L.L., Orvidas, L.J., et al. (2010) Visiting medical student elective and clerkship programs: a survey of US and Puerto Rico allopathic medical schools. *BMC Med Educ.* 10: 41

Murdoch-Eaton, D. (2011) Student selected components. *Med Teach.* 33: 762–764

Murdoch-Eaton, D., Ellershaw, J., Garden, A., et al. (2004) Student-selected components in the undergraduate medical curriculum: a multi-institutional consensus on purpose. *Med Teach.* 26: 33–38

Murdoch-Eaton, D., Drewery, S., Elton, S., et al. (2010) What do medical students understand by research and research skills? Identifying research opportunities within undergraduate projects. *Med Teach.* 32: e152–e60

Murdoch-Eaton, D. and Green, A. (2011) The contribution and challenges of electives in the development of social accountability in medical students. *Med Teach.* 33: 643–648

Murdoch-Eaton, D. and Jolly, B. (2000) Undergraduate projects—do they have to be within the conventional medical environment? *Med Educ.* 34: 95–100

Murdoch-Eaton, D., Redmond, A., and Bax, N. (2011) Training healthcare professionals for the future: Internationalism and effective inclusion of global health training. *Med Teach.* 33: 562–569

Murdoch-Eaton, D. and Whittle, S. (2012) Generic skills in medical education: developing the tools for successful lifelong learning. *Med Educ.* 46: 120–128

Murphy, M.J., Seneviratne, R.DeA., McAleer, S.P., Remers, O.J., and Davis, M.H. (2008) Student selected components: do students learn what teachers think they teach? *Med Teach.* 30: e175–e179

Murphy, M.J., Seneviratne, R.DeA., Remers, O.J., and Davis, M.H. (2009a) Hawks' and 'doves': effect of feedback on grades awarded by supervisors of student selected components. *Med Teach.* 31: e489–e493

Murphy, M.J., Seneviratne, R.DeA., Remers, O.J., and Davis, M.H. (2009b) Student selected components: student-designed modules are associated with closer alignment of planned and learnt outcomes. *Med Teach.* 31: e484–e488

Murphy, M.J., Seneviratne, R.DeA., Cochrane, L, Davis, M.H.and Mires, G.J. (2009b) Impact of student choice on academic performance: cross-sectional and longitudinal observations of a student cohort. BMC *Med Teach.* 13: 26

Neely, D. and Minford, E.J. (2008) Current status of teaching on spirituality in UK medical schools. *Med Educ.* 42: 176–182

Newbegin, R.M., Rhodes, J.C., Flood, L.M., and Richardson, H.C. (2007) Student-selected components: bringing more ENT into the undergraduate curriculum. *J Laryngol Otol.* 121: 783–785

Nicol, D. and Macfarlane-Dick, D. (2006) Formative assessment and self regulated learning: A model and seven principles of good feedback practice. *Studies in Higher Education.* 31: 199–218

Nishigori, H., Otani, T., Plint, S., Uchino, M., and Ban, N. (2009) I came, I saw, I reflected: A qualitative study into learning outcomes of international electives for Japanese and British medical students. *Med Teach.* 31: e196–e201

Office of the Independent Adjudicator for Higher Education (OIAHE) (2004) Annual Report 2004: Resolving Student Complaints. www.oiahe.org.uk/docs/OIA-Annual-Report-2004.pdf Last accessed 29 November 2009

Parker, M. (2006) Assessing professionalism: theory and practice. *Med Teach.* 28: 399–403

Payne, G., Thomson, A., and Flood, C. (2000) Special study modules should be more diverse. *Student BMJ.* 8: 468

Petrosoniak, A., McCarthy, A., and Varpio, L. (2010) International health electives: thematic results of student and professional interviews. *Med Educ.* 44: 683–689

Pulito, A.R., Donnelly, M.B., and Plymale, M. (2007) Factors in faculty evaluation of medical students' performance. *Med Educ.* 41: 667–675

Rees, C. and Shepherd M. (2005) The acceptability of 360-degree judgments as a method of assessing undergraduate medical students' personal and professional behaviours. *Med Educ.* 39: 49–57

Richardson, J. (2009) Factors that influence first year medical students' choice of student selected component. *Med Teach.* 31: e418–e424

Riley, S.C. (2009) *Student Selected Components: AMEE Guide 46. Med Teach.* 31: 885–894

Riley, S.C., Ferrell, W.R., Gibbs, T.J., Murphy, M.J., and Smith, W.C.S. (2008) Twelve tips for developing and sustaining a programme of student selected components. *Med Teach.* 30: 370–376

Riley, S.C., Gibbs, T.J., Ferrell, W.R., Smith W.C.S., and Murphy, M.J. (2009) Getting the most out of student selected components (SSCs): 12 tips for participating students. *Med Teach.* 31: 895–902

Ringsted, C., Hodges, B., and Scherpbier, A. (2012) 'The research compass': An introduction to research in medical education: AMEE Guide No.56. *Med Teach.* 33: 695–709

Robinson, L., Drewery, S., Ellershaw, J., Smith, J., Whittle, S., and Murdoch-Eaton, D. (2007) Research governance: impeding both research and teaching? A survey of impact on undergraduate research opportunities. *Med Educ.* 41: 729–736

Robley, W., Whittle, S., and Murdoch-Eaton, D. (2005). Mapping generic skills curricula: a recommended methodology. *J Further Higher Educ.* 29: 221–231

Ross, M.T. and Cameron, H.S. (2007) Peer assisted learning: a planning and implementation framework. AMEE Guide No 30. *Med Teach.* 29: 527–545

Royal College of Physicians (RCP) of London (2005) *Doctors in society: Medical professionalism in a changing world.* London: RCP London

Sandars, J. (2006) Twelve tips for using blogs and wikis in medical education. *Med Teach.* 28: 680–682

Schonrock-Adema, J., Heijne-Penninga, M., Van Duijn, M.A.J., Geertsma, J., and Cohen-Schotanus, J. (2007) Assessment of professional behaviour in undergraduate medical education: peer assessment enhances performance. *Med Educ.* 41: 836–842

Schor, N.F., Troen, P., Kanter, S.L., and Levine, A.S. (2005). The scholarly project initiative: introducing scholarship in medicine through a longitudinal mentored program. *Acad Med.* 80: 824–831

Schwarz, M.R. and Wojtczak, A. (2002). Global minimum essential requirements: a road towards competence-orientated medical education. *Med Teach.* 24: 125–129

Scottish Doctor (2007) Student Selected Components: a consensus statement on purpose. Scottish Medical School Council of Deans' Curriculum sub-group. http://www.scottishdoctor.org/ Accessed February 2012

Shah, S. and Wu, T. (2008) The medical student global health experience: professionalism and ethical implications. *J Med Ethics.* 34: 375–378

Sharafeldin, E., Soonawala, D., Vandenbroucke, J.P., Hack, E., and Visser, L.G. (2010) Health risks encountered by Dutch medical students during an elective in the tropics and the quality and comprehensiveness of pre- and post-travel care. *BMC Med Educ.* 10: 89

Shehmar, M., Haldane, T., Price-Forbes, A. et al. (2010) Comparing the performance of graduate entry and school-leaver medical students. *Med Educ.* 44: 699–705

Stark, P., Ellershaw, J., Newble, D. et al. (2005) Student-selected components in the undergraduate medical curriculum: a multi-institutional consensus on assessable key tasks. *Med Teach.* 27: 720–725

Stern, D.T. and Papadakis, M. (2006) The developing physician—becoming a professional. *N Engl J Med.* 355: 1794–1799

Tennant, P. and Rowell, G. (2009) Benchmark Plagiarism Tariff: A benchmark tariff for the application of penalties for student plagiarism in higher education. http://www.plagiarismadvice.org/BTariff Accessed 23 July 2012

Thomas, J.C. (2006) Is the pen mightier than the scalpel? *Student BMJ*. 14: 384–385

Van de Ridder, J.M.M., Stokking, K.M., McGaghie, W.C., and ten Cate, O. (2008) What is feedback in clinical education? *Med Educ*. 42: 189–197

van Eyk, H.J. Hooiveld, M.H., and Van Leeuwen, T.N. et al. (2010) Scientific output of Dutch medical students. *Med Teach*. 32: 231–235

Van Tartwijk, J. and Driessen, E.W. (2009) Portfolios for assessment and learning. AMEE guide No 45. *Med Teach*. 31: 790–801

Vieira, J.E., Bellodi, P.L., Marcondes, E., and de Arruda Martins, M. (2004) Practical skills are the most popular elective choice. *Med Educ*. 38: 1013–1016

Violato, C., Lockyer, J.M., and Fidler, H. (2008) Changes in performance: a 5-year longitudinal study of participants in a multi-source feedback programme. *Med Educ*. 42: 1007–1013

West, C.P., Halvorsen, A.J., and McDonald, F.S. (2011) Scholarship during residency training: A controlled comparison study. *Am J Med*. 124: 984–987

West, C.P. and Shanafelt, T.D. (2007) The influence of personal and environmental factors on professionalism in medical education. *BMC Med Educ*. 7: 29

Whittle, S.R. and Murdoch-Eaton, D.G. (2008) Learning about plagiarism using Turnitin detection software. *Med Educ*. 42: 513–543

Willett, T.G. (2008) Current status of curriculum mapping in Canada and the UK. *Med Educ*. 24: 786–793

World Federation for Medical Education (2003) *Basic medical education WFME Global standards for quality improvement*. Copenhagen: WFME. http://www2.sund.ku.dk/wfme/ Last accessed 13 February 2009

World Health Organization, World Federation for Medical Education. WHO-WFME Guidelines for Accreditation of Basic Medical Education (2005) http://www.wfme.org Accessed 1 November 2011

CHAPTER 6

Integrated learning

David Prideaux, Julie Ash, and Anaise Cottrell

'Integration' (pax to the Old Guard!) in the curriculum,
about which there has been much hue and cry in the 'fifties,
is a topic which still arouses both cynicism and fanaticism.

John Spillane

Reproduced from *British Medical Journal*, John D. Spillane,
'New American Medical Schools', 2, p. 778, copyright 1960,
with permission from BMJ Publishing Group Ltd

Why integrated learning

The argument for integrated learning in medical education can be regarded as intuitive. It can be drawn from the work of clinicians as they apply an integrated body of knowledge to patient care. As such it is neither new nor revolutionary. Indeed it is seen as a key element in what Frenk et al. (2010) have defined as the three 'generations of reform' in health professional education.

Frenk et al. defined the first generation as the period from the beginning to the middle of the twentieth century. The dominant discourse of the period centred on the work of Abraham Flexner with his advocacy of overall reform of medical education and William Osler with his emphasis on clinical placements and bedside learning. Flexner's (1910) century old report on medical education in North America, sponsored by the Carnegie Foundation, set directions for reform of medical education worldwide. Flexner argued for the integration of scientific knowledge with practice, encapsulated in the concept of 'bench to bedside'. Ironically, the latter led to medical curricula being based on scientific disciplines in the early years with somewhat less pedagogical attention to integration and application at the bedside. Yet the concept of integration in Flexner's work was so central that it was again emphasized in the follow up Carnegie Foundation review to mark the centennial of Flexner's original work (Cooke et al. 2006).

Flexner and Osler's reforms were centred on the concept of a teaching hospital. Clinical teaching and learning took place in the work context of large comprehensive hospitals but as the hospitals became more specialized it became more difficult to provide integrated learning experiences. In the second generation of reform in the latter part of the 20th century, teaching hospitals were transformed into what Frenk et al. (2010) call academic medical centres with much closer ties with universities and a greater range of health professional programmes. The increased association with universities brought a greater interest in curriculum and pedagogy, the most notable being the development of problem-based learning (PBL) at McMaster University in Canada in the 1960s (Neufeld and Barrows 1974; Neville 2009). PBL provided an integrated approach to teaching and learning the basic sciences underlying medical practice and has been widely adopted. The period was also marked by the introduction of integrated curriculum designs (Benor 1982; Schmidt 1998) which were again widely adopted. Harden et al. (1984) listed integration as one of the hallmarks of an innovative curriculum in their influential paper on the SPICES approach to curriculum planning in medical education. By the end of the period of reform Harden (2000) was able to delineate a ladder or hierarchy of eleven approaches to integrated curriculum design culminating in interdisciplinary or transdisciplinary designs although there is not a clear picture of the extent of the adoption of the various designs.

Frenk et al's (2010) third generation of reforms to mark the 21st century is predictive rather than descriptive. It is based on their analysis of the need for reform to provide relevant and equitable health services. Fundamental to the analysis is the concept of interdependence of health education providers and health services. Integration in this period is driven by transformative learning (Mezirow 2000). Frenk et al. somewhat paradoxically anchor transformative learning in competency-based approaches to medical education. For them integration can be achieved by careful selection of competencies to break down professional silos within medicine and interprofessional silos across the health professions.

The learner and integration

While there has been consistent advocacy of integrated learning through the various phases of medical education the outcomes and effects are largely assumed rather than empirically verified. Statements remain at the grand design level. Ultimately, however, integration must focus on the learner rather than the curriculum or teaching strategies. It is the learner that does the integrating not the curriculum designer.

There are several educational theories relevant to the learner focus on integration. One of the most important is *constructivism*, which has received considerable support in the latter part of the twentieth century in the second generation of reform of medical education. Constructivism has its roots in the active learning concepts of Dewey (1938) and was further developed through Kolb's work on experiential learning (Kolb and Fry 1975). In constructivism learners develop their own understandings from background, culture and social and learning interactions. The responsibility for learning resides with the learners who construct their own meanings, and hence integration, from available learning opportunities (Glasersfeld 1989). Hoffman and Donaldson (2004, p. 451) have used the term 360° learning to describe the learning opportunities provided by encounters with patients and medical and health professional staff in clinical contexts from which students can construct their own learning.

Constructivism has its critics. Cognitive load theorists, for example, argue for the importance of structure in learning environments especially for novice learners (Sweller 1988). Newmann et al. (1996) have claimed that constructivist approaches have sometimes resulted in student engagement for its own end. Their concept of *authentic learning* has particular relevance for integration in medical education. Authentic learning retains an element of construction of learning but also involves structured inquiry and learning, which has value beyond the institutional environment in which the learning takes place. Authentic learning, and hence authentic integration, should take place in real clinical environments with meaningful learning experiences and not just in classroom settings. Separate studies of clinical learning by Jolly (1994) and Dornan et al. (2005) have found that student self-learning from experience in the clinical environment is enhanced when actively supported by clinical teachers.

Authentic learning is related to *situated learning*, in which it is argued that learning is contextual and is embedded in social and physical environments (Lave and Wenger 1991). Regehr and Norman (1996) summarize some of the writings in cognitive psychology that underpin learning in context. First, information is more readily retrieved when combined into meaningful schemata. The second important finding from cognitive psychology is that of context specificity, which has been widely quoted in support of assessment practices in medical education, but which also has important application in understanding integrated learning. Context specificity affects the capacity of a learner to retrieve items from memory. Retrieval depends on the similarity between the context or condition of retrieval and the context or condition in which the item was originally learned. There are at least three implications of this. Learning can be enhanced when knowledge is integrated into wider contexts and when there are repeated opportunities to use information in different contexts. Finally, integrated learning is more likely to be achieved when it takes place in contexts that are as close as possible to integrated clinical practice contexts. These concepts support the idea of teaching basic knowledge in a clinical context through methods such as problem- or case-based learning but also that students need multiple exposures to a wide range of clinical contexts in which they can apply their knowledge.

As indicated previously Frenk et al. (2010) argue that the third period of reform of medical education for the 21st century should be underpinned by *transformative learning* (Mezirow 2000). The key to transformative learning is perspective transformation which, while usually triggered by life crises, may also result from accumulating transformations over time or through construction of transformations by teachers. The key is critical reflection by participants on their current situations. As such it is a holistic approach. Frenk et al. (2010) link transformative education with competency-based

education arguing that the selection of competencies across the health professions provides the best opportunities for relevant integrated learning. While competency-based approaches have gained increasing popularity in medical education (Carraccio et al. 2002; Frank et al. 2010) they focus on breaking down education into smaller measurable components rather than taking a holistic view. A recent critique of competency-based education has focused on the reductionist assumptions of competency-based education and its failure to take account of the important learnings involved in the acquisition of tacit knowledge in clinical settings (Australian Medical Council 2010). Integration may be lost in an accumulation of individual competencies.

Thus, there are at least three important considerations in examining integrated learning from a learner perspective. Learners can achieve integration from constructing learning in real work settings. Learning will be facilitated when there is integration of content beyond the single context into multiple contexts and when the learning contexts are similar those in which information must be retrieved. Finally, integrated learning should be holistic rather than atomistic.

The curriculum and integration

As indicated previously the latter part of the 20th century marked a period of considerable reform at a curriculum level in medical education. Overview papers such as those setting out Harden et al.'s (1984) SPICES model or the later PRISMS approach by Bligh et al. (2001) included reference to the importance of integration (table 6.1).

The curriculum reform approaches included a move away from the advocacy of the use of precise instructional objectives as the basis of curriculum design to the use of outcomes-based designs. The outcomes-based approach aided integration with its emphasis on guiding curriculum development by the determination of broad outcomes which would cross subject and discipline boundaries and would underpin the selection of content, teaching and learning and assessment (Harden 1999; Prideaux 2007). There has been some debate about the specification of outcomes and the need to keep them broad, a message which has not always been heeded as the discourse moved from outcomes to competency-based approaches (Hamilton 1999; Prideaux 2000; Harden 2002). The approaches were driven largely by curriculum questions rather than learner concerns.

Table 6.1 The SPICES and PRISMS models of curriculum

SPICES	PRISMS
A curriculum can be characterized according to its	New strategies for curriculum development for the 21st century
position between the following pairs	**P**roduct-focused
Student-centred ⇔ Teacher-centred	**R**elevant
Problem-based ⇔ Information gathering	**I**nterprofessional
Integrated ⇔ Discipline-based	**S**horter, smaller
Community-based ⇔ Hospital-based	**M**ulti-site
Electives ⇔ Standard programme	**S**ymbiotic (integrated with health services
Systematic ⇔ Apprenticeship-based	

Data from Bligh, J., Prideaux, D. and Parsell, G. (2001) PRISMS; new strategies for medical education. Medical Education, 35(6), 520–1 and Harden, R.M., Sowden, S. and Dunn, W.R. (1984). Educational strategies in curriculum development: the SPICES model. Medical Education, 18(4), 284–97.

Nevertheless, achieving curriculum integration as a technical and socially negotiated process has been an important mechanism for curriculum reform. For example, it has provided a mechanism for the inclusion of non-traditional subjects in the curriculum such as palliative care (Radwany et al. 2011) or domestic violence (Magrane et al. 2000), and for enhancement of the efficiency and relevance of traditional subjects such as anatomy (Klement et al. 2011). More ambitiously it has enabled change of a traditional biomedical curriculum into a biopsychosocial curriculum more consistent with modern healthcare models (Tresoloni and Shugars 1994) including the integration of public health across the entire curriculum (Brill et al. 2011; Campos-Outcalt 2011).

Horizontal integration

Horizontal integration is common in the early years of medical courses. Instead of organizing courses by disciplines such as anatomy, physiology, or biochemistry, the disciplines are combined around concepts or ideas in each year of the course. The most common approach is to use the body systems: cardiovascular, respiratory, renal, gastrointestinal, endocrine, and musculoskeletal as organizational blocks for the course. The various stages in the human lifecycle have also provided the basis for integrated discipline blocks. While it is not always made specific, horizontal integration illustrates the principle of elaborating knowledge in wider contexts. Ideas from disciplines can be linked and elaborated by their association with other disciplines in system, lifecycle or other blocks.

Problem- or case-based learning

Horizontal integration is strongly encapsulated in problem- or case-based learning (PBL, CBL). PBL in particular has been widely adopted internationally since its beginnings in the 1960s. Cases are specifically constructed to become the focus of study for periods of a week to a fortnight. They are located in system, lifecycle, or other organizational blocks and, in themselves, are also integrative. Learners must draw on knowledge from across the disciplines to define and pursue the learning goals driven by the cases.

Schmidt (1983) has outlined the rationale for PBL through three learning principles all of which relate to the learner-centred view of integration. Through PBL learners are able to activate prior learning from across their experiences, learn and retrieve information in the context of a defined case and elaborate and apply their learning to other contexts within a small group environment (Schmidt 1983). Figure 6.1 gives a graphical account of this process. Some medical schools have now introduced the opportunity to elaborate on learning from the single case by consideration of multiple short cases of similar presenting conditions to conclude the case of the week.

There have been three major meta-analyses of PBL where learning outcomes as measured by scores on national board examinations for PBL and non-PBL programmes have been compared (Albanese and Mitchell 1993; Berkson 1993; Vernon and Blake 1993). While these may provide some guide to the learning efficacy of integrated learning, the outcomes show that students in PBL programmes do no better or worse in national examinations than their peers who have not participated in PBL programmes. There is evidence of small gains in clinical skills performance for students in PBL programmes but this may be attributable to overall curriculum effects rather than PBL per se. Comparative studies of PBL performance are beset by methodological problems and it

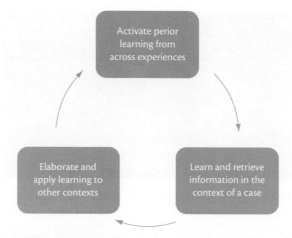

Figure 6.1 PBL and integration.
Data from Schmidt, H.G. (1983). Problem-based learning: rationale and description. *Medical Education*, 17(1): 11–16.

may prove to be impossible to definitively demonstrate the superiority or otherwise of knowledge acquisition in PBL programmes (Norman and Schmidt 2000).

Problem-based learning has been most successfully implemented in the early years of medical courses but it has also been implemented in some programmes as an adjunct to clinical placements. The use of hypothetical paper cases is less frequent when students can interact with patients in clinical settings. Problem-based modules have been taught in parallel to clinical attachments with gains reported in students dealing with uncertainty in clinical practice and recognizing their own limits (O'Neill et al. 2000, 2003). Other schools have centred cases on real patient experience which students then share in a structured manner during tutorials (Barrington et al. 1997). The University of Dundee has adopted task-based learning where clinical tasks provide the bases for integrated learning experiences as students move through discipline-based clinical attachments and facilitate the transfer of basic science knowledge to the clinical years (Harden et al. 1996, 2000).

The often declared challenge of clinical learners is that they find it difficult to integrate their learning of science into the patient context. The development of PBL has provided a mechanism to learn science in the context of a patient case. Whether this helps the transition to learning from clinical experience has not been closely examined.

Vertical integration

Vertical integration has its origins in the work of seminal curriculum writer Hilda Taba (1962) who introduced the term the 'spiral curriculum'. In a spiral curriculum content is introduced at an early level and re-visited in subsequent levels of the spiral where the learning is elaborated and extended. Thus content introduced in one context is reinforced in other contexts.

Vertically integrated designs are aided by the delineation of themes or domains running through all years of the course. Four main themes are common, variously dealing with communication and clinical skills; knowledge in the basic and clinical sciences; social, community, population and public health; and law, ethics and professionalism (fig. 6.2) Content is thus introduced at the varying levels or spirals in the vertical themes.

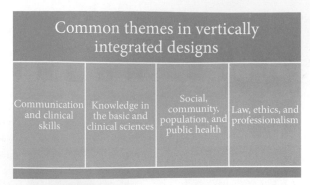

Figure 6.2 Vertical integration.

While Flexner's reforms may have unintentionally resulted in the separation of basic from clinical sciences there are few if any contemporary schools that maintain a strict divide, in intent at least, between the scientific studies of the early years and the clinical studies of the later years. Clinical skills are introduced in the early years and the scientific basis of medicine continues in the clinical years.

The establishment of clinical skills and simulation units in schools has greatly facilitated the vertical integration of communication and clinical skills in medical courses. Students now have opportunities to gain confidence and competence in clinical skills through work with peers, simulated and ambulatory patients, models, manikins, and part-trainers before contact with patients in hospitals. Students in the clinical years can return to skills centres to revise and consolidate skills away from actual patients.

There is evidence of the success of this approach. For example Dent et al. (2001) have demonstrated the integration of patient-based experiences with early learning in their Ambulatory Care Teaching Centre (ACTC). Recent Best Evidence Medical Education (BEME) reviews have demonstrated the gains derived from early clinical learning experiences (Dornan et al 2006; Yardley et al. 2010).

Clinical experience and integration

The clinical years of medical courses provide significant opportunities for integrated learning without the necessity for the organized curriculum structures of the early years. Indeed it was pointed out at the beginning of this chapter that the essential rationale for integrated learning was located in the process of clinicians applying an integrated body of knowledge to patient care. This is contextual integration at its best.

Irby (2011) reports that the 2010 Carnegie Foundation's second recommendation for the reform of medical education in the United States was to integrate formal knowledge with clinical experience. This is a call for integration across the entire medical course and is based on the idea that the expert's clinical pattern recognition comes about by seeing large numbers of clinical cases that require application of formal and best evidence knowledge. Similarly, students' knowledge becomes integrated by actively reasoning through the clinical cases seen during clinical immersion. Medical curricula and learning methods need to support and reinforce this active clinical learning. Irby favours combining formal learning and clinical immersion from the earliest stage to provide contextual relevance to basic knowledge, and maintaining this connection throughout the course so that students concurrently link clinical cases to evidence-based knowledge.

Integrated learning in clinical attachments

Clinical learning typically takes place during attachments that are defined by clinical service disciplines such as medicine, surgery, paediatrics, or general practice. In turn, the curriculum is defined by the disciplines through which the students rotate. However, students in large teaching hospitals may, by necessity, need to be placed with subspecialty team with subsequent concerns about a narrow range of clinical exposure. To overcome this medical schools have supplemented clinical placements with classroom-based programmes. These may be organized within a discipline or through a horizontally integrated core curriculum defined by core problems or patient presentations.

During clinical attachments students' learning is centred on the patients they encounter. This focus on patients has traditionally been the impetus for integration of basic knowledge as applied to the biomedical, psychological and social needs of the patient. The predominant model of learning in clinical placements has been the apprenticeship (Dornan et al. 2005; Ash 2009). The apprenticeship offers students much: regular contact with patients, learning the clinical process with clinicians, a role in patient care as a team member, development of teacher–student relationships and an introduction to the professional clinical community (Ash 2009, 2010). The apprenticeship is a form of situated learning (Lave and Wenger 1991). The concept of supported participation is central in the apprenticeship and has been important in understanding why a supportive student-teacher relationship is essential for student self-learning from clinical practice (Dornan et al. 2007).

The biggest challenge for those responsible for the delivery of the clinical curriculum is how to give students an integrated and generalist clinical learning experience in specialized healthcare settings such as teaching hospitals. While there are some significant positives for learning in these settings, there are well-founded concerns that the traditional block rotations to sub-speciality services result in a limited and fragmented understanding of the broader health needs of society and the role of doctors in healthcare. Key methods of addressing this are: to focus on the needs of clinical learners; to integrate knowledge and reasoning with practice; to understand how students learn from clinical contact; and to recognize how clinicians teach during practice. These are all key characteristics of the apprenticeship.

Medical schools have an important role in developing clinical placements that fit with health services and provide mechanisms for continuity. A key role of the school is the development of an explicit integrated curriculum that provides a guide for students and clinical teachers and determines the mix of clinical experiences across specialties and contexts. It is important that this supports clinical teaching rather than replacing clinical teaching by formal classroom-based sessions aimed at 'covering the content'. An integrated curriculum needs to be built on principles that reinforce supported participation and self-learning. Assessment practices similarly need to reward these.

Longitudinal integrated clinical attachments

The integrated learning drawn from clinical attachments in large teaching hospitals is the legacy that Flexner and Osler left to medical education. Nevertheless, a century later, the nature of teaching hospitals has changed and it is difficult to maintain integrated learning opportunities in their increasingly specialized clinical services. The effect of this on teaching in clinical disciplines such as medicine and surgery has been recognized (Jolly and MacDonald 1989; McManus et al. 1993; Prideaux and Marshall 1994; Stone and Doyle 1996; Leinster 2003; Ramani et al. 2003; Seabrook 2003; Stark 2003; Dornan et al. 2005; Cooke et al. 2006). Many teaching hospitals now focus on tertiary level care. Patients are often admitted through emergency departments and are acutely ill. They frequently undergo complex technological interventions but do not stay in hospital for long periods of time. An increased and appropriate emphasis on respecting patient rights has potentially reduced student access to patients. Finally, clinical staff members are under pressure to increase clinical services and to reduce waiting lists with less time to engage in the facilitation of student learning.

A study of change in clinical education in a surgical setting has exposed the extent to which these changes to healthcare have contributed to disintegration of the traditional clinical apprenticeship (Ash 2010). Surgeons reported a loss of continuity with students, rarely seeing the same student more than once or twice. This seriously disrupted the development of a teacher–student relationship and meant students were unlikely to be given any real or meaningful roles in patient care during their placements. Students had lost their traditional roles of clerking patients prior to surgery. This reduced their opportunity to contribute to patient care, to learn from presenting signs and symptoms and to integrate their knowledge. The disruption of clinical experience was exacerbated by increases in formal teaching sessions including PBL tutorials scheduled during clinical placements (Ash 2010).

Barbara Starfield (2007) has characterized the 20th century teaching hospital as working under a specific disease orientation. In the 21st century health services have to cope with ageing populations and a greater load of chronic and ambulatory care patients. According to Starfield (2007, p. 511) the multimorbidity, chronic disease priorities of care require health services that are 'person-focused, comprehensive and coordinated'. This is likely to be found outside of major teaching hospitals. If students receive the majority of their clinical education in contexts of minimal integration then, according to the principles of contextual learning, they may face difficulties in transferring learning to the contemporary integrated health services.

There is increasing interest in addressing the challenges of integrated curriculum delivery within large teaching hospitals. Hirsh et al. (2007, p. 862) have set out a typology of eight approaches ranging from the kind of discipline-specific attachments discussed previously to fully integrated longitudinal placements. These include placing integrated 'intersessions' between discipline attachments, pursuing longitudinal integrated themes during the attachments, combining two related discipline blocks, or incorporating longitudinal and recurring ambulatory experiences in discipline attachments.

Longitudinal integrated attachments or clerkships (LIC) have been introduced in Australia, Canada, South Africa, and the USA and are gaining support through a group of medical schools known as the Consortium of Longitudinal Integrated Clerkships (CLIC) (Norris et al. 2009). In LIC students are not attached to one discipline for a short period of time. Rather, they follow a panel of patients with presentations from across the disciplines for extended periods of time for up to 12 months or more, under the guidance of a clinician–mentor. Thus they are able to embrace the important concept of continuity in care while at the same time learn essential content from across the core disciplines. Norris et al (2009) claim that this enables a developmental and progressive curriculum which is sequential and responsive to the needs of learners. Hirsh et al. (2007) indicate that LIC illustrate both horizontal and vertical integration. Horizontal integration occurs by linking learning across the specialist clinical disciplines through involvement with patient panels and through learning concepts from ethics and advocacy across the patient experiences. The clinician–mentor fosters vertical integration of biomedical sciences with evidence-based medicine and the application of patient cases to the development of clinical reasoning.

As yet there are no clear findings about the outcomes of LIC for knowledge acquisition (Ogrinc et al. 2002). In a Canadian study McLaughlin et al. (2011) found that students in LIC programmes have higher in-training evaluation report (ITER) ratings than matched peers in non-LIC programmes but lower objective structured clinical examination (OSCE) scores. There is some evidence about reported student learning experiences in LIC. Krupat et al. (2009) have shown how students' patient-centred beliefs were eroded with experience in traditional clinical attachments but not in LIC. Ogur and Hirsh (2009) have produced student narratives from the Harvard Medical School-Cambridge Integrated Clerkship. Students reported more dynamic learning environments, more integrated learning about disease and more experience of illness. They were more connected with patients and more involved in their care. These are important findings given that the central theme of this chapter is that integration must ultimately be achieved in the thinking of the learner.

Community-based longitudinal placements

In response to the increasing specialization of tertiary hospitals some longitudinal experiences have been located in community-based settings in ambulatory care or general practice (Oswald et al. 2001). In Australia longitudinal approaches have been adopted in rural general practice and associated small rural hospitals (Worley et al. 2000; Denz-Penhey and Murdoch 2010). Recently this model has been applied to an outer urban setting in an area of healthcare need (Mahoney et al. 2012). The comprehensive nature of the care provided in these settings has enabled students to readily draw their integrated learning experiences from across the disciplines.

In the Parallel Rural Community Curriculum (PRCC) at Flinders University students are placed in rural general practice and associated small hospitals in the penultimate year of their course. They relocate and live in the small rural communities for the whole year. They are expected to cover the same content in the major clinical disciplines of medicine, surgery, obstetrics and gynaecology, paediatrics, general practice, and psychiatry as their peers undertaking short-term rotations in those disciplines in a larger urban-based teaching hospital. There is evidence of superior performance among students in the PRCC in the end of year written and clinical examinations. There is also evidence that students can learn the content of specialist disciplines in these settings (Worley et al. 2004a, b). Furthermore, students report greater opportunities for patient contact, more time in clinical settings and increased time with clinical supervisors in the PRCC. (Worley et al. 2004c) They make a significant contribution to the general practices and hospitals in which they are located, especially after the first 3 months of placement (Worley and Kitto 2001) and hence engage in the authentic learning approaches previously described by Newmann et al. (1996).

The learning experiences of the PRCC have been fitted into a symbiotic clinical education framework (Prideaux et al. 2007). Symbiotic clinical education, one of the key features of the PRISMS model of medical education, provides a conceptual framework and approach for establishing clinical placement programmes where there are gains for both the university and the health service. Students receive excellent clinical teaching and learning experiences and, in turn, the health service benefits from the students' contribution (Bligh et al. 2001). This has been identified as one of the key features of 21st century medical education and fits with Frenk et al.'s (2010) imperative for greater interdependence between health education and health service providers in the third generation of reform.

Evidence from the PRCC has enabled a model to be built based on four relationships, a personal–professional relationship, a clinician–patient relationship, a university–health service relationship and a government–community relationship (Worley 2002; Worley et al. 2006; Prideaux et al. 2007).

The longitudinal nature of the placements enables students to reconcile their *personal and professional* relationships. In the early years of medical courses students develop a set of personal relationships based on their own learning needs and goals. In clinical contexts these relationships need to be expanded and translated into a set of professional relationships with patients, supervisors and health professionals. In the longitudinal programmes students can develop positive relationships with supervisors over extended time periods and observe them dealing with the reconciliation of personal and professional interests. It has been demonstrated that time is important in developing good social, patient, and supervisor relationships (Oswald et al. 2001; Tolhurst et al. 2006; Ash 2010).

The *clinician–patient* relationship is at the heart of clinical education. Patient-centred models of clinical education are increasingly advocated as a means to achieve integrated learning.

In the *university–health service* relationship it is the responsibility of the health service to provide opportunities for students to construct their own integrated learning under the guidance of supervisors and clinical team members. This should include engagement in 'hot' and 'cold' action which Hoffman and Donaldson (2004, p. 24) have drawn from the original work of Eraut (1994). Hot action requires active participation in patient care as part of a clinical team. Cold action focuses on reflection on learning experiences and integration into overall learning goals under guidance and supervision away from the immediate clinical setting. It is the responsibility of the university to support this (Dornan et al. 2005).

The *government–community* relationship enables students to see how their contribution as members of clinical teams addresses government and community health priorities thus providing contextualization of learning. In the rural programmes this has been achieved through willingness to undertake rural community practice after graduation (Veitch et al. 2006; Worley et al. 2008; Stagg et al. 2009).

Each relationship in the symbiotic model is closely linked to the others. In curriculum design and planning each needs attention. The capacity for clinicians to teach has been shown to be associated with the strength of the relationship between the university and the health services in which students learn (Ash 2010). The teacher's ability to undertake the dual roles of clinician and teacher and the student's ability to learn from having an active role in clinical service is affected by the strength of this relationship.

The recognition that a medical course requires institutional partnerships is essential to creating the capacity for clinical teaching and is relevant in determining the design and delivery of integrated clinical curricula.

Planning an integrated clinical curriculum therefore requires attention to developing the education-service partnership and strengthening commitment to the cross-institutional educational mission. It also involves supporting clinicians, building the capacity for clinical teaching, and examining how continuity can built into students' health services placements. Finally, it means that curriculum outcomes and assessments that support integrated clinical learning must be defined and staff and students must be educated about learning from participation (Ash 2010).

Patient-centred integrated learning

Patient-centred learning has been a key focus of community-based clinical education. It also represents an important means for learners to integrate their own clinical learning. As indicated previously, with the student–patient relationship at the centre of learning students can draw upon the mentorship of all the health professionals involved in patient care as in Hoffman and Donaldson's (2004) concept of 360° learning. Clinical practice requires the application of an integrated body of knowledge to the processes of diagnosis, management and care.

Bleakley and Bligh (2008) have argued that the focus of clinical education should be shifted from the primacy of the doctor-student relationship to the primacy of the student–patient relationship. Traditional doctor-student approaches are characterized by an 'information reproduction' approach. Bleakley and Bligh (2008, p. 91) argue for strong patient-centred models that emphasize collaborative 'knowledge production' obtained through dialogue with patients and with doctors and other health professionals acting as learning resources. This can be achieved through extended placements across clinical services as the patients move through the stages of their care. This has inspired the 'pathways of care' approach in the Peninsula Medical School (Bleakley and Bligh 2008; Brennan and Mattick 2011).

Walters et al. (2011) have proposed four models of interactions between doctor, student and patient in general practice settings:

- the *student–observer model* with the doctor–patient relationship dominant
- the *teacher–healer model* where the doctor's expertise is dominant
- the *doctor–orchestrator* model, akin to Bleakley and Bligh's (2008) approach, where the doctor orchestrates but steps back from the consultation and
- the *doctor–adviser* model appropriate to supervision in postgraduate training.

Walters et al. provide evidence of progression through the first three of these in the longitudinal PRCC programme.

Central to the progress through the three models is the concept of parallel consulting. In this approach a student consults with a patient on his/her own while the supervising GP consults with another patient in another consulting room. Student and doctor then come together with the student's patient before separating again to see further patients. It has been shown that this does not reduce the number of patient consultations by the GP within a consulting session (Walters et al. 2008). Importantly, Walters et al. (2009) found that the activities undertaken by the GPs in the joint sessions were different from those undertaken while consulting alone. In the joint sessions the GPs spent less time on their own patient management tasks, their own physical examination of patients and any associated clerical activities. The additional time was spent on helping students enrich and extend their history taking, to consider contextual factors and to effectively incorporate their findings from the history into the overall patient management plan. Thus the joint sessions became powerful stimuli to integrated learning, as students had opportunities to extend their information over wider sources, to bring the information together and to apply it to patient care.

With a patient-centred focus integrated learning can be facilitated across all clinical contexts and not just in general practice or community-based attachments. The essential process involves following patients for significant periods of time as they access different clinical services. This is akin to horizontal integration. The integration can occur across specialist medical and health professional disciplines. Interprofessional teamwork is a key component of the third generation of health professional education reform. In turn it is a source of much potential integrated learning. Following a patient's progress through a clinical pathway over time also allows for the building and extending of knowledge and skills as in vertical integration. Providing opportunities for students to interact with patients on their own and then jointly with supervisors, as is experienced in parallel consulting, can provide opportunities for extended student history-taking and for further consideration of contextual factors. These can then be incorporated into integrated learning approaches. While the concept of parallel consulting most readily applies to general practice and outpatient clinics, the idea of single then joint patient consultations could also provide a stimulus to learning in inpatient or ward-based clinical attachments.

Integrated learning and integrated assessment

If integrated learning is to be promoted by curriculum design, clinical placement or patient-centred education it must be assessed in an integrated manner. Biggs (1999) has coined the term constructive alignment to describe the process of aligning assessment with learning in curriculum design. If it is accepted that, ultimately, it is learners that are responsible for constructing their own integration, this process of constructive alignment becomes more complex as the curriculum developer has to predict learner outcomes and provide appropriate and relevant assessment. Thus the essential task is to match learning outcomes and assessment. This will require assessment designs that are not top down proceeding from precise objectives or competencies in a lock step manner, but designs that are iterative and fundamentally driven by the matching of broad learning outcomes and assessment (Prideaux 2007). Integration is located in the thinking of learners, and assessment methods will need to tap this. Thus the matching of assessment will require flexibility and some trial and error in the approach.

Schuwirth and van der Vleuten (2011, p. 478) argue that assessment should move from an orientation of assessment *of* learning to assessment *for* learning. In the case of integrated learning, assessment methods must be chosen that will actually promote and encourage students to think in an integrated manner. Assessment

Table 6.2 Integrated assessment

Written assessments	Clinical assessments
MCQs with clinical vignettes	OSCEs
PBL mini-cases	Long cases
Progress testing	Mini-CEX
	Multisource feedback

for learning is fundamentally different, requiring a programmatic approach to assessment, which will provide a range of information from which learners can understand their progress towards learning goals and the assessors can make judgements about readiness for progress. (van der Vleuten and Schuwirth 2005).

The utility of an assessment tool varies according to its psychometric properties, validity and reliability, feasibility and educational impact (van der Vleuten 1996). Rather than relying on single tools, a programmatic approach involves using a combination of assessment tools with different psychometric properties to increase educational impact (van der Vleuten and Schuwirth 2005). Under a programmatic approach the assessment of a single trait or competency is not linked to a single assessment tool but information on student achievement of the trait is gained from the results of several tools (Schuwirth and van der Vleuten 2011). This is important for the assessment of integrated learning as it allows a range of tools to be selected and matched to the learning goals across disciplines and contexts. Table 6.2 shows a number of different forms of integrated assessment.

Integrated written assessments

While the continual theme of this chapter is that learners are ultimately responsible for constructing their own integration it is necessary, if not sufficient, that integrated learning is clearly represented in written assessment blueprints. This implies central test and examination construction at an overall school level rather than at an individual department level. It also implies that written assessment must be of high quality. Written assessments testing application, analysis, synthesis and evaluation are more likely to assess integrated learning than those requiring factual recall. Using well-designed multiple choice question (MCQ) formats is more likely to result in the testing of higher order integrated thinking. Using clinical vignettes as stems enables testing of integrated learning within a specific context (Case and Swanson 2002).

Case-based tools have been developed to test integrated learning within problem-based learning programmes. In effect smaller PBL mini-cases have been constructed to test reasoning, hypothesis formation and identification of learning goals in a sequential manner, similar to modified essay questions (MEQs) (Knox 1989). The limitation of mini-cases is that an individual case requires a longer testing time with potential effects on reliability. In a programmatic approach, however, mini-cases can be included with other formats in an overall balanced assessment programme.

There is growing interest in progress testing (McHarg et al. 2005; Freeman et al. 2010). Students are regularly tested from banks of high quality MCQs set at exit level. Progress towards exit level is then recorded. Progress testing can contribute to assessment of integrated learning through a focus on higher order analysis, application and synthesis by blueprinting items from across the disciplines and by constructing items that require students to draw on knowledge from across disciplines and domains of learning. It is also claimed that progress testing reduces cramming for examinations and an undue focus on single items of recall (Boshuizen et al. 1997).

Integrated clinical assessments

Well accepted assessment formats for the clinical years of medical courses can also be used to assess integrated learning provided they are blueprinted for integration. OSCEs (Harden et al. 1975) can test integrated application and synthesis within a station and can include learning from across the clinical disciplines as well as integration of basic science and clinical knowledge. Traditional long cases have been designed to assess integration and application of learning within a single case. They too require a long testing time with potential reduction in reliability, but can be included in an overall programme of assessment for learning in the clinical years (Wass and van der Vleuten 2004; Wilkinson et al. 2008).

Integrated learning in clinical attachments occurs through patient-centred learning, in authentic integrated work contexts while students make a valued contribution to health services. This emphasis on learning through active participation requires assessment with a purpose that shifts from the base to the apex of Miller's (1990) pyramid of assessment. Fundamentally there should be a move towards assessing what students 'do' and away from Miller's lower levels of 'knows, knows how and shows how'. The mini-CEX represents one such move in this direction. This involves repeated and focused observations of students taking histories, examining and managing patients in real clinical settings (Norcini et al. 2003).

van der Vleuten et al. (2010) note the increasing interest in assessing at the higher levels of Miller's pyramid. They argue for increased attention to workplace-based assessments for assessing the 'does' level at the apex of the pyramid. They locate workplace-based assessment within qualitative frameworks rather than quantitative psychometric frameworks which pervade most assessment in medical education. Thus workplace-based assessment should employ narrative, rich descriptions and triangulation of multiple sources of information. Importantly for assessing integrated learning within longitudinal attachments it should involve assessment over time with trained assessors who have established relationships with students.

As van der Vleuten et al. (2010) point out the development of credible approaches to workplace-based assessment is complex and much work is still to be done. The essence of workplace-based assessment is global judgement by experts in real clinical settings. Experts could include all those in the clinical setting with whom the student has substantive contact. Assessment should be accompanied by feedback. There is some existing use of multisource feedback (MSF) where ratings of performance are gained from colleagues, co-workers and patients, with feedback to the individual assessee (Wood et al. 2006). Portfolios may be used to record the outcomes of workplace-based assessment (Challis 1999).

The development of longitudinal integrated clinical attachments in authentic work-based hospital and community settings has been a challenge in medical education. Yet it is an imperative for the current generation of reform. There is some evidence of the success of these programmes. The next challenge is to develop workplace-based assessment that incorporates the strengths of the relationships between supervisors and learners and enables the latter to

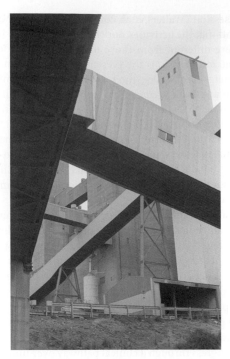

Figure 6.3 Integrated learning provides interconnections between disciplinary silos.
Courtesy of Andrew S. Miller, medical practitioner and keen photographer in South Australia, reproduced with permission

use feedback from multiple clinical teacher judgements to promote the construction of their integrated learning (van der Vleuten et al. 2012) (fig. 6.3).

Conclusions

◆ Deliberately structuring integrated learning into curriculum design is important but is not sufficient on its own.

◆ Integrated learning is likely to be found in clinical attachments particularly in the interprofessional, coordinated, ambulatory and chronic care that is the priority of health services in the 21st century.

◆ Longitudinal clinical placements will enable students to develop the relationships in learning that will assist in the construction of integrated learning.

◆ Patient-centred learning enables students to draw on experiences and resources all around them for integration and application.

◆ Assessment for integrated learning is essential yet complex as it must tap the integration located in the thinking of the learner.

◆ Workplace-based assessment based on multiple expert judgements with feedback is needed for integrated authentic learning in clinical contexts.

References

Albanese, M.A. and Mitchell, S. (1993) Problem-based learning: a review of the literature on its outcomes and implementation issues. *Acad Med.* 68(1): 52–81.

Ash, J.K. (2009) Understanding clinical teaching in times of change. *Clin Teach.* 6(3): 177–180.

Ash, J.K. (2010) A case of meaning: change in clinical education. Unpublished PhD thesis, Flinders University, Adelaide, Australia

Australian Medical Council (AMC) (2010) *Competence-based medical education: AMC consultation paper*. Canberra: Australian Medical Council

Barrington, D., Wing, L., Alpers, J., Latimer, K., and Prideaux, D. (1997) Evaluation of a change from traditional case studies to patient-based, problem-based learning: a case study. *Med Teach.* 19(2): 104–107

Benor, D.E. (1982) Interdisciplinary integration in medical education: theory and methods. *Med Educ.* 16(6): 355–361

Berkson, L. (1993) Problem-based learning: have the expectations been met? *Acad Med.* 68: S79–S88.

Biggs, J. (1999) *Teaching for Quality Learning at University*. Buckingham (UK): SRHE and Open University Press

Bleakley, A. and Bligh, J. (2008) Students learning from patients: let's get real in medical education. *Adv Health Sci Educ.* 13(1): 89–107

Bligh, J., Prideaux, D., and Parsell, G. (2001) PRISMS; new strategies for medical education. *Med Educ.* 35(6): 520–521

Boshuizen, H.P.A., van der Vleuten, C.P.M., Schmidt, H.G., and Machiels-Bongaerts, M. (1997) Measuring knowledge and clinical reasoning in a problem-based curriculum. *Med Educ.* 31(2): 115–121

Brennan, N. and Mattick, K. (2011) Exploring the Map of Medicine's potential in undergraduate medical education. *Med Teach.* 33: e454–e460. http://informahealthcare.com/doi/pdf/10.3109/0142159X.2011.588734 Accessed 19 February 2013

Brill, J.R., Chheda, S.G., Rusch, R.B., and Seibert, C.S. (2011) A mapping process for identifying and enhancing public health education in required medical student clerkships. *Am J Prevent Med.* 41(4 Supp 3): S304–S305

Campos-Outcalt, D. (2011) The integration of public health and prevention into all years of a medical school curriculum. *Am J Prevent Med.* 41(4 Supp 3): s306–s308

Carraccio, C., Wolfsthal, S.D., Englander, R., Ferentz, K., and Martin, C. (2002). Shifting paradigms: from Flexner to competencies. *Acad Med.* 77(5): 361–367.

Case, S.M. and Swanson, D.B. (2002). *Constructing Written Test Questions for the Basic and Clinical Sciences*. Philadelphia: National Board of Medical Examiners (revised ed, first published 1996)

Challis, M. (1999) AMEE medical education guide no 11 (revised): portfolio-based learning and assessment in medical education. *Med Teach.* 21(4): 370–386

Cooke, M., Irby, D.M., Sullivan, W., and Ludmerer, K. (2006) American medical education 100 years after the Flexner Report. *N Engl J Med.* 355: 1339–1345

Dent, J.A., Angell-Preech, H.M., Ball, M-L., and Ker, J.S. (2001) Using the ambulatory care teaching centre to develop opportunities for integrated learning. *Med Teach.* 23(2): 171–175

Denz-Penhey, H. and Murdoch, J.C. (2010) Is small beautiful? Student performance and perceptions of their experience at larger and smaller sites in rural and remote longitudinal clerkships in the rural clinical school of Western Australia. *Rural and Remote Health.* (Online) 10(3), 1470. http://www.rrh.org.au/articles/showarticlenew.asp?ArticleID=1470 Accessed 19 February 2013

Dewey, J. (1938) *Experience and Education*. New York: Kappa, Delta, Pi

Dornan, T., Hadfield, J., Brown, M., Boshuizen, H., and Scherpbier, A. (2005) How can medical students learn in a self-directed way in the clinical environment? Design-based research. *Med Educ.* 39(4): 356–364

Dornan, T., Littlewood. S., Margolis, S.A., Scherpbier, A., Spencer, J., and Ypinazar, V. (2006) How can experience in clinical and community settings contribute to early medical education: a BEME systematic review. *Med Teach.* 28(1): 3–18

Dornan, T., Boshuizen, H., King, N., and Scherpbier, A. (2007) Experience-based learning: a model linking the process and outcomes of medical students' workplace learning. *Med Educ.* 41(1): 84–91

Eraut, M. (1994) *Developing Professional Knowledge and Competence*. London: Falmer

Flexner, A. (1910) *Medical Education in the United States and Canada; A Report to the Carnegie Foundation for the Advancement of Teaching*. New York: The Carnegie Foundation for the Advancement of Teaching

Frank, J.R., Snell, L.S., ten Cate, O. et al. (2010) Competency-based education: theory to practice. *Med Teach.* 32(8): 638–645

Freeman, A., van der Vleuten, C., Nouns, Z., and Ricketts, C. (2010) Progress testing internationally. *Med Teach.* 32(6): 451–455

Frenk, J., Chen, L., Bhutta, Z.A., Cohen, J., et al. (2010) Health professionals for a new century: transforming education to strengthen health systems in an interdependent world. *The Lancet.* 376: 1923–1958

Glasersfeld, E. (1989) Cognition, construction of knowledge and teaching. *Synthese.* 80(1): 121–140

Hamilton, J. (1999) Outcomes in medical education must be wide, long and deep. *Med Teach.* 21(2): 125–126

Harden, R.M. (1999) AMEE medical education guide no14: outcomes-based education: part 1-an introduction to outcomes-based education. *Med Teach.* 21(1): 7–14

Harden, R.M. (2000) The integration ladder: a tool for curriculum planning and evaluation. *Med Educ.* 34(7): 551–557

Harden, R.M. (2002) Learning outcomes and instructional objectives: is there a difference? *Med Teach.* 24(2): 151–155

Harden, R.M., Stevenson, M., Downie, W.W., and Wilson, G.M. (1975) Assessment of clinical competence using objective structured examination. *BMJ.* 1: 447

Harden, R.M., Sowden, S., and Dunn, W.R. (1984) Educational strategies in curriculum development: the SPICES model. *Med Educ.* 18(4): 284–297

Harden, R.M., Laidlaw, J., Ker, J.S., and Mitchell, H.E. (1996) AMEE medical education guide no 7: task-based learning: an educational strategy for undergraduate, postgraduate and continuing medical education part 1. *Med Teach.* 18(1): 7–13

Harden, R.M., Crosby, J., Davis, M.H., Howie, P.W., and Struthers, A.D. (2000) Task-based learning: the answer to integration and problem-based learning in the clinical years. *Med Educ.* 34(5): 391–397

Hirsh, D.A., Ogur, B., Thibault, G.E., and Cox, M. (2007) 'Continuity' as an organizing principle for clinical education reform. *N Engl J Med.* 356: 858–866

Hoffman, K.G. and Donaldson, J.F. (2004) Contextual tensions of the clinical environment and their influence on teaching and learning. *Med Educ.* 38(4): 448–454

Irby, D. (2011) Educating physicians for the future: Carnegie's call for reform. *Med Teach.* 33(7): 547–550

Jolly, B. (1994) *Bedside Manners: Teaching and Learning in the Hospital*. Maastricht: Universitaire Pers, Maastricht

Jolly, B. and MacDonald, M.M. (1989) Education for practice; the role of practical experience in undergraduate and general clinical training. *Med Educ.* 23(2): 189–195

Klement, B.J., Paulsen, D.F., and Wineski, L.E. (2011) Anatomy as the backbone of an integrated first year medical curriculum: design and implementation. *Anatomical Sciences Education.* 43(2): 157–169

Knox, J.D.E. (1989) What is . . . a modified essay question. *Med Teach.* 11(1): 51–57

Kolb, D. A. and Fry, R. (1975) Toward an applied theory of experiential learning. In C. Cooper (ed.) *Theories of Group Process* (pp. 33–58). Chichester: John Wiley & Sons

Krupat, E., Pelletier, S., Alexander, E.K., Hirsh, D., Ogur, B., and Schwartzstein, R. (2009) Can changes in the principal clinical year prevent the erosion of students' patient-centered beliefs? *Acad Med.* 84(7): 582–586

Lave, J. and Wenger, E. (1991) *Situated Learning. Legitimate Peripheral Participation*. Cambridge (UK): University of Cambridge Press

Leinster, S.J. (2003) Medical education in the real world. *Med Educ.* 37(5): 397–398

Magrane, D., Ephgrave, K., Jacobs, M.B., Rusch, R., Donoghue, G.D.,and Hoffman, E. (2000) Weaving women's health across clinical clerkships. *Acad Med.* 75(11): 1066–1070

Mahoney, S., Walters, L., and Ash, J. (2012) Urban community-based medical education: general practice at the core of a new approach to teaching medical students. *Aust Fam Phys.* 41(8): 631–636

McHarg, J., Bradley, P., Chamberlain, S., Ricketts, C., Searle, J., and McLachlan, J. (2005) Assessment of progress tests. *Med Educ.* 39(2): 221–227

McLaughlin, K., Bates, J., Konkin, J., Woloschuk, W., Suddards, C.A., and Regehr, G. (2011) A comparison of performance evaluations of students on longitudinal integrated clerkships and rotation-based clerkships. *Acad Med.* 86: S25–S29

McManus, I.C., Richards, P., Winder, B.C., Sproston, K.A., and Vincent, C.A. (1993) The changing clinical experience of British medical students. *The Lancet.* 341(8850): 941–944

Mezirow, J. (2000) *Learning as Transformation: Critical Perspectives on a Theory in Progress.* San Francisco: Jossey Bass

Miller, G.E. (1990) The assessment of clinical skills/competence/performance. *Acad Med.* 65(9): S63–S67

Neufeld, V.R. and Barrows, H.S. (1974) The 'McMaster Philosophy': an approach to medical education. *J Med Educ.* 49(11): 1040–1050

Neville, A.J. (2009) Problem-based learning and medical education forty years on. *Medical Principles and Practice.* 18: 1–9

Newmann, F.M., Marks, H.M., and Gamorgan, A. (1996). Authentic pedagogy and student performance. *Am J Educ.* 104(4): 280–312

Norcini, J.J., Blank, L.L., Duffy, D., and Fortna, G.S. (2003). The mini-CEX: a method for assessing clinical skills. *Ann Intern Med.* 138: 476–481

Norman, G.R. and Schmidt, H.G. (2000) Effectiveness of problem-based learning curricula: theory, practice and paper darts. *Med Educ.* 34(9): 721–728

Norris, T.E., Schaad, D.C., DeWitt, D., Ogur, B., Hunt, D.D. and members of the Consortium of Longitudinal Integrated Clerkships (2009) Longitudinal integrated clerkships for medical students: an innovation adopted by medical schools in Australia, Canada, South Africa and the United States. *Acad Med.*, 84(7): 902–907

Ogrinc, G., Mutha, S., and Irby, D.M. (2002) Evidence for longitudinal ambulatory care rotations: a review of the literature. *Acad Med.* 77(7): 688–693

Ogur, B. and Hirsh, D. (2009) Learning through longitudinal patient care-narratives from the Harvard Medical School-Cambridge integrated clerkship. *Acad Med.* 84(7): 844–850

O' Neill, P.A., Jones, A., and McArdle, P. (2003). Does a new undergraduate curriculum based on Tomorrow's Doctors prepare house officers better for their first post? A qualitative study of the views of pre-registration officers using critical incidents. *Med Educ.* 37(12): 1100–1108

O'Neill, P.A., Morris, J., and Baxter, C.M. (2000) Evaluation of an integrated curriculum using problem-based learning in a clinical environment: the Manchester experience. *Med Educ.* 34(3): 222–230

Oswald, N., Alderson, T., and Jones, S. (2001) Evaluating primary care as a base for medical education: the report of the Cambridge community-based clinical course. *Med Educ.* 35(8): 782–788

Prideaux, D. (2000) The emperor's new clothes: from objectives to outcomes. *Med Educ.* 34(3): 168–169

Prideaux, D. (2007) Curriculum development in medical education: from acronyms to dynamism. *Teaching and Teacher Education.* 23(3): 294–302

Prideaux, D.J. and Marshall, V.R. (1994) A 'common' surgery curriculum: health care delivery and undergraduate surgical education in Australian teaching hospitals. *World J Surg.* 18: 1–6

Prideaux, D., Worley, P., and Bligh, J. (2007) Symbiosis: a new model for clinical education. *Clin Teach.* 4(4): 209–212

Radwany, S.M., Stovsky, E.J., Frate, D.M., et al. (2011) A 4-year integrated curriculum in palliative care for medical undergraduates. *Am J Hospice Palliative Med.* 28(8): 528–535

Ramani, S., Orlander, J.D., Strunin, L., and Barber, T.W. (2003) Whither bedside teaching? A focus group study of clinical teachers. *Acad Med.* 78(4): 384–390.

Regehr, G. and Norman, G.R. (1996). Issues in cognitive psychology: implications for professional education. *Acad Med.* 71(9): 998–1001

Schmidt, H. (1998) Integrating the teaching of basic sciences, clinical sciences and biopsychosocial issues. *Acad Med.* 73: S24–S31

Schmidt, H.G. (1983) Problem-based learning: rationale and description. *Med Educ.* 17(1): 11–16

Schuwirth, L.W.T. and van der Vleuten, C.P.M. (2011) Programmatic assessment: from assessment of learning to assessment for learning. *Med Teach.* 33(6): 478–485

Seabrook, M.A. (2003) Medical teacher's concerns about the clinical teaching context. *Med Educ.* 76(3): 213–222

Spillane, J.D. (1960) New American Medical Schools. *BMJ.*;2: 778

Stagg, P., Greenhill, J., and Worley, P.S. (2009) A new model to understand the career choice and practice location decisions of medical graduates. *Rural and Remote Health*, (Online) 9, 1245. http://www.rrh.org.au/articles/showarticlenew.asp?ArticleID=1245 Accessed 19 February 2013

Starfield, B. (2007) Global health, equity and primary care. *J Am Board Fam Med.* 20: 511–513

Stark, P. (2003) Teaching and learning in the clinical setting: a qualitative study of the perceptions of students and teachers. *Med Educ.* 37(11): 975–982

Stone, M.D. and Doyle, J. (1996) The influence of surgical training on the practice of surgery: are changes necessary? *Surg Clin N Am.* 70(1): 1–10

Sweller, J. (1988) Cognitive load during problem solving: effects on learning. *Cogn Sci.* 12(2): 257–285

Taba, H. (1962). *Curriculum Development: Theory and Practice.* New York: Harcourt, Brace and World

Tolhurst, H.M., Adams, J., and Stewart, S.M. (2006). An exploration of when urban background medical students become interested in rural practice. *Rural and Remote Health* (Online) 6, 452. http://www.rrh.org.au/articles/showarticlenew.asp?ArticleID=452 Accessed 19 February 2013

Tresoloni, C.P. and Shugars, D.A. (1994) An integrated health care model in medical education: interviews with faculty and administrators. *Acad Med.* 69(3): 231–236

van der Vleuten, C.P.M. (1996) The assessment of professional competence: developments, research and practical implications. *Adv Health Sci Educ.* 1(1): 41–67

van der Vleuten, C.P.M. and Schuwirth, L.W.T. (2005) Assessing professional competence: from methods to programmes. *Med Educ.* 39(3): 309–317

van der Vleuten, C.P.M., Schuwirth, L.W.T., Scheele, F., Driessen, E.W., and Hodges, B. (2010) The assessment of professional competence: building blocks for theory development. *Best Pract Res Clin Obs Gynaecol.* 24: 703–719

van der Vleuten, C.P.M., Schuwirth, L.W.T., Driessen, E.W., et al. (2012) A model for programmatic assessment: fit for purpose. *Med Teach.* 34(2): 205–214

Veitch, C., Underhill, A., and Hays, R.B. (2006) The career aspirations and location intentions of James Cook University's first cohort of medical students; a longitudinal study at course entry and graduation. *Rural and Remote Health* (Online) 6: 537. http://www.rrh.org.au/articles/showarticlenew.asp?ArticleID=537 Accessed 19 February 2013

Vernon, D.T.A. and Blake, R.L. (1993) Does problem-based learning work? A meta-analysis of evaluative research. *Acad Med.* 68(7): 550–563

Walters, L., Prideaux, D., Worley, P., and Greenhill, J. (2011) Demonstrating the value of longitudinal integrated placements to general practice preceptors. *Med Educ.* 45(5): 455–463

Walters, L, Prideaux, D., Worley, P., Greenhill, J., and Rolfe, H.M. (2009) What do general practitioners do differently when consulting with a medical student? *Med Educ.* 43(3): 268–273

Walters, L., Worley, P., Prideaux, D., and Lang, K. (2008) Do consultations in rural general practice take more time when precepting medical students? *Med Educ.* 42(1): 69–73

Wass, V. and van der Vleuten, C. (2004). The long case. *Med Educ.* 38(11): 1176–1180

Wilkinson, T.J., Campbell, P.J., and Judd, S.J. (2008). Reliability of the long case. *Med Educ.* 42(9): 887–893

Wood, L., Hassell, A., Whitehouse, A., Bullock, A., and Wall, D. (2006) A literature review of multi-source feedback systems within and without health services leading to 10 tips for their successful design. *Med Teach.* 28(7): e185–e191

Worley, P. (2002) Relationships: a new way to analyse community-based medical education? (Part 1). *Education for Health.* 15(2): 117–128

Worley, P.S. and Kitto, P. (2001) Hypothetical model of the financial impact of student attachments on rural general practices. *Rural and Remote*

Health. (Online) 1: 83. http://www.rrh.org.au/articles/showarticlenew.asp?ArticleID=83 Accessed 19 February 2013

Worley, P., Silagy, C., Prideaux, D., Newble, D., and Jones, A. (2000) The Parallel Rural Community Curriculum: An integrated curriculum based in rural general practice. *Med Educ.* 34(7): 558–565

Worley, P., Esterman, D., and Prideaux, D. (2004a) Cohort analysis of examination performance of undergraduate medical student learning in community settings. *BMJ.* 328: 207–209

Worley, P., Strasser R. and Prideaux D. (2004b) Can medical students learn specialist disciplines based in rural practice? Lessons from students' self reported experience and competence. *Rural and Remote Health.* [Online] 4,388. http://www.rrh.org.au/articles/showarticlenew.asp?ArticleID=338 Accessed 19 February 2013

Worley, P., Prideaux, D., Strasser, R., March, R., and Worley, E. (2004c) What do students actually learn on clinical rotations? *Med Teach.* 26(7): 594–598

Worley, P., Prideaux, D., Strasser, R., Magery, A., and March, R. (2006) Empirical evidence for symbiotic medical education: a comparative analysis of community and tertiary-based programmes. *Med Educ.* 40(2): 109–116

Worley, P., Martin, A., Prideaux, D., Woodman, R., Worley, E., and Lowe, M. (2008). Vocational career paths of graduate entry medical students at Flinders University: a comparison of rural, remote and tertiary tracks. *Med J Aust.* 188(3): 177–178

Yardley, S., Littlewood, S., Margolis, S.A., et al. (2010) What has changed in the evidence for early experience? Update of a BEME systematic review. *Med Teach.* 32(9): 740–746

CHAPTER 7

Instructional design for medical education

John Sweller and Jeroen J. G. van Merriënboer

To overload the memory with a mass of facts which never become fairly organised into its structure, and which, never being revived, fade gradually but surely into oblivion is a wasteful and exhausting process.

James Cuming

Reproduced from *British Medical Journal*, James Cuming, 'Address in medicine', 2, p. 230, copyright 1892, with permission from BMJ Publishing Group Ltd

Introduction

Until recently, instructional design in medical education, as in most curriculum areas, has tended to proceed without reference to either human cognitive architecture or to quantitative tests of effectiveness. Procedures such as learning-by-doing and 'see one, do one, teach one' are used, not because aspects of human cognition suggested they should be effective, but rather because they have been used traditionally or are attractive to their proponents. In recent years, this situation has begun to change (van Merriënboer and Sweller 2010). There is an increasing realization that instructional procedures should be generated by our enhanced knowledge of human cognition and should be introduced to students only after they have been tested for effectiveness.

In this chapter, we will outline cognitive load theory along with the instructional procedures generated by the theory (Sweller et al. 2011) and also describe an instructional design model: four-component instructional design that is consistent with cognitive load theory principles (4C/ID; van Merriënboer and Kirschner 2012). Cognitive load theory takes an evolutionary view of human cognition. It categorizes knowledge in evolutionary terms, uses biological evolution as an information processing analogue of human cognition, generates instructional procedures and tests those procedures using randomized controlled experiments. We will begin by categorising knowledge from an evolutionary perspective (fig. 7.1).

Categories of knowledge

Knowledge can be categorized in an infinite number of ways. From an instructional perspective, the only categories that are important are ones that require instructional procedures that differ from each other. If a division of knowledge results in categories that require identical instructional procedures, then those categories are irrelevant from an instructional design perspective. One category system that has important instructional consequences was

introduced by Geary (2007, 2008, 2012). He used an evolutionary approach to distinguish between biologically primary and secondary knowledge.

Biologically primary knowledge

Biologically primary knowledge is knowledge we have evolved to acquire over countless generations. It tends to be specific and modular. For example, we have evolved to recognize faces, learn to listen and speak, and solve general problems. These tasks bear little relation to each other. They probably evolved at different times among succeeding human or pre-human populations and so are modular and specific to different skills. They need to be learned but learning primary tasks tends to be automatic in that they do not require specialized instruction, tend to be learned easily, and frequently, are learned unconsciously.

Consider a child learning to listen and speak a first language. The child needs to learn his or her first language and may obtain considerable assistance from parents and others. Nevertheless, key aspects of language are learned but not taught. Children may learn to speak grammatically according to the grammar of their peer group but generally learn grammar without it being taught. Similarly, the complex process of speaking requires a precise coordination of lips, tongue, breath and voice. That knowledge is acquired from adults and other children but tends not to be taught. Despite the lack of tuition, for a normal child, learning to listen and speak a first language requires little more than membership of a functioning society.

The amount of knowledge associated with learning a first language may be larger than most biologically primary knowledge modules but is not unique. Learning to recognize faces, engage in basic social relations or solve problems also results in considerable knowledge but it is knowledge that we learn but do not need to teach. For example, we learn to solve problems using a means-ends strategy (Newell and Simon 1972) according to which we establish

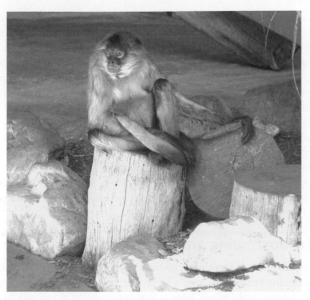

Figure 7.1 The information processing characteristics of cognition can be considered analogously to the information processing characteristics of evolution by natural selection.

our current problem state, establish a goal state, find differences between the two states and attempt to find problem solving operators that reduce those differences. There is no evidence that this ubiquitous strategy is teachable. We all use it without instruction. It can be classified as biologically primary knowledge that is acquired because we have evolved to acquire it.

While primary knowledge is extensive and critical to human cognitive functioning, it is not usually a part of instructional design and so is rarely explicitly taught because we have evolved to acquire it without instruction. In contrast, biologically secondary knowledge belongs to a different category that does require explicit instruction.

Biologically secondary knowledge

We have not evolved to specifically acquire secondary knowledge. It is required for cultural reasons and may vary from culture to culture. We have evolved to acquire secondary knowledge in a general sense rather than the modular manner in which we have evolved to acquire primary knowledge during different evolutionary epochs. We have not evolved to acquire a particular category or module of secondary knowledge but rather, are able to acquire any secondary knowledge in a similar manner. As a consequence, the cognitive processes associated with acquiring biologically secondary knowledge are different from those associated with the acquisition of primary knowledge.

Learning to read and write provides a useful contrast to learning to listen and speak. Reading and writing are biologically secondary skills, unlike the biologically primary skills of listening and speaking a first language. We can learn to read and write but we have not specifically evolved to do so. As a consequence, the manner in which we acquire reading and writing skills is different to the manner in which we acquire listening and speaking skills. While simple membership of a listening or speaking group is all that is required for us to learn to listen and speak, simple membership of a reading or writing group is likely to result in functional illiteracy for most

people. Writing was invented several thousand years ago but during most of that period, and in contrast to listening and speaking, only a minority of privileged individuals learned to read and write. Simple association with someone who knows how to read and write is insufficient for most people to acquire the necessary skills.

Reading and writing only became ubiquitous in some societies with the advent of modern mass education. Most people will not learn to read and write unless they are taught how to do so. Simple immersion in a reading and writing society is insufficient unlike the case of listening and speaking that will result in learning to listen and speak without explicit instruction.

Education was invented to assist people in the acquisition of biologically secondary skills that we have not specifically evolved to acquire but that have become culturally important. Some of that knowledge may have biologically primary components that can be used to assist in the acquisition of biologically secondary knowledge (Paas and Sweller 2012) but in essence, most of the knowledge is likely to be biologically secondary.

Medical education and biologically secondary knowledge

We have not evolved to acquire the knowledge imparted in medical curricula. It is overwhelmingly biologically secondary. There are general instructional consequences for medical education that flow from the distinction between biologically primary and secondary knowledge. If medical information is biologically secondary, it needs to be taught specifically and explicitly. 'Naturalistic' teaching techniques based on observations of the manner in which biologically primary knowledge is acquired may be inappropriate for the bulk of medical curricula. If so, techniques such as 'learning by doing' and 'learning-by-problem solving' may be misguided (Kirschner et al. 2006).

Requiring novice learners to find the solutions to problems that we have evolved to deal with is likely to be effective. It may be ineffective for problems we have not evolved to deal with. Learning to solve medical problems may be domain specific rather than domain general. We may have evolved to solve domain general problems as a biologically primary activity and so teaching learners to solve problems in general may be a futile exercise. We have not evolved to solve the domain-specific problems faced by medical practitioners. The solutions to those problems need to be taught explicitly.

Human cognitive architecture

If the content of medical education consists of biologically secondary knowledge, then the structure of human cognitive architecture associated with the acquisition of secondary knowledge is important. There is a well-defined cognitive architecture associated with biologically secondary knowledge. That architecture can be compared to the architecture that governs information processing during evolution by natural selection (Sweller 2003, 2011, 2012; Sweller and Sweller 2006).

While evolution by natural selection is conventionally considered as a biological theory explaining the creation of biological structures including species, it can also be considered in more general terms as an information processing system that occurs in nature. Human cognition has long been analysed in information processing terms. Furthermore, human cognition presumably

Table 7.1 Natural information processing principles

Principle	Function
Information store principle	Store information
Borrowing and reorganizing principle	Obtain information from other stores
Randomness as genesis principle	Generate novel information
Narrow limits of change principle	Limit the generation of novel information
Environmental organizing and linking principle	Provide unlimited, organized, tested and stored information to determine action appropriate to the environment

evolved using conventional evolutionary principles. We may theorize that the same information processing principles that underpin biological evolution also provide foundations for human cognitive architecture. We will consider human cognition and evolution by natural selection as analogous natural information processing systems that can be described by five basic principles. Table 7.1 summarizes those principles.

The information store principle

Natural information processing systems rely on a large store of information in order to function. We have long known that all genomes rely on an extensive store of DNA-based information, although there is no agreed method for measuring genomic size (Portin 2002; Stotz and Griffiths 2004). That large information store is required to allow organisms to deal with a complex and variable environment. The larger the store of information held in a genome, the better an organism should be able to deal with environmental variations.

The human cognitive system equally relies on a large information store in order to function. Long-term memory provides that store. The centrality of long-term memory to cognition became clear in research on the game of chess carried out by De Groot (De Groot 1965; De Groot and Gobet 1996). Chess is a problem-solving game and at least on the surface, long-term memory appears to play at best, a superficial role in chess expertise. In fact, it is crucial.

In some of the most important experiments on cognitive processes, De Groot demonstrated that chess expertise was critically dependent on long-term memory. His comparison of weekend players with chess grand masters revealed no differences in general problem solving skills. How are chess masters able to choose good moves when their search for such moves appears to be identical to weekend players? De Groot showed both weekend players and masters a board configuration taken from a real game for 5 seconds. He then took the board configuration away and asked the players to reproduce it on a new board. The results were startling. Masters were able to reproduce the recently seen board with an accuracy rate of about 70% while weekend players had an accuracy of about 30%. Chase and Simon (1973) reproduced these results and in addition, demonstrated that they could not be obtained using random board configurations. Both weekend players and masters were equally poor on this task. Masters were only superior on board configurations taken from real games.

These results, which have been replicated in a variety of educationally relevant areas (Chiesi et al. 1979; Egan and Schwartz 1979; Jeffries et al. 1981; Sweller and Cooper 1985) provide us with the source of problem solving skill. We are skilful in an area in which we have extensive, domain knowledge allowing us to recognize problem states and the best moves associated with each state. For substantive areas, it can take 10 years or more to acquire the knowledge associated with high levels of problem solving skills (Ericsson and Charness 1994). That knowledge is stored in long-term memory. A large store of information is just as important to human cognition as to evolution by natural selection. In medical education, the acquisition of that store of biologically secondary knowledge held in long-term memory is the only procedure we have available to us to facilitate problem solving skills.

The borrowing and reorganizing principle

The information store principle indicates that natural information processing systems include a large store of information. The question immediately arises, how is that information acquired? In the case of evolutionary biology, the answer is well known. The vast bulk of the information of any individual genome is borrowed from ancestor genomes via asexual or sexual reproduction. In the case of sexual reproduction, male and female genetic information is combined to produce a new genome that, by necessity, differs from all ancestor genomes and indeed, all other genomes apart from the special case of identical siblings.

The borrowing and reorganizing principle is equally important as a cognitive principle. The vast bulk of the information held in long-term memory is acquired from the long-term memories of other people. We imitate other people (Bandura 1986), listen to what they say, and read what they write. Of course, the information we obtain is not copied exactly as in the case of asexual reproduction. Rather, it is reorganized as in the case of sexual reproduction. Information obtained from others is combined with information already held in long-term memory to provide new, schematic knowledge (Bartlett 1932; Piaget 1928). That knowledge, held in long-term memory, governs most human behaviour, including problem solving.

The borrowing and reorganizing principle is central to all educational endeavour, none more so than medical education. The knowledge medical students must assimilate comes from other people. To some, that may seem self-evident but some more recent reforms of medical education appear to, at least in part, ignore the borrowing and reorganizing principle by placing an emphasis on 'naturalistic' learning and learning through unguided problem solving (Kirschner et al. 2006). Such procedures are appropriate for the acquisition of biologically primary knowledge but inappropriate for the biologically secondary knowledge that constitutes medical curricula. Indeed, there is some evidence that problem-solving can interfere with learning (Sweller 1988).

The randomness as genesis principle

While information can be borrowed from other people, at some point it must be created. The randomness as genesis principle provides the necessary machinery for the creation of novel information.

Under different nomenclature, the randomness as genesis principle has been well-established and accepted in evolutionary biology for a long time. Evolution by natural selection assumes that all variation between individuals and species ultimately can be traced to random mutations. Without those initial random mutations, no biological variation could occur. Of course, in order to be adaptive, random mutation must be coupled with natural selection. Natural selection provides a test of the extent to which a mutation is adaptive with adaptive mutations resulting in increased reproduction rates and maladaptive mutations resulting in extinction.

For human cognitive architecture, problem solving plays the same role as random mutation and natural selection play in biological evolution. The purpose, in both cases, is to generate novelty and creativity (Sweller 2009). 'Random generation and test' provide the core of human problem solving. Ultimately, as is the case with biological evolution, all creative problem-solving depends on random generation of problem-solving moves. The effectiveness of those moves depends on the platform of knowledge provided by the information store principle but once the limits of that knowledge has been reached, no alternative to random generation and test has been discovered. Thus, while most information held in long-term memory is obtained from other people, a small amount of information may be created during problem-solving using a 'generate and test' procedure. If useful, that information may be transmitted to other people via the borrowing and reorganizing principle.

From this analysis, it follows that teaching people to be creative and to solve novel problems would require us to teach them how to engage in a random generation and test procedures while problem solving. Such teaching is likely to be unsuccessful, if only because there is no body of literature indicating that teaching general problem solving techniques applicable to novel problems is effective. Furthermore, there are theoretical grounds for suggesting that such techniques are unlikely to be successful. It may be reasonable to hypothesize that random generate and test when problem solving is a biologically primary skill that is acquired without tuition. If so, attempts to teach students how to engage in random generate and test will fail when dealing with students who have already acquired the technique as biologically primary knowledge. Accordingly, teaching medical students to be good problem solvers when dealing with completely novel problems may be futile. As indicated earlier, problem-solving skill derives from domain specific knowledge held in long-term memory—that knowledge is both teachable and learnable. Domain specific medical knowledge is biologically secondary, is unlikely to have been acquired by novice medical students, and needs to be explicitly taught and learned.

The narrow limits of change principle

The randomness as genesis principle has structural implications for natural information processing systems. If the acquisition of novel information has random components, it is important that information processing systems have structures in place to ensure that the effectiveness of an information store is not compromised by large, rapid, random changes. Changes need to be small and tested for effectiveness before being permanently stored. Both biological evolution and human cognition have the required structure although that structure is better known and better specified in human cognition than in evolutionary biology and so will be discussed first.

Novel, biologically secondary information must be processed by a working memory that has well-known characteristics associated with its severe limitations. We have known at least since Miller (1956) that working memory is limited in its capacity to hold and process novel information. We can hold no more than about seven items of information in working memory and depending on the nature of the items, can process no more than about two to four items of information (Cowan 2001), where processing refers to combining, contrasting or dealing with items in a manner that requires us to relate items in some manner. In addition, we have known at least since Peterson and Peterson (1959) that we cannot retain novel items in working memory for more than about 20 seconds without rehearsal. It needs to be noted that these limitations apply only to novel items. Working memory has different characteristics when dealing with familiar items.

Working memory processes novel information prior to that information being stored in long-term memory. We can see the necessity of a limited working memory when dealing with novel information by considering the consequences of the previous principle, the randomness as genesis principle. Consider the means involved in processing three to four items. There are a limited number of ways in which three to four items can be combined. According to the randomness as genesis principle, if they are novel items they must be combined randomly and tested for effectiveness, assuming no knowledge is held in long-term memory that indicates strategies to be used in determining which combinations are likely to be effective. A working memory that can process a large number of items in this manner would have either no positive consequences or even negative consequences because once more than about seven items are considered, there are millions of possible permutations. It is efficient to process a few items, test them for effectiveness and store effective combinations. It may be impossible to similarly deal with millions of possible combinations. If the amount of information processed in working memory must be small due to capacity and time limitations, all changes to long-term memory must also be small, reducing the chances of a large, catastrophic change that might affect the functionality of long-term memory.

Changes to a genome are similarly small and incremental. Large, rapid changes are likely to be dysfunctional. Genomic changes influenced by the environment are governed by the epigenetic system (Jablonka and Lamb 1995, 2005; West-Eberhard 2003) that may have a similar function to working memory. Both working memory and the epigenetic system act as an intermediary between the environment and the information store. Information from the environment can affect when and where DNA mutations occur with environmental signals facilitating or inhibiting mutations in particular parts of a genome. For example, some organisms increase the number of mutations under stressful conditions in order to ensure sufficient variety for survival of at least some individuals. The epigenetic system, acting as an intermediary between the environment and a genome, facilitates these mutations.

The limitations of working memory are critical to instructional design in all areas, including medical education. While these limitations do not apply to biologically primary information because we have evolved to test appropriate combinations of biologically primary items and so the combinatorial explosions discussed earlier do not apply, medical education is concerned with biologically secondary information where working memory limitations do apply. Cognitive load theory has been used to devise instructional techniques that take into consideration the characteristics of working memory when dealing with biologically secondary information.

The environmental organizing and linking principle

This principle provides a justification and purpose for the preceding principles. Again, it applies equally to biological evolution and human cognition. The epigenetic system not only influences the number and location of mutations, it also switches genetic information held in a genome, on and off. As was the case for the narrow limits of change principle, the epigenetic system again acts as an intermediary between the environment and a genome (Jablonka and Lamb 1995, 2005; West-Eberhard 2003). The profound influence of the epigenetic system can be seen by observing the diverse structures and functions of different cells with identical genetic information. Consider two cells found in different organs of the human body, for example, a skin cell and a liver cell. These two cells differ in both structure and function. Yet for any individual, the genetic information held in their nuclei is identical and so the vast differences between the two cells cannot be established purely by genetic factors. The differences between the cells are determined by the epigenetic system acting as an intermediary between the environment and genetic information. A major function of the epigenetic system is to activate or inactivate genes. Which genes are activated will ensure that the structure and function of any given cell is appropriate for its environment.

Working memory has a similar function in human cognition. At any given time, only a tiny amount of the information held in long-term memory is relevant for a particular set of environmental conditions. Working memory determines which knowledge is brought from long-term memory to appropriately coordinate with given environmental conditions in the same way as the epigenetic system determines which genes are turned on or off depending on the environmental conditions.

The characteristics of information obtained by working memory from long-term memory are different from the characteristics of information obtained from the environment. Unlike environmental information that arrives in working memory in a random and disorganized fashion, information stores such as long-term memory contain information that has already been organized. There is no need for a random generate-and-test process as indicated by the randomness as genesis principle and so there is no need for the information to have capacity or time limits. Accordingly, when information is brought from long-term to working memory, it has no discernible capacity or time limits. The differing characteristics of working memory when it deals with information from the environment as opposed to information from long-term memory has resulted in some theorists proposing a new cognitive structure: long-term working memory, with a much larger capacity and longer time limits than short-term working memory (Ericsson and Kintsch 1995). Long-term working memory provides an example of the purpose and function of the environmental organizing and linking principle.

It is a truism that knowledge changes us. The environmental organizing and linking principle along with the preceding principles on which it relies, indicate how that change occurs. Together, these principles describe a cognitive architecture that can be used to generate instructional procedures. Cognitive load theory uses this architecture to determine instructional procedures, including procedures relevant to medical education.

Element interactivity and categories of cognitive load

The cognitive load imposed on working memory depends on the number of elements of information that must be processed simultaneously while learning (Sweller 2010). In turn, that number is dependent on the extent to which elements interact. Interacting elements must be processed simultaneously and so impose a heavy working memory load while non-interacting elements can be processed individually resulting in a reduced working memory load. There are two basic sources of element interactivity, referred to as intrinsic and extraneous cognitive load along with an ancillary source, germane cognitive load that is closely associated with intrinsic load.

Intrinsic cognitive load

Intrinsic cognitive load is the working memory load that is intrinsic to the information being assimilated. It is immutable in the sense that it cannot be altered other than by changing what is learned or by changing the expertise of the learners dealing with the information.

Consider a student who must learn about the circulation of the blood in the heart, lungs, and body. In order to understand the process, the basic, relevant anatomy along with the appropriate nomenclature must be learned. The student must learn the location and names of the left atrium, the right ventricle, the valves, and the blood vessels. The task can be difficult because there are many separate anatomical structures. While the task may be difficult, it does not impose a heavy working memory load because the name, geometry, and general location of each structure can be learned independently of every other structure. Learning the anatomy of the lungs can be learned independently of learning the anatomy of the ventricles. Because the elements can be considered independently, element interactivity is low and so intrinsic cognitive load is low.

As well as learning the basic anatomy of these systems, the student also must learn the manner in which the blood is circulated. To understand the circulatory system, much of the system must be considered simultaneously because all of its components interact, resulting in high element interactivity. Understanding the function of the mitral valve requires learners to understand the function of the left atrium and the left ventricle. Understanding why the heart has four chambers requires an understanding of how they interact with each other and with the lungs and the rest of the body. All of these interacting elements must be processed simultaneously in working memory resulting in a heavy intrinsic cognitive load. It is a difficult task that historically, took humans a long time to discover, despite knowledge of the basic structures.

While a low element interactivity task such as learning the names and geometry of individual structures may be difficult if there are many structures, a high element interactivity task is difficult for a different reason. Such a task is difficult because it imposes a heavy, working memory load. Learning how the blood circulates in the heart, lungs and body may be difficult due to a high, intrinsic cognitive load. Learning the individual components of the circulatory system may be difficult because of the many elements that must be learned, not because they impose a high working memory load. This distinction has instructional implications.

Once interacting elements have been learned, they combine together into a single schema stored in long-term memory. That schema can be brought into working memory with, as indicated by the environmental organizing and linking principle, minimal working memory load. For someone familiar with the circulation of the blood in the human body, the interacting elements are incorporated in a schema stored in long-term memory. Thus, learning alters the negative consequences of high element interactivity.

Extraneous cognitive load

Differing levels of element interactivity are not only caused by the intrinsic nature of the information being processed. They also are caused by the manner in which the information is communicated to learners. Some forms of communication and some teaching techniques unnecessarily increase levels of element interactivity and so impose an extraneous cognitive load that can be reduced by changing instructional procedures. Here is one example.

Problem-solving is frequently used during instruction. Learners are required to solve problems whenever they are asked to answer a question such as a science question or an essay question. The most common problem-solving strategy used by problem solvers is means–ends analysis (Newell and Simon 1972; Sweller 1988). There are several characteristics of means–ends analysis that are relevant. First, while a means–ends strategy is applied to biologically secondary information, the strategy itself is probably biologically primary. As far as we are aware, there are no examples of successfully teaching the strategy. We all use it automatically because we acquired it as a biologically primary skill. Second, the strategy imposes a heavy, extraneous cognitive load. It requires learners to consider their current problem state, the goal state, differences between the current state and the goal, problem-solving operators that can be used to reduce any difference found, and any sub-goals that have been established. These interacting elements all must be processed simultaneously resulting in high-element interactivity. As a consequence, when dealing with unfamiliar, biologically secondary information, using this strategy can be taxing of working memory resources. Lastly, the use of means–ends analysis is unrelated to learning. It is possible to use the strategy, obtain a problem solution and learn nothing from the exercise because all working memory resources are devoted to dealing with the interacting elements required by the strategy, leaving few resources available for transferring learned information to long-term memory.

Germane cognitive load and the additive effect of intrinsic and extraneous cognitive load

Germane cognitive load refers to the working memory resources devoted to dealing with intrinsic cognitive load. Working memory resources devoted to dealing with intrinsic cognitive load are germane to learning. The more working memory resources can be devoted to the elements of information associated with intrinsic cognitive load, the more is learned. In contrast, the more working memory resources are devoted to the elements of information that are not germane to learning and so cause extraneous cognitive load, the less is learned.

The resources of working memory are devoted entirely to handling intrinsic and extraneous cognitive load, which are additive. Working memory does not distinguish between element interactivity sourced from intrinsic or extraneous cognitive load.

Consequently, any increase in extraneous cognitive load reduces the working memory resources available to handle intrinsic cognitive load resulting in a decrease in germane resources devoted to learning. Instruction should aim to increase the germane resources devoted to dealing with intrinsic cognitive load and decrease the resources that must deal with extraneous cognitive load. Since intrinsic cognitive load cannot be changed except by changing the nature of what is learned or the expertise of the learners, a decrease in extraneous cognitive load is needed to increase the resources devoted to intrinsic cognitive load.

Cognitive load effects and instructional implications

The theory outlined earlier has been used to generate a wide range of instructional procedures, most of which are relevant to medical education. Each instructional procedure is based on a cognitive load theory effect derived from randomized, controlled experiments. In this section, we will describe the cognitive load effects and the instructional procedures that derive from them.

Worked example effect

The worked example effect occurs when showing learners how to solve problems enhances learning compared to having them solve the problems themselves (Cooper and Sweller 1987; Sweller and Cooper 1985). Searching for a solution requires learners to consider a far larger range of interacting elements than being presented with a solution resulting in a large increase in extraneous cognitive load and reduced learning. The effect was discovered using mathematical problems but it has since been demonstrated in a large variety of curriculum areas. In medical education, the worked example effect suggests that learning will be enhanced if learners are provided with demonstrations of problem solutions rather than being required to search for those solutions themselves. For example, one could ask novice students to study or criticize a ready-made treatment plan, rather than having them generate such a plan. Based on the worked example effect, studying a treatment plan should be superior to generating a plan.

Problem completion effect

Rather than present learners with a worked example, they can be presented with a partially completed problem and asked to complete the missing steps (Paas 1992; van Merriënboer 1990; van Merriënboer and de Croock 1992). Learners must carefully study the partial solution because otherwise they will not be able to complete it. Compared to solving entire problems, the problem completion effect is as effective as a worked example. In both cases, the provided solution or partial solution reduces the number of interacting elements with which students must deal. In medical education, one could, for example, let medical interns observe a surgical operation and only perform part of it, rather than having them perform the whole operation independently.

Split-attention effect

Split-attention occurs when, in order to understand information, learners must split their attention between two or more sources of information (Ayres and Sweller 2005; Sweller et al. 1990). For example, a diagram that is unintelligible without text and text that is unintelligible without the diagram must be processed by splitting attention between both. In order to process the information, attention must be devoted to one source, working memory must hold the information, and then the other source of information must be searched in order to find relevant referents. Element interactivity can be high. It can be reduced by integrating the diagram and text. By placing text at appropriate places on the diagram or using alternative means to indicate to students which textual materials refer to which aspects of the diagram, search for referents and element interactivity is reduced (Khalil et al. 2005; Khalil et al. 2008). It should be noted that while diagram/text split-attention is used here as an example, any two or more sources of information that cannot be understood in isolation produce split-attention that can be reduced by integrating the information sources in space or time (Ayres and Sweller 2005). Split-attention applies equally to information that is unnecessarily split in a temporal fashion as well as physically. For example, in medical education you can provide students instructions for operating a piece of medical equipment just-in-time, precisely when they need it, rather than providing the instructions weeks beforehand.

Modality effect

The modality effect occurs using the same categories of information required by the split-attention effect. It requires multiple sources of information that refer to each other and so must be integrated in order to be intelligible. Rather than physically integrating multiple sources of information such as a diagram and text, the textual information can be converted from written to spoken information. A comparison of visual only information in which all sources of information are presented in a visual form with dual modality information in which some of the information is presented in an auditory form indicates an advantage for the spoken information plus the visual (Mousavi, Low, and Sweller 1995; Tindall-Ford, Chandler, and Sweller 1997), resulting in the modality effect.

From a theoretical perspective, the modality effect occurs because presenting all information in a visual form overloads the visual processor. Working memory includes two partially independent processors, the 'visual–spatial sketchpad' that deals with visual information and the 'phonological loop' that deals with auditory information (Baddeley 1986, 1992, 1999). If all information is presented in a visual form, the visual system may become overloaded. By off-loading some of the information to the auditory system, the load on the visual system is reduced and learning may be facilitated. Furthermore, we may have evolved to look at an object while listening to a description of some of its characteristics. In other words, looking at and listening to a description of an object may be biologically primary resulting in biologically primary knowledge being used to facilitate the acquisition of biologically secondary information (Paas and Sweller 2012). There are many potential areas of medical education in which dual mode instruction may be beneficial. For example, one may give students spoken explanations when they study a computer animation of the working of the digestive tract, rather than written explanations on the screen.

Transient information effect

The modality effect has been obtained using relatively short auditory statements. It cannot be obtained using long, complex statements (Leahy and Sweller 2011). When converting written into spoken text, we also are converting permanent into transitory information. When considering a long, complex statement that includes a large number of novel interacting elements, we are unlikely to be able to process that statement in working memory. If the statement is presented in written form, relevant sections can be repeatedly reconsidered without memorizing the entire statement because written statements remain permanently available. In contrast, spoken statements are transient. If a statement is presented in spoken form, the entire statement may need to be memorized in order to be reconsidered because it may be difficult to return to the original version. Accordingly, as statements become longer and more complex, the modality effect is likely to first disappear and then reverse (a result obtained by Leahy and Sweller 2011). Similar results are likely to be obtained using other forms of transient information such as animations. The problem can be alleviated by incorporating pauses in the transient information to reduce the number of interacting elements allowing easier memorization. For example, in medical education, if spoken explanatory text accompanies a long and complex animation showing the working of the human cardiovascular system, it may be helpful to divide the animation into segments or to give the learner the opportunity to stop and replay the animation.

Redundancy effect

The redundancy effect occurs when additional information is presented that is not required for learning. If that additional information is processed in working memory, the additional elements impose an extraneous cognitive load. Whether information is redundant and imposes an extraneous cognitive load or is essential to learning depends on learner expertise and the relation between sources of information. In the section on the split attention effect, we discussed two sources of information, diagrams and text that were unintelligible in isolation. In contrast to two or more sources of information that are unintelligible until they have been integrated, some text merely repeats the information in a diagram and depending on levels of expertise, is redundant because it is intelligible in isolation. Student attempts to mentally integrate the various elements of information are unnecessary and merely impose an extraneous cognitive load. The redundant text with its unnecessary elements should be eliminated rather than integrated with the diagram. There are many forms of redundancy. Diagrams as well as spoken or written text can be redundant. Even the presence of machinery that students are learning how to use can be redundant (Sweller and Chandler 1994). In the medical education sphere, when providing learners with a diagram of the flow of the blood in the heart, lungs, and body, a statement verbally describing the flow is best eliminated (Chandler and Sweller 1991).

Expertise reversal effect

Based on the cognitive architecture discussed previously, all cognitive load effects are likely to be dependent on levels of expertise in a particular area. For novices, instructional technique A may be superior to technique B. With increases in expertise, that difference may reduce, disappear and then reverse resulting in technique B being superior to A and generating the expertise reversal effect (Kalyuga et al. 2003). For example, studying worked examples is superior to solving the equivalent problems, yielding the worked example effect. This effect is obtained with novice learners. As expertise increases, the worked example effect decreases and then reverses resulting in problem solving being superior to worked examples (Kalyuga et al. 2001). In general, the expertise reversal effect applies to all the cognitive load effects discussed in this chapter.

We can explain the expertise reversal effect by assuming that novices, who have not acquired schemas, have to deal with many interacting elements in areas where intrinsic cognitive load is high. Adding additional interacting elements due to the use of, for example, problem-solving rather than worked examples, or materials requiring split-attention rather than physically integrated information, results in extraneous cognitive load that inhibits learning. As expertise increases, the intrinsic cognitive load associated with an instructional area decreases because interacting elements are incorporated in schemas. Providing learners with, for example, detailed instruction such as worked examples may be redundant and increase rather than decrease the element interactivity due to extraneous cognitive load. In other words, once learners have acquired appropriate schemas, providing a worked example to study may be redundant and increase rather than decrease element interactivity and extraneous cognitive load resulting in a reverse worked example effect. Increased expertise has a similar effect for other cognitive load effects (Kalyuga et al. 2003).

Guidance fading effect

From the expertise reversal effect as applied to worked examples, it follows that initial instruction should incorporate many worked examples, those examples then should be replaced by completion problems with their inherent reduction in guidance, and completion problems in turn should be replaced with problems to solve as expertise increases. There are many examples of guidance fading resulting in superior learning when compared to either an emphasis on problems alone or an emphasis on worked examples alone (Atkinson et al. 2003; van Merriënboer 1990; van Merriënboer and de Croock 1992). Van Merriënboer and Kirschner (2012) also describe alternative forms of guidance fading related to the use of process worksheets, performance constraints, and tutor guidance and feedback. As an example in the field of medical education, when students are learning to catheterize, one may first provide them with step-by-step instructions and feedback, then only provide them with feedback, and finally provide no guidance at all.

Imagination effect

The imagination effect occurs when students, asked to imagine a concept or procedure, perform at a higher level than students asked to study the same concept or procedure (Cooper et al. 2001). Students in study groups are provided with instructional material and asked to study it in order to learn the concepts and procedures. Students in imagination groups are presented the same material but instead of being asked to study it, are asked to look at it, before turning away and attempting to imagine it. The imagination effect occurs when imagination instructions are superior to study instructions. Typically, only more expert learners yield the imagination effect with a reverse effect occurring for less expert learners, in accordance with the expertise reversal effect.

The imagination effect occurs because more expert learners need to entrench and automate schemas. They have sufficient working memory to imagine concepts or procedures because they have already acquired the schemas, which incorporate interacting elements. Imagining the information provides an effective form of practice. Less knowledgeable learners are unable to imagine complex concepts or procedures because they must process the large number of interacting elements in working memory, which may exceed working memory capacity and reduce or prevent learning. For less knowledgeable students, studying the material is likely to yield better results than attempting to imagine it, while more knowledgeable students have superior learning outcomes by imagining the information. The imagination effect can be used in medical education, for example, by asking medical students who need to practise physical examination in a skills lab to imagine all the actions that need to be taken before they start to practise. We might expect that having trainee surgeons imagine surgical procedures before practising them should be beneficial.

Intrinsic element interactivity effect

As indicated earlier, all cognitive load effects require a high level of intrinsic cognitive load. If intrinsic cognitive load is low, any increase in element interactivity due to extraneous cognitive load may have no or minimal effects because the increase in extraneous cognitive load may not exceed working memory capacity. Thus, none of the effects discussed in this section apply to areas of study that do not include a high level of element interactivity due to intrinsic cognitive load (Leahy and Sweller 2005; Sweller 1994; Sweller et al. 2011). For this reason, the effects discussed here only apply to some areas of medical education as indicated when discussing intrinsic cognitive load.

Isolated elements effect

This effect relies on altering intrinsic cognitive load rather than altering extraneous cognitive load. Some areas that students must assimilate have exceptionally high levels of element interactivity due to intrinsic cognitive load. That load may exceed working memory capacity. Attempting to assimilate such information may be futile until after schemas have been acquired and stored in long-term memory. Rather than attempting to have students engage in the difficult or perhaps impossible task of processing high element interactivity information, it may be preferable to reduce the element interactivity by only presenting some elements and asking students to learn those elements without connecting them to other, essential elements. Understanding will be compromised by this procedure but understanding can be subsequently acquired by presenting the same information again but this time with all interacting elements included (i.e. a spiral approach to teaching). Pollock et al. (2002) found that presenting high element interactivity information with some of the interacting elements missing followed by the same information with all of the elements was superior to presenting the information with all of the elements twice. As an example in medical education, one could give students tasks that require them to apply the basic physical principles of hydrodynamics, such as pressure–volume and pressure–flow relationships, before giving tasks that require them to apply a full model of how the blood flows through the circulatory system.

Variability effect

Like the isolated elements effect, the variability effect relies on varying intrinsic cognitive load but in this case, rather than reducing the number of elements associated with intrinsic cognitive load, the number of elements is increased. Paas and van Merriënboer (1994) found that if they increased the variability of worked examples, learning was enhanced. Increasing the variability of worked examples increases the number of interacting elements associated with intrinsic cognitive load because the nature of the task is changed. Instead of just learning a particular procedure, students must learn some of the limits of that procedure, such as where and when it should be applied. For example, in the field of medical education, learners learn best about diagnosing a particular disease if the clinical symptoms are demonstrated by patients with different genders, ages, physiques, and medical histories, and if the diagnosis is also illustrated by patients with similar symptoms who do *not* have the disease. Learning the conditions under which a procedure should be applied is obviously useful but it increases the number of interacting elements that learners must process. That increase in interacting elements requires more working memory resources so increasing cognitive load. Of course, to be successful, working memory must be able to handle the increased number of elements. If simply learning how to apply a procedure requires all or most of working memory's resources, then it is likely to be counterproductive to add variability.

Implications for curriculum and course design

Although cognitive load theory offers a useful and research-based set of effects it does not provide a systematic approach to the design of educational programmes, such as courses or curricula. Van Merriënboer's four-component instructional design model (4C/ID-model; van Merriënboer 1997; van Merriënboer, Clark, and de Croock 2002; van Merriënboer and Kirschner 2012) offers such a systematic approach and incorporates most of the cognitive load effects in a whole-task model, that is, a model where the learning process is driven by practice on whole, meaningful tasks (often real-life professional tasks). The central message of the 4C/ID-model is that environments for complex learning can be described by four interrelated blueprint components (see fig. 7.2):

1. *Learning tasks*: authentic whole-task experiences based on real-life tasks that aim to integrate knowledge, skills, and attitudes.

2. *Supportive information*: information helpful for learning and performing non-routine aspects of learning tasks (i.e. problem solving, reasoning, decision-making), explaining how a domain is organized and how problems in that domain are (or should be) approached.

3. *Procedural information*: information prerequisites for learning and performing routine aspects of learning tasks, specifying exactly how to perform these routine aspects.

4. *Part-task practice*: practice items provided to learners to help them reach a high level of automaticity for selected routine aspects.

Learning tasks

In a course or curriculum based on the four components, learners work on learning tasks (see the squares in fig. 7.2) that help them develop an integrated knowledge base in a sub process of schema construction called 'inductive learning', where they gain new knowledge from concrete cases and experiences. Therefore, each learning task should offer whole-task practice confronting the learner with constituent skills important for real-life task performance, together with their associated knowledge and attitudes (van Merriënboer and Kester, 2008). All learning tasks are meaningful, authentic, and representative for the tasks that a professional might encounter in the real world. In this whole-task approach, learners quickly develop a holistic vision of the task that is gradually embellished during the training.

A sequence of learning tasks thus provides the backbone of a training program for complex learning. A first requirement is that all learning tasks differ from each other on all dimensions that also differ in the real world, such as the context or situation in which the task is performed, the way in which the task is presented, the saliency of the defining characteristics, and so forth. For example, if learning tasks require the diagnosis of a particular disease, they should ask the learner to make this diagnosis in different contexts (e.g. hospital, home care), for differently presented tasks (e.g. paper-based case description, electronic virtual patient, simulated patient, real patient), and for different types of patients (e.g. different gender, age, cultural background). Organizing learning tasks in this manner allows learners to abstract more general information from the details of each single task (the *variability effect*). There is strong evidence that such variability of practice is important for achieving transfer of learning—both for relatively simple tasks (Paas and van Merriënboer 1994; Quilici and Mayer 1996) and complex real-life tasks (Schilling et al. 2003; van Merriënboer et al. 2006).

Obviously, the use of whole tasks in combination with high variability of practice will yield a high intrinsic load (van Merriënboer and Sweller 2005). Therefore, it is of utmost importance to make use of cognitive load effects that decrease both intrinsic and extraneous cognitive load. First of all, a course or curriculum will let

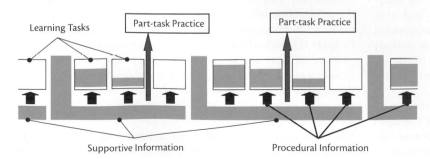

Learning Tasks

Part-task Practice

Part-task Practice

Supportive Information

Procedural Information

Figure 7.2 Instructional design.

learners start work on relatively simple but meaningful tasks and progress toward more complex whole tasks. Categories of learning tasks, each representing a version of the task with a particular level of complexity, are called 'task classes' (in fig. 7.2, the subsets of tasks separated by L-shaped figures). Learning tasks within a particular class are always equivalent in the sense that the tasks can be performed based on the same body of knowledge. A more complex task class requires more knowledge for effective performance than the preceding, simpler task classes in that some of the interacting elements are missing in the first task classes but are gradually added to later task classes. As a result, all tasks throughout the training program will be experienced by the learner as more or less equally difficult because as tasks become more complex, increasingly more knowledge and more embellished knowledge becomes available.

When learners start on learning tasks in a new, more complex task class, it is essential that they receive guidance to coordinate the different aspects of their performance (the *guidance fading effect*; see the grey shading of the squares in fig. 7.2). There are different approaches to fading guidance, such as the use of process worksheets, performance constraints, and tutor guidance (Renkl and Atkinson 2003; van Merriënboer and Kirschner 2012). One particularly effective approach is known as the completion strategy (van Merriënboer 1990; van Merriënboer and de Croock 1992) and has learners work in each task class from worked-out examples, via completion tasks, to conventional problems as they acquire more expertise. When learners begin to work on learning tasks in the first task class, or in a new task class at a higher level of complexity, they first study worked examples or case studies that confront them with useful solution steps (the *worked example effect*). They may answer questions about the effectiveness of the approach taken, possible alternative approaches or the quality of the solution. In a second stage, learners work on completion problems where they study a partial solution that must be completed (the *problem completion effect*). Obviously, they must carefully study the incomplete solution because otherwise they will not be able to correctly complete it. Only in the third and final stage do learners work on conventional problems or tasks. In this stage, they should have sufficient expertise to deal with the conventional problems at the level of complexity that is characteristic of the current task class. As an example in medical education, students who learn to set up treatment plans at a particular level of complexity (e.g. for patients with a single disease) may study and criticize ready-made treatment plans in the first stage, then finish partially completed treatment plans in the second stage, and independently develop whole treatment plans in the final stage. After learners are able to independently perform learning tasks up to the standard, at the given level of complexity, they may continue to the next task class. This process repeats itself until the final learning goals are met. Note that support and guidance thus follow a sawtooth-pattern throughout the whole educational program: They are high at the beginning of each task class and absent at the end of each one.

Supportive information

Most of the skills necessary to perform learning tasks are schema-based processes that are performed in a variable way from situation to situation; experienced task performers can carry out such skills effectively because they possess domain-specific knowledge in the form of cognitive schemas that can be 'interpreted' so as to be able to perform tasks in the task domain. These non-routine skills involve the different use of the same knowledge in a new situation. Obviously, learners need information in order to learn to perform non-routine aspects of learning tasks; this supportive information is what teachers typically call 'the theory' (see the L-shaped figures in fig. 7.2). Because supportive information is relevant to all learning tasks within the same task class, it is best presented before learners start to work on a new set of learning tasks at a higher level of complexity and kept available to them during their work on this task class. Supportive information then explains to learners how the learning domain is organized (aiming at the development of schemas called mental models) and how to systematically approach problems in the domain (aiming at the development of schemas called cognitive strategies). It helps learners to work on the problem solving, reasoning, and decision-making aspects of learning tasks within the same task class.

Instructional methods for the presentation of supportive information should facilitate schema construction such that learners are encouraged to deeply process the new information, in particular by connecting the new information to already existing schemas in memory in a sub process of schema construction called elaboration. Because the learning of supportive information typically yields high element interactivity, it is preferable not to present the supportive information to learners while they are working on the learning tasks (the *intrinsic element interactivity effect* and the *isolated elements effect*). Simultaneously working on a learning task and studying the supportive information would cause cognitive overload. Instead, supportive information is best presented before learners start working on a learning task. In this way, learners can construct a cognitive schema in long-term memory that can subsequently be activated in working memory during task performance. Retrieving the already constructed cognitive schema is expected to be less cognitively demanding than activating the externally presented complex information in working memory during task performance. Other effects that are directly relevant to the presentation of supportive information are the *redundancy effect* and *imagination effect*. Redundant information should be prevented and, especially for learners with higher expertise, instructions to imagine the supportive information might be more effective than instructions to study it.

Procedural information

Supportive information is important for the development of non-routine skills, but other skills necessary to perform learning tasks may be rule-based processes that are performed in the same way from situation to situation. Experienced task performers can carry out such skills fast, without errors, and largely without conscious forethought because they possess knowledge in the form of automated schemas that directly drive particular actions under particular circumstances, such as when the finger movements of a touch-typist are directly driven by reading the text. These routine skills involve the *same use of the same knowledge* in a new situation (i.e. the touch-typist uses the same finger movements regardless of whether the text is a science text or a history text). Obviously, learners need to be told how to perform the routine aspects of learning tasks; this procedural information is what teachers typically call how-to instructions (see the upward pointing arrows in fig. 7.2). Because procedural information specifies how to perform particular routine task aspects, it is best presented just-in-time, precisely when learners need it. For later learning tasks, as learners are able to perform the routine aspects without step-by-step instructions, those instructions can be faded away.

Instructional methods for the presentation of procedural information should facilitate schema automation such that learners construct cognitive rules in a subprocess of schema automation called 'knowledge compilation'. The term compilation is borrowed from computer science, where it refers to the translation of source code, which can be written in a regular word processor into machine code which can be executed by the central processor (cf. cognitive rules) (Anderson 1993). Procedural information has much lower element interactivity than supportive information and the development of cognitive rules requires that relevant information is active in working memory during task performance. Consequently, the *split attention effect* is important for the presentation of procedural information. Procedural information should be presented in such a way that it is optimally integrated with the learning task and the task environment. For example, how-to instructions for operating a particular control are best presented at the moment the control needs to be operated by the learner (just-in-time) and close to the control itself (nearby-in-space). The *modality effect* is also relevant: when learners are working on a visual learning task, how-to instructions are best presented in auditory form, but when learners are working on a verbal learning task, how-to instructions are best presented visually. Finally, the *transient information effect* indicates that for long procedures combined with long and complex how-to instructions, it may be necessary to incorporate pauses or to divide the procedure into segments (Spanjers et al. 2010).

Part-task practice

Learning tasks provide whole-task practice. Such whole tasks help learners construct general cognitive schemas (mental models, cognitive strategies) that may be flexibly interpreted to solve problems, reason, and make decisions in the domain (i.e. non-routine skills). In addition, they also help learners automate cognitive schemas containing cognitive rules that drive particular actions under particular circumstances (i.e. routine skills that need to be used frequently and without conscious control). Although learning tasks train both non-routine and routine skills, there are situations where it may be necessary to include *additional* part-task practice for routine skills in an educational programme. This is usually the case when a high level of automaticity is desired for particular aspects of a task and the learning tasks do not provide enough repetition to reach that level. For those aspects, additional part-task practice may be provided—such as when musicians practise specific musical scales (in addition to playing musical pieces) or surgeons practise on a simulator designed to teach how to operate instruments for minimally invasive surgery (in addition to conducting surgical operations). Instructional methods used for part-task practice facilitate a sub process of schema automation called strengthening, a process where cognitive rules accumulate strength each time they are successfully applied by the learner. Part-task practice for a particular aspect should only begin after it has been introduced in a whole learning task (see fig. 7.2). In this way, the learners start their practice in a fruitful cognitive context. After extensive part-task practice, automated routine skills may decrease the cognitive load associated with performing the whole learning task, making performance of the whole skill more fluid and decreasing the chance of making errors due to cognitive overload.

Conclusions

♦ Understanding human cognitive architecture is an essential prerequisite to effective instructional design in medical education.

♦ The manner in which humans process information is analogous to the manner in which evolution by natural selection processes information. Both are natural information processing systems.

♦ Such systems are used by cognitive load theory to provide an instructional design framework.

♦ In turn, that framework has been used to generate a range of instructional design effects based on randomized, controlled experiments indicating the relative effectiveness of cognitive load theory sourced instruction over alternatives.

References

Anderson, J. R. (1993) *Rules of the mind*. Hillsdale, NJ: Lawrence Erlbaum Associates

Atkinson, R., Renkl, A., and Merril, M. (2003) Transitioning from studying examples to solving problems: Effects of self-explanation prompts and fading worked-out steps. *J Educ Psychol*. 95: 774–783

Ayres, P., and Sweller, J. (2005). The split-attention principle. In: R. E. Mayer (ed.) *Cambridge Handbook of Multimedia Learning* (pp. 135–146). New York: Cambridge University Press

Baddeley, A. (1986) *Working Memory*. Oxford: Oxford University Press.

Baddeley, A. (1992) Working memory. *Science*. 255: 556–559

Baddeley, A. (1999) *Human Memory*. Boston: Allyn & Bacon

Bandura, A. (1986) *Social Foundations of Thought and Action: A Social Cognitive Theory*. Englewoods Cliffs, NJ: Prentice Hall

Bartlett, F. C. (1932) *Remembering: A Study in Experimental and Social Psychology*. Oxford: Macmillan

Chandler, P., and Sweller, J. (1991) Cognitive load theory and the format of instruction. *Cogn Instruct*. 8: 293–332

Chase, W. G., and Simon, H.A. (1973) Perception in chess. *Cogn Psychol*. 4: 55–81

Chiesi, H., Spilich, G., and Voss, J. (1979) Acquisition of domain-related information in relation to high and low domain knowledge. *J Verbal Learn Verbal Behav*. 18: 257–273

Cooper, G., and Sweller, J. (1987). Effects of schema acquisition and rule automation on mathematical problem-solving transfer. *J Educ Psychol*. 79: 347–362

Cooper, G., Tindall-Ford, S., Chandler, P., and Sweller, J. (2001). Learning by imagining. *J Exp Psychol: Appl*. 7: 68–82

Cowan, N. (2001). The magical number 4 in short-term memory: A reconsideration of mental storage capacity. *Behav Brain Sci*. 24: 87–114

Cuming, J. (1892) Address in medicine. BMJ.;2: 230

De Groot, A. (1965) *Thought and Choice in Chess*. The Hague, Netherlands: Mouton

De Groot, A., and Gobet, F. (1996) *Perception and Memory in Chess: Heuristics of the Professional Eye*. Assen, The Netherlands: Van Gorcum

Egan, D.E., and Schwartz, B.J. (1979) Chunking in recall of symbolic drawings. *Memory Cognition*. 7: 149–158

Ericsson, K.A., and Charness, N. (1994) Expert performance; its structure and acquisition. *Am Psychologist*. 49: 725–747

Ericsson, K.A., and Kintsch, W. (1995) Long-term working memory. *Psychol Rev*. 102: 211–245

Geary, D. (2007) Educating the evolved mind: Conceptual foundations for an evolutionary educational psychology. In: J.S. Carlson and J.R. Levin (eds.), *Psychological Perspectives on Contemporary Educational Issues* (pp. 1–99). Greenwich, CT: Information Age Publishing

Geary, D. (2008) An evolutionarily informed education science. *Educ Psychol*. 43: 179–195

Geary, D. (2012) Evolutionary educational psychology. In: K. Harris, S. Graham, and T. Urdan (eds) *APA Educational Psychology Handbook*

(Vol. 1, pp. 597–621). Washington, DC: American Psychological Association

Jablonka, E., and Lamb, M.J. (1995) *Epigenetic Inheritance and Evolution.* New York: Oxford University Press

Jablonka, E., and Lamb, M.J. (2005) *Evolution in Four Dimensions: Genetic, Epigenetic, Behavioral, and Symbolic Variation in the History of Life.* Cambridge, MA: MIT Press

Jeffries, R., Turner, A., Polson, P., and Atwood, M. (1981) Processes involved in designing software. In: J. R. Anderson (Ed.), *Cognitive Skills and Their Acquisition* (pp. 255–283). Hillsdale, NJ: Erlbaum

Kalyuga, S., Ayres, P., Chandler, P., and Sweller, J. (2003) The expertise reversal effect. *Educ Psychol.* 38: 23–31

Kalyuga, S., Chandler, P., Tuovinen, J., and Sweller, J. (2001) When problem solving is superior to studying worked examples. *J Educ Psychol.* 93: 579–588

Khalil, M.K., Paas, F., Johnson, T.E., and Payer, A.F. (2005) Interactive and dynamic visualizations in teaching and learning of anatomy: A cognitive load perspective. *Anat Rec (Part B: New Anatomy).* 286B: 8–14

Khalil, M.K., Paas, F., Johnson, T.E., Su, Y.K., and Payer, A.F. (2008). Effects of instructional strategies using cross sections on the recognition of anatomical structures in correlated CT and MR images, *Anat Sci Educ.* 1: 75–83

Kirschner, P., Sweller, J., and Clark, R. (2006) Why minimal guidance during instruction does not work: An analysis of the failure of constructivist, discovery, problem-based, experiential and inquiry-based teaching. *Educ Psychol.* 41: 75–86

Leahy, W., and Sweller, J. (2005). Interactions among the imagination, expertise reversal, and element interactivity effects. *J Exp Psychol: Appl.* 11: 266–276

Leahy, W., and Sweller, J. (2011) Cognitive load theory, modality of presentation and the transient information effect. *Appl Cogn Psychol.* 25: 943–951

Miller, G.A. (1956) The magical number seven, plus or minus two: Some limits on our capacity for processing information. *Psychol Rev.* 63: 81–97

Mousavi, S.Y., Low, R., and Sweller, J. (1995) Reducing cognitive load by mixing auditory and visual presentation modes. *J Educ Psychol.* 87: 319–334

Newell, A., and Simon, H.A. (1972) *Human Problem Solving.* Englewood Cliffs, NJ: Prentice Hall

Paas, F. (1992) Training strategies for attaining transfer of problem-solving skill in statistics: A cognitive-load approach. *J Educ Psychol.* 84: 429–434

Paas, F., and Sweller, J. (2012) An evolutionary upgrade of cognitive load theory: Using the human motor system and collaboration to support the learning of complex cognitive tasks. *Educ Psychol Rev.* 24: 27–45

Paas, F., and van Merriënboer, J.J.G. (1994) Variability of worked examples and transfer of geometrical problem-solving skills: A cognitive-load approach. *J Educ Psychol.* 86: 122–133

Peterson, L., and Peterson, M.J. (1959) Short-term retention of individual verbal items. *J Exp Psychol.* 58: 193–198

Piaget, J. (1928) *Judgement and Reasoning in the Child.* New York: Harcourt

Pollock, E., Chandler, P., and Sweller, J. (2002) Assimilating complex information. *Learn Instruct.* 12: 61–86

Portin, P. (2002) Historical development of the concept of the gene. *J Med Philosophy.* 27: 257–286

Quilici, J.L., and Mayer, R.E. (1996) The role of examples in how students learn to categorize statistics word problems. *J Educ Psychol.* 88: 144–161

Renkl, A., and Atkinson, R.K. (2003). Structuring the transition from example study to problem solving in cognitive skill acquisition: A cognitive load perspective. *Educ Psychol.* 38: 15–22

Schilling, M.A., Vidal, P., Playhart, R.E., and Marangoni, A. (2003) Learning by doing something else: Variation, relatedness, and the learning curve. *Management Science.* 49: 39–56

Spanjers, I.A.E., van Gog, T., and van Merriënboer, J.J.G. (2010). A theoretical analysis of how segmentation of dynamic visualizations optimizes students' learning. *Educ Psychol Rev.* 22: 411–423

Stotz, K., and Griffiths, P. (2004) Genes: Philosophical analyses put to the test. *History Philos Life Sci.* 26: 5–28

Sweller, J. (1988) Cognitive load during problem solving: Effects on learning. *Cogn Sci.* 12: 257–285

Sweller, J. (1994) Cognitive load theory, learning difficulty, and instructional design. *Learn Instruct.* 4: 295–312

Sweller, J. (2003) Evolution of human cognitive architecture. In: B. Ross (ed.), *The Psychology of Learning and Motivation* (Vol. 43, pp. 215–266). San Diego: Academic Press

Sweller, J. (2009) Cognitive bases of human creativity. *Educ Psychol Rev.* 21: 11–19

Sweller, J. (2010) Element interactivity and intrinsic, extraneous and germane cognitive load. *Educ Psychol Rev.* 22: 123–138

Sweller, J. (2011) Cognitive load theory. In: J. Mestre and B. Ross (eds), *The Psychology of Learning and Motivation: Cognition in Education* (Vol. 55, pp. 37–76). Oxford: Academic Press

Sweller, J. (2012). Human cognitive architecture: why some instructional procedures work and others do not. In: K. Harris, S. Graham and T. Urdan (eds), *APA Educational Psychology Handbook* (Vol. 1, pp. 295–325). Washington, DC: American Psychological Association

Sweller, J. and Chandler, P. (1994) Why some material is difficult to learn. *Cogn Instruct.* 12: 185–233

Sweller, J. and Cooper, G. (1985) The use of worked examples as a substitute for problem solving in learning algebra. *Cogn Instruct.* 2: 59–89

Sweller, J. and Sweller, S. (2006) Natural information processing systems. *Evol Psychol.* 4: 434–458

Sweller, J., Ayres, P., and Kalyuga, S. (2011) *Cognitive Load Theory.* New York: Springer

Sweller, J., Chandler, P., Tierney, P., and Cooper, M. (1990) Cognitive load as a factor in the structuring of technical material. *J Exp Psychol: Gen.* 119: 176–192

Tindall-Ford, S., Chandler, P., and Sweller, J. (1997) When two sensory modes are better than one. *J Exp Psychol: Appl.* 3: 257–287

Van Merriënboer, J.J.G. (1990) Strategies for programming instruction in high school: Program completion vs. program generation. *J Educ Computing Res.* 6: 265–285

Van Merriënboer, J.J.G. (1997) *Training Complex Cognitive Skills.* Englewood Cliffs, NJ: Educational Technology Publications

Van Merriënboer, J.J.G., and de Croock, M.B.M. (1992) Strategies for computer-based programming instruction: Program completion vs. program generation. *J Educ Computing Res.* 8:, 365–394

Van Merriënboer, J.J.G., and Kester, L. (2008) Whole-task models in education. In: J.M. Spector, M.D. Merrill, J.J.G. van Merriënboer, and M.P. Driscoll (eds.) *Handbook of Research on Educational Communications and Technology.* 3rd. edn (pp. 441–456). Mahwah, NJ: Erlbaum/Routledge

Van Merriënboer, J.J.G., and Kirschner, P A. (2012) *Ten Steps to Complex Learning.* 2nd. edn. New York: Routledge

Van Merriënboer, J.J.G., and Sweller, J. (2005) Cognitive load theory and complex learning: Recent developments and future directions. *Educ Psychol Rev.* 17: 147–177

Van Merriënboer, J.J.G., and Sweller, J. (2010) Cognitive load theory in health professional education: Design principles and strategies. *Med Educ.* 44: 85–93

Van Merriënboer, J.J.G., Kester, L., and Paas, F. (2006) Teaching complex rather than simple tasks: Balancing intrinsic and germane load to enhance transfer of learning. *Appl Cogn Psychol.* 20: 343–352

Van Merriënboer, J.J.G., Clark, R.E., and de Croock, M.B.M. (2002) Blueprints for complex learning: The 4C/ID-model. *Educ Technol Res Devel.* 50: 39–64

West-Eberhard, M. (2003) *Developmental Plasticity and Evolution.* NY: Oxford University Press

CHAPTER 8

Using concept maps in medical education

Dario M. Torre and Barbara J. Daley

A concept map is a cognitive networked structure characterized by concepts that take meaning from their interrelatedness.

Dario Torre (personal correspondence, 8th June 2013)

Introduction

According to Novak and Gowin's original work (1984 p. 15) 'a concept map is a schematic device for representing a set of concept meanings in a framework of propositions'. Concept maps are graphic representations that learners draw to depict their understanding of the meaning of a set of concepts. Concept maps are tools for knowledge organization and representation, by which students have the opportunity to summarize and analyse their ideas, visualize their thinking, therefore leading to a deeper understanding of study material. Concept maps demonstrate a student's mastery of a topic's attributes and relationships, for a greater development of holistic understanding. In this chapter we will elucidate the conceptual framework of concept mapping, describe the use of concept mapping in individual and group learning, and discuss issues related to scoring and assessing learning with concept maps.

Assimilation theory and meaningful learning

The theoretical underpinnings of concept mapping encompass the concept of meaningful learning, assimilation theory, and cognitivism.

In the cognitive approach to learning with concept maps, Ausubel's (1968, pp. 24–26) work and his assimilation theory of learning play a key role. Ausubel makes a crucial distinction between meaningful and rote learning. Meaningful learning occurs when learning can be related to previous knowledge and related to a preexisting cognitive framework. Rote learning, on the other hand, is not linked to a cognitive framework and often remains unretained and isolated.

Ausubel believes (1968) there are three types of meaningful learning: representational learning, propositional learning, and concept learning (fig. 8.1). Representational learning 'concerns the meaning of unitary symbols or words' (p. 43) and what they represent. Propositional leaning involves the learning of 'new ideas expressed in propositional form' (p. 43). Thus, in propositional learning the purpose is to learn 'the meaning of verbal propositions that express ideas' (p. 43) where the propositions are created by combining or relating individual words to each other. For propositional learning to occur, it is important to know the meaning of words or terms, and representational learning becomes almost a prerequisite for propositional learning to take place. In concept learning words that are related to form propositions actually constitute concepts, hence 'propositional learning largely involves learning the meaning of a composite idea generated by combining into sentences single words each of which represents a concept' (p. 43).

Finally, learning in a meaningful way involves the development of meaningful relationships among concepts, thus resulting in the creation of 'well integrated, highly cohesive knowledge structures that enable them to engage in the type of inferential and analogical reasoning required for success in the natural sciences' (Mintzes et al. 1998, p. 41). So Ausubel (1968) states that to understand a sentence there are two steps: first, perception of the meaning of the words, and second awareness of the meaning of the relatedness of the words, thus the importance of incorporating 'this perceived potential meaning within existing cognitive structures' (p. 57). This second step is crucial in meaningful learning because it allows the learner to anchor the new perceived proposition or word to ideas in the cognitive structure. Thus, through a meaningful relation of new material to established ideas and concepts in the cognitive structure, the learner is able to use existing knowledge as an 'ideational and organizational matrix for the incorporation, understanding and fixation of large bodies of new ideas' (Ausubel 1968, p. 58). For Ausubel (1968), the efficiency and importance of meaningful learning is related to two main characteristics: 'the non-arbitrariness, and the substantiveness of the learning task's relatability to cognitive structures' (p. 58). The non-arbitrariness of the process allows the learner to internalize new ideas, enabling them to use and exploit their previously acquired knowledge. It is indeed the non-arbitrariness that allows learners to relate new material to an existing cognitive framework in a meaningful way, and it is the

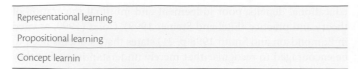

| Representational learning |
| Propositional learning |
| Concept learnin |

Figure 8.1 Three types of meaningful learning.

maintenance of what Ausubel calls 'arbitrary relatability' (p. 59) that extends retention 'through the anchorage of the new meaning to its corresponding established idea' (p. 59). Substantiveness is intended as the assimilation of the substance of ideas rather than the exact words, thus facilitating understanding, processing and retention. Therefore both characteristics are crucial for making new meaning, processing and retaining information.

The principle of assimilation is a key feature in Ausubel's (1968) concept of meaningful learning. Assimilation is intended as part of the process where a new potentially meaningful idea is 'related to and assimilated by an established idea' (p. 91) resulting in an interaction and meaningful product. The term assimilation 'is the hypothesized tendency for the new meaning to be "reduced" to the meaning of the more established idea' (p. 91). The assimilation hypothesis is important for two main reasons: the creation and retention of meaningfully learned concepts and the organization of new knowledge structures. Within the cognitive structures of the meaningful learning process, it is also important to understand the concept of progressive differentiation. Progressive differentiation explains the principles of how subject matter is organized from the most general ideas to more specific and less inclusive concepts. The theoretical basis for progressive differentiation is derived from two assumptions: first, the fact that 'it is less difficult for human beings to grasp the differentiated aspects of a previously learned more inclusive whole than to formulate the inclusive whole from its previously learned differentiated parts' (Ausubel 1968, p. 152). Second, the organization of material in regards to a subject matter in a learner's mind 'consists of a hierarchical structure in which the most inclusive idea occupies a position at the apex of the structure' (p. 5) and tends to progressively subsume less inclusive, more differentiated concepts.

Another important cognitive principle is that of integrative reconciliation. Integrative reconciliation is the explicit exploration of meaningful relationships among ideas, the identification of similarities and differences among ideas and the reconciliation of apparent or true inconsistencies. One of the major benefits of promoting integrative reconciliation is that creating meaningful relationships among ideas allows for discrimination. Thus, the learner can delineate clearly and precisely the similarities and differences between concepts, and might be able, by virtue of an enhanced discriminability, to learn with 'fewer ambiguities, fewer competing meanings, and fewer misconceptions' (Ausubel 1968, p. 157).

Many elements of the cognitive principles of Ausubel (1968), specifically within the framework of meaningful learning, have been applied and further elaborated by Novak and Gowin (1984) with their work on concept mapping. On the basis of Ausubel's cognitive framework, concept maps are a cogent application of meaningful learning in contrast to the rote learning concept where the learner tends to memorize information without relating it to previous knowledge, without creating meaning. Concept mapping facilitates meaningful learning. The learner's knowledge has to be relevant to previous knowledge, must contain concepts and propositions related to previous educational material, and must require the learner to make a conscious choice to learn in a meaningful way, by deliberately choosing 'to relate new knowledge to knowledge the learner already knows in some non-trivial way' (Novak 1998, p 19). In contrast to rote learning meaningful learning has several advantages: first, the knowledge acquired in a meaningful way leads to better retention because the information learned has a meaning, hence facilitating the learning of new related material; second, subsumption of information leads to a greater differentiation of concepts thus additional learning of related material, third; when learning occurs in a meaningful way it is more likely to be transferred to new problems or contexts.

In particular, concept mapping facilitates the student's ability to organize information, assess existing knowledge gains, develop insights into new and existing knowledge and transfer knowledge to new experiences. Also, evident from Ausubel's work, and used in concept mapping, is the opportunity to link new knowledge with previous knowledge, ultimately to not only create meaningful learning, but to contribute to the transfer of knowledge to future problems, thus fostering lifelong learning.

Concept learning and assimilation, as well as, propositional learning previously described, play a major role in scaffolding concept mapping. In concept assimilation 'the meanings for new concept labels are acquired when these labels are associated into propositions containing already known concepts' (Novak 1998, p. 41). In propositional learning the true meaning of concepts is provided by the way they are linked to one another to create a proposition, which becomes the main unit that makes up a meaning within the map. It is important to understand that the highest meaning we have for a concept 'increases exponentially with the number of valid propositions we learn that relate that concept to another concept' (p. 40). It is for this reason that concept maps are a way of representing knowledge frameworks related to meaningful, concept and propositional learning as being a representation of the knowledge structures of a learner.

A component of a constructivist approach (Dewey 1938) is also present in concept mapping, particularly in relation to the work of Novak (1984, 1977, &1998) and his view of human constructivism. Human constructivism is grounded in a number of important assumptions: first, human beings are creators of meaning; thus individuals construct meaning by making connections between new concepts and those that are part of a preexisting knowledge framework. Knowledge is an organized framework of meaningfully related concepts constructed by the learner. Second, teachers are facilitators of meaning making activities and conceptual change. Interaction, reflection, and active participation are learning activities that should be fostered and monitored by teachers to create meaning, sharing, and meaningful learning (Brookfield, 1995). Third, learners are seen as independent, meaning making individuals capable of restructuring knowledge by creating new relationships among concepts when supported by an environment that favors conceptual change and integration of concepts.

From a student's perspective, concept mapping encourages them to think independently, produces more self-confidence and provides an increased awareness of making connections across different areas of knowledge. Teachers reported that concept mapping assisted students to become active learners and organize theoretical knowledge in an integrative manner or conceptual framework (Boxtel et al. 2002; Harpaz et al. 2004).

In summary, Ausubel's concept of meaningful learning is crucial to the theoretical underpinning of concept mapping developed by Novak and Gowin. As previously stated, the goal of concept mapping is to foster learning in a meaningful way (Novak and Gowin 1984). Often, the outcomes of this type of learning are varied and unpredictable. However, the literature cites three main concept mapping outcomes:

1. To provide an additional resource for learning (Qadir et al. 2011)

2. To enable feedback (Anderson 2006) and

3. To conduct learning evaluation and assessments (MacNeil 2007; Roberts 1999).

According to Novak and Gowin (1984, p. 17), 'students and teachers constructing concept maps often remark that they recognize new relationships and enhance new meanings or, at least, meanings they did not consciously hold before making the map' Concept mapping also allows for the students to reflect on their own misunderstandings and take ownership of their learning. Concept mapping has the potential to provide students with an additional educational tool in order to understand the complex and vast amounts of required reading, and allows for the student to demonstrate interrelationships of particular topics to show a holistic knowledge of this understanding (Plotnick 2001). Many literature sources support the use of concept mapping as a beneficial and effective learning method (Novak 1990; Pinto and Zeitz, 1997; McCaghie et al. 2000).

As the medical profession continues to change, so do the educational methods by which students are taught, and concept mapping has been increasingly used in education. Irvine (1995) recognizes concept mapping as a means to promote meaningful learning and as a metacognitive strategy, and provides teachers with insights into misunderstanding, misconceptions or common errors (Boxtel et al. 2002; Edmondson and Smith 1998); Concept maps also provide a valuable tool to medical educators that reveal students' misunderstanding of concepts (West et al. 2002) identifying knowledge gaps or lack of understanding that need to be corrected.

In medical education, concept mapping has been shown to promote critical thinking skills among postgraduate trainees (West et al. 2000). More recently the literature has reported concept maps to be an innovative teaching strategy to facilitate understanding of challenging medical topics such as pathophysiology of fluid and electrolyte disorders (Calderon et al. 2011). They have also been used as an advance organizer to foster learning about a clinical topic such as respiratory failure (Cutrer et al. 2011). Concept maps have been shown to be helpful in educating patients with diabetes (Marchand et al. 2002), in facilitating learning of the pathogenesis of diseases (Kumar et al. 2011), as well as in enhancing retrieval practices when compared to different learning techniques in surgical training (Antonoff and D'Cunha 2011) . In relationship to feedback, concept mapping can assist the student in clarifying a topic; and teachers can use maps to provide feedback and to identify student misunderstandings (Roberts 1999)

Medical students are often enrolled in traditional curricula that use rote learning strategies in their basic science courses (Pinto and Zeitz 1997). However, this methodology will result in educational deficits, poor judgement and minimal integration of theory and practice (Eitel and Steiner 1999). Coles (1990; as cited in Edmondson and Smith 1998 p. 21) states that, 'students need to be encouraged to recognise that merely understanding what they are learning (deep-processing) is not in and of itself, sufficient. Students need to elaborate their knowledge to build up more and more complex networks to structure their knowledge'. When used as a supplemental learning tool, concept maps can potentially promote deep learning in medical and biomedical science education (Laight 2004). Although meaningful learning through concept mapping can be significant and stimulating, it is often difficult for teachers to move away from rote learning to meaningful learning (Harpaz et al. 2004; Novak 1990).

Concept mapping in the medical field allows the student to conceptualize a body of knowledge by identifying numerous cross-links between the concepts, thus serving as a useful tool for selecting and developing learning objectives regarding the topic (Weiss and Levison 2000). Finally, concept maps can help form a bridge from medical school to residency training by integrating new knowledge from the residency program with the knowledge acquired during medical school (Pinto and Zeitz 1997).

Teaching students to use concept maps

Because concept maps have been used to develop knowledge structures of students in the basic sciences as well as in graduate medical education (McGaghie et al. 2000; Gonzalez et al, 2008; West et al. 2000), their use in student and resident education can be a worthy goal to further understand cognitive processes. Often these processes cannot be revealed by traditional standardized tests and as such, the maps measure a student's evolving knowledge framework. According to Kinchin and Hay (2000), concept maps can reveal what each student knows and also can illustrate how the student understands and arranges knowledge in their individual minds. To fully understand the different ways that concept maps can be used in teaching and learning, two main different mapping techniques that are conceptually based on the degree of directedness of the map are presented here (Ruiz-Primo et al. 2004). Directedness of a concept map, which ranges from high to low, means that the concept map is 'characterized along a continuum from high-directed to low directed based on the information provided to students' (p. 101). A low degree of directedness map is characterized by a concept map that is entirely created by the learner in which concepts, linking lines, linking words and structure of the map is provided by the student (Novak and Gowin 1984). A high degree of directedness map is a tool where components of the map are provided by the teacher and the student has the task of filling in the blanks or creating some of the components, but mostly filling in the lines with linking words, or filling the content of nodes (Schau and Mattern 1997). The advantage of a high degree of directedness map is ease of administration and scoring for large-scale assessment where scoring of an entirely student constructed map is time consuming. On the other hand, such a technique of imposing a specific structure on the students' cognitive processes may limit the ability to assess the students' knowledge structures (Ruiz-Primo et al. 2004).

A concept map when used as learning tool may serve a number of purposes: First, maps can facilitate the identification of knowledge gaps, conceptual misunderstanding or misconceptions hence providing the opportunity for feedback focused on a specific domain, topic, knowledge area or mechanism (Roberts 1999; Morse and Jutras 2008; Edmonson and Smith 1998). Second, the cognitive processes associated with concept map development can provide a unique tool for reflection (Novak 1998) and help students reflect on their own learning process, by analysing their own experiences and linking them to previous learning experiences (Coffey et al. 2003; Daley et al. 2007). For example, students can be asked to develop a concept map on a course or clinical rotation that would allow the teacher to further explore aspects of the course that may need changes while encouraging the learner to reflect and think critically about their own learning process; Third, because one of the main premises of concept maps is to promote meaningful learning, learners can develop a concept map on a journal article, a book chapter or a simulated or real clinical scenario. This task helps students to further their understanding of the content, see the interrelationships of multiple themes, create new knowledge based on previous knowledge, and share the meaning of their learning with the teacher (Novak and Gowin 1984). Such processes become beneficial to both learner and teacher because they allow the educator to clearly visualize the knowledge structures of the learner and see the depth of the learner's understanding of a specific problem. Fourth, concept maps can be used in the integration of basic and clinical sciences in curricula. Because the maps focus on developing meaningful connections among concepts or domains, concept maps can be a valuable tool for an integrated curriculum, creating detailed models which allow instructors to combine key elements of basic sciences with clinical sciences in a meaningful way. For example a concept map on congestive heart failure may include the clinical presentation and diagnosis of the disease, the pharmacology related to the drugs needed to treat it, the pathology and physiology related to how the heart fails, as well as the biochemical processes that take place before or during the occurrence of the disease. Such a map allows educators to develop and visualize their integration process, share it with others and eventually communicate it to learners. It may greatly facilitate the process of collaboration in instructional course design and curricular models (Cristea and Okamoto 2001). Fifth, concept maps can be useful learning tools to foster clinical reasoning, critical thinking and problem solving skills (McMillan 2010; Pottier et al. 2010). Regardless of the concept mapping technique used, concept mapping stems from a conceptual framework that encompasses a number of key features of clinical reasoning, such as creation of meaningful and complex relationships, use of critical thinking in the context of ill-structured problems, hypothesis differentiation, information processing and pattern recognition, and use of semantic qualifiers. (Higgs and Jones 2008; Bordage 1994; Norman et al. 1992; Schmidt et al. 1990) As such, concept maps can serve students and residents as a valuable tool to practice and enhance clinical reasoning skills. For example the teacher may ask the student to construct a concept map on a specific topic or to complete a pre-constructed concept map and then ask the student to verbalize their thinking while the learner completes the map. This will shed light into the cognitive process of the learner. Sixth, one of most interesting ways concept maps can be used is to develop knowledge models (Willemsen et al. 2008; Castro et al. 2006) .Teachers may construct a series of concept maps linked together about a specific domain or topic or process that may provide integrated knowledge frameworks which may be particularly helpful to teachers and learners. This application may be useful to create cognitive and performance-based models, which can be applied to medical students' education and or residency training. For example, a number of teachers may develop a knowledge model that can be applied to the clinical performance of professional activities that involve several competencies such as patient care, clinical reasoning, medical knowledge, and professionalism. Concept maps will allow educators and eventually learners to easily visualize the content of the model, to elucidate how, when and where in the model aspects of different competencies can or should be linked to each other, providing opportunities for assessment. The use of concept maps in medical education can be broad and allow creativity. Based on our experiences, we provide some practical ideas and examples of how concept maps can be used.

Before starting any teaching endeavour with concept maps, it is of crucial importance to schedule an introductory session. In this session the instructor should explain the purpose of developing a concept map, how the maps fit into the course or material to be learned, clarify the educational value of the map, and demonstrate on whiteboard or using a computer mapping systems (see: http://cmap.ihmc.us/) how to create a concept map. It is helpful to present the students with an example of a concept map previously developed so that learners can review, ask questions and begin to understand what a concept maps is. Subsequently, students should be given the opportunity to develop a sample concept map, on paper or electronically, and give feedback on it. Such an introductory session may last 1–2 hours and can be repeated if needed. It is also important to keep in mind that it is often during this introductory period that teachers may discover learners' resistance to the use of concept maps and that the method of introduction of the maps can affect students' perceptions of using maps for learning (Santhanam et al. 1998). However, as students become familiar with developing concept maps and the timing and learning context for their introduction improves, students' perceptions of the usefulness of this learning strategy is likely to change (Markow and Lonning 1998; Laight 2004). Once an introduction has been completed, there are several ways (fig 8.1) to use concept maps with students:

1. Develop a concept map from scratch (fig. 8.2). The students can be assigned to develop a concept map on a topic of their choice. Such topics may range from a medical disease, to a complaint (for example difficulty breathing), or a patient they might have seen. The concept maps can be assigned to be developed at home or in class; however, an appropriate amount of time should be allowed. Although there is not a standard time, we believe that 30–60 minutes is a reasonable amount of time to allow students to complete such task. After completion of the concept maps the teacher should review them and use them as they deem appropriate. The teacher can meet separately with each student and ask about links or concepts to be clarified or explained, inquiring about the reasoning behind specific propositions used, concepts included or invalid links. Also the teacher can survey the students about their opinions at the end of the course. In a recent medical clerkship students were asked to develop three concept maps in a period of two months. In a thematic analysis of third year students' perceptions after developing those three concept maps, three themes about concept maps were identified. Students identified that the maps functioned as facilitators of knowledge integration and critical thinking, as a teaching methodology with

Table 8.1 Map techniques, learner and instructor tasks

Component	Learner tasks	Instructor tasks
Map technique and tasks	Develop map from scratch	May or may not assign topic
	Fill in the nodes	Constructs the skeleton of the concept map and may provide a list of concepts or linking words
	Fill in linking words	
	Fill in words and linking words	
	Connect concepts and create linking words	Does not construct the skeleton of the map but provides a list of concepts to be mapped
	Connect concepts by using linking words provided to construct the map	Does not construct the skeleton of the map but provides a list of concepts and linking words to be mapped
	Connect scripts and fill in nodes	Provides scripts and nodes to be filled
Scoring	Structural (hierarchy, propositions)	Scores the map based on Novak and Gowin system
	Relational using a criterion map	Develops with other teachers and experts a criterion map, then compares it
	Combination of structural and relational	Develops scoring based on components of structural and relational (use of a criterion map

great opportunities for feedback, and as a new and helpful learning method. One student stated, 'I think it is valuable in relating the concepts associated with a specific clinical problem. It makes relationships more apparent' (Torre et al. 2007).

2. Provide students with empty nodes to be filled in after a list of concepts was previously provided. This requires the instructor to create a partial map structure in a network of propositions on the basis of what they believe to be most valuable in showing the thinking process or conceptual understanding of a specific topic. Such an approach requires more preparation time on the part of the educator, also because a criterion or reference map should be developed in order to have something to compare with the student map. However, in our experience at times concepts elaborated by the student may still be valid even though they may deviate from the reference map. This type of map requires less cognitive effort on the part of the student.

3. Fill in linking words map. In this type of map the nodes or concepts are provided as well as the lines, yet the student has to fill the lines with linking words. Because the connection among concepts, as previously outlined, determines the meaning and the relatedness of concepts this type of map may give more insight into the mind of the students in relation to mechanisms of disease, provide a greater opportunity for the teacher to inquire about misconceptions, knowledge deficits, or inability to link and connect concepts. Also this technique is more challenging for the teacher who needs to develop a skeleton of the map and also develop a reference map to allow possible scoring or group or individual reviews with the students later on. This technique, similarly to that mentioned earlier, can be used by providing a list of linking words or by letting the learner develop the propositions among concepts on their own.

4. Another interesting technique is a mixed format of fill in the nodes and fill in the linking words (fig. 8.3). The teacher creates the skeleton of the map; however, they do not include or write

in specific concepts and/or linking words. Also the instructor may decide to provide or not provide a list of either concepts or linking words.

5. Another technique is that of a semiscripted concept map where a series of concepts, clusters or scripts are developed and assembled together. The students are provided with nodes that contain medical information specific to the history, physical exam, and diagnostic workup of five diseases that represent a likely differential diagnosis for a presenting complaint. The learner's task is to make the accurate and appropriate connections amongst the nodes (for example, linking a history of aortic dissection with the appropriate physical exam). As more meaningful and accurate connections are made and integrated, a specific diagnosis becomes apparent. The learner then writes the final diagnoses and related treatment in the empty boxes (fig. 8.4). At the top of the map, the age, race and gender of the presenting patient is provided along the presenting complaint. The concepts are vertically structured and ordered within a particular competency domain: for example, patient history, physical examination, or diagnostic work up. All of the concepts are randomly placed and visually displayed on a sheet of paper. The one-dimensional structure provided in the exercise is somewhat similar to the way a patient would present to a physician; namely, with a complaint or problem and a number of clinical components such as history, physical examination, diagnostic work-up, and possible treatment. These are tasks that every physician would generally, yet not always, perform in a specific order or sequence when approaching a patient with a medical problem. Also, distractors or extra concepts, not connected to any of the final diagnoses, can be included. Such concepts represent accurate and plausible information about a disease that could be consistent with the initial presentation. They are randomly placed by the instructor and describe important clinical domains such as history of present illness, physical examination, diagnostic data or work-up, with the final diagnosis to be filled by the learners. In this technique, variations can be added such as leaving some of

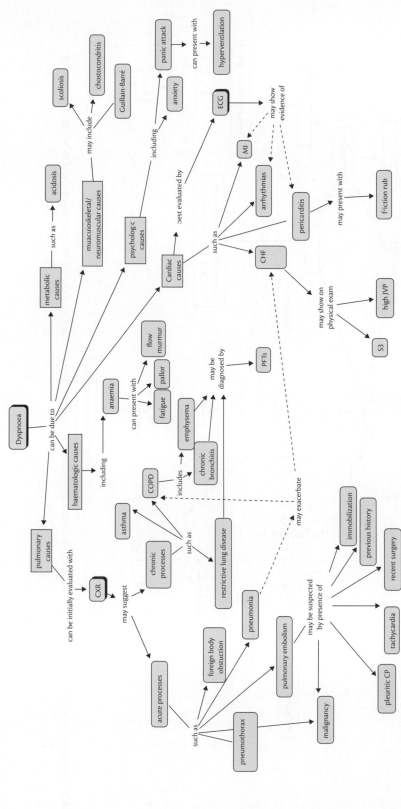

Figure 8.2 A concept map created from scratch by a third year student on the topic of difficulty breathing—a cross link is visible in the centre of the map in dashed lines.

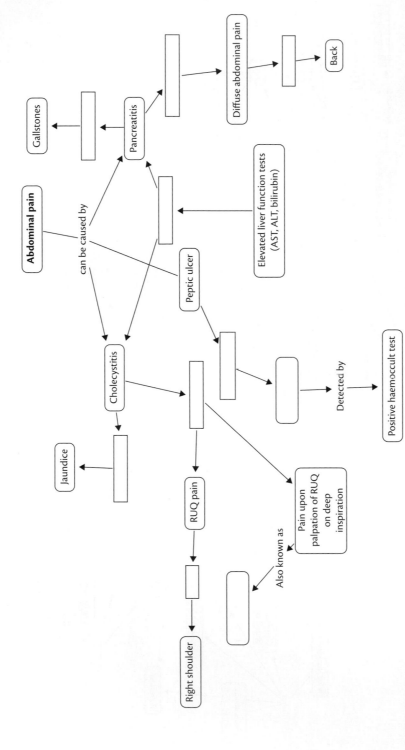

Figure 8.3 A concept map created by the instructor for a junior medical student medicine course—some nodes need to be filled and some linking words also need to be filled by the student.

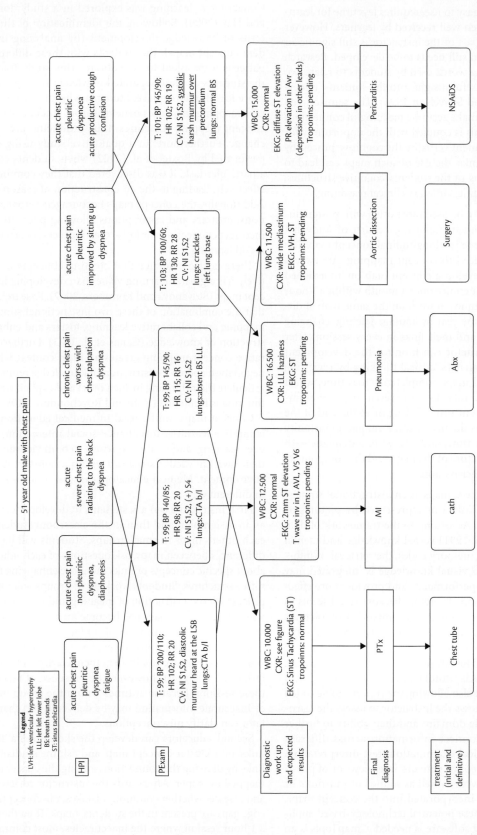

Figure 8.4 A semiscripted concept map developed by an instructor and completed by a second year internal medicine postgraduate trainee—concept scripts are connected (by the learner) and nodes about diagnosis and treatment are filled (by the learner).

the clusters open for learners to write free text—perhaps about a diagnostic workup they would perform in a specific patient. This type of technique is easy to use, requires less time for learners to perform and is often well received by learners. However preparation time on the part of the instructor is still significant and a valid scoring system still needs to be developed. Research has shown that the linking words used by students to relate two concepts can provide a useful insight into the students' understanding (Ruiz-Primo and Shavelson 1996). The semiscripted map requires students to make accurate meaningful connections among concepts; when this is coupled with the opportunity for instructors to hear the student verbalize the cognitive process by which they make those links, the use of such maps can lead to an in-depth understanding of the students' cognitive structures, knowledge gaps, incongruities or faulty clinical reasoning.

6. Another technique that can be used more often with postgraduate trainees or learners who are following a course of study that lasts a longer period of time is a longitudinal concept map. The learners are first introduced to concept mapping. Afterwards each learner begins to develop a concept map on an assigned topic or on a topic of their choice once a month within a 1 hour session. The learner continues to work on the same map at different times throughout the year by adding, deleting, changing and modifying concepts and their links in every session. After several sessions the instructor can monitor the development and progression of the learners' critical thinking by reviewing and comparing the serial maps completed across time, whilst the learner is also able to reflect on the serial maps by examining their work at different times during or at the end of the time assigned. This allows the instructor a unique opportunity to provide feedback over time, and engage in a dialogue with the learner about the structure of the maps and the components elaborated and modified across time.

7. Finally, we have used concept maps as an instructional strategy in which concepts were linked or represented by pictures or photos with annotations. According to the framework of dual code theory (Paivio 1986, 1991) verbal knowledge and mental images are interlinked in memory codes, the retrieval of information, when verbal and visual knowledge is integrated may lead to be more efficient performance and provide more effective retrieval of information. Therefore because recall seems to be more effective when teaching is accompanied by pictures (Baddeley 1992), we have developed concept maps where the image of an electrocardiogram or an x-ray is shown in relation to the text of a concept. The advantage of such practice in the context of a concept maps is twofold; first, images coupled with text allow for better recall also allowing the concept to be coded as an image; second, it allows the instructor to assess the learner's knowledge in multiple domains and their ability to further process, integrate and connect information across different competencies such physical examination, test interpretation, diagnostic reasoning. Videos of patients' interviews or of physical examination manoeuvres as well as sounds of murmurs or lung sounds can also be incorporated into the concept maps. Obviously for many of these potential technology-based applications, concept mapping software is needed. CmapTools is an example of concept mapping software, provided by the Institute for Human and Machine Cognition.

Using concept maps with groups

Collaborative learning was explored in a study done by Kinchin and Hay (2000). Following the identification of three major patterns of knowledge development (by analysing individual student concept maps), the students with these different knowledge patterns were asked to collaborate. This study found that when the students of these separate knowledge structures collaborated, more learning took place. Students who produced 'low end' concept mapping structures benefited from students with 'higher end' concept mapping structures, thus producing greater conceptual change. Furthermore, in a qualitative study using concept maps performed by Boxtel et al. (2002) when students collaborated on a particular task, it was discovered that they communicated more effectively, leading to the co-construction of reason and meaning. Additionally, the concept maps encouraged verbalization of questions, answers and assumptions allowing peers to communicate incorrect connections or links, creating a co-construction of meaningful learning.

There is also evidence that creating concepts maps collaboratively has a greater learning value than developing individual concept maps (Stoyanova and Kommers, 2002). Research also indicates that the combination of these two instructional strategies, concept mapping and collaborative learning, fosters and enhances the construction of knowledge (Canas et al. 2003). Furthermore, collaborative concept mapping creates an ideal context where meaning, negotiation and co-construction of knowledge requires students to articulate their thinking in such overt and explicit ways that critical thinking is facilitated (Roth and Roychoudhury 1993)

Concept maps can be used in medical education to foster collaborative learning, to enhance social interaction, to encourage peer teaching, and to allow learners to both view and reflect about their own knowledge structure within a non-threatening learning environment. Medical educators can use concept maps in groups in different ways.

First, instructors can ask students to develop their concept maps as an assignment and then in the classroom students can review each other's maps in small groups. Students will be able to notice differences between maps, ask questions of each other, and inquire about specific concepts or links therefore enhancing their own cognitive structures. Students working in groups will also engage in a process of co-construction of meaning and mutual understanding, where the concept map may become an anchor for discussion and sharing and communication of understanding. In group concept mapping the students provide explanations for their links and concepts which may eventually help them clarify and learn in a deeper fashion. We suggest, however, the presence of facilitators during these sessions, because at times within the group misconceptions or inaccurate information may be delivered and shared. The facilitator can clarify misconceptions.

Second, educators can develop the skeleton of a 'fill in nodes or links' or a 'cluster concept map' and ask the students to make the links by drawing the connections among the cluster of information mapped on paper. Afterwards the instructor reviews all the maps and assesses whether common mistakes, misconceptions or knowledge gaps are present in the students' maps. Then they can schedule a 1 hour session where the inaccuracies, most commonly found in the maps, are discussed and corrected within the large group. This strategy allows the teacher in collaboration with students to focus

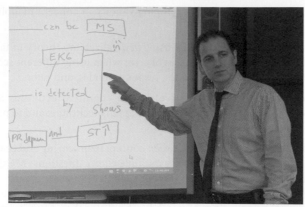

Figure 8.5 Concept mapping in action.

interrelatedness of concepts directly, probing the cognitive processes of other students as well as their own, while reflecting on the whole learning experience of group development of a concept map.

Feedback plays an important role when using concept maps in groups. In a cell biology course students who created maps individually and then discussed them in teams that provided both peer and instructor feedback produced a measurable increase in student problem solving performance and a decrease in failure rates when compared to a control group who did not construct concept maps and to a group that only constructed maps individually (Kinchin 2000; Brown 2003). This study demonstrates how the discussion of concept maps in a group, combined with feedback on the maps provided by the instructor, fosters students' learning and performance (Morse and Jutras 2008). One of the major purposes of concept mapping is to foster the development of shared meaning between instructor and students. As instructors and students discuss, engage in reflection, (Roth 1994) think about and revise concept maps, their learning and shared meaning-making processes deepen

The use of concept maps collaboratively seems to be an effective learning strategy. However, the need for faculty time to develop the appropriate learning environment, the social complexity of working in groups, coupled with the degree of difficulty of the final task and time needed to accomplish it are challenges (Moni and Moni 2008) that need to be acknowledged and examined further.

When using concept maps with groups, concept mapping software is of great value and plays a key role. Concept map software allows the learner to move concepts and links easily thus, facilitating the organization of the maps, creation of links and cross links within the map. Also, concept mapping software allows the instructor to easily visualize the knowledge structures of the student while at the same time giving educators an opportunity to meaningfully integrate audiovisual information to foster student's critical thinking skills.

CmapTools, developed by the Institute for Human Machine and Cognition, is a concept map editing tool that 'is meant to support a concept map centered learning environment' (Daley et al. 2007), and is enriched by a number of features that allow for group concept mapping. CmapTools allows students to access and modify their maps from any location, has features such as annotations and discussion threads which give users the ability to communicate their thinking, peer review each other's maps, and edit their maps in a synchronous way (Novak & Cañas, 2006). CmapTools can also be linked to course management systems thereby allowing students and instructors to access additional content or study material. CmapTools also allows the instructor to compare a previously developed criterion map with that of the students to determine whether all concepts or links provided are included in the final map. CmapTools includes an option to activate a feature called the Cmap recorder which allows a step by step playback of the map construction, in such a way that the instructor can actually follow and assess the process of construction of a specific map done by a group or individual. Through such an environment students or instructors can develop a number of knowledge models collaboratively by linking multiple maps, providing concepts to other students, posing questions or critiquing specific propositions submitted by peers (Hamilton 2001). As an example an instructor can pose a clinical problem or vignette thorough CmapTools to a group of students and then follow the problem-solving process, gauging

on key points, maximize the time for learning, and fill key knowledge gaps that were shown in the maps (fig. 8.5). This strategy can be particularly effective in building and relating new knowledge to existing knowledge, thus adding to what the students already know in an effective and efficient way. For example, if the instructor reviews concept maps about the auscultatory features of heart murmurs in the context of a patient with difficulty breathing, and by the connections made by large number of students realizes that the characteristics of the murmur of aortic insufficiency are being misconstrued, a large group session can then be scheduled. In such a session, the instructor can prioritize the learning by focusing the discussion on the specific topic of aortic insufficiency without having to review the feature of all murmurs depicted in the map as the students have already demonstrated this knowledge.

Third, students can construct concept maps on a medical topic and work together for a longer period of time by developing a map together. This technique is best accomplished with the use of concept mapping software (e.g. CmapTools). The instructor can develop several groups of five to eight students and ask students to select a topic of their choice, or assign one. The group will begin to develop the map and electronically, each member, in an asynchronous or synchronous manner, can access the map and add or modify parts of it. If provided with a discussion board, the students can then communicate with each other and discuss issues that may relate to changes made to the map. Students can also share their thinking within the map itself by developing propositions and labels not yet linked, creating new concepts to be elaborated by others, or sharing their thinking about a specific area of the map. This use of concept mapping can be particularly helpful in professional learning communities, where concept maps may help coordinate learning experiences, group projects, engage students in active learning, and share resources within and across institutions. The instructor also may choose, in agreement with students, to have access at any time during the process to evaluate in real time and in a continuous and progressive manner the work of the students, their level of interaction, and communication (while continually assessing their needs).

Thus using concept maps in groups allows students to engage in group reflection, share their views directly by critiquing the map or specific sections of it, and raise difficult of issues within the group. The concept map also gives each student the opportunity to provide immediate feedback to other students, challenging the meaning or degree of participation, analysing the group work throughout a certain period of time, intervening when and where appropriate. The infrastructure provided by such a rich interconnected electronic platform coupled with the conceptual framework and development of concept maps creates an ideal vehicle for collaborative learning. Ultimately group mapping is capable of promoting more debate and reasoning in the interaction among participating students. Students benefit from the use of group mapping by increasing their exposure to elaborative learning episodes, collaboratively enhancing opportunities for questions, debates and discussions within the discourse generated by the concept map (Baroody and Bartels 2000; Baroody and Coslick 1998). Nevertheless in the medical profession where collaborative work is essential, the use of concept maps is certainly a valuable tool for learners and educators with enormous educational potential for the future.

Assessing learning with concept maps

Finally, concept maps can be used as an assessment tool. When thinking of concept maps as an assessment tool, it is important to keep in mind that concept maps can provide an opportunity to gather information needed to make an assessment of the learner's integrated knowledge structures. Because different mapping techniques evoke different cognitive demands, it is important for educators to be aware and consider the different aspects of the nature of the task, particularly when concept mapping is used as an assessment tool. Nevertheless, we believe that the assessment of the structure and organization of knowledge coupled with the interconnectedness and integration of concepts is of great importance for learners in the medical profession. We argue that the use of the concept maps plays an important and potentially unique role in medical education.

Although concept maps have been used for assessment, further research is needed to better address issues of the validity and reliability of concept maps as an assessment tool (Ruiz-Primo and Shavelson 1996; Ruiz-Primo et al. 2004; Ingec 2009; Nesbit and Adesope 2006). Overall, concept maps have been used more frequently as learning tools than as assessment tools. One of the main challenges in the development of concept maps as a valid and reliable assessment tool is related to three main components (Ruiz-Primo et al. 2004) that inform the use concept maps:

1. *Task*: which entails what type of map technique (such as fill in the nodes or construct a map from scratch) the students are asked to use and whether it is individual or group mapping.

2. *Response*: whether the response is paper or computer based or oral also whether the map is drawn by the teacher or student or both.

3. *Scoring system*: structural, relational with the use of a criterion map or a combination of both. Scoring systems for maps can be based on the map structure and the linkages between concepts created by the student; or the maps can be scored by analysing the relationships between the student map and an expert map.

Such different types of mapping techniques, and scoring systems, coupled with a variety of cognitive and reasoning demands bestowed on the learner, make it challenging to assess the validity and reliability of concept maps in relation to all these components. Nevertheless two main strategies have been proposed to explore the process of developing validity in concept mapping assessment:

◆ One (more quantitative) by using generalizability theory to take into account multiple sources of error when using different scoring systems, maps techniques, response modes, and raters.

◆ The other (more qualitative) where cognitive activities are assessed in relation to the type of mapping technique and to performance scores.

Studies on the relationship between concept map scoring and traditional achievement tests such as multiple choice questions (MCQs) have shown contrasting results (Ingec 2009).

One key issue in the use of concept maps as assessment tools is scoring. However, educators need to be aware that, because map styles and techniques can vary, different scoring methods may need to be developed based on the particular type of map (Roberts 1999; Daley and Torre 2010). Overall there are two main scoring frameworks: structural scoring and relational scoring. Structural scoring was developed by Novak and Gowin, (1984) and assigns points to each of the following four categories:

◆ The hierarchical structure of the maps (from most general to most specific)

◆ The number of valid propositions (linking words or phrases) between concepts

◆ The number of cross links (connections from one side of the map to the other) and

◆ Specific examples related to a concept.

In this scoring system the most points are assigned to valid and significant cross links. The most points are assigned to the cross links category because crosslinks demonstrate a unique ability for creativity, synthesis and accuracy. The structural scoring has been used in concept mapping assessment of medical residents' performance pre- and post-instruction (West et al. 2000; West et al. 2002: Torre et al. 2007).

The relational scoring focuses mainly on propositions, based on the concept that it is the proposition which denotes the depth of understanding (McClure 1999; Ruiz-Primo and Shavelson 1996). Thus such a scoring system assigns points to the number and accuracy of propositions and the overall structure of the map. In this type of scoring the links among concepts, the cross links and examples are scored. The propositions can be further assessed as to whether they represent a valid relationship among concepts and whether they are labeled correctly (Kinchin et al. 2000) .Within relational scoring, propositions can be scored

◆ Quantitatively: thus producing a score that is based on the number or rate of propositions generated or

◆ Qualitatively: which stresses the choice of proposition, where students' cognitive abilities in generating those propositions can be inferred.

Hence, students can be given a number of concepts and asked to create links or propositions between these concepts. Alternatively, the student can be given linking words and concepts and asked to provide the connections. The scoring is then determined by comparing the student map with an instructor or criterion map. When these two relational scoring techniques were compared it seemed that the former technique would be more advantageous to explore and assess the cognitive abilities of students whereas the latter would be better used in the assessment of large number of students (Yin et al. 2005). However, a modification of either scoring system has been used. For example, a scoring system may be developed assigning points to different features of the map by rating:

1. The importance of the relationship between two concepts based on the degree and importance of the relationship (for example congestive heart failure and diuretics would be highly related concepts).

2. The accuracy of the linking words or propositions that describes the meaningfulness of the relationship between concepts and shows learners' understanding.

3. The presence of crosslinks.

Such a scoring system may be considered a hybrid or a modified system, that encompasses features of the two main scoring systems previously described (Srinivasan et al. 2008; Kassab and Hussain 2010; Pottier et al. 2010).

Next we review how concept maps have been used as an assessment strategy:

1. Concept maps have been used in the assessment of critical thinking in medical education (West et al. 2000; Daley et al. 1999). One application is to give the student a brief clinical scenario and ask the student to develop a concept map based on that particular scenario. The teacher may also be more specific in asking the student to map a number of plausible hypotheses or a differential diagnosis for that particular clinical case. These maps can then be scored, and maps from the first part of the semester compared to maps created later in the semester.

2. Concept maps can be used to assess learners' knowledge structure in problem-based learning (PBL) (Kassab and Hussain 2010; Rendas et al. 2006). Concept maps can capture the numerous learning activities involved in PBL such as; identifying knowledge structures of the learners at the beginning and/or the end of the course; assessing how the learner integrates information about knowledge; and discovering aspects of the PBL process that would normally not come to the surface. Also a concept map may be particularly useful to deepen understanding about the self-study part of the PBL process, which usually cannot be observed by the tutor.

3. Concept maps can elicit the knowledge structures of a student in a specific area or topic, allowing the teacher to get inside the mind of the learner. The map, regardless of the technique or scoring method used, provides the teacher with an assessment of the students' cognitive structures in a way that MCQs or other traditional tests may not be able to.

4. Concept mapping can be of great value in the remediation process of a student with academic or personal difficulties. For example, the teacher can use the concept map as an assessment tool in two ways:

    ◆ One way is to asking students to develop a concept map about how they view their performance during a rotation. This allows the teacher to gain a better understanding about the degree of self assessment the learner possesses, furthering understanding into the leaner's' insight.

    ◆ Another use of the maps is to ask the learner to construct a map on a more specific area which may include a clinical question to assess knowledge and understanding. A concept map 'from scratch' may be more appropriate for the former whereas either a map 'from scratch' or pre-constructed could be appropriate for the later. Afterwards, the teacher would review the map, and assess the overall knowledge structure and how that is integrated and organized. The instructor then assesses the links and judges whether they depict a correct or incorrect relationship. Once the teacher has gained a better understanding of the learner's thought process, a time to meet with the student can be scheduled, so that the instructor can question them about specific links or concepts found in the map. This process may help the teacher to identify areas in need of improvement, clarify the thought processes of the learner, identify difficulties not yet discovered, and ultimately plan a focused intervention.

5. Finally, Kinchin et al. (2008) used a qualitative analysis of concept maps created by both students and teachers to demonstrate the occurrence of three morphological types of maps: spokes, chains, and nets. Each of these different types of map depicts a different type and level of thinking demonstrated by the students and/or teacher. Kinchin et al. (2008) believe that the hallmark of expertise is the ability to move back and forth between these different types of thinking as the clinical situation demands. As such, when using this type of qualitative analysis it is possible to make clear to students the knowledge structures and thinking patterns of the instructor and to foster the ability of the student to move from an integrated type of thinking needed for clinical reasoning to a more linear type of thinking needed to implement changes in practice.

Conclusions

◆ It is very important to focus our efforts on understanding the complexity of the thinking processes of learners in complex decisions, most importantly at an early stage in their career.

◆ Concept maps may offer a new framework in which medical educators can develop and assess students' knowledge structures, as well as provide them with opportunities to promote their critical thinking skills.

◆ Physicians will continue to face increasingly complex patient problems with a wealth of new clinical knowledge; as such, the use of a tool that fosters information processing and interrelatedness among knowledge structures is essential.

◆ Concept maps can be used in many ways to foster learning while allowing teachers and curriculum developers to understand how knowledge is arranged in the student's mind, thus creating the premise for innovative and relevant teaching strategies within the appropriate clinical context.

References

Anderson, L.A., Gwaltney, M.K., Sundra, D.L.,. et al. (2006) Using concept mapping to develop a logic model for the Prevention Research Centers Program. [Research Support, US Gov't, PHS]. *Preventing Chronic Disease.* 3(1), A06.

Antonoff, M. B. and D'Cunha, J. (2011) Retrieval practice as a means of primary learning: Socrates had the right idea. *Semin Thoracic Cardiovasc Surg.* 23(2): 89–90

Ausubel, D.P. (1968) *Educational Psychology: A Cognitive View*. New York: Holt, Rinehart and Winston

Baddeley, A. (1992) Is working memory working? The Fifteenth Bartlett lecture. *Q J Exp Psychol.* 44A: 1–31

Baroody, A.J. and Bartels, B.H. (2000) Using Concept Maps to link mathematical ideas. *Mathematics Teaching in the Middle School.* 5(9): 604–609

Baroody, A.J. and Coslick, R. (1998) *Fostering children's mathematical power.* Mayweh, New Jersey: Lawrence Erlbaum Associates

Bordage, G. (1994) Elaborated knowledge: a key to successful diagnostic thinking. *Acad Med.* 69(11): 883–885

Boxtel, C. V., Linden, J. V., Roelofs, E., and Erkens, G. (2002, Winter) Collaborative concept mapping: Provoking and supporting meaningful discourse. *Theory into Practice.* 41(1): 40–46

Brown, D.S. (2003) High school biology: A group approach to concept mapping. *Am Biology Teacher.* 65(3): 192–197

Calderon, K.R., Vij, R.S., Mattana, J., and Jhaveri, K.D. (2011) Innovative teaching tools in nephrology. *Kidney Int.* 79(8): 797–799

Cañas, A.J., Coffey, J.W., Carnot, M.J., et al. (2003) *A summary of literature pertaining to the use of concept mapping techniques and technologies for education and performance support.* Report from the Institute for Human and Machine Cognition, Pensacola, FL

Castro, A,G,, Rocca-Serra. P., Stevens, R., et al. The use of concept maps during knowledge elicitation in ontology development processes—the nutrigenomics use case. *BMC Bioinformatics.* 2006; 7http://www. biomedcentral.com/1471- 2105/7/267 (Accessed 1 April 2012)

Coffey, J.W., Carnot, M.J., Feltovich, P.J., et al. (2003) *A summary of literature pertaining to the use of concept mapping techniques and technologies for education and performance support (Technical Report submitted to the US Navy Chief of Naval Education and Training)* Pensacola, FL: Institute for Human and Machine Cognition

Cristea, A. and Okamoto, T. (2001) Object-oriented collaborative course authoring environment supported by Concept Mapping in MyEnglishTeacher. *Educ Technol Society.* 4(2): 104–115

Cutrer, W.B., Castro, D., Roy, K.M., and Turner, T.L. (2011) Use of an expert concept map as an advance organizer to improve understanding of respiratory failure. *Med Teach.* 33(12): 1018–1026

Daley, B.J., et al. (1999) Concept maps: a strategy to teach and evaluate critical thinking. *J Nursing Educ.* 38: 42–47

Daley, B., Cañas, A. and Stark-Schweitzer, T. (2007) CMAP Tools: Integrating Teaching, Learning and Evaluation in Online Courses. In: Conceição, S. (ed.) *New Perspectives of Teaching Adults Online.* New Directions in Adult and Continuing Education Series. San Francisco: Jossey-Bass, Inc.

Daley, B.J., and Torre, D.M. (2010) Concept maps in medical education: an analytical literature review. *Med Educ.* 44(5): 440–448

Dewey, J. (1938) *Experience and Education.* New York: Collier Books

Edmondson, K.M., and Smith, D.F. (1998) Concept mapping to facilitate veterinary students' understanding of fluid and electrolyte disorders. *Teaching and Learning in Medicine.* 10(1): 21–33

Eitel, F., and Steiner, S. (1999) Evidence-based learning. *Med Teach.* 21(5): 506–513

Hamilton, S. (2001) Thinking outside the box at the IHMC. *Computer.* 34(1): 61–71

Harpaz, I., Balik, C., and Ehrenfeld, M. (2004) Concept mapping: An educational strategy for advanced nursing education. *Nursing Forum.* 39(2): 27–30, 36

Higgs, J., Jones, M.A., Loftus, S., and Christensen, N. (2008) *Clinical reasoning in the health professions.* 3rd edn. Oxford: Butterworth-Heinemann-Elsevier

Ingec, S.K. (2009) Analysing concept maps as an assessment tool in teaching physics and comparison with the achievement tests. *Int J Sci Educ.* 31(14): 1897–1915

Irvine, L. M. (1995) Can concept mapping be used to promote meaningful learning in nurse education?. *Journal of Advanced Nursing,* 21(6), 1175–1179.

Kassab, S.E., and Hussain, S. (2010) Concept mapping assessment in a problem-based medical curriculum. *Med Teach.* 32(11): 926–931

Kinchin, I.M. (2000) Concept mapping in biology. *J Biol Educ.* 34(2): 61–68

Kinchin, I.M., Cabot, L.B., and Hay, D.B. (2008) Using concept mapping to locate the tacit dimension of clinical expertise: towards a theoretical framework to support critical reflection on teaching. *Learn Health Soc Care.* 7(2): 93–104

Kinchin, I.M., Hay, D.B., and Adams, A. (2000) How a qualitative approach to concept map analysis can be used to aid learning by illustrating patterns of conceptual development. *Educ Res.* 42(1): 43–57

Kumar, S., Dee, F., Kumar, R., and Velan, G. (2011) Benefits of testable concept maps for learning about pathogenesis of disease. *Teach Learn Med.* 23(2): 137–143

Laight, D.W. 2004. Attitudes to concept maps as a teaching/learning activity in undergraduate health professional education: influence of preferred learning style. *Med Teach.* 26: 229–233

MacNeil, M.S. (2007) Concept mapping as a means of course evaluation. *J Nurs Educ.* 46(5): 232–234

Marchand, C., D'Ivernois, J.F., Assal, J.P., Slama, G., and Hivon, R. (2002) An analysis, using concept mapping, of diabetic patients' knowledge, before and after patient education. *Med Teach.* 24(1): 90–99

Markow, P.G., and Lonning, R.A. (1998) Usefulness of concept maps in college chemistry laboratories: Students' perceptions and effects on achievement. *J Res Sci Teaching.* 35(9): 1015–1029

McClure, J.R. Sonak, B and Suen, H.K., (1999) Concept map assessment of classroom learning: reliability, validity, and logistical practicality. *J Res Sci Teaching.* 36: 475–492

McMillan J.W. Teaching for clinical reasoning—helping students make the conceptual links. (2010) *Med Teach.* 32: e436–e442

Moni, R.W., and Moni, K.B. (2008) Student perceptions and use of an assessment rubric for a group concept map in physiology. *Adv Physiol Educ.* 32(1): 47–54

McGaghie, W.C., McCrimmon, D.R., Mitchell, G., Thompson, J.A., and Ravitch, M.M. (2000) Quantitative concept mapping in pulmonary physiology: comparison of student and faculty knowledge structures. *Adv Physiol Educ.* 23(1): 72–81

Morse, D. and Jutras, F. (2008) Implementing concept-based learning in a large undergraduate classroom. *CBE Life Sci Educ.* 7(2): 243–253

Mintzes, J.J., Wandersee, J.H., and Novak, J. (1998) *Teaching Science for Understanding: a Human Constructivist View.* London: Academic Press

Nesbit, J.C., and Adesope, O.O. (2006) Learning with concept and knowledge maps: A meta-analysis. *Rev Educ Res.* 76(3): 413–448

Norman, G.R., Coblentz, C.L., Brooks, L.R, and Babcook, C.J. (1992) Expertise in visual diagnosis: a review of the literature. *Acad Med.* 67(10): S78–S83

Novak, J. (1977) *A Theory of Education.* Ithaca, NY: Cornell University Press

Novak, J. (1998) *Learning, creating and using knowledge. Concept maps as facilitative tools in schools and corporations.* London: Erlbaum Associates

Novak, J.D. (1990) Concept maps and Vee diagrams: Two metacognitive tools to facilitate meaningful learning. *Instructional Science.* 19: 1–25

Novak, J.D., and Cañas, A.J. (2006) *The theory underlying concept maps and how to construct them* (Tech. Rep. IHMC CmapTools 2006-01) Pensacola, FL: Florida Institute for Human and Machine Cognition. http://cmap. ihmc.us/Publications/ResearchPapers/TheoryUnderlyingConceptMaps. pdf. Accessed 12 June 2009

Novak, J.D., and Gowin, D.B. (1984) *Learning How to Learn.* New York: Cambridge University Press

Paivio, A. (1986) *Mental Representations: A Dual Coding Approach.* Oxford, UK: Oxford University Press

Paivio, A. (1991) Dual coding theory—retrospect and current status. *Can J Psychol.* 45(3): 255–287

Pinto, A.J., and Zeitz, H.J. (1997) Concept mapping: A strategy for promoting meaningful learning in medical education. *Med Teach.* 19(2): 114–122

Plotnick, E. (2001) A graphical system for understanding the relationship between concepts. *Teacher Librarian.* 28(4): 42–45

Pottier, P., Hardouin, J.B., Hodges, B.D., et al. (2010) Exploring how students think: a new method combining think-aloud and concept mapping protocols. *Med Educ.* 44(9): 926–935

Qadir, F., Zehra, T., and Khan, I. (2011) Use of concept mapping as a facilitative tool to promote learning in pharmacology. *J Coll Phys Surg Pakistan.* 21(8): 476–481

Rendas, A.B., Fonseca, M., and Pinto, P.R. (2006) Toward meaningful learning in undergraduate medical education using concept maps in a PBL pathophysiology course. *Adv Physiol Educ.* 30(1): 23–29

Ruiz-Primo, M.A. and Shavelson R.J. (1996) Problems and issues in the use of concept maps in science assessment. *J Res Sci Teaching.* 33: 569–600

Ruiz-Primo, M.A., Shavelson, R.J., Li, M., and Schultz, S.E. (2011) On the validity of cognitive interpretations of scores from alternative concept mapping techniques. *Educational Assessment.* 7(2): 99–141

Roberts, L. (1999) Using concept maps to measure statistical understanding. *Int J Math Educ Sci Technol.* 30(5): 707–717

Roth, W.M. (1994) Science discourse through collaborative concept mapping—new perspectives for the teacher. *Int J Sci Educ.* 16: 437–455

Roth, W.M., and Roychoudhury, A. (1993) The concept map as a tool for the collaborative construction of knowledge: A microanalysis of high school physics students. *J Res Sci Teaching.* 30: 503–534

Santhanam, E., Leach, C., and Dawson, C. (1998) Concept mapping: How should it be introduced, and is there evidence for long term benefit? *Higher Educ.* 35(3): 317–328.

Schau, C and Mattern, N. (1997) Use of mapping techniques in teaching applied statistics courses. *The American Statistician.* 51: 171–175

Schmidt, H.G, Norman, G.R., Boshuizen, H.P.A. (1990) A cognitive perspective on medical expertise: theory and implications. *Acad Med.* 65(10): 611–621

Srinivasan, M., McElvany, M., Shay, J.M., Shavelson, R.J., and West, D.C. (2008) Measuring knowledge structure: reliability of concept mapping assessment in medical education. *Acad Med.* 83(12): 1196–1203

Stoyanova, N., and Kommers, P. (2002) Concept mapping as a medium of shared cognition in computer-supported collaborative problem solving. *J Interactive Learning Res.* 13: 111–133

Torre, D.M., Daley, B., Stark-Schweitzer, T., Siddartha, S., Petkova, J., and Ziebert, M. (2007) A qualitative evaluation of medical student learning with concept maps. *Med Teach.* 29(9): 949–955

Weiss, L.B., and Levison, S.P. (2000) Tools for integrating women's health into medical education: clinical cases and concept mapping. *Acad Med.* 75(11): 1081–1086

West, D.C., Park, J.K., Pomeroy, J.R., and Sandoval, J. (2002) Concept mapping assessment in medical education: A comparison of two scoring systems. *Med Educ.* 36: 820–826

West, D.C., Pomeroy, J.R., Park, J.K., Gerstenberger, E.A., and Sandoval, J. (2000), Critical thinking in graduate medical education: A role for concept mapping assessment? *JAMA.* 284(9): 1105–1110

Willemsen, A.M., Jansen, G.A., Komen, J.C., et al. (2008) Organisation and integration of biomedical knowledge with concept maps for key peroxisomal pathways. *Bioinformatics.* 24(16): 21–27

Yin, Y., Vanides, J., Ruiz-Primo, M.A., Ayala, C.C., and Shavelson, R.J. (2005) Comparison of two concept-mapping techniques: Implications for scoring, interpretation, and use. *J Res Sci Teaching.* 42(2): 166–184

CHAPTER 9

Creating the learning environment

Rachel Isba

> Man should be master of his environment, not its slave.
>
> Anthony Eden
>
> Speech to the Conservative Party Conference, October 1946

Introduction

Learning can be thought of as a process, not an event. Humans, like other animals, learn by a variety of means, and while much work has been done on how humans learn, much remains to be done. From the first to the last day of life learning forms a vital role in human existence. In the UK, the Department for Education's Early Years Foundation document (2006) states that 'an appropriate environment is key both to safety and to effective learning and development'.

Debate continues as to the nature and theory of adult learning, but it is widely accepted that context plays a role in the process of all human learning. Context is defined by the *Cambridge Dictionary* (2012) as 'the situation within which something exists or happens, and that can help explain it', and context may therefore be made up of a number of elements.

One element of context is the environment, and this learning environment (within which the learners find themselves) may play an important role in the acquisition, development, and consolidation of knowledge. A supportive, positive learning environment may result in the desired outcome, yet equally it may be the case that a less than ideal learning environment has a negative impact on those within it. Learning environments are therefore of interest to those in both undergraduate and postgraduate medical education.

This chapter will discuss what may contribute to a learning environment in medical education, why learning environments are an important aspect of medical education, how learning environments may be evaluated, and will end with an outline of how we can improve learning environments for the benefit of all those within them—learners, educators, and (often) patients.

What is a learning environment?

The learning environment has been identified as educationally important throughout all stages of formal learning. Often interchangeably referred to as the educational climate, educational environment, or learning climate, for the purposes of this chapter I will use the term learning environment as an all-encompassing term to refer to the conditions and surroundings in which learning takes place (physical, emotional, or social). It has been suggested in the wider education community that the learning environment be thought about as having two dominant aspects: the physical and the sociocultural, or the physical and the virtual—with a cross-cutting sociocultural theme (Trevitt and Highton 2011).

While there are descriptions in the medical education literature of the importance of learning environments, there is less exploration of what makes up a learning environment and how they are perceived, particularly by learners (Isba 2009). At first glance, for the educator, the term learning environment may conjure up images of the physical environment, and opportunities to optimize this by providing learners with access to teaching facilities or computers. However, learners are likely to also include emotional and social aspects in their description of what makes a learning environment (Isba 2009), and it is important that we do not neglect these less obvious (and harder to measure and influence) aspects. Learning may also take place outside of the institution, and learning environments may therefore extend beyond the confines of the hospital or medical school, for example with the advent of web-based learning resources and the recent increase in the use of social media.

If you take a holistic view of the curriculum, such as that offered by Harden, 'the curriculum is seen as covering not only what is taught but also how it is taught and learned, how the learning is managed and the overall learning environment' (Harden 2001b p. 335) then it is easy to see how learning environments are of importance within medical education.

The hidden curriculum

As well as the global description already presented, the curriculum can be thought of in several ways, for example, in terms of objectives (the curriculum on paper), teaching (the curriculum in action), learning (that which is experienced by students), and the final goal of assessment (Coles 1985; Dornan et al. 2006). It has also been suggested that the curriculum within a medical school or other institution can be thought of as three parts—formal, informal, and hidden (Hafferty 1998)—or in terms of explicit and implicit elements. Hafferty (1998) describes the formal curriculum as 'the stated, intended and formally offered and endorsed curriculum (e.g. the "what we do curriculum")', the informal as 'an unscripted, predominantly ad hoc, and highly interpersonal form of teaching and learning that takes place amongst and between faculty and students', and the hidden curriculum as 'a set of influences that function at the level of organisational structure and culture'. Figure 9.1 demonstrates the relationship of different components of the curriculum.

Originally coined by sociologist Philip Jackson (1968), and relating to classroom teaching, the term 'hidden curriculum' is now widely understood in undergraduate and postgraduate medical education.

Lempp and Seale (2004) expanded upon Hafferty's definition of the hidden curriculum to describe it as 'the set of influences that function at the level of organizational structure and culture, including, for example, implicit rules to survive the institution such as customs, rituals and taken for granted aspects'. Harden (2001b) described it as 'the values and patterns of behaviour that are acquired, often incidentally'. In their article on the hidden curriculum in continuing medical education, Bennett et al. (2004) draw the parallel between the 3Rs of 'reading', 'riting', and 'rithmetic' and the 'rules, regulations and routines' that make up the hidden curriculum.

As well as providing a description of the hidden curriculum, Lempp and Seale (2004) also identified six processes within it, in the setting of undergraduate medical education:

1. Loss of idealism
2. Adoption of ritualized professional identity
3. Emotional neutralization
4. Change of ethical integrity
5. Acceptance of hierarchy
6. Learning of less formal aspects of good doctoring.

As part of their research they also found that, while medical students were able to identify numerous good teaching experiences and examples of positive role modelling, they also identified a 'hierarchical and competitive atmosphere' and that this had a negative impact on their learning experiences.

In their commentary on the hidden curriculum, D'Eon et al. (2007) warned against the 'perils' of the potential negative aspects of the hidden curriculum and hinted that this may have a detrimental effect on the students and their interactions with patients. This echoes other work which has suggested the potential for the hidden curriculum to convey bad, as well as good, practice (Dobie 2007; Fitz et al. 2007; Glicken 2007; Gofton 2006; Masson and Brazeau-Lamontagne 2006; Turbes 2002).

While cutting across all three of the parts of the curriculum described by Hafferty (1998), learning environments are mostly described as part of the complex, interacting parts of the hidden curriculum (Bennett et al. 2004; D'Eon et al. 2007; Harden 2001b; Hutchinson 2003; Lempp and Seale 2004; Wear 2008). There is much work still to be done to investigate not only the nature of learning environments, but also the particular effects they may exert on the learners within them.

The learning environment

Learning depends on many interrelated factors including those related to the student; the educator; the course or curriculum; and the environment within which learning takes place (Hutchinson 2003). Maslow's (1943) hierarchy of needs for motivating learning postulates that students must feel comfortable and safe, and experience a sense of belonging before being able to learn effectively. Hutchinson (2003) suggested that in order to maximize the educational environment, a number of issues must be addressed, including the arrangement of teaching sessions 'on and off the ward', and the course and curriculum design.

Learning environments and adult learning

Andragogy was a term introduced in 1833 by Alexander Kapp and relates to the teaching of adults. It contrasts with the concept of pedagogy which is used when describing the education of children. It is Malcolm Knowles who introduced the term to modern educational theory—he defines andragogy as being 'the art and science of helping adults learn' (see Kaufman 2003).

Knowles developed a theory of adult learners based on five assumptions he felt differentiated them from child learners:

1. They need to have a concept of self that allows them to become an independent, self-directed learner.
2. They have experience which they are able to use as a resource for learning.
3. They are most interested in learning that relates to, and integrates with, their everyday life or social role.
4. They value learning that is more problem-centred than content-orientated.
5. Their motivational drive is more internal than external.

While there is no explicit statement of the role of the learning environment within this theory, it is possible to hypothesize that the environment in which these processes take place may have a direct influence on them.

Knowles then built on his original core assumptions to develop seven central principles for andragogy. Within these central principles was 'an effective learning climate', or learning environment. In his 2003 paper, Kaufman summarizes Knowles' principles thus:

◆ Establish an effective learning climate, where learners feel safe and comfortable expressing themselves.

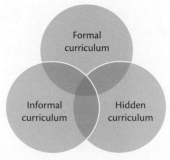

Figure 9.1 The curriculum.

- Involve learners in mutual planning of relevant methods and curricular content.

- Involve learners in diagnosing their own needs—this will help to trigger internal motivation.

- Encourage learners to formulate their own learning objectives—this gives them more control of their learning.

- Encourage learners to identify resources, and devise strategies for using the resources to achieve their objectives.

- Support learners in carrying out their learning plans.

- Involve learners in evaluating their own learning—this can develop skills of critical reflection.

There are many theories to suggest how adults learn, and by extension, how medical students may learn to become doctors. Cognitive approaches are based on theories relating to concepts such as activation of prior knowledge, elaboration, learning in context and information transfer. Social and environmental perspectives include factors such as the dynamic interaction that takes place between the learner and their learning environment and include concepts such as situated learning and self-monitoring (Mann 2002), and have been identified in other fields outside medicine (Billett 2004). Social constructionism suggests that knowledge is 'produced in and through social processes' (Jordanova 1995) and in the case of medical education, many of these social processes may occur within the learning environment.

Learning environments and the learner

Roff and McAleer (2001) suggest that increased interest in learning environments within basic medical education may in part be driven by the changing student population. With increasing numbers of students undertaking medicine as a graduate degree, female-dominated intakes, and greater ethnic diversity, there is an increasing heterogeneity within the medical student body.

If the learners form dynamic interactions with their learning environments, this changing student profile may have an impact on the learning environment, and ultimately the curriculum within an institution. Genn (2001a) similarly identifies studies of climate within an institution as a force for change, and Maudsley (2001) suggested that institutions may benefit from more formal assessment and development of the learning environment.

In addition to a changing student profile, institutions around the world are increasingly delivering the same formal curriculum to students based at different sites within the same parent institution. These different base sites give rise to unique environments within which the students study and learn. These differences in learning environments may result in varying outcomes, and it might therefore be the case that the same formal curriculum may result in contrasting informal and hidden curricula, and that these may affect outcomes. Thus quantifying the learning environment may have implications for those hoping to improve student outcomes.

What makes up a learning environment?

While the literature describes the importance of the learning environment within the curriculum, less work has been done to explore the concept of what makes up a learning environment. While the word environment has synonyms relating to physical space, there are also those that relate to atmosphere. The learning environment

may, therefore, be made up of several elements including physical space and resources, people, and social and emotional components (fig. 9.2). In the case of medical students, learning environments may include the hospital, the library, lecture theatres, fellow students, patients, teachers, equipment and learning opportunities such as clinics and ward rounds. Harden (2001b) suggests that an 'elastic definition' of the hidden curriculum could be stretched to 'include almost everything that happens within the boundaries of an institution, including informal conversations between students in the coffee room'. However, it may also be that the learning environment extends beyond the confines of the medical school, for example with the advent of e-learning resources.

There is little in the medical education literature reporting what educators and learners think a learning environment is—i.e. what the term means to them (Lempp and Seale 2004; Whittle et al. 2007). When this question was explored as part of a qualitative study at Manchester Medical School, both undergraduates and their faculty described an all-encompassing concept that they felt had a large emotional element (Isba 2009). Students and staff seem to interpret the concept of a learning environment as a wide-ranging one that encompasses physical, emotional, and educational aspects, and one in which interpersonal interactions feature heavily, and in which they themselves play an active part. It is possible that emotional aspects represent a common final pathway between the other elements and the holistic learning environment. This is unlikely to be a static relationship, and the learning environment may then 'feedback' with emotion as a final common pathway (Isba 2009). Interestingly, emotional aspects of the learning environment are very much a consideration when we think about the education of children, yet this seems to have less emphasis placed on it in adult learning (from the educator perspective at least).

Some of the elements that make up the learning environment may therefore be more easily quantifiable than others, and tools have been described and validated to enable the measurement of learning environments. However, there may be aspects of these learning environments that are not immediately obvious to those

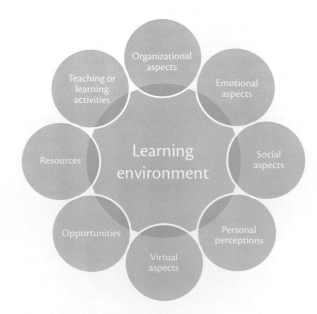

Figure 9.2 The learning environment.

wishing to assess them, but that may be vital to those studying within them.

Organizational aspects

Teaching and learning take place in a whole system, which may be represented by different levels within a single organization. The organizations within which you find learning environments may, therefore, exert particular effects upon them. An organizational culture that values education and educators may result in a learning environment that reflect this value, and will differ from another organization where less value is assigned to educational activities. Learning environments where learners see that educators are rewarded (e.g. by promotion) may encourage the learners themselves to strive to become good teachers. Equally, it is important that those with organizational responsibility for learning environments demonstrate that poor-quality teaching or unprofessional behaviours exhibited by those involved in teaching is not tolerated.

The learners themselves clearly have a role to play in this regulation of the learning environment. By enabling learners to identify positive and negative elements of the learning environment (e.g. by asking them to provide feedback) it may be possible to enable them to actively shape their own micro-learning environments, while also having a greater impact on the holistic environment within their institution.

The learning environment may function at a number of different organizational and hierarchical levels: for example, geographical, undergraduate, postgraduate, or departmental. Each of these levels is subject to a different set of internal and external influences (and potential conflict). It may also be the case that the potential influence exerted by the people within one learning environment upon the development of other learning environments will differ depending on the organizational level of each (Isba and Boor 2011). For example, the medical student may be able to shape their own learning environment, and exert influence upon those of their peers, but will be unlikely to be able to make major changes to the learning environment at an institution-wide level. Equally, the Dean of a medical school is able to exert influence on those learning environments around them and downstream from them, but will be less able to influence learning environments at a national policy level.

Emotional aspects

The qualitative work described earlier in this chapter argues for a much larger influence of emotion in the construction of the learning environment (Isba 2009). While assessment and characterization of learning environments has, to date, included emotional aspects (e.g. selected Dundee Ready Educational Environment Measure (DREEM) items, Roff et al. 1997); it may be that emotion is all-pervasive throughout the learning environment. This has implications for those delivering medical education and who wish to improve learning environments for their learners.

If learners feel that a good learning environment is less about physical aspects and more about emotional aspects, then future interventions to improve the learning environment would need to address this. It is possible that such interventions would be more difficult and time consuming, as they may involve additional training for staff involved in the delivery of teaching. However, aspects such as making medical students feel welcome and valued when they attend activities such as clinics and ward rounds, may involve a cultural shift that will take years.

While resources currently tend to focus on the improvement of physical space and facilities, it may be that learners would rather have a learning environment that supports them more emotionally. The feeling of belonging and being expected that formed part of the description of the learning environment by Manchester medical students (Isba 2009) echoes Lave and Wenger's seminal work on legitimate peripheral participation.

Social aspects

Humans are social creatures, and social interactions play a large part in how we learn. Within the learning environment a learner is likely to have numerous different types of interactions on a daily basis—with fellow learners, educators, patients, and relatives—and some of these interactions may be complex or high-stakes. An interaction that is perceived as having gone well—for example receiving a 'thank you' from a patient—may have a positive impact on a learner. Equally, being humiliated on a ward round may be an interaction that has a negative impact on a learner and their learning.

As well as being involved in interactions, learners are likely to observe interactions too—for example seeing how a senior doctor speaks to patients or other staff. This observed behaviour is also an important part of the learning environment—by acting as a role model (either by intention or accident), the senior doctor is imparting to the learner information about attitudes and skills. Someone in the role of teacher who displays good communication skills, an appropriate bedside manner, and respect for a patient will lead by example, and their behaviour may encourage others to act in a similar manner. Likewise, a display of inappropriate or unprofessional behaviour by a senior may be deemed acceptable by a junior, and assimilated as such. This might be an example of one aspect of the hidden curriculum manifesting as part of the learning environment.

Recently, there has been increased interest in the role of social networks in medical education. A social network is a set of entities and connections, and it is possible to map and quantify these connections. In medical education there are many levels at which social networks may form and function—from two students revising together—to an entire hospital. Recent work has shown that social network formation at medical school is associated with a number of factors, including examination performance (Woolf et al. 2012), and that a school can be thought of as a dynamic but relatively closed system in social network terms, and mapped accordingly (McAleer 2012). It is likely that further exploration of the social networks that exist within medical education will cast additional light on the social aspects of learning environments.

Personal perceptions

In undergraduate medical education, research has shown that students may perceive the learning environment differently depending on their own personal characteristics (e.g. sex and graduate status). It appears that women consistently rate their learning environments more positively than do men (Al-Hazimi et al. 2004a; Bassaw 2003; de Oliveira Filho et al 2005a; Miles and Leinster 2007). However, further work needs to be done to explore the reasons for this observation in more detail, as it may be the case that women perceive their learning environment more positively, or look for different qualities in a learning environment, or simply that they report it more positively.

In contrast, the data relating to graduate status are conflicting, with some work suggesting that graduate students give lower ratings than their undergraduate counterparts, and other work suggesting that there is no difference (Isba 2009; Miles and Leinster 2007). It is also not clear from the relatively limited work in this area if it graduate status that is causing the influence, or if graduate status is acting as a proxy for age.

Other work in undergraduate medical education has shown that students in different years of study, at the same point in time, have different perceptions of the learning environment (Avalos 2007; Dunne et al. 2006; Jiffry 2005; Till 2005). It may be that these differences reflect a difference in the student cohorts in each year, or arise as a result of time spent in the learning environment, or experiences during that time. Preliminary work, however, suggests that perceptions of the learning environment may fluctuate over time, with more students rating it lower in later years than they had previously (Isba 2009). This observation may reflect changes in the learning environment, or in the students themselves, or may simply be due to the test–retest reliability of some of the current learning environment measurement tools. There is little in the literature by way of longitudinal studies of the learning environment and more work in this area might help elucidate changes in the perception of the learning environment over time.

Teaching or learning activities

Teaching and learning activities and opportunities form part of the learning environment and may be an area in which the boundaries between hidden, informal, and formal aspects of the curriculum become blurred. For example, while the content of an activity such as a bedside teaching session may be modelled on the formal curriculum, the way in which it is delivered may fall within the informal curriculum, and the value it is attributed by the person delivering it may be considered as part of the hidden curriculum. Therefore, a consultant who sends students off the ward as they are in the way of a busy ward round, instead of engaging them in a timetabled bedside teaching session, is contributing to the learning environment. As such, while teaching activities are often considered as part of the formal and informal aspects of the curriculum, they are also powerful forces within the hidden curriculum and may have a positive or negative influence on the learning environment via a number of means.

People

In his 1978 book *Social Learning Theory*, Bandura argues that there is an intimate relationship between person, behaviour, and the environment, and that much of what we learn is as a result of modelling. The people part of the learning environment (especially teachers) has been reported by students as important, and this opportunity to model one's own behaviour on the behaviour of teachers fits well within Bandura's framework.

Around the same time as Bandura's social learning theory was being developed, work was being carried out in the US that sought to quantify the learning environment in high schools. This work placed an emphasis on interpersonal relationships—between students, and between pupils and teachers—alongside other aspects such as the subject being taught and the method of learning used (Fraser et al. 1982, p. 7).

It seems, therefore, that people are an important part of the medical learning environment. In this context, the interpersonal relationships are likely to be with peers, teachers, patients (and their carers), and other healthcare professionals. These interwoven and interconnected relationships fit well with Lave and Wenger's (1991, 1999) theories of communities of practice.

Within a medical education learning environment many people factors seem to influence learning, including the mix of patients seen by students, the availability (and quality) of supervision, and the number of students within the learning environment (Dolmans et al. 2002, 2008; Durak et al. 2008). This last observation is of particular importance to those offering the same formal curriculum over multiple sites (Isba 2009).

Resources

Material resources are an obvious, readily quantifiable, and relatively easily alterable, aspect of the learning environment. While no learning environment is likely to be perfect in terms of the resources available to learners, it is important that those with responsibility for this aspect of the learning environment are sensitive to the actual (rather than perceived) needs of those learners. Requirements for material resources are likely to vary depending on the learning environment and the learner, but basic facilities that learners have come to accept as fundamental such as access to libraries, computers or a clinical skills facility are likely to be universal.

However, while the material resources available within a learning environment are an important consideration, supporting learners' basic needs is unlikely to be sufficient, and efforts to improve learning environments must look beyond the physical surroundings in which students find themselves.

Opportunities

Just as teaching activities and material resources are an important part of the learning environment, so too are opportunities—these may be opportunities for supervision; to see and examine patients; for formal and informal teaching activities; for support in times of difficulty; and for feedback. It is possible that this may be an area where there is disparity in perception between learners and educators (Isba 2009)—some staff may see everything within the learning environment as an opportunity, while some students may need opportunities signposted for them. Opportunities within the learning environment are likely to be highly related to other aspects such as teaching activities and it may be possible to quantify (and qualify) them indirectly.

Virtual aspects of the learning environment

Sandars' chapter (Chapter 15) provides an overview of e-learning in medical education, and this is an important consideration when looking at the learning environment. The virtual learning environment (VLE) is increasingly forming part of the learner's experience both in undergraduate and postgraduate medical education. Dewhurst and Ellaway (2005, p. 201) describe the VLE as 'an integrated set of online tools, databases and managed resources that exist as a coherent system, functioning collectively in support of education'. Just as the physical learning environment has aspects that cut across all three parts of the curriculum (formal, informal, and hidden), so too may the virtual learning environment.

As well as VLEs, web resources, and social media such as Facebook (www.facebook.com) and Twitter (https://twitter.com/), it seems that the learning environment in some organizations may also extend beyond the real world into a truly simulated environment. *Second Life* is an avatar-based simulated world that was launched as a place to get away from the real world (www.secondlife.com). However, it seems that the technology is increasingly being used for educational purposes and may provide a novel way of extending the learning environment further (Spooner et al. 2011).

Thinking back to Harden's elastic view of the hidden curriculum (Harden 2001b), it seems that now it could be stretched further to include 'almost everything that happens within *and beyond* the boundaries of an institution, including informal conversations between students in the coffee room *and the online chat room*'.

Why is the learning environment important?

Genn (2001a, b) stated that the learning environment 'is an important determinant of behaviour' and went on to suggest that students will select role models, both positive and negative, and respond to positive and negative aspects of their day-to-day experiences, and that this will be partly responsible for fashioning their development into junior doctors. In 1991, the UK's Standing Committee on Postgraduate Medical Education highlighted the importance of the learning environment in postgraduate medical education. More recently, organizations such as the American Medical Association (AMA, 2008) have published extensive guidance on how to transform the medical education learning environment.

Roff and McAleer (2001) suggested that on entering a new institution, students become aware of the explicit (or documented) curriculum, but also of the '"educational environment" or "climate" of the institution'. They also hypothesized that 'just as there is a "sick building syndrome" there could be a "sick learning environment"'.

Indeed, in medical education, learning environments are increasingly being identified as a potential influence on learning at both undergraduate and postgraduate level. Just as a good or bad teacher may have a positive or negative impact on an individual's learning experience, wellbeing, and motivation, it may be that learning environments exert a similar influence. However, the influence that learning environments (either good or bad) may have on outcomes in medical education is not yet well explored.

Theories of how adults learn form a basis for post-secondary education, and teaching and learning in medical education fits within this. By gaining a better understanding of the environments in which students learn, it may be possible to modify these learning environments and enhance student experiences. Equally, by gaining a better understanding of the environments in which graduates continue to learn (and where the environment is both a learning and a working one), it may be possible to improve training outcomes and even outcomes for patients.

How can we assess learning environments?

While the influence that learning environments may have on outcomes is not well understood, it may be that the learning environment has a profound impact—either intended or not—upon those within it. Therefore, by examining and measuring learning environments it may be possible to identify strengths and weaknesses within them. Having done so, it may then be possible to build on strengths and address weaknesses, in order to optimize learning environments for those within them.

Assessing the learning environment implies that it is measurable in some way. While this is true (and instruments exist for its quantification), it seems increasingly likely that the learning environment is not as fixed and measurable as was previously thought, and that some existing tools for its assessment may benefit from modification. In addition, it may be the case that the learner has a much more dynamic relationship with the development and evolution of their own learning environment. It has also been suggested that, rather than a single quantifiable entity, the learning environment is made up of multiple micro-environments that are intimately related to those experiencing them (Isba 2009). In which case, it may be that quantitative instruments are only able to measure the holistic learning environment, but not the small subtleties or the dynamic interactions within it.

Quantitative analysis

By far the most common way to assess the learning environment is quantitatively. Donnon's chapter (Chapter 53) is an in-depth exploration of the use of quantitative research methods in medical education, and many of the issues encountered elsewhere in medical education research also apply to the science of quantifying the learning environment (Isba and Boor 2011).

Instruments for quantifying the learning environment

Attempting to quantify the learning environment is not a new endeavour. In the 1950s, those with responsibility for educating high school students in the US were trying to develop instruments that would allow them to measure aspects of the classroom social climate by the use of the 'Learning Environment Inventory' (aimed at high school students) and the simplified 'My Class Inventory' (for use with younger children) (Fraser and Fisher 1983; Fraser et al. 1982). Refinement of these instruments went on for decades, perhaps highlighting the difficulties associated with trying to capture such a nebulous and individual experience via 50 to 100 written items. The 1982 version of the Learning Environment Inventory included items such as 'Students who break the rule are penalized', and 'The objectives of the class are not clearly recognized', which have echoes in the instruments used currently to assess learning environments in medical education.

In healthcare education, researchers have been quantifying learning environments for years, with a number of formal instruments developed during this time, such as the Medical School Learning Environment Survey (MSLES, Marshall 1978) and the Clinical Learning Environment Inventory (CLEI, Chan 2002).

In 1997, the DREEM was developed by researchers based in Dundee along with more than 80 collaborators around the world (Roff et al. 1997). The tool was developed 'in response to increasing pressures for assessment and reform in medical education'. DREEM is worth highlighting as it is one of the most widely used instruments in this area.

The College and University Environment Scales (CUES), Pace 1963 and 1969

Classroom Environment Scales (CES), Moos and Trickett 1974

Inventory of College Characteristics (ICCS), Nunnally et al. 1963

Learning Environment Inventory (LEI), Fraser et al. 1982

College and University Environment Inventory (CUCEI), Treagust and Fraser 1986

Medical School Environment Index (MSEI), Hutchins 1961

Institutional Goals Index (IGI), see Peterson 1970

Institutional Functioning Inventory (IFI), Centra et al. 1970

Figure 9.3 Instruments used to measure learning environments.

In their article on the development of DREEM, Roff et al. (1997) described the measure as 'a refinement of established instruments'. These established instruments include those shown in fig. 9.3.

DREEM has been used widely, for example to look at the learning environments:

♦ within and between teaching hospitals (Isba 2009; McKendree 2009;Varma et al. 2005)

♦ within (Al-Hazimi et al. 2004a) and between countries (Abraham et al. 2008; Al-Hazimi et al. 2004a; Roff et al. 2001)

♦ within curricular styles (Al-Hazimi et al. 2004a; Bouhaimed et al. 2009; Till 2004)

♦ in undergraduate (Abraham et al. 2008; Al-Ayed et al. 2008; Al-Hazimi et al. 2004a, b; Avalos et al. 2007; Bassaw et al. 2003; Bouhaimed et al. 2009; Jiffry 2005; Mayya and Roff 2004; McKendree 2009; Roff et al. 1997) and postgraduate medical training (de Oliveira Filho et al. 2005a, b, 2005c)

♦ within a single study module (Varma 2005) and across different stages of undergraduate training (Avalos 2007; Isba 2009)

♦ during times of curricular change (Edgren 2010; Till 2004).

A number of similar instruments have been developed (Isba and Boor 2011), including DREEM's postgraduate counterpart the Postgraduate Hospital Educational Environment Measure (PHEEM, Roff et al. 2005), as well as the Anaesthetic Theatre Educational Environment Measure (ATEEM, Holt and Roff 2004) and the Surgical Theatre Educational Environment Measure (STEEM, Cassar 2004).

Instruments such as these are popular methods of quantitative data collection, although they are not without their drawbacks (Boynton 2004; Boynton and Greenhalgh 2004; Boynton et al. 2004). For example, recent work has suggested that some of the psychometric properties of the scales used to measure learning environments may not be as reproducible as first intended (Hammond 2012; Isba 2009; Jakobsson 2011). Newer scales such as the Dutch Residency Educational Climate Test (D-RECT) have been developed using a variety of approaches that aim to preserve the psychometric properties of the scale, throughout development (Boor et al. 2011; Boor 2009).

Other methods of quantifying the learning environment

Instruments such as DREEM that have been developed in order to help educators quantify learning environments are almost exclusively designed to be filled in by learners. However, other stakeholders, for example those with responsibility for the content and organization of some aspects of the learning environment, can also help with its assessment (Roth 2006; Rotthoff 2011). There has also been a recent call for an exploration of the learning environment and hidden curriculum as experienced by faculty (Hafler 2011).

SWOT analysis

SWOT analysis is an approach that is widely attributed as emerging from Harvard Business School in the 1960s. SWOT stands for 'strengths, weaknesses, opportunities, and threats' and is widely used as an approach in business and management. In medical education, SWOT allows educators to make a rapid assessment of their learning environments, while at the same time planning future changes for quality improvement.

It is also possible to perform a SWOT analysis within a wider evaluation framework. For example, within nursing education, an evaluation tool has been developed that takes the form of a SWOT analysis spread over four domains (experience, resources, mentoring and learning support, and educational approaches) with multiple items under each subheading (Price 2004). This type of approach may allow for a more in-depth analysis, while still resulting in recommendations (under the heading of Opportunities) for improvement.

Other

In addition to the SWOT analysis approach, it may be possible for educators to audit or evaluate learning environments in other ways. For example, the University of Southampton's audit tool for 'practice learning environments in health and social care' is designed to 'assess the quality of learning provision within a particular service, department or directorate' and contains a number of staff-oriented criteria (University of Southampton 2003).

Qualitative analysis

Qualitative methods are increasingly popular in medical education (having long been used in other fields such as social sciences), and focus groups and interviews are commonly used as part of a qualitative methodology (Barbour 2005; Britten 1995). Less work has been done to qualitatively explore the learning environment in medical education research than has been done quantitatively. However, a qualitative evaluation of learning environments may be a much more holistic approach and one that allows the researcher to capture more of the inherent complexity.

Mixed methods

Mixed methods approaches are gaining popularity in medical education research, and have been used widely in other research fields for many years (Morgan 2007). However, few studies have used mixed methods to explore the learning environment, and when they have it has usually been in the form of free text comments at the end of DREEM or focus groups to explore low-scoring DREEM items (Whittle 2007). However, a mixed method approach (that combines quantitative and qualitative methods) is likely to be necessary for anyone intending to assess the learning environment, particularly in order to drive its improvement. Such an approach should also avoid exploring just one perceptual angle (e.g. just asking a group of students from one year and then extrapolating to the whole student body), and should try to include as many stakeholder groups as possible (e.g. learners, teachers, and patients).

As well as allowing for an exploration of the learning environment that would not be possible with either a qualitative or quantitative approach alone, it is also possible to use quantitative data to drive qualitative work, and vice versa.

How can we improve learning environments?

As educators we have a responsibility to be committed to providing an optimal learning environment that will support learners, aid learning, and ultimately improve educational and patient outcomes. Many medical education organizations have formalized this commitment to the learning environment explicitly. For example, in North America, the Liaison Committee on Medical Education introduced a new standard in 2012 that stated 'A medical education program must ensure that its learning environment promotes the development of explicit and appropriate professional attributes in its medical students. . .' The following list serves as a useful framework for improving (and maintaining) the learning environment (AMA 2009):

◆ The medical school and its affiliated clinical teaching sites share responsibility for creating a positive learning environment, and this shared responsibility should be reflected in formal agreements (such as affiliate agreements).

◆ Medical schools should define the professional attributes expected of learners and should inform students of the importance of demonstrating the attributes.

◆ The learning environment should be regularly assessed to determine positive and negative influences.

◆ The school should develop strategies to enhance the positive and mitigate negative influences.

We must also remember that what may be a learning environment for a medical student becomes also a working environment for the medical graduate. Looking again to North America, the Accreditation Council for Graduate Medical Education's (ACGME) Institutional Requirements (2007) reflect the guidelines for medical schools in their commitment to providing a safe and supportive educational and work environment.

What makes up an ideal learning environment?

When evaluating the learning environment in a Canadian chiropractic college, as well as asking how students perceived their environment, Till (2005) went on to use DREEM to see if student perceptions could be used to assist with planning and resource allocation within the same institution by asking what an ideal environment would look like. Work by Miles and Leinster (2007) was similar to that of Till, and sought to characterize the differences between medical students' perceptions of their actual educational environment and what they had expected at the start of their course.

Recent work suggests that the learning environment (or aspects of it) may be fluid, and that students within it may have a key role

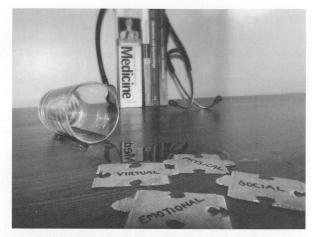

Figure 9.4 Components of the learning environment.
Photograph courtesy of Rhys Jones, reproduced with permission.

to play in its development (Isba 2009). The perceptions and experiences of the same learning environment may not be as stable as was previously thought. However, the concept of what students think makes up an ideal learning environment seems to be more consistent. It might therefore be possible to either administer a quantitative instrument in ideal mode, or engage the learners in a qualitative exploration of what they felt would make an ideal learning environment as a first step in optimization. The concept of what students feel makes an ideal learning environment could also be used as a driving force for future curricular development (fig. 9.4).

Conclusions

◆ The learning environments within which medical education takes place may have a profound effect on the learners within them and are an important part of the hidden curriculum.

◆ Many elements make up the learning environment, including physical, social, emotional, and (increasingly) virtual components. Whilst harder to measure and influence, it may be that positive emotional aspects of the learning environment are the most important for learners.

◆ It is possible to evaluate the learning environment using both quantitative and qualitative approaches, and the evaluation process may be a useful tool for those hoping to optimize the learning environment for their learners.

◆ The learning environment is unlikely to be static, nor experienced in the same way by every learner—educators must therefore be aware of both the 'holistic' learning environment within an organization as well as the micro-learning environments experienced by individual learners.

◆ More work remains to be done to develop more robust tools to allow quantification of the learning environment alongside further research to investigate the impact that learning environments have on learners and on outcomes of educational programmes.

References

Abraham, R., Ramnarayan, K., Vinod, P., and Torke, S. (2008) Students' perceptions of learning environment in an Indian medical school. *BMC Med Educ.* 8: 20

Accreditation Council for Graduate Medical Education (2007) Institutional Requirements. Version 15. http://www.acgme.org/acWebsite/irc/irc_ircpr07012007.pdf Accessed 1 April 2012

Al-Ayed, I.H. and Sheik, S.A. (2008) Assessment of the educational environment at the College of Medicine of King Saud University, Riyadh. *East Mediterr Health J.* 14(4): 953–959

Al-Hazimi, A., Zaini, R., Al-Hyiani, A., et al. (2004a). Educational environment in traditional and innovative medical schools: a study in four undergraduate medical schools. *Educ Health (Abingdon).* 17(2): 192–203

Al-Hazimi, A., Al-Hyiani, A., and Roff, S. (2004 b). Perceptions of the educational environment of the medical school in King Abdul Aziz University, Saudi Arabia. *Med Teach.* 26(6): 570–573

American Medical Association (2008) Strategies for transforming the medical education learning environment. Part 3: Program implementation.

American Medical Association (2009). Report of the council on medical education. Subject: Transforming the Medical Education Learning Environment. CME Rep. 7-A-09. http://www.ama-assn.org/resources/doc/council-on-med-ed/cme-report-7a-09.pdf Accessed 2 April 2012

Avalos, G., Freeman, C., and Dunne, F. (2007) Determining the quality of the medical educational environment at an Irish medical school using the DREEM inventory. *Ir Med J.* 100(7): 522–525

Bandura, A. (1978) *Social Learning Theory*. Upper Saddle River, New Jersey: Prentice Hall

Barbour, R.S. (2005) Making sense of focus groups. *Med Educ.* 39(7):742–750

Bassaw, B., Roff, S., McAleer, S., et al. (2003) Students' perspectives on the educational environment, Faculty of Medical Sciences, Trinidad. *Med Teach.* 25(5): 522–526

Bennett N., Lockyer J., Mann K., et al. (2004) Hidden curriculum in continuing medical education. *J Contin Educ Health Prof.* 24(3): 145–152

Billett, S. (2004) Workplace participatory practices: conceptualising workplaces as learning environments. *J Workplace Learning.* 16: 312–324

Boor, K. (2009). *The clinical learning climate.* PhD thesis. VU Medical Centre Amsterdam

Boor, K., Van Der Vleuten, C., Teunissen, P., Scherpbier, A, and Scheele, F. (2011) Development and analysis of D-RECT, an instrument measuring residents' learning climate. *Med Teach.* 33(10): 820–827

Bouhaimed, M., Thalib, L., and Doi, S.A. (2009) Perception of the educational environment by medical students undergoing a curricular transition in Kuwait. *Med Princ Pract.* 18(3): 204–208

Boynton, P.M. (2004) Administering, analysing, and reporting your questionnaire. *BMJ.* 328(7452): 1372–1375

Boynton, P.M and Greenhalgh, T. (2004) Selecting, designing, and developing your questionnaire. *BMJ.* 328(7451): 1312–1315

Boynton, P.M., Wood, G.W., and Greenhalgh, T. (2004) Reaching beyond the white middle classes. *BMJ.* 328(7453): 1433–1436

Britten, N. (1995) Qualitative Research: Qualitative interviews in medical research. *BMJ.* 311: 251–253

Cambridge Dictionaries Online. http://dictionary.cambridge.org/dictionary/british/ Accessed 2 April 2012

Cassar, K. (2004) Development of an instrument to measure the surgical operating theatre learning environment as perceived by basic surgical trainees. *Med Teach.* 26(3): 260–264

Centra, J.A., Hartnett, R.T., and Peterson, R.E. (1970) Faculty views of institutional functioning: a new measure of college environments. *Educ psychol Measurement.* 30: 405–416

Chan, D.S.K. (2002) Development of the clinical learning environment inventory: using the theoretical framework of learning environment

studies to assess nursing students' perceptions of the hospital as a learning environment. *J Nursing Educ.* 41(2): 69–75

Coles, C.R. and Gale Grant, J. (1985). Curriculum evaluation in medical and health-care education. *Med Educ.* 19(5): 405–422

de Oliveira Filho, G.R., and Schonhorst L. (2005c) Problem-based learning implementation in an intensive course of anaesthesiology: a preliminary report on residents' cognitive performance and perceptions of the educational environment. *Med Teach.* 27(4): 382–384

de Oliveira Filho, G.R., Vieira, J.E., and Schonhorst, L. (2005a) Psychometric properties of the Dundee Ready Educational Environment Measure (DREEM) applied to medical residents. *Med Teach.* 27(4): 343–347

de Oliveira Filho, G.R., Sturm, E.J., and Sartorato, A.E. (2005b) Compliance with common program requirements in Brazil: its effects on resident's perceptions about quality of life and the educational environment. *Acad Med.* 80(1): 98–102

Dewhurst, D. and Ellaway, R. (2005) virtual learning environments. In: Dent, J.A. and Harden, R.M. (eds) *A Practical Guide for Medical Teachers* (pp. 201–210). Edinburgh: Churchill Livingstone

D'Eon M., Lear N., Turner M., and Jones, C. (2007) Perils of the hidden curriculum revisited. *Med Teach.* 29(4): 295–296

Department for Education and Skills (2006) *Early Years Foundation Stage Consultation Document.* Nottingham: DfES Publications (ref. SESCO6_18)

Dobie, S. (2007) Viewpoint: reflections on a well-traveled path: self-awareness, mindful practice, and relationship-centered care as foundations for medical education. *Acad Med.* 82(4): 422–427

Dolmans, D.H.J.M., Wolfhagen, I.H.A.P., Essed, G.G.M., Scherpbier, A.J.J.A., and van der Vleuten, C.P.M. (2002) Students' perceptions of relationships between some educational variables in the out-patient setting. *Med Educ.* 36: 735–741

Dolmans, D.H.J.M, Wolfhagen, I.H.A.P. Heineman, E., and Scherpbier, A.J.J.A. (2008) Factors adversely affecting student learning in the clinical learning environment. *Educ Health.* 21(3): 32

Dornan, T., Muijtjens, A., Hadfield, J., Scerpbier, A., and Boshuizen, H. (2006) Student evaluation of the 'curriculum in action'. *Med Educ.* 40: 667–674

Dunne, F., McAleer, S., and Roff, S. (2006) Assessment of the undergraduate medical education environment in a large UK medical school. *Health Educ J.* 65(2):149–158

Durak, H.I., Vatansever, K., van Dalen, J., and van der Vleuten, C. (2008) Factors determining students' global satisfaction with clerkships: an analysis of a two year students' rating data base. *Adv Health Sci Educ.* 13(4): 495–502

Edgren, G., Haffling, A.-C., Jakobsson, U., McAleer. S., and Danielsen, N. (2010) Comparing the educational environment (as measured by DREEM) at two different stages of curriculum reform. *Med Teach.* 32: e233–e238

Fitz, M.M., Homan, D., Reddy, S., Griffith, C.H. 3rd, Baker, E., and Simpson, K.P. (2007) The hidden curriculum: medical students' changing opinions toward the pharmaceutical industry. *Acad Med.* 82(10 Suppl): S1–S3

Fraser, B.J. and Fisher, D. (1983) Development and validation of short forms of some instruments measuring student perceptions of actual and preferred classroom learning environment. *Sci Educ.* 67(1): 115–131

Fraser, B.J., Anderson, G.J., and Walberg, H.J. (1982). Assessment of Learning Environments: Manual for Learning Environment Inventory (LEI) and My Class Inventory (MCI). Third version. http://www.eric.ed.gov/PDFS/ED223649.pdf Accessed 2 April 2012

Genn, J.M. (2001a) AMEE Medical Education Guide No. 23 (Part 1): Curriculum, environment, climate, quality and change in medical education-a unifying perspective. *Med Teach.* 23(4): 337–344

Genn, JM. (2001b) AMEE Medical Education Guide No. 23 (Part 2): Curriculum, environment, climate, quality and change in medical education—a unifying perspective. *Med Teach.* 23(5): 445–454

Glicken, A.D. and Merenstein, G.B. (2007) Addressing the hidden curriculum: understanding educator professionalism. *Med Teach.* 29(1): 54–57

Gofton, W. and Regehr, G. (2006) What we don't know we are teaching: unveiling the hidden curriculum. *Clin Orthop Relat Res.* 449: 20–27

Hafferty FW. (1998) Beyond curriculum reform: confronting medicine's hidden curriculum. *Acad Med.* 73(4): 403–407

Hafler, J.P., Ownby, A.R., Thompson, B.M., et al. (2011) Decoding the learning environment of medical education: a hidden curriculum perspective for faculty development. *Acad Med.* 86(4): 440–444

Hammond, S.M., O'Rourke, M., Kelly, M., Bennett, D., and O'Flynn, S. (2012) A psychometric appraisal of the DREEM. *BMC Med Educ.* 12: 2

Harden, R.M. (2001a) In: Dent, J.A. and Harden, R.M. (ed.) *A Practical Guide for Medical Teachers*. Edinburgh: Churchill Livingstone.

Harden, R.M. (2001b) The learning environment and the curriculum. *Med Teach.* 23(4): 335–336

Holt, M.C. and Roff, S. (2004) Development and validation of the Anaesthetic Theatre Educational Environment Measure (ATEEM). *Med Teach.* 26(6): 553–558

Hutchins, E.B. (1961) The 1960 medical school graduate: his perception of his faculty, peers, and environment. *J Med Educ.* 36: 322–329

Hutchinson, L. (2003) Educational environment. *BMJ.* 326(7393): 810–812

Isba, R. (2009). *DREEMs, myths, and realities: learning environments within the University of Manchester Medical School*. PhD thesis. University of Manchester, Manchester

Isba, R. and Boor, K. (2011) Creating a learning environment. In: Dornan, T., Mann, K., Scherpbier, A., and Spencer, J. (eds) *Medical Education: Theory and Practice* (pp 99–114). London: Elsevier, Churchill Livingstone.

Jackson P. (1968) *Life in Classrooms*. New York: Holt, Rinehart and Winston

Jakobsson, U., Danielsen, N., and Edgren, G. (2011) Psychometric evaluation of the Dundee Ready Educational Environment Measure: Swedish version. *Med Teach.* 33: e267–e274

Jiffry, M.T., McAleer, S., Fernando, S., and Marasinghe, R.B. (2005) Using the DREEM questionnaire to gather baseline information on an evolving medical school in Sri Lanka. *Med Teach.* 27(4): 348–352

Jordanova L. (1995) The social construction of medical knowledge. *Soc Hist Med.* 8(3): 361–381

Kaufman, D.M. (2003) Applying educational theory in practice. *BMJ.* 326(7382): 213–216

Lave, J. and Wenger, E. (1991) *Situated Learning: Legitimate Peripheral Participation*. Cambridge: Cambridge University Press

Lave, J. and Wenger, E. (1999) *Communities of Practice: Learning, Meaning, and Identity*. Cambridge: Cambridge University Press

Lempp H, Seale C. (2004) The hidden curriculum in undergraduate medical education: qualitative study of medical students' perceptions of teaching. *BMJ.* 329(7469): 770–773

Liaison Committee on Medical Education (2012) Standards for Accreditation of Medical Education Programs Leading to the M.D. Degree. http://www.lcme.org/functions.pdf Accessed 20 March 2013

Mann, K.V. (2002) Thinking about learning: implications for principle-based professional education. *J Contin Educ Health Prof.* 22(2): 69–76

Marshall, R.E. (1978). Measuring the medical school learning environment. *J Med Educ.* 53: 98–104

Maslow, A.H. (1943) A theory of human motivation. *Psychol Rev.* 50: 370–396

Masson, C. and Brazeau-Lamontagne, L. (2006) Paradigms, emperor's clothes syndrome, and hidden curriculum: how do they affect joint, bone, and spine diseases? *Joint Bone Spine.* 73(6): 581–583

Maudsley, R.F. (2001) Role models and the learning environment: essential elements in effective medical education. *Acad Med.* 76(5): 432–434

Mayya, S. and Roff, S. (2004) Students' perceptions of educational environment: a comparison of academic achievers and under-achievers at Kasturba medical college, India. *Educ Health (Abingdon).* 17(3): 280–291

McAleer J. (2012) *What are the medical student interactions within the closed, dynamic system of a small medical school?* MSc (research) Thesis. Lancaster University, Lancaster

McKendree, J. (2009) Can we create an equivalent educational experience on a two campus medical school? *Med Teach.* 31(5): e202–e205

Miles, S., and Leinster, S.J. (2007) Medical students' perceptions of their educational environment: expected versus actual perceptions. *Med Educ.* 41(3):265–272

Moos, R. H., and Trickett, E. J. (1974) *Classroom environment scale manual*. Palo Alto, CA: Consulting Psychologists Press

Morgan, D.L. (2007) Paradigms lost and pragmatism regained. Methodological implications of combining qualitative and quantitative methods. *J Mixed Methods Res.* 1(1): 48–76

Nunnally, J.C., Thistlethwaite, D.L., and Wolfe, S. (1963). Factored scales for measuring characteristics of college environments. *Educ Psychol Measurement.* 23(2): 239–248

Pace, C. R. (1963) *CUES: College and university environment scales: Technical manual*. Princeton: Educational Testing Service

Pace, C.R. (1969) *The College and University Environment Scales*. Institutional Research Princeton, NJ: Program for Higher Education, Educational Testing Service

Peterson, R.E. (1970) *The Crises of Purpose: Definition and Uses of Institutional Goals*. Princeton, NJ: Educational Testing Service

Price, B. (2004) Mentoring learners in practice: evaluating your learning environment. *Nursing Standard.* 19 (5): Number 2

Rhodes James, R. (1987) Anthony Eden. London: Macmillan, . p. 328

Roff, S. and McAleer, S. (2001) What is educational climate? *Med Teach.* 23(4): 333–334

Roff S, McAleer, S., Harden, R.M., et al. (1997) Development and validation of the Dundee Ready Education Environment Measure (DREEM). *Med Teach.* 19(4): 295–299

Roff, S., McAleer, S., Ifere, O.S., and Bhattacharya, S. (2001) A global diagnostic tool for measuring educational environment: comparing Nigeria and Nepal. *Med Teach.* 23(4): 378–382

Roff, S., McAleer, S., and Skinner, A. (2005) Development and validation of an instrument to measure the postgraduate clinical learning and teaching educational environment for hospital-based junior doctors in the UK. *Med Teach.* 27(4): 326–331

Roth, L.M., Severson, R.K., Probst, J.C., et al. (2006) Exploring physician and staff perceptions of the learning environment in ambulatory residency clinics. *Fam Med.* 38(3): 177–184

Rotthoff, T., Ostapczuk, M.S., de Bruin, J., Decking, U., Schneider, M., and Ritz-Timme, S. (2011) Assessing the learning environment of a faculty: Psychometric validation of the German version of the Dundee Ready Education Environment Measure with students and teachers. *Med Teach.* 33: e624–e636

Spooner, N.A., Cregan, P.C., and Khadra, M. (2011) Second Life for medical education. *eLearn Magazine.* September 2011

Standing Committee for Postgraduate Medical Education (1991) *Improving the experience. Good practice in senior house officer training. A report on local initiatives*. London: SCOPME

Till, H. (2004) Identifying the perceived weaknesses of a new curriculum by means of the Dundee Ready Education Environment Measure (DREEM) Inventory. *Med Teach.* 26(1): 39–45

Till, H. (2005) Climate studies: can students' perceptions of the ideal educational environment be of use for institutional planning and resource utilization? *Med Teach.* 27(4): 332–337

Treagust, D.F. and Fraser, B.J. (1986) Validation and Application of the College and University Classroom Environment Inventory (CUCEI). Paper presented at the Annual Meeting of the American Educational Research Association. http://www.eric.ed.gov/PDFS/ED274692.pdf Accessed 2 April 2012

Trevitt, C. and Highton, M. (2011) '*Learning environment'—the context in which learning takes place*. Oxford Learning Institute, University of Oxford. http://www.oucs.ox.ac.uk/ltg/teachingwithtechnology/ learningenvironment.pdf Accessed 2 April 2012

Turbes, S., Krebs, E., and Axtell, S. (2002) The hidden curriculum in multicultural medical education: the role of case examples. *Acad Med.* 77(3): 209–216

University of Southampton (2003) https://www.commonlearning.net/audit/ docs/Learning_Environment_Version_4.pdf Accessed 30 March 2012

Varma, R., Tiyagi, E., and Gupta, J.K. (2005) Determining the quality of educational climate across multiple undergraduate teaching sites using the DREEM inventory. *BMC Med Educ.* 5(1): 8.

Wear, S. (2008) Challenging the hidden curriculum. *J Gen Intern Med.* 23(5): 652–653

Whittle, S.R., Whelan, B., and Murdoch-Eaton, D.G. (2007) DREEM and beyond; studies of the educational environment as a means for its enhancement. *Educ Health (Abingdon).* 20(1): 7.

Woolf, K., Patel, S., Potts, H.W.W., and McManus, I.C. (2012) The hidden medical school: how social networks form and how they influence learning. *Med Teach.* 34(7): 577–586.

PART 3

Identity

CHAPTER 10

Identities, self and medical education

Lynn V. Monrouxe

> Once students are accepted into medical school, a major element in their training is the process of identity development as a doctor.
>
> Cynthia Whitehead
>
> Reproduced from Cynthia Whitehead, 'The doctor dilemma in interprofessional education and care: how and why will physicians collaborate?', Medical Education, 41, 10, p. 1010, copyright 2007, with permission from the Association for the Study of Medical Education and Wiley

Theoretical perspectives of identity

Who are you? This is a seemingly simple and straightforward question, yet its simplicity is deceiving. You hold multiple identities at any one time—these can include biological, personal, familial, societal, historical, professional, situational, and relational identities (Schwartz et al. 2011; Tsouroufli et al. 2011). So, you may be Caucasian, a woman, intelligent, witty and confident, a sister, a mother, a doctor, and so on: each one of these identities lay at a different level and each one intercepts with the other. Sometimes one or more of these identities are salient while others are diminished (fig. 10.1).

When we stop and think about defining the concept of *identity* a number of important conceptual questions arise. Some of these are outlined in box 10.1. These contrasting questions ensue from differing perspectives of what it means to be a social actor in the world. As Smith and Sparkes (2008, pp.5–35) highlight, they can be considered as being on a continuum from *thick individual* (psychological) and *thin social-relational* perspectives of identity and self at the one end, with those that draw on *thin individual* and *thick social-relational* understandings at the other end.

Furthermore, rather than being in opposition to each other, these perspectives can be seen as potentially offering different *levels* of understanding of the same phenomenon: individual, relational and collective (Schwartz et al. 2011)—rather like looking through different lenses of a camera (e.g. macro, wide angle and micro lenses). To put it another way, when talking about the self and identity, Leary (2004, pp.1–3) draws on the metaphors of *self-as-knower*, the *I-self* (self awareness), the *self-as-known*, and the *self-as-decision-maker and doer*—all being set within a relatively thick individual perspective of self and identity—with Bamberg and colleagues (2007, pp. 1–8) preferring the metaphor of *self as-speaker or narrator*.

In order for us to consider the concept of identity within medical education, it is therefore appropriate that we begin by considering these differing levels of understanding identity (fig. 10.2). Without such grounding, the concept of identity within medical education is in danger of becoming an unwieldy catch all and under-theorized concept. Indeed, in other domains it has been argued that the term *identity* has been used to describe such a range of differing concepts that its overuse has resulted in a loss of meaning (Brubaker and Cooper 2000, pp. 1–47).

However, and by way of a caveat, it is impossible to cover all theoretical and empirical approaches to identity in one chapter. There will be omissions. And those aspects that are covered will necessarily be overviews rather than detailed accounts. Furthermore, in addition to drawing on a range of medical education research that includes, or might benefit from, a consideration of identity issues, I draw heavily on my research in this area. This is for no other reason than my own attempts at understanding identity issues within medical education have drawn on a range of different theoretical approaches and so provide concrete examples of these perspectives within medical education. Yet in preparing for this current chapter I now see even more links, connections and future possibilities than I had previously understood. Therefore, it is my hope that this overview will also provide you with some of the clarity it has provided me, amongst the mist and fog in which identity theory and research currently lurks.

Individual perspectives of identity

While this section focuses on theories within individual perspectives of identity and identity formation—in particular the *self as knower* and *as known*—we must not forget the influencing role of social-relational forces. Indeed, it could be argued that Erik Erikson became the forefather of many individual identity theories when he identified his eight phases of chronological ego-growth in his seminal work *identity and the life cycle* (Erikson 1959). However, at each phase of

Box 10.1 Questions about identity

What does it mean to have an identity?

Can we ever *possess* an identity?

Is identity a *product* or a *process*?

Is identity *discovered* by the individual or *created* and *co-created* in social interactional settings?

Is identity a relatively stable and fixed aspect of an individual or is it malleable and changeable according to context?

Is identity primarily related to one's individual self or are one's relational, historical, collective or professional selves equally or more important when defining identity?

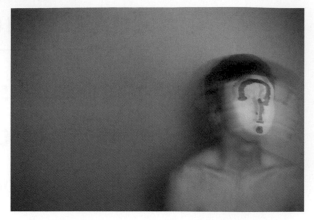

Figure 10.2 Identity.
Figure courtesy of Jasmine Monrouxe, reproduced with permission.

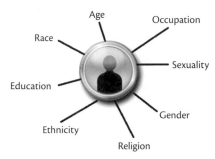

Figure 10.1 Identities.

growth, Erikson stresses the inter-relatedness of the individual and their social milieu and the resulting psychosocial crises. So the social is not just something we adjust to, nor is it a force that shapes us, rather the social and individual are meshed. And this understanding of the individual and the social permeates throughout neo-Eriksonian theories of identity (Blasi 1980, 1983; Marcia et al. 1993).

What renders individual perspectives individual therefore, is not necessarily their claim to psychological over social process, but it is rather the epistemic status of identity—the way in which they treat knowledge and knowing of identity. Individual perspectives of identity suggest that identity resides within a person's head and so can be a *knowable* fact. The challenge for empirical research within this perspective has been how best to measure the presence of certain aspects of identity (dependent upon the specific theory adopted).

Emerging adulthood and identity development: Marcia's 'identity statuses'

Erikson (1968) designated identity versus role confusion as the central crisis of the adolescent stage of life. However, within industrialized societies there is a prolonged period of adolescence: 18 to 25—the so-called period of *emerging adulthood*—during which time most identity exploration appears to take place (Arnett 2000) and a time in which many people make their transition to medical school and becoming a doctor. Within this perspective, identity exploration focuses around the three areas of love, work, and worldviews, as we try out a range of life possibilities, gradually moving toward making lasting commitments.

Marcia (1966, pp. 551–558) developed a semi-structured interview, which he called the *identity status interview,* to examine how

much exploration a person has undertaken in the areas of work and ideological constructs (e.g. religion or politics). From this, four distinct groups of individuals have been classified—people in *identity achievement* and *foreclosure* groups were seen as having a high degree of commitment, with people within *moratorium* and *identity diffusions* groups having a low degree of commitment (Marcia 1966). These four categories are not to be considered as sequential phases, but as different statuses of individuals. Those in the identity achievement group appear to possess a strong, continuous and coherent sense of themselves, achieved through a personal exploratory process: while they are sensitive to others' perspectives, they know who they are, where they are going, and are not easily swayed. These individuals can be contrasted with those classified within the identity status of moratoriums who are given to long periods of rumination as they struggle to define who they are: some may continue this way indefinitely, others move on towards making firm commitments within identity achievement. Individuals classified within the status of foreclosure appear committed within their identity, but the identity they adopt has been prescribed by others around them: they can be seen as being conformists rather than explorers. As they have typically not undergone a period of exploration, they have difficulty in accepting or debating alternative positions. Finally, there are those who are classified within the identity status of diffusion. The commonality amongst such individuals is their lack of exploration combined with a lack of commitment. This enables them to become adaptable and malleable, looking to others for reference, with some feeling a sense of isolation and meaninglessness.

In many countries, medical students start their undergraduate days at the age of 17 or 18. This late adolescent phase into emerging adulthood brings major developmental changes and challenges as young people begin to develop their competencies, attitudes and values, and make their transition into early adulthood within a complex set of social, cultural and historical contexts (Arnett 2000; Erikson 1968). Thus, the developmental tasks for emerging adulthood includes identity formation at both the personal and social levels; the adoption of more demanding roles within society; finding personal meaning and purpose within new roles and making the required life changes to fulfil these roles.

So from an individual perspective, medical educationalists might wish to consider late adolescents' cognitive and social development and how this affects aspects of identity formation—including moral identity. However, only scant attention has been paid to this. The few studies that have been undertaken suggest that at the end of their preclinical years some students' identity status could still be classified as diffuse or as displaying tentative professional identities (Niemi 1997). But by the end of their first year of clerkship (mean age 26.5 years), none are classified as diffuse with around half being in both achievement and foreclosure classifications (Beran et al. 2011). That around 50% of clinical students are classified as being in the foreclosure group might not shock many medical educators, but the consequences of this finding are great. These students appear to have made a commitment to medicine without active exploration of alternative career paths. According to theorists in this area, while these individuals are unlikely to feel anxiety about their career choice, they are at risk of forming less meaningful commitments and of experiencing identity crises in the future (Marcia et al. 1993).

That both statuses of achievement and foreclosure are associated with less personal stress and anxiety than the identity statuses of moratorium or diffusion may well be due to the way in which individuals make sense of their commitments. Underpinning many perspectives of identity, both individual and interactional, is the notion of coherence: individuals are motivated to create a world which seems consistent and which makes logical sense, and in this world they wish to portray themselves as stable and coherent. Individuals experiencing diffusion or moratorium are unlikely to be able to portray themselves as such.

Recently Helmich et al. (2012) used narrative interviewing to examine 17 first-year medical students' experiences of early attachments to nurses in hospitals and nursing homes. Their analysis resulted in four paradigms that displayed differences across emotional talk, meaning and identity, each with similarities to Marcia's identity status paradigms: feeling insecure (relating to identity diffusion), complying (foreclosure), developing (moratorium), and participating (identity achievement). For Helmich and her colleagues, their paradigms go beyond those of Marcia in that they are 'more explicitly taking into account the social and cultural context in which students are developing their nascent professional identities' (Helmich et al. 2012). Indeed, it is imperative that future research examining identities within medical education explicitly considers social and cultural contexts within which students learn.

Self-verification theory and identity negotiation

As mentioned in the previous section, coherence is a central concept within identity formation—it spans many different theoretical approaches. The essence of self-verification theory is that we prefer others to view us as we view ourselves, and we seek to elicit reactions accordingly (Gomez et al. 2009a, b; Swann 2012; Swann et al. 2009, 2000). So, those of us who hold positive self views will seek to reinforce that positivity and those who hold negative self views will seek to reinforce negativity (Swann et al. 2009). Such self-verification is achieved through a process of identity negotiation and it is this interactive process that contributes to the shaping, displaying and preserving of our personal and group identities (Gomez et al. 2009b; Swann 2012).

According to this perspective, as we create our self-verifying social worlds, we might use a number of processes including *identity cues*. These comprise visible signs and symbols of identity such

as the way in which we dress, our mannerisms, and even the way we portray ourselves to others through our online identities (e.g. through the use of consistent labelling of ourselves and the digital organization of social information enabling people to see how trustworthy or eminent we are—a process known as *deep profiling*) (Ma and Agarwal 2007). Recent research investigating medical students' online behaviours revealed the tentative creation of new identities online as students began to develop their professional identities: 'Just because we happen to be entering this profession, we can't completely cut off the person that we are, *but we can just present it in a better way*' (my emphasis: Chretien et al. 2010, p. S69). Thus, we can maintain a consistency and a coherence of our identities through the subtle re-storying of ourselves over time.

This subtle re-storying may go unnoticed even by ourselves, as another process of self-verification is seeing non-existent evidence. Self-views can influence information-processing at the levels of attention, recall and interpretation. For example, experimental research has demonstrated that people with positive self-views spend longer reading evaluations they expected to be positive (and recalled more positive statements) and those with negative self-views behaved similarly with evaluations they expected to be negative (Swann 2012).

However, while these presentational, attentional, encoding and recall processes might serve to stabilize our self-views through consistent confirmatory evidence (Swann et al. 2003), what of the struggling medical student who possesses negative self-views? One area within medical education where we might wish to consider this facet of identity is the process of remediation. While theorizing in this area has drawn on knowledge gained from cognitive, emotional, and socio-cultural domains (Winston et al. 2010) the addition of knowledge developed within identity theory—and in particular the concept of self-verification—will facilitate further understanding, in particular within aspects such as feedback and engagement in the remediation process. This understanding may also help disrupt the self-verifying cycles in which students may be trapped (Swann 1996).

Along with individual outcomes, attending to the issue of self-verification and identities can have interpersonal and societal outcomes. On an interpersonal level, longitudinal research has demonstrated that successful self-verification can lead to increased levels of commitment in small group working and the creation of a safe environment within which to develop creative solutions (Polzer et al. 2002; Swann et al. 2000). This has obvious implications for small-group working within medical educational settings. On a societal level, successful self-verification has been shown to reduce social stereotyping. In this way people are perceived as being individuals rather than as typical members of a social group (Swann et al. 2003).

Personal identity and the moral self

Continuing within the individual perspective but moving into more specific aspects of identity (in particular the *self-as-decision-maker and doer*), moral identity can be seen as being a crucial area for understanding within medical education as it lies at the 'intersection of moral development and identity formation' (Hardy and Carlo 2011, p. 495): one's moral identity is considered to be the motivational force operating between moral reasoning (what it is that we consider to be right or wrong) and behaviour. Indeed, research has shown that moral reasoning is a poor predictor of moral behaviour: one can excel in one's moral reasoning capacities yet commit moral lapses in behaviour. Likewise highly moral acts are committed by individuals whose moral reasoning can be described as being unso-phisticated (Blasi 1980; Colby and Damon 1992). Such findings cast a shadow across current initiatives that rely on Situational Judgment Tests as a measure of moral aptitude and behavior.

Moral behaviour, however, has been linked with both moral iden-tity and social context and has been theorized within individual character perspectives (Blasi 1980, 1983), social cognitive perspec-tives (Lapsley and Narvaez 2004), and sociological interactional perspectives (Hitlin 2011; Mead 1934). According to individual character perspectives, and set within a neo-Erikson framework, Blasi's self model (Blasi 1983, pp. 178–210) sheds light onto the moral reasoning–behaviour disjunction. Blasi highlighted three key aspects that lead to moral behaviour: responsibility, moral identity, and self-consistency. So, before any moral action can occur we must first assume responsibility for the action—not just for the other but also for ourselves. Additionally, our moral identity should be a cen-tral tenet of our self: we see ourselves as moral beings and are driven to live up to that viewpoint through our drive for self-consistency.

According to Blasi, individuals differ regarding the specific issues around which they construct their identities as well as their subjec-tive experiences to their identity (Blasi 1983, pp. 178–210). As our subjective identity matures it becomes more central to our sense of self, more organized, more focused around internal values and goals (rather than external appearances), and we gain a greater sense of agency. As we develop a mature subjective identity, we simultane-ously develop a strong need for self-consistency, with deviations from our ideal resulting in an intense negative affect. Indeed, it has been argued that the strongest form of moral identity can be seen in *moral exemplars* who possess complete unity between their sense of self and moral goals such that their own personal interests are synonymous with their sense of right and wrong, so much so that the 'fulfilment of one implies fulfilment of the other' (Colby and Damon 1992, p. 300).

By contrast to the character perspectives of moral identity, social cognitive perspectives see moral identity as the interplay between cognitive schemas (e.g. representations in our minds of selves, situations and relationships), affective responses and situational influences. From this perspective it is hypothesized that the most accessible schemas may well be those that are most important to us (Lapsley and Narvaez 2004). This accessibility enables us to react automatically to events around us—so-called moral expertise (Narvaez and Lapsley 2005). From this perspective it is argued that moral exemplars are so, not due to the unity of self and moral goals, but the certainty and immediacy of exemplars' moral actions might be due to them having rich systems of accessible moral schemas (Lapsley and Narvaez 2004; Narvaez and Lapsley 2005).

Possible identities and the moral self

Surprisingly, the theoretical concept of *possible identities* has received little attention in the field of medical education. Specific theories focussing on this draw from a range of influences includ-ing neo-Eriksonian, social–cognitive and biographical narrative theoretical perspectives. Within these perspectives, our future identity is considered to be part of our self-concept, focusing on who we might become.

Possible identities comprise the range of working personal the-ories of whom we might be. The likelihood of us holding particu-lar identities of whom we might become is based on whether we think we can become that person given our social–cultural stand-ing, our talents, our personal characteristics, and how hard we are prepared to work in order to make things happen. Thus, future identities move beyond first-person singular *I* identities (who can I aspire to become), and towards more socially situated first-person plural *us* and *we* identities (who *people like me* can aspire to become). From this social perspective, the intersection of gen-dered, racial, sociocultural and socioeconomic identities comes to the fore (Tsouroufli et al. 2011). Furthermore, possible iden-tities can include both positive and negative identities and can influence our identity-based motivational actions. So, in line with the concept of a coherent self, it has been argued that, from this future-oriented perspective of the self, we evaluate our present actions in terms of future identities and that these future identi-ties directly motivate us towards certain actions (Oettingen and Mayer 2002). Moreover, distal future thoughts are likely to acti-vate a strong desire to become like one's *true ideal self*, whereas proximal future thoughts cue more instrumental and pragmatic selves, with the power of the situation having an inhibitory role on whether or not people behave according to their true, inner self (Kivetz and Tyler 2007). Furthermore, research suggests that once a possible identity has been formed, and commitments to this have been made, people are reluctant to revise it downwards or to let go of it completely (Carroll et al. 2009).

So from a possible identities perspective, medical educationalists might wish to consider aspects such as the range of possible identi-ties medical students hold at different times during their under-graduate education, how intersected they are, what the origins of these identities are, and to what extent they are proximal (I want to be an excellent student) or distal (I want to be an excellent sur-geon). Specific questions we might ask within this framework might include: to what extent does attaining their future identity feel linked to students' present action and to what extent do situational factors affect proximal and distal future identities? In other words, how much does a students' future identity cue their identity-based motivational striving and what factors affect the strength of this effect? One specific question in this context would be 'under what situations, and how, do medical students draw on their future iden-tities when explaining their behaviour during events in which they upheld or transgressed professional standards?' (Monrouxe and Rees 2011). More nuanced understandings of the factors underly-ing the expression of ideal future identities might enable medical educators to facilitate students' desires to behave morally during difficult dilemmas. Furthermore, facilitating their moral actions in the face of such dilemmas will not only impact on issues of patient care, but will also have a positive impact on students' wellbeing. Research suggests that *actual* verses *ideal* self discrepancy—acting against ones' ideal future self—can lead to people experiencing neg-ative emotional states such as dejection and agitation (Gramzow et al. 2000). This sheds further light on students' moral distress fol-lowing professionalism dilemmas (Monrouxe et al. in press).

Social or contextual perspectives of identity

While it is impossible to include all theories in this chapter, in the previous section we have considered a range of individual approaches to the concept of identity, mainly within a neo-Eriksonian perspective. And while such theories prioritize the indi-vidual self (in terms of epistemic knowledge) they also acknowledge the inter-relatedness of the individual and the social. We now move further into the social aspect of identities to consider the range of theories that tend to conceptualize identities as being constructed in and through discourse and artefacts, rather than being seen as an essential property of the self. From this perspective identities are not something we *possess*; rather they are something we *do*. This is akin to Bamberg et al.'s (2007, pp. 1–8) metaphor of the *self as speaker or narrator*. Furthermore, due to the primary role of context in the shaping of the self and identity, these concepts are conceptualized in their plural forms: identities and selves. These primarily discourse-based theories conceptualize identities in fluid and dynamic processes of change within which individuals do *identity work*. In other words, an understanding of how people establish their identities is achieved through the analysis of talk.

Narrative approaches to identities

Narrative theories of identity are amongst the most complex. Sometimes, a thick individual and thin social relation perspective is adopted, at other times a thick social relational and thin individual stance is proposed (Smith and Sparkes 2008). Furthermore, individual researchers are often unclear about where they lie along the continuum, and the same researcher will adopt different perspectives at different times and may also fluctuate between perspectives over time (Smith and Sparkes 2008).

Within this tradition there are also differences between researchers about what comprises a narrative: do narratives have to contain certain structural components (Labov 1997; Labov and Waletzky 1967); do they have to be so-called big stories that are autobiographical narratives, frequently collected in interview settings (Frank 1995; Smith 2002; Wengraf 2001); or can they also be the small stories we find in the apparently fleeting moments within interactional settings (Bamberg 2006; Monrouxe 2009a, b; Monrouxe and Rees 2011; Monrouxe and Sweeney in press; Wortham and Gadsten 2006)? Also, while many see the act of narrating both as a cognitive sense-making process and as a means through which we create our identities, narratives are increasingly seen by some to hold a privileged position of holding lives together, providing a sense of coherence to what is in essence a naturally incoherent and unruly set of events.

Narrative coherence is viewed as being artfully crafted in the telling of stories and is beneficial for an individual's wellbeing (Frank 1995; Smith and Sparkes 2002). Furthermore, and possibly related to this notion of wellbeing, not only are biographic narratives considered by some to be self-defining in character, narrative identities become the very 'stories we live by' (McAdams 1993). However, researchers coming from the small-story perspective feel that such a notion overplays the temporal dimension of the sense of self and identity, whilst downplaying interactive and cultural roles of the discursive practice of identities and how identities are co-created interactionally (Georgakopoulou 2006).

Structural theories

We begin this section by considering theories around narrative structure from the field of *narratology*. Narratologists try to understand the internal structure of the narrative in terms of its component parts such as

- Story myths and genres (Frye 1957)

- Regular elements of a narrative plot (e.g. action, scene, actor) (Bruner 1990)

- Temporal structure of regular clauses—so beginning with an explanation of the context and actors, moving on to saying that happened (and why), and ending with evaluations and resolutions to the event (Labov 1972, 1997; Labov and Waletzky 1967) and

- Components of interactional narratives within everyday conversations such as how tellable the story is, whether we are alluding to previous stories we have told or heard, or whether we are deferring our stories for another time (Ochs and Capps 2001).

However, they do so not only to understand the *form* of narrative itself but also to understand the *purpose* behind a narrative, in terms of what narratives tell us about performing and enacting identities. This section focuses on the most well-known account of narrative structure proposed by Labov (Labov 1972; Labov and Waletzky 1967).

In terms of narrative form, Labov suggests that narratives typically begin with an *orientation* which introduces the listener to the actors in the story along with the time, place and initial behaviour of those actors (Labov 1972). Following the orientation, narratives then proceed to the *complicating action*—what happened—and the *most reportable event*. This event is then *evaluated* by the narrator before any *resolution* is found and the listener is brought back to the here and now through a *coda*. Sometimes the narrative is preceded with an *abstract* that summarizes the story and its point (Labov 1972).

Labov (1997, pp. 395–415) elaborates on the issue of narrative form as he further theorizes on the social act of narration and identity formation—that is, what we *do* with narrative—and in particular on issues of

- narrative reportability (how narrators justify the interactional space required for storytelling by generating an interesting enough narrative for their audience)

- credibility (how narrators establish believability)

- causality and

- assignment of praise and blame.

Understanding how narrators assign praise and blame is an important aspect of narrative analysis and interlinks with issues around moral identity. For narratives to be reportable they typically include issues of conflict. In such cases the narrator is frequently driven to portray themselves in a positive light highlighting their own morality, so through their narrative they might concern themselves with the assignment of responsibility for events. One way this is accomplished is through the polarization of characters within the narrative: the protagonist conforms to moral standards (or at least strives to do so) and the antagonist violates them (or attempts to prevent the protagonist from being moral) (Labov 2004; Monrouxe and Rees 2011). Furthermore, these characters are portrayed in subtle ways—for example, through the way narrators put words and thoughts into the mouths of others and themselves and through the way they evaluate events during the act of storytelling (Holt 1996; Labov 1997, 2004).

The perspective of narratology can be used as a starting point for the analysis of medical students' narrative identities (Monrouxe 2009a, 2010; Monrouxe and Rees 2011; Monrouxe and Sweeney in press) as structural theories are more typically used in conjunction with other narrative theories (Riessman 2008).

Autobiographical past and imagined future

Some holistic theorists argue that narrative identity is the evolving story of *the self*: where we have come from and where we are heading. These theoretical perspectives have a similar flavour to the identity theories previously mentioned. However, within a narrative framework, the theoretical focus is on our motivation to *narrate* a coherent life story rather than our motivation to *act* in a coherent manner. Within this framework we are thought to construct a story for ourselves and for others which makes meaning of our lives, and which we subsequently internalize as being our essential self (Diaute and Lightfoot 2004; McAdams 1993; Ricoeur 1992). Our story has a strong temporal dimension reaching backward into our past experiences and forward into our imagined future (Riessman 2003). And we construct our narratives interactively with a particular audience in mind and within a specific context as we draw on 'the well of past stories and flows into future stories' (Ewick and Silbey 2003, p. 1343). As McAdams succinctly writes, 'complete with setting, scenes, characters, plots, and themes, narrative identity combines a person's reconstruction of his or her personal past with an imagined future' (McAdams 2011, p. 100). We provide this personal account of our development along with verbal *explanations* (rather than internal motivations) of our moral commitments—around things such as work and love and who we are and who we will be.

The distinction between the narrative concept of imagined futures and the psychological concept of possible identities is an important one and based on the degree to which each perspective treats the nature of knowledge and knowing. As highlighted earlier, psychological perspectives suggest that we can come to know an individuals' true self whereas narrative approaches tend to focus on how identities are constructed. Therefore, within many narrative perspectives, the drive for narrative coherence is paramount as we try to make links and connections with our pasts, narrating strong moral choices for our futures. And because we cannot see into the future, there is always the possibility of a disruption to our narrative identities. Our lives can be 'ruptured by the *peripeteia*, or the transformative event' (Charon and Montello 2002, p. xi)—the so-called 'narrative wreckage' of an illness as talked about by Arthur Frank (1995). Thus illness is seen as a 'call for stories' where 'stories have to repair the damage that illness has done to the ill person's sense of where she is in life, and where she may be going' (p. 53), restoring a sense of coherence. Additionally, Frank argues that in order to resist the colonization of their bodies as medical territory ('clinical material') (Frank 1995, p. 12), people narrate their stories of illness so as to reclaim their identities as people (rather than patients) with a sense of future-selves.

Likewise, within the field of medical education it has been argued that negative experiences at medical school can be seen as a form of narrative wreckage which might bring forth a call for stories (Monrouxe and Sweeney in press; Shapiro 2009). Such experiences can range from the first time a student witnesses the death of a patient (Monrouxe 2009b; Monrouxe and Sweeney in press) to witnessing or participating in something they feel is immoral or unethical (Monrouxe and Rees 2011; Rees and Monrouxe in press). So a previously held concept of what a doctor is, does and can do—the future that students' hoped for and imagined, including the values and behaviours they aspired to—can be shattered in the face of experience (Monrouxe 2009a, 2010; Monrouxe and Rees 2011; Monrouxe and Sweeney in press; Rees and Monrouxe 2010). Sometimes, students' narratives of troubling experiences help them to make sense of events which conflict with their own personal ideology and can be seen as a way of resisting the flattening out and colonization of students within medical education; bringing to the fore their own individuality and personhood (Shapiro 2009; Takakuwa et al. 2004).

Interactional positioning theories, small stories and discourse

Positioning theorists concern themselves with how people co-construct identities in interaction through the process of offering up their position in relation to particular master narratives or dominant discourses, and how these discourses might be contested by interlocutors (Bamberg 2003; Davies 2001; Wortham and Gadsten 2006). So the positioning of selves and others typically takes place in conversations and through *small stories*—everyday interactional narrative activities, such as stories of ongoing events, future events, hypothetical events, events that are shared by the interlocutors, reminders of past events, deferrals, and refusals to tell (Bamberg 2006; Georgakopoulou 2007; Monrouxe 2009b). Though such activities we explain our positions, we defend and alter them. Furthermore, we position others as we do so, for example others can be wrong, incompetent, immoral or just ignorant. And such positions are established according to an unfolding narrative which enables us to make sense of why the narrator assigns certain positions.

Take for example the medical student's narrative of a consultant surgeon who brutally informs a patient he most likely has an inoperable cancer, resulting in the patient abruptly discharging himself (Monrouxe and Rees 2011). The consultant is positioned as an excellent surgeon (although this is limited to his technical rather than interpersonal skills); the narrator is positioned as a keen, intelligent, knowledgeable, compassionate, and obedient third-year student, who benefits from having an enthusiastic educator; and the patient is depicted as an innocent, naive victim (Monrouxe and Rees 2011). Throughout the narrative these socially known positions are drawn on and maintained through the student's sense-making process of narrating, culminating in her taking the blame for the surgeon's actions (because his teaching of her leads to the neglect of patient care and because she has been taught how to break bad news appropriately while the surgeon has not). This leaves her narrating long-term feelings of regret.

Thus, positioning analysis can help shed light on the way in which people use language within their narrative accounts to lay claim to certain identities for themselves and others. Within narrative accounts, positioning analysis attempts to shift the analytical focus from understanding the specific narrative—the so-called 'discourse' with a little 'd'—towards an understanding of the meaning of that narrative in society—the so-called 'Discourse' with a capital 'D' (Gee 2011; p.34). This happens through the consideration of a number of broad questions: what is the story about? What claims to identity are made? How is this rooted in societal discourse? At one level there is the consideration of how characters are established in the narrative and how they are positioned against each other. Then, focus is turned to what the narrator is attempting to accomplish within their narrative through the linguistic strategies they employ—such as reported talk or metaphor—finally these are drawn together as the analyst considers the question 'who am I vis-à-vis what society says I should be' (Watson 2007, p. 347).

Dramaturgical social theory

Moving away from the concept of narrative identities but remaining firmly within interactional talk, Goffman's dramaturgical theory (1959/1990) argues that the self is not an entity that pre-exists alone—rather it arises in the interactional process of *performance* within everyday social activities. The fundamental unit of analysis for Goffman is not the individual but the *team*, within which roles are co-created through interaction (Mead 1934). Furthermore, performances are primarily about the activity at hand, rather than the characteristic of the performer. So from this perspective, a dramaturgical analysis leads to an understanding of how teams cooperate to create particular impressions of reality though the roles they create for themselves and others, and how these are negotiated and contested interactionally.

Goffman uses terms such as frontstage, backstage, scripts, and roles to describe what is happening within any given scene (Goffman 1959/1990). Three main roles have been identified: team members are *performers* (i.e. directors and actors), acting for an *audience*, and *outsiders*. Goffman also identified *discrepant roles*, including the *non-person*, 'defined by both performers and audience as someone who isn't there' (Goffman 1959/1990, pp. 150–1). While present during the performance, because they are not part of the team, they can be ignored. Goffman cites old people, children and sick people as examples of non-persons (Goffman 1959/1990).

Even with this brief description of Goffman's dramaturgy theory, with his focus on the team, we can see its utility within medical education. From the perspective of dramaturgy we might ask questions such as those outlined in box 10.2.

Within medical education, Monrouxe et al. (2009, pp. 918–930) have considered the concept of team within the triadic doctor–student–patient interaction during bedside teaching activities. They found linguistically bounded backstage talk between doctors and students who used paralanguage—such as shifts in the volume and pace of talk—which rendered the patient as audience. Indeed, participants played multiple roles across and within each encounter including doctors as director and audience, student as actor and audience, and patients as director, audience, and non-person. Furthermore, participants sometimes resisted the passive roles of audience and non-person through the use of laughter and explicit healthy-identity talk in which patients present themselves as their *fit and active* past self rather than their sick present self (Monrouxe et al. 2009; Rees and Monrouxe 2010a).

Box 10.2 The perspective of dramaturgy

How do people present themselves and others within different educational settings?

Who directs the performance at any one time and how is this accomplished?

How are people constructed—as audience or non-person—and how is this resisted?

What happens in the backstage space and how is this accomplished?

To what extent is the patient constructed as a member of the team?

Ethnomethodology: conversation analysis, membership categorization analysis, and discourse analysis

Continuing within the interactional frame of identities, ethnomethodology is a sociological approach to research that originates from the work of Harold Garfinkel (1967). It is the study of the methods through which we assemble and reproduce features of everyday life in situ: as individuals or members of society we continuously make sense of the world and we display our understandings of the world for all to see (Garfinkel 1967). Researchers coming from this perspective take recordings and transcripts of talk from within everyday events—including institutional talk—and analyse people's turn-by-turn interactions with a focus of how conversation works and how identities are interactionally defined (Drew 2005). A number of different theoretical approaches have developed from this background of ethnomethodology; we briefly consider three in this section—conversation analysis, membership categorization analysis, and discourse analysis. Each has its origins in ethnomethodology yet they have been developed to a large degree independently of the other, differing through the relative broadness and inclusivity of the social world within which they analyse talk (they are conceptually similar to the small-d–capital-D of discourse highlighted earlier).

Conversation analysis (CA) is the most stringent approach of all concentrating solely on sequential interaction—rather than individual's talk—and so focusing entirely on the way in which interaction is co-constructed. Furthermore, CA asserts that any claims to identities, and issues of power that might be linked with such claims, must be grounded within specific actualities of talk: 'context and identity have to be treated as inherently locally produced, incrementally developed, and by extension, as transformable at any moment' (Heritage 2005, p. 111). There is no room for the imposition of the academic analysts' political or theoretical agendas onto the data at hand (Schegloff 1992). For some medical educationalists, however, this strict position of not going beyond the data to consider the *so what* questions—in terms of identities, power and resistance, for example—might prove too confining.

While CA focuses entirely on the sequential features of conversational interaction, it has largely ignored social categorical aspects of conversation: the membership categories (social identities) to which speakers are oriented. The focus of membership categorization analysis (MCA) is around the use of membership categories, membership categorization devices (MCD), and category predicates by members (Hester and Eglin 1997). Membership categories are classifications of social types used to describe people: for example, students, nerds, swot, malingerer, daughter, and doctor. Furthermore, collectives (so-called collectivity membership categories) and non-person entities (e.g. institutions) can also be categorized: for example, X hospital, the healthcare system, the middle classes, and socialists. Additionally, within MCA, the concept of category-boundedness is important. This is because category-boundedness constrains the category members' expected activity types, rights, entitlements, obligations, and knowledge.

In the social world, certain activities are expected to be only undertaken by certain members of particular categories. Furthermore, certain characteristics (so-called natural predicates) are associated with certain categories. Take for example the category of *surgeon*. Whatever is known about surgeons can be invoked as being relevant to the individual ascribed with this category label and 'a set of inferential resources by which to interpret and account for past or present conduct, or to inform predictions about likely future behaviour' are activated (Widdicombe 1998, p. 53). Furthermore, category memberships can be ascribed, resisted, avowed, disavowed, displayed, and ignored across different times and places which 'does things as part of the interactional work that constitutes people's lives' (Widdicombe 1998, p. 2).

The final analytic perspective we consider in this section is discourse analysis (DA). While CA and MCA come primarily from sociological theoretical roots, discourse analysis has its origins in psychology. In particular, it challenges the perspectives outlined at the beginning of the chapter whereby identities are seen as being internal to the individual and where language is considered to be an expression of thoughts, desires, attitudes and motivations (Edwards and Potter 1992). Thus language is seen as a performance of inner states with no ontological claims about the basis of that performance being made. From these roots Potter and Wetherell (1987) developed *critical discursive psychology* that advocates a synthetic approach to the analysis of talk in interaction, combining the microanalytical approach of CA with a more macroanalytical attention to cultural–historical contexts. Thus, they urge analysts to begin with the macrosocial or political issues and examine how individuals might orient themselves to—or position themselves against—societal master discourses: so moving from capital-D to small-d discourses. Other researchers have proposed the addition of a Foucauldian approach to discourse analysis (Holstein and Gubrium 2000) thus considering the ideological workings of language and how this serves to construct institutional identities. Drawing on the metaphor of the panopticon—a prison with a guard tower that was always in view although the guards were obscured—Holstein and Gubrium suggest that panopticism represents 'part of the varied discourses we share which, in use, articulate and regulate our subjectivity . . . these discourses also constitute the moral horizons of the self' (Holstein and Gubrium 2000, p. 225). In suggesting this, they wonder 'what degree of choice does panopticism leave for self construction (Holstein and Gubrium 2000, p. 225)?' This is a particularly interesting question for the construction of professional identities.

Directly linked with the ways in which identities are enacted in institutional settings, medical education researchers are beginning to examine the issue of power within workplace learning settings (Monrouxe et al. 2010a; Rees et al. 2013; Rees and Monrouxe 2008). They found that all participants (clinical teachers, students, and patients) employed linguistic and paralinguistic (e.g. using the third person 'she' and laughter) and non-verbal communication strategies (e.g. using medical artefacts) to enact and resist power within bedside teaching activities, so reflecting typical power asymmetries between doctors, students and patients.

Sociocultural perspectives of identities

This final section touches on one of the most popular theories of identity formation found within medical education research: legitimate peripheral participation and communities of practice (LPP and CoP: Lave and Wenger 1991; Wenger 1998). In 1991 Lave and Wenger introduced the concept of LPP 'as a descriptor of engagement in social practice that entails learning as an integral constituent' (1991, p. 35). LPP emphasizes longitudinal

developmental cycles of communities of practices whereby identity formation as a full practitioner is a gradual and relational process of becoming—through a person's ever-changing knowledge, skills and discourse, rather than through the simple development of knowledge and knowing. Knowing entails the newcomer to moving 'centripetally through a complex form of practice [that] creates possibilities for understanding the world as experienced' (Lave and Wenger 1991, p. 123).

Wenger (1998) expands on this description of identity when he asserts that the focus of identity should be the mutual constitution of the individual and community (as it is impossible to understand where one begins and the other ends). Furthermore, he highlights identity as being negotiated (through reification), situated within community memberships, learning trajectories, multimembership categorization and through reconciling our local ways of being (akin to small-d discourses) with global ways of being (akin to capital-D discourses).

While the concepts of LPP and CoP have immediate appeal and a perceived usefulness within medical education, the more nuanced details of the theories often appear to be lost (e.g. the issue of reification, the dimensions of identity through which competence is recognized, the mutual constitution of self and community, and the various types of trajectories that lead us to become legitimate community members). Nevertheless, the concepts of LPP and CoP have been taken up widely within medical education research. LPP is 'attractive as a middle-level theory between structure and agency, which is applicable to and close to actual life and which resonates with detailed ethnographic accounts of how learning happens' (Barton and Tusting 2005, p. 3).

However, while these concepts have been taken up with enthusiasm, they have not been adopted as an a priori theoretical approach whereby researchers examine the nuanced ways in which LPP and CoP play out in medical education (and therefore have not yet contributed to theoretical development). Instead, they have been used in a post-hoc fashion with the concepts being 'bootstrapped' as a way of helping researchers offer theoretical rationales for their data (Balmer et al. 2008). This is not unsurprising for two main reasons. First, it is hard to pin down the various components of the theories—even on close reading the concepts remain 'slippery and elusive' and the critical edge of Lave and Wenger's (1991) original contribution appears to be 'eclipsed and that ideas were being taken over by the certainty and oversimplifications of management training' (Barton and Tusting 2005, p. 6). This oversimplification renders it hard to utilize as a testable theory. Second, and partly due to these oversimplifications, we are left with a high-level description of how people become legitimate members of a community of practice through interactions, placing participation and reification at the core: yet no interactional theory of language and activities is provided through which researchers can examine how meaning is negotiated.

Using these theoretical approaches, the challenge for medical educators is to develop sophisticated research designs to examine the interactional nuances of becoming a legitimate participant within medicine and medical education. Medical educators might ask questions such as

◆ What are the links between language and the other aspects of the social world such as power relationships between doctors, student, patients, and other healthcare practitioners?

♦ What can interactional analyses tell us about the multiplicities of communities within medicine, including where multiple healthcare professionals come together (e.g. within surgical settings)?

♦ To what extent and in what ways do some people not achieve legitimate participation?

This last question challenges Wenger's (1998) 'relatively benign model' (Barton and Tusting 2005: p.10) and delves further into issues of power, conflict and exclusion—concepts such as *illegitimate peripheral participation* and *legitimation conflicts*—where certain individuals may be rendered marginal to practice and in some cases might withdraw (Harris and Shelswell 2005).

Future directions

We have considered a range of identity theories that are being developed and utilized within the social sciences. Necessarily, due to space restrictions, there have been omissions (e.g. gender identities and social identity theory) (Burford 2012; Butler 1988). However, the theories included span the breadth of individual and socially situated approaches, comprising different epistemological ways in which they treat knowledge and knowing of identity. For some, identities are known and knowable, residing in the self. For others, identities are contingent and contextual, ever-present yet fluid in the interactional space that is our social world. Other important theoretical differences include the extent to which identities are individual, relational, or collective, and whether identities are personally or socially constructed. Despite these differences, however, there are similarities. While treated in different ways and afforded different statuses across perspectives, the issue of coherence is a common phenomenon. Furthermore, these different perspectives do not necessarily contradict one another; rather they can be seen as different levels of description (Monrouxe and Poole 2013).

But what does all of this mean to the medical educationalist and to medical education researchers? Ultimately, the richness of social theory is there for us to embrace, synergize and inform as we contemplate the myriad of innovative and practically useful perspectives that identity theories bring to everyday questions (Monrouxe and Rees 2009). Medical education researchers should embrace a range of identity theories and methods, look for synergies within different perspectives, and ask more complex and detailed questions around issues such as leadership, career choice, workplace learning dynamics, gender, and ethnicity, and the complex ways in which these might intersect. As Schwartz and colleagues say 'to truly capture the complexity of this construct [identity], we must move beyond isolated sub-disciplines . . . and design innovative research studies that capture multiple components and processes of identity' (Schwartz et al. 2011: p. 933). The challenge for medical education researchers is to move away from a bootstrapping approach to theory, towards a critical engagement with identity theories at a variety of levels in order to produce high quality research that develops further sophistication for both identity theory and medical education practice.

Conclusions

♦ The concept of identity is of increasing interest to medical educationalists and medical education researchers, although it is still largely under-theorized.

♦ Research within the social sciences currently investigating identities comes from a range of positivist and postpositivist paradigms which can be viewed as providing different levels of understanding.

♦ Engaging with theory from the outset and using theory to drive research questions and methodological design in medical education can bring a critical edge to our work, through which the development of both theory and practice can be better achieved.

References

Arnett, J.J. (2000) Emerging adulthood: A theory of development from the late teens through the twenties. *Am Psychol.* 55: 469–480

Balmer, D.F., Serwint, J.R., Ruzek, S.B. and Giardino, A.P. (2008). Understanding paediatric resident–continuity preceptor relationships through the lens of apprenticeship learning. *Med Educ.* 42: 923–929

Bamberg, M. (2003) Positioning with Davie Hogan—Stories, tellings and identities. In C. Daiute and C. Lightfoot (eds) *Narrative Analysis. Studying the Development of Individuals in Society*(pp. 135–158). London: Sage

Bamberg, M. (2006) 'Stories: Big or small: Why do we care?' *Narrative Inquiry.* 16: 139

Bamberg, M., de Fina, A., and Schiffrin, D. (2007) *Selves and Identities in Narrative and Discourse.* Amsterdam: John Benjamins

Barton, D., and Tusting, K. (eds) (2005) *Beyond Communities of Practice: Language Power and Social Context* Cambridge: Cambridge University Press

Beran, T.N., Hecker K., Coderre S., Wright B., Woloschuk W., and McLaughlin K. (2011) Ego identity status of medical students in clerkship. *Can Med Educ J.* 2: e4–e10

Blasi, A. (1980) Bridging moral cognition and moral action: A critical review of the literature. *Psychol Bull.* 88: 1–45

Blasi, A. (1983) Moral cognition and moral action: A theoretical perspective. *Dev Rev.* 3: 178–210

Brubaker, R., and Cooper F. (2000) Beyond 'identity'. *Theory and Society.* 29: 1–47

Bruner, J. (1990) *Acts of Meaning.* Cambridge, MA: Cambridge University.

Burford, B. (2012) Group processes in medical education: learning from social identity theory. *Med Educ.* 46:143–152

Butler, J. (1988) Performative acts and gender constitution: An essay in phenomenology and feminist theory. *Theatre Journal.* 40: 519–531

Carroll, P, Shepperd, A., and Arkin, R. (2009) Downward self revision: Erasing possible selves. *Social Cognition.* 27: 550–578

Charon, R. and Montello, M. (2002) *Stories Matter: The Role of Narrative in Medical Ethics.* New York: Routledge

Chretien, K.C., Goldman, E.F., Beckman, L., and Kind, T. (2010) It's your own risk: Medical students' perspectives on online professionalism. *Acad Med.* 85(10) Supplement: Proceedings of the Forty-Ninth Annual Conference November 7–November 10, S68–S71

Colby, A., and Damon W. (1992) *Some Do Care: Contemporary Lives of Moral Commitment.* New York: Free Press

Davies, B. and Harre, R. (2001) Positioning: The discursive production of selves. In M. Wetherell, S. Taylor and S.J. Yates (eds) *Discourse Theory and Practice* (pp. 261–271). Thousand Oaks, CA: Sage

Diaute, C., and Lightfoot, C. (2004) *Narrative Analysis: Studying the Development of Individuals in Society.* Thousand Oaks: Sage

Drew, P. (2005) Conversation analysis. In K.L. Fitch and R.E. Sanders (eds) *Handbook of Language and Social Interaction* (pp. 71–102). Mahwah, NJ: Lawrence Erlbaum

Edwards, D., and Potter J. (1992) *Discursive Psychology.* London: Sage

Erikson, E.H. (1959) *Identity and the Life Cycle*, Volume 1. New York: International Universities

Erikson, E.H. (1968) *Identity: Youth and Crisis.* New York: Norton

Ewick, P, and Silbey, S. (2003) Narrating social structure: Stories of resistance to legal authority. *Am J Sociol.* 108: 1328–1372

Frank, A.W. (1995) *The Wounded Storyteller: Body, Illness and Ethics*. Chicago: Chicago University Press

Frye, N. (1957) *Anatomy of Criticism*. Princeton, NJ: Princeton University Press

Garfinkel, H. (1967) *Studies in Ethnomethodology*. Englewood Cliffs, NJ: Prentice-Hall

Gee, J.P. (2011) *An Introduction to Discourse Analysis Theory and Method*. New York: Routledge

Georgakopoulou, A. (2006) Thinking big with small stories in narrative and identity analysis. *Narrative Inquiry*. 16: 122–130

Georgakopoulou, A. (2007) *Small Stories, Interaction and Identities*. Amsterdam: John Benjamins

Goffman, E. (1959/1990) *The Presentation of Self in Everyday Life*. New York: Doubleday

Gomez, A., Brooks, M.L, Buhrmester, M.D., Vazquez, A., Jetten, J., and Swann, W.B. Jr. (2009a) On the nature of identity fusion: Insights into the construct and a new measure. *J Personality Soc Psychol*. 100: 918–933

Gomez, A., D. Seyle, C., Huici, C., and Swann, W.B. Jr. (2009b) Can self-verification strivings fully transcend the self-other barrier? Seeking verification of ingroup identities. *J Personality Soc Psychol*. 97: 1021–1044

Gramzow, R.H., Sedikides, C., Panter, A.T. and Insko, C.A. (2000) Aspects of self-regulation and self-structure as predictors of perceived emotional distress. *Personality Soc Psychol Bull*. 26: 188–205

Hardy, S. A. and Carlo, G. (2011) Moral identity. In S.J. Schwartz, K. Luyckx, and V.L. Vignoles (eds). *Handbook of Identity Theory and Research* (Volumes 1 & 2) (p. 998). New York, NY: Springer Science + Business Media

Harris, S., and Shelswell, N. (2005) Moving beyond communities of practice in adult basic education. In D. Barton and K. Tusting (eds). *Beyond Communities of Practice: Language, Power, and Social Context* (pp. 158–179). Cambridge: Cambridge University Press

Helmich, E., Bolhuis, S., Dornan, T., Laan, R., and Koopmans, R. (2012) Being in medicine for the very first time: emotional talk, meaning and identity development. *Med Educ*. 46(11): 1074–1086

Heritage, J. (2005) Conversational analysis and institutional talk. In K.L. Fitch and R.E. Sanders (eds) *Handbook of Language and Social Interaction* (pp. 103–148). Mahwah, NJ: Lawrence Erlbaum

Hester, S., and Eglin, P. (eds) (1997) *Culture in Action*. Washington, DC: University Press of America, Inc.

Hitlin, S. (2011) Values, personal identity, and the moral self. In S.J. Schwartz, K. Luyckx, and V.L. Vignoles (eds). *Handbook of Identity Theory and Research* (Volumes 1 & 2) (p. 998) New York, NY: Springer Science + Business Media

Holstein, J. and Gubrium, J. (2000) *The Self We Live By*. New York: Oxford University Press

Holt, E. (1996) Reporting on talk: the use of direct reported speech in conversation. *Res Language Soc Interaction*. 29: 219–245

Kivetz, Y. and Tyler, T.R. (2007) Tomorrow I'll be me: The effect of time perspective on the activation of idealistic versus pragmatic selves. *Organizational Behavior and Human Decision Processes*. 102:193–211

Labov, W. (1972) *Language in the Inner City: Studies in the Black English Vernacular*. Philadelphia, PA: University of Philadelphia Press

Labov, W. (1997) Some further steps in narrative analysis. *Journal of Narrative and Life History*. 7: 395–415

Labov, W. (2004) Ordinary events. In C. Fought (ed.) *Sociolinguistics Variation: Critical Reflections* (pp. 31–43).New York: Oxford University Press

Labov, W. and Waletzky, J. (1967) Narrative analysis. Oral versions of personal experience. In J. Helm (ed.) *Essays on the Verbal and Visual Arts* (pp. 12–44). Seattle: American Ethnological Society/University of Washington Press

Lapsley, D.K., and Narvaez, D. (2004) A socio-cognitive approach to the moral personality. In: D.K. Lapsley and D. Narbaez (eds) *Moral Development, Self and Identity* (pp. 189–212). Mahwah, NJ: Erlbaum

Lave, J. and Wenger, E. (1991) *Situated Learning: Legitimate Peripheral Participation*. Cambridge: Cambridge University Press

Leary, M. (2004) Editorial: What is the self? A plea for clarity. *Self and Identity*. 3: 1–3

Marcia, J.E. (1966) Development and validation of ego identity status. *J Personality Soc Psychol*. 3: 551–558

Marcia, J.E., Waterman, A. S., Matteson, R., Archer, S. L., and Orlofsky, J.L. (1993) *A Handbook for Psychosocial Research*. New York: Springer-Verlag

McAdams, D. (1993) *The Stories We Live By*. New York: The Guilford Press

McAdams, D.P. (2011) Narrative identities. In S.J. Schwartz, K. Luyckx, and V.L. Vignoles (eds) *Handbook of Identity Theory and Research* (Volumes 1 & 2) (pp. 99–115). New York, NY: Springer Science + Business Media

Mead, G.H. (1934) *Mind, Self and Society*. Chicago: Chicago University Press

Ma, M., and Agarwal, R. (2007) Through a glass darkly: Information technology design, identity verification, and knowledge contribution in online communities. *Information Systems Research*. 18(1): 42–67

Monrouxe, L.V. (2009a) Negotiating professional identities: dominant and contesting narratives in medical students' longitudinal audio diaries. *Current Narratives*. 1: 41–59

Monrouxe, L.V. (2009b) Solicited audio diaries in longitudinal narrative research: a view from inside. *Qual Res*. 9: 81–103

Monrouxe, L.V. (2010) Identity, identification and medical education: why should we care? *Med Educ*. 44: 40–49

Monrouxe, L.V. and Poole, G. (2013) An onion? Conceptualising and researching identity. *Med Educ*. 47(4): 425–429

Monrouxe, L.V., and Rees, C.E. (2009) Picking up the gauntlet: constructing Med Educ. as a social science. *Med Educ*. 43: 196–198

Monrouxe, L.V. and Rees C.E. (2011) It's just a clash of cultures: Emotional talk within medical students' narratives of professionalism dilemmas, *Adv Health Sci Educ*. 17(5): 671–701

Monrouxe, L.V. and Sweeney, K. (2010) Contesting narratives: Medical professional identity formation amidst changing values. In S. Pattison, B. Hannigan, H. Thomas, and R. Pill (eds) *Emerging Professional Values in Health Care: How professions and professionals are changing* (pp. 61–77). London and Philadelphia: Jessica Kingsley

Monrouxe, L.V. and Sweeney, K. (in press) Between two worlds: Medical students narrating identity tensions. In C.R Figley, P. Huggard, and C.E. Rees (eds). *First Do No Self-Harm: Understanding and Promoting Physician Stress Resilience*. Oxford: Oxford University Press

Monrouxe, L.V., Rees, C.E. and Bradley P. (2009) The construction of patients' involvement in hospital bedside teaching encounters. *Qual Health Res*. 19: 918–930

Monrouxe, L.V., Rees, C.E. Joyce, D., and Wells, S. (in press) Medical and healthcare students' reported experiences of moral distress around professionalism dilemmas: An alternative preceptive on empathy decline.

Narvaez, D., and Lapsley, D.K. (2005) The psychological foundations of everyday morality and moral expertise. In D.K. Lapsley and F.C. Power (eds) *Character Psychology and Character Education* (pp. 140–165). Notre Dame: University of Notre Dame Press

Niemi, P.M. (1997) Medical students' professional identity: Self-reflection during the preclinical years. *Med Educ*. 31: 408–415

Ochs, E., and Capps, L. (2001) *Living Narrative*. Cambridge MA: Harvard University

Oettingen, G. and Mayer, D. (2002) The motivating function of thinking about the future: Expectations versus fantasies. *J Personality Soc Psychol*. 83: 1198–1212

Polzer, J.T., Milton, L.P. and Swann, W.B. (2002) Capitalizing on diversity: Interpersonal congruence in small work groups. *Administrative Sci Q*. 47: 296–324

Potter, J. and Wetherell, M. (1987) *Discourse and Social Psychology*. London: Sage

Rees, C.E., and Monrouxe, L.V. (in press) 'Oh my God uh uh uh': Laughter for coping in medical students' personal incident narratives of professionalism dilemmas. In C.R Figley, P. Huggard, and C.E. Rees (eds). *First Do No Self-Harm: Understanding and Promoting Physician Stress Resilience*. Oxford: Oxford University Press

Rees, C.E., Ajjawi, R. and Monrouxe, L.V. (2013) The construction of power in family medicine bedside teaching: A video observation study. *Med Educ.* 47(2): 154–165

Rees, C.E., and Monrouxe, L.V. (2008) Is it alright if I-um-we unbutton your pyjama top now. *Communication & Medicine.* 5:171–182

Rees, C.E., and Monrouxe L.V. (2010a) "I should be lucky ha ha ha ha": the construction of power, identity and gender through laughter within medical workplace learning encounters. *J Pragmatics.* 42: 3384–3399

Rees, C.E, and Monrouxe, L.V. (2010b) Contesting medical hierarchies: nursing students' narratives as acts of resistance. *Med Educ.* 44: 433–435

Ricoeur, P. (1992) *Oneself as Another.* Chicago: University of Chicago Press

Riessman, C. (2003) Performing identities in illness narrative: masculinity and multiple sclerosis. *Qual Res.* 3: 5–33

Riessman, C. (2008) *Narrative Methods for the Human Sciences.* Thousand Oaks, CA: Sage

Schegloff, E.A. (1992) In another context. In A. Duranti and C. Goodwin (eds) *Rethinking Context: Language as an Interactive Phenomenon*(pp. 191–228). Cambridge: Cambridge University Press

Schwartz, S.J, Luyckx, K., and Vignoles, V.L. (eds) (2011) *Handbook of Identity Theory and Research.* London: Springer

Schwartz, S.J, Vignoles, V.L., and Luyckx, K. (2011) Epilogue: What's next for identity theory and research? In S.J. Schwartz, K. Luyckx, and V.L. Vignoles (eds) *Handbook of Identity Theory and Research* (Volumes 1 & 2) (pp. 933–938). New York, NY: Springer Science + Business Media.

Shapiro, J. (2009) *The Inner World of Medical Students: Listening to Their Voices Through Poetry.* New York: Radcliffe

Smith, B. (2002) The (in)visible wound: Body stories and concentric circles of witness. *Auto/Biography.* 10(1): 113–121

Smith, B, and Sparkes, A.C. (2002) Men, sport, spinal cord injury and the construction of coherence: narrative practice in action. *Qual Res.* 2: 143–171

Smith, B, and Sparkes, A.C. (2008) Contrasting perspectives on narrating selves and identities: an invitation to dialogue. *Qual Res* 8: 5–35

Starr S., Ferguson, W.J., Haley, H.L., and Quirk, M. (2003) Community preceptors' views of their identities as teachers. *Acad Med.* 78: 820–825

Stone, S., Ellers, B., Holmes, D., Orgren, R., Qualters, D., and Thompson, J. (2002) Identifying oneself as a teacher: the perceptions of preceptors. *Med Educ.* 36: 180–185

Swann, W. B. (1996) *Self-traps: The Elusive Quest for Higher Self-esteem.* New York: Freeman

Swann, W.B. (ed.) (2012) *Self-verification theory.* London: Sage

Swann, W.B., Johnson, R.E., and Bosson, J.K. (2009) Identity negotiation at work. *Research in Organizational Behavior.* 29: 81–109

Swann, W.B., Kwan, V.S.Y., Polzer, J.T., and Milton, L.P. (2003) Waning of stereotypic perceptions in small groups: Identity negotiation and erosion of gender expectations of women. *Soc Cogn.* 21(3): 194–212.

Swann, W.B., Milton, L.P., and Polzer, J.T. (2000) Should we create a niche or fall in line? Identity negotiation and small group effectiveness. *J Personality Soc Psychol* 79: 238–250

Swann, W.B., Rentfrow, P.J., and Guinn, J. (2003) Self-verification: The search for coherence. In M. Leary and J. Tagney (eds) *Handbook of Self and Identity* (pp. 367–383). New York: Guilford Press

Takakuwa, K.M., Rubashkin, N., and Herzig, K.E. (eds.) (2004) *What I Learned in Medical School: Personal Stories of Young Doctors.* Berkeley and Los Angeles: University of California Press

Tsouroufli, M., Rees, C.E., Monrouxe, L.V., and Sundaram, V. (2011) Gender, identities and intersectionality in medical education research. *Med Educ.* 45: 213–216

Watson, C. (2007) Small stories, positioning analysis, and the doing of professional identities in learning to teach. *Narrative Inquiry.* 17: 371–389

Wenger, E. (1998) *Communities of Practice.* Cambridge: Cambridge University Press

Wengraf, T. (2001) *Qualitative Research Interviewing: Biographic Narratives and Semi-structured Methods.* London: Sage

Whitehead, C. (2007) The doctor dilemma in interprofessional education and care: how and why will physicians collaborate? *Med Educ.* 41(10): 1010–1016

Widdicombe, S. (1998) 'But don't class yourself': The interactional management of category membership and non-membership. In C. Antaki and S. Widdicombe (eds) *Identities in Talk* (pp. 52–70). London: Sage

Winston, K.A., van Der Vleuten, C P.M., and Scherpbier, A. (2010) At-risk medical students: implications of students' voice for the theory and practice of remediation. *Med Educ.* 44: 1038–1047

Wortham, S. and Gadsten, V. (2006) Urban fathers positioning themselves through narrative: An approach to narrative self-construction. In A. De Fina, D. Schiffrin, and M. Bamberg (eds) *Discourse and Identity* (pp. 315–341). Cambridge, UK: Cambridge University Press

CHAPTER 11

Personality and medical education

Eva Doherty

The 'narrow' and uneducated scientist with no view beyond his specialized horizons is a stock figure of educational mythology. In our desire to produce rounded personalities do not let us fall into the heresy of regarding science as in itself narrowing or as anything less than what it is, one of the great channels by which the human spirit may be enriched.

Eric James

Reproduced from *British Medical Journal*, Eric James, 'General practice and medical education: the education of the scientist', 2, p. 575, copyright 1958, with permission from BMJ Publishing Group Ltd

Personality factors and medical professionalism

Public responses to recent scandals in the corporate, clerical and medical communities attest to an increasing global intolerance of unprofessional behaviour (Kish-Gephart et al. 2010).There is, however, evidence that the personalities of adults born since 1970 are increasingly narcissistic, overly assertive and prone to behaviour problems (Twenge 2009). Regarding medical professionalism, a number of retrospective studies first published 8 years ago revealed that doctors, who were the subject of complaints to medical disciplinary boards, were sources of concern while they were students in medical school (Papadakis et al. 2004, 2005; Teherani et al. 2005). In other words, the unprofessional behaviours reflected difficulties which were longstanding and possibly characterological. Hodgson et al. (2007) reported on the personalities of a small sample of these unprofessional doctors. They were able to obtain personality profiles for 26 doctors from the original cohort. By chance, as part of a test validation study, these individuals completed a measure of personality (California Personality Inventory: CPI) for the test authors as students in medical school between 1951 and 1970. Significant unprofessional behaviours were demonstrated by seven of these individuals while in medical school; the remaining 19 never demonstrated unprofessional behaviours. The CPI profiles of those seven individuals were significantly different from the profiles of the group of 19. Specifically, the CPI subscales; responsibility, communality, well-being and rule respecting and also the total scores were significantly different. In the postgraduate arena, Papadakis and colleagues demonstrated the same related phenomenon—that doctors who were the subject of complaints to disciplinary boards had previously received poor professionalism ratings during their residency training (Papadakis et al. 2008).

Long-standing communication deficits have been shown to be associated with subsequent complaints from the public regarding unprofessional behaviours. In Canada, a cohort study of 3424 physicians who took the national clinical skills examinations between 1993 and 1996 (and who were followed up until 2005) found that subsequent complaints filed to the medical regulatory authorities could be traced back to the doctors' poor communication skills scores in those examinations (Tamblyn et al. 2007; Wenghofer et al. 2009).

Medical educators who are concerned with promoting professionalism in medical schools and postgraduate training will no doubt be aware of the disproportionate amount of time spent supporting students and doctors who despite best efforts continue to struggle and to demonstrate behaviour problems. It is somewhat surprising therefore that so little attention is paid to the relevance of personality factors either in selection procedures or personal and professional development programmes in medical schools (Mitchell et al. 2005; Wear and Aultman 2006).

International recommendations regarding medical competency

A responsible and caring personality is implied in the lists of medical competencies recommended by international medical regulatory bodies and other experts. The CanMEDs framework first initiated by the Royal College of Physicians and Surgeons in Canada in the early 1990s advocated seven medical competencies (The Royal College of Physicians and Surgeons in Canada 2012):

+ medical expert
+ communicator
+ collaborator
+ manager
+ health advocate
+ scholar
+ professional.

Similarly, the Accreditation Council for Graduate Medical Education (ACGME) in the United States identified six domains of medical competence, which encompassed a commitment to patient care, medical knowledge, practice-based learning and improvement, interpersonal and communication skills, professionalism, and systems-based practices (Accreditation Council for Graduate Medical Education 2012). In the United Kingdom, the General Medical Council and the Royal College of Physicians endorsed the importance of ensuring optimal standards of professionalism in doctors (Royal College of Physicians 2005; General Medical Council 2009).Finally, in Australia, Powis et al. (2007, p. 1242) summarized, from available literature, the generic qualities that an ideal doctor must possess:

+ cognitive skills
+ logical reasoning
+ problem solving
+ critical thinking
+ verbal and written communication skills
+ interpersonal skills, including empathy
+ ethical sensitivity and behaviour; integrity
+ flexibility and tolerance
+ conscientiousness and reliability
+ team work and management skills

+ ability to cope appropriately with stress.

All these lists of abilities and attributes imply a broad set of ideal personal qualities. The challenge for medical educators is ensuring that practising doctors possess these qualities.

A guide to personality theory and measurement

The body of knowledge within the science of psychology known as the psychology of individual differences or the psychology of personality is vast and must be baffling to the medical educator without a psychology background. Different theorists have proposed different dynamic systems to explain the phenomenon of personality; these can be difficult to integrate. What follows is a guide to the most commonly recognized theories of personality and the associated instruments (fig. 11.1). The description that follows is not meant to be comprehensive. Interested readers who would like to know more are recommended a recently published textbook, which is easy to read and understand (Cooper 2010), or for a more detailed account, consult Corr and Matthews (2009).

Theoretical approaches to understanding personality

Psychodynamic theories

Sigmund Freud is regarded as one of the fathers of personality psychology, and he began his career studying medicine in Vienna in the late 1800s. He became interested in psychiatry in the 1880s when he went to Paris to study with Charcot, the founder of neurology. Charcot was researching the phenomenon of hypnosis and the power of suggestion. He was interested in the phenomenon of mesmerism (better known as hypnosis) and had noted that hypnotized individuals reported altered sensations in their bodies and were also highly suggestible. Freud began to experiment with hypnosis in a number of his patients who presented with nervous diseases or conditions with physical symptoms with no clear organic basis. These conditions were called the 'hysterias'. The success that Freud achieved and the ensuing insights that he gained led him to postulate a theory of the human mind and an explanation of abnormal behaviour. The theory has been developed and modified since—a comprehensive description of current psychoanalysis is beyond the scope of this chapter. However,

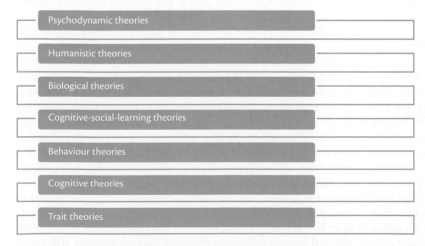

Figure 11.1 The main theoretical approaches to understanding personality.

Psychodynamic theories

Humanistic theories

Biological theories

Cognitive-social-learning theories

Behaviour theories

Cognitive theories

Trait theories

psychoanalysis contributed a number of important key concepts to psychology which have endured. These insights are briefly summarized as it is believed that they might help the medical educator to understand the student or doctor with behaviour problems:

◆ There are two parts to the human mind; the conscious mind and the unconscious mind. We are largely aware of what we think and feel in our conscious mind but mostly unaware of our unconscious mind. The aim of the process of psychoanalysis is to increase our awareness of what is processed in our unconscious mind in order to understand our motives, emotions and behaviours.

◆ Human beings have the capability to 'forget' emotionally painful events which occurred in childhood and may 'bury' them in their unconscious minds. All threats to their recall have to be subsequently resisted in order to preserve a sense of psychological integrity and so individuals develop a system of defence mechanisms which are protective in that they ward off the threat of remembering. The defence mechanism known as projection may be used in this instance to ward off any suggestion of angry feelings and project these feelings out into the minds of others. As a consequence, the individual may perceive him/herself to be surrounded by angry, unfair people while he/she is peace loving, kind, and passive. Such individuals often find themselves in passive–aggressive relationships. Many other defence mechanisms have been identified by psychodynamic theorists and the purpose is always to ward off any reminders of repressed unacceptable emotions.

Psychoanalysis is, of course, much more complex than this brief description. While psychoanalysis does not hold centre stage any longer within contemporary psychology, nevertheless many psychiatrists and psychologists follow a psychoanalytic model in their understanding of human behaviour problems, and many of Freud's ideas and terminologies continue in psychiatric diagnostic manuals and personality instruments.

Jung worked with Freud and developed his own theory of human personality. He added the notion of a collective unconscious, which was passed from generation to generation and which housed common archetypes such as the caring mother or the wise old man. Jung also coined the term *persona*, a term widely used to reflect the idea of a self which we present to the world and which may or may not be a true reflection of the true self. Jung identified that some individuals demonstrated a preference for introspection whereas others for external events and he differentiated between introverts and extroverts, concepts which have been replicated by many personality instruments since.

Personality tests associated with psychodynamic theories

A category of personality tests, known as the projective tests is most closely associated with psychodynamic theories. The Rorschach (Rorschach 1927) and the Thematic Apperception Test (TAT; Murray 1943/1971) are two examples. The Rorschach is made up of 10 cards, each with a different inkblot. Some of the inkblots are black in colour, some are red and black, and some are multi-coloured. The respondent is requested to say what they see in the inkblots and to explain which part of the inkblot prompted each response. The TAT is probably not as well known but uses the same methodology. The cards used in this test are drawings of different scenarios with one or more individuals in ambiguous situations. The respondent is requested to write a story about each picture. Two other different tests of personality, which are paper and pencil tests, are the Myers–Briggs Type Indicator (MBTI; Myers and McCaulley 1985) and the Hogan Development Survey (HDS; Hogan and Hogan 1997). The MBTI is based on the idea of Jungian types (extroversion/introversion, sensing/intuition, thinking/feeling, judgement/perception). Individuals differ in their preferences for each of these types and there are 16 possible combinations. While the reliability and validity of the measure has been criticised, the MBTI is widely used for the purposes of personal development and teamwork training (Pittenger 1993). The HDS comprises 11 scales which were based on Horney's taxonomy of flawed interpersonal tendencies. Finally the Minnesota Multiphasic Personality Inventory (MMPI; Hathaway and McKinley 1983) developed originally in 1939 and since revised (MMPI-2; Butcher et al 1989; MMPI-2-RF; Ben-Porath and Tellegen 2008) is probably one of the most well-known and used tests of personality functioning (Furnham and Crump 2005). It contains 10 clinical scales, 11 validity scales or response style indicators, and 12 supplementary scales. The test can be used to indicate whether an individual is experiencing abnormal levels of depression, somatic concerns, anxiety, bizarre ideation, and social isolation, amongst others. Access to most of these tests is restricted to psychologists who have obtained certain levels of professional training which is controlled by the test distributors.

What can be confusing about these instruments is that while some measure normal personal styles (e.g. MBTI), others focus on abnormality (e.g. HDS) and some are designed to identify both normality and abnormality to different degrees (e.g. Rorschach, TAT, MMPI-2/MMPI-2-RF). The overlap between the normal and the abnormal is an important consideration when assessing personality and in particular with regard to identifying individuals suitable for medical training. Furnham and Crump (2005) discuss these issues within the context of their study which compared the MBTI, the HDS and a measure of normal personality, the NEO Personality Inventory which assesses the 'Big Five' (NEO-PI-R; Costa and McCrae 1992). The 'Big Five' refers to five personality traits, which will be outlined in the section on trait theories. They are neuroticism, extroversion, optimism, agreeableness, and conscientiousness.

Humanistic theories

Rogers was a clinical psychologist who wanted to move away from the 'medical model' approach to behaviour problems and proposed that the way to help people was through genuine empathy and understanding. Rogers developed his theory of personality from ideas first proposed by George Kelly, also a clinical psychologist, who proposed a personal construct theory. Personal construct theory was a theory that moved away from the notion of pathological models of behaviour and instead explained human behaviour in terms of individual constructs, which individuals build of themselves and their world. Rogers emphasized the uniqueness of individuals and maintained that individuals were capable of finding their own solutions if a therapeutic environment of unconditional positive regard could be provided. The role of the self-concept was an integral component, and a measure based on Rogerian theory, the Rosenberg Self-Esteem scale (Rosenberg 1965), may be familiar to the reader. This model of human behaviour underpins contemporary models of counselling. In medical schools, students who are struggling are often referred to counsellors on the basis that counselling will be an effective method of remediation.

Biological theories

Biological theories of personality held that personality was inherited and mediated by differences in the human nervous system. Eysenck postulated the concepts of psychoticism, extroversion and neuroticism each with associated physiological patterns. The theory is briefly included in this guide as readers may have come across the associated personality questionnaire, the Eysenck Personality Questionnaire (EPQ; Eysenck and Eysenck 1975, 1991). Eysenck designed this measure in order to demonstrate that different profiles were associated with different levels of cortical arousal and autonomic nervous system activity. For a comprehensive review of biological theories of personality and associated evidence, the reader is referred to Stelmack and Rammsayer (2008).

Cognitive-social-learning theories

Theories which fall under this category explain personality differences in terms of the relationship between cognitions (perceptions, attitudes, and expectations), learning and the environment.

Behaviour theories

During the early part of the 20th century, another entirely different conceptualization of human behaviour was gaining popularity; this was known as behaviourism, and many behaviourist concepts persist to this day. Behaviourism was founded by Watson and essentially behaviourists believed that only observable behaviour should be studied and that the scientific investigation of any kind of internal processing was not possible. Watson went even further and proposed that individuals were the product of their environment and that an individual's personality was not inherited. A behaviourist perspective maintained that the correct environment could produce the required personality, and human behaviour was the product of the environment. These theories underpin the assumption that given the correct educational milieu, the ideal professional will result.

Other well known behaviourists were Pavlov and Skinner. Their theories postulated that human behaviours were a result of various types of reinforcement patterns (e.g. classical and operant). Classical and operant schedules described the mechanisms of the patterns of reinforcement which maintained behaviours; the theories were attractive because they helped to explain why human beings could behave in apparently self-limiting and confusing ways. The disorder known as obsessive–compulsive disorder, for example, which Freud had explained in terms of a deep-rooted conflict leading to an overwhelming anxiety, the behaviourists explained in terms of the reinforcing effect of rituals. The theory explained that the rituals and obsessions were maintained because the ritualistic behaviours (e.g. hand washing) resulted in the temporary relief from the anxiety triggered by the obsessive preoccupation (e.g. germs). The concept that reinforcement was a powerful motivator proved to be useful as an explanation of individual differences in the world of psychology, medicine, and education. The theory explained why individuals persisted with apparently harmful behaviours—they were experiencing them as reinforcing.

Cognitive theories

In the last 30 years, psychology has come full circle and returned to its roots with a renewal of interest in emotion, cognition and neurobiology—that is internal processing systems, which were of interest to the fathers of psychology in the previous century.

Cognitive theories arose out of dissatisfaction with behavioural theories in the 1960s and it was Ellis who first proposed that people's perceptions and thought patterns had a lot to do with their abnormal behaviours and that these thought patterns could be fundamentally irrational. Beck developed these ideas further and the associated therapy is now known as cognitive-behaviour therapy (CBT). Essentially, CBT identified close links between thoughts and emotions—'we feel the way we think'. Change is facilitated by means of increasing awareness and examination of these links, and the search for the irrational characteristics of the thoughts which are connected to the unwanted emotions. The theories have coincided with an implosion of self-help books, which promise to equip the individual with the skills to control problematic emotions and unhelpful and harmful behaviours. The role of the environment was explained in terms of the initial trigger or stimulus. The advent of powerful functional magnetic resonance imaging techniques has allowed for the investigation of the processing of these thoughts and emotions in the brain and has lent further support to cognitive theories. Tests associated with these theories assess negative thought processes. A good example is Beck's own measure of depression, the Beck Depression Inventory (BDI; Beck et al. 1961).

The branch of psychology known as health psychology embraced many of the cognitive-social-learning theories and there are a multitude of measures available to predict human health-related behaviour. Measures that assess concepts such as locus of control, self-efficacy, optimism, health beliefs, and quality of life are all based on these theories. A recent 10 year longitudinal study demonstrated that a sense of coherence together with levels of anxiety and depression during medical school predicted satisfaction with medicine as a career and quality of life post graduation (Tartas et al. 2011).

Trait theories

Trait theories of personality sit alongside the theories described previously and rely on some of their concepts for support. Trait theories maintained that individuals differed from each other along certain dimensions or traits that were reasonably consistent and permanent and so not a response to an environmental trigger. A distinction was drawn between a *trait* and a *state*. For example, an individual may be high on a *trait* known as anxiety, which is related to the *state* of anxiety they experience in response to a stimulus in the environment—such as an examination. Trait theories relied completely on the measurement of traits and on the use of a statistical procedure called factor analysis to reliably identify categories of traits. Therefore, trait theorists did not theorize about certain phenomena, but rather devised their instruments based on sound theories and used factor analysis to establish whether items were grouped together as predicted.

In order to appreciate what factor analysis can achieve and how important factor analysis is to trait theories, it is necessary to first summarize the concept of what makes a good test: namely reliability and validity. The idea that a psychological test might not be reliable and valid can come as a surprise to some medical educators—especially if they were medically trained and are new to the topic of psychometric testing. Doctors correctly assume that if they test a patient's haemoglobin with a full blood count (FBC) and it is low, it will continue to be so in the short term unless treated. In other words the FBC is reliable. Equally, doctors assume the test is a valid estimate of the concentration of red blood cells in the bloodstream and not indicative of anything else. It can come as a surprise therefore that psychological tests may not be so reliable or valid and that they require rigorous investigation before they can be used. A parent or teacher does not want to hear that an IQ test is so unreliable that if it was administered to the child next week, a different result might be obtained. Unfortunately a lack of appreciation of these basic concepts can sometimes mean that instruments are designed without any attention to whether they are reliable and valid and in some instances educators might be tempted to administer them without validating them first.

Reliability

The first important principle of a good test is that it should measure one dimension and that the items should not be confounded by extraneous variables. For example, a test of anxiety should measure just that and not depression or optimism. The best way to ensure that a test does this is to phrase test items systematically in different ways so that each item is designed to sample the construct from a different angle and the final result is representative of the dimension in common (Cooper 2010). For example, items which enquire about feelings of anxiety in different situations or with respect to different thoughts and behaviours are more likely to measure anxiety than items which ask about anxiety in the one context, phrased using similar language.

All tests are measuring a sample of a reality and so the reliability of the test refers to how good a reflection of that reality the test is. Coefficient alpha is a mathematical calculation of the test's measurement accuracy. For long tests, coefficient alpha (also called 'alpha', 'KR20', 'Cronbach's alpha', or 'internal consistency') can be understood as the square of the correlation between the actual scores obtained on the test and the actual reality. So an alpha of 0.8 indicates a correlation of 0.89. A rule of thumb, which is widely accepted, is that tests should not be used if alpha is less than 0.7 and should not be used at all for high-stakes decisions if alpha is less than 0.9 (Cooper 2010). Tests with few items run the risk of being unreliable because unknown extraneous variables could have a significant effect on the final result. The more test items that sample the trait or state in different ways, the more reliable the test can be as the effect of the extraneous variables cancel each other out. Other threats to the reliability of a test result from using a test which has been validated on a particular sample of individuals (i.e. American university students) in a completely different context (i.e. British doctors). This is why readers will often see Cronbach's alpha reported for a test with a particular sample rather than quoting the alpha scores given in the test manuals. Other methods of assessing the reliability of a test are used which either involve designing two versions of the same test and investigating whether the same alpha is achieved (known as 'alternate forms', 'parallel forms', and 'split-half' reliability) or repeating the test after a short interval to establish whether the same result is obtained (test–retest reliability). Whereas low reliability scores indicate that responses to the test items must have been contaminated by extraneous variables, high reliability does not guarantee that the test is measuring what it is supposed to. Establishing test validity is an entirely different process to establishing reliability and there are many different techniques—some of which can take some time (fig. 11.2). Various types of statistical calculations can be used to estimate validity (consult Cooper (2010) for an explanation).

Validity

Construct validity

Construct validity refers to whether the test results 'behave' in accordance with what was anticipated from the theory used to construct the test. For example, a test of anxiety used to test examination anxiety should demonstrate different scores depending on whether the test is administered before or after the examination.

Divergent validity

Divergent validity refers to whether the test results correlate with characteristics to which they should theoretically be unrelated. For example if the test of anxiety was found to correlate with socioeconomic status or social desirability then it may not be measuring anxiety as such.

Predictive validity

Psychological tests are frequently used to predict behaviours and medical educators are interested in using these tests to identify predictors of future success in a medical career. Establishing the predictive validity of a test can take a substantial length of time depending on the timing of the desired outcome and can be calculated in various ways. Approaches to calculating predictive validity include the identification of score thresholds for a number of different tests which individuals should exceed plus the use of regression equations to estimate the predictive power of any one test (incremental validity) to explain the variance of the desired outcome (e.g. passing the final medicine examination).

Concurrent validity

Concurrent validity is the term used to refer to the investigation of a test with regard to criteria which can be currently measured (e.g. personality scores and grade point average scores).

Factor analysis

The use of factor analysis is an integral component of the design of trait measures of personality. Essentially factor analysis is a sophisticated version of multiple correlation analysis. Correlation coefficients are calculated between all the scores on the items of the test in order to investigate for clusters or factors which can then be conceptualised as subcomponents of the trait being measured. Items on a test designed to measure personality can be factor analysed and for example, may be found to form a number of clusters which can be assigned labels or names (e.g. the 'Big Five'; neuroticism, extroversion, openness, conscientiousness, and agreeableness). Factor analysis can investigate simply for the shared variance of test items (principal component analysis) or it can investigate for the specific as well as shared variance of any test item with the cluster or factor. Readers will often see the term *eigenvalue* being reported, which is

---

Construct validity

Divergent validity

Predictive validity

Concurrent validity

Figure 11.2 Forms of validity of tests of personality.

simply the square of all correlations between an item and a factor added together. This value can then be divided by the number of items to get an estimate of the proportion of variance explained by the factor. Other terms that the reader may see reported are *oblique rotation*, which indicates that factors are correlated with each other or *orthogonal rotation*, which indicates that factors are not related.

Exploratory factor analysis refers to the process of calculating the number of factors to be identified and confirmatory factor analysis and its parent technique structural equation modelling test hypotheses about the number of factors.

Testing tests

Following item construction, tests can be tested by a number of different methods. Criterion keying involves correlating the scores on each of the test items with the desired outcome. This is the method which was used to construct the MMPI and the MMPI-2 (Hathaway and McKinley 1983; Butcher et al. 1989) and the California Personality Inventory (CPI; Gough and Bradley 1996). The method was problematic because frequently, the desired outcome was multifaceted and so the resulting scale measured a number of different things and was also heavily dependent on the type of sample which was used for the validation process. For example, the MMPI and the CPI were validated on psychiatric and medical populations. Factor analysis is another method that can be used; however, a problem arises when items do not load on factors. Classical item analysis involves correlating each item with the total score and systematically removing items with low correlations and then repeating the process with the new total score. The newly constructed test should then be validated using construct validation.

Tests of personality do not have a good public image and criticisms are justified (Millon 2012). Too frequently tests have been used to discriminate between people from different cultures and backgrounds and to instruct high-stakes decisions (Morgeson et al 2007). It is important to limit the impact of bias, which can result from using a perfectly good test, to answer questions that it was not designed to answer. The administration of every test carries measurement error, which can result from factors to do with the administrator of the test, response bias, social desirability factors, cultural and gender factors, test anxiety, and practice effects. Test users need to include consideration of these sources of bias, try to minimize their impact and familiarize themselves with the Code of Fair Testing Practices in Education (Joint Committee on Testing Practices (1988), reproduced in Cooper (Cooper 2010, p. 341–345).

Tests derived by trait theories

Two of the best known personality tests arising from trait theory are the Sixteen Personality Factor questionnaire (16PF) (Cattell and Cattell 1995) and the Revised NEO Personality Inventory (NEO-PI-R), (Costa and McCrae 1992). Cattell spent 10 years devising the 16PF questionnaire. He began with a list of adjectives and confirmed these adjectives by observing corresponding behaviours. Through a series of factor analyses he came up with 15 personality factors and an intelligence factor. Although subsequent factor analyses conducted by other researchers on the questionnaire and other variations of the questionnaire for different age groups failed

to confirm these separate factors, the questionnaire continues to be used widely (see Block 1995, for a critique of Cattell's factors). The 16PF has been rearranged to form a second order structure of five personality factors (extroversion, anxiety, control, independence, and sensitive awareness) in addition to intelligence and this structure has received support from subsequent factor analyses procedures (Hofer et al. 1997).

Costa and McCrae (1976) first identified three personality traits (neuroticism, extroversion, and openness). They subsequently added two more and called them agreeableness and conscientiousness and devised the NEO-PI-R to measure these (Costa and McCrae 1992). The NEO-PI-R has been validated against many other measures and outcomes and remains popular. Briefly, these 'Big Five' are; *neuroticism,* which referred to the degree of negative emotionality (e.g. anxiety, hostility, or impulsivity); *extroversion,* which described the degree of sociability, positive emotions, and the desire to be with people; *openness* was closely associated with intelligence and referred to imaginative abilities and interpersonal sensitivity; the *conscientiousness* trait encompassed orderliness, motivation, degree of self-discipline, and sense of duty; and *agreeableness* referred to the degree of cooperativeness, altruism, and tenderness towards others.

The measure is not without its critics. Two main criticisms were that the initial version of the measure was based on earlier work which did not identify the factors by factor analysis and the second criticism was that the factors were not as orthogonal (unrelated) as Costa and McCrae may have theorized (Vassend and Skrondal 2011). The test is popular because it has been demonstrated to be capable of predicting job performance (Poropat 2009) as well as individuals' abilities to cope with life (Carver and Connor-Smith 2010).

Previously, trait theories and their instruments were not used by clinicians to assess for disorders of personality. The categorization of personality disorders is currently under review within the context of the next revision of the *Diagnostic and Statistical Manual of Mental Disorders* (DSM-5). The new proposals include a dimensional system for the categorization of personality disorders in which criteria are arranged according to trait dimensions instead of categories (Skodal 2012). This represents a merging of two approaches to personality psychology with a model that describes an abnormal personality in terms of varying dimensions of personality traits. The idea is also one which has been adopted by Powis and colleagues in medical education, who have constructed a personality battery for use with medical students (Bore et al. 2009). The measures in the battery have been designed to screen for the presence of extreme manifestations of certain traits (Powis 2009) and will be outlined at the end of this chapter.

Personality and performance

A recent review of the evidence from longitudinal studies concluded that tests of personality factors predict performance both in medical school and in the workplace following graduation (Doherty and Nugent 2011). A comprehensive prospective study of a large cohort of medical students in the five medical schools in Belgium from entry to graduation conducted by Lievens et al. (2002, 2009) demonstrated that overall, high levels of the trait conscientiousness was the most significant indicator of academic success. The researchers administered the authorized Flemish translation of the NEO-PI-R to 80.4% of the total number of registered medical students for 1997 and compared the results to their academic and clinical assessment scores through their medical training. Specifically, they compared the personality assessment results taken at college entry with the students' grade point average (GPA) scores over the 7 years of medical school. To correct for possible bias, they included in their analyses range restriction correlation (μ values) to allow for the reduction in variability in GPAs over the 7 years. Multiple regression analyses demonstrated that personality factors became increasingly able to predict academic success with advancement through the medical curriculum (R^2 for year 1 = 0.22, R^2 for year 7 = 0.56). Conscientiousness, extroversion, and openness became increasingly significant contributors to the relationship between personality and success. The authors concluded that in the first year, GPAs rather than personality factors were the most crucial factors determining student attrition, but personality factors became increasingly important predictors of academic success as the student progressed through medical school.

Ferguson et al. (2003) also measured the 'Big Five' dimensions of personality in 176 students attending Nottingham Medical School in the UK. Sixty-seven percent of the medical school entrants gave their consent to participate. Comparisons were made between personality scores and the results of four academic assessments in years 1 and 2, four assessments in year 3 and ten assessments in years 4 and 5. Once more, the conscientiousness dimension was found to be a significant predictor of academic performance in the preclinical years but not of performance in the clinical years (years 4 and 5) where it was linked with worse performance. No other trait emerged as a significant predictor of performance.

Hojat et al. (2004) administered a series of estimates of personality and assessed their predictive abilities with medical students in the Jefferson Medical College in Philadelphia. Their study was conducted with 1710 students over nine intake years. They used abridged versions of six personality measures. The sample studied represented 82% of the total student population. In addition to personality measures, they asked the groups questions about their relationships with their parents during their childhood and a single question on general health. They compared these assessments taken in year one (with the exception of the 1987 year entrants who were assessed in year two) with faculty global ratings of competence in six third-year clerkships (family medicine, internal medicine, obstetrics/gynaecology, paediatrics, psychiatry, and surgery). These ratings were completed in each clerkship, using a four-point scale ('high honours', 'excellent', 'good', and 'marginal competence'). Data on the psychometrics of these ratings were reported previously (Callahan et al. 2000). Students' personality scores and parental relationship ratings were compared to whether students were allocated to a high/moderate/low level of clinical competence. Results indicated that the students in the low competency group demonstrated significantly poorer levels of self-esteem and sociability, were lonelier, and reported less satisfactory relationships with parents than the other two groups of students.

In Australia, personality characteristics and academic performance were investigated in a cohort of medical students over three years (Knights and Kennedy 2007). The study used the HDS as the measure of personality and compared scores obtained with end-of-year examination grades for years one to three in a sample of 139 students. The students represented three years of students who entered medical school in the years 2000, 2001, and 2002. Borderline/schizoid and narcissistic/antisocial characteristics were found to be negatively correlated with academic success. Scores on one of the subsections of the HDS, the 'Diligent' syndrome was found to be positively related to academic success. The 'Diligent' syndrome is associated with a tendency to be attentive and good with details, orderly, rational, careful and well-organized. The authors acknowledged a number of limitations which included different personality assessment points across the years, however the study added to the evidence demonstrating that once more personality factors were significantly associated with measures of academic success over time and in particular identified a trait, 'Diligent' whose description encompassed characteristics similar to the trait conscientiousness.

Personality factors and stress

There is no doubt that the medical environment both for the student and the doctor is a stressful one. Prevalence rates of stress, depression, and burnout for medical students and doctors have been demonstrated to be unacceptably high. Personality traits have long been recognized as strong predictors of an individual's subjective well-being (Haslam et al. 2009)—especially the 'Big Five' (Horsburgh et al. 2009). Significant levels of stress have been demonstrated in studies of both medical students and doctors (Dyrbye et al. 2006, 2011; Shanafelt 2009; West et al. 2009) and stress and/or depression has been linked to unprofessional behavior in medical students (Dyrbye et al. 2010) and proneness to error in junior doctors (Fahrenkopf et al. 2008; West et al. 2009). A number of significant protective personality factors have been identified. Ferguson et al. (2002) reviewed 15 reports of stress in medical students and concluded that self-actualization, self-awareness and a sense of fulfilment seemed to be protective traits, whereas perfectionism, Type A personality and anger suppression were associated with an increased vulnerability to stress. McManus et al. (2004) followed a sample of 1668 (63.3% of the original sample of applicants) medical students over 12 years and demonstrated that the traits neuroticism and low extroversion were responsible for junior doctors becoming stressed at work. The personality assessment point was at the time of internship and an abbreviated version of the NEO-PI-R was used. Measures of stress were administered at five year's post graduation. Similar to previous research on stress and doctors in the UK, 21.3% of the sample was identified as cases on the General Health Questionnaire (GHQ; Goldberg and Williams 1988). The GHQ is a measure of psychiatric morbidity. Caseness is identified if the individual's total score exceeds a threshold score (usually 4). The concept of caseness is a probabilistic term indicating that mental health difficulties would be identified if the individual was assessed by a healthcare practitioner. The authors used path analysis to investigate whether personality factors could be identified as causes of stress mediating between the doctors' approaches to work practices and learning styles; results confirmed that reported stress was a direct result of personality factors. High levels of neuroticism, low levels of extraversion and low levels of conscientiousness were found to be related to subsequent stress experienced in the workplace.

Mitchell et al. (2005) described a number of studies that investigated the role of personality and doctors' performance during residency training. They conducted a systematic review of personal factors contributing to residents' performance and located four studies which measured personality, only one of which was longitudinal. The studies demonstrated significant associations between results on different personality tests and poor performance and stress. All of the studies were published prior to 2000.

The relationship of vulnerability to stress and conscientiousness has been demonstrated by a number of other longitudinal studies of medical students. In the Karolinska Institute in Sweden, researchers demonstrated that impulsivity (the opposing correlate of conscientiousness), measured at the beginning of the first year in medical school predicted elevated stress levels in medical students when they were in their third year (Dahlin and Runeson 2007). In Norway, Tyssen et al. (2007) investigated the concept of a 'Big Three', assessed with a personality measure called the Basic Character Inventory (BCI) in a longitudinal study of 421 students in four medical schools. The 'Big Three' was combined into eight typologies according to prevalidated methods. The student sample was assessed over the 6 years of training and their perceived level of stress was measured twice using a recognized validated instrument. The findings indicated that 'brooders' who were high on neuroticism and conscientiousness and low on extroversion demonstrated high levels of perceived stress whereas 'hedonists' who were low on neuroticism and conscientiousness and high on extroversion demonstrated low levels of perceived stress.

Emotional intelligence and medical competency

Emotional intelligence (EI) is an emerging topic in personality psychology and also in medical education. EI has been defined both as an ability, a trait, and a mixture of both. The ability definition describes EI as 'the ability to monitor one's own and others' feelings and emotions, to discriminate among them and to use this information to guide one's thinking and actions' (Salovey and Mayer, 1990). Trait theorists define EI as 'a constellation of emotion-related self perceptions and dispositions, assessed through self-report' (Petrides and Furnham, 2003). Mixed model theories define EI as 'an array of non-cognitive capabilities, competencies and skills that influence one's ability to succeed in coping with environmental demands and pressures' (Bar-On, 1997).

Measurement of EI

The trait models and mixed-models advocate the use of self-report as their mechanism of measurement inferring that individuals who state that they function at various levels actually do. Examples of these are shown in fig. 11.3.

The Mayer–Salovey–Caruso Emotional Intelligence Test (MSCEIT V.20; Mayer et al. 2002) is an ability measure of EI and the respondent is requested to interpret emotions in a number of tasks including pictures of faces, abstract designs and landscapes, and interpersonal situations. The MSCEIT V2.0 assesses

- ◆ Emotional Quotient Inventory (EQ-i; Bar-On 1997)
- ◆ Emotional Competence Inventory (ECI; Boyatzis and Burckle 1999)
- ◆ Emotional Intelligence Scale (EIS; Schutte et al.1998)
- ◆ Trait Emotional Intelligence Questionnaire (TeiQue; Petrides and Furnham 2003)

Figure 11.3 Measurement of EI.

the four branches of Mayer and Salovey's emotional intelligence ability model (Mayer and Salovey 1993, 1997) by yielding a profile of scores describing an individual's ability to perceive, use, understand, and manage emotions. The self-report instruments do not correlate with the ability measure indicating they measure different constructs (Mayer et al. 2008, Roberts et al. 2008). Notwithstanding this ambiguity regarding measurement issues, the concept of EI offers the medical educator an attractive tool for the facilitation and development of the 'non-cognitive' abilities of the medical student and doctor (Elam 2000).

EI is recognized to be an important component of the doctor–patient relationship and has been demonstrated to be related to the level of trust and satisfaction felt by the patient towards the doctor (Wagner et al. 2002; Weng 2008; Weng et al. 2008, 2011). Self-rated EI has been shown to be higher in female students at entry to medical school (Carrothers et al. 2000; Austin et al. 2005,) but to deteriorate over the course of medical training (Stratton et al. 2008). The concept of EI has been incorporated into certain interpersonal skills sections of the Australian medical aptitudes test (Carr 2009) and the evidence regarding EI and internationally recognized medical competencies has been recently systematically reviewed (Arora et al. 2010). Self-rated EI has been found to be associated with general academic ability (Barchard 2003; Romanelli et al. 2006, Parker et al. 2004; Qualter et al. 2012). The concept of EI has recently been proposed as an approach to teaching professionalism in postgraduate training programmes (Taylor et al. 2011).

The relationship between EI and stress has been investigated in medical students, and self-report EI scores have been shown to be moderately related in cross-sectional studies (Birks et al. 2009; O'Rourke et al. 2010). In a laboratory based study of EI and stress, 19 medical students were requested to perform an unfamiliar laparoscopic task using a simulator. Heart rate was measured as an objective measure of stress and the State-Trait Anxiety measure was used to assess the subjective stress experience. EI was assessed using a self-report measure. Results demonstrated significant positive associations between both objective and subjective assessments of stress and EI. Students with the highest EI scores also recovered faster than those students with lower EI scores (Arora et al. 2011).

The Personal Qualities Assessment (PQA)

If personality factors and EI are important components of the ability to practise medicine professionally then it follows that the psychometric assessment of these attributes should be included in selection procedures. A comprehensive review of the evidence regarding medical school selection methods is beyond the scope of this chapter (Prideaux et al. 2011). A group of researchers, principally from Newcastle, Australia, have been researching

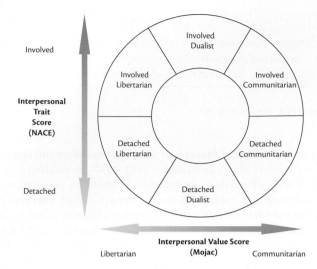

Figure 11.4 Relationship between two of the components of the PQA battery; the involved versus detached (narcissism) and the libertarian versus communitarian (morality) dimensions.

Published with permission from Bore, Munro & Powis, PowerPoint Presentation, 2012.

and publishing the results of their investigations on the topic of personality issues and medical training for more than ten years and recently published a proposal for a new measure and selection process (Bore et al. 2009). The new measure, the PQA was designed to assess a range of both cognitive and non-cognitive attributes for selection into medical school. A version of this new measure was incorporated into the UK Clinical Aptitude Test (UKCAT) and available evidence to date has indicated that it was capable of predicting not only academic scores but also assessments of interpersonal skills in objective structured clinical exams (OSCEs (Dowell et al. 2011). Initial investigations found that the battery did not discriminate between applicants from different socioeconomic backgrounds (Lumsden et al. 2009) and that graduate applicants demonstrated higher levels of conscientiousness, confidence, self-control, and communitarian attitudes compared to school-leavers (James et al. 2009). David Powis, Don Munro, and Miles Bore are the principal designers of this new measure of personal qualities. They described their concept of the 'Big 4' of medical practice (Bore et al. 2009, p. 1069). Briefly these traits are the ability to be:

- involved rather than detached
- emotionally stable rather than vulnerable
- conscientiousness rather than disorderly
- neither overly judgemental nor permissive.

Figure 11.4 illustrates how two of the PQA dimensions (involved/detached; libertarian/communitarian, also called judgemental/permissive) relate to each other. The authors developed two measures to assess these qualities; a measure of narcissism, aloofness, confidence, and empathy (NACE; Munro et al.2005) and a measure of moral orientation (Mojac; Bore 2001; Bore et al. 2005).The area in the middle of the model (dual) represents the individual who is not extreme on either of these dimensions. The other two qualities, conscientiousness and resilience (not shown) are assessed by means of a third

inventory, the Self-Assessment Inventory (SAI; Munro et al. 2008).The PQA contains two further sections; a test of cognitive aptitudes and a lie scale to detect for possible 'faking good'. Thus this battery provides for the assessment of all the personality traits that have been identified to be important predictors of success; in addition, based on their own extensive investigations, the authors have added a moral orientation trait. What is particularly innovative is that the PQA battery is designed to screen out unsuitable candidates rather than to attempt to assess for the ideal medical personality. The authors have recommended that respondents' scores should be categorized according to whether they fall within or outside two standard deviations of the mean. The measure is best used within the context of a comprehensive selection system, which encourages informed self-selection in addition to assessments of prior academic achievement and an interview; either the traditional interview or the multiple mini-interview (Eva et al. 2004). Interested readers should consult Bore et al. (2009) for more details and the accompanying website (Personal Qualities Assessment 2010).

Conclusions

- High levels of conscientiousness predict academic performance.

- Low levels of conscientiousness combined with high levels of neuroticism and low levels of extraversion increased susceptibility to stress.

- While conscientiousness may be advantageous during the early years of medical training, the trait could be disadvantageous later on unless the protective effects of extroversion are present.

- Lievens and colleagues (Lievens et al. 2009, p. 1527) have coined the phrases 'getting ahead' (which is important in the early (often preclinical) years) and 'getting along' (to describe the skills that determine success in clinical training).

- Munro et al. (2008, p. 103) have coined a phrase, 'steady, sane, and nice', which captures their vision of the ideal medical candidate.

References

Accreditation Council for Graduate Medical Education. (2012). Chicago. http://www.acgme.org/acWebsite/irc/irc_compIntro.asp Accessed 24 March 2012

Arora, S., Ashrafian, H., Davis, R., Athanasiou, T., Darzi, A., and Sevdalis, N. (2010). Emotional intelligence in medicine: a systematic review through the context of the ACGME competencies. *Med Educ.* 44: 749–764.

Arora, S., Russ, S., Petrides, K.V., et al. (2011). Emotional intelligence and stress in medical students performing surgical tasks. *Acad Medic.* 86(10): 1311–1317

Austin, E.J., Evans, P., Goldwater, R., and Potter, P.V. (2005). A preliminary study of emotional intelligence, empathy and exam performance in first year medical students. *Personality and Individual Differences.* 39: 1395–1405

Barchard, K.A. (2003) Does emotional intelligence assist in the prediction of academic success? *Educ Psychol Measurement.* 63: 840–858

Bar-On, R. (1997) *Bar-On Emotional Quotient Inventory*: Technical Manual. Toronto: Multi-Health Systems.

Beck, A.T., Ward, C.H., Mendelson, M., Mock, J., and Erbaugh, J. (1961) An inventory for measuring depression. *Arch Gen Psychiatry*. 4: 561–571.

Ben-Porath, Y.S. and Tellegen, A. (2008) *The Minnesota Multiphasic Personality Inventory-2 Restructured Form. Manual for Administration, Scoring and Interpretation*. Minneapolis, MN: University of Minnesota Press

Birks, Y., McKendree, J., and Watt, I. (2009) Emotional intelligence and perceived stress in healthcare students: a multi-institutional, multi-professional survey.*BMC Med Educ.*, 9: 61

Block, J. (1995) A contrarian view of the five-factor approach to personality. *Psychol Bull*. 117(2): 187–215

Bore, M.R. (2001) *The psychology of morality: a Libertarian-Communitarian dimension and a dissonance model of moral decision making*. PhD dissertation, University of Newcastle, Australia

Bore, M., Munro, D., Kerridge, I., and Powis, D. (2005) Not moral 'reasoning': a Libertarian-Communitarian dimension of moral orientation and Schwartz's value types. *Aust J Psychol*. 57; 38–48

Bore, M., Munro, D., and Powis, D. (2009) A comprehensive model for the selection of medical students. *Med Teach*. 31: 1066–1072

Boyatzis, R.E. and Burckle, M. (1999) *Psychometric Properties of the ECI: Technical Note*. Boston: McBer and Company

Butcher, J.N., Dahlstrom, W.G., Graham, J.R., Tellegen, A., and Kaemmer, B. (1989) *MMPI-2: Manual for the Administration and Scoring*. Minneapolis, MN: University of Minnesota Press

Callahan, C. A., Erdmann, J.B., Hojat, M., et al. (2000) Validity of faculty ratings of students' clinical competence in core clerkships in relation to scores on licensing examinations and supervisors' ratings in residency. *Acad Med*. 75(10 suppl): S71–S73

Carrothers, R.M., Gregory, S.W., Jr., and Gallagher, T.J. (2000) Measuring emotional intelligence of medical school applicants. *Acad Med*. 75: 456–463

Carr, S.E. (2009) Emotional intelligence in medical students: does it correlate with selection measures? *Med Educ*. 43: 1069–1077

Carver, C.S. and Connor-Smith, J. (2010) Personality and coping. *Ann Rev Psychol*. 61: 679–704

Cattell, R.B. and Cattell, H.E. (1995) Personality structure and the new 5th edition of the 16PF. *Educ Psychol Measurement*. 55(6): 926–937

Cooper, C. (2010) *Individual Differences and Personality*. London: Hodder Education

Corr, P.J. and Matthews, G. (eds) (2009) *Cambridge Handbook of Personality Psychology*. Cambridge: Cambridge University Press

Costa, P.T. and McCrae, R.R. (1976) Age differences in personality structure: a cluster-analytic approach. *J Gerontol*. 31: 564–570

Costa, P.T. and McCrae R.R. (1992) NEO-PI(R) *Professional Manual*. Odessa, FL: Psychological Assessment Resources

Dahlin, M.E. and Runeson B. (2007) Burnout and psychiatric morbidity among medical students entering clinical training: a three year prospective questionnaire and interview-based study. *BMC Med Educ*. 7: 6

Doherty, E.M. and Nugent, E. (2011) Personality factors and medical training: a review of the literature. *Med Educ*. 45: 132–140

Dowell, J., Lumsden, M.A., Powis, D., et al. (2011) Predictive validity of the personal qualities assessment for selection of medical students in Scotland. *Med Teach*. 33: e485–e488

Dyrbye, L.N., Harper, W., Durning, S.J., et al. (2011) Patterns of distress in US medical students. *Med Teach*. 33: 834–839

Dyrbye, L.N., Massie Jr., F.S. and Eacker, A., et al. (2010) Relationship between burnout and professional conduct and attitudes among US medical students. *JAMA*. 304(11): 1173–1180

Dyrbye, L.N., Thomas, M.R., and Shanafelt, T.D. (2006) Systematic review of depression, anxiety, and other indicators of psychological distress among US and Canadian medical students. *Acad Med*. 81(4): 354–373

Elam, C.L. (2000) Use of 'emotional intelligence' as one measure of medical school applicants' noncognitive characteristics. *Acad Med*. 75: 445–446

Eva, K., Rosenfeld, J., Reiter, H., and Norman, G. (2004) An admissions OSCE: the multiple mini-interview. *Med Educ*. 18: 314–326

Eysenck, H.J. and Eysenck, S.B.G. (1975) *Manual of the Eysenck Personality Questionnaire*. London: Hodder and Stoughton

Eysenck, H.J. and Eysenck, S.B.G. (1991) *Manual of the Eysenck Personality Scale*. London: Hodder and Stoughton

Fahrenkopf, A. M., Sectish, T.C., Barger, L.K., et al. (2008) Rates of medication errors among depressed and burnt out residents: Prospective cohort study. *BMJ*. 336: 488–491

Ferguson, E., James, D., O'Hehir, F., Sanders A., and McManus I.C. (2003) Pilot study of the roles of personality, references, and personal statements in relation to performance over the five years of a medical degree. *BMJ*. 326(7386): 429–432

Ferguson, E., James, D., and Maddeley, I. (2002) Factors associated with success in medical school and in a medical career. *BMJ*. 324: 952–957

Furnham, A. and Crump, J. (2005) Personality traits, types and disorders: An examination of the relationship between three self-report measures. *Eur J Personality*. 19(3): 167–184

General Medical Council (2009) *Tomorrow's Doctors: Outcomes and Standards for Undergraduate Medical Education*. London: General Medical Council

Goldberg, D. and Williams, P.A. (1988) *A User's Guide to the General Health Questionnaire*. Berkshire: NFER-Nelson

Gough, H.G. and Bradley, P. (1996) *CPI Manual*. 3rd edn. Palo Alto, CA: Consulting Psychologists Press

Haslam, N., Whelan, J., and Bastian, B. (2009) Big five traits mediate associations between values and subjective well-being. *Personality and Individual Differences*. 46: 40–42

Hathaway, S.R. and McKinley, J.C. (1983) *Manual for the Administration and Scoring of the MMPI*. Minneapolis MN: National Computer Systems

Hodgson, C.S., Teherani, A., Gough, H.G., Bradley, P., and Papadakis, M.A. (2007) The relationship between measures of unprofessional behaviour during medical school and indices on the California Psychological Inventory. *Acad Med*. 82(10 suppl): S4–S7

Hofer, S.M., Horn, J.L., and Eber, H.W. (1997) A robust five-factor structure of the 16PF: Strong evidence from independent rotation and confirmatory factorial invariance procedures. *Personality and Individual Differences*. 23(2): 247–269

Hogan, R. and Hogan, J. (1997) *Hogan Development Survey Manual*. Tilsa, OK: Hogan Assessment Centers

Hojat, M., Callahan, C.A., and Gonnella, J.S. (2004) Students' personality and ratings of clinical competence in medical school clerkships: a longitudinal study. *Psychol Health Med*. 9(2): 247–252

Horsburgh, V.A., Schermer, J.A., Veselka, L., and Vernon P.A. (2009) A behavioural genetic study of mental toughness and personality. *Personality and Individual Differences*. 46: 100–105

James, D., Ferguson, E., Powis, D., et al. (2009) Graduate entry to medicine: widening psychological diversity.*BMC Med Educ*. 9: 67

James, E. (1958) General practice and medical education: the education of the scientist. *BMJ*. 2: 575

Kish-Gephart, J.J., Harrison, D.A., and Trevino, L.K. (2010) Bad apples, bad cases and bad barrels: meta-analytic evidence about sources of unethical decisions at work. *J Appl Psychol*. 95(1): 1–31

Knights, J.A. and Kennedy, B.J. (2007) Medical school selection: impact of dysfunctional tendencies on academic performance. *Med Educ* 41(4): 362–368

Lievens, F., Coetsier, P., De Fruyt, F., and De Maeseneer J. (2002) Medical students' personality characteristics and academic performance: a five-factor model perspective. *Med Educ*. 36(11): 1050–1056

Lievens, P., Ones, D.S., and Dilchert, S. (2009) Personality scale validities increase throughout medical school. *J Appl Psychol*. 94(6): 1514–1535

Lumsden, M.A., Bore, M., Millar, K., Jack, R., and Powis, D. (2009) Assessment of personal qualities in relation to admission to medical school. *Med Educ*. 39: 258–265

Mayer, J.D. and Salovey, P. (1993) The intelligence of emotional intelligence. *Intelligence*. 17: 433–442

Mayer, J.D. and Salovey, P. (1997) What is emotional intelligence? In: P. Salovey and D. Sluyter (eds) *Emotional Development and Emotional Intelligence: Implications for Educators* (pp. 3–31). New York: Basic Books

Mayer, J.D., Roberts, R.D., and Barsade, S.G. (2008) Human abilities: emotional intelligence. *Ann Rev Psychol*. 59: 507–536

Mayer, J.D., Salovey, P., and Caruso, D. (2002) *Mayer-Salovey-Caruso Emotional Intelligence Test (MSCEIT)*. Toronto: MHS Publ

McManus I.C., Keeling A., and Paice E. (2004) Stress, burnout and doctors' attitudes to work are determined by personality and learning style: a twelve year longitudinal study of UK medical graduates. *BMC Med*. 2: 29

Mitchell M., Srinivasan, M., West, D.C., et al. (2005) Factors affecting resident performance: development of a theoretical model and a focused literature review. *Acad Med*. 80(4): 376–389

Millon, T. (2012) On the history and future study of personality and its disorders. *AnnRev Clin Psychol*. 8: 1–19

Morgeson, F.P., Campion, M.A., Dipboye, R.L., and Hollenbeck, J.R. (2007) Are we getting fooled again? Coming to terms with limitations in the use of personality tests for personnel selection. *Personnel Psychol*. 60: 1029–1049

Murray, H.A. (1971) *Thematic Apperception Test*. Manual. Cambridge, MA: Harvard University Press (original work published 1943)

Munro, D., Bore, M., and Powis, D. (2005) Personality factors in professional ethical behaviour: Studies of empathy and narcissism. *Aust J Psychol*. 57: 49–60

Munro, D., Bore, M., and Powis, D. (2008) Personality determinants of success in medical school and beyond. 'Steady, Sane and Nice'. In: S. Boag, (ed.) *Personality Down Under: Perspectives from Australia* (pp. 103–111). New York: Nova Science Publisher

Myers, I.B. and McCaulley, M.H. (1985) *Manual: A Guide to the Development and Use of the Myers-Briggs Type Indicator*. Paulo Alto, CA: Consulting Psychologists Press

O'Rourke, M., Hammond, S., O'Flynn, S., and Boylan, G. (2010) The medical student stress profile: a tool for stress audit in medical training. *Med. Educ*. 44: 1027–1037

Personal Qualities Assessment, 2010, Newcastle, Australia. http://www.pqa.net.au/files/description.html Accessed 1 April 2012

Papadakis, M.A., Hodgson, C.S., Teherani, A., and Kohatsu, N.D. (2004) Unprofessional behaviour in medical school is associated with subsequent disciplinary action by a state medical board. *Acad Med*. 79(3): 244–249

Papadakis, M.A., Teherani, A., Banach, M.A., et al. (2005) Disciplinary action by medical boards and prior behaviour in medical school. *N Engl J Med*. 353(25), 2673–2682.

Papadakis, M.A., Arnold, G., Blank, L., and Holmboe, R.S. (2008) Performance during internal medicine residency training and subsequent disciplinary action by state licensing boards. *Ann Intern Med*. 148: 869–876

Parker, J.D.A., Summerfeldt, L.J., Hogan M.J., and Majeski, S.A. (2004) Emotional intelligence and academic success: examining the transition from high school to university. *Personality and Individual Differences*. 36: 163–172

Petrides, K.V. and Furnham, A. (2003) Trait emotional intelligence: Behavioural validation in two studies of emotion recognition and reactivity to mood induction. *Eur J Personality*. 17: 39–57

Pittenger, D. (1993) The utility of the MBTI. *Rev Educ Res*. 63: 467–486

Poropat, A.E. (2009) A meta-analysis of the 5-factor model of personality and academic performance. *Psychol Bull*. 135(2): 322–338

Powis, D. (2009) Personality testing in the context of selecting health professionals. *Med Teach*. 31: 1045–1046

Powis, D., Hamilton, J., and McManus, I.C. (2007) Widening access by changing the criteria for selecting medical students. *Teach Teach Educ*. 23: 1235–1245

Prideaux, D., Roberts, C., Eva, K., et al. (2011) Assessment for selection for the health care professions and specialty training: consensus statement and recommendations from the Ottawa 2010 Conference. *Med Teach*. 33: 215–233

Qualter, P., Gardner, K., and Whiteley, H.E. (2012) Ability emotional intelligence and academic success in British secondary schools: a 5 year longitudinal study. *Learning and Individual Differences*. 22(1): 83–91

Roberts, R.D., Schulze, R., and MacCann, C. (2008) The measurement of emotional intelligence: a decade of progress? In: G.J. Boyle, G. Matthews, and D.H. Saklofske (eds). *The Sage Handbook of Personality Theory and Assessment*, Volume 2 (pp. 461–483). London: Sage

Romanelli, F., Cain, J., and Smith, K. M. (2006) Emotional intelligence as a predictor of academic and/or professional success. *Am J Pharm Educ*. 70(3): 69

Rorschach, H. (1927) *Rorschach Test-Psychodiagnostics Plates*. Cambridge, MA: Hogrefe Publ. Corp

Rosenberg, M. (1965) *Society and the Adolescent Self-Image*. Princeton, MA: Princeton University Press

Royal College of Physicians (2005) *Doctors in Society. Medical Professionalism in a Changing World*. Report of a Working Party of the Royal College of Physicians of London. London: Royal College of Physicians

Royal College of Physicians and Surgeons of Canada 2012, Ottawa. http://www.royalcollege.ca/public/resources/aboutcanmeds Accessed 24 March 2012

Salovey, P. and Mayer, J.D. (1990) Emotional intelligence. *Imagination, Cognition and Personality*. 9: 185–211

Schutte, N.S., Malouff, J.M., Hall L.E., et al. (1998) Development and validation of a measure of emotional intelligence. *Personality and Individual Differences*. 25: 167–177

Shanafelt, T.D. (2009) Enhancing meaning in work: a prescription for preventing physician burnout and promoting patient-centred care. *JAMA*. 302(12): 1338–1340

Skodal, A.E. (2012) Personality disorders in DSM-5. *Ann Rev Clin Psychol*. 8: 317–344

Stelmack, R.M. and Rammsayer, T.H. (2008) Psychophysiological and biochemical correlates of personality. In: G.J. Boyle, G.M. Matthews, and D.H. Saflofske (eds). *Sage Handbook of Personality Theory and Measurement*. Volume 1 (pp. 33–56). London: Sage

Stratton, T.D., Saunders, J.A., and Elam, C.L. (2008) Changes in medical students' emotional intelligence: an exploratory study. *Teach Learn Med*. 20: 279–284

Tartas, M., Walkiewicz, M., Majkowicz, M., and Budzinski, W. (2011) Psychological factors determining success in a medical career: A 10-year longitudinal study. *Medi Teach*. 33: e163–e172

Taylor, C., Farver, C., and Stoller, J.K. (2011) Can emotional intelligence training serve as an alternative approach to teaching professionalism to residents? *Acad Med*. 86(12): 1551–1554

Tamblyn, R., Abrahamowicz, M., Dauphinee, D., et al. (2007) Physician scores on a national clinical skills examination as predictors of complaints to medical regulatory authorities. *JAMA*. 298: 993–1001

Teherani, A., Hodgson, C.S., Banach, M., and Papadakis, M.A. (2005) Domains of unprofessional behaviour during medical school associated with future disciplinary action by a state medical board. *Acad Med*. 80(10 suppl): S17–S20

Tyssen, R., Dolatowski, F.C., Røvik, J.O., et al. (2007) Personality traits and types predict medical school stress: a six-year longitudinal and nationwide study. *Med Educ*. 41(8): 781–787

Twenge, J.M. (2009) Generational changes and their impact in the classroom: teaching Generation Me. *Med Educ*. 43: 298–405

Van Mook, W.N.K.A., Gorter, S.L., and de Grave, W.S. (2010) Bad apples spoil the barrel: Addressing unprofessional behaviour. *Med Teach*. 32: 891–898

Vassend, O. and Skrondal, A. (2011) The NEO personality inventory revised (NEO-PI-R): exploring the measurement structure and variants of the five-factor model. *Personality and Individual Differences.* 50(8): 1300–1304

Wagner, P.J., Moseley, G.C., Grant, M.M., Gore, J.R., and Owens, C. (2002) Physicians' emotional intelligence and patient satisfaction. *Fam Med.* 34: 750–754

Wear, D. and Aultman, J.M. (2006) *Professionalism in Medicine: Critical Perspectives.* New York: Springer

Weng, H.C. (2008) Does the physician's emotional intelligence matter? Impacts of the physician's emotional intelligence on the trust, patient–physician relationship, and satisfaction. *Health Care Management Review.* 33: 280–288

Weng, H.C., Chen, H.C., Chen, H.J., Lu, K., and Hung, S.Y. (2008) Doctors' emotional intelligence and the patient–doctor relationship. *Med Educ.* 42: 703–711

Weng, H.C., Hung, C.M., Liu, Y.T., et al. (2011) Associations between emotional intelligence and doctor burnout, job satisfaction and patient satisfaction. *Med Educ.* 45: 835–842

Wenghofer, E., Klass, D., Abrahamowicz, M., et al. (2009) Doctor scores on national qualifying examinations predict quality of care in future practice. *Med Educ.* 43(12): 1166–1173

West, C.P., Tan, A.D., Habermann, T.M., et al. (2009) Association of resident fatigue and distress with perceived medical errors. *JAMA.* 302(12): 1294–1300

CHAPTER 12

Medical education and its context in society

Elise Paradis, Fiona Webster, and Ayelet Kuper

Our profession cannot be and will not be immune from major social change, and history repeatedly shows us that we have a choice: we can either provide leadership that understands society's evolving expectations or have change forced upon us.

Peter Rubin

Introduction

Social institutions are socially constructed, emerging out of a specific sociohistorical context, motivated by sociohistorically defined priorities and organized on sociohistorically sanctioned models of appropriate human behaviour. No institution—be it Church, state, education or the family—takes on a form that is inevitable (fig. 12.1).

Our perspective in this chapter is constructivist (Berger and Luckmann 1989 [1966]). Constructivism is a theory of knowledge (an epistemology) that holds that the reality humans perceive arises out of social, historical and individual contexts (Kuper and Hodges 2011). A constructivist perspective suggests that to understand medical education, we need to see it in the context of the societies that produce it. As noted by Kuper and Hodges (2011), there is nothing inevitable in the current way of doing medical education and organizing medical schools: historical, social, and cultural phenomena shaped them. Seeing medical schools and medical education this way allows us in this chapter to reconsider the relationship they have to society: how they are shaped by history and social factors such as class, gender, lobbies, value systems, and power dynamics, among other things.

In this chapter, we provide an overview of several social scientific studies of Western medical education to show the reader what the field has to offer. We focus on the research paradigms that emerge out of anthropology and sociology and limit ourselves to research on medical education done in the West and in English. We emphasize different theoretical traditions for the world they make visible, building upon a growing literature advocating the conscious use of theory in medical education research (Bordage 2009; Cribb and Bignold 1999; Hodges and Kuper 2012; Kuper and Hodges 2011; Reeves et al. 2008).

For those trained in medicine, the most recent literature is often seen as the best as it builds upon a previously established knowledge base. This is partly because medicine works within a positivistic paradigm: its canonical beliefs include the belief in a 'single truth' that can be discovered using a particular set of methods—the gold standard, most often associated with meta-analyses of randomized controlled trials. For those trained in the social sciences, inspiration comes from publications spanning several decades. Older classics lay the foundations of our understanding; more recent work challenge and illustrate them in a more contemporaneous setting. Neither is seen as inherently more valuable. We thus invite the reader to engage with all of them, and ask: how could I apply these frameworks or methods to my own research interests?

Broader context of medical education: history of medicine and medical education

To understand the sociohistorical context of medical education, we need to examine the sociohistorical context of medicine itself. Indeed, medical education is deeply embedded in the realities of the medical world, and the context within which disease, medical practice and societies' and individuals' relationships to medicine are developed. What we provide here is a brief overview, inspired by a framework that sociologists of medicine have found particularly fruitful: the medicalization of society.

Medicalization of society

Several sociologists have pointed to the medicalization (Conrad 1992; Conrad and Schneider 1992 [1980]) of society over the course of the 20th century. Medicalization is 'the expansion of medical jurisdiction, authority, and practices into new realms' (Clarke

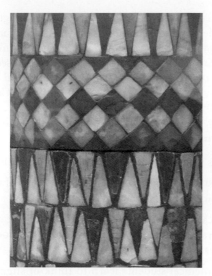

Figure 12.1 Medical education in society.

et al. 2003, p. 161) or, according to another definition, 'a process by which nonmedical problems become defined and treated as medical problems, usually in terms of illnesses or disorders' (Conrad 1992, p. 209).

Medicalization is characteristic of the post-World War II faith in medicine (and science) and the associated rise in medicine's perceived ability to solve social problems ranging from alcoholism to violence. According to medicalization scholars, the rise of the biopsychosocial model of health (Engel 1977) enabled the ever-greater foray of medicine into daily life, replacing law and religion as the main sources of social authority. This displacement led some social theorists to portray medicine not only as a practice or an area of study but as an institution that exerts wide social influence, which some have called social control (Conrad 1992; Freidson 1970; Illich 1976; Zola 1972).

In the late 1970s and early 1980s, voices critical of organized medicine started to be heard more loudly (Calman 2007). As the focus of medicine shifted from infectious diseases toward chronic or human-made diseases, as medical innovations such as immunization and antibiotics were taken for granted, and as for-profit medicine grew, the perceived (moral) authority of medicine declined. Some theorists posited that growing queasiness about medicine's commitment to population health (Ludmerer 1999) and disillusionment with collective solutions to social problems led to the healthist movement and its focus on individual empowerment and individual-level solutions (Cheek 2008; Crawford 1980).

History of medical education

One of the main reasons for medical educators to care about the history of medical education is that it enables us to see that our practices are not inevitable, but rather the result of historical processes of definition and legitimation (Kuper and Hodges 2011). The history of medical education in the 20th century in the West is most often told using the 1910 Flexner Report as a starting point. It is, indeed, a milestone in both the white and grey literatures (Whitehead 2011). The Report, titled *Medical Education in the United States and Canada*, transformed the form and nature of North American medical education, a model later widely copied around the world. It recommended the closure of 124 of 155

schools then in operation, their affiliation with university centres, and a radical transformation of the curriculum. The curriculum Flexner recommended was modelled on that of Johns Hopkins Medical School: 2 years covering the 'six basic biomedical sciences' and 2 years of clinical subjects (Chapman 1974). Flexner also noted the inadequacy of science as a sole basis of professional practice and advocated in favour of preventive medicine (Chapman 1974; Ludmerer 2010). The Flexner Report was not uniformly well received and did not impact every demographic uniformly. Most particularly, it made access to medical education and the medical profession harder for the poor, women, and black people (Beck 2004; Savitt 2006 [1992]).

Between the two World Wars academic medicine was focused on the education of physicians. Several events transformed medical schools. Starting in the 1950s, federal governments funded medical research to unprecedented levels, changing the mission of medical schools such that by the 1960s, research rivalled physician training as the mission of medical schools and their faculty (Ludmerer 1999, p. 196).

In the 1960s, civil rights for black people in the US and women's increased access to higher education changed cohorts of medical students and, thus, medical education (Beagan 2000; Colombotos 1988; Hafferty and Hafler 2011). In the early 1970s, Howard Barrows and his colleagues at McMaster University (Canada) introduced problem-based learning (PBL), suggesting that clinical skills would be best learned through small-group conversations rather than lectures and observations. Harvard Medical School's adoption of PBL helped it gain traction and put medical learners' needs at the core of medical education (Donner and Bickley 1993; Neville 2009).

According to Hafferty and Hafler (2011, pp. 24–5), three interrelated movements emerged out of organized medicine in the 1980s, with broad implications for medical education: first, the professionalism movement; second, the evidence-based medicine movement; and third, the patient safety movement. These three shifts arguably arose out of a struggle for legitimacy and power between physicians and non-physicians (including epidemiologists and other non-clinical scientists) (Amsterdamska 2005).

In the midst of these struggles, medical educators in the early 1990s were increasingly confronted with the public's loss of faith in medicine's commitment to service. The prestige associated with the profession declined and the healthist movement gained momentum (Crawford 1980). The CanMEDS competency framework, introduced in Canada in 2005 and internationally in subsequent years, can be seen as an attempt to address a perceived decline in professionalism among doctors (Frank 2005; Whitehead et al. 2011).

Key social theorists and related work

As noted earlier, our perspective in this chapter is constructivist. The key social theorists whose work we review here have all highlighted the constructed nature of the world, standing in contradistinction to the positivistic functionalist tradition. Functionalism sees norms, traditions and institutions as having a function that enables modern society. The role of medicine within functionalism was most famously described by Talcott Parson in his account of the 'sick role' (Parsons 1951).

In contrast, the social theorists discussed in this chapter were inspired by conflict theory and the linguistic turn. Conflict theorists, inspired by Marx, discussed the power of medicine in society, and its role in maintaining or furthering class, gender and racial inequality. Finally, the theorists we discuss here were all—except for Goffman—inspired by the linguistic turn of the late 1960s, with its emphasis on the importance of language as a structuring agent that creates and legitimates realities and power relations. Each theorist—Goffman, Foucault, Bourdieu, and Smith—will be briefly introduced; their perspective will then be illustrated with specific examples from the medical education literature.

Goffman and symbolic interactionism: presentation of self and negotiation of meaning

Symbolic interactionists believe that the interpretations individuals make of their experiences play an active role in creating their social world (Jacob 1987), and that these interpretations are created by the individual's social interactions. The goal of symbolic interactionist research is to study these interpretations and the meaning that individuals attach to certain things, interactions and ideas: how these interpretations are constructed and evolve; how they are used to make sense of future experiences, especially during interactions. In contrast with functionalists, who see socialization as a relatively ordered process through which students learn to function as doctors and embody their professional role, symbolic interactionists see the socialization of doctors as an active negotiation whereby students interpret and reinterpret social norms, act and react, in light of both previous and current identity, beliefs and experiences.

We will focus here on the work of Goffman, who figures among the most cited sociologists in history. We review briefly three of his books to highlight his contributions to our understanding of social life. Key Goffmanian concepts can be found in table 12.1.

Goffman's Asylums (1990 [1961]) is a series of four essays originating from a study of a Saint Elizabeth's Hospital, a mental health institution in Washington, DC. Through these essays Goffman develops and extends a typology of what he terms the 'Characteristics of Total Institutions' (see table 12.1 and Goffman et al. 1997). The concept of the total institution has been applied previously in educational research and in medical sociology, particularly but not exclusively in the sociology of mental health (e.g. Askham et al. 2007; Egan 1989; Haas and Shaffir 1982b; Malacrida 2005; McEwen 1980; Paterniti 2000).

Next, in his book *The Presentation of Self in Everyday Life*, Goffman (1959) develops an elaborate theatrical metaphor for social life. Goffman compares social action to theatre, discussing script, role, front stage, backstage, props, and audience. According to this metaphor social interactions are scripted; people follow previously defined roles contingent upon their individual characteristics as well as on the specifics of the interactional context; front stage (among strangers) behaviour carefully follows cultural scripts and is thus somewhat deceptive; back-stage behaviour happens among insiders, and sometimes contradicts the cultural norms of the front stage.

Finally, in *Frame Analysis*, Goffman (1986 [1974]) lays out a methodology to investigate the way individuals organize the experiences around them. He uses 'frames' to connote the way life is actively constructed to fit certain prescribed forms or types of stories. Frames can turn a story into 'a joke, a warning, a lesson, an invitation and so on' (Manning 2005, p.338).

Goffman is also seen as a 'radical, corporeal sociologist' for whom action is understood as 'interwoven with the perceptual field of the agent, understood as a visual, sonorous, olfactory, tactile and saporous order' (Crossley 1995, pp. 133, 136). Bodies are seen as critical to the social order: humans analyse information read from others' body idioms and adapt their behaviour accordingly (Crossley 1995; Manning 2005).

Concretely, a Goffmanian or symbolic interactionist orientation would lead researchers to ask questions such as:

1. How does medical school resemble a total institution?

2. How do students make sense of the hardships of medical culture? Which frames do they use?

3. Do medical students participate in face-work (see table 12.1) in their interactions with faculty? If so, how? What does their body idiom give and give off?

4. How do medical students learn to think of stigmatized conditions in medically appropriate ways? How do they learn to interact with stigmatized patients?

5. How do medical students and faculty interact with different types of 'normal' and 'stigmatized' patients (front stage)? Does their behaviour change when patients are not around (back stage)? If so, how?

Exemplars

Socialization

One of the most-cited sociological studies in medical education adopted a symbolic interactionist framework. Becker's (1963 [1961]) *Boys in White* describes the culture of medical school in light of what they see as the main constraints on students' agency: the overwhelming workload. They show how students interact with and adapt to their environment, develop coping strategies and are meanwhile professionalized into a specific worldview. As noted by Laqueur (2002), however, the reality of medical education in the 1950s was incommensurable with that of today; too much has changed in medicine since. A similar study of one of today's medical schools would contribute importantly to the field.

Haas and Shaffir (1982b) analyse the professionalization of medical students using a dramaturgical approach. They convincingly analyse this process using the concepts of audition, costume, props and vocabulary, role, stage fright, dress rehearsal and script. Thirty years later, this study is still one of the most convincing illustrations of the fruitfulness of Goffman's approach.

A later study by Mizrahi (1986) discusses how the requirements of medical education often run contrary to the needs of patients. Her ethnographic study compares house staff attitudes across two different hospitals and illustrates what she calls the 'get-rid-of-patients (GROP) orientation'. House staff, she argues, are made to discharge patients as fast as possible and neglect the least interesting cases by the normative culture and by structural constraints. Mizrahi carefully documents how a combative language positions the patient as an enemy; how students learn to GROP through daily interactions; the strategies that enable house staff to reconcile their mission with the necessity to GROP; and how skilful GROPing helps house staff develop a positive reputation and gain status. The idea of GROPing still has relevance today. Indeed, Ludmerer (1999, p. xxv) writes that in the late 1990s 'medical schools and teaching hospitals could

Table 12.1 Key Goffmanian concepts and their definitions

Concept	Definition	Key Theoretical Texts
Face-work	The work needed for individuals to project a positive image of themselves in interaction with others.	Goffman (2005 [1967])
Total institution	Institution that is segregated from the outside world and is characterized by role dispossession, programming, and identity trimming, dispossession of identity, imposition of degrading behaviour, contaminative exposure, disruption of the relationship between individual and their actions, and restriction on autonomy.	Goffman (1990 [1961]) Goffman, Lemert, and Branaman (1997)
Stigma	An attribute that is deeply discrediting and positions its bearer as being of a less desirable kind. There are three types of stigma: of the body, of character and of race, nationality or religion.	Goffman (1986 [1974])
Body idiom	Information that bodies willingly give and unwillingly give off about self and social relations. This information enables other people's judgement of bodies against conventional standards.	Goffman (1959) Manning (2005)
Front-stage, back-stage behaviour	Front-stage behaviour follows situation and role-appropriate prescriptions. Individuals or teams work to maintain a particular impression of a situation in front of an audience even though they may not believe in this impression themselves. Back-stage behaviour is out of character given the constraints of front-stage prescriptions. Teams or individuals enact it with the expectation that no member of the audience will see or hear it.	Goffman (1959)
Frames	A way of organizing experiences used to identify what is happening around us. Frames can be fabricated to mislead others, either for their own benefit (benign fabrications) or for the fabricator's benefit (exploitative fabrications).	Goffman (1986 [1974]) Manning (2005)

do well financially if patients were admitted and discharged so quickly that learners could no longer profit from their contact with them'. Caldicott (2007) notes how doctors often 'turf' patients to other services to reduce their workload.

Broadhead (1980) analyses how students engage in face work for medical school admission purposes. He shows how students manage their many identities, how they choose to highlight some of them and hide others based on their understanding of the admission process: how they adapt their behaviour to the meaning of medical school. He found that gender was a clearly questionable identity that constrained women's path toward medical school admission.

Learning the proper emotional composure

The study of emotions in medicine started with the pioneering work of Fox (1957, 1980), who first wrote from within a structuralist perspective. A body of literature has since investigated the emotional life of medical students. Hafferty (1988) studied 'cadaver stories': a type of oral culture about a medical school-related practical joke composed of a medical student perpetrator, emotionally vulnerable victims, cadavers or body parts, and reality-anchoring details (Hafferty 1988, p. 347). He argues that these stories help students cope with the new emotions associated with interacting with dead bodies: 'the act of telling cadaver stories (as well as their content) marks the anxious anticipation of anatomy lab, the initial adjustment to lab, and those periods in lab when the cadaver is most likely to appear as a human referent' (p. 349).

Conrad (1986) tells a similar story about emotions and culture through his study of the 'myth of cut-throats' among premedical students at Brandeis University. Conrad found that this myth helped students externalize and explain their failures. It had no clear anchoring into reality, however, with cooperation as the actual dominant mode of interaction at Brandeis.

Foucault: governmentality, discourse and hierarchies of knowledge

Foucault is a theorist of discourse: language is seen as more than merely descriptive, but rather as an agent in the definition and strengthening of power relationships within society, through institutions such as church, (penal) state, medicine and education. Foucault believes that there is 'no external position of certainty, no universal understanding that is beyond history and society' (Rabinow 1991, p. 4). Truth, then, 'is to be understood as a system of ordered procedures for the production, regulation, distribution, circulation and operation of statements' (Foucault 1980, p. 133), rather than as anything objective and universal. Many researchers today adopt a Foucauldian approach to study contemporary language use and practices (Rabinow 1991).

Hodges, Kuper, and Reeves (2008) offer an overview of discourse analysis as it can be applied to medical and medical education research. They group approaches to discourse analyses into three clusters: linguistic, empirical, and critical. Foucault-inspired discourse analyses are 'critical': they are concerned with power and investigate discourse in archives of verbal, text or graphic data. Hodges et al. (2008, p. 570) note how the aim of discourse analyses is thus partly to identify the way language shapes and constrains the way institutions and individuals can think, speak and act.

One of Foucault's main contributions has been to identify three different 'modes of objectification' whereby human beings have been made into subjects (Rabinow 1991, p. 21). The third and most original of these modes is called 'subjectification', the process whereby an individual transforms him or herself into a subject using a range of techniques or operations on one's body, soul, thoughts, and actions (Rabinow 1991, p. 11). Through this lens, researchers can study how students, for example, transform themselves into physicians (table 12.2).

Table 12.2 Key Foucauldian concepts and their definition

Concept	Definition	Key theoretical texts
Power	Something that is performed, a strategy rather than a possession. A web of relationships and practices that subject the individual but also trigger resistance.	Foucault (1980) Mills (2004)
Knowledge	An occurrence that makes sense only within a particular society and history, thus within a specific nexus of power relations.	Foucault (1980)
Normalization	A system of finely graded and measurable intervals within which individuals can be distributed around a mean that defines a social norm.	Rabinow (1991) Clarke et al. (2003)
Regime of truth	The types of discourse that a society accepts and makes function as true and the types of persons who are legitimate bearers of truth.	Foucault (1980)
Discourse	Discourse is not merely text or sign, but practices that produce the object about which they speak.	Foucault (2002 [1972]) Mills (2004)

For Foucault, modern power is something dynamic, evolving and productive rather than sovereign, repressive and inflicted upon helpless people. Power is a web of relationships that permeate society. Individuals are 'the place where power is enacted and the place where it is resisted' (Mills 2004 [2003], p. 35). It is partly for his emphasis on resistance that feminists and critical theorists use Foucault to highlight the possibilities for individuals to resist power (Mills 2004 [2003]).

Using a Foucauldian perspective in medical education research would help us answer questions such as:

1. Historically, how did we come to believe something to be true? Who benefits from having people believe such a thing is true? What function does this thing play in society?

2. Who decides on matters of medical education curriculum and reform? Who has no voice and is forgotten? How do dissidents resist?

3. What are the characteristics of the dominant discourse about certain medical ideas?

4. How does science legitimize the stigmatization of certain bodies and people, and thus serves to subject these people?

5. How did medical ideas evolve? How have they been incorporated into ways of being and ways of doing in medical education?

6. How do medical students and faculty resist socialization or change in their level of autonomy?

Exemplars

Stone (1997) compared the patient-directed and doctor-directed discourses of diabetes care and found that self-care and autonomy were valued in the patient literature, while 'compliance' and 'adherence' were emphasized in the doctor literature. She argues that the compliance-focused discourse of doctors is ultimately driven by economic imperatives and thus partly inhibits the goal of patient empowerment. Speed (2006) revisits the literature on mental health service users to highlight the discursive particularities of framing these users as patients, consumers or survivors. Comparing the discourses as they occur during interviews with mental health service users, Speed shows how these discourses co-exist and enable users to construct their experience of mental

health. Coveney (2008) analyses the discourse surrounding fatness and notes that three 'subject positions' of children condone what he calls the 'government of girth'. These discourses position fat children as sick, anti-social, and/or innocent, and thus as legitimate targets of weight-based intervention.

Hodges (2007), one of the first scholars to bring discourse analysis to medical education research, identifies three discourses around the Objective Structured Clinical Examination: performance, psychometrics and production, each with its own regime of truth. These discourses create specific roles for different types of individuals, and augment the power of different types of institutions.

Whitehead et al. (2011) argue that the construction of the CanMEDS roles and their representation in the form of a daisy can be read as an attempt by the medical profession to defend professional authority: an armour built against threats to medical expertise and autonomy.

Two examples of Foucault-inspired studies in higher education are also worth noting. Gale and Kitto (2003) discuss the marketization of Australian universities and show the individual practices whereby faculty resist and subvert changes that threaten their autonomy. Writing about law school rankings, Espeland and Sauder (2007) argue that the quantification of educational attributes leads to the possibility of comparison, judgement and control and thus enable the conflation of the *statistically* normal with the *morally* normal.

Medical textbooks

Several studies of medical education use discourse analysis to investigate the nature and construction of medical knowledge as it is transmitted to students in medical textbooks. In an early study, Scully and Bart (1973) read and coded 27 gynaecological textbooks across three time periods. They found that textbooks were written from a male viewpoint, portraying men's sex drive as stronger and women as frigid, meanwhile supporting hierarchical gender roles where women's needs were subordinate to men's. One of the most cited examples of such a critical approach to the medical textbook is Martin's (1991) *The Egg and the Sperm*. Martin's description of medical textbooks shows the impact of cultural beliefs about gender in description of biological phenomena, and thus suggests that the scientific objectivity touted to be at the core of medicine is not the full story. The recent study of menopause by Niland and Lyons (2011) shows that textbooks have tended to downplay the complexity of this phenomenon, focusing instead on ideas about hormonal failure and on the likely success of future research in the area. Thus, textbooks reinforce a cultural script that sees medicine as conqueror rather than fundamentally uncertain. Chang and Christakis (2002) investigated the changing norms around body fat in *Cecil's Textbook of Medicine* from 1927 to 2000. They found that obesity shifted from something that people do (a moral failure) to something that people are done to or experience (an environmental press).

Bourdieu: habitus, fields, and capital

Bourdieu's theory of practice seeks to bridge the gap between individualistic and structural theories of human behaviour (Grenfell 2008; Maton 2008). Individualistic theories tend to see humans as rational actors who interpret information and act upon it rationally. Structural theories suggest that human behaviour is partly determined by social factors such as gender, sexual orientation, race, class and education.

Bourdieu's theory views individual practices as the result of a mutually defining relationship between agents' learned dispositions (*habitus*) and their social positions (*capital*) within a specific context (field) (see table 12.3). The individual's subconscious behaviour, in particular, results from such relationships, yielding predictable outcomes at the aggregate social level. In contrast, conscious behaviour in the form of calculated decision-making can sometimes break away from these predictable outcomes (Mullen 2009; Swartz 1997).

Bourdieu's theory of practice discusses social hierarchies in terms of levels of capital (see table 12.3). A person's position in a field depends on their levels of different forms of capital, which include economic, social, cultural, and symbolic capitals (see fig. 12.2).

Bringing Bourdieu to medical education research leads researchers to ask questions about struggles for power (or scientific legitimacy) within medical education. As noted by Albert and Kleinman (2011, p. 266), these struggles 'typically take the form of competition to determine the legitimate ranking of productions and producers, and the principle (or set of criteria) according to which they will be assessed and ranked'.

Concretely, this concern with power would lead researchers to ask questions such as:

1. What are seen as legitimate types and sources of knowledge in medical education?

2. What are the reasons behind medical schools' differences and similarities of organizational form, curriculum, and branding?

3. How do actors in the field perceive legitimate ways of conducting medical research?

4. Upon what factors do hierarchies in medical education depend?

5. How do students from different backgrounds (gender, class, race, sexual orientation) experience medical school differently?

6. What role does gender play in the legitimization of certain ways of being and of hierarchies in medicine?

7. What types of bodies carry symbolic capital? How do these bodies' standards shape admissions and evaluation?

Exemplars

In a 2011 study, Brosnan interviewed students and faculty at two medical schools in the UK to evaluate what is considered as legitimate knowledge in medical education and why. She found that scientific knowledge and the symbolic capital associated with it regularly trumped clinical knowledge for prominence in the curriculum (Brosnan 2011). In an earlier publication, she invited medical educators to conceptualise medical schools as part of a field and to view differences between schools as the result of competition for capital: prestige, students and funding (Brosnan 2010). Albert and his colleagues have a long-standing interest in using Bourdieusian concepts to discuss medical education as a field. Albert (2004) showed how such a conceptualization clarifies the internal debates about what epistemology, methodology, purpose, and quality standards in medical education research hold sway. In a later set of two papers, Albert and colleagues (2009; 2008) have argued that the unequal symbolic capital of different types of research and knowledge production within the health research field put social scientists at the bottom of the hierarchy.

Bourdieu's notion of habitus has been used by Lo and Stacey (2008) to dissect and revisit the idea of cultural competency. The idea of cultural beliefs, they argue, is insufficient to conceptualize the role that culture plays in health encounters. Instead, an understanding of culture as habitus acknowledges the structuring effects of culture meanwhile leaving room for individual and contextual

Table 12.3 Key Bourdieusian concepts and their definition

Concept	Definition	Key theoretical texts
Habitus	'System of durable, transposable dispositions, structured structures predisposed to function as structuring structures, that is, as principles which generate and organize practices and representations that can be objectively adapted to their outcomes without presupposing a conscious aiming at ends or an express mastery of the operations necessary in order to attain them' (Bourdieu 1990, p. 53).	Bourdieu (1990) Bourdieu and Wacquant (1992) Maton (2008) Swartz (1997), Ch. 5
Field	A network or configuration of objective relations between positions. Positions are objectively defined by their present and potential situation in relation to different species of capital whose possession commands access to the profits at stake in the field.	Bourdieu and Wacquant (1992) Swartz (1997), Ch. 6
Capital	Accumulated labour (in its materialized form or incorporated/embodied form) that enables agents or groups to appropriate reified or living labour.	Bourdieu (1986)

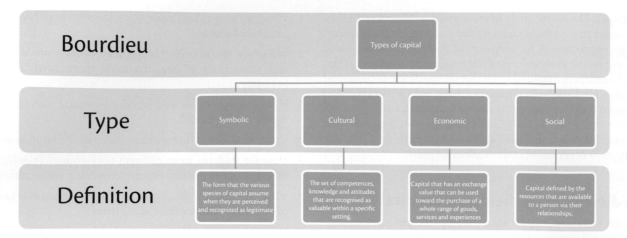

Figure 12.2 Bourdieu's types of capital.

Data from Bourdieu, P. 1986. The forms of capital. In: Richardson, J.G. (ed.) Handbook of Theory and Research for the Sociology of Education. New York: Greenwood Press.

differences. Bourdieu-inspired studies of education more broadly have also yielded critical insights into the way habitus translates into differential experiences and outcomes that are relevant to medical education. Lareau's classic studies, for example, showed the extent to which class transforms youth and parents' experiences with schools through different habitus and relationships to authority (Lareau 1987, 2002). Similarly, Mullen's (2009) interviews with Yale juniors and seniors from different socioeconomic backgrounds highlighted the wide, class-stratified differences in experiences of Yale, and in pathways from high school to Yale. Her studies uncover how successful, lower-class youth broke away from their habitus—applying to Yale on a whim or because of the intervention of a mentor—while upper-class youth took their elite education for granted.

Dorothy Smith and institutional ethnography

Institutional ethnography (IE), developed by feminist sociologist Dorothy Smith, is a method of inquiry that uses people's everyday experiences as the starting point for an exploration of the often invisible social relations that underpin or organize their experiences (Smith 1988, 1999, 2003, 2005, 2006). Smith uses the term institution to denote the complex 'ruling relations' (Smith 2005) organized around specific functions such as education or healthcare. This approach is based on Smith's complex understandings of the social organization of knowledge that makes 'texts' define ruling relations locally in the everyday world. Texts are reports or documents—such as a care pathway or evaluation form—that become activated by those who use them in their work. The materiality of texts enables their replication and shapes people's local activities and ruling relations.

Essential to IE is always actual people, their actual doings, and how the latter are coordinated across different sites. Understanding the social world therefore requires taking up a specific position—for example the standpoint of residents in a first-year program—as a starting point from which to explore, or map, the socially organized conditions of that experience. In this sense, IE samples a process rather than focuses on a population of individuals; it provides an alternative to the highly abstract and theoretical accounts of the world often provided through

mainstream sociology (Smith, 2005). Smith was influenced by George Herbert Mead, Merleau-Ponty, Marx, Bakhtin, Foucault, and Garfinkel, yet she does not identify with any of their theoretical traditions or interpretive procedures. The social strategy she developed is 'constrained by the project of creating a way of seeing, from where we actually live, in the powers, processes and relations that organized and determine the everyday context of that seeing' (Smith, 2005).

A major focus of IE research has been people's everyday lives as sites of interface between individuals and a vast network of institutional relations, discourses and work processes. Institutional ethnography also emphasizes people's work and how it is coordinated with that of others. Work refers to what people actually do in particular places, under definite conditions and with definite resources (Smith 2003). So defined, 'work' eliminates the paid/unpaid dichotomy and includes activities that we do not normally consider part of work, such as waiting (Diamond, 1992).

IE researchers use the notion of 'problematic' to denote and investigate a puzzling aspect of the taken-for-granted everyday world rather than what those in a local setting describe as a 'problem'. The problematic is what defines and gives rise to the series of 'puzzles' the researcher wishes to explore. IE has been increasingly used in healthcare-focused research over the past two decades. Examples of the types of questions institutional ethnographers might ask include:

1. How do physicians, or other clinicians, integrate hospital or government policies, such as waiting time strategies, into the clinical work that they perform?

2. How do medical educators take up the pressure to adopt psychometric measurement strategies in their everyday practices with residents?

3. How is the patient's everyday experience of pain management organized textually and discursively through the increasing emphasis on self-management?

4. How do medical students adapt their learning strategies to the types of assessment they will undergo?

5. How do undergraduate medical faculty understand and implement competency frameworks?

Exemplars

Diamond's (1992) ethnography of seniors' residences in Chicago is an extraordinary account of the experience of both working in and being a resident of a nursing home. Diamond became a certified nursing assistant in a nursing home in the Chicago area in order to take up the standpoint of nursing home workers. Diamond explores how nursing care is institutionally organized and how this coordination contributes to efforts at ongoing healthcare reform as they are being practiced in the United States and elsewhere: with an emphasis on efficiency.

Rankin and Campbell's (2006) book *Managing to Nurse* focuses on nurses' participation in Canadian healthcare reform. Among the important contributions of this book is an emphasis on how the accounting logic that permeates current healthcare reform changes the caring work that nurses perform. In addition, Campbell has conducted several IE studies aimed at explicating the role of nursing work in healthcare delivery and healthcare reform (Campbell 2001; Campbell and Jackson 1992; Campbell and Manicom 1995). Rankin's recent work has also used the theoretical framework of institutional ethnography to explore the practices of nursing educators as they evaluate students, thus explicating some of the troubling practices of evaluation work (Rankin et al. 2010).

McCoy (2005) undertook a study of the doctor–patient relationship from the standpoint of women and men who live with human immunodeficiency virus (HIV) in conditions of economic and social marginality. She draws on focus group and interview conversations with 79 HIV-positive individuals in southern Ontario to offer a close reading of patients' descriptions of good doctoring in light of their specific needs and life circumstances.

Focusing on a high-profile research report on hospital length-of-stay, Mykhalovskiy (2001) conducted an ethnographic study of the production of health services research and how this research is taken up by hospital administrators. In Mykhalovskiy's analysis, the discourse of 'efficiency' and its role in hospital restructuring is rendered visible.

Webster (2009) explored the positivist discourse of evidence-based medicine as it is taken up by community physicians charged with implementing 'best-practice' acute stroke care in Ontario, Canada. Through her work, the discourses of evidence-based medicine and knowledge translation come into view as managerial tools designed to control the delivery of care rather than as designed to improve patient care. She uncovers some of the assumptions and hidden priorities underlying these discourses.

Other theorists worth reading

Given space constraints, we have focused on four theorists out of a large number of possibilities. Here we introduce briefly four other theorists whose theoretical contributions could fruitfully inspire medical education research.

♦ Through his research, Bruno Latour has shown how scientific facts are created (Latour and Woolgar 1986 [1979]) and suggested a methodology for studying scientists (Latour 1987). He emphasizes the role of rhetoric in the scientific community and in the processes of adoption of scientific innovations (Latour 1993).

♦ Ian Hacking, who is a philosopher of science, argued that a 'looping effect' transforms patients and medical diagnoses, particularly

in the case of mental health (Hacking 1990; Hacking 1998), and forced social scientists to reconsider what they mean when they say that something is 'socially constructed' (Hacking 1999).

♦ The international, comparative research of John W. Meyer, Francisco Ramirez and colleagues at Stanford University provides a compelling theoretical framework for the investigation of diffusion processes in higher education as in other organizational fields (Drori et al. 2003; Frank and Meyer 2007; Meyer et al. 1997).

♦ Sandra Harding is a feminist pioneer in studies of science. Harding (1986) asked: can the sciences, with their Western, bourgeois, masculine history and worldview, ever serve women? She also argues that Western science has led to the development of Western society and culture at the expense of those she calls 'others' (Harding 1991): developing world peoples, women, the poor and nature.

Hot topics of social scientific study in medical education

The hidden curriculum

As noted in a key text by Hafferty and Castellani (2009, p. 16), the hidden curriculum can be both a theoretical framework and a 'particular process of student learning' characterized by the socialization into particular attitudes, values, beliefs, and behaviours.

Early studies of the hidden curriculum included Haas and Shaffir's (1982a) study of student socialization and Hafferty and Franks' (1994) discussion of ethics teaching within medical education. The former notes the import of relationships in the development of students' sense of competence. The latter conceptualizes medical training as 'a process of moral enculturation, and that in transmitting normative rules regarding behaviour and emotions to its trainees, the medical school functions as a moral community' (Hafferty and Franks 1994, p. 861). Sinclair (1997) highlights the socialization process inherent to medicine, the learning of attitudes, values and behaviours, most particularly the loss of idealism and the acceptance of a ritualized professional identity.

Hafferty and Castellani (2009) argue that two main factors led to the rising interest in the hidden curriculum as a theoretical framework among medical educators in the 1990s: first, new information technologies enabled different studies of healthcare quality and medical training; second, a way to be critical of the old way of doing things that would not alienate the old guard needed to be found. The hidden curriculum framework suggested that even if the formal curriculum were of high quality, something *else* was being taught in medical education. Several studies have shown how medical students are indoctrinated into a culture that makes them more cynical and less caring or empathetic when they graduate than they were when they started, most particularly in how they see or relate to patients (Anspach 1988; Becker and Geer 1958; Mizrahi 1986; Newton et al. 2008). A study of when and where values are taught within an internal medicine training programme highlighted the importance of informal learning spaces: those outside the structured teaching times such as rounds and lectures (Stern 1998). Two studies suggest that clinical learning is particularly to blame for this loss of idealism: White et al. (2009) note the conflicting messages medical students receive through the formal (preclinical) and informal (clinical, via role modelling) curricula; Hojat et al.'s (2009) longitudinal study confirms that the 'devil is in the third year'. Other studies emphasise the import of the student–teacher relationship in the transmission of the hidden curriculum of medicine (Haidet and Stein 2006) and find gendered patterns of appreciation of role models: men were valued for their knowledge, professional power and authority, women for their tolerance, integrity, respectfulness and support (Lempp and Seale 2004).

Professionalism

The literature on professionalism in medicine and in medical education is large and spans several decades. Freidson (1970), in *Profession of Medicine*, argued that professionalism is as much a function of the knowledge and skills of practitioners as it is a function of the environment within which professionals learn and practice. While technical definitions of professionalism have been broadly used and, while educating 'professionals' could be seen as merely a technical challenge, a few sociologically inspired studies have forced medical educators to step back and consider the assumptions built into their research and practice.

Several authors have noted how conceptualizations of professionalism do not connect clinical practice with the abstract concepts they advocate, such as altruism, duty, and honesty (Wear and Kuczewski 2004). Too abstract, these attributes of the 'truly professional doctor'—what Whitehead (2011) calls 'the Good Doctor'—are not anchored in actual behaviour. To complicate matters, according to Connelly (2003), professionalism applies both to medicine as a whole and to individual practice. Wear and Kuczewski (2004) use discourse analysis to reflect upon a decade of medical school efforts at developing professionalism among their students. They note the arbitrariness of curricular efforts and suggest that relationships (between doctors across professions, with patients) be the focus of professionalism education in an effort to transform abstractions into ways of doing.

Martimianakis et al. (2009) write: 'professionalism is an extremely value-laden term with societal, institutional, historical and contextual expectations built into it' (p. 830). Understanding, as social scientists, that a construct such as 'professionalism' is an interactional process inextricable from the political, social and economic dimensions of medicine broadens its scope—in terms of how it can be researched and taught. For example, as argued by Wear (1998), certain symbols of medical professionalism—the white coat in particular, a symbol of care hierarchies, of social and economic dominance, and of exclusivity—carry meaning with them. Hodges et al. (2011) also use discourse analysis to identify dominant notions about professionalism. They found that discourses varied along two main dimensions: epistemology (positivist–objectivist and subjectivist–constructivist) and scope (individual, interpersonal, and social or institutional). Each perspective thus identified was found to be fruitful in illuminating certain elements of professionalism and potential means of assessment.

Globalization of medical education

The social sciences have paid scant attention to the globalization of medical education to date. One exception comes from Bleakley et al. (2008, p. 266; see also Chapter 12 in Bleakley et al. 2010), who invite medical educators to consider their attempts to spread 'Western curricula, educational approaches and teaching technologies' in light of postcolonial theory. Similarly, Hodges et al. (2009, p. 910) argue that globalization discourse and its claim to universality have to be reconsidered given the 'differences and discontinuities in goals, practices and values that underpin medical competence'.

For decades now, researchers have documented gaps between the discourse of adoption of Western medical education standards and actual practices (Gallagher 1988; Gukas 2007; Rao 2006). Altbach and Knight (2007) contextualize these findings and discuss how internationalization efforts are borne out of academic capitalism (Slaughter and Leslie 1997) and provide a regional overview of initiatives around the world. An Australian study by Hawthorne et al. (2004) highlights the impact of globalization on medical education and notes how changing financial imperatives have dramatically changed the composition of the student body, raising several questions about the content and delivery of medical education.

A recent review of the broader education literature by Dolby and Rahman (2008) reviews six different approaches and unearths their historical roots, assumptions, strengths, and weaknesses. It will also serve as a great introduction to this growing field.

Future research

The role of the social sciences in medical education research is to broaden the discourse, to suggest alternative ways of viewing the world, to situate today's reality within a social, cultural and historical perspective, and to problematize and make strange the world that medical educators, students and clinicians have come to take for granted. We believe that future research would benefit immensely from more theoretically driven research studies.

Some areas where social scientific approaches would be most valuable have already been noted. Yet we would like to suggest others. First, contributions of the social sciences to our understanding of medical school culture and its impact on diversity will become more important as institutions move to recognize the chilly climate experienced by students and faculty who are women or who come from racial, ethnic, religious, or sexual minorities. Time has come to reopen the black box of medical student socialization and of harmonizing forces. Second, studies of medical education that build upon the broader higher education research literature would add some important contextual elements and fresh theoretical perspectives. Third, international, comparative studies of medical education would yield interesting insights into cultural beliefs and assumptions, including with respect to the rise of new technologies, and help develop locally appropriate approaches to medical education. Finally, studies that put front and centre issues of power within medical education—among faculty, among students, as well as between faculty and students, among ways of knowing (epistemologies) and ways of doing, across disciplines and types of disciplinary expertise—would be of high import.

Conclusions

◆ The social sciences have a critical role to play in the reconceptualization of medical education as a dynamic space where history, culture and social processes come to define medicine, health and illness.

◆ Using sociological theory enables researchers to ask different types of research questions and to see the world differently.

◆ Seeing medicine and medical education as social constructions helps deconstruct their apparent objectivity and unavoidability.

◆ Sociologically inspired studies are particularly well suited to discuss issues of power: between areas of knowledge; among students or faculty; or between students and faculty.

References

Albert, M. (2004) Understanding the debate on medical education research: a sociological perspective. *Acad Med.* 79: 948–954

Albert, M. and Kleinman, D. (2011) Bringing Pierre Bourdieu to Science and Technology Studies. *Minerva.* 49: 263–273

Albert, M., Laberge, S., and Hodges, B.D. (2009) Boundary-work in the health research field: biomedical and clinician scientists, perceptions of social science research. *Minerva.* 47: 171–194

Albert, M., Laberge, S., Hodges, B.D., Regehr, G., and Lingard, L. (2008) Biomedical scientists' perception of the social sciences in health research. *Soc Sci Med.* 66: 2520–2531.

Altbach, P. G. and Knight, J. (2007) The internationalization of higher education: Motivations and realities. *J Studies Internat Educ.* 11: 290

Amsterdamska, O. (2005) Demarcating epidemiology. *Sci Technol and Human Values.* 30: 17–51

Anspach, R.R. (1988) Notes on the sociology of medical discourse: the language of case presentation. *J Health Soc Behav.* 29(4): 357–375.

Askham, J., Briggs, K., Norman, I., and Redfern, S. (2007) Care at home for people with dementia: as in a total institution? *Ageing Society.* 27: 3–24

Beagan, B.L. (2000) Neutralizing differences: producing neutral doctors for (almost) neutral patients. *Social Sci Med.* 51: 1253–1265

Beck, A.H. (2004) The Flexner Report and the standardization of American medical education. *JAMA.* 291: 2139–2140

Becker, H.S. (1963) [1961]. *Boys in White: Student Culture in Medical School.* Chicago: University of Chicago Press

Becker, H.S. and Geer, B. (1958) The fate of idealism in medical school. *Am Sociol Rev.* 23: 50–56

Berger, P.L. and Luckmann, T. (1989) [1966]. *The Social Construction of Reality: A Treatise in the Sociology of Knowledge* New York: Anchor Books

Bleakley, A., Bligh, J., and Brice, J. (2010) *Medical Education for the Future: Identity. Power and Location.* New York: Springer Verlag

Bleakley, A., Brice, J., and Bligh, J. (2008) Thinking the post-colonial in medical education. *Med Educ.* 42: 266–270

Bordage, G. (2009) Conceptual frameworks to illuminate and magnify. *Med Educ.* 43: 312–319

Bourdieu, P. (1986) The forms of capital. In: Richardson, J.G. (ed.) *Handbook of Theory and Research for the Sociology of Education.* New York: Greenwood Press

Bourdieu, P. (1990) *The Logic of Practice.* Stanford, CA: Stanford University Press

Bourdieu, P. and Wacquant, L.J.D. 1992. *An Invitation to Reflexive Sociology.* Chicago: The University of Chicago Press

Broadhead, R.S. 1980. Individuation in facework: theoretical implications from a study of facework in medical school admissions. *Symbolic Interaction.* 3: 51–68

Brosnan, C. (2010) Making sense of differences between medical schools through Bourdieu's concept of 'field'. *Med Educ.* 44: 645–652

Brosnan, C. (2011) The significance of scientific capital in UK medical education. *Minerva.* 49: 317–332

Caldicott, C.V. (2007) 'Sweeping up after the parade': professional, ethical, and patient care implications of 'turfing'. *Perspect Biol Med.* 50: 136–149

Calman, K.C. (2007) *Medical Education: Past. Present. and Future: Handing on Learning.* Edinburgh, New York: Churchill Livingstone

Campbell, M.L. (2001) Textual accounts, ruling action: the intersection of knowledge and power in the routine conduct of community nursing work. *Studies in Cultures. Organizations and Societies.* 7: 231–250

Campbell, M.L. and Jackson, N.S. (1992) Learning to nurse: plans, accounts, and action. *Qual Health Res.* 2: 475–496

Campbell, M.L. and Manicom, A. (1995) *Knowledge. Experience and Ruling Relations: Studies in the Social Organization of Knowledge.* Toronto: University of Toronto Press

Chang, V.W. and Christakis, N. A. (2002) Medical modelling of obesity: a transition from action to experience in a 20(th) century American medical textbook. *Sociol Health Illness.* 24: 151–177

Chapman, C.B. (1974) 'The Flexner Report' by Abraham Flexner. *Daedalus.* 103: 105–117

Cheek, J. (2008) Healthism: a new conservatism? *Qual Health Res.* 18: 974–982

Clarke, A., Shim, J.K., Mamo, L., Fosket, J.R. and Fishman, J.R. (2003) Biomedicalization: technoscientific transformations of health, illness, and US biomedicine. *Am Sociol Rev.* 68: 161–194

Colombotos, J. (1988) Continuities in the sociology of medical education: an introduction. *J Health Soc Behav.* 29: 271–278.

Connelly, J.E. (2003) The other side of professionalism: doctor-to-doctor. *Camb Q Health Ethics.* 12: 178–183

Conrad, P. (1986) The myth of cut-throats among premedical students—on the role of stereotypes in justifying failure and success. *J Health Soc Behav.* 27(2): 150–160

Conrad, P. (1992) Medicalization and social control. *Ann Rev Sociol.* 18: 209–232

Conrad, P. (2005) The shifting engines of medicalization. *J Health Soc Behav.* 46: 3–14

Conrad, P. and Schneider, J.W. (1992) [1980]. *Deviance and Medicalization: From Badness to Sickness.* Philadelphia: Temple University Press

Coveney, J. (2008) The government of girth. *Health Sociol Rev.* 17: 199–213

Crawford, R. (1980) Healthism and the medicalization of everyday life. *Int J Health Services.* 10: 365–388

Cribb, A. and Bignold, S. (1999) Towards the reflexive medical school: The hidden curriculum and medical education research. *Studies in Higher Education.* 24: 195–209

Crossley, N. (1995) Body techniques, agency and intercorporeality: on Goffman's relations in public. *Sociology.* 29: 133–149

Diamond, T. (1992) *Making Gray Gold: Narratives of Nursing Home Care.* Chicago, IL: University of Chicago Press

Dolby, N. and Rahman, A. (2008) Research in international education. *Rev Educ Res.* 78: 676

Donner, R.S. and Bickley, H. (1993) Problem-based learning in American medical education: an overview. *Bull Medical Library Ass.* 81: 294

Drori, G.S., Meyer, J.W., Ramirez, F.O., and Schofer, E. (2003) *Science in the Modern World Polity.* Stanford, CA: Stanford University Press

Egan, J.M. (1989) Graduate-school and the self—a theoretical view of some negative effects of professional socialization. *Teaching Sociology.* 17: 200–208

Engel, G.L. (1977) The need for a new medical model: a challenge for biomedicine. *Science.* 196: 129–136

Espeland, W.N. and Sauder, M. (2007) Rankings and reactivity: how public measures recreate social worlds. *Am J Sociol.* 113: 1–40

Foucault, M. (1980) *Power/Knowledge: Selected Interviews and Other Writings, 1972-1977.* New York: Pantheon Books

Foucault, M. (2002) [1972]. *Archaeology of Knowledge.* New York: Routledge

Fox, R.C. (1957) Training for uncertainty. In: R.K. Merton, G.G. Reader, and P.L. Kendall (eds) *The Student Physician: Introductory studies in the sociology of medical education* (pp. 207–241). Cambridge, MA: Harvard University Press

Fox, R.C. (1980) The evolution of medical uncertainty. *The Milbank Memorial Fund Quarterly. Health and Society*: 1–49

Frank, D.J. and Meyer, J.W. (2007) University expansion and the knowledge society. *Theory Society.* 36: 287–311

Frank, J. (2005) The CanMEDs 2005 physician competency framework: better standards, better physicians, better care. The Royal College of Physicians and Surgeons of Canada. [Online] http://www.royalcollege.ca/portal/page/portal/rc/common/documents/canmeds/resources/publications/framework_full_e.pdf Accessed 20 March 2013

Freidson, E. (1970) *Profession of Medicine: A Study of the Sociology of Applied Knowledge.* New York: Dodd, Mead

Gale, T. and Kitto, S. (2003) Sailing into the wind: New disciplines in Australian higher education. *Br J Sociol Educ.* 24: 501–514

Gallagher, E.B. (1988) Convergence or divergence in Third World medical education? An Arab study. *J Health Soc Behav.* 29: 385–400

Goffman, E. (1959) *The Presentation of Self in Everyday Life.* Garden City, NY: Doubleday Anchor Books

Goffman, E. (1986) [1974]. *Frame Analysis: an Essay on the Organization of Experience.* Boston: Northeastern University Press

Goffman, E. (1990) [1961]. *Asylums: Essays on the Social Situation of Mental Patients and Other Inmates.* New York: Anchor Books

Goffman, E. (2005) [1967]. *Interaction Ritual: Essays in Face-to-face Behavior.* New Brunswick, NJ: Aldine Transaction

Goffman, E., Lemert, C.C., and Branaman, A. (1997) *The Goffman Reader.* New York: John Wiley & Sons, Inc..

Grenfell, M. (ed.) (2008) *Pierre Bourdieu: Key Concepts.* Stockfield, UK: Acumen

Gukas, I.D. (2007) Global paradigm shift in medical education: issues of concern for Africa. *Med Teach.* 29: 887–892

Haas, J. and Shaffir, W. (1982a) Ritual evaluation of competence—the hidden curriculum of professionalization in an innovative medical-school program. *Work and Occupations.* 9: 131–154

Haas, J. and Shaffir, W. (1982b) Taking on the role of doctor: A dramaturgical analysis of professionalization. *Symbolic Interaction.* 5: 187–203

Hacking, I. (1990) Making up people. In: Stein, E. (ed.) *Forms of Desire: Sexual Orientation and the Social Constructionist Controversy* (pp. 67–88). New York: Garland Publications

Hacking, I. (1998) *Rewriting the Soul: Multiple Personality and the Sciences of Memory.* Princeton, NJ:Princeton University Press

Hacking, I. (1999) *The Social Construction of What?* Cambridge, MA: Harvard University Press

Hafferty, F.W. (1988) Cadaver stories and the emotional socialization of medical students. *J Health Soc Behav.* 29: 344–356

Hafferty, F.W. and Castellani, B. (2009) The hidden curriculum: A theory of medical education. In: Brosnan, C. and Turner, B.S. (eds) *Handbook of the Sociology of Medical Education* (pp. 15–35). New York: Routledge

Hafferty, F.W. and Franks, R. (1994) The hidden curriculum, ethics teaching, and the structure of medical-education. *Acad Med.* 69: 861–871

Hafferty, F.W. and Hafler, J.P. (2011) The hidden curriculum, structural disconnects, and the socialization of new professionals. In: Hafler, J.P. (ed.) *Extraordinary Learning in the Workplace* (pp. 17–35). Dordrecht, the Netherlands: Springer.

Haidet, P. and Stein, H.F. (2006) The role of the student–teacher relationship in the formation of physicians. *J Gen Intern Med.* 21: S16–S20

Harding, S.G. (1986) *The Science Question in Feminism.* Ithaca, NY: Cornell University Press

Harding, S.G. (1991) *Whose Science? Whose Knowledge? Thinking from Women's Lives.* Ithaca, NY: Cornell University Press

Hawthorne, L., Minas, I. H., and Singh, B. (2004) A case study in the globalization of medical education: assisting overseas-born students at the University of Melbourne. *Med Teach.* 26: 150–159

Hodges, B.D. (2007) A Socio-historical study of the birth and adoption of the Objective Structured Clinical Examination, PhD dissertation. Ontario Institute for Studies in Education, University of Toronto, Toronto

Hodges, B.D., Ginsburg, S., Cruess, R., et al. 2011. Assessment of professionalism: Recommendations from the Ottawa 2010 Conference. *Med Teach.* 33: 354–363

Hodges, B.D. and Kuper, A. (2012) Theory and practice in the design and conduct of graduate medical education. *Acad Med.* 87: 25–33

Hodges, B.D., Kuper, A., and Reeves, S. (2008) Discourse analysis. *BMJ.* 337: 570–572

Hodges, B.D., Maniate, J.M., Martimianakis, M.A., Alsuwaidan, M., and Segouin, C. (2009) Cracks and crevices: Globalization discourse and medical education. *Med Teach.* 31: 910–917

Hojat, M., Vergare, M.J., Maxwell, K., et al. (2009) The Devil is in the third year: a longitudinal study of erosion of empathy in medical school. *Acad Med.* 84: 1182–1191

Illich, I. (1976) *Medical Nemesis : The Expropriation of Health.* New York: Pantheon Books

Jacob, E. (1987) Qualitative research traditions: A review. *Rev Educ Res.* 57: 1

Kuper, A. and Hodges, B.D. (2011) Medical education in its societal context. In: Dornan, T., Mann, K., Scherpbier, A., and Spencer, J. (eds) *Medical Education: Theory and Practice* (pp. 39–49). Oxford: Elsevier

Laqueur, T. (2002) Boys in white: student culture in medical school. *BMJ.* 325: 721

Lareau, A. (1987) Social class differences in family-school relationships: the Importance of cultural capital. *Sociol Educ.* 60: 73–85

Lareau, A. (2002) Invisible inequality: Social class and childrearing in black families and white families. *Am Sociol Rev.* 67: 747–776

Latour, B. (1987) *Science in Action.* Cambridge, MA: Harvard University Press

Latour, B. (1993) *The Pasteurization of France.* Boston, MA: Harvard University Press

Latour, B. and Woolgar, S. (1986) [1979]. *Laboratory Life: The Construction of Scientific Facts.* Princeton, NJ: Princeton University Press

Lempp, H. and Seale, C. (2004) The hidden curriculum in undergraduate medical education: qualitative study of medical students' perceptions of teaching. *BMJ.* 329: 770–773

Lo, M.C. and Stacey, C.L. (2008) Beyond cultural competency: Bourdieu, patients and clinical encounters. *Sociol Health Illn.* 30: 741–755

Ludmerer, K.M. (1999) *Time to Heal: American medical education from the turn of the century to the era of managed care.* New York: Oxford University Press

Ludmerer, K.M. (2010) Commentary: understanding the Flexner report. *Acad Med.* 85: 193–196

Malacrida, C. (2005) Discipline and dehumanization in a total institution: institutional survivors' descriptions of time-out rooms. *Disability Society.* 20: 523–537

Manning, P. (2005) Erving Goffman. In: Ritzer, G. (ed.) *Encyclopedia of Social Theory* (pp. 333–338). New York: Sage Publications, Inc.

Martin, E. (1991) The egg and the sperm: how science has constructed a romance based on stereotypical male-female roles. *Signs.* 16: 485–501

Maton, K. (2008) Habitus. In: Grenfell, M. (ed.) *Pierre Bourdieu: Key Concepts* (pp. 49–63). Stockfield, UK: Acumen

Mccoy, L. (2005) HIV-positive patients and the doctor-patient relationship: Perspectives from the margins. *Qual Health Res.* 15: 791

Mcewen, C.A. (1980) Continuities in the study of total and nontotal institutions. *Ann Rev Sociol.* 6: 143–185

Meyer, J.W., Boli, J., Thomas, G., and Ramirez, F.O. (1997) World society and the nation state. *Am J Sociol.* 103: 144–181

Mills, S. (2004) *Discourse.* London; New York: Routledge

Mills, S. (2004) [2003]. *Michel Foucault.* London; New York: Routledge

Mizrahi, T. (1986) *Getting Rid of Patients: Contradictions in the Socialization of Physicians.* New Brunswick, NJ: Rutgers University Press

Mullen, A. (2009) Elite destinations: pathways to attending an Ivy League university. *Br J Sociol Educ.* 30: 15–27

Mykhalovskiy, E. (2001) Troubled hearts, care pathways and hospital restructuring: Exploring health services research as active knowledge. *Studies in Cultures. Organizations and Societies.* 7: 269–296

Neville, A.J. (2009) Problem-based learning and medical education forty years on. *Med Principles Pract.* 18: 1–9

Newton, B.W., Barber, L., Clardy, J., Cleveland, E., and O'Sullivan, P. (2008) Is there hardening of the heart during medical school? *Acad Med.* 83: 244

Niland, P. and Lyons, A.C. (2011) Uncertainty in medicine: Meanings of menopause and hormone replacement therapy in medical textbooks. *Social Sci Med.* 73: 1238–1245

Parsons, T. (1951) Illness and the role of the physician: A sociological perspective. *Am JOrthopsychiatry.* 21: 452–460

Paterniti, D.A. (2000) The micropolitics of identity in adverse circumstance—a study of identity making in a total institution. *J Contemp Ethnogr.* 29: 93–119

Rabinow, P. (1991) *The Foucault Reader.* London: Penguin Books

Rankin, J.M. and Campbell, M.L. (2006) *Managing to Nurse: Inside Canada's Health Care Reform.* Toronto: Univ of Toronto Press

Rankin, J.M., Malinsky, L., Tate, B., and Elena, L. (2010) Contesting our taken-for-granted understanding of student evaluation: insights from a team of institutional ethnographers. *J Nursing Educ.* 49: 333

Rao, R.H. (2006) Perspectives in medical education: 1. Reflections on the state of medical education in Japan. *Keio J Med.* 55: 41–52

Reeves, S., Albert, M., Kuper, A., and Hodges, B.D. (2008) Why use theories in qualitative research? *BMJ.* 337, 949

Rubin P C. (2008) Formative years: not what we used to be? *BMJ.* 337: 2905

Savitt, T. (2006) [1992]. Abraham Flexner and the black medical schools. *J Natl Med Ass.* 98: 1415

Scully, D. and Bart, P. (1973) A funny thing happened on the way to the orifice: women in gynecology textbooks. *Am J Sociol.* 78: 1045–1050

Sinclair, S. (1997) *Making doctors: an institutional apprenticeship.* Oxford: Berg

Slaughter, S. and Leslie, L.L. (1997) *Academic Capitalism: Politics, Policies. and the Entrepreneurial University.* Baltimore: Johns Hopkins University Press

Smith, D.E. (1988) *The Everyday World as Problematic: A Feminist Sociology.* Toronto: University of Toronto Press

Smith, D.E. (1999) *Writing the Social: Critique, Theory, and Investigations.* Toronto: University of Toronto Press

Smith, D.E. (2003) Making sense of what people do: A sociological perspective. *J Occ Sci.* 10: 61–64

Smith, D.E. (2005) *Institutional Ethnography: A Sociology for People.* Lanham MD: AltaMira Press

Smith, D.E. (2006) *Institutional Ethnography as Practice.* Lanham MD: Rowman and Littlefield Pub Inc.

Speed, E. (2006) Patients, consumers and survivors: a case study of mental health service user discourses. *Social Sci Med.* 62: 28–38

Stern, D.T. (1998) Culture, communication, and the informal curriculum: in search of the informal curriculum: when and where professional values are taught. *Acad Med.* 73: S28–S30

Stone, M.S. (1997) In search of patient agency in the rhetoric of diabetes care. *Tech Commun Q.* 6: 201–217

Swartz, D. (1997) *Culture and power: the sociology of Pierre Bourdieu.* Chicago: University of Chicago Press

Wear, D. (1998) On white coats and professional development: the formal and the hidden curricula. *Ann Intern Med.* 129: 734

Wear, D. and Kuczewski, M.G. (2004) The professionalism movement: can we pause? *AmJ Bioethics.* 4: 1–10

Webster, F. (2009) *The social organization of best practice for acute stroke: An institutional ethnography.* Unpublished PhD dissertation, University of Toronto

White, C.B., Kumagai, A.K., Ross, P.T., and Fantone, J.C. (2009) A qualitative exploration of how the conflict between the formal and informal curriculum influences student values and behaviors. *Acad Med.* 84: 597–603

Whitehead, C.R. (2011) The Good doctor in medical education 1910–2010: a critical discourse analysis. Toronto, ON: Leslie Dan Faculty of Pharmacy, University of Toronto

Whitehead, C.R., Austin, Z., and Hodges, B.D. 2011. Flower power: the armoured expert in the CanMEDS competency framework? *Adv Health Sci Educ* 16: 681–694

Zola, I.K. (1972) Medicine as an institution of social control. *Sociol Rev.* 20: 487–504

PART 4

Delivery

CHAPTER 13

Small group learning

Joy Rudland

The use of small groups to encourage active participation and deep learning as well as learning group skills and the ability to express and defend new ideas is well established in medical education.

Honor Merriman

Reproduced from Merriman H, 'Clinical governance for primary care teams: how useful is a learning set for individuals from different teams?' Education for Primary Care, 14, pp. 189–201, © Radcliffe Publishing, 2003, with permission

Theories associated with small group work

Learning theories can confuse, overlap and lack obvious applicability to practice. However, consideration of learning theories is important to determine why and when certain educational approaches such as small groups benefit learning (Johnson et al. 2007) and can positively affect learners' performance (Roseth et al. 2008). Appreciating some of the underpinning theories may result in more appropriate use of small group learning.

A transmission or instructional model, in which a teacher or lecturer transmits information to learners, has dominated medical education over the past century. The past couple of decades may have seen a shift from the transmission model to more learner-centred theories that promote learners playing an active role. The learner-centred model shifts the roles of teacher and learner, with the teacher collaborating with learners to help the learner construct meaning. Learning becomes a reciprocal experience for the learners and teacher.

No single underpinning theory explains why small group collaborative learning is beneficial (Springer et al. 1999), but some social and cognitive theories are relevant to small group learning.

Social theory underpinning small group work

Social theory contends that new ways of knowing develop in a social sphere. Social learning relies on learners communicating, questioning and sharing a common issue or task or problem. Social theory precedes cognitive theories as it proposes that cognition only develops through socialization (Vygotsky 1987). Vygotsky's concept of the proximal zone of child development has been more recently considered relevant in both tertiary (Harland 2003) and medical education (Kneebone et al. 2004), with Harland (2003, pp. 263–272) linking it to problem-based learning. It is proposed that learning, specifically high level cognitive

processing, is social and begins with how people internalize social events, with consciousness and cognition being the end product of socialization and social behaviour. Individuals can learn more when they collaborate than when learning alone. Chalkin (2003, p. 135) described Vygotsky's premise as 'an interaction of a more competent person and a less competent person, such that the less competent person becomes independently proficient at what was initially a jointly accomplished task'. While this can be applied to other aspects of learning within the small group setting, the varied developmental abilities of both learners and tutor promote this development.

The importance of imitation, not as simple copying but involving appreciation of how action results in a problem being solved, is also a key component of learning (Vygotsky 1977). Imitation is initiated through observation and modelling (Bandura 1977). This can occur through situated learning where there is an authentic activity and context (Lave and Wenger 1990). Small group learning in the context of the work environment or simulated alternatives should emphasize this authenticity. Current research on the development of doctors, particularly on forming professional identity (Devos 2010) and developing communities of practice (Wenger 2000), suggests other researchers share similar lines of thought.

Wenger summarizes communities of practice as 'groups of people who share a concern or a passion for something they do and learn how to do it better as they interact regularly' (Wenger 2006). Within the undergraduate setting these communities are often artificially devised by forming small groups looking at health problems (simulating working scenarios); in the postgraduate setting they represent the structures within which healthcare is delivered. Recent work on professional identity formation suggests that the relation between students' learning experience and their anticipated practice in professional working life is important (Reid et al. 2008). The development of small groups, representing communities of practice, may be an obvious learning strategy in developing professional identity.

The social aspect of learning emphasizes enhanced motivation, social cohesion and the development of social norms and cultural values.

Motivation

Motivating the individual's desire to learn is vital for education; other learners in a small group can motivate and there is also the motivation engendered through interaction (Slavin 1996).

Motivation to learn is ideally intrinsic. However, social relatedness and autonomy are required to develop this intrinsic motivation, (Deci and Ryan 2000). The coexistence of autonomy and social relatedness has been challenged; they may even be competing (Vallerand and Ratelle 2002). The rebuttal to this argument is that, in this case, the issue of autonomy relates to self-organization of an experience (Deci and Ryan 2000).

Social cohesion

Motivating others and being motivated though interactions with others are the other facets of motivational theories. These suggest that cooperative learning is maximized when the group cannot succeed in its task unless all the members work together (Gillies 2004). Just placing learners into a group will not necessarily result in cooperative learning; they may feel that they can learn as efficiently on their own or learn from others while doing little work. Cooperative learning requires that all work together for mutual benefit—so they must develop a degree of cohesion. Two conditions are considered indispensable for this cohesion: positive interdependence and individual accountability (Antil et al. 1998). The challenge is how we engender these attributes in the small group setting through both tutor attributes and the learning activities devised.

Development of social norms and values

It has been proposed that the development of meaning comprises two dimensions: 'habits of mind' and resulting 'points of view' (Wiessner and Mezirow 2000, p. 345) allowing individuals to gain insight into how and why they think and behave in a certain way (Gravett 2004). These allow for the possibility of critiquing and modifying assumptions and considering alternative views. Small groups are seen as an ideal learning opportunity for transformation. This may involve changing views, or reinforcing and providing foundations for attitudes or behaviours already held, thus developing social norms and values.

Cognitive theory of small group work

Cognitive theory proposes that learners within small groups learn through activating prior knowledge and elaborating to acquire new knowledge (Schmidt 1993). This can be achieved within social activity, in this case small group learning, through actively selecting and constructing new understanding (Biggs 1996).

Elaboration is a form of higher-order thinking, which generates new ideas by connecting new information with existing knowledge and by combining new ideas. It leads to deep levels of information processing (Craik and Lockhart 1972) and is assumed to inhibit forgetting, because it produces a richer memory structure (Reder 1980). Elaboration requires two fundamental skills, the ability to listen and the ability to explain, which are required not only for learning but also in interactions with patients.

Underpinning the cognitive elaborative perspective is the theory that learners process information at deeper levels when they learn collaboratively (O'Donnell 2006). There is evidence that learning strategies that promote elaboration through communication in collaborative settings enhance academic achievement (O'Donnell et al. 1985).

The role that members of the group play in teaching each other, termed teaching expectancy, involves explaining and elaboration. Explaining to others is one of the main components of elaboration, as it positively affects long-term memory (van Blankenstein et al. 2011). However, current research findings on teaching expectancy differ, with one study reporting a positive relationship between cognitive involvement and teacher expectancy (Benware and Deci 1984) and one finding no correlation (Renkl 1995).

Social and cognitive learning theories explain why small group work is well positioned for the associated transformation required in becoming a doctor. Equally, social aspects of learning enhance the cognitive development necessary to underpin practice. The social aspects of small groups are likely to motivate learning, allowing learners to test assumptions linked with prior knowledge and elaborate on their understanding, thus developing themselves and each other.

Factors influencing effective small group work

Many factors influence the success of small group work. This section starts by describing five main inter-related factors affecting the effectiveness of small group learning (fig. 13.1). These factors include the learning outcomes, the tutor, the learners, the learning environment and the learning activity (Beetham and Sharpe 2007). The remaining text specifically covers the issue of small group dynamics influenced by these factors.

The learning outcomes
The tutor
The learners
The learning environment
The activity

Figure 13.1 Factors influencing small group work.

The learning outcomes

The learning outcomes expected should be a main starting point in considering any educational experience required. Small group learning should only be used when it aligns to the outcomes specified (Shuell 1986). A small group should never exist just for a tutor to impart information; a large group format or paper-based material may be more cost effective for this purpose.

The strengths of small groups lie in social and cognitive development through collaborative learning. The small group setting lends itself to five broad outcomes: the development of critical thinking; knowledge acquisition; attitudinal and transformational learning; teamwork; and skills development.

Critical thinking

Medical education must balance the learner's amassing of factual knowledge with developing the process of critical thinking. An onus on factual knowledge offers a framework for the immediate moment; critical thinking may offer a framework for ongoing development. Both are important. Small group learning is particularly useful in developing critical thinking (Norman 1992; Wood 2003).

Cognitive gains

Critical thinking cannot be achieved in a vacuum; it must be attached to some declarative knowledge. The ability to amass content or knowledge should not be underestimated, even if it is a lower level purpose of small groups.

Small group learning may not necessarily equate with improved outcomes in knowledge-based examinations. Comparisons of didactic lectures versus small group learning began in earnest in the 1980s. Where such comparison was possible, the studies have differed on whether small group learning improves test scores (Costa et al. 2007; Fischer et al. 2004) or does not improve them (de Jong et al. 2010). A recent study found that exam scores improved with a move from didactic to small group learning, although learners reported spending more time preparing for small groups than lectures (Cendan et al. 2011). While one may speculate that the results would be comparable if learners spent as much time preparing for didactic learning, it is reasonable to expect that better results will follow situations where the learner's participation in the learning approach will expose their preparation or lack thereof. However, the findings point to the motivation of small groups as an advantage over the less social and more didactic approaches.

Attitude formation and transformational learning

Small group learning is considered to promote social skills, a humanistic approach, and professional skills (Peters et al. 2000). Small group learning can offer an opportunity to make sense of and challenge attitudes, which develop most readily and meaningfully within a social context, and may be changed through experience and persuasion. Research attests that small group learning influences learner attitudes to the treatment of alcoholism (Martin et al. 1988)—more so than lectures. Nurturing transformational educational opportunities requires learners to place themselves in the role of others, whether it is as a more advanced practitioner or the recipient of care, sometimes simulating clinical scenarios that may arise in future practice.

Working as a team

The relationship between learning in small groups and subsequent team-working behaviour is poorly researched. While small group learning may be considered a method for developing skills for working in professional teams, small group learning and teamwork may not be synonymous. Real healthcare teams often include many different people, depending on rosters and rotation of training staff. While successful teams demonstrate the ability to integrate new team members, generating stable, formed teams that maximize cognitive development, this aspect may not always be built into small group learning, especially at undergraduate level.

However, small groups and teamwork share many important features. The collaborative and cooperative skills required and developed in small groups could be replicated usefully within the team setting. Research into effective teamwork in the intensive care setting identified the following crucial factors: stable teams, leadership, trust between team members and team reflexivity (Richardson et al. 2010). These aspects can be engendered in the small group setting.

Skill development

Small groups are frequently used to develop skills, for example clinical and communication skills (Perez et al. 2009; Harden et al. 1997). This is often a credible alternative to one-to-one supervision that can be logistically difficult to achieve, especially given numbers in the undergraduate setting.

The benefit of small group learning in developing clinical skills is not just restricted to the clear benefit of efficiency (more learners per tutor). The value is again in the collaborative aspects: learners can share the experiences of developing a skill with an emphasis on avoiding the pitfalls, maximizing the advantageous approaches, and developing a community of practice. Small groups can operate at the bedside or in more protected environments like clinical skills centres. Specialized units focusing on skills development have become popular both in undergraduate (du Boulay and Medway 1999) and postgraduate environments (Grant and Marriage 2012). Many units track, video, or observe the learner undertaking an interaction prior to offering feedback. Involving groups in feedback, rather than only the individual, can raise educational engagement.

The tutor

The tutor (also known as facilitator) is essentially a member of the group assigned to ensure that it meets the intended outcomes of small group learning and that the group works as cohesively as possible. Many tutors like small group learning as it allows communication with the learner within an environment that enables assessment of the learner's knowledge base, judgement, and reasoning (Cendan et al. 2011).

The literature on content expert and non-expert tutors in health professional education generally compares generalists with specialists. Some studies found no difference in learner performance between groups led by experts and those led by non-experts (Davis et al. 1994), while others found that specialist tutors were better and that their students did better in examinations (Davis et al. 1992; Schmidt et al. 1993). Evidence suggests that some learners in small groups prefer staff they perceive to be content experts (Peets et al. 2010) and feel more confident with these tutors, although no difference (Davis et al. 1994) and the reverse has also been found (de Grave et al. 1999). The structure and focus of the small group work may be a contributing factor explaining these mixed findings.

However, learners do appear to perform better with tutors who attend to the process of small group facilitation (Peets et al. 2010; Silver and Wilkerson 1991). Tutors possessing group-dynamic skills were more highly rated by learners than tutors who lacked these skills (Dolmans et al. 2001a).

Irrespective of the required outcomes, the tutor's two main roles in small group learning are to facilitate the learners' attainment of the outcomes (possibly related to a specific task), and to ensure the cohesion of the group to maximize learning.

An ability to enhance group cohesion through collaboration and cooperation has been found to be more important than an ability of the tutor to explain (Chng et al. 2011). In addition, giving learners time and permission to think is an important aspect in all types of small group learning (Amin et al. 2009). At these times the tutor needs the discipline to remain silent (Brookfield and Preskill 1999) even when this is uncomfortable.

In problem-based learning sessions learners appreciated tutor characteristics including facilitating thinking and problem-solving where this facilitation was non-threatening, encouraged interaction, did not involve lecturing, and ensured clinical relevance (Steinert 2004).

Tutors should be good at stimulating and formulating good questions. Many questioning frameworks can be used but the emphasis should be on questions that promote critical thinking and reasoning (Myrick and Yonge 2002). Questioning in small groups is often at the lower level of cognition: for example, recall, rather than higher levels like analysis or synthesis (Profetto-McGarth et al. 2004). Tutors should also encourage students to formulate questions, as this has also been shown to be effective in learning (Bobby et al. 2007).

In considering the social interactions of group work, it is important to appreciate how responses to verbal and non-verbal cues regulate the flow of discourse—especially where engagement and participation are advocated (Sacks et al. 1974). Members who speak either self-select or are selected by the current speaker, often by verbal and non-verbal signs (Sacks and Jefferson 1974). The three crucial features to consider are speaking time, the participant's eye gaze and the listener's eye gaze. Attention is gained when the listener's gaze is directed to the speaker, and is lost when it is averted from the speaker (Stiefelhagen and Zhu 2002). The tutor, who wishes attention from all the members of the group, with the possibility of interruption, should include all the members in their gaze.

Sometimes learners fail to participate or participate inappropriately, for example, dominating the session. The tutor is responsible for encouraging the quiet participants and reducing the input of the dominant members. Appropriate methods to address such problems are strongly predicated on the expectations that the group establishes. At the start of group work *ground rules* should be generated, indicating the norms and behaviours expected of the group, including the expectations of the tutor. Revisiting ground rules when problems arise in the group is an appropriate mechanism for reminding learners of expected behaviour. Ground rules can be added to or removed as experience dictates. Lists of ground rules can be accessed elsewhere (Crosby 1996); each group should devise and take ownership of its rules.

Due to the social nature of the experience, difficult situations will vary and different solutions may be appropriate. If 'problem' students continue to obviously breach the established ground rules, more decisive action may need to be taken. For example, dominance may be reduced through seating, non-verbal and verbal cueing, or agreed reduction of the learner's input. There are many different ways to address problem students—tutors should ask institutional support staff, either other tutors, or dedicated medical educators.

If one of the outcomes of small group learning is that groups learn to work independently of a tutor, self-regulating and managing the group they work in, active strategies need to be taken to move the responsibility from the tutor to the members of the group. This should occur explicitly, otherwise it might appear like abandonment.

The specific skills required of tutors depend on the outcome expected of the learners. For example, developing clinical skills may well need a tutor competent (through experience) in both demonstrating and observing skills and in giving constructive feedback. If the intended outcome is to develop the learners' thinking, then the tutor's facilitation skills will be important.

The learners

The learner has to take responsibility for being a member of a group. They are as responsible as the tutor for making small group learning effective, if not more so. Learners must be willing to listen, to contribute, to respect others' contributions and to prepare for sessions appropriately. In some situations, educating learners about a collaborative social learning environment may be necessary. The small group process needs to be continually reinforced and where possible supported by appropriate assessments. Where social, learner-centred small group learning coexists with individual or teacher-centred approaches, care must be taken to emphasize the purpose of the small group learning approach to avoid undermining the method.

In many other learning contexts, such as e-learning or large group learning, the learner is deemed an individual. In these contexts, other learners may have little impact on learning. But in small groups, the other learners are what make the learning opportunity. The number of learners, their levels of ability and the age and gender mix can influence the effectiveness of the learning.

Culture, gender and age are interesting variables. The limited research on gender indicates that females are less likely than males to take a leadership role within groups but are equally capable when asked to assume the role (Wayne 2010). If leadership skills are desirable, tutors may need to be active in ensuring females take this role.

The cultural composition of groups may also affect the group dynamics and complex thinking (Antonio et al. 2004). In the UK setting, cultural diversity has been found to have a variety of effects (Brodbeck et al. 2011). Some cultures are characterized by willingness to contribute and challenge, other by quietness and reservation. Certainly culture has been cited as a perceived reason from other learners for lack of participation of some members of the group (Gill et al. 2004). Cultural diversity may be useful in sharing different perspectives (van Knippenberg and Schippers 2007).

The age demographic of the learners, especially in the undergraduate setting, could also be considered. Older learners can bring a more motivated, experienced perspective but it is unknown whether group members who have completed a first degree (graduates in undergraduate medical courses) make a difference to group dynamics. Research has found that age-related experience rather than a previous degree influences performance (Wilkinson et al. 2004).

Real life seldom gives us the luxury of balanced groups or teams. In education, engineering a heterogeneous or homogeneous group may be desirable, depending on the outcomes.

The learning environment

In this context the learning environment relates to the physical resources and the ambience of the group.

Physical resources

Physical resources include aspects like temperature, light, and seating arrangements. The placement of the tutor and learners within a space can significantly influence how members of the group interact (Saran 2005), so the tutor should consider seating options carefully. Small group learning often assumes a flatter hierarchy than for other learning opportunities. A tutor in a hierarchical position (i.e. at the head of table or at the apex of a horseshoe) may engender an expectation of leadership, or a tendency to direct answers to or through the tutor. A dominant position may be required when giving instructions but a less obviously hierarchal position may be required to enhance self-efficacy and self-regulation of the learners. Tutors should position themselves so they can observe all participants and encourage responses.

As well as the physical space, thought needs to be given to appropriate resources required to complete small group tasks (Engle and Conant 2002).

Resources may include things like a whiteboard, useful for the link between visual perception and thinking (Arnheim 1980). Illustrations can enhance external memory by drawing on both the visual and spatial working memory system (Baddeley 1998). In design, visual representation (sketching) is used to develop and clarify ideas (Buxton 2007). The whiteboard can also be used for sharing of information and as an aide memoir for the group. Its utility depends somewhat on legibility, accuracy and brevity. One issue is who writes on the board. Learners should be encouraged to take turns to undertake this task, not least because it allows the facilitator to focus on the group.

Ambience

Perhaps unsurprisingly it has been found that feeling tired or tense results in less commitment to listening and contribution (Bramesfield and Gasper 2008) and feeling happy or calm is related to positive group interactions (Linnenbrink-Garcia et al. 2011) with improved effort and persistence (Frenzel et al. 2007). The learner should be refreshed and positive in order to maximize small group learning. This affirms the necessity to consider the timing of the group work and the need to engender a positive group atmosphere. Tutors who fail to espouse and support the principles on which small group learning is based and manifest a negative attitude will undermine the value of small group work.

The activity

How a small group functions is strongly influenced by how well its activities have been planned and constructed. Studies have found that the structure of an activity can reduce the necessity for tutors to use a content-focused approach (Regehr et al. 1995). Small group learning cannot succeed unless all members of the group work together (Gillies 2004), so attention must be paid to how group collaboration relates to fulfilling the stated objectives.

Small group learning frequently involves producing stimulus material: a clinical scenario for a problem-based learning session, questions relating to a case or instructions, and equipment for completing physical examinations. Engle and Conant (2002, p. 404) state that the material needs 'problematizing'—staging as a problem to be solved or problems to be identified by the learner. The activity needs to:

* require collaboration for completion
* be clearly relevant
* be challenging but possible
* be timed appropriately.

The activity should not be too easy and should include a disorientating element if transformative learning is desired. Mezirow (1995, p. 50) mentions major life events as disorientating, but transition periods in medicine can also be considered disorientating, and teachers should seize the opportunity to take learners out of their comfort zone (Torosyan 2007). A disorienting dilemma is especially useful in stimulating reflection.

Effective small group learning requires integrating all these components. However, there are other important factors, specifically engagement in learning and group interaction.

Engagement in learning

The learner's engagement in the group is a necessary requirement for learning in small groups. However, some small group learning also requires preparation prior to or after the small group activity. This section raises the difficulty of lack of engagement prior to and during the sessions.

Preparation by the learners

One aspect can be the requirement that members of small groups prepare before the formal class. The learners and tutor should have a clear expectation of the learning activity and an appreciation of the necessary preparation; resources may also need to be available for completion of preparation work.

The idea of learners preparing before a session in order to maximize formal small group time is often poorly thought out. Research has shown that preparation can increase participation in the formal setting (Chizmar 2005). Learners have themselves identified preparation as an important determinant for small group participation (Karp and Yoels 1976). Despite this, research indicates that learner preparation can be reported by tutors as being be poor (Gill et al. 2004; Burchfield and Sappington 2000) with one study finding that 66% of the learners demonstrated lack of preparation (Gill et al. 2004). Although some research considers that older learners prepare best (Dolmans 2006) and preparation skill develops over time (Gill et al. 2004; Burchfield and Sappington 2000) the issue of preparation requires greater examination.

If there are no consequences to lack of preparation and the learning can continue without this preparation, either through poor activity design or rescuing by the tutor, this may perpetuate the rationale in the learner's mind that preparation is not required. If preparation and the associated outcomes, for example taking responsibility for one's own learning, are important, this situation has to be appropriately managed. This is intended not to embarrass the learners but to clarify the expectations for learning.

Active learning

Engaging in a small group does not necessarily mean that the learner is actively learning. Problem based learning is not immune from issues of ritual behaviour, where learners give the impression of fulfilling the remit of learning but are not actually meeting the small group expectations (Dolmans et al. 2001b).

Dolmans et al (2001b, pp. 886–887) give examples of ritual behaviour including: new ideas being introduced without connection to prior ideas; lack of clarity or relevance regarding what needs to be learnt; and an inability to link independent learning to the task or problem—possibly just reading from notes.

To counteract this, the design of the learning activity should include clear expectations, reinforced by tutors not accepting ritual behaviour.

Another phenomenon is social loafing, where a learner reduces their effort and relies on other learners (Woodman et al. 2011), leading to disengagement with the task (Karau and Williams 1995). The design of small group activities and the facilitation of the group should minimize social loafing. Research points to identifying individual contributions as one mechanism for combating it (Williams et al. 1989). Where the tutor is unable to accurately appraise individual efforts, using peer assessment to identity individual contributions may be the most valid approach. Self-selection into groups has also been found to reduce social loafing (Oakley et al. 2007), but this brings other challenges especially if sharing diverse opinions is desired.

Another aspect of engagement to consider is the educational paradigm of the learners and if necessary how this paradigm can be altered. It is important to consider where learners currently lie in their learning paradigm and how to move them to the desired paradigm (Bogaard et al. 2005).

Group interaction

How the group interacts and functions depends on the number and characteristics of the learners and the abilities of the tutor.

The number of learners that can function as a group has been widely debated. Numbers from 6 to 12 are often quoted (Walton 1997); some people ask whether a dyad is a group (Williams 2010). Learning will exist where there is meaningful social interaction allowing for engagement, collaboration and cooperation amongst learners. This is most often seen in the small group (6–12) setting but some skilled teachers can engender these elements in larger groups. The differentiation should perhaps not be defined by quantity but by social function through motivation and performance. Even a large group setting can effectively adopt some of the principles of small group work, especially when broken down into subgroups.

Numbers are also often dictated by logistics, the ratio of tutors to learners, what is expected of the learners.

The interactions of members in small groups change over time (Sweet and Michaelsen 2007) and many models have described this phenomenon. Perhaps the most validated, Wheelan's model of the group development process (Wheelan 2004), is based on the life-cycle model initially described by Tuckman (Tuckman 1965). Both models contend that groups develop in a sequential manner and share many of the same characteristics. The Tuckman and Jensen model names the stages forming, storming, norming, performing, and adjourning (Tuckman and Jensen 1977). This development may not always be predictable: some groups may fail to reach specific stages or regress under stress, with some failing to reach their full potential (Sweet and Michaelsen 2007).

Groups failing to attain the stage of performing (Wheelan and Lisk 2000) may need help to move through the stages. This help ideally comes from the tutor, but an external facilitator may also be required to observe the group and make suggestions on improving cohesion. Course organizers should resist changing group members during the storming phase.

Some authors rightly place great emphasis on the initial meetings of groups—this is especially pertinent when time with the learners is limited. This involves developing ground rules, as previously mentioned, but group familiarity can also be accelerated through appropriate icebreakers (West 1976).

Associated with group function is how long you keep a group together; this is debatable and should be influenced by the expected outcomes. Groups are more likely to achieve the performing stage if they are together for a period of time that correlates with meeting frequency, the functioning of the group and the nature of the tasks, rather than for a specific time. Familiarity tends to heighten trust in the group and identification of the group goals. With greater familiarity members are willing to disagree with each other, using open discussion to resolve conflict (Birmingham and McCord 2004).

Preparing and developing staff and learners to work in groups

The challenge of small group learning can be considerable for some staff and learners. While both may need support, support appears to focus on staff more than students.

Learners

Collaborative, cooperative learning appears an intuitive activity for young children, but the educational system may erode the acceptance of this type of learning. It has been found that students' expectations of the group process can be diverse (Gill et al. 2004), which may disrupt the effectiveness of the group learning.

The common perception that education, even at tertiary level, involves the learner consuming, perhaps uncritically, what is placed before them, is potentially damaging. Didactic sessions, however well presented, emphasize the consumption paradigm. A different paradigm is the learner as a producer, making connections and developing ideas through a critical approach. While it is important to develop students' understanding of small group learning, it should be done in a curriculum that aligns its outcomes to teaching methods and assessment. If assessment only values retention of individual knowledge and facts, small group learning should focus on this outcome. However this belies the value of education and the benefits of small group learning.

If there is a real commitment to small group learning, then time must be spent:

◆ Setting the expectations of a learner's role within the group. Giving learners authority to address problems and holding learners accountable for their learning has been found to be important (Engle and Conant 2002). If this is not evident to learners it is unlikely that they will meet expectations.

◆ Educating learners about skills and behaviours required in a group. This involves attention to ground rules.

◆ Reviewing with the students what is happening in the group and the relevant ground rules.

◆ Devising assessment that aligns with the products of small group work.

Learner support to embrace small group learning can be easily undermined if staff fail to advocate and model the underpinning philosophy.

Staff

For some tutors, teaching is seen to be imparting the knowledge they have acquired. Research suggests that moving from the more traditional lecturing role to the role of a facilitator of learning can be challenging (Hitchcock and Mylona 2000). Some tutors may consider helping learners to think, question, and elaborate in the small group setting more difficult than giving information. In addition, while staff often like being a small group tutor, they do not always like the amount of time required to effect learning (Cendan et al. 2011).

The Best Evidence Medical Education (BEME) systematic review is perhaps the best guide on initiatives to improve teaching effectiveness (Steinert et al. 2006). The BEME guide reports many examples of courses and workshops, which aim to enhance tutor skills; however, it mostly reports on the participant's opinion of such courses. The evidence indicates that staff are satisfied with teacher support and training, positively change their attitudes, and self report changes in teaching behaviour. However, there is little conclusive evidence of the benefit of teaching training on the learners' outcomes (Steinert et al. 2006). If the outcome of teacher training in medical education is poorly evidenced, what implications does this have for staff support for a small group tutor?

The lack of evidence for effective staff development may be due to the complexity of learning and the inability to distil and examine a single factor (the tutor). The importance of staff training may be inherent in how we value staff and the modelling they convey. Failure to acknowledge and support the tutor's role in small groups may inadvertently undermine the educational approach. Certainly development of facilitation skills may be at least served by first appreciating the skills.

Plenty of resources explain the small group process: dynamics of groups; tips on running small groups; and how to cope with problem students. However, small groups require practical, interpersonal skills and require tutors to learn through reflection and deliberative practice. From experience, some of the best development sessions for staff have been those allowing staff to exchange their ideas and the outcomes of differing approaches.

Another way of supporting staff is to seek the opinions of learners and feed the findings back. This approach may identify poorly performing tutors, but its main focus should be on improvement of the tutor.

Supporting staff in developing learning activities related to small group learning is often addressed poorly. Teachers may be expected to develop cohesive, authentic problems or scenarios with related learning tasks. This content or practice input is imperative, but needs to include attention to the educational construct of the activity. Teachers responsible for designing small group material should be offered support in developing the required skills of instructional design and educational cohesion.

Small group techniques

Various techniques can be adopted to improve collaboration and cooperation between learners (fig. 13.2). A purist attitude with small groups is unnecessary; the emphasis should be on creativity, modifying and combining techniques that align with the outcomes expected. A session may include several specific techniques.

Discussion group

A discussion group requires that learners consider questions—either individually before the session or in the actual group with

Discussion group
Tutorial
Seminar
Buzz groups
Snowballing
Integrated panel
Goldfish bowling
Role play
Problem-based learning (PBL)

Figure 13.2 Small group techniques.

the tutor and other group members. Alternatively it may involve raising a topic for immediate discussion. It can involve breaking into subgroups, allocating tasks and may rely on experience already gained or resources supplied to answer the questions. Discussion groups often need careful facilitation to keep on track.

Tutorial

Perhaps the most traditional of small group approaches—the tutorial—requires the learners to be given set questions and coming together to explain their answers to the rest of the group. With well-prepared students and a tutor adopting a facilitatory approach, this can engender strong learning, utilizing the cognitive theories of small group work. The main risk is that it deteriorates into a small-scale didactic group in which the tutor provides the answers.

Seminar

The traditional seminar relies on the learners reading the same text and then coming together as a group to discuss the material, often in a free discussion; questions can be raised and debates conducted (Billings and Fitzgerald 2002). The seminar approach is a popular method and has been advocated for the development of teachers (Steinert et al. 2006).

Buzz groups

Buzz groups, which originated in large group settings, can be used as a sub-approach within a small group. A small discussion group set up specifically to generate ideas and or solve problems within a specific period of time period, a buzz group breaks up larger numbers of learners into smaller numbers, often dyads. Discussing a specific topic seldom poses problems in small numbers. This approach can break up previous patterns of a session and introduce new thoughts. The discussion question must still be carefully thought out and the approach must contribute positively to the overall outcomes of a session.

Snowballing

Snowballing interaction takes place when subgroups combine with other groups to share their understanding—ultimately resulting in the whole class discussing the topic (fig. 13.3). The number in the group will determine the number of iterations.

Integrated panel

An integrated panel (sometimes called a crossover group) aims to maximize the panel's sharing of understanding. Similar to snowballing, it has the added benefit of directed 'teacher expectancy', where the participants are expected to teach members of the group. In this excellent and under-utilized technique, the group breaks into smaller groups—for example, a group of 12 may break up into three groups of four. Each member in the group is assigned a number (in this case 1 to 4—see fig. 13.4). In their group they attempt a task before breaking that group to reform with those members from the other groups assigned the same number, sharing with the second group the output of the previous group's discussion. This technique's advantages appear in the second round of group work. The expectation that all members will teach appears to heighten the first group attention and the seeking of

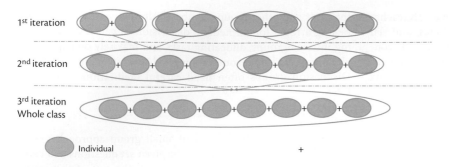

Figure 13.3 Snowballing.

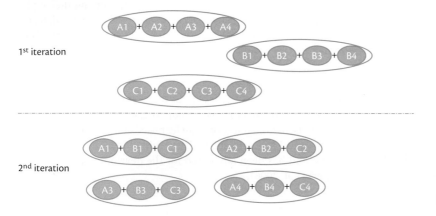

Figure 13.4 Integrated pane.l

clarification—so that the first group's information can be imparted to the second group. The integrated panel works best if this expectation is clearly stated.

Goldfish bowling

Goldfish bowling focuses on sharing an experience and critical analysis; it is often used effectively in clinical skills acquisition. Some group members undertake an activity; the rest of the group observes. The whole group then unites to talk about the experience and observation. Adopting positive strategies for constructive feedback is crucial to maximize the safety of the individuals conducting the activity.

It is important not to make the watched activity too long and to give the observers clear guidance on what they are observing. This technique hones observational, reflective, and feedback skills among those watching; it also makes those being watched more attentive to their actions.

Role play

Role play can be part or all of a small group session (Steinert 1993). The focus on role playing here is on experiencing interactions that one may be involved with in practice; it is also used to engender empathy. A scenario is generated with members of the group taking roles, which can be scripted or free-formed. Role play can often be successfully combined with goldfish bowling.

Problem-based learning (PBL)

Any chapter on small groups would be remiss without some mention of PBL, sometimes described as a curriculum philosophy as a well as a small group approach (for more detail see Chapter 3) (fig. 13.5).

Challenging environments

Some environments can be challenging for small group teaching.

The clinical environment is often the best place for learning for healthcare professions. It is authentic and social. The challenge here is considering the three critical parties: the tutor, the learner, and the patient, who are all required to participate in the educational encounter (Kroenke et al. 1997). The dual focus of bedside interactions with patient care and educational provision can easily alter the dynamics of small group work. The presence of family members can further compound the challenge (Cox et al. 2011). It has been found that learners need more reassurance in the bedside setting, but reinforcing their autonomy and ensuring that they are part of the learning process remains critical (Williams et al. 2008).

Articles regarding small groups in the operating theatre tend to focus on the process of small groups already described (Lipp and Holmes 2009). However, research highlights the tensions and limitations of the operating theatre, specifically poor communication and collaboration (Lingard et al. 2002). As such it may not be an appropriate small group learning environment, but rather an opportunity for appreciation of practice.

Research into online groups and whether small groups can be socially mediated within a virtual environment is embryonic. It is unclear whether the social aspects of cooperation, collaboration, motivation, and elaboration can be replicated when individuals are geographically distanced. It is known that 90% of undergraduate learners use virtual spaces like Facebook (King et al. 2009); this high proportion suggests that the online environment needs greater exploration.

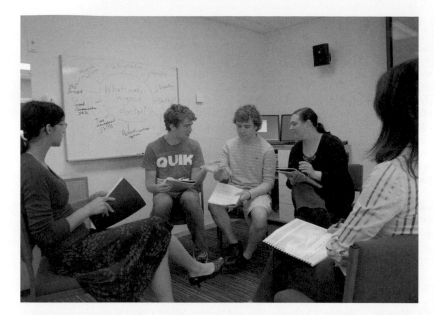

Figure 13.5 Small group learning in action.

Technology may be employed in an online environment or video conference. Video conferencing seems to be more intuitively aligned to the challenges presented by groups located apart. Further challenges may be how facilitation takes place across the medium and how to include all participants.

Evaluating small group learning

As with any interaction with learners, the formula of what went well and why, what could be improved, and how and what could be changed (Jones 2007) could be adopted. A tutor who evaluates small group function on a regular basis is seen by the learner as performing better than a tutor who does not (Dolmans et al. 2001a).

Various evaluation models can be used to frame evaluation of any intervention. Kirkpatrick's model of evaluation (Kirkpatrick 1975) outlines four levels: reaction, learning, behaviour, and results.

Much evaluation seems to concentrate on the first level where learners describe or rate their experience in small groups. Carefully constructed, this may give insights to whether the tutors are fulfilling the perceived aims of the small group philosophy. In focusing on the tutor's skills, other aspects may be ignored that potentially influence the success of the learning. The nature of the evaluation and questions asked can also be dictated by the nature of the outcomes expected (e.g. acquisition of clinical skills or cognitive gains).

The difficulty in applying Kirkpatrick's model is the onus on learning as an isolated event. There is a danger of simplifying learning in this way. Learning is an ongoing, formal and informal process, sometimes happening when we least expect. Unravelling learning and attributing it to one distilled factor can be fraught with difficulties and may yield irrelevant answers.

One area of small group evaluation that appears rather neglected is *how* constructing learning activity in small groups promotes the attainment of the outcomes. Does the activity require collaboration and preparation; does it allow opportunities for transformative learning; or the time to acquire basic clinical skills?

Conclusions

◆ Learning in small groups is an invaluable approach to enhance learning, being predicated on the social theory of learning and the importance of collaboration and cooperation.

◆ Many factors influence the successful attainment of outcomes of small group learning. These include the learners and how they interact, the tutor, the activity devised to structure the learning, the learning environment and the expected learning outcomes.

◆ Attention needs to be paid to ensure that the learners are fully engaged in the learning process, recognizing particularly how groups develop over time.

◆ The tutor must ensure that the outcomes are met and the group functions in a cohesive manner. However the learners also need to take responsibility for the effective functioning of their group.

References

Amin, Z., Tani, M., Eng, K.H., Samarasekara, D.D., and Huak, C.Y. (2009) Motivation, study habits, and expectations of medical students in Singapore. *Med Teach.* 31: e560–e569

Antil, L.R., Jenkins, J.R., Wayne, S.K., and Vadasy, P.F. (1998) Cooperative learning: prevalence, conceptualizations, and the relation between research and practice. *AmEduc Res J.* 35: 419–454

Antonio, A.L., Chang, M.J., Hakuta, K., Kenny, D.A., Levin, S., and Milem, J.F. (2004) Effects of racial diversity on complex thinking in college students. *Psychol Sci.* 15: 507–510

Arnheim, R. (1980) A plea for visual thinking. *Critical Inquiry.* 6: 489–497

Baddeley, A. (1998) Recent developments in working memory. *Curr Opin Neurobiol.* 8: 234–238

Bandura, A. (1977) *Social Learning Theory.* New York: General Learning Press

Beetham, H. and Sharpe, R. (2007) *Rethinking Pedagogy for a Digital Age: Designing and Delivering e-learning.* Abingdon: Routledge

Benware, C.A. and Deci, E.L. (1984) Quality of learning with an active versus passive motivational set. *Am Educ Res J.* 21: 755–765

Biggs, J. (1996) Enhancing teaching through constructive alignment. *Higher Educ.* 32: 347–364

Billings, l. and Fitzgerald, J. (2002) Dialogic discussion and the Paideia Seminar. *Am Educ Res J.* 39: 907–941

Birmingham, C. and McCord, M. (2004) Group process research: implications for using learning groups. In L.K. Michaelsen, A.B. Knight, and L.D. Fink (eds) *Team-based Learning: A Transformative Use of Small Groups in College Teaching* (pp. 73–93). Sterling, VA: Stylus Publishing

Bobby, Z., Koner, B.C., Sridhar, M.G., et al. (2007). Formulation of questions followed by small group discussion as a revision exercise at the end of a teaching module in biochemistry. *Biochem Molec Biol Educ.* 35: 45–48

Bogaard, A., Carey, S., and Dodd, G. (2005) Small group teaching: perceptions and problems. *Politics.* 25: 116–135

Bramesfield, K. and Gasper, K. (2008) Happily putting the pieces together: a test of two explanations for the effect of mood on group-level information processing. *Br J Soc Psychol.* 47: 285–309

Brodbeck, F.C., Guillaume, Y.R.F., and Lee, N.J. (2011) Ethnic diversity as a multilevel construct: the combined effects of dissimilarity, group diversity, and societal status on learning performance in work groups. *J Cross-Cultural Psychol.* 42: 1198–1218

Brookfield, S.D. and Preskill, S. (1999) *Discussion as a Way of Teaching.* Buckingham: Open University Press

Burchfield, C.M. and Sappington, T. (2000) Compliance with required reading assignments. *Teach Psychol.* 27: 58–60

Buxton, B. (2007) *The Anatomy of Sketching.* San Francisco, CA: Morgan Kaufmann

Cendan, J.C., Silver, M., and Ben-David, K. (2011) Changing the student clerkship from traditional lectures to small group case-based sessions benefits the student and the faculty. *J Surg Educ.* 68: 117–120

Chalkin, S. (ed.) (2003) *The Zone of Proximal Development in Vygotsky's Analysis of Learning Instruction.* Cambridge: Cambridge University Press

Chizmar, J. (2005) The effectiveness of assignments that utilize a time-efficient grading scheme. *J Excellence Coll Teach.* 16(1): 5–21

Chng, E., Yew, E.H.J., and Schmidt, H.G. (2011) Effects of tutor-related behaviours on the process of problem-based learning. *Adv Health Sci Educ.* 16: 491–503

Costa, M., Van Rensburg, L., and Rushton, N. (2007) Does teaching style matter? A randomised trial of group discussion versus lectures in orthopaedic undergraduate teaching. *Med Educ.* 41: 214–217

Cox, E.D., Schumacher, J.B., Young, H.N., Evans, M.D., Moreno, M.A., and Sigrest, T.D. (2011) Medical student outcomes after family-centered bedside rounds. *Acad Pediatr.* 11: 403–408

Craik, F.I. M. and Lockhart, R.S. (1972) Levels of processing—framework for memory research. *J Verbal Learning Verbal Behav.* 11: 671–684

Crosby, J. (1996) AMEE Medical Education Guide 8: Learning in small groups. *Med Teach.* 18: 189–202

Davis, W.K., Nairn, R., Paine, M.E., Anderson, R.M. and Oh, M.S. (1992) Effects of expert and nonexpert facilitators on the small-group process and on student performance. *Acad Med.* 67: 470–474

Davis, W.K, Oh. M.S., and Anderson, R.M. (1994) Influence of a highly focused case on the effect of small-group facilitators' content expertise on students' learning and satisfaction. *Acad Med.* 69(8): 663–669

De Grave, W.S., Dolmans, D., and van der Vleuten, C.P.M. (1999) Profiles of effective tutors in problem-based learning: scaffolding student learning. *Med Educ.* 33: 901–906

De Jong, Z., Van Nies, J.A.B., Peters, S.W.M., Vink, S., Dekker, F.W., and Scherpbier, A. (2010) Interactive seminars or small group tutorials in preclinical medical education: results of a randomized controlled trial. *BMC Med Educ.* 10 [Online] http://www.biomedcentral.com/1472-6920/10/79 Accessed 20 March 2013

Deci, E.L. and Ryan, R.M. (2000) The 'what' and 'why' of goal pursuits: Human needs and the self-determination of behavior. *Psychol Inquiry.* 11: 227–268

Devos, A. (2010) New teachers, mentoring and the discursive formation of professional identity. *Teach Teach Educ.* 26: 1219–1223

Dolmans, D., Wolfhagen, I., Scherpbier, A., and van der Vleuten, C.P.M. (2001a) Relationship of tutors' group-dynamics skills to their performance ratings in problem-based learning. *Acad Med.* 76: 473–476

Dolmans, D., Wolfhagen, I., and van der Vleuten, C.P.M. (1998) Motivational and cognitive processes influencing tutorial groups. *Acad Med.* 73: S22–S24

Dolmans, D., Wolfhagen, I., van der Vleuten, C.P.M., and Wijnen, W. (2001b) Solving problems with group work in problem-based learning: hold on to the philosophy. *Med Educ.* 35: 884–889

Dolmans, D. and Schmidt, H.G. (2006) What do we know about cognitive and motivational effects of small group tutorials in problem-based learning? *Adv Health Sci Educ.* 11: 321–336

Doucet, M.D., Purdy, R.A., Kaufman, D.M., and Langille, D.B. (1998) Comparison of problem-based learning and lecture format in continuing medical education on headache diagnosis and management. *Med Educ.* 32: 590–596

Du Boulay, C. and Medway, C. (1999) The clinical skills resource: a review of current practice. *Med Educ.* 33: 185–191

Edmunds, S. and Brown, G. (2010) Effective small group learning: AMEE Guide No. 48. *Med Teach.* 32: 715–726

Engle, R. and Conant, F. (2002) Guiding principles for fostering productive disciplinary engagement: explaining an emergent argument in a community of learners classroom. *Cognition Instruction.* 20: 399–483

Epstein, R.J. (2004) Learning from the problems of problem-based learning. *BMC Med Educ.* 4: 1

Fischer, R.L., Jacobs, S.L., and Herbert, W.N.P. (2004) Small-group discussion versus lecture format for third-year students in obstetrics and gynecology. *Obstet Gynecol.* 104: 349–353

Frenzel, A. C., Pekrun, R., and Goetz, T. (2007) Perceived learning environment and students' emotional experiences: A multilevel analysis of mathematics classrooms. *Learning Instruction.,* 17: 478–493

Gill, E., Tuck, A., Lee, D., and Beckert, L. (2004) Tutorial dynamics and participation in small groups: a student perspective in a multicultural setting. *N Z Med J.* 117(1205) [Online] http://journal.nzma.org.nz/journal/117-1205/1142/ Accessed 20 March 2013

Gillies, R. (2004) The effects of cooperative learning on junior high school students during small group learning. *Learn Instruct.* 14(2): 197–213

Grant, D.J. and Marriage, S.C. (2012) Training using medical simulation. *Arch Dis Childh.* 97: 255–259

Gravett, S. (2004) Action research and transformative learning in teaching development. *Educ Action Res.* 12: 259–272

Harden, R.M., Davis, M.H., and Crosby, J.R. (1997) The new Dundee medical curriculum: a whole that is greater than the sum of the parts. *Med Educ.* 31: 264–271

Harland, T. (2003) Vyotsky's zone of proximal development and problem based learning: Linking a theoretical concept with practice through action research. *Teach Higher Educ.* 8: 263–272

Hesselgreaves, H. and MacVicar, R. (2012) Practice-based small group learning in GP specialty training. *Educ Primary Care.* 23: 27–33

Hitchcock, M.A. and Mylona, Z.H. (2000) Teaching faculty to conduct problem-based learning. *Teaching Learning Med.* 12: 52–57

Jacques, D. (2000) *Learning in Groups.* New York: Kogan Page

Johnson, D.W., Johnson, R.T., and Smith, K. (2007) The state of cooperative learning in postsecondary and professional settings. *Educ Psychol Rev.* 19: 15–29

Jones, R.W. (2007) Learning and teaching in small groups: characteristics, benefits, problems and approaches. *Anaesth Intensive Care.* 35: 587–592

Karau, S.J. and Williams, K.D. (1995) Social loafing—research findings, implications, and future-directions. *Curr Directions Psychol Sci.* 4: 134–140

Karp, D.A. and Yoels, W.C. (1976). College classroom—some observations on meanings of student participation. *Sociol Soc Res.* 60: 421–439

King, I., Jiexing, L., and Kam Tong, C. (2009) A brief survey of computational approaches in social computing. In: *Proceedings 2009 International Joint Conference on Neural Networks* (IJCNN 2009—Atlanta).

Kirkpatrick, D. (1975) Techniques for evaluating training programs. In D. Kirkpatrick (ed.) *Evaluating Training Programs—A Collection of Articles from the Journal of the American Society for Training and Development* (pp. 119–142). Alexandria, VA: ASTD

Kneebone, R.L., Scott, W., Darzi, A., and Horrocks, M. (2004) Simulation and clinical practice: strengthening the relationship. *Med Educ.* 38: 1095–1102

Kroenke, K., Omori, D.M., Landry, F.J., and Lucey, C.R. (1997) Bedside teaching. *S Med J.* 90: 1069–1074

Lave, J. and Wenger, E. (1990) *Situated Learning: Legitimate Peripheral Participation.* Cambridge, UK: Cambridge University Press

Lingard, L., Reznick, R., Devito, I., and Espin, S. (2002) Forming professional identities on the health care team: discursive constructions of the 'other' in the operating room. *Med Educ.* 36: 728–734

Linnenbrink-Garcia, L., Rogat, T.K., and Koskey, K.L.K. (2011) Affect and engagement during small group instruction. *Contemp Educ Psychol.* 36: 13–24

Lipp, A. and Holmes, A. (2009) Facilitating small group learning in the operating department. *J Periop Pract.* 19: 148–152

Martin, A., Burra, P., Martines, D., Sturniolo, G.C., and Naccarato, R. (1988) Educational value of small-group work and lectures on changing medical students attitudes towards alcoholism. *Ital J Gastroenterol.* 20: 21–23

Merriman H. (2003) Clinical governance for primary care teams: how useful is a learning set for individuals from different teams? *Educ Prim Care.* 14: 189–201

Mezirow, J. (1995) Transformation theory of adult learning. In M.R. Welton (ed.) *Defense of the Lifeworld* (pp. 158–172). New York: SUNY Press

Myers, S., Bogdan, L., Eidsness, M., et al. (2009) Taking a trait approach to understanding college students' perception of group work. *Coll Student J.* 43: 822–831

Myrick, F. and Yonge, O. (2002) Preceptor questioning and student critical thinking. *J Profess Nursing.* 18: 176–181

Norman, GR. and Schmidt, HG. (1992) The psychological basis of PBL. A review of the evidence. *Acad Med.* 67: 557–565

O'Donnell, A. (ed.) (2006) *The Role of Peers and Group Learning.* Mahaw, NJ: Lawrence Elbraum Associates

O'Donnell, A., Dansereau, D.F., Rocklin, T.R., et al. (1985) Effects of elaboration frequency on cooperative learning. *J Educ Psychol.* 77: 572–580

Oakley, B.A., Hanna, D.M., Kuzmyn, Z., and Felder, R.M. (2007) Best practices involving teamwork in the classroom: Results from a survey of 6435 engineering, student respondents. *IEEE Trans Educ* 50: 266–272

Peets, A.D., Cooke, L., Wright, B., Coderre, S., and McLaughlin, K. (2010) A prospective randomized trial of content expertise versus process expertise in small group teaching. *BMC Med Educ.* 10

Perez, D., Rudland, J.R., Wilson, H., Roberton, G., Gerrard, D., and Wheatley, A. (2009) The revised 'Early Learning in Medicine' curriculum at the University of Otago—focusing on students, patients, and community. *N Z Med J.* 122: 61–70

Peters, A.S., Greenberger-Rosovsky, R., Crowder, C., Block, S.D., and Moore, G.T. (2000) Long-term outcomes of the new pathway program at Harvard medical school: A randomized controlled trial. *Acad Med.* 75: 470–479

Profetto-McGarth, J.B., Smith, K., Day, R.A., and Yonge, O. (2004) The questioning skills of tutors and students in a context based baccalaureate nursing program. *Nurse Educ Today.* 24: 363–372

Reder, L.M. (1980) The role of elaboration in the comprehension and retention of prose—a critical review. *Rev Educ Res.* 50: 5–53

Regehr, G., Martin, J., Hutchison, C., Murnaghan, J., Cusimano, M., and Reznick, M. (1995) The effect of tutors' content expertise on student learning, group process, and participant satisfaction in a problem-based learning curriculum. *Teach Learning Med.* 7: 225–232

Reid, A., Dahlgren, L.O., Petocz, P., and Dahlgren, M.A. (2008) Identity and engagement for professional formation. *Studies Higher Educ.* 33: 729–742

Renkl, A. (1995) Learning mathematics from worked-out examples: Analyzing and fostering self-explanations. *EurJ Psychol Educ.* 14: 477–488

Richardson, J., West, M.A., and Cuthbertson, B.H. (2010) Team working in intensive care: current evidence and future endeavors. *Curr Opin Crit Care.* 16: 643–648

Roseth, C.J., Johnson, D.W., and Johnson, R.T. (2008) Promoting early adolescents' achievement and peer relationships: The effects of cooperative, competitive, and individualistic goal structures. *Psychol Bull.* 134: 223–246

Sacks, H., Schegloff, E.A., and Jefferson, G. (1974) A simplest systematics for the organization of turn-taking for conversation. *Language.* 50: 696–735

Saran, A. (2005) *Environmental Psychology.* Delhi: Anmol Publications

Schmidt, H.G. (1993) Foundations of problem-based learning—some explanatory notes. *Med Educ.* 27: 422–432

Schmidt, H.G., van der Arend, A., Moust, J.H.C., Kokx, I., and Boon, L. (1993) Influence of tutors subject-matter expertise on student effort and achievement in problem-based learning. *Acad Med.* 68: 784–791

Shuell, T. J. (1986) Cognitive conceptions of learning. *Rev Educ Res.* 56: 411–436

Silver, M. and Wilkerson, L.A. (1991) Effects of tutors with subject expertise on the problem-based tutorial process. *Acad Med.* 66: 298–300

Slavin, R. (1996). Research on cooperative learning and achievement: what we know, what we need to know. *Contemp Educ Psychol.* 21: 49–36

Springer, L., Stanne, M.E., and Donovan, S.S. (1999) Effects of small-group learning on undergraduates in science, mathematics, engineering, and technology: a meta-analysis. *Rev Educ Res.* 69: 21–51

Steinert, Y. (1993) 12 tips for using role-plays in clinical teaching. *Med Teach.* 15: 283–291 Steinert, Y. (2004) Student perceptions of effective small group teaching. *Med Educ.* 38: 286–293

Steinert, Y., Mann, K., Centeno, A., et al. (2006) A systematic review of faculty development initiatives designed to improve teaching effectiveness in medical education: BEME Guide No. 8. *Med Teach.* 28: 497–526

Stiefelhagen, R. and Zhu, J. (2002) Head orientation and gaze direction in meetings. In: CHI EA '02 CHI '02 *Extended Abstracts on Human Factors in Computing Systems* (pp. 858–859). New York, NY: ACM

Sweet, M. and Michaelsen, L.K. (2007) How group dynamics research can inform the theory and practice of postsecondary small group learning. *Educ Psychol Rev.* 19: 31–47

Torosyan, R. (2007) *Teaching for Transformation: Integrative Learning, Consciousness Development and Critical Reflection.* Unpublished manuscript. Columbia University, New York

Tuckman, B.W. (1965) Developmental sequence in small groups. *Psychol Bull.* (63)6: 384–399

Tuckman, B.W. and Jensen, M.C. (1977) Stages of small-group development revisited. *Group Organization Management.* 2: 419

Vallerand, R.J. and Ratelle, C.F. (2002) Intrinsic and extrinsic motivation: a hierarchical model. In R.M. Ryanand E.L. Deci (eds) *Handbook of Self-determination Research* (pp. 37–63). Rochester, New York: University of Rochester Press

Van Blankenstein, F.M., Dolmans, D.H.J.M., van der Vleuten, C.P.M., and Schmidt, H.G. (2011) Which cognitive processes support learning during small-group discussion? The role of providing explanations and listening to others. *Instructional Sci.* 39: 189–204

Van Knippenberg, D. and Schippers, M.C. (2007) Work group diversity. *Ann Rev Psychol.* 58: 515–541

Vygotsky, L. (1987) *The Collected Works of LS Vygotsky. Vol 4. The History of the Development of Higher Mental Function.* New York: Plenum Press

Walton, H. (1997) Small group methods in medical teaching. *Med Educ.* 31: 459–464

Wayne, N.L., Vermillion, M., and Uijtdehaage, S. (2010) Gender differences in leadership amongst first-year medical students in the small-group setting. *Acad Med.* 85: 1276–1281

Wenger, E. (2000) Communities of practice and social learning systems. *Organization.* 7: 225–246

Wenger, E. (2006) Communities of practice, a brief introduction. http://www.ewenger.com/theory/ Accessed 22 February 2013

West, E. (1976) *201 Icebreakers: Group Mixers, Warm-Ups, Energizers and Playful Activities.* New York, NY: McGraw-Hill

Wheelan, S. (2004) *Group Processes: A Developmental Perspective.* Boston: Allyn and Bacon

Wheelan, S.A. and Lisk, A.R. (2000) Cohort group effectiveness and the educational achievement of adult undergraduate students. *Small Group Research.* 31: 724–738

Wiessner, C.A. and Mezirow, J. (2000) Theory building and the search for common ground. In J. Mezirow (ed.) *Learning as Transformation* (pp. 329–358). San Francisco: Jossey-Bass

Wilkinson, T.J., Wells, J.E., and Bushnell, J.A. (2004). Are differences between graduates and undergraduates in a medical course due to age or prior degree? *Med Educ.* 38: 1141–1146

Williams, K.D. (2010) Dyads can be groups (and often are). *Small Group Research*. 41: 268–274

Williams, K.D., Nida, S.A., Baca, L.D., and Latane, B. (1989) Social loafing and swimming—effects of identifiability on individual and relay performance of intercollegiate swimmers. *Basic Appl Soc Psychol*. 10: 73–81

Williams, K.N., Ramani, S., Fraser, B., and Orlander, J.D. (2008) Improving bedside teaching: findings from a focus group study of learners. *Acad Med*. 83: 257–264

Wood, D. (2003) ABC of learning and teaching in medicine. *BMJ*. 326: 328–330

Woodman, T., Roberts, R., Hardy, L., Callow, N., and Rogers, C.H. (2011) There is an 'I' in TEAM: narcissism and social loafing. *Res Q Exerc Sport*. 82: 285–290

CHAPTER 14

Large group teaching

Janet Tworek, Rachel Ellaway, and Tim Dornan

People have nowadays... got a strange opinion that everything should be taught by lectures. Now, I cannot see that lectures can do so much good as reading the books from which the lectures are taken. Lectures were once useful; but now, when we can all read, and books are so numerous, lectures are unnecessary.

Samuel Johnson
(Boswell 1791)

Introduction

Large group teaching is one of the most common and least well-regarded forms of contemporary medical education practice. The lecture is the archetypal form of large group teaching and much has been written on how to lecture in general (e.g. Aarabi 2007; Exley and Dennick 2004; Race 2001), how to lecture in medical education (Brown and Manogue 2001; Long and Lock 2010), and in particular, how to overcome the problems of lecturing (Matheson 2008). Despite all this attention, most authors consider no more than one or two components of the complex educational method that makes up large group teaching. Recognizing the potential complexity of this topic we have reviewed historical, cultural, and organizational aspects of large group teaching in medical education as well its behavioural and cognitive dimensions. This chapter presents a multidimensional analysis of the activities that make up large group teaching in the health professions, their uses and impacts, and their interactions with the sociocultural contexts in which they take place.

How large is 'large'?

For the purposes of this chapter, we will define a large group as involving more learners than can engage meaningfully in educational activities that need smaller groups such as problem-based and simulation-based learning. In practice, a large group can be defined for teaching purposes as having 15 participants or more. Defining a higher threshold is a little more complex. The primary underlying reason for teaching large groups would seem to be one of efficiency. It is tacitly assumed that material can be more efficiently covered by presenting it to a whole class in a single session, than to smaller groups in several sessions. The size of the large group is therefore linked to the class size, which may be a whole academic year (particularly in preclinical stages) or a cohort within a year such as a

group of clerks on a particular clinical rotation. The maximum size of medical classes is typically limited by the number of clerkships a school can provide. Courses that do not have an experiential component are less restricted in the size of their classes, especially if they take place online. The larger the group, however, the less the opportunity for individuals to interact with the lecturer; the upper boundary for large group teaching can therefore be defined as the point at which the opportunity to interact becomes too diffused.

The lecture

The lecture is such an ancient form of teaching it could be viewed as the *ur-form* of organized education. The lecture has long been institutionalized as the primary form by which a structured and definitive body of knowledge is imparted to large groups of learners, growing as it did from the practices of teachers in medieval universities who summarized, read, and critiqued canonical texts for their students' edification (Haskins 1957).

Two texts stand out in the appraisal and critique of lecturing as a generic higher educational practice in the modern age. McLeish's (1968) meta-analysis was grounded in broader academic discourses around knowledge, cognition, and the social construction of the lecture. Bligh's (1971) monograph was both a meta-analysis and a commentary on earlier meta-analyses that compared the effectiveness of lecturing with other instructional methods. Both authors criticized the research available to them for its confounding factors and its artificiality. McLeish (1968) also linked modern practice to traditions where the lecturer was the only available source of knowledge on a given subject, and linked the then growing dissatisfaction with the lecture with broader sociocultural changes in higher education demographics and practice. McLeish identified the primary function of lectures as inspiring students rather than transferring knowledge, that short-term retention of lecture material was limited, while long-term retention was virtually impossible to test, and that there are critical differences between lecturing as a system of education and lecturing as an educational method. Although he did not use the term, McLeish noted a co-creating relationship between a 'hidden curriculum' of lecturing and the episteme of the material being taught.

Bligh (1971) saw lectures as best suited to knowledge acquisition but far less suited to stimulating thinking or changing attitudes. He emphasized that lectures alone could not provide a well-rounded educational experience, and they therefore needed to be combined with other activities. Bligh also noted a number of procedural issues around lecturing, including a three-phase sequence of activities: planning, presentation, and follow up.

Building on the foundations laid by McLeish and Bligh, we identified seven key themes around which contemporary lecturing and other forms of large group teaching can be understood:

1. *Large group teaching involves interacting with learners' cognitive states*: there are conflicting opinions as to whether lectures should be primarily about knowledge transfer or other cognitive benefits such as motivating learners or summarizing topics and themes.

2. *Large group teaching involves a sequence of distinct activities*: Planning and preparing the presentation, delivering or performing the presentation, and follow-up.

3. *Large group teaching involves participating in the discourse of a particular domain*: Lectures function both as narratives and meta-narratives on the material being taught.

4. *Large group teaching is both an educational method and a systematic approach to program delivery*: Educational methods, such as lectures, that are relatively inefficient at transmitting information are still widely used for that purpose in programmes that define their curricula in terms of lectures.

5. *Large group teaching is constructed by the affordances of available technologies*: Lectures are both enabled and constrained by the physical and technical capabilities of the spaces in which they take place and of the participants they involve.

6. *Large group teaching is constructed by the affordances of the educational ecologies in which it takes place*: Large group teaching is also defined by learning objectives, other educational activities, and the milieu of the curricula and programmes in which they take place.

7. *Large group teaching involves a broad range of activities*: Large group teaching can involve a lot more than didactic presentations, particularly when using online technologies to extend the range and temporality of participants' involvement.

Reviewing the literature

In order to ground these themes in evidence, we searched the ERIC, EMBASE, EBSCOHost, and PsychInfo databases using the keywords 'large group teaching', 'lecture', and 'large group learning'. We aggregated the results of the searches and eliminated duplicates. This search identified 1193 papers published between 2002 and 2011. These were then reviewed by title and abstract to identify potentially informative empirical research that had been conducted in the context of health professional education. All articles were retrieved in full text and reviewed. Articles were included in the evidence synthesis only if they fulfilled all of the following criteria:

◆ Fifteen or more participants physically located in a single physical space with a nominated individual (lecturer) leading the event

◆ Empirical research conducted within a vocational programme of health professions education

◆ Single events or programmes of events where the context and intervention were sufficiently well described to inform the review

◆ Findings judged 3 or higher on the Best Evidence Medical Education (BEME) 1–5 scale for 'strength' as judged in relation to the purposes of this review (http://www.bemecollaboration.org/; Yardley and Dornan 2012). The points on the scale are anchored as follows: 1 = 'no clear conclusions can be drawn', 2 = 'results are ambiguous', 3 = 'conclusions can probably be based on the results', 4 = 'results are very likely to be true', 5 = 'results are unequivocal'.

The evidence synthesis followed realist principles, as described by Wong et al. (2012). The seven themes set out in the previous section were used as a programme theory of how large group teaching works, for whom, and under what conditions. The contents of the papers were coded to an analytical framework, which expanded the programme theory into 17 free-text coding fields. Finally, the coders identified trustworthy (using the BEME strength scale) causal links between one or more conditions or processes, and outcomes. Because the purpose of the review was to explore how lectures could be given most effectively, experimental research that compared lectures with other instructional designs (most of which treated 'traditional lectures', which had not been optimized, as the control condition for a novel intervention), or experiments that gave no information about the conditions and processes that went on within lectures, were excluded from analysis. This review identified 26 publications, which are cited in the following discursive analysis of large group teaching in medical education.

Large group teaching and cognition

Lectures have long been criticized in research publications and the general discourse of medical education. Brown and Edmunds (2009), for instance, recognized that many lecturers failed to succinctly review complex material, motivate learners, and stimulate reflection because they provided no more than standard texts, kept learners passive, and relied overmuch on their authority to manage the educational event. Powell (1970, p. 199) observed that lectures could help learners to acquire knowledge, but not to foster their higher-level cognitive processes:

> the lecture is the best technique we have for passing on factual information, but…it is much less suited to the development of high-level intellectual skills and attitudes.

Other authors have taken different positions. For instance, lecturers can show learners how to organize their thoughts in general or around a specific topic (McKeachie 2006); MacNeil (2007) for example, showed how learners' concept maps could be enriched by lectures.

Ambrose et al. (2010) synthesized a large body of research and showed the importance of making the organization of lectures explicit to learners, making clear connections between concepts, using contrasting and boundary cases, and getting learners to map out and share their understanding of the subject matter presented to them. Kessler et al. (2011) noted the need for lecturers to work from a strong understanding of the material they were presenting and to be confident and enthusiastic in their approach. Copeland and colleagues (2000) noted effective lecturers were 'engaging'. Cosgrove et al. (2006) showed how simple visual imagery could make physiology more comprehensible and increase learners' interest, motivation, and knowledge. Gülpinar and Yegen (2005) designed a lecture using cognitive principles to optimize learning, including using a template of the material being taught, segmenting, and sequencing the material, and periodically stopping to reinforce messages and allow learners to integrate what they had encountered.

Ensuring that learners are learning what the lecturer had intended is another recurring issue. Several studies have found that learners' lecture notes do align well with lecturers' expectations (Hartley and Cameron 1967; Kiewra 1985; Kiewra et al. 1988, 1991). This is not just a matter of direct transfer but also one of social compliance. Cavenagh (2011) showed how learners adapt and normalize their learning approach to the environments in which they find themselves, learning only what they are directed to engage with, thereby diffusing the role of the lecturer as the ultimate arbiter of what constitutes good learning.

In summary, large group teaching can afford a range of cognitive benefits including knowledge transfer, synthesis of existing knowledge, and affective aspects such as motivation. The extent to which these benefits are realized, however, depends on other factors.

Large group teaching as activity

Educational events such as lectures are rarely a single unitary activity but rather constructs of multiple interconnected activities (Ellaway et al. 2005). Large group teaching can generally be considered as having at least three distinct phases: planning and preparation; the execution of the event itself; and follow-up (see fig. 14.1).

Preparation

The preparation of a large group teaching event involves many factors. Some of these are logistical or curricular in nature, such as the allocated time, the capabilities of the allocated room, and the learning objectives to be attained. Others, such as the learners' previous experiences, the nature of the subject matter and how it relates to the curriculum as a whole are more pedagogical. The lecturer must understand and be able to apply pedagogical principles to ensure that the event and their learners' experiences be consistent with the content, epistemology, and the professional context of the programme as well as the practical organization of their lecture.

Kessler et al. (2011) showed that exemplary lecturers prepared their presentations by: mastering the subject matter on which they planned to speak; defining clear objectives; being clear about the scope of the presentation; using novel elements and case-based examples to increase interest and applicability; and, by thoroughly rehearsing their presentations ahead of time.

Brown and Manogue (2001) identified various ways of organizing lecture material including: 'classical' (proceeding from broad concepts to increasing detail); 'problem-centred'; 'sequential reasoning'; 'comparative' (two or more contrasting perspectives); and 'thesis' (presenting a particular perspective then proving or disproving it). Hartley and Cameron (1967) recommended accommodating learners' limited attention spans by breaking lectures

into sections, changing pace, style and presentation method within them, interjecting questions and so on. Responding to learner needs may also involve extending activity beyond the traditional bounds of a lecture. Johnson and Mighten (2005), for example, provided nursing students with comprehensive notes before a lecture and then used the lecture to discuss the material. van Dijk et al. (2001) posted scenarios in advance and invited students to choose appropriate laboratory tests. Canfield (2002) posted questions, which were discussed when the class met and Richardson (2011) sent questions by text message to students' phones.

Technologies have also had a significant influence on the preparation of large group teaching. The widespread use of computer-generated slides (in particular Microsoft's near-ubiquitous PowerPoint) has collapsed the design of the lecture as a whole and the design of the materials used within them into a single activity. It is even arguable that the ability to prepare lecture slides has become a proxy for being ready to teach from them and in doing so it has perhaps changed teachers' ideas about what it means to lecture. For instance, many lecturers now post their slides online for learners to access in lieu of preparing handouts. Technical planning is not just about the creation of slides as it is about making sure that the various technical resources needed to present them are in place and working properly—this has become another task that lecturers must accommodate in their planning (Mishra and Koehler 2006).

Presentation

There have been many studies on the lecture as a performance (Brown et al. 1984; Brown and Manogue 2001; Harden and Crosby 2000; Matheson 2008). Presentation skills, particularly good pacing and time management, are of paramount importance (McKeachie 2006). There are a number of strategies that can be used to engage learners more effectively including grabbing an audience's attention (Kessler, et al. 2011), using an appropriate narrative style and a clear voice with variation in annunciation (Visioli et al. 2009), and displaying enthusiasm, passion, humour, confidence, and humility throughout the presentation (Kessler et al. 2011; Melamed et al. 2006). Lectures also benefit from having clear goals, keeping subject matter appropriate to the objectives, and encouraging learners' independent thinking (Melamed et al. 2006). Yet another strategy is to pause or change methods every 8-15 minutes (Cain et al. 2009; Gulpinar and Yegen 2005) so as to allow learners to reflect on what has been said, and take notes.

Not only do teachers need to be trained to be lecturers, learners also need to be well-prepared to make good use of the lecture format. Some preparation is practical in terms of completing pre-lecture reading or activity and coming equipped to take notes. Some preparation is more strategic; including deciding how active or passive they will be during the event, or indeed whether it is in their best interests to attend at all. Westrick et al. (2009) found students chose to attend lectures when they wanted to take their own notes and needed help in mastering what they considered to be difficult course material. Lecturers' attributes, such as being known to care about students and being good at highlighting important content, also influenced learner decisions on whether or not they should attend a lecture.

We found evidence of many ways lecturers could increase learner participation during the event, including asking learners to answer questions, find information, or read material before the event (Canfield 2002; Gulpinar and Yegen 2005; Johnson 2005; Van Dijken et al. 2008). Audience response systems have been used to foster group cohesion (Cain et al. 2009), explore differences in perspective between students from different disciplines (Williams et al. 2011), as well as sometimes just providing an alternative to learners raising their hands (Liu et al. 2010).

There are many ways to make didactic learning more active. Video accompanied by spoken commentary may encourage learners to relate material to their real life experiences (Bye 2009). Splitting the lecturer role into two, using a content expert and a discussant of the content expert's presentation, could provide a clear presentation of content along with a secondary voice for critical appraisal of the subject matter (Ochsendorf et al. 2006). Student participation can be made more active, for example by having students volunteer as clinicians and family members, as a previously unannounced simulation event unfolds in the lecture theatre, where learners jointly manage the patient (Fitch 2007). Introducing team-based learning to what had been previously been a particularly didactic lecture can foster greater dialogue and improved knowledge acquisition amongst learners (Thomas and Bowen 2011). Not only can such events make large group events more interactive, they can also transfer a certain amount of control and responsibility to learners. However, learner autonomy is not always welcome. In one study, a quarter of the students did not favour moving away from teacher-centred to learner-centred modalities (Canfield 2002). Despite the many ways large group teaching can be enhanced, it may still not meet the needs of all learners; indeed, another study found a significant proportion of learners did not want to attend large group events at all (Westrick 2009). The value of attendance or non-attendance is still under debate.

Follow up

Follow up, like preparation and performance, requires different participants to do different things. Lecturers review learner evaluations to improve subsequent iterations of their lectures although student satisfaction ratings may be limited in their ability to provide useful information for quality improvement (Bligh 1971). Furthermore, large group teaching may be linked to other teaching events, such as problem-based learning (which may depend on lectures having covered key concepts), clinical skills training, or bedside teaching. The lecture may therefore be evaluated as a part of a system of interlinked events rather than as a standalone event.

Learners provide the evaluations on their experiences and consolidate and exchange what they have learned and apply it as part of their developing practice. They will also be assessed on the material at some point. Assessment is clearly a follow-up activity, but is usually displaced in time, typically to the end of a module, course, or semester, and aggregated with the evaluations of other lectures and teaching events. It is often hard, therefore, to gauge the long-term impact of a single large group teaching event. Most experimental studies, therefore, only evaluate short-term retention (Kao 1976).

Variations on large group teaching activities

The traditional lecture can be enhanced in many ways. Some hybrid variations on large and small group teaching have been developed, such as team-based learning (Hills 2001; Michaelsen et al. 2008) where large groups divide into smaller groups for collaborative activities before coming back together as a larger group. Various studies have shown beneficial effects on learning from such mixed group size methods (Antepohl and Herzig 1999; Doucet et al. 1998; Nandi et al. 2000; Smits et al. 2010), while others have been less conclusive (Norman and Schmidt 1992).

Large group teaching can have many components with many different interactions. The ability to map out these designs indicating who does what, in what order, and in what contexts is an important part of appraising them individually and collectively. 'Use cases' or sequence diagrams (Ellaway 2008), which are routinely used in designing computer software, can fulfil that function. Figure 14.1 is a simple sequence diagram showing the roles played by teachers and learners at different phases. Figure 14.2 shows how that approach can be expanded to represent some of the other components we have described. Variations on the basic lecture pattern can also be illustrated; for example, fig. 14.3 shows a variation where a didactic component is separated from the discursive component.

In summary, there are many potential ways of organizing large group teaching events. Different activities can be described using mapping techniques to provide a common notation to compare different designs and to identify differences between apparently similar learning designs that might be otherwise overlooked.

Large group teaching as discourse

An often-overlooked function of lectures is the way they allow learners to 'participate in the discourse' of a particular domain (Northedge and MacArthur 2009). The language, values, and attitudes of a discipline can constitute the 'discursive repertoires' (Trowler 2009) through which disciplines understand and reproduce themselves. Murphy (2007, pp. 9–16) saw such engagement in disciplinary discourse as ensuring the relevance of the material being presented and sustaining learners' motivation. Lectures therefore have an essential role to play in the early stages of medical education in inducting learners to these discursive repertoires as well as at key points in learners' subsequent professional development when cultural orientation to new professional contexts is required.

Disciplinary discourses are defined by the ways in which they diverge from each other. Large group teaching would therefore be

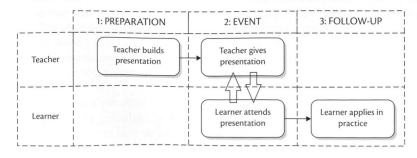

Figure 14.1 A basic three-phase, two-participant model of large group teaching. Teachers prepare presentations on their own, present them to their learners, and these learners then make use of what was presented.

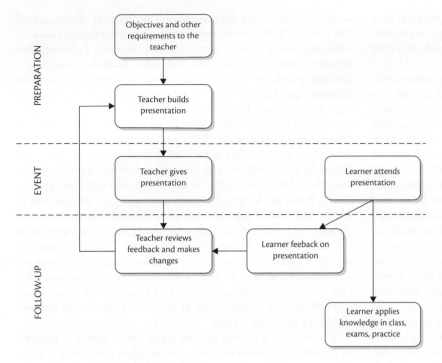

Figure 14.2 Extended three-phase, two-participant model of large group teaching. The teacher prepares their presentation based on curriculum objectives and prior experience and then presents to learners, who make use of what they have heard and give feedback on the lecture performance, which allows the lecturer to refine their presentation.

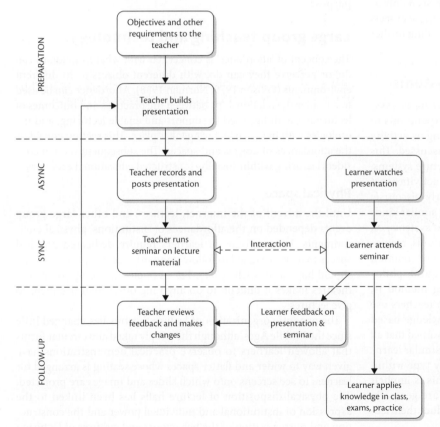

Figure 14.3 Sequence diagram of the 'inverted lecture' or 'flipped classroom' large group teaching activity design. The teacher prepares a presentation based on curriculum objectives and prior experience and records it. Learners watch the recorded presentation in their own time (asynchronously with other learners). Lecturer and learners come together for an interactive seminar on the material presented (synchronous). Learners use what they have learned, feed back on the lecture, and the lecturer changes their presentation.

expected to differ according to the philosophies and approaches of the presenters' disciplinary culture. A teacher's disciplinary perspective may be as important as what they are teaching. For example, one study found that basic science lectures concentrated on the structure and clarity of factual content while illustrative narratives

and insights dominated lectures in the social sciences (Brown and Manogue 2001). Disciplinary discourses may go further than the boundaries of specific academic disciplines to include patient perspectives. Balandin and Hines (2011, pp. 436–445) described lectures given by people with disabilities to students in a speech and language pathology program. These 'expert patient' lecturers were able to function as both the medium and the message of the presentation which in turn was reported as having a more enduring impact on the audience.

Engagement with disciplinary discourses may also extend beyond the lecture event. Rong et al. (2011, p. 36) described how a lecture on depression was augmented with a self-directed learning intervention, in which students conducted research, organized a half-day advocacy event, and used their creative and artistic talents to express understanding of life with depression. Tulsky et al. (2011, pp. 593–601) reinforced a discourse of empathic caring by augmenting a lecture with video clips of physicians' communication behaviours. Learners' observed communication behaviours improved as a result—which had a positive impact on patients' health. Williams et al. (2011, pp. 337–350) used an audience response system to engage students of various health professions into an interprofessional curriculum discourse while Ventura and Onsman (2009, pp. 662–664) used video clips from popular movies to form a link with societal discourses around diseases illustrated in them.

In summary, large group teaching can function as a narrative on a particular subject, a meta-narrative on disciplinary discourses about the subject, and a meta-meta-narrative on how that discourse is constructed and renewed. That these higher functions go largely unnoticed may explain why lectures are often seen only as a medium for knowledge transfer. Whether making these aspects more explicit can improve learning is another area needing further exploration.

Lecturing methods and lecturing systems

A dialectic between lecturing as a method and lecturing as a system has been observed (McLeish 1968). We can expand this to three levels: activity, method, and system. Lecturing as activity (what participants actually do) has already been discussed. This section therefore considers lecture methods and lecture systems. Educational methods are 'collections of educational activities that share common attributes' that emerge from scholarly discourse, often as shorthand ways of identifying and grouping similar kinds of educational activities (Ellaway 2012) Educational systems, on the other hand, are 'functional organizations of methods, regulations, resources and participants around the pursuit of common goals' (Ellaway 2012) embodying common procedural, philosophical, and political perspectives. The lecturing method is, therefore, that set of educational activities in which teachers use didactic techniques to present predominantly knowledge-based material to large groups of learners. It is generally assumed that all activities within an educational method will afford similar learning experiences and outcomes and that one activity type within a method should be substitutable for any other. This is implicit in the case of lecturing as a method, as lecturers are generally afforded significant autonomy to organize and conduct their lectures as they will.

Considering lecture systems provides a lens to analyse how lecturing is constructed within broader medical education contexts. For instance, lecturing as a system is typically based around assumptions that faculty are the primary and largely autonomous designers and presenters of lectures. This can be somewhat self-reinforcing as lecturers can gain considerable security from teaching something they have predefined and which they alone control (McKeachie 2006). However, lecturing as a system is not only about increasing lecturer autonomy and authority. Lecturing also appeals to academic managers in times of budgetary constraint, increasing student numbers, and other administrative stressors (Spencer and Pearson 2010). Lecturing may, therefore, be serving other interests. Indeed, the lecture has been characterized by some as an imposed rather than an educationally driven format (Hogan and Kwiatkowski 1998). Lecturing may be described as a recurrent practice that is 'habitual and unconsidered' and reinforced by promotion criteria and social conventions rather than something deliberately selected for its desirable qualities (Trowler 2009). While the lecture system is taken to be an efficient use of faculty and student time (Brown and Belfield 2002), there may be cheaper but less effective modes (textbooks only) and more costly but more effective modes (personal tuition). Lecturing seems to occupy a perceived 'sweet spot' where cost and effectiveness are well balanced, at least in many contemporary programmes. That cost is an administrative concern and effectiveness an academic one reflects the intertwining of different educational cultures within the lecturing system.

In summary, a lecture system, perspective makes it possible to unpack the reasons why lectures, which are relatively ineffective for transferring knowledge, are still so widely used for that purpose.

Large group teaching and technology

The concept of 'affordance' is concerned with what individuals can do, or perceive they can do, with different objects or in different environments (Gibson 1979; Norman 1988). Affordance can be used to consider the relationships between the practices and outcomes of lecturing, the things used to support and enable lecturing, and the ecologies with in which lecturing takes place. This section considers the affordances of objects and spaces. The subsequent section considers lecturing within socially-constructed educational ecologies.

Physical space

Until the advent of the internet, lectures, and other large group events depended on the affordances of institutions' physical environments. Large groups of learners require dedicated physical spaces that are designed to follow standard preconceptions of what should happen in such spaces. For example, the design of lecture theatres makes it difficult to do anything other than use them to give lectures.

The panoptic organization of lecture theatres has changed little since the Middle Ages, although the steeply raked and circular forms that allowed learners to observe practical demonstrations have given way to wider and flatter spaces whose seating is arranged for learners to see screens onto which slides and images are projected. The physical disposition of lecture halls has been linked to the expression of institutional and individual power and the construction and normalization of the behaviours and cultures of lecturing (Bourdieu et al. 1994). Even when teachers wish to cede aspects of their control to students for group interaction, the physical spaces they have available to them limit how far such deviation from the standard lecture format can be supported. Some medical schools have recognized these limitations and have changed the traditional physical model to accommodate other kinds of educational activity.

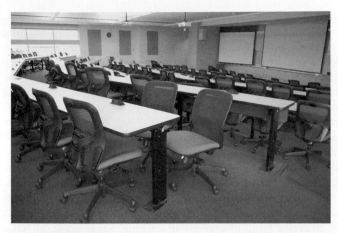

Figure 14.4 Lecture theatre at the University of Colorado School of Medicine. Each row of seating is comprised of two long sets of tables. The chairs are on casters that students may reorganize into smaller groupings as the learning scenario requires.

Queen's University in Canada and University of Colorado School of Medicine in the United States, for example, installed two rows of 360-degree rotating chairs and tables per tier to give students the flexibility to move in and out of smaller groups as directed within large group sessions (University of Colorado 2011; see fig. 14.4).

Lecture theatres are not the only spaces used for large group teaching events in medical education. Others include dissecting rooms and laboratories, particularly in more traditional schools that have had both large classes and the funds to construct these dedicated large spaces for them. Although their physical organization differs significantly from lecture theatres, the layout and design of these large group teaching spaces again follows preconceptions about how space should and will be used and in doing so allows for little variance from these originally conceived uses.

The increasingly widespread use of webinars and other online large group methods requires an internet-based environment where many people can assemble and interact. Large group web-based tools like Elluminate, Connect, and Wimba provide various tools for slide presentation, desktop sharing, lecturer control over learners' ability to talk, and other analogs of face-to-face events. Online spaces for large group teaching are also designed to support certain ways of organizing and running multiparticipant activities and can be similarly enabling of certain kinds of learning activity, and limiting of others.

Audiovisual technologies

Many technologies, including chalkboards, whiteboards, overhead projectors, 35-mm slides, live patients, cadavers, charts, and models have been used in support of large group teaching over the years. Teaching has changed as the technologies have changed. Activities that would once have used a chalkboard now use whiteboards or digital 'smart' boards. Visuals that were presented in the form of posters, wax models, and other fixed forms are now shown using PowerPoint (or similar tools) and a data projector. Since preparing a lecture became synonymous with creating a PowerPoint slide deck, the ability to design audiovisual materials, in particular PowerPoint slides, has become an essential teaching skill. The field of instructional design identifies ways in which slides can be better designed, in particular the interaction between cognitive load and multimedia design (Mayer 2009). Mayer's multimedia principles for redesigning

lecture materials may be a way to improve understanding and knowledge retention by medical students (Issa et al. 2011).

Mayer's multimedia learning principles are based on aspects of cognitive load theory and focus on improving the efficacy of educational materials by reducing extraneous cognitive load (minimizing distraction) and improving germane load (improving instructional design). These include reducing extraneous load by removing unnecessary content (the coherence principle), adding cues so learners understand how the material is organized (the signalling principle), using just pictures and narration rather than pictures and narration and text (the redundancy principle), putting corresponding words and images adjacent to each other (the spatial principle), presenting corresponding words and images at the same time (the temporal principle). They also include improving germane load by presenting paced segments rather than a single bolus of information (the segmenting principle), putting key concepts first (the pretraining principle), using words and pictures together (the multimedia principle), adopting a conversational style (the personalization principle) and using a real human voice rather than a machine-generated voice (the voice principle) (Mayer 2009).

Preparing slides can also raise intellectual property and copyright issues. Although the use of the internet makes it increasingly easy to use third-party materials in lecture presentations, lecturers may be breaking the law if they do so without regard to whether they have the right to do so. Different legal jurisdictions have different laws regarding these issues so a single set of lecture slides that may be considered legal in one jurisdiction may be considered illegal in another. This is exacerbated by publishing slides containing third party content online, as this is in essence a form of republishing.

Lecturers who have full ownership of their original presentation content may also post their slides to a public online repository (such as SlideShare or Scribd) or a peer-reviewed portal (such as MedEdPortal) for others to use. Alternatively they may use more generic media sites such as YouTube, TeacherTube, Prezi, or iTunesU. Copyright is not the only concern arising from publishing slides online as there are also ethical and legal consequences for disclosing confidential medical materials or content that lay people may construe as medical advice.

Some newer technologies, such as podcasting or vodcasting, allow lecturers to prerecord their presentations and allow learners to access them in their own time. Live lectures may likewise be webcast or captured for subsequent viewing. Some lecture capture systems permit students to annotate the recordings, communicate with the professor or fellow students, or complete quizzes embedded between sections of lecture material.

Fike et al. (2009, p. 88) showed how remote synchronous participation in lectures could achieve comparable learning outcomes to face-to-face participation. Moving from synchronous to asynchronous forms of presentation can be less well received, however, if the greater convenience of being able to view a lecture in one's own time is offset by not being able to interact with the lecturer or other learners (Moridani 2007). On the other hand, simply making recordings of lectures available after a lecture can reduce student stress (Pilarski et al. 2008) and the simple expedient of being able to control playback speed increased learners' capacity to 'attend' from an average of 1.9 lectures per day to 2.6 lectures per day (Cardall et al. 2008).

Large group teaching in educational ecologies

Large group teaching exists within educational programmes defined by learning objectives, other educational activities, and curricular and institutional cultures within which it takes place and is thereby shaped and constructed by what we can consider to be educational ecologies. Cultural expressions of academic disciplines may inform the conduct and design of the teaching and learning carried out within them (MacArthur 2009). Examples of such academic cultural factors include lectures being assumed to be intrinsic to medical education (tacit assumptions), lecturers seeing teaching as being about knowledge transfer (implicit theories), lecturers feeling that they should 'fit in' with the local way of doing things (conventions of appropriateness), lecturers feeling that since they have lecture halls they should use them (codes of signification), and lecturing as a way of reinforcing the authority of the lecturer (power relations) (MacArthur 2009).

The ecologies of lecturing and the different roles of lecturers and learners within them are socially constructed. Students' expectations are directly linked to their academic and professional development and their interpretations of what teachers tell them (Kinzie 2010). Many medical students organize into groups that divide labour, some learners taking lecture notes and sending them to their group, others specializing in searching libraries and the internet, and others interpreting and synthesizing material. As a result, lecturers may not always be able to rely on attendance as a measure of which learners they are reaching.

Educational ecologies are not neutral environments. For instance, lecture system ecologies see lectures as axiomatically sufficient for learners' needs; any problems learners have are due to their failure to learn properly (Northedge and MacArthur 2009). These kinds of power relations are also reflected in terms of various 'control strategies', which emphasize a lecturer's control of the lecture process and procedures, and 'independence strategies' where students have more say and influence in how and what learning occurs (Gibbs and Jenkins 1992). One further ecological factor to consider is the interdependence of large group teaching with the specific ecologies of medical education. For instance, the traditional preclinical/clinical divide dictates the educational methods used at either stage, particularly the central role of lectures in preclinical knowledge-based curricula (Cavenagh, 2011). The key question becomes 'how do we make lectures better?' rather than 'are lectures the best method to use?'

Beyond the lecture

Although the lecture is the dominant form of large group teaching, there are many other large group teaching formats including: small group learning within large groups (e.g. peer instruction (Crouch and Mazur 2001), team-based learning (Hills 2001; Michaelsen et al. 2008; Parmelee and Michaelsen 2010), synchronous non-co-located learning events (e.g. web-based conferences, videoconferences), or asynchronous captured content (e.g. podcasts, lecture recordings). The inverted classroom model has students reading or listening to recordings of knowledge content in advance of time with a faculty member 'expert' (Gannod et al. 2008; Lage and Platt 2000).

The growing range of variations on large group teaching highlights the role of technology and the need for student-teacher engagement. The ability to engage learners remotely and asynchronously has marked a major change in how large group teaching can be designed and enacted. Table 14.1 reflects some variations in location and temporality in large group teaching.

Blurring of the lecture with other formats is reflected in the use of study groups, notes from past classes, tutor guides, and peer-led tutorials (Zhang et al. 2011). Students also engage in sharing digital resources from lectures, using third party web-based applications, or content repositories (Gallagher 2011; Rubio Carbó and Serrat Antolí 2011). These may represent one aspect of optimal learner behaviour (Brown and Czerniewicz 2010), although this remains a relatively unexplored phenomenon and as such deserves further investigation.

This chapter began by asking what 'large' means in the context of large group teaching. Orthodox forms are now being challenged by emerging forms of large group teaching. For example, MOOCs (massively open, online courses) are purposefully designed to connect large numbers of participants (often 500 or more) in open online education. They use various combinations of synchronous web conference sessions alongside asynchronous postings on social media (e.g. blogs, Twitter or wikis , or forums in online portals (e.g. discussion boards in learning management systems)). Each of these forms of participation are registered with the MOOC and aggregated into regular postings to students (de Waard et al. 2011; Kop et al. 2011). Participants may also connect and proximally share or mentor, even teach, sessions. The lecture is being reinvented in some quarters in the format of video-based education such as the Khan Academy, YouTube Education, and Vimeo. These forms are 'new' in that they utilize a web-based form to facilitate independent learning, but 'old' in combining didactic instruction with embedded assessment. It is interesting to note that the contents of most videos and tutorials are profoundly didactic and subject to the same criticisms as traditional lectures. Each of the seven themes that were identified earlier can also be applied to these newer forms of large group teaching. Understanding how cognition, activity design, ecologies of learning, disciplinary discourse and the opportunities and limitations of physical and virtual spaces are still essential for ensuring effective and meaningful learning experiences.

In summary, large group teaching is no longer a self-contained undertaking. Technology has changed how teachers and learners

Table 14.1 Different temporal and spatial organization of large group teaching with examples from medical education

Learners and teacher colocated and working synchronously	Methods include: breaking the large group into smaller groups and then bringing their deliberations back to the larger group (Michaelsen et al 2008; Hills, 2001); using individual learner response systems such as keypads or clickers (Premkumar and Coupal 2008); individual writing activities such as the one minute paper (Wilson 1986); and debates (McKeachie 2006) and voting.
Lecturer and group not colocated but working synchronously	Many forms of distance or distributed medical education (Snadden and Bates 2005) including webcasts and web-conferencing (Salmon 2002; Horton 2006).
Lecture and group working asynchronously	Prerecorded lectures in the form of podcasts (audio), vodcasts (video) or more interactive web-based lecture modules.

interact (Clark 1994) and given tool designers important roles (Ellaway et al. 2006; Smythe and Hughes 2008). Technology may also be a replacement for existing practice, such as using clickers in place of asking class members to raise their hands. In these cases, although technology provides an instructional tool, it may not significantly change the abstract interactions between teachers, learners and educational materials (Kozma 1991).

Conclusions

◆ Lecturing is most effective when both teachers and learners are well trained and supported.

◆ Lecturing involves a sequence of different activities that lead up to and include a 'performance' as well as subsequent follow up activities.

◆ Lecturing allows learners to participate in disciplinary discourses. What is said may be less important than how it is said or who says it.

◆ Lecturing is both an educational method and a systematic approach to programme delivery. However, these are not necessarily congruent and one may at times contradict the other.

◆ Lecturing is determined in part by the affordances of the technologies available to support it.

◆ Lecturing is determined in part by the affordances of the educational ecologies within which it takes place.

◆ Large group teaching can take many more forms than traditional and didactic lectures. Internet-based technologies, in particular, afford new forms that transcend traditional spatial and temporal limitations but which may be more or less satisfying than face-to-face encounters.

References

Aarabi, P. (2007) *The Art of Lecturing: a Practical Guide to Successful University Lectures and Business Presentations*. Cambridge: Cambridge University Press

Ambrose, S., Bridges, M., DiPietro, M., Lovett, M., and Norman, M. (2010) *How Learning Works*. San Francisco: Jossey-Bass

Antepohl, W., and Herzig, S. (1999) Problem-based learning versus lecture-based learning in a course of basic pharmacology: a controlled, randomized study. *Med Educ*. 33(2): 106–113

Balandin, S., and Hines, M. (2011) The involvement of people with lifelong disability and communication impairment in lecturing to speech-language pathology students. *Int J Speech-Language Pathol*. 13: 436–445

Bligh, D.A. (1971) *What's the Use of Lectures?* London, UK: Penguin

Boswell, J. (1791). The Life of Samuel Johnson LLD. http://ebooks.adelaide.edu.au/b/boswell/james/osgood/ Accessed 22 February 2013

Bourdieu, P., Passeron, J.C., and de St Martin, M. (eds) (1994) *Academic Discourse*. Stanford, CA: Stanford University

Brown, C., and Belfield, C. (2002) How cost-effective are lectures? A review of the experimental literature. In: H. Levin and P. McEwan (eds) *Cost-Effectiveness and Educational Policy* (pp. 139–153). Larchmont, NY: Eye on Education

Brown, C., and Czerniewicz, L. (2010) Debunking the 'digital native': beyond digital apartheid, towards digital democracy. *J Computer Assisted Learning*. 26(5): 357–369

Brown, G., Bakhtar, M., and Youngman, M. (1984) Toward a typology of lecturing styles. *Br J Educ Psychol*. 54(1): 93–100

Brown, G., and Edmunds, S. (Eds.). (2009). *Lectures: A Practical Guide for Medical Teachers*. Edinburgh, UK: Churchill Livingstone

Brown, G., and Manogue, M. (2001) AMEE Medical Education Guide No. 22: Refreshing lecturing: a guide for lecturers. *Med Teach*. 23: 231–244

Bye, A.M.E, Connolly, A.M., Farrar, M., Lawson, J.A., and Lonergan, A. (2009) Teaching paediatric epilepsy to medical students: A randomised crossover trial. *J Paediatr Child Health*. 45: 727–730

Cain, J., Black, E.P., and Rohr, J. (2009) An audience response system strategy to improve student motivation, attention, and feedback. *Am J Pharm Educ*. 73: 21

Canfield, P.J. (2002) An interactive, student-centered approach to teaching large-group sessions in veterinary clinical pathology. *J Vet Med Educ*. 29: 105–110

Cardall, S., Krupat, E., and Ulrich, M. (2008) Live lecture versus video-recorded lecture: Are students voting with their feet? *Acad Med*. 83: 1174–1178

Cavenagh, P. (ed.) (2011) *The Effects of Traditional Medical Education: the Changing Face of Medical Education*. Oxford, UK: Radcliffe

Clark, R. (1994) Media will never influence learning. *Educ Technol Res Devel*. 42(2): 21–29

Copeland, H.L., Longworth, D.L., Hewson, M.G., and Stoller, J.K. (2000) Successful lecturing: a prospective study to validate attributes of the effective medical lecture. *J Gen Intern Med*. 15: 366–371

Cosgrove, J.F., Fordy, K., Hunter, I., and Nesbitt, I.D. (2006) Thomas the Tank Engine and Friends improve the understanding of oxygen delivery and the pathophysiology of hypoxaemia. *Anaesthesia*. 61: 1069–1074

Harden, R.M. and Crosby, J. (2000) AMEE Guide No 20: The good teacher is more than a lecturer—the twelve roles of the teacher. *Med Teach*. 22(4): 334–347

Crouch, C.H., and Mazur, E. (2001) Peer instruction: ten years of experience and results. *Am J Phys*. 69(9): 970–977

de Waard, I., Abajian, S., Gallagher, M.S., et al. (2011) *Using mLearning and MOOCs to understand chaos, emergence, and complexity in education. Int Rev Res Open Distance Learn*. 12(7) http://www.irrodl.org/index.php/irrodl/article/view/1046 Accessed 9 April 2013

Doucet, M.D., Purdy, R.A., Kaufman, D.M., and Langille, D.B. (1998) Comparison of problem-based learning and lecture format in continuing medical education on headache diagnosis and management. *Med Educ*. 32(6): 590–596

Ellaway, R. (2008) 'What I meant was...' —the power of use cases. *Med Teach*. 30(1): 112–113

Ellaway, R. (2012) Educational Methods, Educational Systems. *Med Teach*. 34(5): 428–430

Ellaway, R., Dewhurst, D., Mills, E., Hardy, S., and Leeder, D. (2005) ACETS: Assemble, Catalogue, Exemplify, Test and Share. JISC Final Project Report *JISC Development Programmes*. Newcastle-upon-Tyne: The Higher Education Academy Subject Centre for Medicine, Dentistry and Veterinary Medicine

Ellaway, R., Begg, M., Dewhurst, D. and MacLeod, H. (2006) In a glass darkly: identity, agency and the role of the learning technologist in shaping the learning environment. *E-Learning*. 3(1): 75–87

Exley, K., and Dennick, R. (2004) *Giving a lecture: from presenting to teaching*. London: Routledge

Fike, D.S., McCall, K.L., Raehl, C.L., Smith, Q.R., and Lockman, P.R. (2009). Achieving equivalent academic performance between campuses using a distributed education model. *Am J Pharm Educ*. 73: 88

Fitch, M.T. (2007) Using high-fidelity emergency simulation with large groups of preclinical medical students in a basic science course. *Med Teach*. 29: 261–263

Gallagher, M.S. (2011) Open badges and acknowledging decentralized activity in learning. Retrieved from http://michaelgallagher.posterous.com/open-badges-and-acknowledging-decentralized-a Accessed 22 February 2013

Gannod, G.C., Burge, J.E., and Helmick, M.T. (2008) *Using the inverted classroom to teach software engineering*. Paper presented at the Proceedings of the 30th International Conference on Software Engineering, Leipzig, Germany

Gibbs, G., and Jenkins, A. (1992) *Teaching Large Classes in Higher Education: how to Maintain Quality with Reduced Resources*. London: Kogan Page.

Gibson, J.J. (1979) *The Ecological Approach to Visual Perception*. Boston: Houghton Mifflin

Gulpinar, M.A., and Yegen, B.C. (2005). Interactive lecturing for meaningful learning in large groups. *Med Teach.* 27: 590–594

Hartley, J., and Cameron, A. (1967). Some observations on the efficiency of lecturing. *Educ Rev.* 20(1): 30–37

Haskins, C.H. (1957). *The Rise of Universities*. Ithaca: Cornell University Press

Hills, H. (2001) *Team-based Learning*. Farnham UK: Gower.

Hogan, D., and Kwiatkowski, R. (1998) Emotional aspects of large group teaching. *Human Relations.* 51(11): 1403–1417

Horton, W. (2006) *E-Learning by Design*. San Francisco: Pfeiffer

Issa, N., Schuller, M., Santacaterina, S., et al. (2011) Applying multimedia design principles enhances learning in medical education. *Med Educ.* 45(8): 818–826

Johnson, C.G. (2005). Lessons learned from teaching web-based courses: the 7-year itch. *Nursing Forum.* 40(1): 11–17

Johnson, J.P., and Mighten, A. (2005) A comparison of teaching strategies: lecture notes combined with structured group discussion versus lecture only. *J Nursing Educ.* 44: 319–322

Kao, H.S.R. (1976). On educational ergonomics. *Ergonomics.* 19(6): 667–681

Kessler, C.S., Dharmapuri, S., and Marcolini, E.G. (2011) Qualitative analysis of effective lecture strategies in emergency medicine. *Ann Emerg Med.* 58(5): 482–489.e7

Kiewra, K.A. (1985) Learning from a lecture: An investigation of notetaking, review and attendance at a lecture. *Human Learning: J Pract Res Appli.* 4(1): 73–77

Kiewra, K.A., DuBois, N.F., Christian, D., and McShane, A. (1988) Providing study notes: Comparison of three types of notes for review. *J Educ Psychol.* 80(4): 595–597

Kiewra, K.A., Mayer, R.E., Christensen, M., Kim, S.-I., and Risch, N. (1991) Effects of repetition on recall and note-taking: strategies for learning from lectures. *J Educ Psychol.* 83(1): 120–123

Kinzie, J. (2010) Student engagement and learning: experiences that matter. In: J. Cnristensen Hughes and J. Mighty (eds) *Taking Stock: Research on Teaching and Learning in Higher Education* (pp. 139–154). Kingston, ON: Queens University School of Policy Studies

Kop, R., Fournier, H., and Mak, J.S.F. (2011) *A pedagogy of abundance or a pedagogy to support human beings? Participant support on massive open online courses. Int Rev Res Open Distance Learn.* 12(7) http://www.irrodl.org/index.php/irrodl/article/view/1041 Accessed 9 April 2013

Kozma, R.B. (1991) Learning with media. *Rev Educ Res.* 61: 179–211

Lage, M.J. and Platt, G. (2000). The internet and the inverted classroom. *J Econ Educ.* 31(1): 11–11

Liu, F.C., Gettig, J.P., and Fjortoft, N. (2010) Impact of a student response system on short- and long-term learning in a drug literature evaluation course. *Am J Pharm Educ.* 74: 6

Long, A., and Lock, B. (2010) Lectures and large groups. In: T. Swanwick (ed.) *Understanding Medical Education: Evidence, Theory and Practice* (pp. 139–150). Oxford: Association for the Study of Medical Education

MacArthur, J. (2009) Diverse student voices within disciplinary discourses. In: C. Kreber (ed.) *The University and its Disciplines* (pp. 119–128). London: Routledge

MacNeil, M.S. (2007) Concept mapping as a means of course evaluation. *J Nursing Educ.* 46: 232–234

Matheson, C. (2008) The educational value and effectiveness of lectures. *Clin Teach.* 5: 218–221

Mayer, R. (2009) *Multimedia Learning*. 2nd edn. New York, NY: Cambridge University Press

McKeachie, W.J. (2006) McKeachie's teaching tips: strategies, research and theory for college and universty teachers. Belmont CA: Wadsworth

McLeish, J. (1968) *The Lecture Method*. Cambridge: Cambridge Institute of Education

Melamed, Y., Ophir, G., Nechama, Y., Abramovitzh, R., Notzer, N., and Apter, A. (2006) Resident psychiatrists as assessors for lectures in continued medical education in psychiatry. *Ind J Med Sci.* 60: 514–519

Michaelsen, L.K., Parmelee, D.X., and McMahon, K.K. (2008) *Team-based Learning for Health Professions Education: a guide to using small groups for improving learning*. Steerling VA: Stylus Publishing

Mishra, S.P., and Koehler, M.J. (2006) Technological pedagogical content knowledge: a framework for teacher knowledge. *Teachers College Record.* 108(6): 1017–1054

Moridani, M. (2007) Asynchronous video streaming vs. synchronous videoconferencing for teaching a pharmacogenetic pharmacotherapy course. *Am J Pharm Educ.* 71: 16

Murphy, G. (2007) *The 'Dreaded Lecture'. Strategies for Healthcare Education*. Oxford: Radcliffe Publishing, pp. 9–16

Nandi, P.L., Chan, J.N.F., Chan, C.P.K, Chan, P., and Chan, L.P.K. (2000) Undergraduate medical education: comparison of problem-based learning and conventional teaching. *Hong Kong Med J.* 6: 301–306

Norman, G.R. (1988) Problem-solving skills, solving problems and problem-based learning. *Med Educ.* 22, 279–286.

Norman, G., and Schmidt, H. (1992) The psychological basis of problem-based learning: a review of the evidence. *Acad Med.* 67(9): 557–565

Northedge, A., and MacArthur, J. (2009) Guiding students into a discipline. In: C Kreber (ed.) *The University and its Disciplines*. London: Routledge

Ochsendorf, F.R., Boehncke, W.H., Sommerlad, M., and Kaufmann, R. (2006) Interactive large-group teaching in a dermatology course. *Med Teach.* 28: 697–701

Parmelee, D.X., and Michaelsen, L.K. (2010). Twelve tips for doing effective team-based learning (TBL). *Med Teach.* 32(2): 118–122

Pilarski, P.P., Johnstone, A.D., Pettepher, C.C., and Osheroff, N. (2008) From music to macromolecules: Using rich media/podcast lecture recordings to enhance the preclinical educational experience. *Med Teach.* 30: 630–632

Premkumar, K., and Coupal, C. (2008) Rules of engagement–12 tips for successful use of "clickers" in the classroom. *Med Teach.* 30(2): 146–149

Powell, J. (1970) University teaching methods. *Educ Res Britain.* 2: 193–206

Queens' University (2011). Our new medical school building. http://meds.queensu.ca/home/building Accessed 22 February 2013

Race, P. (2001) *The Lecturer's Toolkit: a Practical Guide to Learning, Teaching and Assessment*. New York: Routledge

Richardson, A., Littrell, O.M., Challman, S., and Stein, P. (2011) Using text messaging in an undergraduate nursing course. *J Nursing Educ.* 50: 99–104

Rong, Y., Glozier, N., Luscombe, G.M., Davenport, T.A., Huang, Y., and Hickie, I.B. (2011) Improving knowledge and attitudes towards depression: a controlled trial among Chinese medical students. *BMC Psychiatry.* 11: 36

Rubio Carbó, A., and Serrat Antolí, N. (2011) Online students initiate informal learning practices using social tools *eLearning Papers* (Vol. 26). http://www.elearningpapers.eu Accessed 22 February 2013

Salmon, G. (2002) *E-tivities: The Key to Active Online Learning*. London: Kogan Page

Shulman, L.S., and Shulman, J.H. (2004) How and what teachers learn: a shifting perspective. *J Curriculum Studies.* 36(2): 257–271

Smits, P.B., de Buisonjé, C.D., Verbeek, J.H.A.M., van Dijk, F.J.H., Metz, J.C.M., and ten Cate, O.J. (2010) Problem-based learning versus lecture-based learning in postgraduate medical education. *Scand J Workplace Env Health.* 36: 488–498

Smythe, G. and Hughes, D. (2008) Self-directed learning in gross human anatomy: Assessment outcomes and student perceptions. *Anat Sci Educ.* 1: 145–153

Snadden, D. and Bates, J. (2005) Expanding undergraduate medical education in British Columbia: a distributed campus model. *Can Med Ass J.* 173: 589–590

Spencer, J., and Pearson, J. (2010) Cost-effective face-to-face learning. In: K. Walsh (ed.) *Cost Effectiveness in Medical Education* (pp. 48–59). Abingdon: Radcliffe Publishing

Thomas, P.A., and Bowen, C.W. (2011) A controlled trial of team-based learning in an ambulatory medicine clerkship for medical students. *Teaching Learning Med.* 23: 31–36

Trowler, P. (2009) *Beyond Epistemological Essentialism: Academic Tribes in the Twenty-First Century. The University and its Disciplines*. London: Routledge

Tulsky, J.A., Arnold, R.M., Alexander, S.C., et al. (2011) Enhancing communication between oncologists and patients with a computer-based training program: a randomized trial. *Ann Intern Med.* 155: 593–601

Van Dijk, L.A., Van Der Berg, G.C., and Van Keulen, H. (2001) Interactive lectures in engineering education. *Eur J Engng Educ.* 26(1): 15–28

Van Dijken, P.C., Thevoz, S., Jucker-Kupper, P., Feihl, F., Bonvin, R., and Waeber, B. (2008) Evaluation of an online, case-based interactive approach to teaching pathophysiology. *Med Teach.* 30: 131–136

Ventura, S., and Onsman, A. (2009). The use of popular movies during lectures to aid the teaching and learning of undergraduate pharmacology. *Med Teach.* 31: 662–664

Visioli, S., Lodi, G., Carrassi, A., and Zannini, L. (2009). The role of observational research in improving faculty lecturing skills: A qualitative study in an Italian dental school. *Med Teach.* 31: e362–e369

Westrick, S.C., Helms, K.L., McDonough, S.K., and Breland, M.L. (2009) Factors influencing pharmacy students' attendance decisions in large lectures. *Am J Pharm Educ.* 73: 83

Williams, B., Lewis, B., Boyle, M., and Brown, T. (2011) The impact of wireless keypads in an interprofessional education context with health science students. *Br J Educ Technol.* 42: 337–350

Wilson, R. (1986) Improving faculty teaching: effective use of student evaluations and consultants. *J Higher Educ.* 57(2): 196–211

Wong, G., Greenhalgh, T., Westhorp, G., and Pawson, R. (2012) Realist methods in medical education research: what are they and what can they contribute? *Med Educ.* 46: 89–96

Yardley, S., and Dornan, T. (2012) Kirkpatrick's levels and education 'evidence'. *Med Educ.* 1: 97–106

Zhang, J., Peterson, R., and Ozolins, I. (2011) Student approaches for learning in medicine: What does it tell us about the informal curriculum? *BMC Med Educ.* 11: 87

CHAPTER 15

E-learning

John Sandars

> In my view it is in our interest as e-learners that those who design e-learning should understand contemporary learning theory, that is to say, they should understand what they are doing.
>
> Alex Jamieson

Reproduced from Jamieson A, 'E-learning', Work Based Learning in Primary Care, 1, 2, pp. 137–146, © Radcliffe Publishing, 2003, with permission

Introduction

There are several definitions of e-learning but the essential aspect is the use of technology to enhance teaching and learning. Technology has become increasingly sophisticated and is now readily available in a wide variety of types, with a vast range of different devices (the computing hardware), software (to enable the hardware to perform its intended functions), and connectivity (how the devices and software can connect to other technology, including the internet or mobile telephony networks). Technology can enhance the essential interactions between learner and content, learner and learner, and learner and tutor. It is easy to become seduced by the latest technology and this applies to all stakeholders, from learners to educational developers to educational providers. The exciting educational opportunities that technology can create will only be realized if there is careful attention to its perceived usefulness to the users, its perceived usability by the users and its cost-effectiveness.

Most of the literature about e-learning in medical education has been concerned with whether it improves learning, especially the extent to which knowledge-based learning outcomes have been increased by the use of e-learning compared with alternative approaches to medical education (Cook et al. 2008). It is reassuring to know that several systematic reviews have consistently shown that e-learning is at least as effective as more traditional approaches but there are wide differences in the learning impact between the various approaches to e-learning (Childs et al. 2005; Curran and Fleet 2005; Cook et al. 2008; Wutoh et al. 2004). This is hardly surprising when often there appears to be little critical appreciation about when and how best to use technology to enhance teaching and learning.

Research suggests that there are some common themes about how and when to use technology, especially in medical education. Childs et al. (2005) identified several common difficulties in the implementation of e-learning from the evaluation of their project and an associated systematic review of the literature. They noted that many e-learning packages were poorly designed, that

the available technology to learners was inadequate, that learners preferred a component of face-to-face teaching and that e-learning required learners' time but that there was a lack of protected time for learning.

The focus of this chapter will be the practical implementation of e-learning in medical education so that its potential impact on learning outcomes can be realized. Many of the issues that will be highlighted about e-learning interventions, whether an entire programme or a more discrete package (such as a web site or podcast), are also typical of the implementation of any aspect of medical education, such as understanding the needs of the learner, choosing appropriate methods of delivery and being aware of the context in which learning will occur. Although there are many similarities between educational delivery using e-learning and more traditional approaches, more attention is required in this field since the technology is an additional mediating influence on the process of learning. Technology has many advantages, such as allowing access at any time and any place, but this can also create difficulties since providing education at a distance may reduce opportunities for tutor to learner interactions or may be best by difficulties with internet connectivity.

A framework for the implementation of effective e-learning

Implementation of e-learning in medical education can be a rewarding, yet challenging, experience for any educator. Careful planning at each stage of the development and implementation process is essential. A general framework that can practically guide the educator in a structured process is the DDD-E model: Decide, Design, Develop, and Evaluate (Ivers and Barron 2010).

Decide

The Decide phase is an essential first step before embarking on any intended e-learning project. The educational challenge should be clearly identified. This challenge will usually be based on the intended learning outcomes, such as what new knowledge, skills and/or attitudes are expected to be acquired by the learner. However, an important consideration that is often neglected concerns the process by which the learner will be expected to achieve these outcomes.

A vision of how the learner is intended to engage with the learning resource should be an essential guiding principle and is dependent on the underlying 'pedagogic models and concepts' (Dabbagh and Bannan-Ritland 2005). There is increasing interest in developing life-long learners to effectively respond to the demands of our complex world and professional practice. This requires an educational approach that encourages individual and collaborative inquiry, information-seeking and reflection. Creating an e-learning approach that merely provides lists of information can be easily provided but ensuring that there is active collaborative can be a major challenge.

Other essential factors to consider are the competence and confidence of the learner in using the intended technology, the availability of technology within a specific context and the connectivity of the chosen technology to the various types of networks. Designing an e-learning intervention for delivery on an institutional system, with its capability for fast and reliable internet access that can cope with large file sizes, may be inappropriate for another audience, such as learners who are in remote and rural settings where internet access is by dial-up telephony networks.

It is often a salutary experience for the e-learning enthusiast that the use of technology to address the educational challenge may not be the most appropriate response and that more traditional approaches are to be preferred or that the two approaches are best blended together. It is better to make this important design decision at the earliest possible stage in the development and implementation process so that effort and valuable resources are not wasted.

Design and develop

The Design phase involves the careful consideration and alignment of several essential factors: the content to be delivered, the learner, the instructional design to maximize the learning experience, the technology to deliver the learning experience; and the context within which the learning experience will be utilized by the learner (Zaharias and Poylymenakou 2009).

Authoritative content is an important aspect but this depends on the intended learning outcomes. For example, the intended learning outcome may be that the learner can identify, analyse and synthesize a wide range of information sources that have variable quality. In this situation, the content is less important but the learning process is paramount. The initial design phase is followed by the develop phase in which the factors are translated into an e-learning educational intervention, from either a single and small learning package, such as a website or podcast or app, to a large and complex e-learning module (fig. 15.1).

The learner

Understanding the learner requires an appreciation of not only what they want or need to learn but also how they prefer to learn. The identification of learning needs and the establishment of intended learning outcomes are essential educational principles for any effective teaching and learning but are beyond the remit for

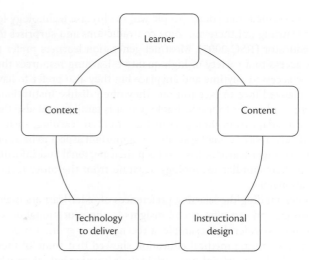

Figure 15.1 The essential factors for effective e-learning.

Data from Zaharias, P. and & Poylymenakou, A. (2009) Developing a usability evaluation method for e-learning applications: beyond functional usability. International Journal of Human–Computer Interaction, 25, 75–98.

this chapter. However, understanding learning preferences is essential, especially the use of technology for educational purposes by young people.

The concept of the 'net generation' learner has extensively influenced the use of technology in all areas of education, including medical education. The net generation are those young people who have grown up in a world in which they have been constantly surrounded by technology (Tapscott 2009). The assumption is that these 'digital natives' have not known a life without computers, the internet and mobile phones (Prensky 2001). It has been suggested that the net generation have a different approach to learning compared with previous generations, with a preference for multimedia rich environments (especially visual and audio), active engagement in learning tasks with a self-directed inquiry approach and collaboration with others (Tapscott 2009). It has even been suggested that the brains of net generation learners are 'hard-wired' differently to previous generations.

A critical appreciation of the net generation is warranted since there are many generalizations about their use of technology (Bennett et al. 2008). There is widespread use of technology by most young people but there are exceptions, especially related to gender, cultural and financial factors. It is important to be aware that only a limited range of the available technology is used by young people and that its use is mainly to support their social life (Sandars et al. 2008). There is high use of social network sites (such as Facebook), media sharing sites (such as YouTube), games and mobile devices. There is also high use of the internet to surf web sites for information to answer queries but they tend to mainly rely on the first ten sites retrieved by Google and appraisal of the quality of the information that they find is often low (CIBER/JISC 2008; Kingsley et al. 2011). There are similar concerns about their use of social network sites. For example, medical students and junior doctors often do not appear to appreciate the public nature of popular social network sites and that they reveal unprofessional behaviours and can breach patient confidentiality (Thompson et al. 2008).

It is assumed that young people will readily use technology for their learning but there are some contradictions and surprises for the educator (JISC 2007). Most net generation learners prefer to have access to a variety of high quality e-learning resources that can be accessed anytime and anyplace but they also prefer to have personalized face to face tuition. They often dislike institutional systems and prefer to use technology that is familiar and also that they can adapt from their personal use to their learning, such as social networks or e-mail systems. An important aspect to be aware is that younger learners wish to keep their personal and informal use of their familiar technology separate from the more formal educational use.

Understanding the learning preferences of older learners is also important and can offer useful insights to the educational developer and provider. For example, a recent survey of high users of online continuing medical education showed that some of these learners had a superficial approach to their learning but others who had a preference for a deeper approach were high users since they were attempting to balance busy work and family lives (Sandars et al. 2010). These deep learners valued the opportunity to revisit content at a convenient time. Using e-learning can also be an isolating experience and some older learners actively engage in providing feedback about modules they have completed in an attempt to create a community of learners (Sandars and Walsh 2009).

In conclusion, there is no 'typical' learner but understanding the intended audience for any e-learning intervention is an essential aspect of the first phase in design and development.

The instructional design

Instructional design is a nebulous concept but it is concerned with how the intended educational impact of an educational intervention can be realized. In essence, it is the 'design for learning' and translates the theoretical 'pedagogic models and concepts' into practical 'instructional strategies' (Dabbagh and Bannan-Ritland 2005). The most widely used instructional design approach in e-learning has a focus on the individual learner since e-learning is usually an individual and isolated endeavour. In this circumstance, cognitive aspects of learning are paramount and are widely used to inform the design of e-learning interventions. A more general approach to instructional design is that proposed by Gagne and another, as proposed by Mayer, concentrates on the application of specific cognitive principles when using multimedia. The social aspects of e-learning interventions are often not fully appreciated or implemented, mainly because of the difficulty in creating effective online social learning spaces. This aspect will be discussed later in this chapter.

Gagne (1965) proposed a theory of 'nine events of instruction' based on the assumption that different instructional approaches will stimulate different types of learning. These 'events' include:

1. Gain attention, such as by using a title or introduction that puts the topic into immediate practical relevance and provides a focus for the learner.

2. Inform learners of objectives by informing them of what they can expect to learn when they have completed the intervention.

3. Stimulate recall of prior learning, such as by an initial quiz or reflection exercise. It is expected that the self-directed learner will be both motivated and more focused in their learning when they appreciate that there is a discrepancy between what they presently know and what they should know.

4. Present the content. This is where the skilful use of Mayer's theory of multimedia learning is essential.

5. Provide learning guidance, such as differentiating between essential and recommended reading or activities.

6. Elicit performance, for example by a final quiz, to help the learner identify if the intended learning objectives have been met by the intervention.

7. Provide feedback to help the learner understand their level of performance and how they can make changes.

8. Assess performance, such as comparing the score of the final quiz with the initial quiz. This can help consolidation of learning but also to stimulate further study if there is a discrepancy between what they know and what they should know.

9. Enhance retention and transfer to practice, for example by encouraging reflection on how the new learning can be applied to practice.

The theory of multimedia learning proposed by Mayer (2001) more specifically considers how to maximize the learning by the effective presentation of content, with particular emphasis on the cognitive aspects of working memory and cognitive load for the processing of new information. The technology used in e-learning readily creates an opportunity for the senses of the learner to be bombarded with a variety of different media. It is often thought that 'more the better' is the design feature for e-learning, for example as provided through online games or simulations. However, a series of experimental studies have led to several practical recommendations to ensure that learning is most effective:

1. Multiple representation principle: It is better to present an explanation in words and pictures than solely in words.

2. Contiguity principle: When giving a multimedia explanation, presenting corresponding words and pictures together rather than separately is important.

3. Split-attention principle: When giving a multimedia explanation, presenting words as an auditory narration rather than as a visual on-screen series of text messages.

4. Coherence principle: When giving a multimedia explanation, using fewer rather than many extraneous words and pictures. This is essentially 'keeping it simple'—too much information can detract from the main intended message.

In conclusion, instructional design provides the essential process in which underlying 'pedagogic models and concepts', which theoretically inform how content should be presented to produce effective learning, interact with the 'instructional strategies' that operationalize the theory into practice.

The technology

A wide range of technology is potentially available to any medical educator who wishes to use e-learning but the reality is that there are likely to be restrictions due to the availability of hardware, software and connectivity.

The use of institutionally provided technology, such as virtual learning environments (VLEs) or managed learning environments

(MLEs), may have the advantage of secure and stable delivery platforms but they often have restricted access to users, lack interoperability with mobile devices and limit the variety of approaches in which content can be presented to the learner. These large institutional systems are expensive to initially purchase and maintain, being out of reach to many developing countries. However, for many medical educators the VLE or MLE is likely to be the main avenue by which they can provide e-learning.

Mobile devices, such as the recent smartphones (iPhones and Android devices) and tablet devices (such as the iPad), have the advantage of being familiar to many learners and are almost always constantly at hand (Chatterley and Chojecki 2010). This has an intuitive appeal for use in busy clinical environments but their potential use may be limited since there are often concerns about interference with equipment and the response by both clinical staff and patients to what they consider to be a social communication device that is inappropriate for learning (Sandars and Dearnley 2009). The current market place for mobile devices has several key players and there may be problems with compatibility between the main operating systems and their applications.

Sophisticated software to produce e-learning packages, which can range from modules to single podcasts, requires not only financial investment for licences or technical development but also the technical expertise to make meaningful use of the software. More cost-effective approaches, such as using freely available open source software may overcome some of these difficulties, especially in developing countries, but usually the available functionality is reduced. Another approach is to share e-learning packages or to download preprepared content, such as with the recent phenomenal growth in the available number of 'apps' for mobile devices.

Connectivity to networks is an important consideration, even in countries that have well developed mobile phone or Wi-Fi internet networks since they may be blocked within clinical environments. In most developing countries, traditional cable-based broadband networks have been bypassed by the use of mobile networks but this can severely limit access to e-learning packages that can only be delivered from VLEs or MLEs.

In conclusion, an awareness of the types of technology that are available to both the learner and provider of any proposed e-learning intervention is an essential aspect that needs to be considered early in the design and development phase before more widespread implementation.

The context

Understanding where and how e-learning is intended to be used is essential if all of the hard work in producing the e-learning package is to be successfully implemented. Many of the barriers have already been highlighted in the previous sections but a wider appreciation of how any proposed intervention will fit into the wider curriculum is essential. A case study by Grant et al. (2011) highlights the range of difficulties associated with implementing an online undergraduate teaching package on evidence-based medicine. Despite the modules being well liked by the learners there was less than optimal uptake. The experience led to several important recommendations to guide further design and development. It was recommended that the whole of the curriculum should be mapped to identify the most appropriate place for the new resource, that competing resources in the existing pool of resources that are used in the curriculum should be identified, that the preferred learning

approaches of the students with the intended use of the resources should be identified and that an understanding of the strategic aims of the students for learning, especially their priorities when under time constraints and the pressure of impending examinations, was essential.

The readiness of the intended organization in which e-learning is to be implemented is an important consideration, especially the organization's cultural readiness (Broadbent 2002). Any e-learning intervention has the potential to disrupt existing patterns of activity within an organization, from its conception of learning and training to its approaches of assessment of learners to how it provides technical support for learners using technology for learning. These disruptions may lead to positive changes that can enhance teaching and learning but often they highlight underlying tensions that exist in the organization. For example, within a healthcare context, technical support tends to be concerned with information systems instead of educational systems and this can lead to difficulties with online security, such as blocking of social network or other websites, or lack of appreciation that many online learners will want access outside normal office hours.

In conclusion, a thorough appreciation of the likely barriers to implementation and how they can be realistically overcome is an essential part of the design and development phase. This aspect is ignored at the peril of the e-learning designer and provider.

Evaluate

The design and subsequent implementation of any e-learning intervention, from a whole online programme to a standalone e-learning package to an individual podcast or app, is a complex process. It may go smoothly and produce the desired educational impact—equally it may not. An iterative process of evaluation is an essential component of any e-learning project but, unlike most evaluations of e-learning that only occur after full implementation, it should be performed at each of the main phases of the project. A crucial time for evaluation is at the early design and development phase, ensuring that prototypes are fit for purpose before more resources are committed to their development.

The use of action research in the development of e-learning has been well described by McPherson and Nunes (2004). The Educational Management Research (EMAR) Model is based on the extensive experience of its authors and highlights the importance of actively involving the learners at each stage of the evaluation process. This model allows iterative development though cycles of evaluation and refinement, in which the opinions of the learners are incorporated into the design and development of the e-learning intervention.

Most evaluation has a focus on the learner's perceived usefulness of the e-learning intervention. However, usability testing is an essential component of any evaluation for any e-learning intervention since the main components for effective learning are perceived usefulness and usability (Davis 1989). The key features of usability and usability testing will be discussed later in this chapter.

Two detailed case studies are now presented to illustrate how careful attention to the essential design, development and evaluation phases can produce an effective learning experience.

The first case study is a biostatistics module in a postgraduate online masters in public health—described by Gemmell et al. (2011). The module was delivered within the constraints of an institutional VLE with learners who were widely dispersed across the world, including developing countries. Each module and weekly topic commenced with an introduction and list of learning objectives, recall of prior knowledge was facilitated by a writing style that prompted students to think about the content, there were frequent points in the text to stimulate reflection, short animated presentations were used to clarify difficult statistical concepts and at the end of each module was a short quiz with answers so that students could check their understanding. Consolidation of learning and further transfer of new knowledge to practice was enhanced by the weekly online discussion boards. There was a constant awareness of the need to ensure that any student with a reasonably strong internet connection should be able to fully utilize all of the features used in the module. Student feedback was regularly sought by evaluation to ensure that the module had both high usefulness and usability.

The second case study is the use of digital storytelling for reflective practice on a first-year undergraduate medical student personal and professional development module (Sandars and Murray 2009). The educational challenge was to engage the 'net generation' students with reflection. A questionnaire survey of the students noted that their learning preference was not for text based but for more active approaches. Digital storytelling is an active and creative process in which digital photographs (taken by mobile devices) can be assembled into a visual narrative using standard software on university computers. The students varied in their competence to use the technology and additional training was provided. An evaluation noted that the students enjoyed the new approach to reflective practice but, more importantly, their reflective ability increased.

Social software and the rise of informal e-learning

The original vision of the web was that of a vast network in which widely dispersed individuals, both in time and place, could be rapidly and easily connected to form virtual networks and communities in which knowledge was collaboratively produced in a 'bottom—up' active process (Berners-Lee and Fischetti 1999). However, the available technology was not widely accessible and the supply of information was provided by a limited number of providers, including professional bodies, pharmaceutical companies and commercial organizations. In the last few years, this situation has started to dramatically change with the introduction of a wide range of new social software. This user dominated phenomenon has been called Web 2.0 to clearly differentiate it from the previous 'top-down' provider approach (O'Reilly 2005).

Social software is a collective term that covers a wide range of approaches that have the intention of allowing individuals to be connected through the web (Kamel Boulos and Wheeler 2007). The main approaches that have educational potential include:

- Blogs. These are personal web sites that allow rapid updating by the author. Examples include Blogger (www.blogger.com) and Wordpress (www.wordpress.com). Content can be easily created and shared by making the blog accessible to others.
- Wikis. These are similar to blogs but allow the text on the web site to be edited by others, with the creation of a common document that can be shared between individuals. Examples include Wikispaces (www.wikispaces.com) and Wetpaint Central (www.wetpaintcentral.com)

- Media sharing. Visual media can be uploaded and stored on a web site, such as Flickr (www.flickr.com) for photographs and YouTube (www.youtube.com) for videos. These media can then be shared with others.
- Social networking sites. Several of these approaches can be combined in these sites, such as Facebook (www.facebook.com) and Twitter (www.twitter.com). In these sites there are opportunities to blog, communicate by instant messaging and share a variety of media.
- Social bookmarking. Favourite web sites can be 'book marked' and stored on a website. Examples include Delicious (www.delicious.com) and Digg (www.digg.com). These bookmarks can be shared with others.

Social software offers an exciting approach to informal learning (Cross 2006). In the post-modern world, with its multiple competing perspectives on issues, responding to the complexities of professional practice cannot be met by simple prepackaged educational resources.

The educational potential of social software is that individuals can begin to actively share information and opinions but also offer mutual support and validation of performance. Social software can provide information though blogs, wikis or media-sharing sites. Opinion and support can be provided through social network sites and blogs. The outcome is the creation of a rich and personalized learning experience that is highly relevant to practice (Sandars and Haythornthwaite 2007). This approach to learning has been called a 'learner-centric ecological approach' since there are multiple and different learning resources spread across a learning landscape and, using the analogy of ecology, learning occurs when these resources are uniquely assembled to produce the learning experience (Luckin 2008). For example, a junior doctor may be interested in how to manage a middle-aged man with a rare genetic disorder. In this theoretical scenario, information from the main medical information websites and Google provide important background information, but there appears to be conflicting views about early screening and its impact on patients. A range of different opinions can be obtained from a variety blogs written by specialist geneticists, ethicists, patients and members of their families. There may be keynote presentations from world renowned speakers on YouTube. All of these findings could be shared with other doctors on social network sites, either general ones or those created specifically for doctors, such as doc2doc (http://doc2doc.bmj.com).

Creating content can be a useful learning experience and it has never been easier with the latest technology. Individuals can create their own content but they can also work collaboratively with others. For example, a blog can support an exam study group. At the simplest level, text can be added and web links provided but with a bit more sophistication podcasts and videos can be easily added as well (Sandars 2006 a). Wikis provide a unique shared space, which allow content to be constantly edited. The equivalent of an interactive textbook can be created that is relevant to the needs of users. YouTube and other media sharing sites also offer an alternative for uploading created content, including audio and visual media files produced by learners (Sandars 2009a).

Using existing content to enhance teaching and learning avoids the necessity of creating content. There are millions of blogs, videos and podcasts that can be freely accessed with ease. The content is of variable quality but social bookmarking software allows annotated lists to be made and shared with others so that the most useful content can be quickly identified. Links to existing content can be used within VLEs but more innovative approaches include online projects where learners can be directed to a range of different content so that a variety of viewpoints can be considered. For example, the learning task could be to compare the differing perspectives of policy makers, pressure groups, epidemiologists, urologists, oncologists and the public about the dilemma of screening asymptomatic middle-aged men for prostate cancer.

The rise of social networking has been attributed to the ease with which these sites can allow individuals to connect with numerous other individuals. These sites are extensively used by millions of medical students and junior doctors, although mainly for informal social interaction. However, a recent survey from Australia noted that 25% of medical students regularly used Facebook for education related reasons and another 50% said they were open to doing so (Gray et al. 2010). The students could easily set up an informal online study group in preference to the institutional-provided VLE. There are increasing numbers of social network sites that are restricted to doctors and many professional organizations are launching these sites.

Using social software as an e-learning approach in medical education is not without problems. The informal nature can create difficulties with the group dynamics required for collaborative learning since there are often tensions between social and academic functions. There are also wider concerns about the use of Facebook and unprofessional behaviour. Medical educators can creatively respond to these challenges by developing the 'digital competences' of both themselves and also their learners (Sero Consulting 2007). The concept of 'digital competences' includes the skills to effectively create online content for social software or to form online learning communities, as well as an understanding of the legal and ethical issues of sharing personal information and uploaded content online.

Ensuring that online collaborative e-learning is effective

Opportunities for face to face collaborative learning are becoming restricted in all areas of medical education and the attraction of online methods is that learners can have the opportunity to share information and collaboratively learn despite the group not being physically present. This is particularly important when learners are widely geographically distributed and when there are varying times when learners can meet.

Discussion boards are probably the most widely used approach in both formal and informal settings. This format allows all messages to be threaded so that the sequence of postings can be easily identified. Newer social software, such as social network sites and blogs, are also becoming increasingly used for collaborative learning, including that within formal educational settings. Most discussions are not real-time or simultaneous (synchronous) but occur over a period of time (asynchronous).

The use of online discussions for collaborative learning has exciting potential but often there are low levels of active participation and engagement with this approach (Sandars and Langlois 2006). Online approaches appear to be most effective when learners cannot easily meet face to face and a blended approach, in which online discussions are used as an integral part of other educational provision, is more likely to be effective.

Online discussions are a social process and the development of mutual trust between group members is essential. This can be most effectively achieved by face to face meetings, especially at the beginning of the online group, but also at regular intervals. An initial meeting is also useful to introduce learners to the technology. Although face to face meetings may be impossible, the initial development of the learners into a social group is still important. This can be achieved online by providing an opportunity for learners to introduce themselves and share their hopes and expectations for the group.

Research suggests that some learners want to engage in an active discussion about a topic but others only want a quick answer to a question and do not wish to enter a discussion (Sandars and Langlois 2005). These two aspects may need to be incorporated into the design. Many learners also like to have structured discussions, in which there are a series of clearly defined steps that guide the learner to consider important aspects of the topic under discussion, and often this requires a facilitator. The facilitation of an online discussion, often called e-moderation, requires an appreciation of the unique aspects of this approach (Salmon 2005). Great care has to be taken in the writing of messages. It is important that the meaning intended by the facilitator is clearly conveyed to the reader and that any instructions are as specific as possible. The presence of a facilitator can also reduce the possibility of 'flaming' and 'lurking' by quickly identifying these behaviours and taking appropriate action, similar to group leadership in face to face environments. Flaming occurs when a group member begins to post aggressive messages to other group members. The consequence of this behaviour is that there is loss of mutual trust and the group activity begins to dramatically fall. Prompt action by the facilitator includes online comments, offline contact by email or phone and blocking message posts. Lurkers read messages but do not post, and this results in the breakdown of reciprocity in which members who post messages expect them to be replied to by other group members. The facilitator can make online comments about the importance of participation by all group members and also comments by email or phone.

Facilitation of online discussions, especially those that are asynchronous and with a more formal educational function, require careful attention to ensure that the discussions are keeping on task (Sandars 2006b). This can be difficult for the facilitator but useful techniques include periodic summarizing of discussions with a question to prompt further discussion and a summary as a closure at the end of a sequence of discussions.

The importance of usability for e-learning

Usability is an essential aspect of any e-learning intervention. It is unlikely that the user will find an intervention useful (to enhance their learning) if they find it difficult to use (the usability). Usability refers to the ease with which a person can use a product in a particular set of circumstances (Dumas and Redish 1999).

Usability testing is widely employed in the development of software and information systems but it appears to be rarely used for e-learning, especially in medical education. The focus of usability testing is always the user and it attempts to systematically identify usability problems at an early stage in the design and development process so that they can be rectified before the intervention is more widely implemented (Sandars and Lafferty 2010). The main areas to consider for usability testing of the technological approach (how the e-learning is delivered and accessed) are the ease of navigation, learnability of the various commands, ease of accessibility if disabilities, consistency in the style of presentation, and visual design (including colour schemes and font formats). These aspects are concerned with the ease of use of the technology by the learner and all are vital components required to motivate learners and to facilitate their engagement with both the learning content and the instructional design. The usability of the instructional design (how e-learning tools reinforce the learning) can likewise be considered and include interactivity, content and resources, use of multimedia, learning strategies design and learner guidance and support.

The experience in other areas of product development, such as software, can offer additional guidance about how to effectively perform the testing (Chisnell and Rubin 2008). The characteristics of the target group of learners and the context in which the e-learning intervention is intended to be used should be identified at the earliest possible stage so that the interrelated aspects of the technological approach and instructional design can be fully informed about any possible constraints. A commonly used method for usability testing in other areas of product development is think-aloud protocols in which the user verbalizes their thoughts as they use the product under the conditions in which it is expected to be used. This method has the advantage of immediately capturing usability problems that are identified by the user as they interact with the product. This is in contrast to the inevitable incomplete recall of problems if the user is questioned after use. The importance of usability testing in the intended context can be illustrated by the following example. A mobile device appears to the designer to be perfectly adequate to deliver an online learning package in the test laboratory but the screen size is too small to be clearly seen in the clinical setting. Although there is no 'typical' learner, research suggests that 95% of usability problems that will become apparent with wider implementation of a product can be quickly identified with only five or six randomly identified potential users. An interesting approach that is also sometimes used in usability testing is the 'least competent user', with the assumption that if an identified user who has poor computer skills or low internet connectivity can use the product then the 'typical user' should have fewer problems.

Usability testing allows an iterative and user-centred product design model to be implemented. This model is widely used in product development and typically consists of four or five rapid cycles of test–rectify–retest before a product is launched. A series of prototypes are systematically and thoroughly tested for usability to ensure that they are fit for purpose rather than relying on evaluation following widespread use.

The importance of the tutor in e-learning

It is easy to forget the essential role of the tutor in e-learning. The skill of the tutor is to craft the learning experience so that there is effective learning (Slabbert et al. 2009). This role may be readily apparent when there is a more formal and systematic e-learning project but it is equally important for the optimization of informal learning experiences, such as using the internet for inquiry based learning or online collaborative learning.

The key aspects of the 'e-tutor' role include creating the learning task and the necessary conditions to allow this task to be achieved by the learner. There is also the essential debriefing after the learning experience to ensure that the learner has achieved the intended learning outcomes and to consolidate the learning for the future, with a clear plan for future learning.

An example of the role of the tutor for inquiry based learning is the webquest approach (Sandars 2005a). The tutor sets the parameters for the learning task but the learner is encouraged to identify a range of internet resources that are not only relevant to the task but also build on their existing knowledge and interests. This structure avoids aimless 'surfing' or 'Googling'. A personalized learning experience can be created and the learning can be enhanced by specifying higher-level learning outcomes that require appraisal and synthesis instead of the simple recall of information.

The tutor may also provide face to face tuition in addition to an e-learning intervention. This so-called 'blended approach' has many advantages and is often preferred by learners. Creative 'blending' of the two interventions could include an online discussion between face to face seminars, an e-learning package followed by a face to face seminar or a lecture followed by a student-led Facebook group.

The tutor is crucial to the success of using technology for self-directed learning (Sandars 2009b). It is essential that tutors have well-developed information and digital literacy skills but also that they feel confident and competent in crafting worthwhile learning opportunities in a complex and unstructured learning environment. It is only too easy in these circumstances for tutors to revert back to tightly structured didactic teaching methods. The role of the tutor becomes that of a coach who can guide and support the self-directed learner on all the stages of the their learning journey, including the use of appropriate resources, critical appraisal of what they find and help in making sense of the information so that it can be applied to their own practice.

The challenge of continuing medical education and e-learning

Maintaining the competence of the medical workforce is essential if high quality patient care is to be achieved and this is a challenge to the providers of continuing medical education (CME) since the audience is widely dispersed and has different learning needs. The use of online approaches has attractions for the many providers and users of CME; it can deliver a wide range of educational experiences to a vast and diverse audience of learners who are trying to balance the busy demands of professional, home and social lives.

The predominant approach for online continuing medical education is the delivery of information. A typical approach to online continuing medical education and an evaluation of its impact is that described by Walsh et al. (2010). Over 5000 users completed an interactive module with pre- and post-tests. The evaluation noted a significant increase in knowledge between the pre- and post-test but the only indicator of measure of change in practice were self-reported claims that they had or intended to change practice. A systematic review of 86 studies of online continuing medical education by Curran and Fleet (2005) noted that most studies were also limited to participant satisfaction and only a few studies demonstrated performance change in practice. No studies were found that demonstrated an impact on patient or health outcomes. A qualitative review attempted to identify the factors that enhanced the learning experience of online continuing medical education and noted five key themes:

* peer communication
* flexibility
* support
* knowledge validation
* course presentation and
* design (Carroll et al 2009).

Scales et al. (2011) highlighted the importance of a social and collaborative learning component in online continuing medical education for its impact on patient care. This was a multifaceted intervention that included a video-conference-based forum with audit and feedback, expert-led educational sessions and dissemination of algorithms. The findings of these studies on online continuing medical education resonate with the results from several systematic reviews of traditional CME, in which interactive techniques, including collaborative learning in small groups, produce the greatest impact on care outcomes compared with didactic approaches that merely provide information (Bloom 2005).

Professional practice is characterized by dealing with complex situations that require the skilful integration of explicit (external) and tacit (internal) knowledge (Eraut 1994). Generalized information is often of little practical value for effectively dealing with the 'messy' and unique situations that professionals face in their daily practice (Schon 1983). In such circumstances, greater value is found in the tacit knowledge, either from individual experience or from the experience of others who have faced similar situations. Research in healthcare shows that new knowledge is actively constructed by exchanging information and opinion within social networks (Gabbay and Le May 2004). The resultant 'practical knowledge' is an amalgam of both explicit and tacit knowledge, thereby allowing professionals to make strategic sense of the complex situations that they face and to effectively change their thinking and behaviours to improve care.

The provision of online continuing medical education requires a shift in both policy and practice to emphasize the importance of online social and collaborative learning. There is also the need to structure the learning experience to ensure that effective online discourse occurs between the various members of the online discussion (including facilitators, experts and practitioners) so that the complexity of practice can be grasped and practical solutions proposed, implemented and refined.

The use of e-portfolios in medical education

An e-portfolio, as its name suggests, is a combination of two dimensions: technology and the portfolio approach (Woodward and Nanlohy 2004). A portfolio is a collection of materials (often called artifacts) by the learner. Some of these artifacts will represent important personal learning opportunities, such as reflections on a critical incident, but others may be required to demonstrate achievement of specific standards, such as descriptions of attended educational events.

The most basic use of technology is to create a file that stores the chosen artifacts. This may be a simple text file, like a standard Word document, but it can also contain multimedia. This simple approach is typical of that used by many postgraduate accreditation agencies and professional bodies. However, there are further

exciting opportunities—for example giving and obtaining feedback from peers or a mentor or linking groups of learners to create communities of learners (Sandars 2005b).

Future developments

The main future developments are likely to be determined by both the rapid changes in technology but also increasing concern about the financial constraints (fig. 15.2).

Ubiquitous learning

The rapid developments and widespread use of mobile devices has allowed both content delivery and connectivity to the internet to be available to any user at anytime and anyplace (So et al. 2008). The recent increased market for both apps and e-readers (such as Kindle) offer unrivalled opportunities to access learning content in the workplace. There are now an enormous variety of apps for the main formats of mobile devices (iPhones/iPads, Android, and Blackberry), but there is little crossover between devices. The apps provide access to key information sources (such as guidelines and clinical tools) and both apps and e-readers offer immediate access to clinical textbooks. The potentially universal internet access is likely to occur with the widespread introduction of cloud computing (Vouk 2008). The computing power resides in only one master computer and this allows the mobile devices 'under the cloud' to become cheaper, lighter and smaller. The possibility is that e-learning can become truly mobile and constantly available. This increased mobility of learning can also be linked to global positioning systems so that information can be targeted to specific contexts, such as while walking around a ward. These advances in technology have the potential to offer learners new and exciting learning opportunities, especially in their immediacy and relevance (fig. 15.3).

Immersive learning environments

Interactive games, simulations and virtual patients can add significant value to the learning experience since the learner becomes engrossed in an environment where the virtual world becomes indiscernible from the actual world (Hansen 2008). The virtual world is perceived as physically real since the main senses (visual, auditory, and tactile) are replaced by digital technology. This phase of intense immersion is highly motivating to the learner and is a key aspect of flow experience that is associated with significant learning (Csíkszentmihályi 1975). Immersive technology is costly in resources and requires significant design and computing power to deliver meaningful learning experiences. This approach to the future curriculum is likely to be

---

Ubiquitous learning

Immersive learning environments

Sharing online resources

Understanding the processes required for effective e-learning

Learning analytics for the assessment of e-learning

Cost effectiveness of e-learning

Research in e-learning

Figure 15.2 Future developments in e-learning

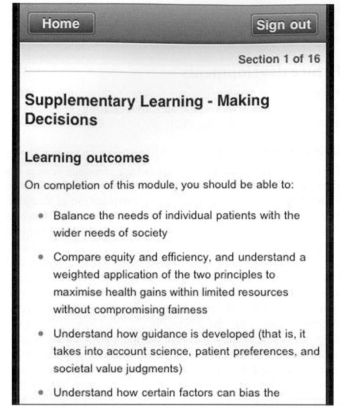

Figure 15.3 Ubiquitous learning.

Reproduced with permission from MedHand.

limited to a few important areas, such as surgical skills training (Harders et al. 2006).

Sharing online resources

There has been increasing interest in sharing resources with other e-learning developers and providers since the creation of high quality learning resources is both time consuming and expensive. This has led to the concept of a 'reusable learning object' (RLO) that can vary in size from a small animation to a module (Schoonenboom et al. 2009). These RLOs can then be assembled to create a larger e-learning package. Two of the major difficulties have been the copyright of the produced material and technical interoperability. However, there have been several international ventures, such as collaborative production (for example, IVIMeds) or creative commons, to try and overcome these difficulties. It is likely with the globalization of medical education that there will be increasing ventures to support e-learning, especially in developing countries.

Understanding the processes required for effective e-learning

Over the last decade there has been increasing interest in how different learners approach their learning, including e-learning. An important perspective has been that of self-regulated learning (SRL), which regards all learners as being active participants in their own learning. The effective self-regulated learner sets clear goals and then selects, monitors and adapts a range of different strategies to ensure that their learning goals are met (Artino 2007). The choice of an appropriate strategy to meet the demands of the learning task is an important predictor of increased interest in and satisfaction with e-learning. This finding is important since both interest in the topic and satisfaction are important factors in motivation to learn online, leading to increased engagement with the learning content and more effective learning. Users of the latest type of e-learning modules, in which recent advances in technology can offer the learner a choice of different multimedia learning resources, are likely to benefit from more developed SRL skills that they can use to enhance their learning (Azevedo et al. 2004). Learners using a more learner centric generated approach to learning face a similar situation and are also likely to benefit from the development of their SRL skills. A short training module on the essential SRL processes that are required for effective learning before commencing an e-learning module can increase the impact on learning (Azevedo and Cromley 2004). Prompting learners to reflect on their use of essential SRL processes during an e-learning module has also been shown to impact on learning (Sitzmann and Ely 2010).

Learning analytics for the assessment of e-learning

Learning analytic technology can track the process of learning to provide formative data to inform teaching and learning (Zhang and Almeroth 2010). For example, essential SRL processes can be identified by noting the sequence of choice of different resources during a learning task and by asking the learner to explain what they are doing at the same time as they are making their choices. These explanations can be collected either as written free-text comments or as audio-recorded talk-aloud thoughts (Hadwin et al 2007). The collected data provides a profile of the SRL processes that the learner has used during an authentic learning task. This insight can provide feedback to the learner about how they approach learning. The most effective feedback has a focus on the process of learning, especially the use of SRL (Butler and Winne 1995).

Cost effectiveness of e-learning

The recent global financial situation has focused attention on the potential cost-effectiveness of e-learning compared with more traditional approaches (Sandars 2010). At the present time, there is little research evidence to guide medical educators in this area.

The commercial world has embraced the use of technology for training purposes and there are numerous case studies of how global companies have achieved substantial financial savings. However, the savings are often based on comparisons with expensive alternative approaches, such as the costs associated with sending employees to national or international conferences and the additional costs related to their loss of productivity while attending these conferences. Calculating the true cost of using technology for training, and also for medical education, is likely to be significantly underestimated since usually there are substantial additional costs that are often not fully appreciated by both the provider and the user. The initial cost often only considers the input from content developers and learning technologists but the hidden costs invariably includes the purchase, depreciation and service costs of all of the technology that is required to develop and deliver the learning resource to the user, including hardware and software. Often the learner will access the resource using their own equipment and

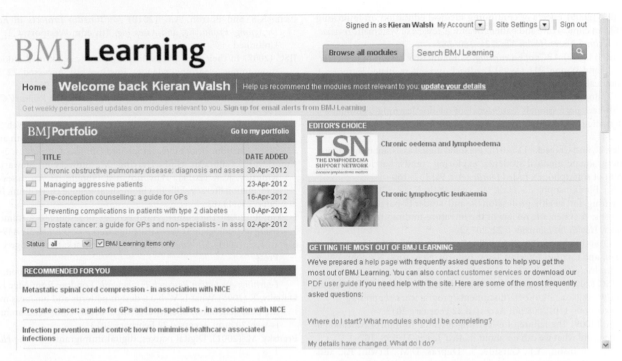

Figure 15.4 E-learning.

Reproduced with permission from BMJ Learning.

in their own time, thereby passing on additional costs that are not appreciated by the educational provider. A comprehensive calculation of the total costs is rare.

Ensuring that technology can produce effective learning requires careful instructional design. The most effective educational interventions to change behaviour are usually complex and include a mix of cognitive and social approaches to learning (fig. 15.4). These approaches are likely to be expensive compared with merely uploading a presentation to a website or VLE. Education, using technology that fails to provide an effective learning experience, is poor value for money. The challenge for all medical educators is to design educational interventions that can fully exploit the potential that technology can offer to the learning experience and to evaluate the effectiveness of these interventions.

Research in e-learning

Most research about e-learning in medical education has concentrated on comparing no-intervention with e-learning or between e-learning and traditional instructional approaches (Cook 2009). A meta-analysis has shown e-learning has a similar effect to more traditional approaches and is better than no intervention but there is little understanding of when and how to use technology for effective teaching and learning (Cook et al 2008). It is essential to recognize the complexity of most e-learning interventions, with numerous variables, and this requires more sophisticated approaches to e-learning research. These approaches include similar methods to researching complex health care interventions (which seek to explore the complex relationships between variables) and the increasing use of transdisciplinary collaboration (which develop new conceptual frameworks based on a combination of different perspectives).

Conclusions

◆ The use of e-learning has rapidly become an established component for medical education, from undergraduate to continuing.

◆ The quest to achieve the potential benefits of e-learning for the enhancement of teaching and learning has yet to be fully realized and there is no 'one size fits all'.

◆ Technology will continue to evolve and provide new and exciting opportunities for education but there are still fundamental aspects that need to be addressed related to the notion of what is e-learning, with the distinction between the provision of content and the social/collaborative construction of knowledge.

◆ A structured process is required that can carefully align the needs of the learner, the content, the instructional design, the technology and the context.

References

Artino, A.R. (2007) Self-regulated learning in online education: A review of the empirical literature. *Int J Instructional Technol Distance Learning*. 4: 3–18

Azevedo, R. and Cromley, J.G. (2004) Does training on self-regulated learning facilitate students' learning with hypermedia? *J Educ Psychol*. 96: 523–535

Azevedo, R., Guthrie, J.T., and Seibert, D. (2004) The role of self-regulated learning in fostering students' conceptual understanding of complex systems with hypermedia. *J Educ Computing Res*. 30: 87–111

Bennett, S., Maton, K., and Kervin, L. (2008) The 'digital natives' debate: A critical review of the evidence. *Br J Educ Technol*. 39: 775–786

Berners-Lee, T. and Fischetti, M. (1999) *Weaving the Web: The Original Design and Ultimate Destiny of the World Wide Web by its Inventor*. New York: HarperOne Imprint of Harper Collins

Bloom, B.S. (2005) Effects of continuing medical education on improving physician clinical care and patient health: A review of systematic reviews. *Int J Technol Assess Health Care*. 21: 380–385

Broadbent, B (2002) *ABCs of e-Learning*. San Francisco: Jossey-Bass/Pfeiffer

Butler, D.L. and Winne, P.H. (1995) Feedback and self-regulated learning: A theoretical synthesis. *Rev Educ Res*. 65: 245–281

Carroll, C., Booth, A., Papaioannou, D., Sutton, A., and Wong, R. (2009) UK health-care professionals' experience of on-line learning techniques: a systematic review of qualitative data. *J Continuing Educ Health Prof*. 29: 235–241

Chatterley, T., and Chojecki, D. (2010) Personal digital assistant usage among undergraduate medical students: exploring trends, barriers, and the advent of smartphones. *J Med Library Ass*. 98: 157–160

Childs, S., Blenkinsopp, E., Hall, A., and Walton, G. (2005) Effective e-learning for health professionals and students-barriers and their solutions. A systematic review of the literature-findings from the HeXL project, *Health Inf Libraries J*. 22: 20–32

Chisnell, D. and Rubin, J. (2008) *Handbook of Usability Testing: How to Plan, Design, and Conduct Effective Tests*. 2nd edn. New York, NY: John Wiley & Sons, Inc.

CIBER/JISC (2008) Information behaviour of the researcher of the future http://www.jisc.ac.uk/media/documents/programmes/reppres/gg_final_keynote_11012008.pdf Accessed 22 February 2013

Cook, D.A. (2009) The failure of e-learning research to inform educational practice, and what we can do about it, *Med Teach*. 31: 158–162

Cook, D.A., Levinson, A.J., Garside, S., Dupras, D.M., Erwin, P.J., and Montori, VM. (2008) Internet-based learning in the health professions: a meta-analysis. *JAMA*. 300: 1181–1196

Cross, J. (2006) *Informal Learning: Rediscovering the Natural Pathways That Inspire Innovation and Performance*. San Francisco, CA: Jossey Bass

Curran, V.R. and Fleet, L. (2005) A review of evaluation outcomes of web-based continuing medical education. *Med Educ*. 39: 561–567

Csíkszentmihályi, M. (1975) *Beyond Boredom and Anxiety*. San Francisco, CA: Jossey-Bass

Dabbagh, N. and Bannan-Ritland, B. (2005) *Online Learning*. Upper Saddle River, NJ: Pearson

Davis, F.D. (1989) Perceived usefulness, perceived ease of use, and user acceptance of information technology. *MIS Quarterly*. 13: 319–340

Dumas, J.S. and Redish, J.C. (1999) *A Practical Guide to Usability Testing*. 2nd edn. Bristol, UK: Intellect

Eraut, M. (1994) *Developing Professional Knowledge and Competence*. London Routledge/Taylor and Francis

Gabbay, J. and LeMay, A. (2004) Evidence based guidelines or collectively constructed 'mindlines?' Ethnographic study of knowledge management in primary care. *BMJ*. 329(7473): 1013

Gagné, R.M. (1965) *The Conditions of Learning*. New York: Holt, Rinehart and Winston

Gemmell, I., Sandars, J, Taylor, S., and Reed, K. (2011) Teaching science and technology via online distance learning: the experience of teaching biostatistics in an online Master of Public Health programme. *Open Learning*. 26:165–171

Grant, J., Owen, H., Sandars, J., et al. (2011) The challenge of integrating new online education packages into existing curricula: a new model. *Med Teach*. 33: 328–330

Gray, K., Annabell, L., and Kennedy, G. (2010) Medical students' use of Facebook to support learning: Insights from four case studies. *Med Teach*. 32: 971–976

Hadwin, A.F., Nesbit, J.C., Code, J., Jamieson-Noel, D.L., and, Winne, P.H. (2007) Examining trace data to explore self-regulated learning. *Metacognition and Learning*. 2: 107–124

Hansen, M.M. (2008) Versatile, immersive, creative and dynamic virtual 3-D healthcare learning environments: a review of the literature. *J Med Internet Res* [online], 10:e26. (www.jmir.org)

Harders, M., Bajka, M., Spaelter, U, Tuchschmid S, Bleuler, H., and Szekely, G. (2006) Highly-realistic, immersive training environment for hysteroscopy, *Studies in Health Technology and Informatics*. 119: 176–181

Ivers, K.S. and Barron, A.E. (2010) *Multimedia Projects in Education: Designing, Producing, and Assessing*. 4th edn. Westport, CT: Libraries Unlimited

JISC (2007) In their own words. http://www.jisc.ac.uk/media/documents/programmes/elearningpedagogy/iowfinal.pdf Accessed 22 February 2013

Jamieson A. (2003) E-learning. *Work Based Learning in Primary Care*. 1(2): 137–146

Kamel Boulos, M.N. and Wheeler, S. (2007) The emerging Web 2.0 social software: an enabling suite of sociable technologies in health and health care education. *Health Information and Libraries Journal*. 24: 2–23

Kingsley, K., Galbraith, G.M., Herring, M., Stowers E., Stewart, T., and Kingsley, K.V. (2011). Why not just Google it? An assessment of information literacy skills in a biomedical science curriculum. *BMC Med Educ*. 25(11): 17

Luckin, R. (2008) The learner centric ecology of resources: A framework for using technology to scaffold learning. *Computers Educ*. 50: 449–462

Mayer, R.E. (2001) *Multimedia Learning*. New York: Cambridge University Press

McPherson, M.A. and, Nunes, J.M. (2004) *Developing Innovation in Online Learning: An Action Research Framework*. London: Routledge Falmer

O'Reilly, T. (2005) What Is Web 2.0 design patterns and business models for the next generation of software. http://oreilly.com/web2/archive/what-is-web-20.html Accessed 22 February 2013

Prensky, M. (2001). Digital natives, digital immigrants. *On the Horizon*. 9: 1–6

Salmon, G. (2005) *E-moderating: The k=Key To Teaching And Learning Online*. 2nd edn. London: Kogan Page

Sandars, J. (2005a) Using Web Quests to enhance work based learning. *Work Based Learning in Primary Care*. 3: 210–217

Sandars, J (2005b) Electronic portfolios for GPs: the beginning of an exciting future, *Educ Primary Care*. 16: 535–539

Sandars, J (2006b) Twelve tips for effective online discussions in continuing medical education. *Med Teach*. 28: 591–593

Sandars, J. (2006a) Twelve tips for using blogs and wikis in medical education. *Med Teach*. 28: 680–682

Sandars, J (2009a) Twelve tips for using podcasts in medical education. *Med Teach*. 31: 387–389

Sandars, J. (2009b) Developing competences for learning in the age of the internet. *Education for Primary Care*. 20: 337–422

Sandars, J. (2010) Cost-effective e-learning in medical education. In K. Walsh (ed.) *Cost Effectiveness in Medical Education* (pp. 40–47). Oxford: Radcliffe Publishing

Sandars, J. and Dearnley, C. (2009) Twelve tips for the use of mobile technologies for work based assessment. *Med Teach*. 31: 18–21

Sandars, J. and Haythornthwaite, C. (2007) New horizons in medical education: ecological and Web 2.0 perspectives. *Med Teach*. 29: 307–310

Sandars, J., Homer, M, Pell, G., and Crocker, T. (2008) Web 2.0 and social software: the medical student way of e-learning. *Med Teach*. 30: 308–312

Sandars, J. and Lafferty, N. (2010) Twelve tips on usability testing to develop effective e-learning in medical education. *Med Teach*. 32: 956–960

Sandars, J. and, Langlois, M. (2005) On-line learning networks for general practitioners: evaluation of a pilot project. *Education for Primary Care*. 16: 688–696

Sandars, J. and Langlois, M. (2006) Online collaborative learning for healthcare continuing professional development: lessons from the recent literature. *Education for Primary Care*. 17: 584–592

Sandars, J, and Murray, C. (2009) Digital storytelling for reflection in undergraduate medical education: a pilot study. *Education for Primary Care*. 20: 441–444

Sandars, J. and, Walsh, K. (2009) The use of online word of mouth opinion in online learning: A questionnaire survey. *Med Teach*. 31: 362–364

Sandars, J., Walsh, K., and Homer, M. (2010) High users of online continuing medical education: a questionnaire survey of choice and approach to learning. *Med Teach*. 32: 83–85

Scales, D.C., Dainty, K., Hales, B., et al. (2011) A multifaceted intervention for quality improvement in a network of intensive care units: a cluster randomized trial. *JAMA.* 305: 363–372

Schoonenboom, J., Sligte, H., and, Kliphuis, E. (2009) Guidelines for supporting re-use of existing digital learning materials and methods in higher education. *ALT-J, Research in Learning Technology.* 17: 131–141

Schon, D. (1983) *The Reflective Practitioner. How Professionals Think in Action.* London, UK: Temple Smith

Sero Consulting Ltd. (2007) Next generation user skills: a report for digital 2010 the SQA. http://www.sqa.org.uk/sqa/files_ccc/HNComputing_NGUSReport_NextGenerationUserSkills.pdf Accessed 22 February 2013

Sitzmann, T. and Ely, K. (2010) Sometimes you need a reminder: the effects of prompting self- regulation on regulatory processes, learning and attrition. *J Appl Psychol.* 95: 132–144

Slabbert, J.A., de Kock, M.A., and Hattingh, A. (2009) *The Brave 'New' World of Education: Creating a Unique Professionalism.* Cape Town: Juta Academic

So, H.J., Kim, I. S., and Looi, C. K. (2008) Seamless mobile learning: possibilities and challenges arising from the Singapore experience. *Educ Technol Int* 9: 97–121

Tapscott, D. (2009) *Growing Up Digital: How the Net Generation is Changing Your World.* New York: McGraw-Hill

Thompson, L.A., Dawson, K., Ferdig, R., et al. (2008) The intersection of online social networking with medical professionalism. *J Gen Intern Med.* 23: 954–957

Vouk, M.A. (2008) Cloud computing—issues, research and implementations. *J Computing Inf Technol.* 4: 235–246

Walsh, K., Sandars, J., Kapoor, S.S., and Siddiqi, K. (2010) NICE guidelines into practice: can e-learning help? *Clinical Governance: An International Journal.* 15: 6–11

Woodward, H. and Nanlohy, P. (2004) Digital portfolios: fact or fiction. *Assessment and Evaluation in Higher Education.* 29: 227–238

Wutoh, R., Boren, S.A., and Balas, E.A. (2004) eLearning: A review of Internet-based continuing medical education. *J Continuing Education Health Prof.* 24: 20–30

Zaharias, P. and Poylymenakou, A. (2009) Developing a usability evaluation method for e-learning applications: beyond functional usability. *Int J Human–Computer Interact.* 25: 75–98

Zhang, H. and Almeroth, K. (2010) Moodog: tracking student activity in online course management systems. *J Interact Learning Res.* 21: 407–429

CHAPTER 16

Simulation-based medical education

Margaret Bearman, Debra Nestel, and Pamela Andreatta

Simulation should be viewed as a parallel universe which mirrors and augments actual practice; it should place the learner at the centre of the process while ensuring patients do not experience avoidable harm.

Roger Kneebone

Introduction

Simulation is, in plain terms, an educational method. While it has several modalities and diverse applications, its fundamental role in medical education is to enhance learning. In this chapter we use David Gaba's definition of simulation as, 'a technique to replace or amplify real experiences with guided experiences, often immersive in nature, that evoke or replicate aspects of the real world in an interactive fashion' (Gaba 2004, p. 2). Simulation-based education (SBE) has particular features that we explore in this chapter, but we commence with a caveat, that it is always important to select the most appropriate educational method for the particular purpose that you are trying to achieve.

Simulation is prominent in most high-reliability industries such as aviation, the military, and nuclear power generation. As part of these industries' workplace cultures, simulation is used for training and assessment in full-scale immersive simulation environments such as cockpits, battlefields, and control rooms. SBE has a centuries-old tradition in healthcare (Owen 2012) but only in the last few decades has SBE re-emerged as a significant influence in medical education. This is partially due to advances in the genesis and integration of computing and material technologies that facilitate the creation of realistic clinical encounters. There continues to be wide variation in the uptake of SBE in undergraduate, postgraduate and continuing medical education, although the trend appears to be for more rather than less simulation.

In the UK, simulation has been identified by the Chief Medical Officer as one of five significant challenges for health services in this decade (Donaldson 2009). In Australia, a federal government agency has a national simulated learning environments program for the health workforce (Health Workforce Australia n.d.). In the United States the contributions of simulation to quality and safety in healthcare are seen as irrefutable (Institute of Medicine 2001). Governing and regulatory agencies such as the Agency for Healthcare Research and Quality (AHRQ) have acknowledged its importance by funding research evaluating its role in improving the safety and quality of healthcare delivery (Henriksen 2011). Accrediting bodies such as the Accreditation Council for Graduate Medical Education (ACGME) have recognized that simulation allows healthcare practitioners to safely acquire the valuable skills and experience they need—without putting patients at risk—and have included simulation-based experience as a requirement for residency programmes (ACGME 2008). More tellingly in a society with privatized healthcare, provider networks such as the Banner Health Network have invested in simulation infrastructure, equipment and personnel to further a mandate towards improving clinical and team performance in their affiliated hospitals and ambulatory care centres (Banner Health Network n.d.).

This chapter is relevant to all types of simulation, but we focus most upon issues pertaining to skills trainers and manikin modalities. However, it is important that simulation modalities are not viewed in isolation but are integrated across a range of modalities and educational methods. As an example, consider the role of hybrid simulations in which simulated patients are aligned with skills trainers for procedural skills training (Kneebone et al. 2002).

The chapter will discuss:

- the range of simulation modalities
- drivers for simulation education
- learning in SBE
- the evidence underpinning SBE
- how to design SBE programmes.

The range of simulation modalities

Simulation in medical education means different things to different people. Simulation is associated with procedural skills, where simulators are frequently used to support the development of psychomotor skills; for assessment of competence; to learn new techniques; and to revisit challenging ones. For example, medical students now usually learn simple suturing on a skin pad before attempting to suture a wound on a real patient. A surgical trainee is likely to learn basic instrument handling and simple manoeuvres for laparoscopy on a 'box trainer' before attempting any laparoscopic skills on a real patient. For new technologies such as robotic surgery, surgeons will usually be certified in a robotic simulator before being allowed to practice. Simulation is also often used in 'crisis resource management' (Flanagan et al. 2004; Maran and Glavin 2003; Bradley 2006) and in the learning of teamwork, leadership, decision-making, and communication skills. However, the term simulation can also be used to refer to cases used in problem-based learning; role-play with other students to develop patient-centred communication skills; or a station in a high stakes examination. The extent to which these examples meet the definition of simulation by David Gaba varies according to the simulation design, the setting in which the simulation takes place, and the participants engagement in the simulation.

Simulation can mean

- Simulated patients (see Chapter 17)
- Role-play: 'where learners take on their own role or another (patient, relative or a healthcare professional) in a scenario'
- Hybrid simulations: 'a blending of simulation modalities such as simulated patients with skills trainers'
- Anatomical simulation skills or 'part-task' trainers: 'models or devices that replicate only a part of the real thing, or part of the body, to teach specific tasks or skills'
- Manikins: 'full body patient manikins of various degrees of capability/sophistication with which the learners must interact'
- Virtual reality: 'parts or all of the patient and environment are presented to the user via two or three-dimensional visual and audio representations, with or without "touch" (haptics) to create a more "immersive" experience'
- Computer simulation: 'learner interaction is mediated by a computer interface'
- Written scenario: 'based on a healthcare scenario that requires the learner/s to think about potential problems, issues and actions as if the scenario was real'
- Environmental simulation: 'contextually situated drills conducted with the intention of measuring, identifying or evaluating clinical or procedural factors related to patient care'.

(Flanagan et al. 2007)

Drivers for the uptake of SBE

The drivers for the expansion of SBE are well documented. They include ethical imperatives, restricted working times, patient empowerment, the patient safety movement, and the need for learner-centred education (Aggarwal 2006; Ziv et al. 2003; Reznick and MacRae 2006; Kneebone and Nestel 2010). The latter is compromised in real clinical settings where there is inherent tension between the primary need for clinicians to be patient-centred and yet also respond to trainees in a learner-centred way (Kneebone et al. 2006). It is not possible to be both patient- and learner-centred in the same space (Kneebone and Nestel 2010). Simulation permits learner-centeredness while remaining patient-focused (Kneebone and Nestel 2010). Box 16.1 summarizes some of the drivers for SBE.

Learning in simulation-based environments

To understand learning in SBE, it is helpful to think of SBE as a series of phases, only one of which involves the actual simulation (Sprick et al. 2012).

1. *Preparation*, where the educator/administrator organizes logistics, briefs faculty, and ensures all equipment is ready for use.

2. *Briefing*, where the educator orients learners and faculty to the simulation environment and to the learning activity itself.

Box 16.1 Drivers for uptake of simulation-based education

Humanistic drivers

- Ethical imperative of causing no harm to patients
- Raised profile of patient perspectives and patient empowerment

Educational drivers

- Increased numbers of medical and health professional students
- Growing evidence of simulation as an effective educational method
- Mounting evidence that effective health professional/patient communication is key to patient and clinician (learner) satisfaction and reduced litigation
- Development of national assessments
- Facilitates a systematic approach to curriculum activities
- Assures students have direct/indirect exposure
- Allows for adjustment in the level of challenge
- Identifies boundaries of competence
- Provides access to technical, communication and other professional skills essential for safe clinical practice
- Enables rehearsal of infrequently occurring events

External drivers

- Working time directives
- Prominence of the patient safety movement
- Reduced hospital stays

Adapted from Nestel *et al.*, 'Key challenges in simulated patient programs: An international comparative case study,' *BMC Medical Education*, 11, 69, p. 2, with permission from the authors, copyright 2011.

3. *Scenario or encounter*, where the learner interacts within the simulated environment.

4. *Debriefing/feedback*, where the learner receives feedback, often through a structured debrief on the performance within the simulated environment.

5. *Reflection*, where the learner considers further how to integrate the feedback into future practice.

6. *Evaluation*, where the educator gathers data regarding the success of the learning exercise and reframes for future practice.

The educational use of simulation is well supported by learning theories, and it is important to understand how learning theory frames SBE in order to make cogent, informed, and creative educational designs across these six phases. There is a diverse body of theories that influence how simulation is used to teach. Theories are helpful because they provide explanatory frameworks for understanding when, where, and how learning occurs. Effective educational design is about deep thought and considered decisions, not about following recipes.

Sometimes those new to educational practice struggle with the range of theoretical perspectives, which are not always complementary. Sfard (1998, pp. 4–8) coined two metaphors for learning, which are not exclusive to each other: *acquisition* and *participation*. 'Learning as acquisition' is the metaphor in which we are used to working; there is knowledge to be acquired and we learn it. 'Learning as participation' may be less familiar. It is the learning that healthcare professionals find through the relationships with their peers, teachers, senior colleagues, and patients. Some learning theories align more readily with one metaphor than another, and it may be helpful when thinking about or working with simulation design, to consider which metaphor is dominant.

Learning theories intersect in multiple ways but for simplicity we present three broad themes (fig. 16.1):

- learning by 'doing'
- learner-centred simulation and
- simulation as a 'bridge' to clinical practice.

Learning by 'doing'

One of the key attributes of simulation is that it provides learners with the opportunity to learn through concrete experience ('doing') but without impacting upon patients. This capacity to learn from experience without causing harm is seen as a 'moral imperative' (Ziv et al. 2003) as it is unique to the simulation modality. Simulation also provides safety for learners, as they can practice

at the right level of challenge without the variability and stresses of the clinical environment.

There is a simple notion at the heart of experiential learning theory, and this is that experience forms a central role in learning. The Lewinian experiential learning model (Kolb 1984) proposes an idealized circle of experience: a learner has an experience, which promotes observation and reflection, this in turn, transforms into abstractions which are actively tested by the learner. Finally, this leads on to further experience (Kolb 1976; Kolb and Fry 1975). This cycle assists us to view the simulation in light of a larger circle of understanding and helps explain why debriefing and feedback are so important, as they help shape the learner's higher order understanding of the experience, which in turn will shape how they practice. Additionally, this theory draws attention to the needs of the 'observer' in simulations, where the experience is one of scrutiny of another's performance.

Deliberate practice is another learning theory, the primary focus of which is upon 'doing'. This is highly relevant to SBE. Deliberate practice is a theory of expert performance based on the observation of the development of highly performing musicians and other 'experts' (Ericsson 2004; Ericsson 2005). This theory proposes that deep expertise is developed through motivated learners engaging in concentrated repetitive practice on a well-defined problem. With feedback and guidance from an expert coach, and active refinement by the learner, there is incremental improvement until mastery is achieved, and then the goals are redefined to challenge the learner further. A 2011 systematic review strongly suggests that this approach is more effective than traditional clinical environments for learning procedural skills (McGaghie et al. 2011). This is the domain in which deliberate practice is often used, but the features of repetition, feedback, motivation, and clear challenges at the right level of difficulty are useful to understanding many types of learning. The parallels between deliberate practice and mastery learning, which is an instructional design methodology presented later in this chapter, are strong. Both of these sit within the 'learning as acquisition' metaphor.

Learner-centred simulation

Learner-centred educational theories place the locus of control with the learner. In doing so, this type of framework acknowledges the learner's prior experiences and already developed skills and knowledge. This frames learning as a socially constructed act, although the focus tends still to be individual. This 'constructivist' view holds that knowledge is interpreted and created rather than regarded as an absolute truth (Biggs 1996). Learner-centred pedagogy is often contrasted to the 'transmission' model of education, where the learner replicates the teacher's knowledge set. Broadly speaking, learner-centred theories are relevant to the design of the simulation encounter. A learner-centred approach to debriefing ensures that learners will be asked what they wish to focus upon (Kneebone and Nestel 2005; Arora et al., 2012) and is intended to facilitate understanding and reflective practice. In a nutshell, a learner-centred approach promotes the agency of the individual. That is, the learner is given the opportunity to take responsibility for their learning.

'Reflective practice' is a broad concept, and the term is used in many different ways (Boud and Walker 1998). In general, reflective practice revolves around the learner deliberately exploring their

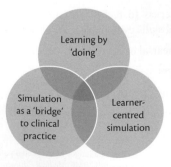

Figure 16.1 Themes that underlie learning theories in simulation.

own experiences in order to learn from them. Schon linked reflection to professional development, describing both

- ◆ Those considered reflections to adjust practice during the practical experience (reflection-in-action) and
- ◆ Those reflections which are made post hoc (reflection-on-action) (Schon 1983, 1987).

Both of these notions underpin simulation facilitation techniques. 'Reflection-in-action' may be cultivated through the judicious use of pauses in scenario development. Recent research has indicated however that this approach is less effective than 'reflection-on-action', and certainly provision of feedback is associated with the effectiveness of a simulation (McGaghie et al. 2010; McGaghie 2009; Issenberg et al. 2005).

Boud and Walker (1998) warn against the dangers of uncritical use of reflective practice to frame learning. Specific concerns revolve around loose and unframed reflection; the emotional nature of reflective practice; and the need for educators to manage the micro-contexts of reflection when learning is taking place in a group. These are timely reminders for simulation practice. First, briefing provides the opportunity to frame both the scenario and the debriefing experiences in a way that will maximize the learning experience. Second, one of the great advantages to simulation is that emotions are part of the learning process; however, this must be planned for and processes set in place to guard against learners becoming unduly stressed. Finally, another of the great advantages of simulation is that it most often occurs in a group context. Debriefing is, by nature, a social practice and can be considered a process whereby a group develops shared meaning of their experience (Dieckmann et al. 2009; Dieckmann 2009). The micro-context of the debrief is sensitive, and the educator has the complex but rewarding task of facilitating the group dynamic to ensure that there is group as well as individual learning.

Self-regulatory learning is a learner-centred framework, which has made significant impact in the medical education literature and which is also relevant to SBE. Zimmerman refers to self-regulatory learners as those able to self-observe, self-assess, and self-react to performance outcomes (Zimmerman 1990). This has obvious application in SBE with the opportunity for performance, audiovisual recording, reflection, feedback, and debriefing. Nestel et al. 2012) discuss self-regulatory learning in the context of SBE, with a focus on feedback or debriefing. Hattie and Timperley (2007, pp. 86–97) describe a model of feedback to enhance learning. Their basic premise is that feedback is intended 'to reduce discrepancies between current understandings and performance and a goal'. They propose that feedback must answer three questions: 'Where am I going? How am I going? Where to next?' and argue that an important role for teachers is 'to create a learning environment in which students develop self-regulation and error detection skills'. They describe feedback at four levels—task, process, self-regulation, and self—each of which is accessible through SBE. Nestel et al. (2012) build on Nicol and Macfarlane-Dick's (2006) work, proposing seven principles of feedback practice that support self-regulation. These include: defining good performance, facilitating self-assessment, delivering high quality feedback information, encouraging teacher and peer dialogue, encouraging positive motivation and self-esteem, providing opportunities to close the gap (between actual and desired performance), and using feedback to improve teaching. These have direct relevance in the SBE

environment; SBE may provide a critical link to promoting self-regulatory learners.

Simulation as a 'bridge' to clinical practice

A significant driver for the use of simulation, particularly in continuing professional education, comes from developments in the patient safety movement, with its focus on reduction of risk to patients. Simulation is incorporated into risk management processes in industries such as aviation and nuclear power (Ziv et al. 2003). The terms 'crisis resource management' or 'crew resource management' stem from this imperative, where the focus is on learning to manage complex crisis situations through emphasis on such skills as communication, leadership, metacognition, situation awareness, teamwork, and leadership (Flanagan et al. 2004b). There is a body of work which considers the professional skills required for safe practice, drawing heavily from human factors and organizational psychology domains (Glavin and Flin 2012). The use of SBE to improve patient safety is based on an understanding that simulation can replicate clinical environments with sufficient realism to capture the complexity of practice.

In these instances, SBE can be thought of as learning within a specific and authentic context. This resonates with the concept of 'situated learning', which argues that learning is contextual and socially mediated (Lave and Wenger 1991). This sociocultural perspective is a different frame altogether from the notions of deliberate practice, or of experiential learning, where the emphasis is on individual improvement and experience. In this view of learning, the learner is part of a complex system of practice and learning is constantly occurring, from interactions with peers, educators, senior clinicians and the physical environment. Here, we are in the territory that Sfard (1998) would consider learning as 'participation'. Experience itself is part of a broader social, political, and cultural landscape, where patterns that we take for granted shape every aspect of the way we learn (Boud and Walker 1998).

However, authenticity is not about fidelity. Kneebone and colleagues discuss 'circles of focus'—the elements of a simulation required for verisimilitude (Kneebone et al. 2010). Additionally, sociocultural learning theories underpin the notion that even simple simulations are building professional identity and cultures of practice. Care must be taken in all instances to ensure that unintended side-effects of simulation do not translate into poor practice. Being too reductionist and task-oriented may impede the learning of appropriate patient-centred practice (Kneebone 2011). Theories such as 'transformative learning' and 'threshold learning' suggest that simulation can offer a space where learners can tackle difficult challenges, through engaging with complex, affective domains (Kneebone 2011), what Schon would term the 'swampy lowlands of practice'.

Evidence underpinning SBE programmes

SBE in healthcare has been studied in detail, with a number of published systematic reviews looking at simulation effectiveness in general (Cook et al. 2011; Marinopoulos et al. 2007; Issenberg et al. 2005; McGaghie et al. 2010) and a number looking more closely at specific features or domains such as fidelity (Norman et al. 2012), deliberate practice (McGaghie et al. 2010), surgical training (Sutherland et al. 2006), and virtual reality training in endoscopic and laparoscopic surgery (Walsh et al. 2012; Gurusamy et al. 2009). Cook et al (2011) concluded from their meta-analysis of technology-enhanced simulation across all professions that:

> In comparison with no intervention, technology-enhanced simulation training in health professions education is consistently associated with large effects for outcomes of knowledge, skills, and behaviors and moderate effects for patient-related outcomes.

Against this backdrop of studies, including those which demonstrate improvements to patient care (Draycott et al. 2008; Zendejas et al. 2011; Bruppacher et al. 2010), it is worth noting that there are few studies which provide evidence of the effectiveness of teamwork training in improving patient care. This is irrespective of whether the training is provided through simulation or other modalities.

Issenberg et al.'s 2005 systematic review is helpful because it focuses upon features of effective, high-fidelity, simulations. Drawing from this and also from literature published in the last 7 years, key features of simulation will be discussed in the next section. We will do so in three categories: features which are most relevant when designing an overall programme; features which are most relevant to simulation resources, including faculty; and features which are most relevant to the design of the simulation encounter itself.

Programme design level

Curriculum integration is identified by Issenberg et al. (2005) as a feature of successful simulation design, and by Cook et al (2011) as being a prevalent feature of many successful simulation studies. Curriculum integration is generally an excellent principle for any teaching modality or episode of teaching, which should not be 'stand alone' or isolated, but part of an overall programme. McGaghie et al. (2010) identify other features of effective simulation that revolve around programme design. These are: repetitive practice within the SBE; multiple exposures to the SBE; and the encountering of an increasing range of difficulty within the SBE. Interestingly, these features taken together form the foundations of a deliberate practice or a mastery learning approach. McGaghie et al.'s (2011) review of general SBE using deliberate practice indicates that SBE with deliberate practice is 'superior to traditional clinical medical education in achieving specific clinical goals'.

Simulation environment level

Some features of effective learning through simulation in Issenberg et al.'s (2005) paper focus on the environment, including simulators which can adapt to multiple learning strategies (e.g. small group, large group, instructor-led, or student-led), and which can provide a range of clinical variation. McGaghie et al. (2010) also identify the need for teachers who have been trained to educate via SBE. They argue that teaching via SBE can be challenging and that 'clinical experience is *not* a proxy for simulation instructor effectiveness, and simulation instructors and learners need *not* be from the same health care profession'.

Simulation encounter level

The simulation encounter level can be considered the single episode of simulation and its associated phases. Some of the important features of SBE are noteworthy at this level. Issenberg et al. (2005) identified feedback as the foremost feature of effective learning in high-fidelity SBE. This is not surprising as feedback is a vital component of effective education generally (Hattie and Timperley 2007). As noted earlier, SBE feedback is often framed in a debriefing phase, which includes other elements. We expand upon feedback, briefing and debriefing in a later section.

Other elements at the simulation encounter level include presenting the learner with a safe or controlled learning environment, in which all learners are actively engaged in standard equivalent activities with clearly defined outcomes at a suitable level. There is a need for activities to have face validity to match the real clinical environment (Issenberg et al. 2005). Nestel et al. (2011a) capture this with their analysis of the procedural skills SBE literature: 'learning is more likely to occur when there is alignment of the learner, instructor, simulator, setting, and simulation'. They note some of the variables influencing the impact of SBE in procedural skills learning, including:

- skill or topic, including the nature of topic and the level of complexity

- learner and instructor characteristics, such as learning styles, motivation, preparation, orientation, training, prior experience, and physical limitations

- simulator and setting characteristics, such as the modality and the degree to which the simulator and setting represent real practice

- instructional design characteristics, such as the defining of learning objectives, feedback mechanisms, and underlying theory

- contextualizations, which provide an understanding of how SBE integrates scenario tasks within broader curricula

- transferability, or how the learning translates to practice at a learner, programme, profession, institution, and government level

- access and scalability, including issues of cost-effectiveness.

Designing SBE programmes

There is no single right way to design a SBE programme. In general, we recommend a good understanding of learning theories—to provide a strong foundation for designing SBE instructional frameworks. We present here some general principles of instructional design, followed by a description of a mastery learning approach, which is associated with empirical successes and clear theoretical frameworks. In this example, the notion of learning aligns with Sfard's (1998) metaphor of learning as 'acquisition'—i.e. acquisition of knowledge and skills. It emphasizes the curriculum integration, repetition, and deliberate practice elements, which are associated with measurably improved outcomes in learning.

An overview of instructional design

The first step in instructional design is to establish the overarching goal of the specific instruction. For example, an instructional goal could be to teach medical students how to manage a cardiopulmonary arrest. After the primary goal is established, detailed instructional objectives that collectively lead to the achievement of the instructional goal can be written. These learning objectives should be explicit and measurable, stating what the learners should be able to do, the context they should be able to do it in, and the expected standard of successful performance (Gagne 1985; Mayer

2001). Learning objectives should be written for each relevant performance domain (cognitive, psychomotor, affective, system-level) and encompass the entire content domain associated with the instructional goal. A sample learning objective for intubating a patient simulator might be: 'Upon completion of this instruction the learner will be able to correctly place an endotracheal tube in a manikin simulator in less than 1 minute, given the correct equipment, instruments, and supplies'. Learning objectives associated with an instructional goal do not have to include all requisite abilities, but any prerequisite abilities that will be required for learners to be successful should be made explicit.

After the learning objectives are defined, the next steps involve creating instructional events. Instructional events are activities and assessment opportunities designed to help learners engage with the content domain and to progressively acquire competency (Gagne et al. 2004). Here, the relevant theoretical underpinnings are valuable because the performance domain referenced by the learning objective can be compared against the learning theories germane to SBE. For example, the instructional approach for helping learners achieve an objective with significant psychomotor factors will benefit by considering the theoretical construct of deliberate practice. Similarly, an objective with strong relational cognitive integration may benefit from experiential learning theory. Instructional events should be sequenced in accordance with a natural progression of competency, from lesser to more complex abilities within the content domain.

Here again, drawing on the relevant learning theories will help determine the type of activities that best serve the progressive accumulation of abilities and the optimal location of assessments to inform the learner's progress. For example, formative feedback that is delivered between instructional activities will allow learners the benefits of naïve exploration favoured by experiential learning theory, while providing them with the opportunity to reflect on their performance with constructive feedback that subsequently informs their performance in succeeding activities. This is illustrated well through typical SBE instructional events that include the progressive sequencing of simulation-based activities, followed by debriefing and successive re-engagement with other simulation-based activities. The iterative cycle of instructional events leading to the acquisition of all relevant abilities specified by the learning objectives can be served through the mastery learning model of instruction. We further discuss this model later, but it is essentially learning facilitated by the progressive sequencing of content, providing a roadmap for learners to acquire mastery over time.

Assessment events may be formative (providing feedback designed to help improve learner performance and inform further practice and learning within the content domain) or summative (providing concrete evidence that the learner has achieved the learning requirements) (Black and William 2004). Formative assessment may be formal or informal, but always includes elements that provide the learner with specific information that will allow them to modify their performance in a way to further enhance their abilities. Formative assessment may be sequenced within the instruction. Summative assessment is almost always more formal in that it is considered a form of terminal evaluation that confirms the acquisition of performance objectives within the specified content domain. Summative assessment is typically sequenced at the end of an instructional programme, but can also occur at the logical point where all content has been addressed by the instructional activities.

The next consideration will be to define and secure the resources required to facilitate the instructional events. These typically include physical space, simulators, ancillary equipment, feedback protocols, assessment instruments, supplies and other material, and human resources that are necessary to implement the programme of instruction. Finally, it is necessary to develop and implement an evaluation plan for the instruction itself.

Mastery learning

The mastery learning approach puts the impetus on the learner to achieve the requisite cognitive, psychomotor, or affective objectives under the guidance and supervision of an instructor. The learner progresses through sequenced content and activities designed to help them master specific objectives that are deliberately assessed to a defined performance standard; the learner may not progress to the next level without mastering the prior steps (Levine 1987; Slavin 1989; Guskey and Pigott 1988). This approach is well considered within constructivist learning theories, and easily accommodates multimethod instructional strategies because it is pedagogically independent. That is, mastery learning processes relate solely to the acquisition of knowledge, skills, and attitudes that are independent from the methods used to achieve them. They can be equally achieved through independent study, team-based activities, e-learning modules, or simulation-based environments. The dependency factor for the mastery learning approach is the assessment of whether or not learning objectives are achieved at each sequential step, not the instructional methodology. To facilitate an effective mastery learning model of instruction, standards of performance must be defined for each sequential step (Levine 1987; Slavin 1989; Guskey and Pigott, 1988).

Prior to the development of SBE platforms it was virtually impossible to exploit mastery learning in medical education because of the lack of specific and measurable performance standards. Performance metrics in any given domain are defined through repetitive performance measurement by experts in the domain of interest (Cizek et al. 2004). The commonly implemented apprenticeship model of training must prioritize ethical and optimal patient care over performance repetition for learners. SBE provides a foundation from which performance can be measured because the contextual aspects of patient care may be replicated without the necessary prioritization of a real patient's needs. SBE facilitates the repetitive acquisition of performance data, while controlling for extraneous variables (such as comorbidities) that may impact performance in the real patient care environment. The acquisition of data is essential for deriving and validating the rigorous performance standards that establish the foundation of mastery learning. Simulation facilitates the ability to establish standards of performance, and allows for the derivation of performance curves to be established for the acquisition and degradation of abilities in the content domain. Once those standards are defined, they can be used to support a multilevel learning context that includes data driven and repeated feedback, evidence of progress towards achieving the delineated standards (mastery), identification of areas of performance strength, and identification of areas where targeted remediation is merited to achieve the specific training objectives.

The mastery learning model requires that learners are given specific feedback about their progress at regular intervals in order to identify what they have learned well and what they have not learned well (Slavin 1989; Levine 1987; Guskey and Pigott 1988). Learners may then spend additional time in those areas where they need to improve so that they are fully prepared to move to the next level. The feedback provided to learners that facilitates this iterative approach is referred to as formative assessment. Formative assessment identifies areas that were insufficiently learned so that more time or a different instructional approach may be tried to achieve mastery. The intention of the mastery learning approach is for all learners to achieve proficient performance in the content domain. Therefore, summative assessment is useful upon completion of a mastery learning-based programme to confirm performance achievement within the instructional domain.

Novice learners demonstrate higher achievement with the mastery learning approach than with more traditional instructional methods, largely because the rate of cognitive, psychomotor and affective understanding is controlled by the learner (Block and Burns 1976). Whereas time is held constant with traditional instruction, the mastery learning model allows time to vary in favour of learner performance (Robinson 1992). In the ideal situation, mastery learning is independent of time and learners can move through the progressive steps towards mastery of the content domain at their own pace. In practice, it is challenging to accommodate this within the prescribed curricular frameworks of most academic institutions. Still, there are numerous advantages associated with the mastery learning approach for any content domain.

Mastery learning in simulation-based programmes

To design a mastery learning programme that includes simulation-based instructional methods, clear definitions of the instructional goals and learning objectives must be established. The learning objectives must be specific and must include explicit definitions of what the learners will be expected to be able to do, in what contexts, and to what standard of performance they will be evaluated. After these numerous learning objectives have been delineated, the course content should be segmented into modules of similar concepts that are sequenced in a logical progression so that introductory concepts precede more advanced ones. Formative assessment points should be defined within and between course modules to help learners and instructors organize progression through the content.

Next, instructional strategies must be developed to help learners move through the course modules. This is the area where simulation-based experiential activities can help expedite the achievement of contextually driven learning objectives in a way that would be impossible in the applied clinical context. The simulated environment facilitates the iterative performance-feedback loop that is necessary for developing abilities through deliberate practice. This is especially beneficial for the acquisition of psychomotor skills, high order cognitive processing and critical thinking, and team-based practice behaviour. A simulated clinical environment that adequately reflects the contextually relevant factors influencing performance of the learning objective will optimally support transfer of the acquired abilities to the real clinical environment (Schunk 2004; Cree and Macaulay 2000). The degree of contextual fidelity that is required for the transfer of these abilities is an active area of research. The degree of requisite contextual elements directly impacts the materials and resources that will be required to implement the instructional activity, and all instructional events will need to be assembled and tested prior to the instruction.

Traditional instruction assumes that the learner is prepared to move through the content with prerequisite abilities; however, the mastery learning approach necessitates that prerequisite abilities be demonstrated before progressing with the instructional sequence (Block and Burns 1976). Therefore, the instructional design process must include the explicit identification of expected pre-course cognitive, psychomotor, and affective abilities in the content domain. With the prerequisite abilities identified and the expected performance outcomes defined through the learning objectives, assessment instruments can be designed and validated. Prerequisite assessment instruments will provide learners with information about their readiness for the course content and indicate areas where pre-course remediation may be required. Formative assessment instruments will provide performance metrics and feedback to the learner about how well they are progressing towards the performance standards. Summative assessment instruments will provide performance metrics to the learner and course director.

In sum, the important features of a mastery learning-designed programme will include pre-instruction verification of prerequisite abilities; a modular approach to content dissemination; explicit definition of objectives for each module that includes performance standards; learner-paced achievement of the course objectives; specific feedback intervals to guide learning; formative assessment to identify areas of proficiencies, and deficiencies requiring remediation; and valid and reliable summative assessments to evaluate learner performance against predefined standards.

Challenges of the simulation-based instructional environment

Simulation-based training events have clear advantages over traditional training activities in medicine; however, there are several disadvantages as well. An advantage of the apprentice model of learning is that it embeds affective contextual elements that may be absent in a simulated context. That is, given that a real, living patient is an integral component of the apprenticeship learning context, and given that the demands of clinical care within an institutional system place extraordinary affective demands on the learner, inclusive and apart from cognitive and psychomotor demands, the learning context includes those real factors that must be accommodated during the instructional process. In the absence of those affective factors within the simulated environment, the learner can focus exclusively on the cognitive and psychomotor competencies that comprise the learning objectives for any given procedure, task, or other clinical competency. The difficulty arises when the learner must transfer those acquired cognitive and psychomotor competencies from the simulated context to the applied environment, inclusive of affective factors that have not been integrated in the learning environment. Arguably, affective overload is one of the most challenging aspects of providing clinical care and yet is largely overlooked in the medical education literature. This is reasonable if an apprenticeship model of learning is implemented because these factors are embedded in the learning environment. However, in simulated learning environments these factors must be conscientiously considered and built into the instruction so that transfer from the less stressful learning context (simulation) to the more stressful context (applied patient care) is seamless (Hassan et al. 2006; Andreatta et al. 2010; Prabhu et al. 2010).

The optimal way to facilitate this is to address and accommodate multimodal instructional pedagogy so that cognitive, psychomotor, and affective elements are all incorporated in the simulated learning context. The methodology for this must be carefully considered, but several are well documented in the literature for training in other performance contexts where affective overload has the potential to abate effective training in affectively charged contexts (Inzana et al. 1996; Smith and Nye 1989; Mitchell 1983). In those circumstances, it is best to train within an affectively neutral environment so that knowledge and skills may be mastered away from affective stimuli that may overload and disrupt the optimal learning processes for cognitive and psychomotor skills. However, the affective domain must eventually be accommodated within the training environment in order to facilitate optimal transfer to the applied context. Stress management and affective integration training is well documented in military, law enforcement, and other domains where hazardous duty is a part of professional responsibility.

Simulation as social learning

Not all SBE takes place within a mastery learning context. SBE can also be designed to evoke the chaotic affective domain of clinical practice, enabling a kind of social learning. As noted previously, it is important not to place learners in situations where the challenge is too intense. However, it is worth drawing upon simulation as a medium to introduce some of the complexity of practice. This does not mean that learners should be poorly prepared for practice. It is important to ensure there is reasonable proficiency in the psychomotor or cognitive aspects of practice, as performance in these will be stressed under social challenges. It is also helpful to have a simulation that draws on the authentic nature of practice. Hybrid modalities are helpful here, particularly those which employ simulated patients or faculty. These hybrid modalities enable practitioners to integrate the complex sets of skills required for safe clinical practice. For procedural skills, this may involve the alignment of a skills trainer (e.g. suture pad) with a simulated patient in a simulated setting enabling the practitioner to practice psychomotor and communication skills together.

Measuring improvements in the human factors components of performance is difficult. It is hard to say whether the lack of direct evidence linking teaching these skills to patient care improvements is due to measurement difficulties or lack of impact. However, this is a major use of simulation. Providing situations with social challenges—including difficult or emergency situations where learners must work together outside of their normal patterns—provides training in the skills required to manage difficult situations. This opportunity to include affective and social dimensions in a relatively controlled environment cannot be underestimated, as it is difficult to achieve in an otherwise safe manner, both for learners and for patients. The skill of the educators becomes particularly pertinent in this type of learning.

Briefing, debriefing, and feedback

Feedback is critical to successful SBE. Its role in the mastery learning curriculum is well described. Likewise briefing, because it outlines the expectations of the learner, and frames the expectation of what can occur. However, in a complex simulation, educators must set up a learning environment in which the learner feels supported within the affective domain. In an affective, socially oriented simulation, briefing and debriefing can take on certain intensity. The issue of the group dynamic becomes more important, and this is amplified again if teamwork is part of the focus of the exercise and if colleagues come to a simulation with longstanding attitudes that they need to work on.

Feedback here needs to be more sensitive because professional identities are at stake. The many debriefing models, which embed feedback into practice, offer multiple ways of supporting effective feedback processes. Debriefing generally offers learners: an opportunity to divest themselves of tensions and emotions; an environment for feedback conversations; and a chance to come as a group to a shared understanding of what has just taken place. In a sense these three things roughly match to what Fanning and Gaba (2007) describe as the natural tendency of debriefing to go through three phases: 'description, analogy/analysis, and application'.

In short, it is probably sufficient to note that debriefing and facilitation in SBE are skilful activities. Some simulations may require specific feedback on performance, in other cases feedback may be conversational, in others still it may focus on transfer to practice. The variations of learners, topics, simulators, and educators require nuanced and adaptive debriefing practices. This is where training of simulation educators is vital. Simulation educators must be comfortable with a range of tools at their disposal, in order to sensitively manage a range of debriefing situations.

Case studies: SBE in practice

We present two case studies here, which illustrate how careful educational design in SBE can build learner skills through application of instructional design/or and mastery learning principles. Both case studies also describe affective or social elements in their SBE through use of simulated patients and both also exemplify how SBE should be integrated into the practice environment. Although these two case studies are set in undergraduate and continuing medical education environments, they still draw on similar principles.

Case study 1: Simulation-based Training for Enhancement of Procedural Skills (STEPS)

The STEPS program is underpinned by principles of instructional design (van Merrienboer and Kirschner 2007). The programme was designed by one of the chapter's authors (Debra Nestel) for medical students at Monash University in Australia. Box 16.2 illustrates the elements of STEPS. The approach is illustrated with the procedure of inserting a peripheral intravenous cannula. The first part consists of a training module in which a small group of students view an illustrative DVD followed by practical simulation experience. In the DVD students are provided with requisite knowledge of the procedure including: anatomy, physiology, indications, safety issues, patient-centred communication, and documentation of the procedure. Finally, students listen to patients talk about their experiences of the procedure. Students then work in pairs to practise the technique on a benchtop model.

Observation and feedback of paired students is encouraged. After 30 minutes, students perform the procedure in a scenario-based assessment (contextualized simulation, which introduces the challenge of a simulated patient)—see fig. 16.2. The boundaries of the procedure extend from the initial approach to the patient, through performing the procedure, completing paper work, and leaving the clinical environment. All students complete one scenario and observe a colleague in a different scenario. All are expected to use a generic rating form, the Direct Observation of Procedural Skills (DOPS) (Modernising Medical Careers 2007) to assess and guide post-scenario discussion. Simulated patients (SPs) participate in the discussion offering their perspective on the student's performance. In the second part, students are given the opportunity to perform intravenous cannulation on real patients. Clinical teachers supervise students and use the DOPS form to provide structured feedback; promote reflection; and develop self-awareness and self-regulation.

Box 16.2 Elements of Simulation-based Training for Enhancement of Procedural Skills (STEPS): Intravenous cannulation

PART 1

Students view a DVD as a group (about seven to eight students), discuss issues as they arise (30 minutes), practice in simulation on bench top models (30 minutes) and then with simulated patients (60 minutes).

DVD—Audiovisual and commentary from experts

◆ Overview of intravenous cannulation

◆ Essential knowledge for intravenous cannulation

◆ Introduction to simulator and equipment

◆ Demonstration of technical elements of the procedure in simulation

◆ Overview of DOPS

◆ Demonstration of the procedure in hybrid simulation

◆ Patient safety

◆ Communication

◆ Feedback from patients on their experiences

Practice in simulation

◆ Perform procedure on bench-top model

◆ Hybrid simulation: perform procedure using bench-top model integrated with simulated patient (SP)

◆ Receive expert feedback (technical and SP)

◆ Receive peer feedback

◆ Observe peer in hybrid simulation, provide peer feedback

◆ Reflect on progress

PART 2

Students complete at least two procedural skills in real clinical settings assessed by a clinical teacher using the DOPS rating form. Patients are invited to provide feedback. Each observation takes up to 25 minutes.

◆ Practice under supervision in real clinical settings

◆ Receive expert feedback

◆ Reflect on progress

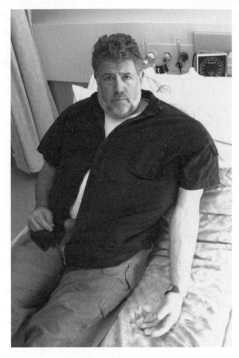

Figure 16.2 Simulated patient aligned with skills trainer for peripheral intravenous cannulation in a patient-focused (hybrid) simulation.

Case Study 2: Instructional design process for an interdisciplinary code team training programme

An example of a purposeful instructional design process tied to mastery learning principles is the paediatric and neonatal mock code programme at the University of Michigan in the United States. The programme was designed by one of this chapter's co-authors (Pamela Andreatta) after the institution expressed the desire to improve paediatric and neonatal survival rates from cardiopulmonary arrest. The goal was to improve outcomes (survival rates) by providing routine experiential instruction and deliberate practice opportunities for clinicians and trainees. The learning objectives were defined for five performance categories: recognition and assessment of atypical rhythms, application of the correct clinical response protocols, execution of tasks, team-related behaviours and protocols, and contextual management (e.g. management of the family). The mastery learning model was implemented to ensure competency was reached by the participants after each training session. This eliminated the need to track individual performance in favour of tracking team-based performance in applied practice. Instructional activities and formative assessment opportunities were designed around three phases: rhythms without a pulse, rhythms with a pulse, and with both types of rhythms. Activities included randomly called mock codes built around a case library of 24 clinical cases where all code team members were required to respond in the same way as they would to an actual code. Formative assessment and mastery learning conditions were built in to debriefing events after each mock code. Materials and resources included the patient room features, furnishings, equipment, instruments, and ancillary supplies used in the actual clinical environment. Patients were represented by manikin simulators (neonatal, infant, or child) and parents were represented by standardized patient actors. Summative evaluation included institutional patient survival rates from cardiopulmonary arrest for all rhythm types. The outcomes from this program demonstrated an overall correlation of 0.87 between the number of mock codes (deliberate practice opportunities) and clinical survival rates, with a 1.00 correlation between content (pulseless, pulse, both) and survival rates. Specific details associated with these outcomes are reported elsewhere (Andreatta et al. 2011), but the overall success of the programme is attributable to the detailed instructional design, tied to mastery learning principles that facilitated the control of potentially confounding individual performance factors.

Implementing a simulation education programme

A simulation education programme does not exist in isolation. Although we provide an example of designing SBE with a mastery learning approach, there are often many barriers to implementing such an approach. Sometimes the broader landscape curtails all but the most ad hoc curricula. A recent national study of current simulation use within Australian medical schools indicates some of the important organizational factors, which may promote or prevent the use of simulation in medical education (Sutton et al. 2010). This study indicates that access to simulation facilities, the cost of simulation resources, and the number of appropriately trained staff all have significant impact on how simulation can be used.

As we have consistently indicated, integrating simulation into the overall curriculum is ideal. This is true for medical school programmes as well as hospital-run postgraduate training. However, simulation elements of curricula or training are often managed in stand-alone centres, or through the advocacy of simulation champions. These arrangements sometimes cause difficulties as various organizations and individuals can have competing priorities. We argue that embedding simulation into curricula starts with good governance of programmes and facilities, clear lines of reporting, and opportunities for collegiate exchange of information. This also lays the foundation for effective sharing of simulation resources across sites and disciplines.

The need to share resources stems from the reality that many simulation modalities are expensive. Organizations often must make high capital investments and there is significant need for ongoing maintenance. This is why the discussion regarding the need for high versus low fidelity and high versus low technology is so important (Norman et al. 2012) as this is a question of cost-benefit as much as education. There have been some discussion regarding the cost-benefit of simulation (Ker et al. 2010) but much further work is needed. Furthermore, sharing resources is not as straightforward as it sounds. The Australian experience indicates that resources are not always readily shared (Sutton et al. 2010). This may be because one of the most difficult issues in planning simulation at the undergraduate level is the sheer number of students. Rotations through simulation centres and the necessary scheduling are complex and time-consuming to organize. Other sorts of logistical pressures affect continuing professional development, in particular the release of clinicians to attend SBE events (even when they are held in the clinicians' working environments). These types of logistical considerations, coupled with unclear governance lines, can create challenges.

Participants in the Australian study also described significant amounts of expensive equipment which was not used optimally (Sutton et al. 2010). There was a deficit of specialist simulation educators who could work in this modality. The need for extensive training has been recognized by the Australian government who has funded significant training programmes (Health Workforce Australia). The purpose of these programmes is to introduce the fundamental principles of SBE as well as promoting best practice in the use of simulation across different modalities.

This investment in simulation educators is taking place against a global backdrop of a growing professional identity for simulation educators. National simulation societies are an important aspect of this growth (e.g. the Association of Simulated Practice in Healthcare in the UK, the Society for Simulation in Healthcare in the USA, and the Australian Society for Simulation in Healthcare). Through attendance and presentation at conferences, simulation practitioners develop a sense of identity and craft.

As simulation education moves towards being an accepted professional pathway, quality assurance and research agendas become increasingly important as part of everyday simulation-education practice. As the evidence attests, simulation is relatively well studied, although there are still gaps in our understanding. However, the integration of research and evaluation to educational practice at the coalface is perhaps less well articulated. Evaluation is a fundamental part of good simulation practice, as it informs improvement and can incorporate new research evidence into practice.

Conclusions

- Simulation is an educational methodology, which provides distinctive benefits to learners.

- In medical education, it is important to remember that SBE contains a broad range of modalities, and a distinctive cycle of educational activities, including briefing and debriefing, to support the simulation encounter.

- Instructional design methodologies and a mastery learning approach can assist in developing effective programmes.

- SBE is well placed to encourage the learning of social and affective aspects of practice, but these must be carefully considered so as not to overwhelm the learner.

- While logistical and organizational aspects of SBE can provide considerable challenges, there is no question that simulation is an increasingly important educational tool in the medical education landscape.

References

ACGME (2008) *ACGME Program Requirements for Graduate Medical Education in General Surgery.*[Online] http://www.acgme.org/acWebsite/downloads/RRC_progReq/440_general_surgery_01012008_07012012.pdf Accessed 12 July 2012

Aggarwal, R. (2006) Technical-skills training in the 21st century. *N Engl J Med.* 355: 2695

Andreatta, P.B., Hillard, M.L., and Krain, L.P. (2010) The impact of stress factors in simulation-based laparoscopic training. *Surgery.* 147: 631–639

Andreatta, P.B., Saxton, E., Thompson, M., and Annich, G. (2011) Simulation-based mock codes improve pediatric patient survival rates. *Pediatr Crit Care Med.* 12: 33–38

Arora, S., Ahmed, M., and Paige, J. et al. (2012) Objective Structured Assessment of Debriefing (OSAD): bringing science to the art of debriefing in surgery. *Ann Surg.* Online

Biggs, J. (1996) Enhancing teaching through constructive alignment. *Higher Educ.* 32: 347–364

Black, P. and William, D. (2004) Assessment and classroom learning. *Assessment in Education.* 5: 7–74

Block, J.H., and Burns, R.B. (1976) Mastery learning. *Rev Res Educ.* 4: 3–49

Boud, D. and Walker, D. (1998) Promoting reflection in professional courses: the challenge of context. *Studies in Higher Education.* 23: 191–206

Bradley, P.P. (2006) The history of simulation in medical education and possible future directions. *Med Educ.* 40: 254–262.

Banner Health Network (n.d.) *About Banner Health.* [Online] http://www.bannerhealthnetwork.com/NR/rdonlyres/EDDA527D-3BCC-4544-B7F2-1DB6038C1D3A/58558/BannerHealthNetworkFactSheet.pdf Accessed 12 July 2012

Bruppacher, H.R., Alam, S.K., Leblanc, V.R. et al. (2010) Simulation-based training improves physicians' performance in patient care in high-stakes clinical setting of cardiac surgery. *Anesthesiology.* 112: 985–992

Cizek, G.J., Bunch, M.B., and Koons, H. (2004) An NCME instructional module on setting performance standards: Contemporary methods. *Educ Manage: Issues Pract.* 2: 31–50

Cook, D.A., Hatala, R., Brydges, R. et al. (2011) Technology-enhanced simulation for health professions education: a systematic review and meta-analysis. *JAMA.* 306: 978–988

Cree, V. and Macaulay, C. (2000) *Transfer of Learning in Professional and Vocational Education.* New York: Routledge

Dieckmann, P. (ed.) (2009) *Using Simulations for Education, Training and Research,* Lengerich: PABST

Dieckmann, P., Molin Friis, S., Lippert, A., and Ostergaard, D. (2009) The art and science of debriefing in simulation: Ideal and practice. *Med Teach.* 31: e287–e294

Donaldson, L. (2009) *150 Years of the Chief Medical Officer's Annual Report 2008.* London: Department of Health

Draycott, T.J., Crofts, J.F., Ash, J.P. et al. (2008) Improving neonatal outcome through practical shoulder dystocia training. *Obstet Gynecol.* 112: 14–20

Ericsson, K. (2004) Deliberate practice and the acquisition and maintenance of expert performance in medicine and related domains. *Acad Med* 79: S70

Ericsson, K. (2005) Recent advances in expertise research: A commentary on the contributions to the special issue. *Appl Cogn Psychol.* 19: 233–241

Fanning, R.M., and Gaba, D.M. (2007) The role of debriefing in simulation-based learning. *Simulation in Healthcare.* 2, 115–125

Flanagan, B., Clavisi, O., and Nestel, D. (2007) *Efficacy and effectiveness of simulation based training for learning and assessment in health care.* Melbourne, Victoria: Department of Health

Flanagan, B., Nestel, D., and Joseph, M. (2004) Making patient safety the focus: Crisis Resource Management in the undergraduate curriculum. *Med Educ.* 38: 56–66

Gaba, D.M. (2004) The future vision of simulation in health care. *Quality Safety Health Care*: 13 Suppl 1): i2–i10

Gagne, R.M. (1985) *The Conditions of Learning and Theory of Instruction.* New York: Holt, Rinehart and Winston

Gagne, R.M., Wagner, W.W., Golas, K., and Keller, J.M. (2004) *Principles of Instructional Design.* Belmont, CA: Wadsworth Publishing

Glavin, R. and Flin, R. (2012) Review article: The influence of psychology and human factors on education in anesthesiology. *Can J Anesth.* 59: 151–158

Gurusamy, K., Aggarwal, R., Palanivelu, L., and Davidson, B. (2009) Virtual reality training for surgical trainees in laparoscopic surgery. Cochrane Database of Systematic Reviews. 1: CD006575

Guskey, T. and Pigott, T. (1988) Research on group-based mastery learning programs: A meta-analysis. *J Educ Res.* 81: 197–216

Hassan, I., Weyers, P., Maschuw, K., and Al, E. (2006) Negative stress-coping strategies among novices in surgery correlate with poor virtual laparoscopic performance. *Br J Surg.* 93: 1554–1559

Hattie, J. and Timperley, H. (2007) The power of feedback. *Rev Educ Res.* 77: 81–112

Health Workforce Australia (n.d.) *Simulated Learning Environments (SLEs)* [Online], http://www.hwa.gov.au/work-programs/clinical-training-reform/simulated-learning-environments-sles Accessed 18th July 2012

Henriksen, K. (2011) Improving patient safety through simulation research: Funded projects AHRQ Pub. No. 11-P012-EF. Rockville MD: Agency for Healthcare Research and Quality

Institute of Medicine (2001) *Crossing the Quality Chasm.* Washington DC: National Academy Press

Inzana, C., Driskell, J., Salas, E., and Johnston, J.H. (1996) Effects of preparatory information on enhancing performance under stress. *J Appl Psychol.* 81: 429–435

Issenberg, S.B., McGaghie, W.C., Petrusa, E.R., et al. (2005) Features and uses of high-fidelity medical simulations that lead to effective learning: a BEME systematic review. *Med Teach.* 27: 10–28

Ker, J., Hogg, G., and Maran, N. (2010) *Cost-effective simulation. Cost-effectiveness in Medical Education* (pp. 61–71). Oxford: Radcliffe

Kneebone, R.L. (2009) Practice, rehearsal, and performance: an approach for simulation-based surgical and procedure training. *JAMA.* 302(12): 1336–1338

Kneebone, R. (2011) Simulation. In H. Fry and R. Kneebone (eds) *Surgical Education: Theorising an Emerging Domain* (pp. 37–54). London: Springer.

Kneebone, R., and Nestel, D. (2005) Learning clinical skills—the place of simulation and feedback. *Clin Teach.* 2: 86–90

Kneebone, R. and Nestel, D. (2010) Learning and teaching clinical procedures. In S.E. Dornan (ed.) *Medical Education: Theory and Practice* (pp. 171–192). Edinburgh: Elsevier

Kneebone, R., Kidd, J., Nestel, D., et al. (2002) An innovative model for teaching and learning clinical procedures. *Med Educ.* 36: 628–634

Kneebone, R., Nestel, D., and Wetzel, C. et al. (2006) The human face of simulation: patient-focused simulation training. *Acad Med.* 81: 919–924

Kneebone, R., Arora, S., King, D. et al. (2010) Distributed simulation—accessible immersive training. *Med Teach.* 32: 65–70

Kolb, D. (1976) *The Learning Style Inventory: Technical Manual.* Boston, MA: McBer

Kolb, D. (1984) *Experiential Learning, Experience as the Source of Learning and Development,* Englewood Cliffs, NJ: Prentice Hall

Kolb, D. and Fry, R. (1975) Toward an applied theory of experiential learning. In C. Cooper, (ed.) *Theories of Group Process* (pp. 33–58). Chichester: John Wiley & Sons Ltd

Lave, J. and Wenger, E. (1991) *Situated Learning: Legitimate Peripheral Participation,* Cambridge: Cambridge University Press

Levine, D.U. (1987) *Improving Student Learning Through Mastery Learning Programs* San Francisco: Jossey-Bass

Maran, N. and Glavin, R. (2003) Low- to high-fidelity simulation—a continuum of medical education? *Med Educ.* 37: 22–28

Marinopoulos, S., Dorman, T. Ratanawongsa, N., et al. (2007) Effectiveness of continuing medical education. *Evid Rep Technol Assess (Full Rep).* 149: 1–69.

Mayer, R.E. (2001) Rote versus meaningful learning. In L.W. Anderson and D.R. Krathwohl (eds) *A Taxonomy for Learning, Teaching, and Assessing:*

A Revision of Bloom's Taxonomy of Educational Objectives. New York: Longman 226-232.

McGaghie, W.S.V., Mazmanian, P. and Myers, J. (2009) Lessons for continuing medical education from simulation research in undergraduate and graduate medical education: Effectiveness of continuing medical education: American College of Chest Physicians evidence-based educational guidelines. *Chest.* 135(3 Suppl): 62S–68S

McGaghie, W.C., Issenberg, S.B., Cohen, E.R., Barsuk, J.H., and Wayne, D.B. (2011) Does simulation-based medical education with deliberate practice yield better results than traditional clinical education? A meta-analytic comparative review of the evidence. *Acad Med.* 86: 706–711

McGaghie, W.C., Issenberg, S.B., Petrusa, E.R., and Scalese, R.J. (2010) A critical review of simulation-based medical education research: 2003–2009. *Med Educ.* 44: 50–63

Mitchell, J.T. (1983) When disaster strikes…the critical incident stress debriefing process. *J Emerg Med Services.* 8: 36–39

Modernising Medical Careers (2007) Foundation Programme. http://www.foundationprogramme.nhs.uk/pages/home/training-and-assessment [Accessed 7 March 2013]

Nestel, D., Groom, J., Eikeland-Husebo, S., and O'Donnell J, M. (2011a) Simulation for learning and teaching procedural skills: the state of the science. *Simul Healthc: J Soc Simul Healthc.* 6(Suppl): S10–S13

Nestel, D., Tabak, D., and Tierney, T. et al. (2011b) Key challenges in simulated patient programs: An international comparative case study. *BMC Med Educ.* 11: 69

Nestel, D., Kneebone, R., and Bello, F. (2010) Feedback to learners in healthcare simulations. In E. Molloy and D. Boud (eds) *Effective Feedback in Higher and Professional Education: Understanding it and doing it well.* London: Routledge

Nicol D. and Macfarlane-Dick, D. (2006). Formative assessment and self-regulated learning: A model and seven principles of good feedback practice. *Studies Higher Educ.* 31: 199–218

Norman, G., Dore, K., and Grierson, L. (2012) The minimal relationship between simulation fidelity and transfer of learning. *Med Educ.* 46: 636–647

Owen, H. (2012) Early use of simulation in medical education. *Simul Healthc.* 7: 102–116

Prabhu, A., Smith, W., Yurko, Y., Acker, C., and Stefanidis, D. (2010) Increased stress levels may explain the incomplete transfer of simulator-acquired skill to the operating room. *Surgery.* 147: 640–645

Reznick, R. and Macrae, H. (2006) Teaching surgical skills—changes in the wind. *N Engl J Med.* 355: 2664–2669

Robinson, M. (1992) Mastery learning in schools: some areas of restructuring. *Education.* 113: 121–126

Schon, D. (1983) *The Reflective Practitioner: How Professionals Think in Action*, London: Temple Smith

Schon, D. (1987) *Educating the Reflective Practitioner.* San Francisco: Jossey-Bass

Schunk, D. (2004) *Learning Theories: An Educational Perspective.* Upper Saddle River, NJ: Pearson

Sfard, A. (1998) On two metaphors for learning and the dangers of just choosing one. *Educ Res.* 27: 4–13

Slavin, R.E. (1989) On mastery learning and mastery teaching. *Educ Leadership.* 46: 77–79

Smith, R. and Nye, S. (1989) Comparison of induced affect and covert rehearsal in the acquisition of stress management coping skills. *J Counsel Psychol.* 36: 17–23

Sprick, C., Jolly, B., Nestel, D., Bearman, M., Owen, H., and Freeman, K. (2012) AusSETT program: Module C2. Health Workforce Australia

Sutherland, L., Middleton, P., and Anthony, A. (2006) Surgical simulation: a systematic review. *Ann Surg.* 243: 291–300

Sutton, B., Bearman, M., Jolly, B., et al. (2010) *Simulated Learning Environments Medical Curriculum Report* [Online] http://www.hwa.gov.au/sites/uploads/simulated-learning-environments-medical-curriculum-report-201108.pdf Accessed 8 Feb 2012

Van Merrienboer, J. and Kirschner, P. (2007) *Ten Steps to Complex Learning: A Systematic Approach to Four Component Instructional Design.* New Jersey: Lawrence Erlbaum Associates

Walsh, C., Sherlock, M., Ling, S., and Carnahan, H. (2012) Virtual reality simulation training for health professions trainees in gastrointestinal endoscopy. *Cochrane Database of Systematic Reviews.* 6: CD008237.

Zendejas, B., Cook, D. A., Bingener, J., et al. (2011) Simulation-based mastery learning improves patient outcomes in laparoscopic inguinal hernia repair: a randomized controlled trial. *Ann Surg.* 254: 502–511

Zimmerman, B. (1990) Self-regulated learning and academic achievement: An overview. *Educ Psychol.* 25: 3–17

Ziv, A., Wolpe, P., Small, S., and Glick, S. (2003) Simulation-based medical education: an ethical imperative. *Acad Med.* 78: 783–788

CHAPTER 17

Simulated patients in medical education

Jennifer Cleland, Keiko Abe, and Jan-Joost Rethans

> For the junior student in medicine and surgery it is a safe
> rule to have no teaching without a patient for a text, and the
> best teaching is that taught by the patient himself.
>
> William Osler
>
> (Osler 1905)

Introduction

Sir William Osler's assertion is embedded within the rhetoric of
modern medical education. Patient contact is seen as essential to
learning medicine by teachers, enjoyed by medical students and
enjoyed by the patients themselves (Collins and Harden 1998;
Hoppe 1995).

Historically, the role of the patient in medical education was
passive—an interesting case, to be goggled at by a group of students following a consultant on the ward round, or as the basis for
anecdotes to illustrate particular learning points. Patients are now
much more actively involved in the education of doctors and other
healthcare professionals (e.g. physiotherapists [Lane and Rollnick
2007], dieticians [Beshgetoor and Wade 2007], pharmacists
[Watsonet al. 2006]), and there is an extensive literature on how
to involve patients in medical education (Spencer and McKimm
2010). This chapter focuses on one broad area of patient involvement—involvement as simulated patients.

The chapter considers the evidence base for the use of simulated patients, explains the theoretical foundations that underpin
their use and gives a comprehensive account of how to implement
simulated patient programmes in medical education. It introduces now well-established uses and emerging trends in the use
of simulated patients. Before doing so, however, it is important
to define what a simulated patient is, and give an overview of the
societal, political, clinical and educational influences which drove
this development.

What is a simulated patient?

Barrows (1987, p. 17) defined a simulated patient (SP) as 'a person who has been carefully coached to simulate an actual patient
so accurately that the simulation cannot be detected by a skilled
clinician. In performing the simulation, the SP presents the gestalt
of the patient being simulated; not just the history, but the body
language, the physical findings, and the emotional and personality

characteristics as well'. Thus, broadly speaking, a simulated patient
is a lay person who has been trained to portray a patient with a
specific condition in a realistic way (Wind et al. 2004) usually by
learning a preprepared scenario. The first known effective use
of simulated patients was by Barrows and Abrahamson (1964,
pp. 802–805), who used them to appraise students' performance in
clinical neurology examinations.

You will also see the term 'standardized' patients in the literature.
With a simulated patient the emphasis is on *simulation* (presenting the symptoms and signs of an actual patient); whereas, with
a standardized patient, the emphasis is on consistency, on standardization of the simulation process (Norman et al. 1982). Thus,
standardized patients are trained to give a consistent presentation
that does not vary from student to student and does not vary from
standardized patient to standardized patient. On the other hand,
simulated patients (presenting the same case) may well show variation. An example of guidance for a simulated patient role is given
in box 17.1. Collins and Harden (1998, pp. 515–516) provide a
description of different types of simulated patients, which illustrates a continuum of training and preparation.

- Those who are only given an outline of what is expected of them
  such as in a situation like a physical examination or a procedure where the interaction between the student and patient is
  minimal.

- Those who are given a short brief or scenario with which they
  must become familiar, but beyond which they are free to respond
  as they wish. This may mean that roles are adjusted to the
  patient's own background or personal experience. For example, a
  simulated patient in this type of role may learn to present a particular set of symptoms and drug history but their occupational
  and family circumstances may be their own.

- Finally, there is the person who is extensively trained and whose
  every response is carefully thought through and rehearsed (the
  standardized patient).

Box 17.1 An example of guidance for a simulated patient role

Patient: You are in your late twenties, and have a sedentary job in IT support

Why you have come to the doctor?

+ You have a cough

+ You've had it for about 3 months

+ It's getting worse

+ It's worse at night

+ You are coughing up white phlegm

+ You have also lost weight

What you think the problem is?

+ You have just spent a year working on a project in Zimbabwe and you are worried that you might have picked up something there

+ You are worried about HIV/AIDS but would not divulge this unless the doctor was easy to talk to

Social history

+ You are living at home with your parents.

+ You don't smoke and only drink occasionally.

+ You usually play a lot of sport but can't at the moment.

Health beliefs/other treatments

+ You've taken cough syrup but it doesn't work.

+ You've seen an acupuncturist in the past.

Currently, 'standardized patient' is the terminology of choice in the United States (where SPs are much used for high-stakes assessment), whereas 'simulated patient' is used more in Asian and European countries.

In this chapter, we use the term simulated patient (SP) to indicate any individual who is trained to play a patient role in medical education.

Why use simulated patients?

Early clinical contact is now a prerequisite of much medical training (GMC 2009). This presumes the need for patient participation in teaching and learning but the availability of patients for teaching and learning medicine has been influenced, first, by changes in healthcare delivery. A reduction of inpatient beds, multiple comorbidities and increased acute illness in those patients who are in hospital, and a shift to care in the community and reduced average hospital admission period for patients have all had a major impact on the availability of patients to take part in the training of healthcare professionals. Care has shifted from acute settings to community settings and there are fewer opportunities for students to learn from a breadth of real patients in a teaching hospital (McManus et al. 1998). Clinical teaching time has been squeezed with learners receiving less time on direct bedside teaching. Increased emphasis on patient safety and protecting patients from unnecessary harm

(Ziv et al. 2003) places limits on the nature of patient contact, particularly for relatively inexperienced learners; so learners need to be prepared for practice to an acceptable level before being let loose on patients. Additionally, increased consumerism and a less unquestioning stance have seen a growing reluctance from patients to contribute to the training of medical students (Ker et al. 2005)—although it is still enjoyed by those who do contribute (Collins and Harden 1998). There is also now significant evidence of the failure of traditional 'apprenticeship' approaches to medical education (Cartwright et al. 2005; Maguire and Rutter 1976): using SPs offers a feasible alternative for learning clinical, procedural, and communication skills in safe, learner-centred environments (Ker et al. 2003; Kneebone et al. 2002).

SPs also have a key role in assessment within medical education. World-wide, undergraduate and postgraduate medical education is now planned within an outcomes-based model using competency-based curricula (Accreditation Council for Graduate Medical Education 1999; GMC 2009). A student's clinical competency must be assessed to see if they have achieved the necessary outcomes to progress to the next stage of training or to complete training. Doing so involves the measurement of a wide range of inter-related skills including clinical communication and examination. The bedside clinical examination was the traditional method for assessing a student's skills and knowledge. However, wide variations in the level of difficulty presented by different (real) patients, compounded by variation in the objectivity of examiners, led to problems with reliability in clinical exams (Collins and Harden 1998).

Thus, as a consequence of these changes in healthcare delivery, patient attitudes, educational teaching and assessment models and approaches, and ethical issues, alternative approaches to using real patients in teaching medicine were sought in the 1960s (Barrows and Abrahamson 1964).

The use of SPs within undergraduate, postgraduate, and continued healthcare education is now widely established and accepted (Bowman et al. 1992; Gerner et al. 2010; Lane and Rollnick 2007), not just for the reasons outlined earlier but because they also have various advantages over real patients. For example, SPs are available as and when required. They can be trained in a broad range of clinical cases, thus giving students a variety of experiences that they may not encounter in real patients. On-demand learning can be facilitated as scenarios can be created as required (Gordon et al. 2004). SPs are willing and ready to undergo scenarios many times. Their behaviour is predictable. They can be used in situations where the use of a real patient would be inappropriate (e.g. practising sensitive communication skills such as giving a terminal diagnosis or first attempts at clinical examination). They can be trained to match their role to the student's level of experience and thus provide a safe, learner-centred environment (Ker et al. 2005). They can play the same role again and again while the student practises and learns specific skills. Unlike real patients, they can be trained to give specific behavioural feedback to students (Kurtz et al. 2005). Their use in teaching has been found to be more effective than didactic teaching for learning consultation skills (Madan et al. 1998). Finally, the use of SPs is accepted and liked by medical practitioners (Bowman et al., 1992) and students (Rees et al. 2004), who prefer working with SPs compared to role-playing with colleagues (Lane and Rollnick 2007; Rollnick et al. 2002).

There are, of course, disadvantages to using SPs. Mostly, these centre on authenticity—SPs are not 'real' patients. However, much research shows that well-trained SPs are not usually distinguished from real patients. Beullens et al. (1997) reviewed rates of detection in a number of divergent studies using SP methodology. They found SPs were detected by only 0–18% of the physicians. Detection is reduced where there is a lengthy period between doctors' consent to participate in studies using SPs and the actual visit, and where the SP uses authentic supporting materials (e.g. simulated health insurance cards) (Rethans et al. 2007a).

The second obvious disadvantage of using SPs over real patients is cost. Training and managing a group of SPs, often referred to as an SP Programme, involves dedicated staff (see Cleland et al. [2009, 2010]) for a detailed overview of the roles and activities required from staff working with SPs). Another cost is that of paying SPs for their time or at the least, any travel expenses incurred in travelling to the medical school. It is useful here to explain that SPs may be volunteer or paid laypersons, or professional actors. Obviously, volunteer SPs, who are unpaid, although usually reimbursed for expenses, are a relatively low-cost resource. On the other hand, using professional actors as SPs can incur substantial costs (Ker et al. 2005).

In the UK, some medical schools use only professional actors. Others, such as Aberdeen, use a combination of volunteers and professional actors: volunteer SPs are used for most teaching purposes other than when more complex specialist (e.g. psychiatric) simulations are needed; in these cases, professional (paid) actors are used (Eagles et al. 2007). In contrast, in Maastricht only lay SPs are used in teaching and assessment purposes. Similarly, medical schools differ in terms of whether or not they pay non-professional, volunteer SPs more than expenses. Some medical schools have different tiers of SPs, with some SPs being paid.

While there is much evidence that simulated patients cannot be reliably discriminated from real patients by experienced clinicians (Rethans et al. 2007a), there are few published comparisons or evidence as to the superiority of paid, volunteer, or professional SPs over each other. To the best of our knowledge, only two studies have compared real patients with an SP (a professional actor) (Eagles et al. 2001; Bokken et al. 2010). In the first study, responses between groups differed only on one question, where students rated their experience with the actor as significantly better than that with the real patient with regard to their acquisition of interview skills. However, the actor had come out of role after the interview, and gave students feedback as to his experience of the interview. Thus, the differences between groups could have been due to different student experiences rather than differences between a real patient and an actor. The second study showed that students preferred SPs compared to real patients because of the quality of SP feedback.

It seems that historical and financial reasons dictate what type of SP is used by an individual medical school. Given the reduced access to real patients but ongoing requirements for early clinical contact, using SPs is necessary, and medical schools must anticipate their needs and stance on payment, and plan their resources accordingly.

Theoretical underpinnings

Medical education is more than the acquisition of knowledge, skills and attitudes. It is now viewed as the transformation of an applicant to medicine from a lay person to a professional who is prepared for lifelong learning (Mann 2011). This perspective influences how to plan learning as well as what to teach. In terms of simulation and, specifically, simulated patients, it is useful to take a moment to consider the learning theories relevant to this perspective.

First, practising communication, clinical, or procedural skills with an SP comes into the category of experiential learning, a principle of adult learning. Confucius once said, 'I hear, I forget; I see, I remember; I do, I understand'. Learning from real-life experiences has been important for thousands of years. Experiential learning is an active process in which the learner constructs knowledge by linking new information and new experiences with previous knowledge and understanding (Kolb 1984). Learners can work with SPs to acquire the required knowledge and skills. In reference to socio-cognitive theory, through experience and observing the actions of others, an individual acquires skills and knowledge and develops a sense of self-efficacy, or perception of agency and ability to perform specific tasks and achieve certain goals.

However, there is more and more evidence, including from medical education, that learning is always inextricably tied to its context and to the social relations and practices there—so-called situated learning. (to read further on situated learning, see contemporary interpretations of Vygotsky's zone of proximal development (ZPD) such as Guile and Young, 2001, and Etienne Wenger's body of work on situated learning, e.g., Wenger 1998). Mann (2011) proposes that situated learning and experiential learning complement each other by framing the exploration of, and reflection on, individual experience within the community's norms, values, and activities. This reminds us that experience of working with an SP must be coupled with aims and objectives, and specific feedback, to contribute to reflection, and that an individual's learning goes beyond individual feedback—the situation itself is a learning experience.

Kneebone et al. (2005) argue that simulations which mirror clinical reality, allow students to make the best use of their clinical experience and improve the quality of the care they provide. This assertion is based on evidence that the acquisition of expertise requires sustained deliberate practice over a number of years (Ericsson et al. 1993) and the conditions under which learning takes place exert a powerful effect (Arthur et al. 1998). The best way to support learners is to plan teaching in such a way to ensure that simulations and real-life clinical environments are as similar as possible, while still supporting learners to work at their own pace, and learn from failures without putting themselves or patients at risk. Thus, simulated patients must be used in a way to facilitate skills acquisition and practice, in a way that models real life clinical practice.

Gerner et al. (2010) give a useful recent example of this. Their aim was to achieve effective training to help GPs deliver effective healthy family advice for families with obese children. They selected the approach of practice visits by SPs to achieve this balance, rather than taking the GPs to workshops for training; hence, situating learning completely in practice. Watson et al. (2007) used a similar approach in pharmacist communication skills training. While in situ learning is not always feasible with students, planning the learning environment so it reflects real-life practice as closely as possible can be done (Ker et al. 2003).

In short, the use of SPs is not just a means to circumvent practical issues, such as a lack of willing and able real patients, but a way of supporting effective learning.

Using SPs in teaching and assessment

Most medical schools now have a SP bank of individuals who have been trained in a number of teaching and assessment roles. Here, we review the well-established uses and emerging trends in the use of SPs. In teaching, SP roles span consultation skills, clinical skills and procedural skills, team-working and inter-professional education (IPE). SP involvement in assessment focuses on clinical examinations and assessing the performance of doctors. The involvement of SPs in giving feedback to learners is also discussed.

Consultation skills

Comprehensive evidence exists to guide the modern practice of communication skills teaching and learning (Kurtz et al. 2005), and over 30 years of accumulated research linked to outcomes has guided the choice of communication domains, tasks, skills, and issues to teach and learn (Makoul 2003; Simpson et al. 1991; Stewart et al. 1999). There are a number of tasks to learn in terms of gaining competency in the process of carrying out a consultation. These tasks include: initiating the session; gathering information/history taking; giving information (including explaining a diagnosis, giving test results, and planning treatment); closing the consultation; communication skills (Friedman et al. 1991).

The skills required for successfully carrying out these tasks include using open and closed questions, facilitation (of the patient's response and questions), responding to verbal and non-verbal cues, summarizing information, and closing the session (von Fragstein et al. 2008).

SPs have a long history of involvement in the teaching and learning of communication skills in medicine and other health professions; role-playing scenarios, which enable the authentic simulation of doctor–patient consultations. Students interact with SPs as though they were taking a history, giving a diagnosis, or explaining a management plan with a real patient. An SP role may cover part of the consultation (e.g. giving a history) or all components of a full consultation, including physical examination.

In keeping with the model of helical learning, in addition to these core consultation skills, SPs have also been used successfully to train more senior learners in more complex consultation skills; for example, discussing medical error (Halbach and Sullivan 2005), sexual history-taking and human immunodeficiency virus (HIV) counseling (Haist et al. 2004), and identifying and exploring domestic violence issues (Haist et al. 2003). SPs can also be trained to portray patients who would probably decline to see students in real life but who have common problems, such as alcohol dependency (Eagles et al. 2001). Thus, many different scenarios or roles are needed if SPs are employed throughout a communication skills curriculum. These will range from straightforward history-taking scenarios for early skills training to complex presentations for more senior learners.

Similarly, the approaches to roles for which an SP may be trained also range widely from, for example, being reasonably passive (being examined by a learner with little interaction on the part of the SP) or giving a relatively straightforward, well-defined history, to acting the role of a 'vague' historian where the student has to be quite skilled to elicit necessary information, or asking challenging questions or demonstrating complex emotional reactions such as crying or anger.

In teaching, the use of SPs is mostly 'single-case'; a student has repeated but unconnected consultations with SPs. An important shortcoming of these single-case encounters is the lack of opportunity for students to learn about continuity of care. With the rapidly growing prevalence of chronic illness, there have been calls to improve the training of students in chronic care (Darer et al. 2004; Pham et al. 2004). This training requires extensive, longitudinal patient encounters rather than snapshot, single-case encounters (Diederiks et al. 2006). However, where longitudinal SP encounters have been used, student evaluations are generally positive (Brown et al. 2003; Linssen et al. 2008; Linssenet al. 2007; Rull et al. 2006). Furthermore, compared to single-case encounters, SPs found the longitudinal SP encounters more realistic, developed a more familiar relationship with the students and were able to provide the students with more detailed feedback (Linssen et al. 2007, 2008). Longitudinal encounters are also popular with students and staff (Bokken et al. 2009). However, such programmes require detailed planning in terms of training, management, and the logistics of matching SPs to students.

Also of relevance is the concept of psychological fidelity. This is the degree to which the skill or skills in the real task are captured in the simulated task (Druckman and Bjork 1994). The level of fidelity required depends on the type of task and stage of training. A complex scenario presented in an emotionally distraught manner by a highly trained SP is not appropriate where a young student is learning the basic skills involved in history taking. However, at advanced levels of training, complex tasks can be supported by use of SPs trained to give the correct cues to support high-level clinical decision-making.

Interprofessional education

SP involvement in teaching communication skills extends beyond the doctor–patient dyad to learning to communicate and work effectively in teams. Teamwork is critical to patient safety; poor staff communication and teamwork, as well as system failures, are greater contributors to medical error than poor individual performance (Mann et al. 2006). To be authentic, learning about teamwork in healthcare has to involve all those who work together, rather than each professional group separately. IPE, defined as occurring 'when two or more professions learn with, from and about each other to improve collaboration and the quality of care' (Center for Advancement of Interprofessional Education 2002), is considered an educational strategy that has potential benefit for improving teamwork and collaboration in practice, leading to improved patient outcomes (Irajpour et al. 2006). IPE simulation can create a risk-free and error-tolerant environment that is similar to clinical settings, where students from different professions can learn from and about each other to improve teamwork and quality of care, often using role play and SPs to deliberately practise teamwork and understanding of roles. A recent multidisciplinary study (Hobgood et al. 2010) involved SPs in the simulation of handover—looking at how best to support medical and nursing student acquisition of teamwork skills, knowledge, and attitudes. Students participated in a standardized patient exercise designed to elicit teamwork skills. Each participant was provided essential information needed by the team in order to treat the patient successfully and do a handover from Nurse A/Doctor A to Nurse B/Doctor B. Participants shared their information with the team, completed a focused patient history and physical exam, and completed orders for the patient.

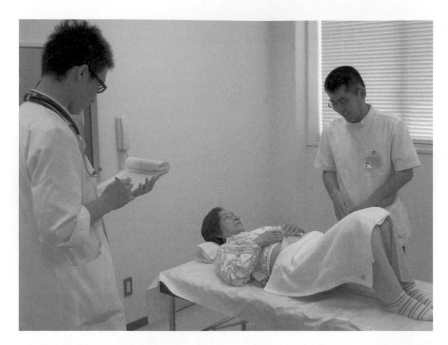

Figure 17.1 Medical students carrying out physical examination with a simulated patient.

Physical examination

Physical examination skills are a basic competency of clinical method. It is common practice for SPs with normal signs to be involved in early years teaching and learning of physical examination, where the teaching covers the basic techniques of physical examination or procedural skills. If you walk round a clinical skills centre on a teaching day, many rooms will contain learners trying to develop proficiency in examination skills by practising on SPs (fig. 17.1).

SPs are also involved in teaching sensitive physical examinations, most notably gynaecological and rectal examinations. Embarrassment, anxiety, fear of causing pain, and lack of confidence, hinder students in performing these examinations. In situations such as these, it is particularly important for students to learn and integrate their clinical skills in a safe environment that allows them to gain confidence and competence before encounters with real patients. The use of specialist groups of SPs (women who volunteer to undergo vaginal examinations and who are trained to provide feedback on technical and communication skills) was first reported in 1974 (Godkins et al. 1974) and is now well established in some medical schools, predominantly in the United States, Australia, and the Netherlands. Teaching programmes with these specialist SPs have been shown to be superior to training on plastic models in terms of developing students' skills in pelvic examination and interpersonal communication compared with controls, who received practical training only on clinical patients (Kleinman et al. 1996). Research also shows that students, teachers, and the SPs themselves view this training as of great value (Wanggren et al. 2005). However, it is difficult to recruit patients to these programmes, not just because of the nature of the examination but because women in the required age range (usually 20–40) are usually working or have other responsibilities (Van Ravesteijn et al. 2007).

If the purpose is measure a student's ability to identify important physical signs then real patients with these signs will usually, but not always, be required. Barrows stated that 'the only limitation for

topics/cases to be simulated by SPs is in one's mind' and described more than 50 physical findings that can be simulated (Barrows 1999). His list included all pain symptoms and pain syndromes. Barrows showed that even neurological signs such as, for example, loss of tendon reflexes, can be simulated by training the SP to exaggerate the reflexes on their 'healthy side'. However, Stillman (1993) emphasizes the need for considerable expertise if SPs are going to be trained to simulate signs and symptoms realistically. Clearly, training SPs to simulate physical signs and symptoms is quite an undertaking and usually real patients are used where real signs and symptoms are required.

Procedural skills

Opportunities to develop procedural skills (e.g., intravenous injection, urinary catheterization, gastroendoscopy) without harming real patients tended, until relatively recently, to focus on the use of stand-alone manikins or inanimate models. This meant that students learned communication skills and procedural skills separately. However, this did not mean that they could combine these technical and interpersonal skills with ease and safely perform the procedure on a live patient. Kneebone et al. proposed that simulation must be realistic, patient-focused, structured, and grounded in an authentic clinical context that recreates key components of the clinical experience (contextualized learning). They pioneered a combination of SPs and inanimate models as a means of heightening realism during simulated procedures (Kneebone 2005; Kneebone et al. 2002, 2005, 2007). This is referred to as hybrid simulation. They started with simple situations: imagine an SP lying on a surgery bed waiting to get an intravenous injection in the left arm. All the materials are there: syringes, patches, and vials. However, the SP's left arm is hidden under a sheet and instead of this real arm a phantom arm is visible for the doctor. This arm is placed in such a way that it looks as if this were the real arm. When the doctor touches this phantom arm, the SP reacts by saying something authentic such as 'ouch, it hurts when you touch my arm in that way'. In another situation, that of a male patient waiting for an urinary catheter procedure after being unable to void for 24 hours after surgery, clear use of sheets means the SP is positioned with a urinary tract model plus fake legs placed in such a way that it looks as if the patient is lying on the bed with only his penis uncovered, waiting for the doctor with the cathether. Again, the SP is trained to express pain and discomfort in a realistic way.

These simulations provide learners with an opportunity to integrate technical, communication and other professional skills essential for effective practice with real patients. They involve quite complex simulated patient training, however, which, for example, must includecd knowledge of key aspects of the procedure to ensure appropriate responses (e.g. time taken for a local anaesthetic to work).

It is important to ensure that patient preference for the extent of their role(s) is taken into account. Some SPs may be perfectly happy to be involved in physical examination and procedural skills training, others may wish only to take on consultation skills roles (Abe et al. 2005, 2009) Furthermore, where SPs indicate willingness to take on roles which involve physical examination, it is essential to explicitly find out what examinations they will consider, and if extra training is required. For example, in Maastricht, if SPs are willing to undergo genital or rectal examination, they are referred to specialist programmes. SPs may also have preferences for consultation skills scenarios: for example, we have found that SPs who smoke find roles involving being given a diagnosis of lung or mouth cancer or chronic obstructive pulmonary disease (COPD) emotionally difficult.

Objective structured clinical exams (OSCEs)

In assessment, SPs are used most commonly in the context of formal examinations, often in the form of objective structured clinical examinations (OSCEs) (Harden 1990; Harden and Gleeson 1979). OSCEs consist of multiple, standardized task-based stations, which mainly assess clinical and communication skills. The OSCE format is used extensively in healthcare education at undergraduate, postgraduate, and professional examination levels of training. In stations using SPs, learners may be expected to perform a physical examination or procedure, take a history, or give bad news. These exams provide a means of assessing clinical and communication skills in a systematic, standardized, and measurable way.

In assessment, SPs are trained not only to present the same case or symptoms, but to present the same emotional responses or attitudes towards their illness and symptoms, to provide consistent verbal and non-verbal responses during the consultation, and in response to questions and actions on the behalf of the learner. As such they are akin to the standardized patient described by Collins and Harden (1998).

SPs must present in a consistent, standardized manner to ensure that all students face the same test situation and to minimize variation in the examination (Ladyshewsky 1999). Additionally, multiple standardized patients can be trained to play the same patient role with relatively little measurement error (van der Vleuten and Swanson 1990). This is helpful in these days of many students and doctors in training sitting clinical exams, often over multiple sites at the same time. It also overcomes the difficulties of using real patients for assessment purposes as, while they may have the same condition and similar signs, these may change and/or their condition may deteriorate; or medication may preclude them from taking part.

For most exams, it is likely that a combination of real patients, with clearly abnormal findings, and simulated patients, with normal signs and predictable, standardised roles, will work best—depending on the purpose of the examination and the availability of suitable, real patients.

In situ assessment

The use of SPs for educational or assessment purposes, however, is no longer limited to medical schools or licensing bodies. SPs are being used increasingly to assess the performance of practising doctors, believing that performance under actual practice conditions differs from performance in structured examination conditions (Rethans et al. 2002). Simulated patients have been used successfully in this capacity, particularly in general practice. SP involvement in this type of assessment can be overt (Allen et al. 1998; Gerner et al. 2010) but SPs can also be used to measure candidate performance in real-life practice incognito. Practitioners who are visited by these incognito SPs are unaware that the consulting patient is not a real patient (Owen and Winkler 1974). Rethans et al. (2007a) found that more than 21 research projects have been carried out using incognito SPs. The majority of those projects were conducted in primary care but Gorter et al. (2002) demonstrated that it is feasible to use incognito SPs undetected in secondary care. In their study, when simulating rheumatic disease, accompanied by fake X-rays and fake laboratory results, incognito SPs were retrospectively identified in only 1% of hospital visits.

In short, studies examining the face validity of SPs have indicated that they have high face validity and usually candidates cannot discriminate between real and simulated patients. It is worth reinforcing at this point that validity can only be achieved by good training and preparation of SPs: it is likely that validity would be compromised where SPs were not prepared appropriately. Furthermore, ensuring standardization is critical when training and using SPs for assessment purposes. This may mean training a number of SPs to play the same role in exactly the same way, including what questions they ask the candidate, what information they should divulge when asked particular questions, and their emotional reactions. It is crucial that SPs play identical cases with minimal variation so all candidates are faced with exactly the same patient case and, hence, level of difficulty. A detailed, standardized script is required when using SPs for assessment purposes, whether this assessment is a formal examination or in practice. Wallace (2007) provides a detailed scenario for training SPs for assessment purposes. She describes the content of the training sessions, the areas to be addressed, and an estimated timetable for training. Other quality control procedures include recording SP performance in OSCE stations, then reviewing these tapes with the SP after the exam using structured checklists to provide the SP with constructive feedback. The Maastricht Assessment of Simulated Patients (MaSP) (Wind et al. 2004) checklist can also be used to assess SP performance.

Developing a bank of suitable scenarios plus guidance notes for the SP for teaching and assessment purposes is another time-consuming task, one which requires the involvement of appropriate clinical colleagues. For example, if developing a respiratory scenario for consultation skills teaching within the respiratory system semester, it is important to have input from one of the local respiratory physicians in terms of the focus of the scenario (e.g. asthma), relevant clinical content (what questions the student is likely to ask, and hence what answers the SP needs to learn), and some guidance as to how particular patients are likely to present (e.g. a teenager with asthma may be quite laissez-faire about self-management, which can be a challenging consultation requiring quite advanced communication skills from the doctor).

Feedback

Simulated patients can be trained not just to deliver a role for teaching or assessment purposes but also to assess the student's performance and provide feedback to the student (Blake et al. 2006, 2000). This may be in the form of a feedback sheet or checklist of the precise actions performed by the students during the encounter. Specific, skills-based feedback is a valuable and unique method for helping learning (Kurtz et al. 2005). The accuracy of SPs in recording checklist items has been found to be good and consistent (van der Vleuten and Swanson 1990).

Many centres are now expanding the role of SPs by using them to teach and/or assess clinical skills, initiatives that have been shown to be cost effective (McGraw and Connor 1999). There is an obvious practical advantage to this: reduced need for physician involvement in teaching and examination processes. However, training SPs to record student behaviours is quite a different task from training them to give feedback. This is a much more complex task, which depends on knowing the expected level of competence in students at different levels of training.

There is concern, however, that SPs may not be adequately trained or sufficiently experienced to teach or examine students to the appropriate professional standard, or to have the background knowledge to identify acceptable variations of students' skills. In addition to this, SPs may not have the skills to deliver adequate or appropriate feedback to students. The literature in this area of medical education is limited and conflicting (Rothman and Cusimano 2000) although there is evidence that reliability is related to the amount of training raters receive and the degree to which the measurement instruments and scoring procedures are standardized (Connell et al. 1993; Stillman et al. 1990; Vu et al. 1987, 1992). There is a need for further research into the validity and reliability of SPs as examiners.

Indeed, on a cautionary note, much of the research assessing SP input to teaching or assessment has been in the form of small studies using non-validated, subjective or questionable measures, or not reporting sufficient information in terms of, for example, SP training (Watson et al. 2006 for a notable exception). Lane and Rollnick's (2007) review of the use of simulated patients and role play in communication skills training, while not a critique of simulated patient methodology per se, highlights numerous other methodological issues, such as small sample sizes, in studies of this approach to teaching and learning.

Who can be a simulated patient?

Ability, suitability, and credibility must be considered.

Ability

Realistically and consistently presenting a role in the same way has been said to require both above-average intelligence and emotional maturity (Bowman et al. 1992). A SP must be able remember their role(s): including a number of medical facts, maintain focus, or concentration on delivering their roles over the time required; and realize the importance of sticking to the script provided. It is

relatively easy for an SP who is allowed to adjust the role to their real life situation, like family status and previous medical records. However, being asked to deliver a standardized performance, such as in an examination, is more demanding in terms of the sheer number of facts and instructions to remember.

Some roles are more emotionally complex and demanding than others but evidence suggests that SPs playing such roles, who follow a detailed script (and who do not bring their own experiences and characteristics to a role), suffer few negative emotional effects (McNaughton et al. 1999). Playing emotionally charged roles may, however, be something that only some SPs are comfortable with.

Where the SP is involved in giving feedback to the learner they must have the ability to manage the dual task of performing the role on the one hand, and remembering the students' performance at the same time. They must then be able to give appropriate feedback to the learner. In examination situations where SPs contribute to the assessment of a learner's performance, they must be trained in the criteria for judging performance and how these are applied.

Suitability

It is important to determine why the individual wishes to be an SP. You do not want to recruit a SP who has a negative attitude, or a personal crusade, towards the medical profession, or the healthcare profession with which you wish them to help in training. Your priority is to protect the students' safety while trying to maximize their educational experience and develop their confidence—so screening potential SPs is necessary (Ker et al. 2005).

Conscientiousness is also important: someone who commits to a teaching session or a clinical exam but then fails to attend without notice is worse than useless. To underpin conscientiousness, it is important to explicitly outline the responsibilities of being a SP at the time of recruitment. This may be something along the lines of 'being available for five sessions over an academic term'. Being explicit about what is required from a simulated patient is helpful for both parties (fig 17.2).

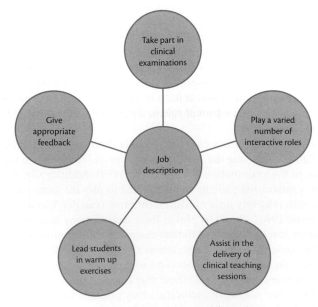

Figure 17.2 A typical example of the main responsibilities of a simulated patient.

Credibility

Inevitably, in any discussion of simulation, the term fidelity will be used to describe some aspect of the reality of the experience. Fidelity is the extent to which the appearance and behaviour of the simulator or simulation match the appearance and behaviour of the simulated system (Farmer et al. 1999). In terms of SPs, a more appropriate term might be credibility. Your SP must be credible in the role they are playing. For example, it is important that the SP appears like the actual patient being simulated.

Children can be SPs. Lane et al. (1999) reported that children as young as seven years of age, trained to present a clinical case, were good role-players. Brown et al. (2005) found that children as young as nine could play psychiatric roles. One method of using young children as SPs is to recruit a 'parent and child pair' who play themselves. We used this approach in Aberdeen and found it worked well, particularly with young children. Trained adolescents have been used to allow medical students to practise communication about topics such as risk-taking activities and confidentiality (Blake and Greaven 1999; Blake et al. 2000, 2006, ; Bokken et al. 2010b) and have also been successfully used as SPs in the training and assessment of doctors (Hardoff and Schonmann 2001; Lane et al. 1999).

Many SPs are people who have retired from work and thus have time to volunteer for tasks which interest them, such as helping train medical students. Younger SPs are usually students, who can be recruited through university administration or college societies. While it is critical to strive for authenticity and credibility, it can be difficult to recruit SPs aged between 25–50 years as people in their middle-years are usually fully engaged in employment and/or home responsibilities. In practice, it can sometimes be difficult to match required scenarios with the SP pool available in an authentic way.

No matter how good a SP, quality assurance and training are ongoing processes. Do not expect to train a SP in a role(s) and not have to assess and address training needs over time (Adamo 2003). A single SP can only perform a limited number of encounters before they begin to make mistakes. Training, and retraining SPs, is one of the resource costs involved in having an SP programme.

On being a simulated patient

The emphasis on research into simulated patients has mostly concerned the validity, reliability, consistency, feasibility and costs of the use of SPs (Barrows and Abrahamson 1964; Rethans 1998; Stillman et al. 1990, van der Vleuten and Swansen 1990). Only recently has the impact of simulating a patient role on an individual been explored. Research has focused on examining either the effect of simulating a patient role or the impact of doing so on the individual's subsequent contact with healthcare professionals.

McNaughton et al. (1999) used focus groups to explore the impact on SPs of performing affective psychiatric roles. The majority of the SPs mentioned negative effects, consisting predominantly of stress symptoms like exhaustion, irritability, sleeping problems and physical complaints. The number of patient roles and amount of experience as an SP influence the probability of an SP experiencing such symptoms (Woodward 1998; Woodward and Gliva-McConvey 1995). Debriefing after playing a role seems important (van Ments 1999). Reassuringly, however, any symptoms of stress identified as a result of being an SP seem to be short-lived and to do not affect SPs' enjoyment of the work (Bokkenet al. 2006; Naftulin and Andrew 1975).

Studies have also looked at the impact of performing a patient role for adolescent SPs and identified no negative findings (Blake and Greaven 1999; Bokken et al. 2006; Hanson et al. 2002). This may be attributable to the careful selection of adolescent SPs in these studies.

Of interest is a study from Japan (Abe 2007). The SPs in this study reported that feelings of stress connected with performance and involvement in assessment decreased over time but stress about giving feedback did not. This suggests that giving feedback is a different task to role play, and one where we need more information as to how we can best support SPs.

Other studies have looked at the long-term effects on being an SP on subsequent contact with healthcare professionals. These found that SPs developed a more balanced view of healthcare professionals, developed better communication skills and became more tolerant of others during the course of their contact with healthcare professionals (Woodward 1998; Woodward and Gliva-McConvey 1995). Wallach et al. (2001) reported that SPs had a better understanding of medical history taking and physical examination, showed improved communication with healthcare professionals and were more comfortable with healthcare visits, especially regarding physical examination.

Thus, it seems that being an SP may bring short-term stressors, which can be minimized by careful management of SP roles, training and debriefing, but long-term benefits in terms of healthcare communication and understanding.

Conclusions

- ◆ Simulated patients are indispensible in medical and healthcare education.

- ◆ Use of SPs is theoretically robust, mapping onto theories of experiential learning, deliberate practice and situated learning.

- ◆ This immensely valuable resource circumvents many of the present day difficulties in accessing and using real patients, enables safe, early clinical contact in medical training, as well as innovative and yet replicable and standardized training and assessment at all stages of medical education.

- ◆ Students report that feedback from SPs is particularly valuable.

- ◆ There has been much research into the use of SPs in medical education but the need remains for robust, well-designed studies into their use and impact on teaching and assessment in order to maximize our understanding of best practice and ensure best-evidence medical education.

Further resources

The Association of Standardized Patient Educators http://www.aspeducators.org/

References

Abe, K., Mukohara, K., and Ban, N. (2005) Qualitative analysis of how simulated patients perceive physical examinations. *Jap J Med Educ.* 36: 107–111

Abe, K., Suzuki, T., Fujisaki, K., and Ban, N. (2007) Demographic characteristics of standardized patients and their satisfaction and sense of burden in Japan: The first report of a nationwide survey. *Jap J Med Educ.* 38: 301–307

Abe, K., Suzuki, T., Fujisaki, K., and Ban, N. (2009) A national survey to explore the willingness of Japanese standardized patients to participate in teaching physical examination skills to undergraduate medical students. *Teaching and Learning in Medicine*, 21, 240–247.

Accreditation Council for Graduate Medical Education (1999) ACGME Outcome Project. Accreditation Council for Graduate Medical Education. Chicago: Illinois

Adamo, G. (2003) Simulated and standardized patients in OSCEs: achievements and challenges 1992–2003. *Med Teach*. 25: 262–270

Allen, J., Evans, A., Foulkes, J., and French, A. (1998) Simulated surgery in the summative assessment of general practice training: results of a trial in the Trent and Yorkshire regions. *Br J Gen Pract*. 48: 1219–1223

Arthur, W., Bennett, W., Stanush, P.L., and McNelly, T.L. (1998) Factors that influence skill decay and retention. A quantitative review and analysis. *Hum Perf*. 11: 57–101

Barrows, H.S. (1987) *Simulated (Standardized) Patients and Other Human Simulations*. Chapel Hill (NC): Health Sciences Consortium

Barrows, H.S. (1999) *Training Standardized Patients to have Physical Findings*. Springfield: Southern Illinois: Illinois University School of Medicine

Barrows, H.S. and Abrahamson, S. (1964) The programmed patient: a technique for appraising student performance in clinical neurology. *J Med Educ*. 39: 802–805

Beshgetoor, D. and Wade, D. (2007) Use of actors as simulated patients in nutritional counselling. *J Nutr Educ Behav*. 39: 101–102

Beullens J., Rethans J.J,, Goedhuijs J., and Buntinx F. (1997) The use of standardized patients in research in general practice. *Fam Pract*. 14: 58–62

Blake, K. and Greaven, S. (1999) Adolescent girls as simulators of medical illness. *Med Educ*. 33: 702–703

Blake, K., Mann, K.V., Kaufman, D.M., and Kappelman, M. (2000) Learning adolescent psychosocial interviewing using simulated patients. *Acad Med*. 75(10 Suppl): S56–S58

Blake, K.D., Gusella, J., Greaven, S., and Wakefield, S. (2006) The risks and benefits of being a young female adolescent standardised patient. *Med Educ*. 40: 26–35

Bokken, L., Linssen, T., Scherpier, A., van Der Vleuten, C., and Rethans, J.J. (2009) The longitudinal simulated patient program: evaluations by teachers and students and feasibility. *Med Teach*, 31: 613–620

Bokken, L., Rethans, J.J., Jobsis, Q., Duvidier, R., Scherpbier, A., and van Der Vleuten, C. (2010) Instructiveness of real patients and simulated patients in undergraduate medical education: a randomized trial. *Acad Med*. 85: 148–154

Bokken, L., Van Dalen, J., and Rethans, J.J. (2006) The impact of simulation on people who act as simulated patients: a focus group study. *Med Educ*. 40: 781–786

Bokken, L., Van Dalen, J., and Rethans, J.J. (2010b) The case of 'Miss Jacobs': adolescent simulated patients and the quality of their role playing, feedback, and personal impact. *Simul Healthc: J Soc Simul Healthc*. 5: 315–319

Bowman, M.A., Russell, N.K., Boekeloo, B.O., Rafi, I.Z., and Rabin, D.L. (1992) The effect of educational preparation on physician performance with a sexually transmitted disease-simulated patient. *Arch Intern Med*. 152: 1823–1828

Brown, A., Anderson, D., and Szerlip, H.M. (2003) Using standardized patients to teach disease management skills to preclinical students: a pilot project. *Teach Learn Med*. 15: 84–87

Brown, R., Doonan, S., and Shellenberger, S. (2005) Using children as simulated patients in communication training for residents and medical students: a pilot program. *Acad Med*. 80: 1114–1120

Cartwright, M.S., Reynolds, P.S., Rodrigues, Z.M., Breyer, W.A., and Cruz, J.M. (2005) Lumbar puncture experience among medical school graduates: the need for formal procedural skills training. *Med Educ*, 39: 437

Centre for Advancement in Interprofessional Education (CAIPE 2002) *Interprofessional education. Defining IPE*. http://www.caipe.org.uk/resources/ Accessed 19 February 2012

Cleland, J., Abe, K., and Rethans, J.J. (2009) The use of simulated patients in medical education: AMEE Guide No 42. *Med Teach*. 31: 477–486

Cleland, J.A., Abe, K., and Rethans, J.J. (2010) *The use of simulated patients in Med Educ. AMEE Teaching and Learning Guide no. 10*. Dundee: Association for Medical Education in Europe (AMEE)

Collins, J.P. and Harden, R.M. (1998) AMEE Medical Education Guide No. 13: real patients, simulated patients and simulators in clinical examinations. *Med Teach*. 20: 508–521

Connell, K.J., Sinacore, J.M., Schmid, F.R., Chang, R.W., and Perlman, S.G. (1993) Assessment of clinical competence of medical students by using standardized patients with musculoskeletal problems. *Arthritis Rheum*. 36: 394–400

Darer, J.D., Hwang, W., Pham H.H., Bass, E.B., and Anderson, G. (2004) More training needed in chronic care: A survey of US physicians. *Acad Med*. 79: 541–548

Diederiks, J.P., Bosma, H., Van Eijk, J.T., Van Santen, M., Scherpbier, A., and van Der Vleuten, C. (2006) Chronic patients in undergraduate education: Didactic value as perceived by students. *Med Educ*. 40: 787–791

Druckmann, D. and Bjork, R. (eds) (1994) *Learning. Remembering. Believing. Enhancing Human Performance*. Washington, DC: National Academic Press

Eagles, J.M., Calder, S.A., Nicoll, K.S., and Walker, L.G. (2001) A comparison of real patients, simulated patients and videotaped interview in teaching medical students about alcohol misuse. *Med Teach*. 23: 490–493

Eagles, J.N., Calder, S.A., Wilson, S., Murdoch, J.M., and Sclare, P.D. (2007) Simulated patients in undergraduate education in psychiatry. *Psychiatr Bull*. 31: 187–190

Ericsson, K.A., Krampe, R.T., and Tesch-Romer, C. (1993) The role of deliberate practice in the acquisition of expert performance. *Psychol Rev*. 100: 363–406

Farmer, E., Van Rooig, L., Riemersma, J., Joma, P., and Morall, J. (1999) *Handbook of Simulator Based Training*. Aldershot, UK: Ashgate

Friedman, M., Sutnick, A.L., Stillman, P.I., et al. (1991) The use of standardised patients to evaluate the spoken English proficiency of foreign medical graduates. *Acad Med*. 66: S61–S63

General Medical Council (2009) *Tomorrow's Doctors: recommendations on undergraduate medical education*. General Medical Council: London

Gerner, B., Sanci, L., Cahill, H., et al. (2010) Using simulated patients to develop doctors' skills in facilitating behaviour change: addressing childhood obesity. *Med Educ*, 44: 706–715

Godkins, T.R., Duffy, D., Greenwood, J., and Stanhope, W.D. (1974) Utilisation of simulated patients to teach the 'routine' pelvic examination. *J Med Educ*, 49: 1174–1178

Gordon, J.A., Oriol, N.E., and Cooper, J.E. (2004) Bringing good teaching cases to life: a simulator-based medical education service. *Acad Med*. 79: 23–27

Gorter, S., Van Der Heijde, D.M., Van Der Linden, S., et al. (2002) Psoriatic arthritis: performance of rheumatologists in daily practice. *Ann Rheum Dis*. 61: 219–224

Guile, D. and Young, M. (2001) Apprenticeship as a conceptual basis for a social theory of learning. In: Paechter C, Preedy M, Scott D, Soler J (eds) *Knowledge. Power and Learning* (pp.56–73). London: Paul Chapman Publishing

Haist, S.A., Griffith, C.H., Hoellein, A.R., Talente, G., Montgomery, T., and Wilson, J.F. (2004) Improving students' sexual history inquiry and HIV counselling with an interactive workshop using standardized patients. *J Gen Intern Med*. 19: 549–553

Haist, S.A., Wilson, J.F., and Pursley, H.G. (2003) Domestic violence: increasing knowledge and improving skills with a four-hour workshop using standardized patients. *Acad Med*. 78: S24–S26

Halbach, J.L. and Sullivan, L.L. (2005) Teaching medical students about medical errors and patient safety: evaluation of a required curriculum. *Acad Med*. 80: 600

Hanson, M., Tiberius, R., Hodgens, B., et al. (2002) Adolescent standardized patients: method of selection and assessment of benefits and risks. *Teach Learn Med*. 14: 104–113

Harden, R.M. (1990) *The OSCE—a 15 year perspective*. Montreal: Can-Heal Publications

Harden, R.M. and Gleeson, F.A. (1979) Assessment of clinical competence using an objective structured clinical examination (OSCE) *Med Educ*. 13: 41–54

Hardoff, D. and Schonmann, S. (2001) Training physicians in communication skills with adolescents using teenage actors as simulated patients. *Med Educ*. 35: 206–210

Hobgood, C., Sherwood, G., Frush, K., Hollar, D., and Maynard, L. (2010) Teamwork training with nursing and medical students: does the method matter? Results of an inter-institutional, interdisciplinary collaboration. *Quality Safety Health Care*. 19: e25

Hoppe R.B. (1995) Standardized (simulated) patients and the medical interview. In: M. Lipkin Jr, S.M. Putnam, and A. Lazare (eds) *The Medical Interview*. New York: Springer Verlag

Irajpour, I., Norman, P., and Griffiths, P. (2006) Interprofessional education to improve pain management. *Br J Community Nursing*. 11: 29–32.

Ker, J.S., Dowie, A., Dowell, J., et al. (2005) Twelve tips for developing and maintaining a simulated patient bank. *Med Teach*. 27: 4–9

Ker, J., Mole, L., and Bradley, P. (2003) Early introduction to interprofessional learning: a simulated ward environment. *Med Educ*, 37: 248–255

Kleinman, D.E., Hage, M.L., Hoole, A.J., and Kowlitz, V. (1996) Pelvic examination instruction and experience: a comparison of laywomen-trained and physician-trained students. *Acad Med*, 71: 1239–1243

Kneebone, R. (2005) Evaluating clinical simulations for learning procedural skills: a theory-based approach. *Acad Med*. 80: 549–553

Kneebone, R., Kidd, J., Nestel, D., Asvall, S., Paraskeva, P., and Darzi, A. (2002) An innovative model for teaching and learning clinical procedures. *Med Educ*. 36: 628–634

Kneebone, R.L., Kidd, J., Nestel, D., et al. (2005) Blurring the boundaries: scenario-based simulation in a clinical setting. *Med Educ*. 39: 580–587

Kneebone, R., Kidd, J., Nestel, D., and Darzi, A. (2007) Complexity, risk and simulation in learning procedural skills. *Med Educ*, 41: 808–814

Kolb, D.A. (1984) *Experiential Learning: Experience as the Source of Learning and Development*. Englewood Cliffs, NJ: Prentice Hall

Kurtz, S., Silverman, J., and Draper, J. (2005) *Teaching and Learning Communication Skills in Medicine* (3rd edn). Oxford: Radcliffe Medical Press

Ladyshewsky, R. (1999) Simulated patients and assessment. *Med Teach*. 21: 266–269

Lane, C. and Rollnick, S. (2007) The use of simulated patients and role play in communication skills training: A review of the literature to August 2005. *Patient Educ Counselling*. 67: 13–20

Lane, J.L., Ziv, A., and Boulet, J.R. (1999) A pediatric clinical skills assessment using children as standardized patients. *Arch Pediatr Adolesc Med*. 153: 637–644

Linssen, T., Van Dalen, J., and Rethans, J.J. (2007) Simulating the longitudinal doctor-patient relationship: experiences of simulated patients in successive consultations. *Med Educ*. 41: 873–878

Linssen, T., Bokken, L., and Rethans, J.J. (2008) Return visits by simulated patients. *Med Educ*. 42: 536

Maguire, G.P. and Rutter, D.R. (1976) History taking for medical students. 1. Deficiencies in performance. *Lancet*. 2: 556–558

Madan, A.K., Caruso, B.A., Lopers, J.E., and Gracely, E.J. (1998) Comparison of simulated patient and didactic methods of teaching HIV risk assessment to medical residents. *Am J Prevent Med*. 15: 114–119

Makoul, G. (2003) The interplay between education and research about patient-provider communication. *Patient Educ Counselling*. 50: 79–84

Mann, S., Marcus, R., and Sachs, B. (2006) Lessons from the cockpit: How team training can reduce errors on LandD. *Contemp Obstet Gynecol*. 51: 34–42

Mann, K.V. (2011) Theoretical perspectives in medical education: past experience and future possibilities. *Med Educ*, 45: 60–68

McGraw, R.C. and O'Connor, H.M. (1999) Standardized patients in the early acquisition of clinical skills. *Med Educ*, 33: 572–578

McManus, I., Richards, P., and Winder, B. (1998) Clinical experience of UK medical students. *Lancet*. 351: 802–803

McNaughton, N., Tiberius, R., and Hodges, B. (1999) Effects of portraying psychologically and emotionally complex standardised patient roles. *TeachLearn Med*. 11: 135–141

Naftulin, D.H. and Andrew, B.J. (1975) The effects of patient simulations on actors. *J Med Educ*. 50: 87–89

Norman, G.R., Tugwell, P., and Feightner, J.W. (1982) A comparison of resident performance on real and simulated patients. *J Med Educ*. 57: 708–715

Osler, W. (1905) The hospital as a college. In: H.K. Lewis (ed.) *Aequanimatus. and Other Addresses*. H.K. Lewis: London, Chapter XVI

Owen, A. and Winkler, R. (1974) General practitioners and psychological problems. An evaluation using pseudopatients. *Med J Aust*. 2: 393–398

Pham, H.H., Simonson, L., Elnicki, D.M., Fried, L.P., Goroll, A.H., and Bass, E.B. 2004. Training U.S. medical students to care for the chronically ill. *Acad Med*. 79: 32–40

Rees, C.A., Sheard, C., and McPherson, A. (2004) Medical students' views and experiences of methods of teaching and learning communication skills. *Patient Educ Counselling*. 54: 119–121

Rethans, J.J. (1998) Needs assessments in continuing medical education through standardised patients. *J Cont Educ Health Prof*. 18: 172–178

Rethans, J.J., Gortor, S., Bokken, L., and Morrison, L. (2007) Unannounced standardised patients in real practice: a systematic literature review. *Med Educ*. 41(6): 537–549

Rethans, J.J., Norcini, J., Baron-Moldonado, M., et al. (2002) The relationship between competence and performance: implications for assessing practice performance. *Med Educ*. 36: 901–909

Rollnick, S., Kinnersley, P., and Butler, C. (2002) Context-bound communication skills training: development of a new method. *Med Educ*. 36: 377–383

Rothman, A. and Cusimano, M. (2000) A comparison of physician examiners', standardized patients', and communication experts' ratings of international medical graduates' English proficiency. *Acad Med*. 75: 206–211

Rull, G., Rosher, R.B., McCann-Stone, N., and Robinson, S.B. (2006) A simulated couple aging across the four years of medical school. *Teach Learn Med*. 18: 261–266

Simpson, M., Buckman, R., Stewart, M., et al. (1991) Doctor-patient communication: the Toronto consensus statement. *BMJ*. 303: 1385–1387

Spencer, J and McKimm, J. (2010) Patient involvement in Med Educ. In: Swanwick, T. (ed) *Understanding Medical Education: evidence. theory and practice* (pp. 181–194). Oxford: John Wiley and Sons

Stewart, M., Brown, J.B., Boon, H., Galagda, J., Meredith, L., and Sangster, M. (1999) Evidence on patient-doctor communication. *Cancer Prev Control*. 3: 25–30

Stillman, P.L., Regan, M.B., Philbin, M., and Haley, H.L. (1990) Results of a survey on the use of standardized patients to teach and evaluate clinical skills. *Acad Med*. 65: 288–292

Stillman, P.L. (1993) Technical issues: logistics. AAMC. *Acad Med*. 68: 464–468

van der Vleuten, C. and Swanson, D. (1990) Assessment of clinical skills with standardised patients: state of the art. *Teach Learn Med*. 2: 58–76

Van Ments, M. (1999) *The Effective Use of Role Play*. 2nd edn. London: Kogan Page

Van Ravesteijn, H., Hageraats, E., and Rethans, J.J. (2007) Training of the gynaecological examination in the Netherlands. *Med Teach*. 29: e93–e99

von Fragstein, M., Silverman, J., Cishing, A., Quilligan, S., Salisbury, H., and Wiskin, C. (2008) UK consensus statement on the content of communication curricula in undergraduate medical education. *Med Educ*. 42(11): 1100–1107

Vu, N.V., Steward, D.E., and Marcy, M. (1987) An assessment of the consistency and accuracy of standardized patients' simulations. *J Med Educ*. 62: 1000–1002

Vu, N.V., Marcy, M.M., Colliver, J.A,, Verhulst, S.J., Travis, T.A., and Barrows, H.S. (1992) Standardized (simulated) patients' accuracy in recording clinical performance check-list items. *Med Educ*, 26(2): 99–104

Wallace, P. (2007) *Coaching Standardized Patients for use in the Assessment of Clinical Competence*. New York: Springer Publishing

Wallach, P.M., Elnick, M., Bognar, B., et al. (2001) Standardized patients' perceptions about their own health care. *Teach Learn Med.* 13: 227–231

Wanggren, K., Pettersson, G., Rgycsemiczky, G., and Gemzell-Danielsoon, K. (2005) Teaching medical students gynaecological examination using professional patients—evaluation of students' skills and feelings. *Med Teach.* 27: 130–135

Watson, M.C., Cleland, J.A., Francis, J., Inch, J., and Bond, C.W. (2007) Communication skills training for medicine counter assistants to improve consultations for non-prescription medicines. *Med Educ,* 41: 450–459

Watson, M.C., Norris, P., and Granas, A.G. (2006) A systematic review of the use of simulated patients and pharmacy practice research. *Int J Pharmacy Pract.* 14: 83–93

Wenger, E. (1998) *Communities of Practice. Learning. Meaning and Identity.* Cambridge: Cambridge University Press

Wind, L.A., Van Dalen, J., Muijtjens, A.M., and Rethans, J.J. (2004) Assessing simulated patients in an educational setting: the MaSP (Maastricht Assessment of Simulated Patients) *Med Educ.* 38: 39–44

Woodward, C.A. (1998) Standardised patients: a fixed role therapy experience in normal individuals. *J Construct Psychol.* 11: 133–148

Woodward, C.A. and Gliva-McConvey, G. (1995) The effect of simulating on standardized patients. *Acad Med.* 70: 418–420

Zhang, C., Thompson, S., and Miller, C. (2011) A review of simulation-based interprofessional education. *Clin Simul Nursing.* 7: c117–e126

Ziv, A., Wolpe, P.R., Small, S.D., and Glick, S. (2003) Simulation-based Med Educ: an ethical imperative. *Acad Med.* 78: 783–788

CHAPTER 18

Work-based learning

Clare Morris and Martina Behrens

One of the key problems in developing learning is how to recognise and accredit learning undertaken in the workplace.

Nigel Oswald

Reproduced from Oswald N, 'Agenda for Change: agenda for learning change', Education for Primary Care, 16, pp. 644–647, © Radcliffe Publishing, 2005, with permission

Introduction

Medicine has a long tradition of recognizing the workplace as a significant site for learning. The emphasis on hospitals as a prime focus for this learning can be traced back to the French revolution, with the Hôtel-Dieu in Paris being regarded as the birthplace of clinical medicine (Calman 2006). From then on, clinical medicine has been practised and learnt at the bedside all across the globe. Throughout the centuries, debates arise about the best ways to combine book knowledge with practical experience; as medicine moved into European universities, differences in the preparation of the magister medicinae and medicus (scholarly physician versus craftsman) were the focus (Calman 2006). Six centuries later, in the UK, echoes of the past remain. The General Medical Council (GMC) articulates distinct outcomes for doctors as scholars and scientists, as practitioners and as professionals (GMC 2009a). Between medical schools, differences are observed in the ways in which theoretical and practical elements are combined. Some favour traditional preclinical/clinical models, which frontload knowledge. Others embrace problem- and system-based models, seeking to integrate different types of professional knowledge and experience. Whichever model is adopted, and no matter how rapidly medical knowledge and contexts change, learning in, for and from practice remains an essential part of the work of medical professionals (fig. 18.1). It is this learning that is the focus of this chapter—work-based learning—argued by Evans (2012, p. 6) as 'best understood as learning that derives its purposes for the contexts of work'. Current conceptualizations of work-based learning are varied and wide, exploring 'relationships between the two fundamental human and societal processes of learning and working' (Evans et al. 2011, p. 149).

How this relationship is to be explained depends on the observer's viewpoint; a singular answer to the question cannot be expected. However, to build a bigger picture from influencing disciplines (such as psychology and sociology) offers an inclusive way of thinking about work-based learning, described by Siebert (2012, p. 115) as being 'in the face of ambiguity and uncertainty, plurality and contingency'.

In this chapter we adopt an inclusive definition, viewing learning as:

> …the combination of processes whereby the whole person—body (genetic, physical, and biological) and mind (knowledge, skills, attitudes, values, emotions, beliefs, and senses)—experiences a social situation, the perceived content of which is then transformed cognitively, emotively or practically (or through any combination) and integrated into the person's individual biography resulting in a changed (or more experienced) person

Jarvis 2006, p. 13.

Consider the junior doctor, coming towards the end of a night shift, who is faced with an acute medical emergency (the 'social situation'). In this critical moment, they make a rapid decision for action, based on their prior knowledge, experience and skill ('mind'). Their decision to call for help is shaped by this and their affective response (encompassing, for example, fatigue, levels of confidence, and self belief). It may, of course, also be shaped by wider contextual issues such as organizational protocol, curriculum requirements, and the type of relationship they have with their supervising clinician. The actions they take in this moment have consequences not only for the patient, but also in the learning that arises from the transformation of their response to the situation. Cognitively, they may further develop their understanding of the particular disease process. Emotionally they may discover new insights into the ways in which they function in stressful circumstances. Practically, they may hone skills as part of the resuscitation team. Given that no two junior doctors will be the same (in terms of personality, biography, experience, or situation) the learning arising for each will be different.

It is not only individuals who learn in such a situation, but also the organization and wider societal system. Those working alongside the junior doctor gain new knowledge about their performance and the expertise they might bring to their shared work. They may realize that their handover practices could be further developed, but be reassured they handle medical emergencies well as a team. Alternatively, they may identify causes for concern, around

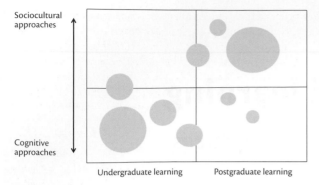

Figure 18.1 Approaches to work-based learning in the medical education literature.

level of medical cover, to feed back into organization practices. The relationships between learning and working are undoubtedly complex. In the next section we review how they are understood within the medical education literature.

Working and learning relationships in the medical education literature

The terms 'work-based' and 'workplace' learning are argued to have 'entered the lexicon of higher education' in the 1980s (Evans et al. 2011) when the move to integrate learning based on work activity, within higher education, was seen as attempt to 'engage seriously with the economic, social and educational demands of our era' (Boud and Solomon 2001, p. 3). Learning based on work activity has long been a feature of professional education, medicine included. The timing and duration of such learning is influenced by factors such as: the choice of curriculum model; the capacity of the workplace to support placements, and regulator requirements. In our exploration of the medical education literature, we notice a number of tendencies in the ways in which working–learning relationships are understood and articulated.

The first tendency observed, is that the literature is skewed towards early professional formation and concerns about graduates' readiness for medical work. Fewer studies offer insights into the continuous, work-related learning which underpins the development of medical practice. The ways in which more experienced workers continue to learn for and from work activity is marginalized, or reduced to an account of hours of continuing professional development. If work-based learning, however, is to be understood as the relationship between the 'two fundamental human and social processes of working and learning' (Evans 2012, p. 6), the consequence is that every worker learns through and for work, throughout their working lives. Work-based learning does not become the domain of particular groups of workers (e.g. medical professionals) or workers at particular stages of their working lives (e.g. new graduates). An emphasis on the learner status of particular workers runs the risk of decoupling learning and work, seeing them as distinct rather than mutually constitutive activities. We learn for work and we learn from work; artificial distinctions between time for service and time for educational activity downplay this. A more nuanced account of the nature of working and learning relationships, throughout the lifespan of a medical professional is warranted.

The second tendency is an emphasis on teaching and assessment methods, rather than learning per se. It is perhaps because of the

emphasis on undergraduate education and related gatekeeping functions that this occurs. We note, however, that the faculty development literature, concerned with the development of doctors as educators, have perhaps rather too closely followed the approach '...of handing out recipes and models to be followed in teaching' (Dewey 1916, p. 170). Scant attention is paid to the conceptions of learning that may underpin pedagogic practices. Some commentators express go so far as to dismiss educational discourse as futile: 'faculty members want simple messages, concepts and directions, and it is our responsibility to avoid complexity and promote practicality' (Steinert 2000, p. 48).

This position is countered by those who are critical of the a-theoretical nature of much medical education research. They argue the need to broaden conceptions of learning in order to make sense of and develop educational practices, a position we support (Swanwick 2005; Bleakley 2006; Bordage 2009; Morris and Blaney 2010).

A final tendency is the limited educational discourse about the nature of working and learning relationships in medicine. This is surprising, given the long and rich traditions of medical apprenticeship. Professions such as medicine have, historically, self-regulated how knowledge is created, how experiences are to be gained, and have adapted curricula accordingly. Medical apprenticeship practices are perhaps so deep seated that the need to make them explicit only arises when they cease to be sustainable or when regulatory relationships change.

Beck and Young (2005, p. 183) provide a powerful commentary on the challenges to professional autonomy, knowledge and identity experienced in recent years—exploring the consequences 'particularly with regard to their relationship to knowledge, to clients, and the organisational structures within which most of them work'.

Changing relationships between the medical profession, state and society are perhaps most readily observed in increasing regulation of working and training practices. One such example in the UK was the 'modernization' of medical careers, which lead to a public inquiry into the purposes and practices of postgraduate medical education (Tooke 2007). This and the most recent edition of *Tomorrow's Doctors* (GMC 2009a) reflect current policy preoccupations with professional standards and accountability, wrapped up in concerns for patient safety. The need to show 'evidence' of safe working practice has perhaps hastened a move to the competency-based training models seen across the globe. Whilst the intent behind such changes may be benign, the consequences for work-based learning may be less so. For example, clinicians operating in an increasingly risk-averse context may be less likely to delegate aspects of work activity to their more junior colleagues. If working and learning are integrally related, this narrows opportunities for development. This may make the practice of junior colleagues more, rather than less risky, when they are carrying responsibility for patient care without close supervision. In limiting the educational discourse in this area, doctors fail to equip themselves with the theoretical and conceptual resources to challenge policymakers' beliefs about the best ways to educate and train doctors.

Our brief exploration of accounts of working–learning relationships in medical education identifies a need to develop thinking about work-based learning on three levels; first, to offer a more nuanced account of medical working and learning relationships throughout a professional lifespan; second, to provide access to key educational debates, in order to broaden current conceptions of learning; and finally, to offer up conceptual tools that may allow the medical profession to respond meaningfully to rapidly changing work-based learning contexts.

Changing approaches to medical education and training

We have suggested that work-based learning comes into focus when traditional methods of medical apprenticeship (starting with theoretical inputs) are challenged. New regulatory arrangements hold previously closed practices up to external scrutiny and changed work patterns make apprenticeship difficult to sustain. The introduction of shift working in medicine, for example, weakens training relationship bonds. Apprenticeship is supported by stable societal, organizational and personal systems; global examples of this can be readily identified. The Flexner reforms created a coherent, shared approach to medical training in the USA and Canada, influencing training across the world (Flexner 1910). The creation of the UK National Health Service in 1947 provided the conditions to plan medical training, ensuring it was the responsibility of its senior medical staff. Apprenticeship is undermined in times of uncertainty and the types of system reform, which fragment or reduce healthcare provision and resources (Morris 2011; Dornan et al 2011). For example, advances in medical practice alongside changing population demographics (e.g. increased prevalence of chronic disease) support a move to community-based healthcare. This creates tensions in a system relying on teaching at the hospital bedside. The number of available bedsides is reduced and the patients occupying these beds have increasingly complex medical needs, going beyond those that can be managed by trainees.

Forms of apprenticeship have evolved over the centuries but can be seen as an approach that seeks to bring together theoretical and practical elements. The apprentice develops both subject-specific and work-based knowledge, bringing together the magister medicinae and medicus of old. Apprenticeship, based upon strong relationship ties, unsurprisingly contributes to the identity building of individuals and the profession itself.

These processes of socialization into the profession, encompassing ways of thinking, feeling and acting, are often referred to as the hidden curriculum of medicine. Seven centuries ago, such elements were visible, with students of the medical school of Vienna being required to obey rules of practice that related to their approaches to learning and practice and extended into personal conduct (Calman 2006). Whilst we may find the guidance on the characteristics of a suitable wife archaic, the caution to avoid party going and to 'be aloof of civil cares' (Calman 2006) has resonances with the fitness to practise discourse that begins on day 1 of undergraduate medical education in the UK:

> students must be aware that their behaviour outside the clinical environment, including in their personal lives, may have an impact on their fitness to practise...behaviour at all times must justify the trust the public places in the medical profession (GMC 2009b, p. 7).

This expectation that students behave as if already doctors signals a shifting rhetoric from that of the Todd Inquiry, which posits that 'the aim of the undergraduate course should be to produce not a finished doctor but a broadly educated man who can become a doctor by further training' (Todd 1968, p. 23).

We propose that undergraduate medical education continues to function as a starting point for later development of increasingly specialist practice, under the guidance of those already deemed to be expert practitioners. In the undergraduate years, learning is best understood as learning *for* work. Time spent in the workplace offers glimpses into future working lives and practices and provides a rich contextualization for knowledge acquired in the university. Whilst clinical attachments may offer authentic opportunities to rehearse ways of thinking and acting, students are not workers in the employment sense. Throughout periods of postgraduate training, as a worker, the 'broadly educated' graduate becomes a doctor through further training. Here, learning can be understood as both *for* work and *from* work. Knowledge is put to use in work activity, which becomes the curriculum for training. Knowledge, here, means every kind of knowledge that is stored in the memory of an individual, from factual (what you know) to practical knowledge (what you know to do), based upon prior experience, skills, and sensitivities (e.g. how it feels and strategies for successful solutions to problems). Trainees bring knowledge to the workplace and are gradually exposed to greater levels of responsibility and complexity in the medical work they undertake. The affordances of the workplace and more experienced practitioners determine the types of work experiences to be delegated and the supervisory practices that are needed. The requirements of practice are invariably both practical and theoretical and 'can only become work in the pedagogic sense of the term if it stems from intellectual effort that has been invested beforehand and is taken up anew throughout the course of its performance' (Kerschensteiner 1950, p. 55).

If work is conceptualized as gradual development, the more experienced, expert practitioners, continue to learn for and from work. Complex cases, changing work practices, new clinical protocols and a rapidly changing knowledge base provide the stimulus for the development of professional practices. Here, new knowledge derives from such work practices, disseminated through collegiate discussion, education and research activity.

In turning to the learning literature, ways of conceptualizing distinctions between working and learning relationships at different points in a medical career can be found. A starting point is Sfard's account of two contrasting metaphors for learning: learning-as-acquisition and learning-as-participation (Sfard 1998). The learning-as-acquisition metaphor emphasizes individual learners and the acquisition of knowledge and skills. Learning-as-acquisition is a powerful guiding metaphor for undergraduate medical education. Students, through assessment processes, demonstrate that they have gained the necessary knowledge and skills allowing them entry into the medical profession, where they put acquired knowledge to use. In contrast, learning-as-participation has a collective focus, framing learning in terms of processes of becoming and belonging, emphasizing full participation in the work of community. Learning-as-participation, in contrast, is a key guiding metaphor for postgraduate training, which has, as its intended end point full participation in the work of medical communities. It is perhaps in the later stages of a medical career that learning-as-participation becomes the dominant guiding metaphor for professional learning, with medical practice developing through full participation in the work of medical communities.

We have already noted an apparent reluctance to engage in an educational discourse about work-based learning in medicine. We do not share this reluctance, believing that the development of such a discourse is pivotal to both sustaining and developing high quality work-based learning opportunities at all stages of a medical career. A detailed and sustained critique of the work-based learning literature is beyond the scope of this chapter and can be found elsewhere (see, for example, the collection of works edited by Malloch et al. 2011). However, in order to make sense of, and enhance the learning value of medical work, it is necessary to understand key debates. In the following section, trends in the conceptualization of work-based learning will be traced and illustrated with reference to medical learning. In so doing, ways of rethinking and enhancing medical learning will emerge.

Making sense of work-based learning

Sfard's (1998, pp. 4–13) metaphors map to two broad schools of educational thought found within the work-based learning literature. These have been described as historical trends, moving from individual to collective accounts (Hager 2011). Individualized accounts of learning, captured in the *learning-as-acquisition* metaphor, have their origins in psychology and can be seen to bring together behaviourist and cognitive theories. Hager notes the early influence of behaviourism where 'learning is understood and explained only in terms of what is directly observable', going on to posit that 'the notion that job performance can be fully specifiable in advance remains a seductively attractive one. This false hope has underpinned much of the support that competency-based training has garnered in recent times' (Hager 2011, p. 18).

Illeris (2011) notes a move away from concerns about professional qualifications to those of professional competence, arguing that the latter has a much broader basis, capturing what a person is actually able to do. In this way, competency encompasses prior knowledge, skills and experiences, and how someone applies this to their work activity. The recent but widespread move toward competency-based postgraduate medical training has attracted criticism and fostered debate about the nature of medical training (ten Cate and Scheele 2007). Concerns have been raised about the reductionist nature of a competency-based curriculum (Talbot 2004); the need to foster excellence rather than competence in medical professionals (Tooke 2007); and the tick-box culture arising from the assessment of multiple competencies on multiple occasions (Collins 2010). Distinctions between competency as a theoretical concept, capturing the 'broad general attributes of a good doctor' (ten Cate and Scheele 2007), sit in tension with the operationalization of the concept, seen in the concrete delineation of competencies and the associated assessment 'machinery'. A recent analysis of how the term is used in healthcare education (Fernandez et al. 2012) highlights the importance of such conceptual and operational distinctions, leading some to argue a shift from conceptions of competence to that of 'entrustable professional activities' (ten Cate and Scheele 2007). In identifying the types of work we are willing to entrust to another, we signal recognition of the associated competency.

Behaviourist principles are difficult to apply to unobservable actions (like thinking); this is where the contributions of *cognitive* theories are seen. Hager (2011) notes that some of the earliest theories of work-based learning come from this school of thought, citing the work of Chris Argyris and Donald Schon (1978). Schon's (1983, 1987) accounts of reflection in and on action arose from Dewey's (1916) work. Dewey's concept of reflexive experience

captures the consequences of confusion: careful analysis, problem definition, and the formulation of hypotheses lead to a plan for action. This account has immediate resonances with descriptions of clinical reasoning practices. Other, popular accounts of work-based learning in medicine draw upon Kolb's description of an experiential learning cycle (Kolb 1984) and Knowles' explanation of adult learning or andragogy (Knowles 1973). Bleakley et al. (2011) note the lack of close and critical readings of such primary texts in the medical education literature, arguing these lead to over-simplified accounts, lacking the explanatory power necessary to capture the complexity of collaborative clinical activity. Schon, for example, offers up a counter critique to the notion of technical rationality, where practitioners are assumed to apply theory to practice. His accounts of reflective practice were part of a sustained critical stance, drawing attention to the messy realities of complex professional work. He explores the professional artistry of experts, who are able to reflect in action, adapting their responses in the moment, when things do not go by the book. This feels far removed from the obligatory reflection on action and completion of reflective portfolios. Schon's work becomes just one example of complex educational ideas, which are lost in translation.

A criticism to be levied at behavioural and cognitive accounts of work or experience-based learning is that they present learning as unsituated and unmediated. Learning is discussed without explicit consideration of the shaping or constraining forces of the environment or the presence of more experienced or expert others who determine and shape the experiences made available. Here, Vygotsky's contributions become helpful, providing a way of conceptualizing the contributions of 'more knowledgeable others' and how they mediate learning through the use of symbolic and other tools (Vygotsky 1978). Vygotsky's contributions move thinking beyond the ways in which individuals make sense of the world around them, to those which explain how this knowledge is coconstructed with others, be it peers, seniors, or teachers. So whilst a trainee may not yet be able to undertake a procedure from start to finish, completely independently, they may be able to do so with the support of a more knowledgeable other who is able to guide and safety net if need be. This provides an account of individual learning within a social context (social-constructivism). Sociocognitive theories also offer ways of understanding interactions with the environment itself. Bandura's work, for example, looks at the dynamic interplay between the personal, cognitive, and environment (reciprocal determinism) arguing that together these determine an individual's self-efficacy and subsequent behaviour (Bandura 1977, 1997). Part of the trainees' ability to work independently will be determined by their sense of self-efficacy and the support readily available in the environment, should a need arise.

Sociocognitive theories consider the interplay between learners and their environment; the focus of the explanation of learning is on the internal processes of an individual. Transfer of learning, from one setting to another, is assumed as a given and, on the whole, treated as unproblematic. Contexts of knowledge generation, acquisition and subsequent use are therefore dealt with as separate from the learner (and learning). Psychological-type theories dominate the learning literature, even though research to support claims to transfer is sparse. Bransford and Schwartz (1999) highlight strategies to increase the likelihood of direct transfer. These include ensuring deep rather than surface learning; presenting concepts in multiple contexts (so they are not strongly tied to one in particular);

engaging students in problematizing ('what if' thinking) and emphasizing metacognition, particularly reflection and the development of problem-solving strategies. The emphasis on problem-based learning, case-based discussion, the strong advocacy of 'reflection', and the development of clinical reasoning skills in medical education appear supportive of transfer. However, Colliver (2004) cautions that neither large- (curriculum scale) or small-scale studies of transfer in medical education are conclusive. Indeed, it is argued that there are 'enough examples of transfer failure to consider positive transfer to be at least a relatively rare event' (Bransford and Schwartz 1999, p. 66).

However, the same authors go on to argue that perhaps the issue is the research focus on direct transfer, perhaps missing valuable elements of transfer captured in their term 'preparation for future learning'. Here, they refer to a person's ability to learn in a knowledge-rich environment, making use of the resources available to them (in documents, texts, and colleagues) in order to rapidly adapt to their new environment. This position may lead us to rethink the preparedness literature, a point that will be returned to later. Despite the potential limitations of these viewpoints on learning, they do allow a debate about transfer. The position at the other end of the internal—external continuum explaining learning is found in sociocultural accounts. These see all learning as being situated, essentially silencing accounts of the ways in which people take knowledge and practices from one work context to another.

Sociocultural accounts

Hager's (2011) second category of work-based learning draws upon sociology and social-anthropology. In sociocultural theories of learning, learning is framed not in terms of an individual's success in acquiring knowledge, rather in the extent to which they are able to become full participants in the work of the communities they enter. Becker et al.'s (1997) study of American medical training in the 1950s and Sinclair's (1997) more contemporary analysis of British medical training provide rich accounts of the ways in which individuals are socialized into the medical profession, developing professional identities and practices as a result. Arguably, one of the most influential contributions made to understanding workplace-based learning in these terms, is made by Lave and Wenger (1991, p. 29), who set out 'to rescue the idea of apprenticeship'. They offer up an analytic viewpoint on work-based learning through the use of two linked concepts: *legitimate peripheral participation* in *communities of practice*. The first focuses attention on the ways in which newcomers to a community (for example a school leaver joining the medical course at university, or a trainee joining a medical team) are engaged in increasingly purposeful activity, moving towards full participation in work activity. The considered allocation of work activity becomes a pedagogic strategy, drawing the new worker into the complex, shared practices of the community.

In using the term community, Lave and Wenger (1991) signal the technical knowledge of communities as well as the social relations that bind them. In this way they talk not of experts and novices, rather of *newcomers* and *old-timers*, outlining the ways in which a newcomer into a community will change some activities, with the development of practice being multidirectional between workers at all stages of careers. Their work invites a reconsideration of the status of work-based learning: work is seen as the curriculum for learning and learning is embedded in everyday work. It also offers up the possibility of analysing the work-based learning

opportunities for experienced workers who move into new work roles, teams or organizations.

Lave and Wenger's work has been influential in rethinking work-based learning, but is not without its critics (Hughes et al 2007; Cairns 2011). Lave and Wenger themselves acknowledge that the concept of communities of practice is underdeveloped and it is difficult to delineate the lifecycle of a community of practice, creating challenges for researchers who struggle to find an appropriate unit of analysis (Matusov 2007).

Communities of practice are framed in benign terms, failing to make explicit emotional dimensions of learning (Turnbull 2000) or the ways in which power-relations may skew the types of work activity newcomers gain access to, which in turn may restrict the learning. Whilst their work is particularly helpful in analysing how newcomers gain access to the work of a community, it is less developed in thinking about the ways in which expert practitioners move across communities. Others argue that the concept itself is conservative, best used to explain how stable working practices can be reproduced over time, through incremental developments, rather than looking at the rapid expansion of practices in times of change (Engestrom 2001; Hager 2005; Fuller 2007). This may limit the concept's usefulness in developing novel practices.

Perhaps the greatest value of sociocultural theories of learning is that they lead to explicit consideration of the ways in which the workplace and work activities can support learning (Hager 2011). Further meaning to the concept of communities of practice has been added by Wenger (1998), who looks at the ways in which social practices support processes of 'belonging and becoming' (of relevance when considering the ways in which a workplace supports identity formation). Billett (2002, 2004) invites consideration of the invitational qualities and affordances of particular workplaces and how individual agency shapes the extent to which workers seek out and engage with work-based learning opportunities. These ideas may help us consider the ways in which certain workers are afforded richer work-based learning opportunities than others. One example might be that trainees have rich and varied working practices scripted into their jobs whereas those in non-training grades may have more restricted work practices and therefore restricted learning opportunities.

Alternatively, concerns about competency may mean that more experienced workers in non-training grades, are entrusted with a broader or more complex range of work activity than less experienced workers with trainee status. The idea of restricted learning arising from restricted working practices is picked up and elaborated in Fuller and Unwin's (2004) account of a restrictive–expansive continuum of apprenticeship. They provide a useful analytic tool that encourages consideration of the opportunities for learning scripted into everyday working practices and, as a result, may reveal unintended favouring of some types of workers over others.

Within the medical education literature it is possible to find examples of research that implicitly, if not explicitly, explores issues aligned with these sociocultural perspectives. There is a notable growth in published ethnographic studies of medical workplace learning; several have, for example, looked at the ways in which students and residents engage with the learning opportunities arising from different types of rounds. These studies explore the extent to which different participants are able to recognize the learning inherent in morbidity and mortality rounds (Kuper et al 2010), the learning potential of paediatric rounds (Balmer, et al 2010), and strategies necessary to activate this potential (Prado et al 2011). Together, the studies raise questions about the extent to which trainees are able to recognize and access the learning inherent in workplace activities and how these can be made more explicit. Other studies have explored the extent to which it is possible to conceptualize postgraduate rotations and undergraduate placements as times spent in communities of practice (Cornford and Cornford 2006; Morris 2012). Both of these studies note limits to the extent to which trainees and students are afforded opportunities to become full participants in the work of the communities they join, a point underlined by a recent study of medical graduate preparedness for first posts (Illing et al 2008). Roberts (2009) notes the tendency for such transitions to greater medical responsibility to be conceptualized in terms of preparedness, inviting a reconsideration of the situated nature of work and questioning whether it is ever possible to be fully prepared. Whilst sociocultural perspectives may offer rich, situated accounts of learning from work, they do not offer up an account of the ways in which practices (and learning) are taken from one context to another. Whichever standpoint on learning we adopt, the 'problem' of transfer invites further consideration.

Overcoming the problem of transfer

The different viewpoints on learning encompassed within Hager's (2011) categories or Sfard's (1998) metaphors both invite critique and have added value when we draw upon both, rather than favouring one over another. In the field of professional education, there are limits to the contributions either currently offer in understanding the notion of transfer. Individual theories treat transfer as a relatively unproblematic concept. Sociocultural theories see learning as situated and do not deal with the issue of how learning generated in one context may be taken and put to use in another. We see this tension in the medical education literature. For example, Brown (2010) provides an account of how such views of learning have shaped the teaching of clinical communication skills and how processes of transfer (from classroom to clinical workplaces) are inherently problematic, requiring work-based support and supervision. Recent concerns about medical graduates preparedness for medical practice (Illing et al 2008) and a growing literature about transitions to greater medical responsibility (Roberts 2009; Kilminster et al 2011; Tallentire et al 2011) invite a reconsideration of the assumptions of transfer.

Eraut (2000, 2004) has made helpful contributions to the thinking about the types of knowledge that professionals access and put to use in their work activities. He provides a breakdown of the interrelated stages in knowledge transfer, which involve the practitioner recognizing which aspects of previously acquired knowledge might be transformed to fit the new situation (Eraut 2004). Such connections are not automatically made, because of the different logics and contexts of knowledge generation. A classic example is the lament that 'medical students don't know anything these days'. In reality, highly knowledgeable students may struggle to recognize which aspects are relevant to the observed, complex situations they encounter in the workplace.

The ways in which knowledge is put to work, in a range of professional contexts, including nursing and pharmacy, has been the subject of a number of research studies, exploring the concept of recontextualization (Harris et al 2007; Evanset al. 2011). This research leads to a helpful rethinking of work-based learning, based upon a four-mode typology, which captures the ways in which

knowledge is recontextualized as learners move between different sites of learning (Harris et al 2007; Evans et al 2011).

Content recontexualization is seen when codified knowledge (typically subject or discipline based) is selected (and often simplified) for inclusion in a formal learning programme. For example, in an undergraduate curriculum this relates to choices made about what is included, the order in which it is offered and so on. Debates about what should (or should not) be included in periods of initial professional formation are contestable, often reflecting wider sociopolitical and professional debates. For example, the first inclusion of teaching skills in the undergraduate curriculum in the UK was seen in 2003, following the GMC (1999) *Doctor as Teacher* publication. This addition to the curriculum arose during a period described as the professionalization of medical education (Swanwick 2008) and coincided with the introduction of more structured, formalized postgraduate training programmes as a part of *Modernising Medical Careers* (DoH 2004).

A second form of recontextualization is termed *pedagogic recontextualization* and happens when teachers make decisions about how to bring together discipline-based and practice-based knowledge; here, choices are made about teaching, learning, and assessment practices. The place and approach to anatomy teaching in undergraduate medical education is one exemplar. The reliance on cadaver dissection at Cambridge University (Blackman 2006) sits in contrast to a decision to use living and surface anatomy at Peninsula Medical School (Mclachlan and Regan De Bere 2004) and to use three-dimensional anatomy imaging techniques at Durham (Patten 2007). Each centre puts forward a rationale for adopted approaches, extending from the pedagogic to the sociopolitical. Whilst tradition may account in part, for the continued use of cadaver dissection in one institution, a desire to teach anatomy the way it is encountered in clinical practice guides the other. The second, in particular, suggests explicit consideration of the ways in which the practices and contexts from which anatomical knowledge is generated will shape how it is put to use. Other examples of approaches to pedagogic recontextualization in medicine might be seen in the adoption of integrated, systems-based, and problem-based curricula, each reflecting a desire to bring together discipline- and practice-based knowledge. Likewise, the widescale adoption of simulation could be recast as an attempt to create a space where learners and workers may put different types of knowledge to use, bridging gaps between formal learning spaces and the workplace.

Workplace recontextualization is understood in terms of how workplace activity supports knowledge development and how this is supported through the guidance, supervision, coaching and mentoring offered by other workers. Whilst the extent to which clinical placements or attachments offer authentic work-based learning experiences is open to debate, their long inclusion in initial professional formation says something of the ways in which they help learners put knowledge to use. A live example of this can be found by tracing through three editions of the curriculum guidance offered to medical schools in the UK by the General Medical Council (GMC 1993, 2003, 2009a). Each offers a particular steer with regards to the timing, nature, and organization of clinical experience elements for medical students. The most recent guidance stipulates the need to include at least one student assistantship where each student works alongside a junior doctor, in the hope of increasing their preparedness for working life as a new doctor.

Workplace recontextualization does not only need to happen at points of transition into the workplace however. As workers move into new teams, new organizations, or more senior roles, they often encounter periods of discomfort where they seek to make sense of workplace practices and identify how they may rapidly make a meaningful contribution to these. A growing emphasis on the ready availability of educational supervision, coaching or mentoring perhaps reflects the need of an increasingly transient, mobile healthcare workforce. Finally, *learner/employee recontextualization* refers to the ways in which the worker (whether new entrant or experienced practitioner) brings all their prior knowledge together to make sense of, develop and reshape work activities and identities (Evans et al. 2011). Links can be seen here to Bandura's accounts of self-efficacy or Billett's of individual agency. Learner recontextualization can be witnessed in the sense-making practices of individuals, often in dialogue with others workers around them, often out with formalized support structures.

In reviewing debates in the work-based learning literature, distinctions between different educational schools of thought have been outlined. Cognitive-behavioural accounts enable us to analyse the learning trajectories of individuals, allowing us to talk about the ways in which knowledge generated in one context may be put to use in another. Caveats arise from the learning literature on transfer, which suggests that these processes are complex and non-linear. Sociocultural accounts provide ways of understanding how learning is developed in context, arising through participation in the work of communities of practice. The emphasis on situated learning effectively silences debates about transfer. Recent work looking at how knowledge is put to work bridges these two schools, providing a helpful typology of recontextualization, which in turn leads us to examine pedagogic strategies that may support the development of professional practice throughout a doctor's working life. Exemplars from different points of a medical professional's career have been used to illustrate the ways in which learning theory may shed light on existing practices. In offering these exemplars, questions are raised about the extent to which work-based learning is explicitly valued and supported. In this final section we revisit three stages of a medical career: initial professional formation; postgraduate training; and continuing professional development. At each stage we consider how knowledge of these ideas about learning can be put to work, allowing a rethinking of ways to support learning for, and from, medical work. Table 18.1 outlines some selected theoretical contributions from the work-based learning literature.

Enhancing learning for and from medical work

Initial professional formation

UK medical students study in medical schools within universities and primarily undertake work-related learning in National Health Service (NHS) contexts. The GMC offers guidance and advice on clinical placements—arrangements where students, either as

Table 18.1 Selected theoretical contributions from the work-based learning literature; questions arising for clinical educators

Selected theoretical contributions	Questions arising for clinical educators?
Linking knowledge and experience	Are current notions of reflective practice congruent with original accounts?
Concept of 'reflective experience', which arises from perplexity or confusion leading to careful analysis, problem definition and development of a hypothesis as a plan for action (Dewey 1916).	Is it possible to 'capture' reflective thought and to turn it into plans for future action (and are these then realized)?
Work (in a pedagogic sense) seen as on-going intellectual effort, which guides work and fosters possibility of self-review (Kerschensteiner 1950).	What kinds of work activities encompass 'reflective experience'?
Accounts of professional practice as professional artistry, underpinned by both knowledge-in-action and reflection-in-action (Schon 1983).	Does reflection necessarily lead to change (learning)?
Linking knowledge and practice	How do we make use of different forms of knowledge when we move between different sites of learning and practice?
Work involves processes of putting different forms of knowledge, underpinned by different values and logics, to use. Processes of recontextualization are at play, and can be supported by different pedagogic strategies (Harris et al. 2007, Evans et al. 2011).	What types of curriculum and pedagogic strategies, within the academy and workplace, help bring subject-based and work-based knowledge together?
	What kinds of work activity support knowledge development and use? How can (co) workers support this type of development?
Learning situated in practice	To what extent do we organize work activity to foster transitions to full participation and support newcomers to achieve this? How can we make our workplaces equally invitational to all newcomers and ensure equitable opportunities to learn through fair distribution of work activity?
Linked analytical concepts of legitimate-peripheral-participation in communities of practice (Lave and Wenger 1991; Wenger 1998) invite an exploration of the ways newcomers become full participants in the shared, purposeful activity of a community. Work becomes the learning curriculum.	To what extent do we recognize and make explicit the inherent learning value of work activities (to ourselves and others)? How might we do this more effectively?
The invitational qualities of workplaces and the distribution of workplace affordances vary considerably. Individual agency influences the extent to which learners and workers recognize, value, and engage with work-based learning opportunities (Billett 2002, 2004).	How might we change the structure of different forms of work activity to enhance the learning value of work activity?
Apprenticeships vary along a restrictive–expansive continuum; the ways in which working practices are organized, distributed, and supported, shapes the extent to which they offer rich learning opportunities for current and future roles (Fuller and Unwin 2006).	What factors seem to foster the engagement of individual workers (or otherwise) and how might we promote this?
	To what extent are our workplaces inherently restrictive or expansive in terms of the opportunities they offer to all workers?

observers or contributors to patient care, are 'present in an environment that provides healthcare or related services' (GMC 2011a, p. 2).

Student assistantships and *shadowing* are particular types of clinical placement, where students, close to graduation, work alongside junior doctors, assisting them in their daily work. All types of placements are expressed in terms of helping students prepare for first medical posts and therefore foreground the rehearsal of clinical skills and increasing involvement in the work of medical teams (GMC 2011a). These times spent in the workplace allow familiarization with healthcare environments, insights into working practices, and some opportunities to rehearse aspects of early work activity.

A close reading of GMC guidance on undergraduate medical education (GMC 2009a, 2011a) reveals a broadly cognitive framing of learning. *Tomorrow's Doctors* advocates an outcomes-based curriculum, which enables students to 'link theory and practice' (GMC 2009a, p. 51). Graduate outcomes under the heading 'reflect, learn and teach others', place an emphasis on students being able to acquire, apply and integrate their knowledge through systematic and continuous reflection, throughout their professional lives, translating this reflection into action where necessary (GMC 2009a). The endpoint of undergraduate education, however, has sociocultural framings, promoting increasing participation and integration into medical workplaces, teams and practices. There is a tension to be found in these guidelines; the primary responsibilities of medical schools are outlined in terms of protecting patients from any risk of harm (when patients are involved in student training). This, along with the emphasis on rehearsal and preparation lead us to question the authenticity and meaningfulness of some student placement activity.

How then, might work-based learning be enhanced during periods of initial professional formation? Content and pedagogic recontextualization are key here. Evans et al. (2011) suggest that *gradual release* is a vital supporting principle, drawing attention to the sequencing and integration of knowledge and workplace elements. This supports a move away from curriculum models that frontload knowledge, to those providing an ongoing interplay between knowledge and practice elements—as with problem-based, spiral, and integrated curriculum models. Gradual release into the workplace is equally important. Clinical teachers become knowledge brokers, able to help students make explicit connections between their learning in formal settings and the practices observed on placement (fig. 18.2).

Pedagogic recontextualization begins from a position where transfer is seen as problematic and actively explored. The use of clinical data, narratives, paper cases, and case-based discussion may help develop the types of conceptual understandings that go beyond the original context of knowledge generation. Rethinking the use of simulation, seeing it as a mediating environment between the classroom and workplace, is another supporting strategy. Rather than seeing simulation as a place to rehearse future practice, it may be seen as a place to revisit experiences, considering the ways in which knowledge is put to use and how practice may be further developed. Traditional bedside teaching methods, actively rehearsing students in thinking through diagnosis, management and prognosis, are also valuable here. Opportunities to be part of a medical team can be meaningful, if this involves active participation in patient care activity, with the support of more knowledgeable others. Planning for participation means taking time to consider aspects of work that students may undertake independently, albeit with support. These strategies invite shared responsibility for aspects of work activity, increasing the value of clinical placements.

Postgraduate training

Postgraduate medical training in the UK is shaped and supported by royal colleges, the GMC and postgraduate deaneries and can be loosely divided into three stages: foundation, core, and specialty training. There are over 60 medical specialties; it is beyond the scope of this chapter to undertake a full contextual analysis of curriculum documents and operational frameworks. The following commentary offers a degree of thematic analysis, capturing trends in thinking and practice.

The major shift in the organization of postgraduate medical education in the UK has been from a time-served apprenticeship to a time-measured competency-based model (Tooke 2007; Morris 2011). This could be seen as move away from sociocultural

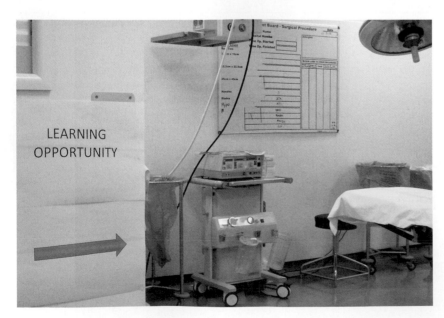

Figure 18.2 Work-based learning opportunities.

to cognitive-behavioural orientations in postgraduate learning. Postgraduate training programmes adopt outcomes-based, competency-assessed practices, originating from the introduction of the foundation years curriculum, the first 2 years after medical school. All specialties and stages have adopted or extended their use of work-based assessments, which combine formative and summative functions. The original intent behind training reform was to make explicit and capture the learning arising through work. The operationalization of the curriculum, however, focuses attention on ensuring that the workplace allows trainees to achieve specified competencies. The distinction, whilst subtle, is important; in the former, the workplace is the curriculum, in the latter a curriculum is imposed upon the workplace.

This training reform has been the subject of significant political and professional scrutiny; formal reviews and evaluations provide a situated account of the ways in which the operationalization of new curriculum models may lead to the skewing of trainer and trainee work activity, creating a tick-box culture to meet regulator requirements (Tooke 2007, Collins 2010). The tension here is that the formalization of the work-based curriculum shifts attention from the learning arising *through* working, to the demonstration of learning arising *while* working, inadvertently downplaying the learning value of work. This point is underlined by research illustrating the difficulties trainees have in recognizing the implicit learning value of work activity (Swanwick and Morris 2010). How might the learning value of work be enhanced in postgraduate stages?

Gradual release continues to be a supporting principle, moving the trainee towards full participation in the work of the communities they join. This involves consideration of the ways in which work activity can be systematically delegated, to support trainee learning and development as they take on work of increasingly responsibility or complexity. Similar principles underpin the idea of 'graded responsibility' involving 'careful increased exposure to practice that the trainee is capable of undertaking; first under supervision and then independently' (PMETB 2008, p. 36).

Gradual release and graded responsibility are easiest to envisage in relation to procedural skills, but can be applied to the development of judgement and problem-solving, through strategies such as case-based discussion. It is worth noting that whilst formal documentation supports incremental growth in workload and responsibilities, the reality is often different (Roberts 2009; Kilminster et al 2011). Moving thinking beyond competence to one concerned with extending the range of 'entrustable professional activities' supports this approach. Likewise, the forthcoming move away from work-based assessments, to 'supervised learning events' during foundation training, reinforces the originally intended formative functions of these tools.

Workplace recontextualization is a critical component of clinical and educational supervision. The role of clinical supervisors can be understood in terms of making the learning arising through working explicit. This involves briefing activity (e.g. 'during the ward round this morning, think about the ways in which results of investigations lead us to adjust planned management strategies') and debriefing (e.g. 'talk me through your management of this case, showing how you have adapted your approach in light of new information arising'). It includes feedback, and clinician 'think aloud' techniques, where the clinical supervisor verbally shares their diagnostic reasoning processes. It also includes mentoring techniques, enabling trainees to come to their own solutions to problems.

Educational supervision can be understood in terms of structuring work activities to ensure a rich, expansive apprenticeship (Fuller and Unwin 2006). This can be supported through the facilitation of faculty or supervisory groups, which recognize that trainee development is supported by a range of colleagues, including those out with their own professional grouping. Recognizing points of transition to greater medical responsibility as critically intensive learning periods requiring formal support and incremental increases in responsibility are also important (Kilminster et al 2011).

Continuing professional development

The GMC have regulatory responsibility for UK doctors' continuing professional development (CPD). Every doctor is expected to actively develop their practice, with recent draft guidance (GMC 2011b) stipulating that some of this development activity should target improvement in team or organizational practices. The GMC is in the process of reviewing CPD drawing upon a systematic review of international practices and literature (GMC 2011c). Their emphasis is clear; CPD should ensure that doctors offer safe and effective care for patients. The CPD guidance points to a range of ways in which this might happen; the learning arising through working is explicitly foregrounded as being of particular value. There is a strong emphasis on reflection being the learning process of choice, but, in this case, triangulated through collegiate discussion and engagement with published and grey literature (GMC 2011b).

In the UK at least, the ways in which doctors develop work practices through work activity has received much less attention than other stages of a doctor's career. Yet it is here, outwith the demands of a formal training curriculum and assessment regimen that the workplace offers the richest learning opportunities. The assumption that doctors activate the potential of the learning arising through working informally is being countered by a growing emphasis on appraisal processes and moves toward revalidation. Such approaches require explicit evidence of the professional development activity that has enhanced the doctor's practice over a given time period. Inadvertently, this may downplay the value of rich, opportunistic learning moments, where, for example a chance conversation with a coworker or an in-the-moment thought, offers new and significant insights into one's professional practice. How can work-based learning be enhanced throughout a doctor's working life?

Workplace recontextualization continues to be important—supervision or mentoring beyond training grades would be of value. Where informal opportunities for professional dialogue become squeezed by workloads and increasing fragmentation of teams, more formal scripting of these opportunities may be necessary. For example, moving beyond regulatory functions of appraisals to reclaim them as an opportunity for rich peer dialogue supporting the development of practice is one way forward. Opportunities for occasional joint clinics or arranged visits to other institutions may offer chances to review practice and learn from others. Valuing handovers and team briefing and debriefing as conversations that can support the development of individual and shared practices is key—a 5 minute summary of lessons learned can make these more explicit to oneself and others.

The diversification of work activity throughout a career in itself brings rich learning opportunities. Change stimulates learning for work and offers new opportunities to learn from that work. In agreeing to cover for colleagues or to undertake sessions in a new work environment, insights into different team working practices may arise and shape practice in the usual work environment. In electing to undertake an explicit educational or clinical leadership role, new development opportunities present themselves. Likewise, active participation in audit, governance and research activity may lead to the generation of new knowledge that can be put to work.

Learning for medical work revisited

In this chapter we have explored the nature of working and learning relationships throughout a medical career. We have looked at how these relationships are shaped by personal, organizational, and societal factors. We have argued that to develop work-based learning in medicine, an educational discourse is imperative. This discourse has to move beyond accounts of curriculum models and pedagogic strategies to one that engages with the key debates in the learning literature. In so doing, it is possible to rethink work-based learning in the current period where previously sustainable apprenticeship practices are threatened by changed regulatory relationships and work contexts. Strategies to overcome the problem of transfer have been proposed, along with those to explicitly value and mobilize the learning arising through work. Finally, in tracing through the stages of a medical career, ways to extend the value of work-based learning have been suggested. Medicine has a long tradition of recognizing the workplace as a significant site for learning; the future of medicine relies upon a revitalization of working-learning relationships throughout a medical career.

Conclusions

◆ Learning that derives its purposes for the context of work is work-based learning. Health professionals work throughout their career in changing contexts of work. Hence, work-based learning constitutes an essential part of the work of medical professionals at all stages of their careers.

◆ Cognitive accounts of learning are predominately drawn upon in the context of undergraduate medical education and socio-cultural accounts within postgraduate training and continuing professional development. An inclusive understanding of work-based learning in medical education can only arise if we bring together these complementary orientations towards learning, at all stages of a medical career.

◆ Throughout a career as a health professional, the individual gains experience and knowledge by moving between different sites of employment and learning. Further exploration of the ways in which connections are made between factual and practical knowledge, skills, and sensitivities is merited. Conceptions of recontextualization may help such an exploration.

◆ The discourse about what is the relationship between working and learning varies through the different stages of a medical career, often aligned to competence and improving practice according to a new set of demands. Learning that derives its purpose for the context of work is concerned with wider aspects such as learning how to do the current job, how to do the next job, or learning to work in different contexts. Thus, the discourse on work-based learning needs to be widened to take up the long tradition of medicine recognising the workplace as a significant site for learning for the profession.

References

Argyris, C. and Schon, D. (1978) *Organisational Learning: A Theory of Action Perspective*. Reading, MA: Addison-Wesley

Balmer, D., Master, C., Richards, B., Serwint, J., and Giardino, A. (2010) An ethnographic study of attending rounds in general paediatrics: understanding the ritual. *Med Educ.* 44: 1105–1116

Bandura, A. (1977) *Social Learning Theory*. New York: Prentice Hall

Bandura, A. (1997) *Self-efficacy: The Exercise of Control*. New York: W.H. Freeman

Beck, J. and Young, M. (2005) The assault on the professions and the restructuring of academic and professional identities: A Bernsteinian analysis. *Br J Sociol Educ.* 26(2): 183–197

Becker, H., Geer, B., Hughes, E. and Straus, A. (1997) *Boys in White*. 5th edn. New Jersey: Transaction Publishers

Billett, S. (2002) Workplace pedagogic practices: co-participation and learning. *Br J Educ Studies.* 50(4): 457–481

Billett, S. (2004) Learning through work: Workplace participatory practices. In H. Rainbow, A. Fuller, and A. Munroe (eds) *Workplace Learning in Context* (pp. 109–125). London: Routledge

Blackman, H. (2006) Anatomy and embryology in medical education at Cambridge University, 1866–1900. *Med Educ.* 40: 219–226

Bleakley, A. (2006) Broadening conceptions of learning in medical education: the message from team-working. *Med Educ.* 40: 150–157

Bleakley, A., Bligh, J., and Browne, J. (2011) *Medical Education for the Future. Identity, Power and Location*. London: Springer

Bordage, G. (2009) Conceptual frameworks to illuminate and magnify. *Med Educ.* 43(4): 312–319

Boud, D. and Solomon, N. (2001) *Work-based Learning: A New Higher Education?* Buckingham: SRHE and OUP

Bransford, J. and Schwartz, D. (1999) Rethinking transfer: a simple proposal with multiple implications. *Rev Res Educ.* 24(1): 61–100

Brown, J. (2010) Do the communication skills of medical students transfer to the workplace? *Acad Med.* 85(6): 1052–1059

Cairns, L, (2011) Learning in the workplace: communities of practice and beyond. In M. Malloch, L. Cairns, K. Evans, and B.N. O'Connor, (eds) *The Sage Handbook of Workplace Learning* (pp. 73–85). London: Sage

Calman, K. (2006) *Education, Past, Present and Future. Handing on Learning*. Edinburgh: Churchill Livingstone

Collins, J. (2010) *Foundation for Excellence: An Evaluation of the Foundation Programme*. London: Medical Education England

Colliver, J. (2004) Full-curriculum interventions and small-scale studies of transfer: implications for psychology-type theory. *Med Educ.* 38(12): 1212–1214

Cornford, C. and Cornford B. (2009) A qualitative study of the experiences of training in general practice: a community of practice? *J Educ. Teach.* 32(3): 269–282

Department of Health (2004) *Modernising Medical Careers—the next steps. The future of Foundation, Specialist and General Practice Training Programmes*. Department of Health: London

Dewey, J. (1916) *Democracy and Education. An introduction to the philosophy of education* (1966 edn), New York: Free Press

Dornan, T., McKendree, J., and Robbé, I. (2011) Commentary: medical education in a time of complexity, uncertainty and reflection. A coda to the Flexner Report. *Med Educ.* 45(1): 2–6

Engestrom, Y. (2001) Expansive learning at work: toward an activity theoretical reconceptualization. *J Educ Work.* 14(1): 133–156

Eraut, E. (2000) Non-formal learning and tacit knowledge in professional work. *Br J Educ Psychol.* 70: 113–136

Eraut, M. (2004) Transfer of knowledge between education and workplace settings. In H. Rainbird, A. Fuller and H. Munro (eds) *Workplace Learning in Context* (pp. 201–221). London: Routledge.

Evans, K., Guile, D., and Harris, J. (2011) Rethinking work-based learning: for education professionals and professionals who educate. In M. Malloch, L. Cairns, K. Evans, and B.N. O'Connor (eds) (2011) *The SAGE Handbook of Workplace Learning* (pp. 149–161). London: Sage

Evans, K. (2012) Introduction: working to learning in clinical practice. In V. Cook, C. Daly and M. Newman (eds) *Work-based Learning in Clinical*

Settings. Insights from socio-cultural perspectives (pp. 5–18). Abingdon: Radcliffe

Evans, K., Guile, D., and Harris, J. (2011) Rethinking work-based learning: for education professionals and professionals who educate. In M. Malloch, L. Cairns, K. Evans, and B.N. O'Connor, (eds) *The SAGE Handbook of Workplace Learning* (pp. 149–161). London: Sage.

Fernandez, N., Dory, V., Ste-Marie, L., Chaput, M., Charlin, B., and Boucher, A. (2012) Varying conceptions of competence: an analysis of how health sciences educators define competence. *Med Educ.* 46: 357–365

Flexner, A. (1910) *Medical Education in the United States and Canada* (The Flexner report) [online]. New York: Carnegie Foundation for the Advancement of Learning. http://www.carnegiefoundation.org/publications/medical-education-united-states-and-canada-bulletin-number-four-flexner-report-0 Accessed 14 April 2012

Fuller, A. and Unwin, L. (2006) Expansive and restrictive learning environments. In Evans, K., Hodkinson, P., Rainbird, H., and Unwin, L. (eds) *Improving Workplace Learning* (pp. 27–48). London, Routledge.

Fuller, A. (2007) Critiquing theories of learning and communities of practice. In J, Hughes, N. Jewson, and L. Unwin (eds) *Communities of Practice: Critical Perspectives* (pp. 17–29). London: Routledge.

General Medical Council (1993) *Tomorrow's Doctors: recommendations on undergraduate medical education.* London: GMC

General Medical Council (1999) *The Doctor as Teacher.* London: GMC

General Medical Council (2003) *Tomorrow's Doctors.* London: GMC

General Medical Council (2009a) *Tomorrow's Doctors: outcomes and standards for undergraduate medical education.* London: GMC

General Medical Council (2009b) *Medical Students: professional values and fitness to practice.* London: GMC

General Medical Council (2011a) *Supplementary Advice: clinical placements for medical students.* London: GMC

General Medical Council (2011b) *Draft CPD Guidance for Consultation.* London: GMC

General Medical Council (2011c) *Continuing Professional Development: the international perspective.* London: GMC

Hager P. (2005) Current theories of workplace learning: a critical assessment. In N. Bascia A. Cumming, A. Dannow, et al. (eds) *International Handbook of Educational Policy* (pp. 829–846). London: Kewer

Hager, P. (2011) Theories of workplace learning. In M. Malloch, L. Cairns, K. Evans, and B.N. O'Connor, (eds) *The Sage Handbook of Workplace Learning* (pp. 17–31). London: Sage.

Harris, J., Evans, K., and Guile, D. (2007) Project report: Putting Knowledge to Work: Integrating Work-based and Subject-based Knowledge in Intermediate-level qualifications (1)—An orientation and a Framework. [online]. http://www.wlecentre.ac.uk/cms/files/projects/reports/PR_Harris-Evans-Guile_2007.pdf Accessed 9 August 2012

Hughes J., Jewson N., and Unwin L. (eds) (2007) *Communities of Practice: Critical Perspectives.* London: Routledge

Illing, J., Morrow, G., Kergon, C., et al. (2008) How prepared are medical graduates to begin practice? London: GMC. [online] http://www.gmc-uk.org/FINAL_How_prepared_are_medical_graduates_to_begin_practice_September_08.pdf_29697834.pdf Accessed 9 August 2012

Illeris, K. (2011) Workplaces and learning. In M. Malloch, L. Cairns, K. Evans, and B.N. O'Connor, (eds) (2011) *The SAGE Handbook of Workplace Learning* (pp. 32–45). London: Sage

Jarvis, P. (2006) Towards a Theory of Human Learning. London: Routledge

Kilminster, S., Zukas, M., Quniton, N., and Roberts, T. (2011) Preparedness is not enough: understanding transitions as critically intensive learning periods. *Med Educ.* 45: 1006–1015

Kerschensteiner, G. (1950) *Der Begriff der staatsbürgerlichen Erziehung* [The concept of civic education]. Munich. Cited in: UNESCO: International Bureau of Education (1993) *The quarterly review of comparative education.* Paris, vol. XXIII, no. 3/4, 1993, p. 807–822

Knowles, M. (1973) *The Adult Learner. A Neglected Species.* (4th edn. Houston: Gulf Publishing

Kolb, D. (1984) *Experiential Learning.* Englewood Cliffs, NJ: Prentice Hall

Kuper, A, Nedden, N, Etchells, E., Shadowitz, S., and Reeves, S. (2010) Teaching and Learning in morbidity and mortality rounds: an ethnographic study. *Med Educ.* 44(6): 559–569

Lave, J. and Wenger, E. (1991) *Situated Learning: Legitimate Peripheral Participation.* Cambridge: Cambridge University Press

Malloch, M., Cairns, L., Evans, K. and O'Connor, B.N. (eds) (2011) *The SAGE Handbook of Workplace Learning.* London: Sage

Matusov, E. (2007) In search of 'the appropriate' unit of analysis for sociocultural research. *Culture Psychol.* 13: 307–332

McLachlan, J. and Regan De Bere, S. (2004) How we teach anatomy without cadavers. *Clin Teach.* 1(2): 49–52

Morris, C. and Blaney, D. (2010) Work-based learning. In T. Swanwick (ed.) *Understanding Medical Education* (pp. 69–82). Chichester: John Wiley & Sons Ltd

Morris, C. (2011) *From time-served apprenticeship to time-measured training: new challenges for postgraduate medical education.* Thesis presented in partial fulfilment for EdD, Institute of Education, University of London

Morris, C. (2012) Re-imagining 'the firm': clinical attachments as time spent in communities of practice. In V. Cook, C. Daly, and M. Newman (eds) *Work-based Learning in Clinical Settings. Insights from socio-cultural perspectives* (pp. 11–25). Oxford: Radcliffe

Oswald N. (2005) Agenda for change: agenda for learning change. *Educ Prim Care.* 16: 644–647

Patten, D. (2007) What lies beneath: the use of three-dimensional projection in living anatomy teaching. *Clin Teach.* 4: 10–14

PMETB (2008) *Educating Tomorrows Doctors. Future models of medical training; medical workforce shape and trainee expectations.* [online]. http://www.gmc-uk.org/Educating_Tomorrows_Doctors_working_group_report_20080620_v1.pdf_30375087.pdf Accessed 9 August 2012

Prado, H., Falbo, G., Falbo, A., and Figueiroa, J. (2011) Active learning on the ward: outcomes from a comparative trial with traditional methods. *Med Educ.* 45: 273–279

Roberts, T. (2009) *Learning responsibility? Exploring doctors' transitions to new levels of medical responsibility: Full Research Report.* ESRC End of Award Report, RES-153-25-0084. Swindon: ESRC

Schon, D. (1983) *The Reflective Practitioner.* New York: Basic Books

Schon, D. (1987) *Educating the Reflective Practitioner: Towards a new Design for Teaching and Learning in the Professions.* San Francisco: Jossey-Bass

Sfard, A. (1998) On two metaphors for learning and the dangers of choosing just one. *Educ Res* 27(2): 4–13

Siebert, H. (2012) Sustainability communication: a systemic-constructivist perspective. In J. Godemann and G. Michelsen, G. (eds) *Sustainability Communication. Interdisciplinary Perspectives and Theoretical Foundations* (pp. 109–115). London: Springer.

Sinclair, S. (1997) *Making Doctors. An Institutional Apprenticeship.* Berg: Oxford

Steinert, Y. (2000) Faculty development in the new millennium: key challenges and future directions. *Med Teach* 22(1): 44–50

Swanwick, T. (2005) Informal learning in postgraduate medical education: from cognitivism to 'culturism'. *Med Educ.* 39(8): 859–865

Swanwick, T. (2008) See one, do one, then what? Faculty development in postgraduate medical education. *Postgrad Med J.* 84: 339–343

Swanwick, T and Morris, C. (2010) Commentary: Shifting conceptions of learning in the workplace. *Med Educ.* 44: 538–539

Talbot, M. (2004) Monkey see, monkey do: a critique of the competency model in graduate medical education. *Med Educ.* 38(6): 580–581

Tallentire, V., Smith, S., Skinner, J., and Cameron, H. (2011) Understanding the behavior of newly qualified doctors in acute care contexts. *Med Educ.* 45: 995–1005

ten Cate, O. and Scheele, F. (2007) Viewpoint: competency-based postgraduate training: can we bridge the gap between theory and clinical practice? *Acad Med* 82(6): 542–547

Todd, T. (1968) *Report of the Royal Commission on Medical Education.* London: HSMO

Tooke, J. (2007) *Aspiring to excellence. Findings and Recommendations of the Independent Inquiry into Modernising Medical Careers*, London: MMC Inquiry.

Turnbull S (ed.) (2000) The role of emotion in situated learning and communities of practice. Working Paper 59. *Productive Learning at Work*. Sydney, Australia: Lancaster University Management School, University of Technology

Vygotsky L (1978) Tool and symbol in child development. In M. Cole, V. John-Steiner, S. Scribner, and S. Souberman (eds) *Mind in Society: the development of higher psychological processes* (pp. 19–30). Cambridge, MA: Harvard University Press,

Wenger, E. (1998) *Communities of Practice: Learning, Meaning and Identity*. Cambridge: Cambridge University Press

CHAPTER 19

Learning in ambulatory care

John Dent

Most patients in most disciplines are managed at home unless they are very seriously ill, and teaching of clinical method must be organised to take account of this and use outpatient, day patient, and domiciliary arenas.

DJ Jolley

Introduction

The reason for our interest in medical education might be explained by both a desire to help students to learn and a willingness to help clinician colleagues to teach. Doctors and other healthcare professionals in general have what has been called a teaching instinct (Hesketh and Laidlaw 2002), which serves as the bedrock on which further instruction in teaching and staff development activities can be built. Although doctors often have a lifetime's experience of teaching in the inpatient situation our experience in the ambulatory care environment may be more limited and, if thinking of teaching in the context of a busy outpatient clinic, may be tainted with memories of time-pressures and inconvenience. As Skeff has said (1988 p. S31):

> Many faculty members have an intrinsic desire and enthusiasm for teaching, but they are drawn in several directions with various responsibilities. Without clear emphasis on the importance of clinical teaching in the ambulatory setting, they will understandably spend less time concentrating on this role.

In 2000 Fields and colleagues wrote:

> Current physicians, just as society as a whole, must not abandon the important role of ensuring the quality of the medical education of future physicians. When implemented properly, ambulatory education is uniquely suited to meet the needs of students, practicing physicians and most importantly, the patients.

> Fields et al. (2000)

This chapter asks six fundamental questions to help us develop opportunities for ambulatory care teaching:

1. Why should we teach in ambulatory care?

2. What can be taught and learned in ambulatory care settings?

3. Where are there venues for ambulatory care teaching?

4. How can we help students to learn in ambulatory care settings?

5. When should we teach students in ambulatory care?

6. Who can teach students in ambulatory care settings?

We should also ask:

- How can we assess students in ambulatory care settings?

- How can we evaluate teaching in ambulatory care settings?

Why should we teach in ambulatory care?

'Ambulatory care refers to any place where patients are seen in hospital without being admitted as inpatients' (Dent 2005 p. 302). It can provide experiences in which clinicians, patients and students meet, in what can be ideal teaching situations. Changes in hospital practice have resulted in there being fewer inpatients available that are suitable for undergraduate teaching, while at the same time there are an increasing number of students to teach. From 1970 to 1990, the duration of inpatient stay for acute specialties reduced from 11.3 to 6.1 days, with 70% of hospital patient contacts now in ambulatory settings (Lawson and Moss 1993). Inpatients are acutely unwell, in the midst of active clinical care or investigations or represent medical problems beyond the scope of the core undergraduate curriculum. In brief 'the inpatient area [may be] less representative of actual medical practice and a less desirable place for students to glean the fundamentals of clinical care and problem-solving than in the past' (Fincher and Albritton 1993). As long ago as 1986 Pergoff recognized these challenges to inpatient teaching and called for a major change in resources for the financing and organization of more ambulatory care teaching. Dealing with these problems requires innovative programmes to be created in alternative venues (Bentley et al. 1989). If hospital wards no longer present a balanced overview of patterns of health and disease then, as the King's Fund review concluded, 'increased use of out-patient and general practice for teaching is essential to reflect the true spectrum of health and disease in the community' (Towle 1991). 'When new facilities are being built, ambulatory teaching space should be incorporated into plans' (Krackov et al. 1993). If ambulatory care is to become a key facet of modern medical practice then it is important that 'teaching follows the patient' (Lawson and Moss 1993).

Almost 20 years later the problem remains the same. Tertiary hospitals have a decreasing number of suitable inpatients for student teaching and increasing numbers of students to teach. According to Parry et al. (2002) clinical teaching will need to expand from this traditional venue to develop teaching opportunities in district general hospitals. More recently the UK General Medical Council (GMC) has directed that clinical education 'must provide experience in a variety of environments including hospitals, general practices and community medical services' (GMC 2009a).

Some studies have found that ambulatory care experiences were effective in improving both students' knowledge and skills (Frye et al. 1998) and in some studies were preferable to inpatient experiences (Lynch et al. 1999). While McLeod and colleagues (1997) reported that inpatient experiences were preferable for learning clinical skills and making diagnoses, Kalet and colleagues (1998) found that students had better relationships with patients and teachers in ambulatory care. However, although clinical timetables appear to provide an adequate amount of patient contact with both inpatients and outpatients, the actual time students spend with patients is probably less than suggested (McKergow et al. 1991; Davis and Dent 1994).

The benefits of ward-based teaching are often compromised by there being only a small number of suitable patients available for students to see, by the opportunistic nature of the clinical conditions available and by the pressure of service commitments on the staff. In contrast, outpatient facilities can offer large numbers of patients with common medical conditions who are more representative of general medical practice (Butterfield and Libertin 1993). Unlike inpatients, patients seen in ambulatory care are not acutely unwell and unlike simulated patients have their own clinical histories and maybe ongoing physical findings. Finally, there is now a substantial body of literature indicating that undergraduate medical education can safely be delivered in ambulatory or community settings without compromising academic standards (Worley et al. 2004a; Lyon et al. 2006).

What can be taught and learned in ambulatory care settings?

Stearns and Glasser (1993) suggested that while opportunities for student learning with inpatients is usually focused on aetiology,

history, physical examination, laboratory tests, and therapy; ambulatory care settings can also include opportunities for students to gain experience in:

◆ continuity of care

◆ context of care

◆ resource allocation

◆ health education

◆ patient responsibility.

Students experience continuity of care and integration of interdisciplinary healthcare with basic and clinical sciences; there are opportunities for collaborative and self-directed learning and they can observe doctor–patient communication as well as the doctor relating to other healthcare professionals (Irby 1995; Fields et al. 2000), see fig. 19.1.

Although some of these outcomes may seem 'soft' they are important; for instance, complaints against doctors can often be traced to a lack of appropriate communication with colleagues or adequate explanation to patients and relatives. Practically all learning outcomes can be indicated or experienced in the ambulatory care teaching venue (Harden et al. 1997; Simpson et al. 2002). Finally, 'ambulatory-based teaching can also provide multiple exposures to the same clinical problem allowing learners to build more complex and transferable knowledge', as a result (Sprake et al. 2008). It is probably more likely that opportunities for student reflection, tutor feedback, and formative assessment will be taken up in the ambulatory care setting than in ward-based teaching sessions.

Where are the venues for ambulatory care teaching?

Opportunities for students to learn with ambulatory care patients exist in both tertiary care teaching hospitals and district general venues.

Traditional venues

Medical school undergraduate clinical teaching in a tertiary care teaching hospital is traditionally based on inpatients; any exposure to learning in an ambulatory context is usually limited to visits to outpatient clinics as part of attachments in medical and surgical specialties.

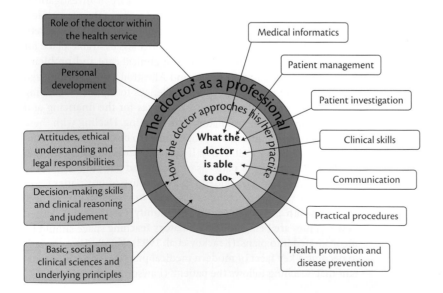

Figure 19.1 The 12 learning outcomes of the Scottish doctor.

J.G. Simpson, J. Furnace, J. Crosby et al., 'The Scottish doctor—learning outcomes for the medical undergraduate in Scotland: a foundation for competent and reflective practitioners', Medical Teacher, 2002, 24, 2, pp. 136–143, copyright © 2002, Informa Healthcare. Reproduced with permission of Informa Healthcare.

Additional venues

Opportunities for students to visit additional outpatient venues tend to depend on personal arrangements made by individual clinical teachers or a proactive approach from enthusiastic students, and are subject to serendipity rather than the presence of a timetabled, structured programme. Possible additional ambulatory care teaching venues where teaching opportunities could be developed may include:

- Visits to patient-treatment activities with physiotherapists, occupational therapists, speech therapists, dieticians, or orthotists.

- Screening clinics such as the antenatal clinic, well-baby clinic, or paediatric day unit.

- Interprofessional clinics—for instance a diabetes clinic may provide students with exposure to a variety of allied health professionals including the specialist nurse, dietician, podiatrist, and optometrist.

- Clinical investigation unit—an endoscopy suite may offer experiences in upper and lower GI endoscopy as well as cystoscopy, which may be led by doctors or nurse-practitioners.

Other venues include radiology departments, renal dialysis units, blood transfusion units, child development centres, and day surgery units.

So it is worthwhile thinking widely to identify new ambulatory venues which might be suitable for teaching. Interestingly, when suitable opportunities for student access to children were difficult to find, the paediatric ward play areas and outpatient waiting areas were found to provide purposeful child–student contact (Bardgett and Dent 2011).

Wherever you identify a suitable location, developing a structured comprehensive approach to teaching and learning is most important. The following tips might be helpful:

- identify available spaces and resources

- approach enthusiastic colleagues working there

- create a structured programme for teaching and learning

- timetable an appropriate number of students to the sessions

- provide staff development opportunities and listen to feedback

- give ownership of the programme to the providers.

The day surgery unit programme

After reviewing the types of surgical procedure being carried out in the day surgery unit (DSU), Dunnington (1990) suggested that there was a distinct body of clinical experience which could only be observed in the ambulatory surgery setting.

Changes in healthcare delivery over the last 20 years have reduced the number of surgical patients attending inpatient settings by 25–50% (DaRosa et al. 1992). As earlier hospital discharge and an increase in day surgery operating has become possible following advances in surgical procedures and anaesthesia there has been a growth in day surgery procedures. This provides an incentive to focus resources on the restructuring of surgical teaching in the day surgery unit especially as increasing specialization in teaching hospitals means that inpatients are often unrepresentative of patients seen in general medical practice (Schwartz 1992; Dunnington and DaRosa 1994).

Despite these incentives, Seabrook and colleagues (1997) reported the DSU as an underutilized venue for ambulatory care teaching. In a survey of 227 DSUs they found only 45% were used for teaching and only 7% had students present for more than one day per week. Teaching tended to be unstructured, theatre-based and centred on shadowing the surgeons present.

This possibly underutilized learning resource can be looked at from the perspective of skills training. Nakayama and Steiber (1990) reported that often basic surgical skills had not been practised by students prior to graduation. Both Lossing and Groetzsch (1992) and Seabrook and colleagues (1998a) reported the positive benefits of introducing technical skills instruction in scrubbing, gowning, gloving, instrument handling, suturing, cutting, and stapling to students, and were able to demonstrate improved performance in these skills after training. In 2009 Kellet and colleagues reported how a theatre etiquette course teaching small groups of students to scrub, gown, and glove could be delivered to a whole class of 160 third-year medical students in one day using available operating theatre space.

Student-centred, structured learning programmes for day surgery units have been developed to include experiences in preoperative assessment, diagnosis, anaesthetic, and surgical procedures and interprofessional postoperative recovery and follow-up (Seabrook et al. 1998a; Hannah and Dent 2006). Importantly in today's working environment such teaching programmes have not been found to impact negatively on patient care (Rudkin et al. 1997) and in fact there is a mean waiting time of 3 hours before surgery when patients are available for teaching (O'Riordan and Clark, 1997).

Innovative venues

Teaching clinics

Patients with particular problems relevant to students' learning needs are specifically selected from routine GP referral letters and asked to attend a special teaching clinic. They are advised that there will be students present and that their appointment will be longer than usual. They will however be seeing a specialist about their clinical problem and there will be an opportunity to speak privately at the end of the consultation if requested.

Simulated outpatient clinic

Simulated patients may be used for practising clinical skills in the ambulatory care setting. Encounters with simulated patients (SPs) may be followed by a feedback session using a video of the event (Myung et al. 2010).

In one study third year medical students were given either a four hour encounter with standardized vascular patients or with unselected patients attending a routine outpatient clinic. Standardized vascular patients were found to be more effective for teaching problem-solving and clinical skills and promoted more student satisfaction and confidence than traditional patients (Sullivan et al 2000).

Ambulatory or community care programmes

Latta and colleagues (2013) describe a programme for fourth and fifth year students in nine medical disciplines based in a simulated outpatient clinic adjoining the clinical skills laboratory. The programme includes clinical skills revision and teaching with invited ambulatory patients (and is integrated with ward-based teaching). A model to structured student learning has been described by Kurth and colleagues (1997) to help students adapt to an ambulatory or community clinical environment by promoting active, self-directed learning. They report that the model enhances the standardization of learning across a variety of clinical sites and increases the cost-effectiveness of teaching.

Station clinics

In the leg ulcer clinic of a dermatology department, waiting room space and multiple side rooms were used for an OSCE-like learning progression through various stations including: revision of learning material, taking a patient history, nurse-led examination, video learning, peer-supported skills practice, and computerized self-assessment (Stewart 2005).

Ambulatory care teaching centre (ACTC)

This is a specially developed facility created to provide structured clinical teaching activities with clinical tutors and non-acute patients from a bank of clinical volunteers (Dent et al 2001b).

Diagnostic and treatment centre (DTC)

Facilities in these regional centres may include a variety of ambulatory care opportunities for students including outpatient consultations, rehabilitation and therapy sessions, attendances for clinical investigations and day surgery (Dent et al. 2007).

An ambulatory care teaching centre programme

The ACTC was developed to meet identified curriculum needs including practice at physical examination, integration of clinical and basic sciences, and critical thinking and judgement. In a systems-based programme the sessions are based on selected clinical volunteers and invited tutors with the whole programme coordinated by an ACTC administrator. Building up a bank of volunteer patients to support the clinical teaching programme is crucially important. These 'ex-patients' have real clinical histories and may have physical findings but are not acutely unwell or requiring hospital treatment. Patients with different clinical problems can be invited to attend in rotation, as appropriate for the students' learning requirements. Travel expenses and some recognition or appreciation go a long way

to rewarding these volunteers for their involvement. A patient bank coordinator is required to recruit, select, train and categorize these volunteers and then to invite them to teaching sessions as required, to reimburse them and to keep a record of their attendance.

An ambulatory care centre administrator is required to:

♦ oversee the day-to-day running of the facility and take bookings for its use

♦ produce a summary of the patients' clinical history and management

♦ gather and set out the additional teaching material required for each day to complement the programme and support integrated learning

♦ be based in the ambulatory care teaching facility.

Students may attend one ACTC session during each week of a systems-based course seeing one or two system-specific patients each time

A DTC programme

In the UK some district general hospitals have been recommissioned to provide diagnostic and treatment facilities at a regional level and so avoid tertiary hospital referral for ambulatory patients (Mail online 2002; Walters 2003). This new ambulatory care resource may be available for student teaching (fig. 19.2).

A clinical elective attachment in a rural centre DTC near Dundee gave final year students 4 weeks of ambulatory experience in a range of outpatient, rehabilitation and day surgery clinics (Henderson 2005). Clinical staff in a variety of disciplines acted as tutors and supplementary clinical teaching sessions were provided for a further two sessions per week by clinical skills tutors and GPs

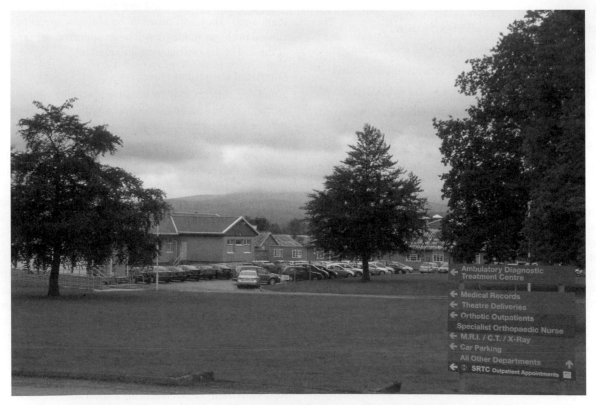

Figure 19.2 An ambulatory care centre.

(Dent et al. 2007). Worley and colleagues (2004b) in particular have argued that such community-based, ambulatory care placements are credible alternatives to clinical attachments in traditional teaching hospitals.

How can we help students learn in ambulatory care settings?

An ambulatory care venue, which is the workplace of a group of healthcare providers, will of necessity be focused on patient care; so at first impression may not appear welcoming to student visitors. Barriers to teaching encountered in such a managed care environment may include: a large patient workload, time pressures, inadequate space for students to see patients independently, and the unpredictability of the patient problems presenting. Difficulties with providing teaching may include orientating students to the workplace, observing students' performance and giving appropriate feedback.

Strategies will need to be developed to balance service and teaching commitments. Good teaching practice includes, creating a welcoming environment, promoting direct communication between students and patients, observing learners' performance, giving timely feedback, and encouraging learners to take an increased responsibility for their own learning both during and after the event (Sprake et al. 2008; Ashley et al. 2008).

In the outpatient clinic

According to Feltovich et al. (1987) 'it appears that in most cases students have been fitted into existing clinics or patterns of teaching with insufficient effort given to achieving the maximum educational benefit for the student'. Fully integrating students into the routine of the outpatient department can be helped by prior learning on the part of the students, reviewing their current learning competences before they start, and creative scheduling of patient appointments. Parallel booking of patients for learners, and patients for clinicians, can be one way to help with this (Regan-Smith et al. 2002).

A clinical teacher may have to orient learners prior to attendance so that they are prepared for the expected learning opportunities and to discuss the learning strategies with them; these may include self-directed learning, post-clinic conferences or a small study project to stimulate further learning. None of these activities should negatively impact the normal duration of the clinic.

Ever increasing student numbers mean that less time is available in the clinic for individual student-patient contact. Five strategies have been described by Ferenchick and colleagues (1997), which go some way to helping this situation by using creative ideas for both students and tutors:

1. 'Wave' scheduling of patient appointments
2. Orienting learners to patients
3. Having learners do their case presentation in the consulting room
4. Employing the microskills of the one minute preceptor (Lipsky et al. 1999)
5. Effectively reflecting on one's teaching in order to develop effective teaching scripts for future use.

A busy outpatient clinic can, however, be overwhelming. As Meadows observed (1979), 'it is sad that this area where teaching is of the greatest importance is also the one where the needs of the patient and the needs of the student conflict most'. In such circumstances it is helpful to have a variety of models available to help manage the student group to maximal advantage. So, thinking of the outpatient department, what simple strategies can be used to help teaching? The following models for managing clinical teaching sessions with various numbers of students have been described (Dent 2009).

Grandstand

All students attending observe the clinician's consultation but are not usually able to interact with the patient in this crowded situation.

Breakout

Students observe the whole consultation with a patient and then take turns to see the patient independently in another room.

Supervising

Students interview selected patients independently before being visited by the clinician to supervise their performance.

Report back

Students see patients independently before presenting the case to the clinician in the main consulting room.

Figure 19.3 shows models for managing students in the outpatient clinic.

Ultimately the most appropriate choice of teaching model depends on:

- the number of clinicians attending
- the number of rooms available
- the number and prior experience of the students present
- the number of patients expected.

Other ideas for effective teaching in busy ambulatory care settings include (Sprake et al. 2008):

- Hot seating: teachers hand over the second part of a patient interview to the students and observe the student's performance.
- Directed observation: the learner is given specific parts of the doctor's history and physical examination to observe while watching the whole consultation. They discuss these parts afterwards.
- Productive diversion: students interview a new patient from lower down the clinic list and present them to the clinician once their appointment time is reached.
- Educational prescriptions: specific questions are left with the students to research and to present their answers at a later date.
- Hot review: be ready to give immediate feedback and answers to questions.

In more detail Ashley and colleagues (2008) identified 18 practical recommendations to support students in the outpatient clinic or GP surgery (see fig. 19.4).

In the clinical investigations suite

Radiology, vascular assessment and endoscopy may all be available to provide students with learning opportunities with ambulatory patients. Learning may be helped by structured logbooks where students record the patients and conditions seen or with workbooks

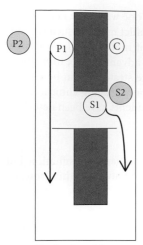
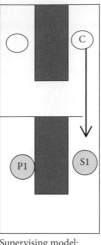

Break out model:
Students take turns to see a
patient independently after the
initial consultation

Supervising model:
Students see selected patients
unger supervision

Report back model:
Students see patients
independently and report back
to clinician

C = Clinician   P = Patient   S = Student

Figure 19.3 Models for managing students in the outpatient clinic.

This figure was published in A Practical Guide for Medical Teachers, JA Dent and RM Harden, Copyright Elsevier 2009.

- Regard students as people who are scared of you and patients as people who feel warm towards students.
- Be approachable and friendly, not dictatorial.
- Consider that students may be more comfortable attending in pairs.
- Tell them what to expect from you and what you expect of them.
- Obtain every patient's consent for a student to be present and ensure the student knows you have done so.
- Orientate students to patients before consultation begins.
- If time and space permits, have them interview patients on their own first.
- Brief them or give them a written template to guide their interview/examination.
- Arrange the furniture to make everybody feel included and promote good eye contact.
- Use your interactions with students to create a comfortable and relaxed climate for patients.
- Encourage direct verbal interactions with patients that makes students active participants in the consultation.
- Handle sensitive consultation carefully so you involve students to patient' benefit rather than harm.
- Have students perform any hands-on procedures they are capable of on your behalf.
- Use physical examination to help them connect with patients.
- Allow them to practice presenting cases.
- Find out, conversationally, their level of knowledge and meet their learning need.
- Help them understand your questions if they seem to have difficulty answering them.
- Debrief at the end, summarise, and reinforce take home messages.

Figure 19.4 Tips on supporting a medical student in an outpatient clinic or surgery.
J Ashley , P. , Rhodes , N. , Sari-Kouzel , H. , Mukerjee , A. , and Dornan , T., 'They've all got to learn'. Medical students' learning from patients in ambulatory (outpatient and general practice) consultations', Medical Teacher, 2009, 31, 2, pp. 1–8, copyright © 2009, Informa Healthcare. Reproduced with permission of Informa Healthcare.

where they answer patient-management problems (Dent et al. 2007).

In the day surgery unit

Students can follow the patient journey from presentation in an outpatient clinic, through interaction with the multidisciplinary team in preoperative assessment and preparation, during the operative procedure itself with anaesthetists and surgeons, and into postoperative care with the planning of discharge and follow-up care back in the community (O'Driscoll et al. 1998; Seabrook et al. 1998a; Hannah and Dent 2006).

The operating theatre may present a difficult environment for students (Lyon 2003). Challenges include:

- the physical environment and emotional impact of surgery
- the educational tasks for the students
- social relations with operating theatre staff.

The 12 tips shown in fig 19.5 for delivering a clinical teaching programme in the DSU may help to avoid these issues (Dent 2003).

Dunnington (1990) suggests that surgical departments must move towards structured learning modules for ambulatory surgery that are provided either as a block experience or integrated into the existing surgical clerkship. Seabrook and colleagues (1998b) reported the positive view of students, teachers and managers to these new teaching initiatives in the DSU.

In the ACTC

Experience has shown that tutors in the ACTC feel more comfortable if additional resources for teaching are readily available. These might include edited case notes or summaries giving a précis of the part of the patient volunteer's history relevant for the current session; laboratory reports of pertinent investigations to be used in the discussion of patient management; images—radiographs, scans, and clinical photographs; videos may be useful if a review of the school's preferred approach to clinical examination is required; and diagnostic equipment for students to practise basic clinical skills (Dent et al. 2001a).

Tutors should take the opportunity to help students integrate their clinical experience in the ambulatory care programme to material they have learned elsewhere.

Vertical integration can be provided by reference to material from earlier years in the students' programme. Horizontal integration may include reference to patients seen elsewhere in concurrent clinical attachments.

Preparation

1 Identify the learning objectives that students can achieve in the DSU

2 Secure institutional support and form an implementation / steering group representing all parties involved

3 Decide which year of the course will most benefit from the programme and how many students can be accommodated

4 Identify a method for selecting appropriate patients

5 Identify space for student/patient consultations

6 Reserve space in a skills training unit

7 Provide staff development opportunities

Delivery

8 Provide a study guide/logbook

9 Employ a DSU-based tutor/supervisor

10 Provide opportunities for student reflection, tuition and assessment

Evaluation

11 Evaluate feedback from students, tutors and DSU staff

12 Discuss research and development opportunities with all parties involved

Figure 19.5 12 tips for delivering a clinical teaching programme in the DSU. Data from Dent, J.A. (2003) Twelve tips for developing a clinical teaching programme in a day surgery unit. Med Teach. 25: 364–367.

Educational strategies for maximizing learning opportunities

The key to a successful ambulatory care teaching programme is to have a structured approach to teaching. 'Appropriate instructional strategies must be selected and developed to facilitate student learning and maximize the resources and opportunities provided by these ambulatory venues' (Dent 2005). Strategies are required both to facilitate student learning and to identify gaps in student experience which may occur in both the breadth and depth of their patient encounters (Gruppen et al. 1993). Educational strategies may include those shown in fig. 19.6.

Structured logbook

Learning can be structured to follow the curriculum learning outcomes or domains (Dent and Davis 1995). The EPITOMISE logbook (Dent 2009), based on the 12 learning outcomes of the Scottish Doctor (Harden et al. 1997; Simpson et al. 2002), has been used to focus student learning on the opportunities related to the various patients seen in ambulatory care. With every patient they meet students are invited to ask themselves three questions:

Structured logbooks and portfolios (Patil and Lee 2002; Buckley et al. 2009)

Integrated learning

Study guide (Mires et al. 1998; Roth et al. 1997; Latta et al. 2013)

Task-based learning (Harden et al. 1996)

Record of clinical achievement

Learning contracts (Parsell 1997; Chan and Chien 2000)

Microskills for students (Lipsky et al. 1999)

Learner-centred approach (Wolpaw et al. 2003)

Patient journey record books (Hannah and Dent 2006)

Focused discussion (DaRosa et al. 1997)

Figure 19.6 Educational strategies.

- ◆ What did you see?
- ◆ What did you do?
- ◆ What did you learn?

The EPITOMISE acronym helps students to look for all learning outcomes in any patient encounter:

E ethics and enquiry (communications skills)

P physical examination

I investigations and interpretation of results

T technical procedures

O options of diagnosis (clinical judgement)

M management and multidisciplinary team

I information handling

S sciences, basic and clinical

E education of the patient and yourself.

Students record their interactions and learnings with each patient and then reflect on what they need to do next to develop their learning further.

Study guide

The University of Otago has a structured workbook for students to document their learning and procedural skills during their integrated ambulatory medicine programme (Latta et al. 2013).

The University of Minnesota medical school has described a 'Worksheet for Ambulatory Medicine', a one-page form including learning objectives, which students and tutors complete during each patient encounter (Roth et al. 1997). The University of Dundee has described a two-part study guide (Mires et al. 1998) for use in Obstetrics and Gynaecology attachments. It provides Topics, Programme, Issues for learning, Clinical tasks, and Assessment (the TOPICAL approach). In the second part, the response book, students submit a structured case report.

Task-based learning (TBL)

TBL helps students in the clinical phase of the course to learn by understanding the concepts and mechanisms underlying various prescribed tasks (Harden et al. 1996).

Record of clinical experience tick-book

Students are required to demonstrate competence in a series of prescribed tasks. Good examples of this type of logbook have several detailed descriptors for each task by which the individual student's competence on successive occasions can be rated.

Learning contracts

Parsell (1997) describes a handbook for junior hospital doctors incorporating a learning contract between trainees and tutors based on an agreed curriculum of learning objectives and a mechanism for formal review. In a nursing degree course this strategy was found to increase student autonomy and motivation and to promote sharing between students and clinical tutors (Chan and Chien 2000).

Microskills for students

Lipsky and colleagues (1999) describe how students can take the initiative both before and after the outpatient event to facilitate their own learning.

Learner-centred approach

Wolpaw et al. (2003) describe the 'SNAPPS' approach. Students are asked to:

- summarize the history
- narrow the differential diagnosis
- analyse the differential diagnosis
- probe the preceptor with questions
- plan management
- select a case-relevant issue for self-directed learning.

Patient journey record book

In the day surgery unit students describe the learning points from their interaction with patients in the outpatient department and in preoperative assessment; during the surgery; and in postoperative recovery and subsequent patient follow-up in the clinic.

Focused discussion

Timetabled pre- and postclinic discussion with the clinical teacher can be used to stimulate the students in higher order thinking about issues related to the patients seen.

Additional resources

Virtual patients

This approach provides computer-based clinical scenarios in an interactive format and can be especially good for promoting clinical reasoning skills (Cook and Triola 2009). In the Rural Clinical School of Western Australia the virtual patient cases are presented either on line or by DVD to fill gaps in the students' clinical experience while they are working in remote or rural locations. Their further use with a follow-up seminar adds to the value of this resource (Edelbring et al. 2012).

Video recording a student–patient consultation

Video recording of a student–patient interview or of a clinical examination can be viewed in real time by the student group and tutor and later reviewed by the student. Sympathetically presented peer critique and tutor feedback followed by self-review of the video is a powerful learning experience for the individual student (Dent and Preece 2002).

When should we teach students in ambulatory care?

The extent of a student's learning in ambulatory care activities can be placed on a spectrum beginning with observing an outpatient consultation, progressing to being supervised in practising skills and finally active participation in an ambulatory care event. Ambulatory care attachments have something to offer students at whatever stage of learning they have reached. For junior students early clinical contact is a valuable feature of an innovative curriculum (Harden et al. 1984) providing them with insight, experience and excitement—which often motivates learning. For intermediate students the ACTC can act as a bridge between learning through simulation in the Clinical Skills Centre to learning from real patient encounters in real clinical venues. Finally, senior students are able to adopt an apprenticeship approach and participate with clinicians in a working ambulatory care environment,

perhaps by using parallel consulting rooms (Worley et al. 2000; Lake and Vickery 2006; Phinney and Hager 1998).

Who can teach students in ambulatory care settings?

To take advantage of educational opportunities as they present in ambulatory care, clinical tutors must acquire the mental agility required to 'capture the teachable moment' as it presents (Bowling 1993). Enthusiasm and good-will go a long way to making a good clinical teacher.

Not all of the teaching or supervision in the ambulatory care teaching programme, especially in the ACTC, needs to be done by a content expert or specialist clinician.

Teaching fellows

Trainees with an interest in teaching may be able to contribute. Some centres appoint teaching fellows for a limited period who may enrol in a Certificate or Diploma course in Medical Education while continuing their clinical training. Such appointments may become part of a move towards an emerging academic career.

Other healthcare professionals

Colleagues from other healthcare professions may be able to illustrate aspects of patient care relevant to the clinical problem from their own perspective, for example the physiotherapist or paediatric nurse educator (Bardgett and Dent 2011).

Peer-assisted learning scheme (PALS)

Senior students can be invited to train as peer tutors to contribute to the programme by assisting junior students in physical examination procedures and history taking sessions with clinical volunteers (Ross and Cameron 2007).

Clinical tutor

GPs and hospital doctors from any discipline should be able to help students practise clinical history taking and examination. Sessional work by a senior or retired clinician can give a valuable lead to a teaching programme especially in the ACTC. A DSU teaching firm has been described which focussed on active learning and skills development by using a multiprofessional team of tutors, led by an expert in medical education (Seabrook et al. 1998b).

Patients

With appropriate briefing and consent patients from a variety of sources may be available to contribute to the programme (Howe and Anderson 2003) (as shown in table 19.1).

Staff development

While much depends on individual enthusiasm and motivation for teaching, several ancillary factors of effective teaching have been described (Irby et al. 1991); knowledge of the medical school's curriculum and learning objectives and of how the presenting clinical experience may fit into students' prior knowledge; organization and clarity; group instructional skills, clinical supervision skills; clinical competence; role modelling and professional characteristics.

Anderson et al. (1997) conducted a survey of 14 medical educators involved in faculty development for ambulatory care

Table 19.1 Patients and ambulatory care teaching

New patients

New patients attending outpatient clinics may be seen at the time that the students are present. However, these patients bring a largely unselected variety of clinical problems, not all of which may be appropriate for the students' current learning needs.

Selected patients

Appropriate patients with conditions relevant for the students' current learning needs can be selected from those newly referred by their GP for outpatient appointments and invited to a special teaching clinic.

Bank patients

A 'bank' of previous patients may be built up from volunteers whose clinical condition no longer requires acute medical care. These bank patients can be categorised by the body system affected and, in a systems-based curriculum, be invited to attend during the appropriate part of the student programme (Brush and Moore, 1994, Dent et al. 2001b)

Standardized or simulated patients—standardized or simulated patients may be used in dedicated teaching clinics to demonstrate particular features and allow students to practise particular skills (Myung et al. 2010)

education. Programmes were largely conducted as workshops and emphasized the teaching encounter. They recommended that programmes should emphasis the role of preinstruction and planning, should teach faculty how best to use postinstructional learning such as reflection and train learners and other clinical staff to collaborate with faculty in the learning process. However, other methods of information sharing such as briefing handouts and posters may be more popular with clinicians than attending additional meetings (Ker and Dent 2002). The '*Getting started...*' series of booklets from Dundee, recently commended by the GMC in their QABME report on the medical school (GMC 2009b), provide easily accessible briefings on how to facilitate clinical teaching sessions in a variety of locations (Dent and Davis 2008).

A comprehensive, inclusive approach to staff development is emphasized by Schofield et al. (2010). This approach recognizes that ownership of medical student teaching is not the prerogative of the medical school alone but should be shared with clinical staff from a variety of other healthcare professions all of whom participate to various extents with student teaching. This broader approach to staff development involving all stakeholders is becoming increasingly appropriate as funding for staff development becomes available from a variety of sources.

How can we assess students in ambulatory care settings?

Logbooks and e-logbooks provide a means of continuous assessment of learning, encourage interaction of students with tutors and provide feedback to evaluate learning activities (Patil and Lee 2002). A summary of the literature is provided by Denton and colleagues who state that 'the ideal logbook should be inexpensive, feasible, and acceptable to students and should allow rapid collation of accurate, relevant data for timely analysis and feedback to the student and clerkship director' (Denton et al. 2006).

Buckley and colleagues (2009) provide a comprehensive overview of portfolios; e-portfolios help to reduce paperwork and promote immediacy and effectiveness of feedback (Duque 2003).

Focus scripts (Peltier et al. 2007) have been used to help students learn history taking and physical examination skills.

A formal mini-CEX takes between 15 and 25 minutes and so may be difficult to fit into a routine clinic. However, students appreciate the immediate feedback, which helps them to identify strengths and weaknesses and improve skills (Norcini et al. 2003).

Direct observation of procedural skills (DOPS) is a method of assessment developed specifically for assessing practical skills. The learner is directly observed while carrying out a procedure on a real patient. Specific components of the procedure are assessed against a checklist and feedback given (Wilkinson et al. 1998; Norcini and Burch 2007).

Video review provides opportunities for self review, peer critique and tutor feedback (Dent and Preece 2002).

Figure 19.7 shows some options for the assessment of learners in ambulatory care.

How can we evaluate teaching in ambulatory care settings?

A comparison of ambulatory and inpatient experiences was reported by East Carolina University (Lynch et al. 1999). Evaluation questionnaires were gathered from 72 students in five clerkships over 12 months. These showed that experiences in ambulatory venues were more welcoming and less threatening; they had better scheduling, improved clarity of student roles and responsibilities, and more supervised teaching. Other studies have suggested that medical students see a broader range of patient problems in ambulatory care venues than in inpatient teaching (McLeod et al. 1997) and score the educational value more highly (McLeod et al. 1999). Hajioff and Birchall (1999) found that 92% of students preferred to see patients alone.

To what extent does the delivery of teaching activities impact on patient care and clinical efficiency? In the managed care environment it is important that any new teaching requirement does not negatively impact on patient wellbeing or physician and practice productivity. Models of teaching which standardize learning and emphasize student self-directed learning can increase the cost effectiveness of teaching in ambulatory care (Kurth et al 1997). Clinic patients were not adversely affected in terms of patient consulting time when students were present (Hajioff and Birchall 1999; Usatine et al. 2000; Walters et al. 2008) nor was patient satisfaction reduced (Simon et al. 2000).

On reviewing final year student logbooks Davis and Dent (1994) showed that students learned more from attending the outpatient

Logbooks and e-logbooks
Portfolios and e-portfolios
Focus scripts
Mini-CEX
DOPS
Video review

Figure 19.7 Assessment in ambulatory care

clinics than ward rounds although they did not make the full use of the learning potential of either situation. The different settings did not prejudice the balance of learning outcomes experienced, although surgical complications were more likely to be seen in ward rounds. Papadakis and Karawa (1993) found that problem -solving and therapeutic skills in particular were less like to be taught in the ambulatory care environment.

Questionnaire feedback in the ACTC found that intermediate students appreciated the focussed atmosphere and the opportunities to see real patients rather than simulated ones and also the personal tuition and feedback. Tutors were happy to teach if they had prior knowledge of the patient problems presenting and if additional learning resources were available. Patients enjoyed contributing to the teaching programme and the chance to talk to students about their illness and experiences (Dent et al. 2001a). Stewart and colleagues (2005) found that students preferred the ACTC venue to the routine outpatient department although each venue demonstrated individual strengths with regard to giving students exposure to different learning outcomes.

Questionnaire review of the DTC programme found that senior students appreciated opportunities for learning in small groups and that the whole experience prepared them well for their first clinical posts. Clinicians particularly enjoyed the stimulus of having students with them. A problem highlighted by student attachments in this venue was the need for access to reliable IT facilities to support independent learning (Dent et al. 2007).

Parry and colleagues (2002) found that students perceived district hospitals as having a friendlier and more supportive learning environment than the traditional teaching hospital and that they offered an increased chance of hands-on practical experience.

Conclusions

To help us consider aspects of learning in ambulatory care we can ask ourselves six questions:

◆ Why should we teach in ambulatory care?
For various reasons tertiary referral teaching hospitals have a decreasing number of inpatients suitable for student teaching, but an increasing number of students to teach. Medical schools should now recognize the extended role played by ambulatory care facilities in patient care and take advantage of the teaching opportunities that they provide.

◆ What can be taught and learned in ambulatory care settings?
As outcome based education opens up a range of competencies that may not have previously been included in curricula, it becomes apparent that a number of these can be more readily taught in ambulatory care facilities

◆ Where are there venues for ambulatory care teaching?
Traditional ambulatory care teaching venues such as outpatient clinics or therapy departments are easy to find. Additional venues such as endoscopy and radiology suites or day surgery units are also usually available for teaching. In some situations a dedicated ambulatory care teaching centre or ambulatory care teaching programme can be created.

◆ How can we help students to learn in ambulatory care settings?
Management strategies are necessary to facilitate student attendance in the working environment. A variety of educational strategies can be used to maximize student learning opportunities. These may include structured logbooks, study guides, and online support.

◆ When should we teach students in ambulatory care?
Junior students benefit from early contact with patients with a variety of common clinical problems. For intermediary students the ambulatory care teaching centre can act as a bridge between learning through simulation in the clinical skills centre to learning in real clinical venues. Senior students are able to adopt an apprenticeship approach, and participate with clinicians in a variety of ambulatory care venues.

◆ Who can teach students in ambulatory care settings?
A variety of healthcare professionals and trainees may be available to help with teaching but all will benefit from a staff development programme.

References

Anderson, W.A., Carline, J.D., Ambrozy, D.M., and Irby, D.M. (1997) Faculty development for ambulatory care education. *Acad Med.* 72: 1072–1075

Ashley, P., Rhodes, N., Sari-Kouzel, H., Mukerjee, A., and Dornan, T. (2008) 'They've all got to learn'. Medical students learning from patients in ambulatory (outpatient and general practice) consultations. *Med Teach.* 31: e24–e31

Bardgett, R.J.M. and Dent, J.A. (2011) Teaching and learning in outpatients and beyond: how ambulatory care teaching can contribute to student learning in child health. *Arch Dis Child Educ Pract Ed.* 96: 148–152

Bentley, J.D., Knapp, R.M., and Petersdorf, R.G. (1989) Education in ambulatory care—financing is one piece of the puzzle. *N Engl J Med.* 320: 1531–1534

Bowling, J.R. (1993) Clinical teaching in the ambulatory care setting: how to capture the teachable moment. *J Am Osteopath Ass.* 93: 235–239

Brush, A.D. and Moore, T.G. (1994) Assigning patients according to curriculum: a strategy for improving ambulatory care residency training. *Acad Med.* 69: 717–719

Buckley, S., Coleman, J., Davison, I. et al. (2009) The educational effects of portfolios on undergraduate student learning: a Best Evidence Medical Education (BEME) systemic review. BEME Guide No. 11. *Med Teach.* 31: 281–298

Butterfield, P.S. and Libertin, A.G. (1993) Learning outcomes of an ambulatory care rotation in internal medicine for junior medical students. *J Gen Intern Med.* 8: 189–192

Chan, S.W. and Chien, W.T. (2000) Implementing contract learning in a clinical context: report on a study. *J Adv Nursing.* 31: 298–305

Cook, D.A. and Triola, M.M. (2009) Virtual patients: a critical literature review and proposed next steps. *Med Educ.* 43: 303–311

DaRosa, D.A., Dunnington, G.L., Sachdeva, A. J., et al. (1992) A model for teaching medical students in an ambulatory surgery setting. *Acad Med.* 67(10 Suppl): S45–S47

DaRosa, A.D., Dunnington, G.L., Stearns, J., Ferenchick, G., Bowen, J.L., and Simpson, D.E. (1997) Ambulatory teaching 'lite': less clinic time, more educationally fulfilling. *Acad Med.* 72: 358–361

Davis, M.H. and Dent, J.A. (1994) Comparison of student learning in the outpatient clinic and ward rounds. *Med Educ.* 28: 208–212

Dent, J.A. (2003) Twelve tips for developing a clinical teaching programme in a day surgery unit. *Med Teach.* 25: 364–367

Dent, J.A. (2005) AMEE guide Number 26: Clinical teaching in ambulatory care settings—making the most of learning opportunities with outpatients. *Med Teach.* 27: 302–315

Dent, J.A. (2009) Ambulatory care teaching. In J.A. Dent and R.M. Harden (eds) (2009) *A Practical Guide for Medical Teacher.* 3rd edn. pp. 104–112. Edinburgh: Elsevier.

Dent, J.A. and Davis, M.H. (1995). Role of ambulatory care for student-patient interaction: the EPITOME model. *Medical Education* 29:58–60

Dent, J.A. and Davis, M.H. (2008) *Getting started... a practical guide for clinical teachers.* 3rd edn. Dundee: Centre for Medical Education, University of Dundee

Dent, J. and Preece, P. (2002) What is the impact of participating students of real-time video monitoring of their consultations skills? *Br J Educ Technol.* 33: 349–351

Dent, J.A., Angell-Preece, H. M., Ball, H.M., and Ker, J.S. (2001a) Using the ambulatory care teaching centre to develop opportunities for integrated learning. *Med Teach.* 23: 171–175

Dent, J.A., Ker, J.S., Angell-Preece, H.M., and Preece, P.E. (2001b) Twelve tips for setting up an ambulatory care (outpatient) teaching centre. *Med Teach.* 23: 345–350

Dent, J., Skene, S., Nathwani, D., Pippard, M., Ponnamperuma, G., and Davis, M. (2007) Design, implementation and evaluation of a medical education programme using the ambulatory diagnostic and treatment centre. *Med Teach.* 29: 341–345

Denton, G.D., DeMott, C., Pangaro, L.N., and Hemmer, P.A. (2006) Narrative review: use of student-generated logbooks in undergraduate medical education. *Teach Learn Med.* 18: 153–164

Dunnington, G.L. (1990) The outpatient clinic as a critical setting for surgical clerkship training. *Teach Learn Med.* 2: 212–214

Dunnnington, G.L., and DaRosa, D.A. (1994) Changing surgical education strategies in an environment of changing healthcare delivery systems. *World J Surg.* 18: 734–737

Duque, G. (2003) Web-based evaluation of medical clerkships: a new approach to immediacy and efficacy of feedback and assessment. *Med Teach.* 25: 510–514

Edelbring, S., Brostrom, O., Henriksson, P., et al. (2012) Integrating virtual patients into courses: follow-up seminars and perceived benefit. *Med Educ.* 46: 417–425

Feltovich, J., Mast, T.A., and Soler, N.G. (1987) A survey of undergraduate internal medicine education in ambulatory care. *Proceedings of the Annual Conference of Residents in Medical Education.* 26 137–141

Ferenchick, G. Simpson, D. Blackman, J. DaRosa, D., and Dunnington, G. (1997) Strategies for efficient and effective teaching in the ambulatory care setting. *Acad Med.* 72: 277–280

Fields, S.A., Usatine, R., and Steiner, E. (2000) Teaching medical students in the ambulatory setting. *JAMA.* 283: 2362–2364

Fincher, R.M.E. and Albritton, T.A. (1993) The ambulatory experience for junior medical students at the Medical College of Georgia. *Teach Learn Med.* 5: 210–213

Frye, E.B., Hering, P.J., Kalina, C.A., Grodinsky, D.J., Lloyd, J.S., and Nelms, D.S. (1998) Effect of ambulatory care training on third-year medical students' knowledge and skills. *Teach Learn Med* 10: 16–20

General Medical Council (2009a) *Tomorrow's Doctors.* London: General Medical Council

General Medical Council (2009b) *Quality Assurance of Basic Medical Education. Report on Dundee Medical School, University of Dundee.* November, pp. 7 and 11. London: General Medical Council

Gruppen, L.D., Wisdom, K., Anderson, D.S., and Woolliscroft, J.O. (1993) Assessing the consistency and educational benefits of students' clinical experiences during an ambulatory care internal medicine rotation. *Acad Med.* 9: 674–680

Hajioff, D. and Birchall, M. (1999) Medical student in ENT outpatient department: appointment times, patient satisfaction and student satisfactions. *Med Educ.* 33: 669–673

Hannah, A. and Dent, J.A. (2006) Developing teaching opportunities in a day surgery unit. *Clin Teach.* 3: 180–184

Harden, R.M., Davis, M.H., and Crosby, J.R. (1997) The new Dundee medical curriculum: a whole that is greater than the sun of the parts. *Med Educ.* 31: 264–271

Harden, R.M., Laidlaw, J.M., Ker, J.S., and Mitchell, H.E. (1996) Task-based Learning: An Educational Strategy for Undergraduate, Postgraduate and Continuing Med Educ. AMEE Education Guide No. 7 (Association for Medical Education in Europe)

Harden, R.M., Sowden, S., and Dunn, W.R. (1984) Some educational strategies in curriculum development: the SPICES model. *Med Educ.* 18: 284–297

Henderson, J. (2005) Featured day surgery units: Developing an ambulatory surgical unit within Stracathro hospital, Tayside. *JOne-Day Surg.* 15: 45–47

Hesketh, E.A. and Laidlaw, J.M. (2002) Developing the teaching instinct. *Med Teach.* 24: 239–240

Howe, A. and Anderson, J. (2003) Involving patients in medical education. *BMJ.* 327(7410): 326–328

Irby, D.M. (1995) Teaching and learning in ambulatory care settings: a thematic review of the literature. *Acad Med.* 70: 898–931

Irby, D.M., Ramsay, P.G., Gillmore, G.M., and Schaad, D. (1991) Characteristics of effective clinical teachers of ambulatory care medicine. *Acad Med.* 66: 54–55

Kalet, A., Schwartz, K.A., Capponi, L.J., Mahon-Salazar, C., and Bateman, W.B. (1998) Ambulatory versus inpatient rotations in teaching third year medical students internal medicine. *J Gen Intern Med.* 13: 327–330

Kellet, C.F., Stirling, K.J., McLeod, R., Dent, J. and Boscainos, P. (2009) Development of an undergraduate medical student theatre etiquette course. *Int J Clin Skills.* 3: 70–72

Ker, J.S. and Dent, J.A. (2002) Information-sharing strategies to support practicing clinicians in their clinical teaching roles. *Med Teach.* 24: 452–465

Krackov, S.K., Packman, C.H., Regan-Smith, M.G., Birskovich, L. Seward, S.J., and Baker, S.D. (1993) Perspectives on ambulatory programs: barriers and implementation strategies. *Teach Learn Med.* 5: 243–250

Kurth, R.J., Irigoyen, M., and Schmidt, H.J. (1997) A model to structure student learning in ambulatory care settings. *Acad Med.* 72: 601–606

Lake, F.R. and Vickery, A.W. (2006) Teaching on the run tips 14: teaching in ambulatory care. *Med J Aust.* 185: 166–167

Latta, L., Tordoff, D., Manning, P., and Dent, J. (2013) Enhancing clinical skill development through an ambulatory medicine teaching programme: an evaluation studya, Med Teach. in press

Lawson, M. and Moss, F. (1993) *Sharing good practice:* innovative learning and assessment. 26th November. London: King's Fund Centre

Lipsky, M.S., Taylor, C.A., and Schnuth, R. (1999) Microskills for students: twelve tips for improving learning in the ambulatory care setting. *Med Teach.* 21: 469–472

Lossing, A. and Groetzsch, G. (1992) A prospective controlled trial of teaching basic surgical skills with 4th year medical students. *Med Teach.* 14: 49–52

Lyon, P. (2003) Making the most of learning in the operating theatre: student strategies and curricular initiatives. *Med Educ.* 37: 680–688

Lyon, P., McLean, R., Hyde, S., and Hendry, G.D. (2006) The student experience of learning in a rural clinical environment. AMEE 2006, Genoa, Italy, Conference Abstracts, September 2006, p. 38

Lynch, D.C., Whitley, T. W., Basnight, L., and Patselas, T. (1999) Comparison of ambulatory and inpatient experiences in five specialties. *Med Teach.* 21: 594–596

Mail Online (2002) £68M boost for day surgery. [online] www.dailymail.co.uk/health/article-133698/68m-boost-day-surgery.html Accessed 3 April 2012

Meadows, S.R. (1979) The way we teach... Paediatrics. *Med Teach.* 1: 237–243

McKergow, T., Eagan, A.G., and Heath, C.J. (1991) Student contact with patients in hospital: frequency, duration and effects. *Med Teach.* 13: 39–47

McLeod, P.J., Meagher, T., Tamblyn, R.M., and Zakarian, R. (1997) Are ambulatory care-based learning experiences different from those on hospital clinical teaching units? *Teach Learn Med.* 9: 125–130

McLeod, P.J., Meagher, T.W., and Tamblyn, R. (1999) How good is the ambulatory care clinic for learning clinical skills? Students' and residents' opinions differ. *Med Teach.* 21: 315–317

Mires, G.J., Howie, P.W., and Harden, R.M. (1998) A 'topical' approach to planned teaching and using a topic-based study guide. *Med Teach.* 20: 438–441

Myung S.J., Kang, S.H., Kim, Y.S., et al. (2010) The use of standardised patients to teach medical students clinical skills in ambulatory care settings. *Med Teach.* 32: e467–e470

Nakayama, D.K. and Steiber, A. (1990) Surgical interns' experience with surgical procedures as medical students. *Am J Surg.* 150: 341–343

Norcini, J.J., Black, L.L., Duffy, F.D., and Fortna, G.S. (2003) The mini-CEX a method of assessing clinical skills. *Ann Intern Med.* 138: 476–481

Norcini, J. and Burch, V. (2007) Workplace-based assessment as an educational tool: AMEE Guide No. 3. *Med Teach.* 29: 855–871

O'Driscoll, M.C.E., Rudkin, G.E., and Carty, V.M. (1998) Day surgery: teaching the next generation. *Med Educ.* 32: 390–395

O'Riordan, D.C. and Clark, C.L. (1997) Potential availability of patients in a short stay ward for medical student teaching. *Ann Roy Coll Surg Engl.* 79(1): Suppl, 15–16

Papadakis, M.A. and Kagawa, M.K. (1993) A randomized, controlled pilot study of placing third-year medical clerks in a continuity clinic. *Acad Med.* 68: 845–847

Parry, J., Mathers, J., Al-Fares, A., Mohammad, M., Nandakumar, M., and Tsivos, D. (2002) Hostile teaching hospitals and friendly district general hospitals: final year students' views on clinical attachment locations. *Med Educ.* 36: 1131–1141

Parsell, G. (1997) Hand books, learning contracts and senior house officers: a collaborative enterprise. *Postgrad Med.* 73: 395–398

Patil, N.G. and Lee, P. (2002) Interactive logbooks for medical students; are they useful? *Med Educ.* 36: 672–677

Peltier, D., Regan-Smith, M., Wofford, J., Wheton, S., Kennebecks, G., and Carney, P.A. (2007) Teaching focused histories and physical exams in ambulatory care: multi-institutional randomised trial. *Teach Learn Med.* 19: 244–250

Pergoff, G.T. (1986) Teaching clinical medicine in the ambulatory setting. An idea whose time may have finally come. *N Engl J Med.* 314: 27–31

Phinney, A.O. and Hager, W.D. (1998) Teaching senior medical students in an office setting: the apprentice system revisited: a cardiologist's perspective. *Connecticut Med.* 62: 37–41.

Regan-Smith, M., Young, W.W., and Keller, A.M. (2002) An effective and efficient teaching model of ambulatory education. *Acad Med.* 77: 593–599

Roth, C.S., Griffiths, J.M. and Fazan, M.J. (1997) A teaching tool to enhance medical student education in ambulatory internal medicine. *Acad Med.* 72, 440–441.

Ross, M.T. and Cameron, H.S.C. (2007) AMEE Guide 30: Peer assisted learning: a planning and implementation framework. *Med Teach.* 29: 527–545

Rudkin, G.E., O'Driscoll, M.C.E., and Carty, V.M. (1997) Does a teaching programme in day surgery impact on efficiency and quality care? *Aust N Zeal J Surg.* 67: 883–887

Schofield, S.J., Bradley, S., Macrae, C., Nathwani, D., and Dent, J. (2010) How we encourage faculty development. *Med Teach.* 32: 883–886

Schwartz, R.W., Donnelly, M.B., Young, B., Nasj, P.P., Witte, F.M., and Griffen W.O. Jr. (1992) Undergraduate surgical education for the twenty-first century. *Ann Surg.* 216: 639–647

Seabrook, M.A., Lawson, M., and Baskerville, P.A. (1997) Teaching and learning in day surgery units: a UK survey. *Med Educ.* 31:105–108

Seabrook, M. A., Lawson M., Malster, M., Jolly, J., Rennie, J., and Baskerville, P.A. (1998a) Teaching medical students in a day surgery unit: adapting medical education to changes in clinical practice. *Med Teach.* 20: 222–226

Seabrook, M.A., Lawson, M., Woodville, S., and Baskerville, P.A. (1998b) Undergraduate teaching in a day surgery unit: a 2-year evaluation. *Med Educ.* 32: 298–303

Simon, S.R., Peters, A.S., Christiansen, C.L., and Fletcher, R.H. (2000) The effect of medical student teaching on patient satisfaction in a managed care setting. *J Gen Intern Med.* 15: 457–461

Simpson, J.G., Furnace, J., Crosby, J., et al. (2002) The Scottish doctor—learning outcomes for the medical undergraduate in Scotland: a foundation for competent and reflective practitioners. *Med Teach.* 14: 136–143

Skeff, K. (1988) Enhancing teaching effectiveness and vitality in the ambulatory setting. *J Gen Intern Med.* 3(Mar/Apr Supplement): S26–S33

Sprake, C., Cantillon, P., Metcalf, J. and Spencer, J. (2008) Teaching in an ambulatory care setting. *BMJ.* 337: 690–692

Stearns, J. A. and Glasser, M. (1993) How ambulatory care is different: a paradigm for teaching and practice. *Med Educ.* 27: 35–40

Stewart, C.I.L, (2005) Getting started in the ambulatory care teaching centre. In J.A. Dent and M.H. Davis (eds.) *Getting started…A Practical Guide for Clinical Teachers* (pp. 6–7). 2nd edn. Dundee: Centre for Medical Education, University of Dundee

Stewart, C.I.L., Preece, P.E., and Dent, J.A. (2005) Can a dedicated teaching and learning environment in ambulatory care improve the acquisition of learning outcomes? *Med Teach.* 27: 358–363

Sullivan, M.E., Ault, G.T., Hood, D.B., et al. (2000) The standardized vascular clinic: an alternative to the traditional ambulatory setting. *Am J Surg.* 179: 243–246

Towle, A. (1991) *Critical Thinking: the Future of Undergraduate Medical Education.* London: King's Fund Centre

Usatine, R.P., Tremoulet, P.T., and Irby, D.I. (2000) Time-efficient preceptors in ambulatory care settings. *Acad Med.* 75: 639–642

Walters, L., Worley, P., Prideaux, D., and Lange, K. (2008) Do consultations in rural general practice take more time when practitioners are precepting medical students? *Med Educ.* 42: 69–73

Walters, R. (2003) Diagnostic and treatment centres: the future of healthcare? Architects for Health [online] 13 May, 1–3. http://www.architectsforhealth.com/2003/05/diagnostic-and-treatment-centres-the-future-of-healthcare/ Accessed 21 March 2013

Wilkinson, J., Crossley, J., Wragg, A., Mills, P., Cowan, G., and Wade, W. (1998) Implementing workplace-based assessment across the medical specialties in the United Kingdom. *Med Educ.* 42(4): 364–373

Worley, P., Silagy, C., Prideaux, D., Newble, D., and Jones, A. (2000) The parallel rural community curriculum: an integrated clinical curriculum based on rural general practice. *Med Educ.* 34: 558–565

Worley, P., Esterman, A., and Prideaux, D. (2004a) Cohort study of examination performance of undergraduate medical students learning in community settings. *BMJ.* 328: 207–209

Worley, P., Prideaux, D., Strasser, R., March, R., and Worley, E. (2004b) What do medical students actually do on clinical rotations? *Med Teach.* 26: 589–590

Wolpaw, T.W., Wolpaw, D.R., and Pap, K.K. (2003) SNAPPS: a learner-centred model for outpatient education, *Acad Med.* 78: 893–898

CHAPTER 20

The humanities in medical education

John Spicer, Debbie Harrison, and Jo Winning

Medicine is my lawful wife but literature is my mistress.
When I am bored with one I spend a night with the other.

Anton Chekhov

(Chekhov 1888)

Medical humanities and education theory

Educational objectives

In this chapter we set out the theory behind medical humanities, but our overarching aim is to 'show not tell'. Through our examples and short narratives we demonstrate the ways in which students can be challenged to construct new ways of understanding identity and other culturally freighted paradigms, such as health and sickness, normal and diseased, and cure and healing.

The medical humanities are relevant to all stages in public healthcare, including the clinical encounter, the development of policy, and the effective design and delivery of services. Its study helps students in three crucial developmental areas as shown in fig. 20.1.

The development of the clinician's expertise is experiential; increasingly so now that the training pathway represents a continuum from the position of undergraduate student to the role of skilled and knowledgeable practitioner. Our emphasis here on experience reinforces the essential acquisition of knowledge and skills in the classroom and skill centre, as presented in certain models, such as the experiential learning cycle (Kolb 1984) and its related theory (Honey and Mumford 1982; Hudson 1967).

The environments in which clinicians work involve real people in real situations, but the skills they bring will depend on their own cultural and social background, as well as what they have been taught, and the ways in which they have been encouraged to develop. Within the classical experiential learning cycle, convergent knowledge is located between the pragmatist and theorist learning styles: the active experimenter versus the abstract conceptualizer. Typically, this is where the scientist is most comfortable. Conversely, divergent knowledge lies between the activist and the reflector: the domain of the concrete experiencer and the reflective observer. Typically, this is the domain of the artist.

While this model is not uncontested (Race 2005), it has proved to be useful and persistent in medical education where the convergent/divergent paradigm serves as a theoretical authentication for the argument that consideration of the arts augments the more formal scientific education (Halperin 2010). To conclude, we draw attention to the meaning of curriculum. Traditionally curriculum has described a list of contents or a syllabus, and this is evident in references to UK postgraduate curricula. A more fruitful and progressive understanding of curriculum, alluded to by Stenhouse (1975), describes the entire learning journey from needs assessment, through delivery, to final assessment and evaluation. The metaphor of the journey connects the clinician and patient experience.

To date medical humanities has concentrated on specific ways of enhancing the teaching and learning experience, which rely in turn on the engagement of the teacher. This is unnecessarily restrictive. As a discipline, the medical humanities are perfectly aligned with the more progressive (literal and metaphorical) concept of lifelong learning as a journey or voyage of discovery.

Educational drivers

What then are the regulatory and organizational drivers for the development of medical humanities, as core content in medical curricula? In the UK, medical training at an undergraduate and postgraduate level is governed by the General Medical Council (GMC), which issues guidance to universities and postgraduate deaneries. *Tomorrow's Doctors* (GMC 1993), in guidance to UK universities, endorsed the special study module (SSM) curricular content as follows: 'It is hoped that the student of tomorrow may be drawn towards…opportunities to study a language, or to undertake a project related to literature, or the history of medicine'. The 1993 guidance proposed that this area of the curriculum should be optional, but this changed in 2003 (GMC 2003) to a requirement for a specified proportion of student-selected components (SSCs) for study. Of the one-quarter to one-third of curricular time considered appropriate for SSCs, two-thirds, 'must be in subjects related to medicine, whether laboratory-based or clinical, biological or behavioural, research-orientated, or in humanities related to medicine'.

There was no specific reference to the medical humanities in the 2009 guidance (GMC 2009), apart from the proposal that SSCs

To engage with abstract concepts that enable them to challenge and explore evidence more holistically

To develop critical analytical skills that enable them to understand multilayered narratives

To participate more actively and fully in discursive narrative-based patient accounts or case histories, as partners on the journey

Figure 20.1 How medical humanities can help learners.

should promote the 'intellectual development of students through exploring in depth a subject of their choice' and that this should accommodate not less than 10% of curricular time. Nevertheless, the implicit value of the study of medical humanities is acknowledged at various points in the text by reference to clinical communications, professionalism and diversity.

At postgraduate level in the UK, curricular content is defined by the Foundation curriculum (which covers the first two years of training after qualification) and the specialist training curricula, which were adopted following a fundamental review of medical career pathways implemented in 2007.

From the documents described earlier, three salient issues arise. First, we should take seriously the natural relationship between science and art in the context and content of medical training. The science–arts discourse, which foregrounds an illogical dichotomy, has been framed in different ways. One of the most accessible is the differentiation between evidence-based medicine and values-based medicine (RCGP 2007). While evidence-based practice demands an understanding of statistical methodology, critical appraisal, and population health outcomes, among other facets, the argument that medical practice should also integrate knowledge of the personal and patient-held values that inform decision making is gaining momentum.

As qualitative concepts, notions of value are impossible to capture in rigorous quantitative analysis and therefore require a different knowledge and skill set, together with different ways of measuring outcomes. Above all, qualitative concepts place demands upon the most challenging aspect of medical activity, which relates to the attitudinal dispositions of the practitioner. From the theoretical perspective this is the most persuasive reason for the inclusion of the humanities in the curricula described previously: it develops the practitioner's humanism, which is essential if we are to treat patients as complex human beings rather than cases (Shapiro et al. 2009). Humanism, in the context of medical education, denotes qualities essential to the clinical encounter: compassion, dignity and empathy.

Second, we argue that the elective role of medical humanities content within curricula is counterintuitive, given that the development of conceptual analytical and empathetic qualities is held to be a universally required criterion for the doctor skilled in values-based medicine. The medical humanities can perform a vital role in developing humanism within the integrated curriculum and so a degree of obligation over SSCs or other elective components is required (Oyebode 2010). Ultimately, the medical humanities should be regarded as part of the *core* curriculum of medical study (Grant 2002).

Third, the location of the medical humanities in the medical curriculum requires careful reexamination in relation to other areas of enquiry. Medical humanities should not be treated as generic term that denotes all the disciplines that do not form part of the scientific core. Art, critical theory, history, law, literature, music, philosophy, and theology fall under the mantle of medical humanities (fig. 20.2)—an educational structure that is observed in certain US

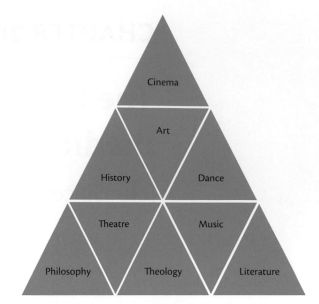

Figure 20.2 Humanities that can be used in medical education.

universities but in general does not necessarily pertain in Europe (AMEE 2011; Friedman 2002). Yet the concept is far from new. In all curricula, the study of medical law and ethics is universal and compulsory: both subjects develop ways of thinking that are qualitatively different from the scientific disciplines that underlie pre-clinical areas. Medical humanities deliver this qualitative mode of analysis and incorporate medical law and ethics as part of a much broader and more powerful discipline. However, if the medical humanities are incorporated into medical education, there needs to be a rebalancing of traditional medical curricula (fig. 20.3).

Before we examine teaching content and methods, we explore briefly the significance of this discipline for medical practitioners, in terms of personal and professional development—and we start with the language of illness and suffering.

Metaphor: the primary language of thoughts and feelings

The humanities teach us that metaphor is the natural language of illness and suffering because it is the primary language of thought and feelings. As Donald Freeman (2012) observes:

metaphors project structures from source domains of schematised bodily or enculturated experience into abstract target domains. We conceive the abstract idea of life in terms of our experiences of a journey, a year, or a day.

Freeman continues:

we do not understand Robert Frost's 'Stopping by Woods on a Snowy Evening' to be about a horse-and-wagon journey but about life. We understand Emily Dickinson's 'Because I Could Not Stop for Death' as a poem about the end of the human life span, not a trip in a carriage.

This understanding of metaphor explains why patient care is so frequently described or perceived as a journey with a clear narrative structure: the first consultation (chapter one) and the history (flashback), through to the diagnosis (detection), therapeutics (journey towards resolution), and a satisfactory or unfortunate prognosis (the happy or sad ending). By sharing this concept of the journey with the patient, clinicians mirror the universal metaphor, that life itself

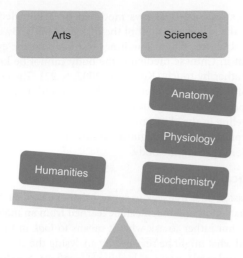

Figure 20.3 Medical curricula?

is a journey on which each individual constructs and reconstructs their own narrative and respond to meta-narratives that describe human experience in the broader cultural and historical context.

The use of shared metaphor embeds empathy within the clinical encounter and facilitates a common sense of meaning in relation to what has passed, what lies ahead, and the obstacles that must be faced and, hopefully, surmounted: the patient is no longer travelling alone along a dangerous and frightening road towards an unknown destination. The shared metaphor creates an empathetic connection between the patient's account and the clinical interpretation, and it authenticates the clinician's ability to *listen*, as well as to hear.

The disconnections between clinical and patient modes of expression are not insurmountable, but without the empathetic connection crucial information can be lost in translation, due to the way medical students are taught to interpret and then to convert an emotionally charged patient narrative that is rich in imagery and metaphor, into a medical narrative based on aetiology, diagnosis, pathology, treatment, and prognosis.

Cognitive linguists explain that metaphors serve to facilitate the understanding of one conceptual and abstract domain (illness and suffering) by reference to imagery that is more concrete and vivid. In Sarah Kane's play about depression, *4:48 Psychosis*, (Kane 2001) this is what the unnamed character means when she says 'the defining feature of a metaphor is that it's real'. Kane uses metaphor to devastating effect, but so too does J.K. Rowling (1999) in her physical embodiment of depression in the Harry Potter books for children. Dementors literally feed on fear and misery. They turn the victim's world cold and grey, and with their devouring kiss they suck out the soul, leaving behind an empty shell; alive but devoid of all feeling except desolation.

The importance of listening to metaphor in the clinical setting is demonstrated by the work of the pioneering psychiatrist and psychotherapist Alexis Brook. Brook, who first trained as a physician, then as a psychiatrist, and finally as a psychoanalyst, devoted his clinical career to the connections between language and the body. His published and unpublished papers on disorders of the gut and eye demonstrate a unique attunement to the complex relationship between psyche and soma, as well as to the insightful recording of the bodily metaphors and symbols which permeate his patients' narratives.

In 1995 Brook published a clinical paper on the psychological aspects of disorders of the eye. The paper emerged from his work as

a psychoanalytic psychotherapist in the Eye Department of Queen Alexandra Hospital in Portsmouth and the Well Street GP Practice in East London. Brook set out to study 'psychological aspects of disorders of the eye' and based his findings on interviews with 50 patients, aged nine to 81. Two-thirds of the cohort was female. The eye disorders represented fall into two distinct groups: those suffering from inflammatory disorders of the eye and those for whom there were no physical changes in the eye but who were experiencing severe eye pain.

The eye, for Brook, is a crucial organ for the human subject; one that is central in the subject's relationship with external reality. 'The eye', he says, 'is not just an organ of vision but is one of the most significant organs through which an individual makes contact with the world'. According to Brook:

> Everyday language indicates that it is inherently recognised that the eye and the mind are very much equated. *I see* means 'I understand.' We visualise a problem. *To have one's eyes open* is to be emotionally and intellectually aware of what is going on. But if there is something we do not want to acknowledge, because it may be unacceptable, we *turn a blind eye*. The eye can reflect aspects of one's personality. We can *look with love* but we can *look with hate*. We can go in to *a blinding rage* and *looks can kill*. To make *eye contact* means making a relationship, and seeing *eye to eye* means experiencing mutual understanding. *Giving insight* means giving internal sight with the eyes to the mind.

Brook's attention to idiom and metaphor, and the way in which both express the correlation between psyche and soma, is evident in his clinical work. In the Department of Gastroenterology at St Mark's Hospital he continues to listen closely to the language of his patients and in his 1991 paper, 'Bowel distress and emotional conflict', he illustrates his findings with direct quotations from patients' accounts, for example:

> Mrs. D, a 40-year-old glamorous, successful, fun-loving woman who had a 10-year history of mild abdominal symptoms, had, for the past year, been suffering from intractable constipation and abdominal pain'. Brook interprets these symptoms via a 'reading' that would not be out of place in the field of literary analysis: 'It seemed that her constipation was the expression of her intense need to keep everything inside her under control. Many women experience this as "being afraid of letting go" or "afraid of the bottom falling out of my world" [patients' word]. One woman complained of severe constipation, which began shortly after the death of her small child; in verbalizing her feelings about this tragedy she pointed to her lower abdomen saying "I held it in."' Here Brook interprets the last patient's description as a refusal to let go of the dead child, so that loss as an *embodied* thing, is articulated through a physical symptom. The lower abdomen contains the bowel, but also the *womb*. In an unpublished paper 'Gut language of somatising patients', Brook (2008) collects quotations from gastroenterology patients: 'My whole gut is in rebellion', says one woman, 'my abdomen is screaming and complaining' says another. A third says 'Fighting is going on in my abdomen, like there are a whole lot of people fighting. My whole system is rebelling, my gut is boiling up'. Brook's notion of gut language suggests that the gut—that corporeal entity—has its own language or mode of expression. His fundamental premise in clinical work is that if the physician starts to think about metaphor, to analyse the figurative language that is embedded within patient narrative, somatic truths will be yielded up.

The ability to understand metaphor is a gift with which many medical professionals are naturally blessed, as devotees (and often practitioners) of the arts, music, and literature. But not all clinicians have a natural affinity for metaphor, which is why the medical humanities have such a crucial role to play in medical education. Through an interdisciplinary approach to the humanities and medicine, it is possible to *teach* empathy through the development of conceptual analytical and critical thinking skills.

Such skills are essential for young doctors preparing for a career in an environment in which diversity can be confrontational and shocking—what is described within ethics as relativism. Relativism—arguably the most complex and paradoxical aspect of moral philosophy—is the theory that each community has its own morality, and that there are no universal moral imperatives. Today a relativist position would accept as morally neutral: female circumcision in Somalia, termination of pregnancy in Northern Europe, and the avoidance of porcine insulin in Muslim communities. Yet such practices are challenged by those who adopt a different religious or secular position.

Today female genital mutilation (FGM) is condemned throughout most of the world and is regarded as an infringement of a universal moral rule. Students can learn, formally, the law in UK forbidding FGM (Female Genital Mutilation Act 2003) or the professional rules from the General Medical Council (2008). However, a more thoughtful insight will be gained where the student interrogates the social and moral context of current and historic practices. For this the student will need to consult the first-person narratives of experience, the anthropological literature, and the history of western medicine—and there they might discover that Victorian surgeons performed female circumcision in the UK on young middle-class women, to spare them (and their families) the shame of what was perceived as an excessive sexual appetite.

To see and to say

Ways of 'knowing' the body

Andreas Vesalius, the 16th-century Flemish physician–anatomist, took the radical step of contesting the dominant paradigms of the human body in Galenic medicine and undertook the extensive dissection practice that led to the ground-breaking publication of *De humani corporis fabrica* in 1543. What drove Vesalius to challenge orthodoxy seems to have been an overwhelming desire to *look*, and indeed to look *more deeply* into the material truths of the human body and its functions than had previously been the practice. As Shigehisa Kuriyama demonstrated, the need to 'know' and conceptualize the body through dissection fundamentally shapes Western biomedical practice in a way that is divergent from Eastern understandings of the body and models of medical practice (Kuriyama 2002).

To illustrate this point Kuriyama uses the example of feeling the pulse, which he notes is 'a passionate interest' shared by both Western and Eastern medical traditions alike. In the Western context, after the multiple pronouncements on the anatomy of the nerves, arteries and muscles offered by various anatomists, including Galen, Kuriyama argues that 'anatomy framed the very possibility of imagining the pulse'. He argues that having built knowledge of the body upon the concrete fact of dissection; having *seen* and conceptualized the heart and the arteries, 'anatomy shaped how and what the fingers felt'. Thus a Western clinician's interpretation of haptic experience is always modified by a knowledge base built upon the privileged sight of the dissected body. By contrast, Kuriyama observes, 'Chinese writings testified that the eyes were wrong', that in Chinese medicine, the body cannot be known by sight but rather by touch (Kuriyama 2002, p. 22). The conceptualization of the pulse, therefore, is far broader and more complex, while the practice of taking the pulse requires a more sophisticated sense of feeling in the clinician's fingers because subtle nuances of pulse and pulsation offer diagnostic information about, it is held, all the major organs in the body.

The medical 'gaze'

This discussion does not seek to suggest that one medical tradition is better than another—much can be learned from an intercultural approach—but rather to ask what it means to *look* in the clinical setting, and what might be revealed by analysing the affects, power structures, and implications of looking at a patient, as a doctor.

The seminal analysis of medical perception is *The Birth of the Clinic* (1963), by Michel Foucault (2007), in which the 20th-century social theorist provides an 'archaeology' of the history of the 'act of seeing, the gaze' in clinical practice. Describing the 'loquacious gaze' of the doctor, Foucault reveals the connection between the act of *seeing* and the production of knowledge and, by implication, power. Foucault's description, 'loquacious gaze', encapsulates the way in which a look—the kind of look epitomized by Vesalius' dissecting practice—might produce a great deal of speech or interpretation about diagnosis, but also about the lived experience of the diseased body. Theoretically, the power of this loquacious gaze is such that it can subsume or even eliminate the patient's voice from the clinical experience.

Responses to Foucault partly depend upon the claim to truth and authority made by biomedical science. Foucault argues that we might understand the growing confidence of biomedical science in the 19th century as the result of an increasing conflation of the medical gaze and the production of language; by the 'new alliance [being] forged between words and things'. Being able to *see* confers upon the doctor both the right and the confidence to *say*, with authority and power—to articulate the 'truth' of a patient's condition more accurately than the patient.

Foucault's analysis questions the way the relation between seeing and saying is enacted within clinical practice. Among the formative phenomena that shaped Western medicine during the nineteenth century, the French physician–philosopher Georges (Canguilhem (1994) identifies the rise of 'the physiological point of view' and the quest for further refinement of the detail upon which the clinical gaze fixes. Physiology focuses 'on disease at the tissue level' and then uses new technology to 'focus even more sharply on the cell' (Canguilhem 1994, pp. 134–135). Canguilhem concludes that the process changes the patient from *subject*—a person with agency and autonomy—to *object*; a clinical case to be investigated, diagnosed and treated. His conclusion is that 'the 'object has a human form, that of a living individual who is neither the author nor the master of his own life and who must, in order to live, sometimes rely upon a mediator' (Canguilhem 1994, p. 157).

As this example demonstrates, the medical humanities can apply the apparently abstract insights of critical theory to clinical care and practice—here to demonstrate the power of the clinical gaze in relation to the patient's sense of identity. This point can also be illustrated with reference to the visual arts. In 2003, the photographer

Deborah Padfield, herself a chronic pain sufferer, undertook a collaborative project with Dr. Charles Pither, Consultant Pain Specialist at the INPUT pain management unit at St. Thomas' Hospital, London. Padfield worked with a group of chronic pain patients to produce a collection of photographic images that articulated their experience of pain more fully and accurately than verbal language. These images, together with short patient narratives, were published in *Perceptions of Pain* (Padfield 2003). Padfield says that pain can 'take us back to a primal space where words have not yet formed' (Padfield 2003, p. 18). Where verbal language fails us, she argues, 'visual language' which can 'contact the unconscious in maker and viewer' offers a far more insightful mode of communication and connection (Padfield 2003, p. 18) Padfield describes this process as 'the bridge between the private suffering of an individual and a medical and collective understanding' (Padfield 2003, p. 18).

Nell Keddie, a patient in Padfield's collection, suffered a crushing injury to her lumbar spine, which resulted in increasing and unremitting pain. One of Keddie's images uses the symbolism of cracked glass to represent the internal experience of her pain. The composite image, the radiating fractures in the sheet of glass laid over the photograph of Keddie's back, symbolically shifts the invisible, the internal reality of pain, into the visible realm (fig. 20.4). The making of the image was therapeutic for Keddie: 'When I wake up at night in pain, instead of being controlled and overwhelmed by it, I think about how I might represent it visually'. Keddie's own gaze is of paramount importance; in making an image, she can effect a kind of separation from her pain. As Padfield notes, 'by connecting us to an unconscious or pre-verbal part of ourselves, but translating that part into an objective, "readable" object, the photograph simultaneously brings us closer to our experience, and distances us from it'.

Charles Pither considers what such images might mean to the clinician and says that once a patient has described their pain and given an account of their story, 'the physiology and pathology now take precedence over the subjective experience: the person takes second place to the disease' (Pither 2003, p. 125). Following Canguilhem, Pither describes this shift in perception of the patient from subject to object and the impact it has upon patient–clinician communication. What is lacking, Pither observes, is 'a transaction between the lived experience of the sufferer and the non-judgmental acceptance of these offerings by the physician'.

How, then, might the introduction of a visual image into the consultation change this dynamic? Pither argues that 'the addition of a visual dimension can aid this process because it can allow both parties to imagine and share the problem from a second person perspective'. The image is conceptualized through the *patient's* gaze to produce a visualization of the subjective, embodied experience of pain and disease. As a focal point for discussion it empowers the patient, while simultaneously providing the clinician with a practical tool that aids diagnosis and treatment.

To listen to a story

Patient narratives and metanarratives

The patient's narrative is the focal point of most aspects of medical practice. Clinicians learn to listen to and interpret the patient's story, but frequently this subjective narrative is converted into a formulaic account, where the clinician translates the patient's words into a recognizable *medical* narrative (the medical history)

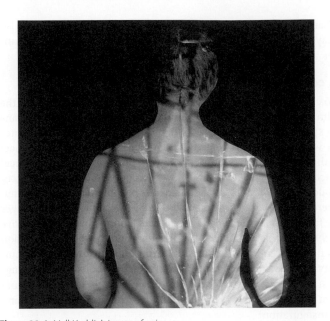

Figure 20.4 Nell Keddie's image of pain.

Reproduced by kind permission of Dewi Lewis Publishing and Deborah Padfield.

for the senior clinician on a ward round, for example. This process of translation raises important issues in relation to interpretation. What is lost in medical translation might be the key to diagnosis (Brody 1994).

The more students of medicine listen to and understand how patients *construct* their narratives, the better they will understand how to alleviate the distress presented (Engel et al. 2008). In modern medical faculties listening and interpreting are usually dealt with under communication skills, where students are asked to explore how the patient's narrative conforms to certain diagnoses, pathologies, or interventions. The construction of the story, or to be more accurate, the co-construction (Launer 2002) within the medical encounter, is the primary material that forms the diagnostic and therapeutic relationship.

Patients' stories frequently reflect their encounters with medical professionals and these encounters can indicate positive and negative experiences, partly shaped by the empathetic or disconnected clinical environment. But they are also shaped by broader cultural, social, and theological metanarratives (Posen 2005). Brody (2007) produced a model in which illness narratives are embedded within a series of metanarratives and this can help students to recognize how to locate and contextualize the patient's story. So the story of the patient's illness fits within the story of the patient's life which fits within the wider narrative of the society and culture within which the patient lives.

This brief section illustrates the powerful analytical tools that emerge in interdisciplinary analysis by re-forging connections between the patient's *biographical* narrative and the doctor's *biotechnical* case history—between the biopsychosocial (holistic) and the arguably more precise but restricted scientific interpretation. One fruitful way in which medical humanities explores these different narratives is through historical artist-as-patient analysis: for example we might consider how the music of composers reflects and interprets their pathologies: the deafness of Beethoven, the hallucinations of Chopin or the mental state of Robert Schumann

(Caruncho 2010; O'Shea 1990; Jensen 2001). But music can also play a defining role in our analysis of the modern clinical encounter, as the next section demonstrates.

A confusion of tongues, music, and the third space

To contextualize our analysis of the play *Wit* (Edson 2010) and the film version of *Wit* (Nicolls 2001) we first consider what it means to speak as a patient and as a doctor within a clinical encounter in which delineated roles might limit communication. Michael Balint's (1957) mid-20th-century model envisages the clinical encounter as a 'polyglossic' space, a place in which the 'speech acts' of doctor and patient do *not* meet; a place in which, to quote Balint, there is a 'dangerous confusion of tongues'. This model re-emerges in Judith Butler's *Excitable Speech: A Politics of the Performative* (1997), in which the author argues that any act of speech, as soon as it is uttered, immediately places the subject within 'a community of speakers'. But while the concept of community might suggest stable affective or social bonds and cohesion, Butler argues that in practice this space is always 'volatile' or open to change and transfiguration.

Butler's book, written in the sociopolitical context of the late 1990s, is about hate speech, as Homi Bhabha describes it: 'the dark heart of a world where words wound, images enrage, and speech is haunted by hate' (Bhabha 1997). As such, it would seem an unlikely theoretical frame to help access the way speech and language work between doctor and patient. However, Butler's interrogation of what speech can *do* is instructive with reference to Balint and Foucault. Butler's phrase 'linguistic vulnerability', when applied to the clinical encounter, enables us to perceive the space in which doctor and patient become a community of speakers and simultaneously a space in which linguistic vulnerability might be both enacted by the doctor and embodied within the patient.

Margaret Edson's play *Wit*, first performed in California in 1995, dramatizes this power relationship in the clinical encounter (Edson 2010). It centres on the experiences of Vivian Bearing, a professor of 17th century poetry, who is diagnosed with Stage IV metastatic ovarian cancer, for which she undergoes aggressive chemotherapy. Speaking 'the part' in *Wit* is problematized by the shortcomings of the clinical encounter, but more broadly and philosophically by the failure of human language to convey concrete meaning. In an early scene, when Dr Harvey Kelekian breaks the news of her advanced metastatic cancer to Bearing, the split text on the page literally enacts the way in which doctor and patient retreat into their own consciousness; they *hear* each other but do not—cannot—*listen*. Partly out of emotional defence, and partly out of scholarly habit, Bearing picks up single words used by Kelekian and ponders their etymology and composition. Kelekian says: 'the antineoplastic will inevitably affect some healthy cells, including those lining the gastrointestinal tract from the lips to the anus, and the hair follicles. We will of course be relying on your resolve to withstand some of the more pernicious side effects'. Simultaneously, Bearing thinks: 'Antineoplastic, Anti: against. Neo: new. Plastic. To mould. Shaping. Antineoplastic. Against new shaping. [. . .] Hair follicles. My resolve. [. . .] Pernicious. That doesn't seem—'(Edson 2010, pp. 3–4).

Bearing *hears* Kelekian but her thought process—and her affective, emotional process—interacts and also runs parallel with his speech act. The seemingly strange juxtaposition—'hair follicles.

My resolve'—enacts the precise moment in which Bearing takes in the truth of her embodied state; her disease and what will be required to fight it. But Kelekian's speech takes little or no account of Bearing's affective state. In turn, he hears but does not listen to the patient's process, her assimilation of bad news: in fact he misses it altogether. What the dramatic form records so usefully here is the complexity of speech, communication, and meaning-making in the highly charged moment of the clinical encounter: this particular 'community of speakers' fractures.

The breaking of bad news is *not* the same thing as hate speech, yet there are similarities here in the sense of violence inflicted upon the patient; what she is expected to absorb and understand in the speech directed *at* her. Her linguistic vulnerability is real but it is also a metaphor for her physical vulnerability. Kelekian's refusal to move beyond speech constituted from the discourses of biomedical science turns Bearing into a vulnerable subject—indeed an object of the clinical gaze. Her own speech—internal of course, but in the script literally enacted—is cut across, stopped, by the clinician. The space of the page—the fractured and truncated sentences—symbolizes the way in which the space of communication becomes a binary opposition; doctor and patient reduced to delimited roles and miscommunications.

Yet, as much as we might say that the text of *Wit* is a perfect rendition of Balint's notion of the confusion of tongues in the clinical encounter, the play pushes into deeper territory related to language, and the difficulties of meaning-making, even in the act of literary analysis: a realm in which it seems possible to capture deep and true meaning, and fix it concretely. This scene, in which Kelekian consents Bearing, is followed immediately by a flashback in which Bearing remembers her tutor—the 'great E.M. Ashford'—the scholar who inspired Bearing's own rigor and passion for the complex devotional poetry of John Donne. Ashford teaches Bearing to attend to the Donne's nuances and metaphysical complexities by *reading* his language properly, accurately, returning to the source. The sonnet used in the script is Donne's Holy Sonnet 6. Ashford directs Bearing to the most rigorous scholarly edition and asks her to look to the simple punctuation of the concluding two lines:

> Gardner's edition of the Holy Sonnets returns to the Westmoreland manuscript source of 1610—not for sentimental reasons, I assure you, but because Helen Gardner is a *scholar*. It reads: 'And death shall be no more, *comma*, Death thou shalt die. Nothing but a breath—a comma—separates life from life everlasting.' With the original punctuation restored, death is no longer something to act out on a stage, with exclamation points. It's a comma, a pause.

This memory creates an epiphany for the dying Bearing. At last able to *listen* to the advice Ashford gives her—to go and live—she realizes that she has sacrificed her emotions in the service of her intellect. It is a forceful and deliberate parallel with the model of clinical practice: Bearing's scholarly drivenness mirrors the drivenness of biomedical discourse, research and practice. They are one in the same. Like Kelekian, Bearing is so locked into intellectual interpretation that she misses the deepest metaphysical truth of all: that life and death coexist, separated only by a pause—a comma—the small punctuation mark of human experience and time.

The medium of film, as it develops from its early silent form, uses sound—most commonly music—either scored specifically, or identified by the filmmaker as an apposite choice to enhance the visual material. This is different from stage production: the director of the film *Wit* has a wealth of music at his disposal and his choice is instructive because it suggests that deeper communication might be achieved in forms beyond linguistic structures.

In his book *Listening Subjects*, David Schwarz (1997) argues that music affects us viscerally because it functions as a 'sonorous envelope'; beyond linguistic form it creates an oceanic feeling in which 'the boundary separating the body from the external world seems dissolved or crossed in some way'. For Schwarz this embodied pleasure resurrects early infantile memories of enveloping and containment by the maternal body. Moreover, 'threshold crossing', as he puts it, creates listening as a *space*. Beyond Schwarz's formulation we can say that it creates an internal space into which affect or emotion might move. In film it represents a third enveloping space between the spectator and the projected image on the screen.

Music speaks in and through the body in a way linguistic structures do not. The music theorist David Lidov (2005) argues that music offers a 'semiotic transcendence' that begins in, and does not entirely leave, the body: 'In speech we see predominantly the final extreme of the abstractive process' (by which he means 'meaning-making', in structuralist terms, locking signified to signifier). In music we can observe every part of the spectrum 'from immediate physiological expression to the purest play of form'. He argues that musical experience starts in the body. Unlike speech, which abstracts corporeal meaning, music arises from and communicates with the body most fully.

The music in the film *Wit* is *Spiegel im Spiegel* (literally 'mirror in the mirror') by Pärt. The piece is used throughout the film to intensify moments of deepening revelation and epiphany. The effect is to invite an empathic response in the audience: the spareness of the musical form creates a space in which the spectator creates their own affective meaning. Pärt understood the response to this piece: 'I could compare my music to white light which contains all colours. Only a prism can divide the colours and make them appear; this prism could be the spirit of the listener' (Pärt 1999).

Spiegel im Spiegel is written for single piano and violin, although in its definitive recording, used in *Wit*, the string voice is also played by cello. The piece is built of tonic triads (three-chord notes): the piano playing rising triads while the strings play rising and falling scales. The triad embeds the notion of thirdness as a principle of construction. In the same way, the two musical voices of piano and strings evoke the sense of a conversation, an encounter and a communication, which involves a dyad but which creates a third.

From 1976, Pärt was experimenting with what he called the tintinnabulation technique. 'Here', Pärt explains, 'I discovered the triad series, which I made my simple, little guiding rule'. He describes tintinnabulation as an attempt to isolate deep truth, which is felt in the purity of the repetition of the triad:

> Tintinnabulation is an area I sometimes wander into when I am searching for answers—in my life, my music, my work. In my dark hours, I have the certain feeling that everything outside this one thing has no meaning. The complex and many-faceted only confuses me, and I must search for unity. What is it, this one thing, and how do I find my way to it? Traces of this perfect thing appear in many guises—and everything that is unimportant falls away. Tintinnabulation is like this…. The three notes of a triad are like bells. And that is why I call it tintinnabulation.

What Pärt seeks is the space of the third and this is of crucial importance in the clinical encounter. The psychoanalyst Jessica Benjamin (2004) writes: 'To the degree that we ever manage to grasp two-way directionality, we do so only from the place of the *third*, a vantage point outside the two' (Benjamin 2004, p. 7). Her analytical model transfers well to the clinical encounter. For Benjamin, as for many contemporary psychoanalysts, speaking as 'a two' therapeutically requires the acknowledgement of the intersubjectivity of our human interactions. 'Thirdness', she writes, 'is anything one holds in mind that creates another point of reference outside the dyad' (Benjamin 2004, p. 7). In Benjamin's view of thirdness, 'recognition is not first constituted by verbal speech; rather, it begins with the early nonverbal experience of sharing a pattern, a dance, with another person' (Benjamin 2004, p. 16). In addition to the notion of dance, Benjamin also writes of the third metaphorically as 'the harmonic or musical dimension' (Benjamin 2004, p. 18).

To return to the misaligned speech acts of Kelekian and Bearing's clinical encounter, we can apply Benjamin's model to the pattern of their dialogue and the way they break into and occlude the other's speech. From the perspective of the audience we can imagine the page—the script—rewritten with the concept of a third in mind. This creates an 'in-between space' and reveals the deeper meaning, so that the rigid binary oppositions and roles—doctor/patient, speaker/spoken to, healthy/sick—begin to break down and new patterns of speaking and listening emerge across the seeming divide of the white space in between.

Medical models of normality

The biopsychosocial versus the biomedical model

Earlier in this chapter we discussed the distinction between narratives that are biomedical in form and those that reference the more holistic view of a patient's experience. Having considered story telling through various modes, we now return to this theme and to medical writing.

One of the most stylized examples of reductive medical writing is where the patient's history is transformed into a segmented presentation for the ward round or clinic, the context of which is described memorably as 'doing a can-can in a marsh' (Tallis 2004). Students of medicine are taught how to extract the clinically salient highlights from a narrative, at speed, in order to deliver to a senior the core narrative required to determine the best management of the condition. The environment of over-work and under-staffing (the marsh) drives clinicians to execute their can-can as expeditiously as possible. However, where fuller narratives can be shared between clinician and patient a richer biographical account emerges, partly where there is a continuity of relationship between the two (or more) participants. Patients' stories are rarely explored fully in a single encounter: the multiple layers become evident over time and in one-to-one sessions, in which empathy and trust has been previously established. Stories change, too, with the passage of time.

For the student of medicine it is instructive to compare the stylized biomedical account of illness with the biographical account that emerges over time (Shapiro 2011; Newman 2003). Both accounts are valid in the clinical environment, but this comparison raises students' awareness of the differences. Biographical accounts are more patient-centred, or at least more consistent with the demonstration of patient-centred care, which is part of the care of the generalist physician (Reeve 2010). Health, under a biomedical paradigm, has been described as a normal set of process markers (Gillies 2010); the story told by the patient is checked for normality, or otherwise, against a population derived from numerical values of average, which here denotes function. The contrast with a view of patients as part of their more complex biographical account is obvious and converts that rather rigid and technical perception of normality into a narrative that can enhance their care. This is not to devalue the need for a scientific approach, but simply to locate it in a longitudinal and holistic account of suffering and experience.

The parallels with fictional examples of suffering are clear because the reader or viewer creates that third space, learning much more about the patient than is conveyed in the dialogue with a medical practitioner—as in the case of *Wit*. In the third space we share the sufferer's journey. The hermeneutics of narratives, therefore, can be revealed to the student through a parallel study of the biomedical and biographical accounts in conjunction with a fictional example.

The reflective practitioner

The capacity to be reflective is regarded as a key skill among clinicians. Donald Schön (1983) describes reflection as 'the capacity to reflect on action so as to engage in a process of continuous learning'. The humanities develop this powerful teaching mode further through the study of conceptual analysis and critical thinking.

We explore this point through a worked example; one that haunts practice in manifold ways. Consider this story—a composite fictionalized narrative based on clinical practice—from the care of a patient at the end of his life (box 20.1).

In stories like this care is provided in a complex and emotionally challenging environment. Here we consider the doctor's response because empathy can at times be painful. We are told that Bill's pain was refractory—that is, he did not respond to analgesia. Dr Jeremay would know that in terminal care 5–10% of pain is refractory, but this might not help him to rationalize his personal and professional response to dealing with a dying patient in pain. Nor would it help him to understand the nature and purpose of suffering in this context. A religious perspective may be of value (Williams 2001) and there is no shortage of theologically inspired writing on end of life. As a reflective practitioner, Dr Jeremay will no doubt discuss with his colleagues the progress of Bill's illness and, with hindsight, consider whether there might have been scope for other interventions, which may help in future patients. The personal perspective is more complicated. Dr Jeremay is troubled by the coincidences between Bill and his own life experiences. Locating the suffering of his patient in ways that go beyond the pathological process may be helpful to Dr Jeremay and, by extension, to his future patients.

We have already discussed music as a powerful mode of thought and expression. Dunn (2006) compares pain at the end of life to the sufferings of the characters in the opera *Parsifal* and implies that Wagner's art allows us to discern truths not otherwise accessible. J. S. Bach, in his *Chaconne* from the 2nd Violin Partita, gives us an extended meditation on the nature of bereavement, composed, it is thought, as a response to the death of his first wife, Maria Barbara. The structure of the music is a theme and variations in the style of an antique Spanish dance, mainly but not exclusively in a sombre minor key. As such it could be held to mirror the classical stages of bereavement—from shock to acceptance. Through the repetitive form of a passacaglia it is also a study in elaboration and variation of melody and structure, providing multiple perspectives of

Box 20.1 Worked example—the reflective practitioner
Dr Jeremay made a house call to the family of a patient, Bill Doggins, for whom he had cared through his terminal carcinomatosis. Bill had been an accountant, 45 years old when he received his diagnosis. He then underwent chemotherapy and surgery, which gave him an extra 2 years of life. His final illness lasted a month and was characterized by refractory pain, among other symptoms. He had, at least, been able to die at home, supported by his family and a full primary care team. Dr Jeremay was calling to see how the family were coping, but he was thinking too about the coincidence that he was Bill's age and, like Bill, had lost his father a couple of months ago.

musical structure and function and a comparison with the emerging perspectives experienced by grieving relatives. That such connections can be suggested may seem fanciful, but they have a broad and illuminating scholarship and are potentially useful to the medical learner (Bicknell, 2002)

There is a rich body of music that is manifestly associated with the end of life: virtually all the great composers have written requiems as part of Christian worship, but all cultures identify forms of music particular to, and appropriate for, death and dying. The question here is how this body of knowledge can help Dr Jeremay to understand his patient's experience of dying and his empathetic pain?

That this chapter is formed in words and print clearly precludes examples from musical extracts, but we know that listening to music can be therapeutic, both for the patient approaching death (O'Kelly 2002) and also for an attendant physician like Dr Jeremay. Music can facilitate the analytical process, in the sense that the *Chaconne* might resonate with the process of bereavement described in classical accounts. It might also be both heuristic and experiential by provoking reflection and the pursuit of further knowledge on the part of clinicians who deal with end of life care (Stein 2004).

These clinicians. in turn. might teach younger doctors a skill that is based as much on experience and wisdom, as it is on scientific expertise. For while this chapter has focused primarily on the doctor-in-training, nevertheless, the themes explored are relevant throughout the professional journey and beyond. The doctor in retirement is in an ideal position to reflect on their lifetime experience of clinical practice and to pass on to the doctors of the future their experience and wisdom in relation to compassion, dignity, and empathy.

Teaching the medical humanities

In this final section we draw attention to the variety of teaching methods and to the range of experience and expertise required to deliver a successful medical humanities programme. Collectively these aspects can be considered part of the wider interpretation of curriculum. We would stress here that incorporating the medical humanities into the curriculum requires good teaching skills; it does not necessarily require specific training. Having said that, it is our experience that medical teachers interested in the humanities can benefit from—and also enjoy—such training.

Pedagogical aims, methodologies, and environments

In the context of this chapter, traditional pedagogy, with its intrinsic bias towards didactic teaching, is less useful than Knowles's (1980) version of andragogy. Knowles's six principles of adult learning stress, *inter alia*, that content should be relevant, reasoned and driven by experience. Several authors (Knight 2006; Friedman 2002) have commented on the difficulties of obtaining 'a positive view of the relevance of [some] medical humanities material'. This chapter demonstrates how carefully-selected material can relate directly to medical education and is well-aligned with the thoughts of Shapiro et al. (2009), who argue that the consideration of the suffering patient drives the development of a specific set of methods and concepts from the humanities, which student doctors can use to enhance understanding and reflection.

Teaching methods ideally should be consistent in the way they help learners to make meaning of the material to which they are exposed. Irrespective of the teaching methodology, the potential for individual or shared reflection on such material should be maximized. Teaching styles can move between *didactic* and *facilitative* depending on context. A formal lecture on the many possible causes of Mozart's death (Karhausen 2010) is of value in itself, but infinitely more so when considered with Milos Forman's 1984 film *Amadeus*, a listening of the *Requiem* and accounts of the composer's mental state. These examples from the interpretation of the life and works of Mozart can also illustrate the value of *heuristic* learning.

A further style is relevant with reference to the 'personal' in Fenwick's (2000) statement, namely the exploration of students' *emotional* responses to a patient's experience. By any reference, learners need to understand and calibrate their own reactions to patients' lived experiences, and there is no better way of doing so than directly learning from individual patients on clinical attachments. We would argue that facilitated exposure to any of the humanities can assist this understanding. In making this statement we acknowledge that learning is partially cognitive and partially affective Music, for example, can evoke a visceral, purely affective, response, often bypassing cognitions, which makes it a valuable resource in considering this aspect of learning (Levitin 2008; Newell and Haines 2003; Blood and Zatorre 2004; Panksepp et al. 2002).

Traditionally, after the lecture theatre and laboratory, clinicians in training move on to learn from and with patients in wards and clinics. These spaces represent essential teaching environments, the significance of which should be interrogated to understand better how space shapes the clinical encounter. Beyond these conventional environments, teachers might also consider the art gallery, theatre, concert hall, and cinema, as spaces where legitimate learning can take place and be evaluated.

Expected objectives and assessment

The rigour with which objectives and assessments are implemented will depend on the degree to which the humanities are integrated into the medical curriculum. For example, where the syllabus is delivered by problem-based learning, it is relatively straightforward to work objectives into cases that explore literature or drama as parallel themes (Grant 2002).

A second method is to align the medical humanities component with more traditional aspects of the curriculum. To pursue the example of Mozart, a reflective piece of work on his symphonies or operas can introduce core psychology or neurophysiology content (Sloboda 1985). This enables teachers to approach these subjects

from an innovative and unexpected angle, which is likely to engage the learner more readily (Rauscher et al. 1995; Schellenberg 2005; Levitin 2009). In our experience the 'Mozart effect' (the demonstration that listening to Mozart can increase the IQ of certain listeners) provides an introduction with which students engage enthusiastically, irrespective of their knowledge of classical music (Jenkins 2001).

To date, formal assessment of humanities projects, as part of undergraduate or postgraduate programmes, has been inconsistent. This is partly because medical humanities itself represents such a diverse field but also because it can be difficult to assess more abstract and conceptual disciplines, including those identified as humanistic at the beginning of this chapter. Nevertheless, the traditional models of formative and summative assessment, such as essays, assignments, and presentations, are all valid, as are more modern modes of writing that may demonstrate reflection, such as portfolios and medical blogs. In drawing up a scheme of assessment, the medical humanities add the potential for learners to present original creative work, written, composed or created, as responses to other curriculum material or experiential work with patients. This can be accommodated within formative or summative assessment.

One of the challenges for medical humanities is to overcome the perception that all knowledge assessment should conform to current statistical analysis (Swanwick 2010). The engagement between humanistic development and professional practice *can* be assessed, provided the item descriptors are clearly identified. Reference to the rubrics used to assess the work of humanities students will be helpful here but assessors should bear in mind that the primary purpose of medical humanities is the contribution to professional development as a doctor and not, valuable as it may be, towards an artistic role.

The study of medical humanities can be introduced with relative ease at the lower levels of enquiry by gathering reactive material in relation to a session or course. As students move on to higher levels of education, it is more challenging to assess outcomes using conventional medical educational methods—and this is one area where assessment methodologies from the humanities (such as essays in which the student determines the thesis, with the teacher's approval) will be helpful.

Conclusions

- The literature on medical humanities education delivery is now vast, diverse and fascinating.

- The humanities deliver a different cognitive and affective experience to that of science and provide innovative teaching techniques.

- Over the past 50 years medical education has grown from the lecture theatre and laboratory to the problem-based learning centre and community clinic, introducing different learning environments and formats. The humanities extend this transition further and assist the constructivist process of personal meaning-making.

- According to Naughton (2000), undergraduate students on a humanities course were more critical and less accepting of unsupported information; laudable outcomes for the development of the enquiring medical mind. Equally important from a humanities perspective, is the role of group- and self-evaluation, which must always be overseen by a trained teacher, but which develops independently-minded practitioners, who can engage with—and also challenge—the clinical environments in which they work.

References

Association of Medical Educators of Europe (AMEE) Conference (2011) Vienna Austria. AMEE 2011 Abstract Book p. 434

Balint, M. (1957) *The Doctor, His Patient and the Illness.* London: Pitman Medical Publishing Co. Ltd,), p. 26

Benjamin, J. (2004) Beyond doer and done to: An intersubjective view of thirdness. *Psychoanal Q.* 73: 5–46

Bhabha, H. (1997) In J. Butler (ed.) *Excitable Speech: A Politics of the Performative* London: Routledge

Bicknell, J. (2002) Can music convey a semantic content: a Kantian approach. *J Aesthetics Art Criticism.* 60(3): 253–261

Blood, A.J. and Zatorre, R.J. (2001) Intensely pleasurable responses to music correlate with activity in brain regions implicated in reward and emotion. *Proc Natl Acad Sci USA.* 98(20): 11818–11823

Brody, H. (1994) My story is broken, can you help me fix it: medical ethics and the joint construction of narrative. *Literature and Medicine.* 13: 79–92

Brody, H. (2007) Narrative ethics. In R.E. Ashcroft, et al. (eds) *Principles of Health Care Ethics* (pp. 151–158). Chichester: John Wiley & Sons Ltd

Brook, A. (1991) Bowel distress and emotional conflict. *J Roy Soc Med.* 84: 41

Brook, A. (1995) The eye and I: psychological aspects of disorders of the eye. *J Balint Soc.* 23: 13

Brook, A. (2008) Gut language of somatizing patients. Quoted in Julian Stern, 'Keeping the Gut in Mind', presented at 'Psychotherapy, Medicine and the Body: Alexis Brook Memorial Conference', Tavistock Clinic, London, 31st October. (Our thanks to Dr. Julian Stern for his generous sharing of this material)

Butler, J. (1997) *Excitable Speech: A Politics of the Performative.* London: Routledge

Canguilhem, G. (1994) The epistemology of medicine. In: *A Vital Rationalist: Selected Writings from Georges Canguilhem* (p. 135). New York: Zone Books

Caruncho, M.V. and Fernandez, F.B. (2011) The hallucinations of Frederic Chopin. *Med Humanities.* 37(1): 5–8

Chekhov A. Letter to Suvorin, 1888

Donne, John., (1572-1631), Holy sonnet XIV. [Online] http://www.luminarium.org/sevenlit/donne/sonnet14.php Accessed 26 February 2013

Dunn, K.L. (2006) Sickness, healing and opera: Wagner's Parsifal. *J Med Humanities.* 32: 7–10

Edson, M. (2010) *Wit.* London: Nick Hern Books

Engel, J.D. Zarconi, J., Pethtel, L.L., and Missimi SA. (2008) *Narrative in Health Care.* New York: Radcliffe Publishing

Evans, M. (2007) Medical humanities: an overview. In *Principles of Health Care Ethics,* Chapter 26. Chichester: JohnWiley & Sons Ltd

Female Genital Mutilation Act (2003) [Online] http://www.legislation.gov.uk/ukpga/2003/31/section/1 Accessed 26 February 2013

Fenwick, T.J. (2000). Expanding conceptions of experiential learning: a review of five contemporary perspectives on cognition. *Adult Educ Q.* 50(4): 243–272

Freeman, D. (2012) *Linguistics and Literature.* Linguistic Society of America. http://www.lsadc.org/info/ling-fields-lit.cfm Accessed 30 May 2012

General Medical Council (1993) *Tomorrow's Doctors.* London: GMC, para 29

General Medical Council (2003) *Tomorrow's Doctors.* London: GMC, para 41

General Medical Council (2008) *Personal beliefs and medical practice—guidance for doctors.* London: GMC, para 12–16

General Medical Council (2009) *Tomorrow's Doctors.* London: GMC, para 96

Gillies, J. (2010) Annual Conference report. Royal College of General Practitioners, Liverpool

Grant, V.J. (2002) Making room for medical humanities. *Med Humanities.* 28: 45–48

Halperin, E.C. (2010) Preserving the humanities in medical education. *Med Teach.* 32: 76–79

Foucault, M. (2007) *The Birth of the Clinic: An Archaeology of Medical Perception* (p. ix) (1st edn. 1963). London: Routledge

Friedman, L.D. (2002) The precarious position of the medical humanities in the medical school curriculum. *Acad Med.* 77(4): 320–322

Jenkins, J.S. (2001). The Mozart Effect. *J Royal Soc Med.* 94: 170–172

Jensen, E.F. (2001) *Schumann.* Oxford: Oxford University Press

Kane, S. (2001) *4:48 Psychosis.* In: *Complete Plays* (pp. 203–245). London: Methuen.

Karhausen, L.R. (2010). Mozart's 140 causes of death and 27 mental disorders. *BMJ.* 341: 1328–1329

Knight, L.V. (2006) A silly expression: consultants' implicit and explicit understanding of medical humanities: a qualitative analysis. *Med Humanities.* 32: 119–124

Knowles, M. (1980). *The Modern Practice of Adult Education: From Pedagogy to Andragogy.* Chicago IL: Follet

Kolb, D. (1984) *Experiential Learning.* Englewood Cliffs NJ: Prentice Hall, pp. 21–31

Kuriyama, S. (2006) *The Expressiveness of the Body and the Divergence of Greek and Chinese Medicine.* New York: Zone Books

Launer, J. (2002) *Narrative Based Primary Care: A Practical Guide.* Oxford: Radcliffe Press

Levitin, D.J. (2009) The neural correlates of temporal structure in music. *Music and Medicine.* 1(1): 9–13

Levitin, D.J. (2008) *This is Your Brain on Music.* London: Atlantic Books

Lidov, D. (2005) *Is Language a Music? Writings on Musical Form and Signification.* Bloomington, IN: Indiana University Press, p. 146

Naughton, J. (2000) The humanities in medical education: context, outcome and structures. *Med Humanities.* 26: 23–30

Newell, G.C. and Hanes, D.J. (2003) Listening to music: the case for its use in teaching medical humanism. *Acad Med.* 78(7): 714–719

Newman, T.B. (2003). The power of stories over statistics. *BMJ.* 327: 1424–1427

Nicolls, M. (dir.) (2001) *Wit* (HBO)

O'Kelly, J. (2002) Music therapy in palliative care: current perspectives. *Int J Pall Care Nurs.* 83): 130–136

O'Shea, J. (1990) *Music and Medicine.* London: Dent, p. 39 et seq

Oyebode, F. (2010) The medical humanities: literature and medicine. *Clin Med.* 10(3): 242–244

Padfield, D. (2003) *Perceptions of Pain.* Stockport: Dewi Lewis Publishing

Panksepp, J. and Bernatzky, G. (2002) Emotional sounds and the brain: the neuro-affective foundations of musical appreciation. *Behav Processes.* 60: 133–155

Pärt, A. (1999) CD liner notes for *Alina.* ECM Records

Pither, C.E. (2003) Unspeakable pain. In D. Padfield(ed.) , *Perceptions of Pain* (p. 125). Stockport: Dewi Lewis Publishing

Posen, S. (2005) *The Doctor in Literature: Satisfaction or Resentment.* Abingdon: Radcliffe Press

Race, P. (2005) *Making Learning Happen : A Guide for Post Compulsory Education.* Thousand Oaks CA: Sage, Chapters 1 and 3

Rauscher, F.H., Shaw, G.L., and Ky, K.N. (1995) *Listening to Mozart enhances spatio temporal reasoning: towards a neurophysiological basis. Neurosci Lett.* 185: 44–47

Reeve, J. (2010) *Interpretive Medicine: Supporting Generalism in a Changing Primary Care World.* London: RCGP

Royal College of General Practitioners (UK) (2007) section 3.3 [now updated 2012 at section 2.10] http://www.rcgp.org.uk/gp-training-and-exams/~/media/Files/GP-training-and-exams/Curriculum-2012/RCGP-Curriculum-2-01-GP-Consultation-In-Practice.ashx Accessed 28 March 2013

Rowling, J.K. (1999) *Harry Potter and the Prisoner of Azkaban.* London: Bloomsbury.

Schellenberg, E.G. (2005). Music and cognitive abilities. *Curr Dir in Psychol Sci.* 14(6): 317–320

Schön, D. (1983) *The Reflective Practitioner, How Professionals Think In Action.* New York: Basic Books

Schwarz, D. (1997) *Listening Subjects: Music, Psychoanalysis, Culture.* Durham, NC: Duke University Press

Shapiro, J. (2011) Illness narratives: reliability, authenticity and the empathic witness. *J Med Humanities.* 37(2): 68–72

Shapiro, J., Coulehan, J., Wear, D.,. and Montello M. (2009) Medical Humanities and their discontents: definitions, critiques and implications. *Acad Med.* 84(2): 192–198

Sloboda, J. (1985) *The Musical Mind: the Cognitive Psychology of Music.* Oxford: Clarendon Press

Stein, A. (2004) Music, mourning and consolation. *J Am Psychoanal Ass.* 52(3): 783–811

Swanwick, T. (ed.) (2010) *Understanding Medical Education: Evidence, Theory and Practice.* Chichester: John Wiley & Sons Ltd

Tallis, R. (2004) *Hippocratic Oaths: medicine and its discontents.* London: Atlantic Books

Williams, R. (2001) Living well, dying well (2). In M. Marinker (ed) *Medicine and Humanity* (pp. 117–124). London: Kings Fund

CHAPTER 21

Study skills

Raja C. Bandaranayake

"Do not just read, memorise or imitate, but so that you
realise the principle from within your own heart study hard
to absorb these things into your body."

Miyamoto Musashi

Introduction

Study skills are an essential component of the armamentarium of
the medical student to prepare him or her for lifelong practice.
While many guides to study skills are available, today's medical student has special needs brought about by the many changes taking
place the world over in healthcare practices. This chapter will:

1. Outline some of these changes which impact on the educational
   process of the medical student

2. Discuss the effects of these changes on the study skills that the
   student must acquire and

3. Suggest ways in which the medical teacher can facilitate the
   development of these skills.

The latter two sections of this chapter will be underpinned by some
generic developments that have taken place in our knowledge of
how students learn, and relate these developments to the specific
needs of medical students.

Trends in healthcare

Growth of knowledge

The growth of knowledge in the health professions has had a profound effect on the manner in which healthcare is delivered to the
public. The perpetual extension of the frontiers of knowledge and
the unending search for better ways of preventing and curing illness continue to influence the practice of medicine—so that it is no
longer possible to expect the health professional to be cognizant of
all the facts and skills needed for effective practice.

Growth of knowledge in the physical and chemical sciences
has resulted in technological and pharmacological developments
applied to investigative and therapeutic aspects of medical practice. It would not be an exaggeration to surmise that a medical
graduate who qualified for the practice of medicine even a couple of decades ago would not be able to do so effectively in the
current context, had steps not been taken to update skills and
knowledge in line with intervening developments. Hence, the
need has grown for the continuing education of the physician and
mandatory processes of recertification to ensure that the practitioner has taken the necessary steps to do so.

Escalating healthcare costs

A second trend in healthcare that has affected the education of
the medical student, and indirectly the study skills to be developed, is the escalating costs of healthcare. As a result, hospital stays
by patients in tertiary care teaching hospitals, for long the main
locus of clinical training of the student, have become increasingly shorter. Thus the medical student is exposed to only a brief
part of the patient's total illness, and is denied the opportunity to
learn from the continuity of care that is given to the patient by the
healthcare team. However, it is this continuity of care that becomes
necessary for the newly graduated physician in the real world of
practice. To overcome this major disadvantage in training, countries have employed different strategies depending on their contexts. Ambulatory care settings are commonly used for training in
North American medical schools, while community hospitals and
general practices are used in many other countries in the developed
world. In developing countries, on the other hand, the use of primary care and community settings has been a trend that has been
growing ever since the Alma Ata Declaration of 1978 (WHO 1978).
Training in each of these settings has necessitated the development
of particular sets of study skills if the medical student is to benefit
from such experiences.

Increasing public awareness

A third trend that is becoming increasingly evident in healthcare
stems from increasing public awareness of their rights to the best
possible care available. While increasing literacy and education has
been the main force leading to this trend, developments in information technology have also contributed. The marked increase in
medical litigation, particularly in countries of the developed world,
is one consequence of this trend. Another is the increasing tendency for self-therapy on the part of patients. The effects of these
tendencies on the education of medical students, and necessarily
on the nature of study skills that need to be inculcated in them, are
discussed next.

Developments in education for healthcare

Approaches to learning

Studies on student learning, starting from the early work of Entwistle (1975) and Marton and Säljö (1976a, b), have increased our understanding of the learning approaches used by students in self study. The two main approaches identified were the surface and deep approaches, the former associated with passive acquisition of knowledge (Morgan 1993), while the latter involved understanding of what is learned. Deep learning is an active process, involving 'relating new ideas to what was already known, examining evidence and the logic of the material, and creating an integrated whole' (Entwistle and Entwistle 1992, p. 10). Undoubtedly, the deep approach to learning is preferred even though much of the basic facts on which the practice of medicine is based are learned through passive acquisition. Particularly important to the development of effective study skills is the finding that the learning approach adopted by the learner in a given situation depends on the nature of the learning task. An example will be given to illustrate how even factual knowledge can be acquired through a process of understanding without memorizing, through the judicious prescription of learning tasks by the teacher.

A strategic approach was later identified whereby a student strives to obtain the best possible grade, for instance, by using a combination of surface and deep approaches in study (Laurillard 1979; Ramsden and Entwistle 1981).

Self-directed learning

Self-directed learning (SDL) includes:

♦ setting goals for learning

♦ identifying strategies directed towards those goals as efficiently as possible

♦ monitoring the effects of implementing those strategies through self-testing as learning progresses

♦ making modifications, either to the objectives or to the strategies when obstacles are encountered (Butler and Winne; 1995; Winne 1995).

While SDL has always been a *sine qua non* of medical studies, the need for it has increased exponentially with knowledge explosion and the inability of the formal medical curriculum to cover all the content that the medical student is required to learn. Students must, therefore, acquire a set of self-study skills which will stand them in good stead, not only while in medical school but also through post-graduate and continuing medical education.

Knowles (1990) has stressed the importance of diagnosing one's learning needs in relation to future practice in formulating objectives as performance outcomes. Once appropriate learning strategies have been identified and implemented, evidence must be collected of the achievement of the objectives by the learner.

Studies have shown that SDL and intrinsic motivation are mutually dependent: SDL increases intrinsic motivation, while intrinsic motivation encourages the student to be more independent in learning (Corno and Mandinach 1983).

The teacher's role in SDL is not passive, but one which facilitates the student to achieve these skills. In postgraduate training, and even more so in continuing medical education, the importance of SDL is obvious, as the degree of teacher facilitation decreases progressively. Continuing education activities are mandatory now in most countries, and recertification procedures are in place in many. Thus it is most important for the medical student to develop skills of SDL during the phase of undergraduate medical education.

Distance learning

Another trend becoming increasingly evident in medical education is distance learning, particularly in the continuing education of the physician. This has important repercussions for the education of the medical student. In addition to the skills of SDL, proficiency in the skills associated with advances in information technology must be developed during undergraduate medical education. Furthermore, confronted with a vast amount of information, the student must develop skills of critical review and judicious selection of what is to be read. Evaluation of the literature requires prior knowledge, which is not as extensive in the student as in the teacher. Even the presence of a prior knowledge base is by itself insufficient for evaluation; it must be related to the new knowledge that is presented in the literature (Pressley et al. 1997). Thus, critical review of the literature, while an important skill, is difficult to learn. However, it is a skill which must be developed in medical school and not postponed for later professional life. Recognition of its importance has led to courses in critical review of literature being increasingly incorporated into undergraduate medical curricula.

Unlike students who come face-to-face with their teachers, distance learners develop learning skills on a trial-and-error basis. The prescriptive nature of most distance learning manuals goes against the grain of SDL. Prescription undermines the learner's inherent self directedness (Knowles 1980; Candy 1990).

Morgan et al. (1998) have identified higher order generic skills desirable for the distance learner as:

♦ thinking and reasoning skills: critical, analytical, evaluative thinking

♦ research skills: literature searching, purposeful reading, thesis building

♦ written communication skills: coherent essay structuring and representation of convincing argument.

While these skills must be developed in the undergraduate medical student, most medical curricula pay scant attention to them. The testing of lower order cognitive skills, mostly through the use of multiple choice questions, and the paucity of opportunities for the development of skills of creativity and inquiry, do not foster these higher order generic skills in the medical student.

Computer-assisted learning

Computer-assisted learning (CAL) involves a set of skills, which most students currently entering medical school possess to an adequate degree. They are usually particularly adept in the use of computers, and only a minority may require training to acquire this skill. However, online learning involves more than the use of computers. Many students do not possess the skills to effectively access and evaluate information, a set of skills referred to as information literacy, involving cognitive, psychomotor and attitudinal components (see table 21.1). Cognitive skills include those of recall (of bibliographic sources), comprehension (of physical layout), and critical thinking (analysis, synthesis and evaluation of information

Table 21.1 Objectives related to information literacy

Domain	Learning objective
Cognitive	Recall bibliographic sources and library services available
	Select appropriate terminology for content
	Understand scope of information and resources needed
	Formulate search strategy
	Analyse, synthesize and evaluate information
	Apply information to problem at hand
Psychomotor	Use a variety of search methods
	Use a variety of appropriate media
	Use information sources with dexterity
Affective	Accept personal deficiencies in use of resources
	Be willing to request aid when necessary
	Persevere with searches
	Accept legal and ethical issues surrounding access of information
	Accept copyright and intellectual property laws

presented); psychomotor skills include handling of equipment; affective skills include acceptance of deficiencies, willingness to request aid, and perseverance.

Elective study

A significant development in education for healthcare has been the increasing tendency to afford students an opportunity to exercise their choice of what they would like to study, in addition to what they are required to study, in an at least a part of the curriculum. The growth of elective programmes has steadily increased over the last half century, partly as a result of exhortations by educational philosophers such as Illich (1984) and Friere (1982) to give students the freedom to decide what to learn and how to learn it. This freedom to learn has been tempered to some extent by the need to inculcate in all medical students certain abilities that are essential for the safe practice of medicine. The skills of SDL have been promoted by such elective programmes.

Problem-based learning

Many of the skills described earlier come into play in the most significant development in education for healthcare over last decades, namely problem-based learning. The student is called upon to engage in deep learning in a problem-solving session when confronted with the problem for the first time. Pooling existing knowledge with that of peers in the tutorial group identifies deficiencies in knowledge, which impede the group from solving the problem. Each student is then called upon to undertake self-study on assigned topics, and the resulting new learning is presented at the next group meeting. The student thereby develops skills of teamwork, SDL and teaching, in addition to that of problem-solving.

The developments in education for healthcare described in the previous sections have had a significant effect on the nature of study skills that should be acquired by the medical student in order to successfully meet the requirements of undergraduate medical education. These skills will now be dealt with.

Study skills required by the 21st century medical student

The theory underpinning study skills is the result of research in all areas of education, which has contributed to our knowledge of how learning takes place most effectively. Some of this research has been referred to earlier. Much research has also been undertaken in the field of distance learning, which many undergraduate students may not be called upon to undertake. Nevertheless, these research findings are important for two reasons:

◆ Students must be equipped with distance learning skills in order to prepare them for the subsequent phases of medical education.

◆ The findings of these studies can be applied to developing SDL skills in any context.

The study skills dealt with in this chapter are categorized under the three headings shown in fig. 21.1.

Skills in developing a study plan

Constantly faced with an array of new areas for learning, it is critically important for the medical student to develop a regular study plan over a limited period of time, such as a week or a fortnight, if they are to successfully negotiate the task of mastering the required knowledge during undergraduate training. This requires skills in planning study, taking into account various factors personal to the student.

Identification of what to study

One of the main skills is identification of priorities for learning, which is partly determined by individual circumstances. Priorities for study should be based, not on expediency, but on importance of subject content, difficulty, and timeliness (Bandaranayake 2009). Importance, in turn, is dependent on the extent to which the content is: (i) useful for future practice; (ii) continuous with previous learning; and (iii) required to be understood for further learning. Difficulty depends on: (i) the degree of prerequisite learning acquired by the student; (ii) the abstractness of the content; and (iii) prior exposure of the student to the topic. Difficulty is coloured by

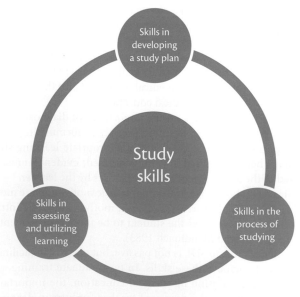

Figure 21.1 Study skills.

the predilection of the student for the subject. Timeliness depends on factors beyond the control of the student, who must learn to plan study according to the timing of activities laid down by the teachers—through timetabling, sequencing, synchronization of subjects, and assessment.

The first prerequisite for becoming an effective self-directed learner is the ability to identify one's weaknesses on which to focus self-study. One way of identifying such weaknesses is from individual feedback provided to the student as a result of formative assessment by the teacher. Another way is through discussion among peers, during which the student realizes learning deficiencies in certain areas in comparison to peers. A third way is through self-realization when attempting to solve problems or to apply learning to novel situations.

Identification and accession of learning resources

The self-directed learner's next task is to develop a strategy to correct those deficiencies. This may involve a set of learning methods to achieve the objectives. In order to be able to do so, however, the student must be aware of the resources which are available for learning. A recent personal experience was quite illuminating. Many years after anatomy dissection was replaced by prosected specimens in one medical school, a small group of students requested the author for permission to undertake cadaver dissection by themselves outside the scheduled timetable. Following the principle that students vary in the way in which they learn best, the students' request was willingly granted, quite to their surprise, as they were unaware that this was a mode of study available to them. The students willingly undertook dissection by themselves after hours, and undoubtedly learned from the experience.

Skills in retrieval of information extend beyond identification of resources for learning. While information is readily available from a variety of resources at present, the effective self-directed learner must possess technical skills to utilize those resources. If necessary, students must be shown how to access information through library networks or the internet. Locating information from different sources includes the skills of using library filing systems, referring to indices, scanning reading materials to determine relevance and importance, and referencing for subsequent easy retrieval (Saunders et al. 1985).

Effective self-directed learners 'set realistic goals and utilise a battery of resources' (Paris and Byrnes 1989, p. 169). Through trial and error they identify which strategies suit them best and pursue them in self-study. Gorsky et al. (2004) found that, in a distance education course in physics, students usually undertook independent study first, and only when that failed or proved to be inadequate did they engage in collaborative study with peers, and interaction with teachers. When confronted with a new learning situation, the self-directed learner's ability to utilize relevant strategies is related to the amount of reflective awareness possessed by the learner (Prawat 1989). Thus, it is important for the self-directed learner to engage in individual reflection on the identified deficiencies before embarking on group studies or seeking help from the teacher.

Critical review of retrieved information

Critical thinking is an important ability to be developed in the medical student. The flood of information that is available to medical practitioners in the present age requires them to critically consider what they are confronted with, before making therapeutic decisions. Thus students must be deliberately exposed to situations where they are required to exercise and develop their critical thinking abilities. Self-directed students also need to think critically when they are confronted with a flood of information from different sources, to enable them to select that which best suits their particular needs. Critical thinking can only occur in those who already have some knowledge about a particular topic. As students lack the extensive background knowledge and experience that the expert has, their critical thinking ability may be impeded. However, it is important that this ability is developed early in their training if students are to undertake their studies efficiently and effectively.

Students can be given training in critical thinking through assignments which require them to undertake critical review of relevant literature. Conscientious students will take steps not only to review such literature, but also to fill in gaps in their knowledge on the content they encounter in such assignments. As a result deep learning is promoted and long-term retention enhanced.

Management and storage of relevant information

It would be well-nigh impossible for students to store in their memory all the information they learn during self study. They must develop a system of identifying key points for storage in memory and of summarizing and storing relevant material for ready reference in the future. An easy way out, and a common practice, is to photocopy identified literature for later use without adequate discrimination. This practice should be avoided. If for logistic reasons, such as time or availability of the original material, a student is compelled to copy material which has not been reviewed, it should be studied as soon as possible, highlighting important points and taking notes on index cards. This would avoid wading through piles of accumulated photocopied material during critical study periods. The practice of summarizing content also requires prior understanding.

Skills in the process of studying

Learning with understanding

In the medical field a vast amount of information must be retained by students. While mnemonics, such as anagrams, keywords, and imagery, are effective in simple retention of facts (Hattie et al. 1996), they are learned without the understanding necessary for use in professional practice. The following example helps to illustrate this.

The vagus nerve nuclei in the brainstem are complicated. The student of anatomy may use a simple mnemonic to remember their positions, without understanding the rationale for their positions. In practice, the student may recall these positions by applying the mnemonic. On the other hand, a student who undertakes deep learning, may not be able to recall the positions immediately, but can determine them by relating the positions of functional nuclear groups in the alar and basal laminae of the developing neural tube (including changes in the region of the fourth ventricle) to the functions of the vagus nerve.

This knowledge would help the latter student to determine the positions of the central connections of all the cranial nerves (fig. 21.2). If a congenital defect of the neural tube in the region of the fourth ventricle exists, this student would be able to deduce where the vagus nerve nuclei are likely to be placed in the abnormal part of the brain stem. In other words, the student is able to apply existing learning to a new context, while the surface learner, who used mnemonics to aid retention, will not be able to do so. It is important for the student to understand, not merely recall, what needs to remembered, whenever possible, even in a subject, such as anatomy, where many facts must be recalled. This is one reason why 'useful' anatomy extends beyond issues of relevance, as understanding may require learning content which is not by itself directly applicable to practice (Bandaranayake 2010).

It is more effective for the student to develop the skills of determining how certain facts could be understood, without the teacher's explanation. An additional advantage of achieving such understanding is that the student learns to integrate knowledge from different disciplines, a skill which is essential for practice. In the example of the cranial nerves, in order to achieve understanding, the student is called upon to integrate knowledge of gross anatomy, embryology and physiology.

Reflecting on what is learned

Boud et al. (1985, p. 19) define reflective learning as: 'those intellectual and affective activities in which individuals engage to explore their experiences in order to lead to new understandings and appreciations'. Students often complain of the tedious nature of basic science courses, partly due to issues of relevance. Lack of time and opportunity for reflection may also contribute to dissatisfaction. If students are to develop the practice of reflecting on the subject matter they learn, they must be shown ways in which it can be connected with what they already know and be able to summarize new learning in their own words (Bandaranayake 2011, p. 71).

The importance of perceiving learning as internal to the learner, for understanding and dealing with issues in the real world, must be emphasized. Clinical students who, for example, have just examined a patient with cirrhosis of the liver may then learn about this condition and its consequences through self-study. In reflection, they should now attempt to explain the symptoms and signs of the patient just examined, through the new learning acquired through self-study. They may even reflect further upon

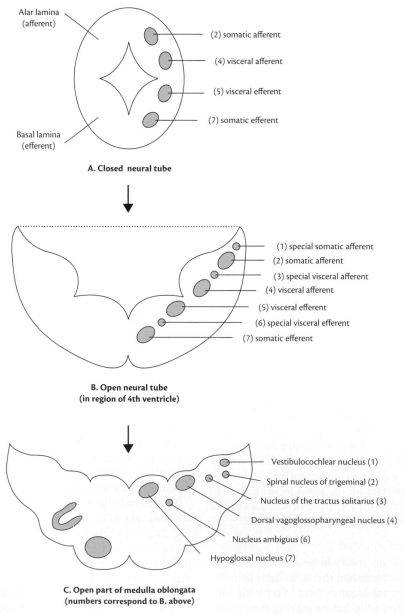

Figure 21.2 Central connections of cranial nerves in the medulla oblongata.

their own life habits and relate them to this new learning. The reflective student is one who sees the connection between learning and living.

Student portfolios are effective in encouraging reflective evaluation of student learning, in addition to providing a permanent record of study activities for subsequent teacher evaluation (Buckley et al. 2009). For this purpose portfolios should not contain mere descriptions of experiences, but should include the student's reactions to each experience.

Application and problem-solving

The skill of applying new learning to novel situations is one which is often practised by children in assignments set to them by teachers. In mathematics this skill is practised through numerical problems, which the student has not encountered previously. Medical students see application in practice in the hospital ward and in ambulatory care, as every patient's illness is a novel situation. They observe clinicians applying their learning to each novel situation in formulating a management plan. Clinical students emulate them each time they clerk a patient. The same practice can be effectively undertaken in self-study. Currently, there are many textbooks, reference books, and journals in the field of medicine that encourage learners to apply what they learn to problems related to each content area. Attempting to solve those problems reinforces the learning just acquired and facilitates its transfer into long-term memory.

Marton and Säljö (1984, p. 48) found that questions in the text, which required the learners to revisit knowledge just acquired, encouraged surface rather than deep learning, as they 'invented a way of answering the interspersed questions *without* engaging in the kind of learning that is characteristic of a deep approach'. Finding answers to the questions became the important task, rather than relating those answers to the substance of the text. They suggested, instead, that the learner be invited to relate the material they are learning to some aspects of the real world. If questions or activities which interrupt the text are to be included, it is necessary to frame them in such a way that they require learners to apply what they read to their own or other situations, rather than merely recall what they are learning. This is of particular importance in distance learning manuals. It should be remembered, however, that the ability of a student to transfer knowledge to a novel situation does not guarantee transfer of the same knowledge to a different, but relevant, situation (Bransford et al. 1986). Thus a student who learns facts pertaining to bilirubin formation in the body may be able to explain jaundice in a patient with haemolytic jaundice, but not in a patient with obstructive jaundice.

Integration of learning

Integrated learning is when learning from different components of the curriculum, be they disciplines, organ systems or phases, are linked by the learner in a meaningful and relevant manner (Bandaranayake 2011, p. 2). While linking by the teacher facilitates the student's ability to integrate, learning is most effective if the integration is undertaken by the student. Pace (1958) points out the integrative nature of the objectives that call upon critical thinking. Skills of integrated learning and critical thinking are complementary. On the one hand, the student who consciously seeks meaningful relationships between isolated bits of information has gone a long way towards developing skills of creative thinking; on the other, the creative student is always searching for links between even seemingly unrelated content, and thereby develops skills of integrative thinking. In the example pertaining to haemolytic jaundice, the student who is able to apply knowledge of bilirubin formation to explain the pathogenesis of haemolytic jaundice, is bound to develop integrative skills if existing knowledge is consciously linked to new knowledge on the anatomical arrangement of the biliary tree to explain the pathogenesis of obstructive jaundice.

In self-study students should not be satisfied with only studying content that is being learned in the classroom at that point of time. They should relate such learning to what has been learned previously in other segments of the curriculum, whenever possible. For example, while studying the functions of the different parts of the nephron, students should link the function of each part with its histological structure, even if the latter was studied some time previously, and explain how histological structure is related to function. They would then develop skills of horizontal integration. In addition, they should find out how this knowledge could explain derangement of function of each part. Similarly, clinical students should, in self-study, revisit the normal and abnormal structure and function, which has been studied in previous segments of the curriculum, to explain the clinical aspects of kidney disease. Vertical integration is facilitated by both these activities.

Integration helps learning according to two well-accepted principles of learning (Bandaranayake 2011, p. 33):

♦ 'perception of relevance motivates and enhances learning'

♦ 'immediate application enhances long-term memory'.

An effective method to exercise the skills of integration is to develop concept maps (Novak and Cañas 2006). A concept map is a diagrammatic representation of the concepts related to a particular content area, showing the relationships among them. The learner can draw such maps during self study in order to bring to the fore the relationships among the new concepts in the particular area under study. While the concepts themselves are not difficult to construct, the mental activity involved in explaining the relationships among them is what results in effective learning. Novak and Cañas argue that the teacher may even provide some of the concepts on which mapping is undertaken by the student, without detracting from the integrative activity which the learner engages in, although such provision may inhibit creative thinking.

Creative thinking skills

Creative thinking skills call upon the learner to relate seemingly unrelated items to come up with something new. Koestler (1964) coined the term 'bisociation' for this type of mental activity. If two separate experiences are grouped together, they may take on added significance, stimulating creativity through the process of bisociation. Creativity is considered a high level of meaningful learning (Novak and Cañas 2006). Integration develops the creative thinking of students if it encourages them to form their own opinions and insights about issues of importance. The development of this attribute depends on the nature of the learning experience: if it is teacher-dominated, creativity is suppressed even though integration is enhanced.

Creative thinking is an important attribute of the physician and should be a major educational objective of medical education.

Skills in assessing and utilizing learning

Self-assessment

The process of SDL is incomplete until self-assessment takes place. Although generally considered the final step, learners are, in reality, assessing their own learning, albeit unconsciously, throughout the process of learning. One can, in fact, refer to formative and summative assessment of learning during SDL. When learners seek and obtain feedback, by themselves or from others, during the process of learning, they are engaging in formative self-assessment. The assessment of one's ability to apply learning at the end of the process of learning is akin to summative assessment. Both types of self assessment are essential for effective SDL.

The self-directed learner should engage in self explanation of what has just been learned. While this is one form of reflection, it is also a useful means of assessing one's learning. Self-explanation positively affects use of material read to solve subsequently presented problems (Bielaczyc et al. 1991). Problem-solving involves the application of learned material to new situations, and is aided by the understanding that is necessarily involved in self-explanation.

Research on CAL has shown that learners granted full control of what they learn, without feedback during the instructional process, often failed to achieve mastery before exiting instruction, while peers provided with feedback about their knowledge during the instructional process were more likely to persist until mastery was achieved (Steinberg 1989). The importance of feedback will be considered further in relation to the teacher's role in developing study skills.

Teaching and discussing with peers

An effective way of assessing one's learning is the ability to teach one's peers. Teaching has the further advantage that the medical student practises a role, which is bound to be undertaken in later professional life, in teaching patients, community, and other members of the team.

Group interaction greatly enhances individual learning through awareness of expected standards and identification of knowledge gaps. The interpersonal communication that occurs in groups meeting physically aids all group members. A student who is required to explain a difficult concept or process to peers is more likely to take particular care to understand it first, as questions and comments are bound to be forthcoming in the discussion which takes place in the group. As Brown and Campione (1986, p. 1066) point out, 'the burden of explanation is often the push needed to make him or her evaluate, integrate and elaborate knowledge in new ways'. Integration, elaboration and self-assessment are stimulated during self-study under such circumstances. In problem-based learning, the second tutorial, in which students share with each other their gains from self-study of the learning needs identified in the first tutorial, is when teaching skills can be practised.

A student who has the task of teaching a peer group on a particular topic should not only prepare for such teaching but rehearse it, through self-explanation, using the necessary aids to teaching. The active learning involved in the process of planning and implementing peer teaching enhances long-term retention of the content taught.

In situations where regular group meetings at appointed times may prove to be difficult, the 'asynchronous discussion system', a text-based computer communication tool, can support collaborative learning across time and distance (Kear 2004). While this has been used as a distance learning technique, a recent experience (Inuwa et al. 2011) in applying an adaptation of this technique to the study of anatomy amongst students has met with a high degree of acceptance amongst first-year students. Learning takes place independent of the tutors in peer-supported forums through an electronic communication system. Evans and Nation (1989) point out the importance of dialogue among students to fill gaps in their knowledge, to encourage deep learning and to seek information such as the nature of impending examinations.

Peer discussion also has the effect of motivating the student to learn in order to be on level terms with peers during discussion. The competitive spirit in some students stimulates them to contribute more than their peers. Others may be averse to displaying their ignorance in the peer group, and study to avoid embarrassment. Still others may genuinely wish to contribute their share to the group activity. Irrespective of the reason, self-study, which precedes peer discussion, would benefit the student, and should be capitalized on by the teacher in the manner in which interactive classes are arranged for their students.

The teacher's role in developing self-study skills

Though self-study is undertaken by the student, the teacher is not absolved from responsibility. On the contrary, teachers have an important role to play in developing self-study skills in their students.

Fostering deep learning skills

If teachers want their students to develop deep learning skills in self-study, they can facilitate this in various ways.

First, the teacher must correct, if necessary, the student's conception of learning. Säljö (1979) found that adult students had different conceptions of learning: an increase in knowledge, memorizing, acquisition of facts, skills, and methods for use when required, relating parts of the subject matter to each other and interpreting and understanding reality in different ways. The teacher must advise students that the mere accumulation of knowledge is by itself inadequate and inefficient, and that they must learn to integrate what they study by identifying links among the component parts of the subject in order to apply learning to problems in the real world. The teacher can provide examples to the students as to how knowledge is integrated and applied.

A second way in which the teacher can foster deep learning is through appropriate course design. Courses that are designed in a way where teachers systematically cover all that the students are required to know, do not provide space for the students to develop their own skills of deep learning. Instead they encourage surface learning through revision of notes taken by the students during exposition of the subject by the teacher. Courses should be designed in a way so that exposition is interspersed with opportunities for self study of uncovered topics. For example, a lecture where some questions are left unanswered provides students with opportunities for self-study. To promote deep learning, it is imperative that the objectives related to the unanswered areas are spelt out clearly and framed in a manner which extends beyond recall.

Deep learning is also encouraged by setting assignments that require the student to integrate disciplines and provoke thought. Linking one subject to another requires deeper understanding of facts from each, unless the linking has already been done for the students by the teacher. Assignments on questions unanswered during lectures stimulate deep learning. For distance learners, Holmberg (1986) suggests promoting deep learning through assignments that require summaries, critical appraisal, justifying conclusions, and establishing links between concepts.

Many workers have found that multiple choice questions in assignments and examinations tend to produce surface learners, while well constructed open-ended questions are more likely to promote deep learning (Thomas and Bain 1984; Scouller 1998). Unfortunately, many poorly constructed open-ended questions do not call upon the student's ability to link concepts, but promote surface learning, as they can be replaced by multiple choice questions of the recall type. Even multiple choice questions can be constructed to test ability to link content areas. If questions are set in assignments, they should test understanding, application and problem solving, rather than recall. When such assignments are set, however, the teacher must ensure that they are reviewed and feedback given to the student.

Increase students' self-efficacy beliefs

Bandura (1977) defined self-efficacy as one's belief in one's ability to succeed in specific situations. Prat-Sala and Redford (2010) concluded that focusing on self-efficacy beliefs among students may be beneficial in improving their study approach. Students with high levels of self-efficacy view a difficult task as a challenge to be mastered, while those with low levels generally shun difficult tasks. Some of the latter may be stimulated to study more to overcome their perceptions of low efficacy. Thus in some situations having a low perception of one's efficacy may be helpful for learning.

The teacher's role in improving students' perceptions of their own efficacy is to help them set goals for themselves for study, and to provide feedback on the efforts of their study. Goals, in addition to giving directions for self study, provide a yardstick against which students can measure achievement. Knowledge of success in achieving even short-term goals helps improve students' perceptions of efficacy.

Increasing SDL

Self-direction displayed by a student depends on a number of factors, which include the approach taken by the teacher (Pratt 1988). Candy (1990, p. 244) states that 'adult learners judge and evaluate the demands of learning situations and...adjust their learning strategies to what they perceive to be the demands of the task'. Teachers can influence the learning strategy by addressing the nature of the task assigned to students and by minimizing the degree of control exerted on them in undertaking the task. If the expectations are clear, the teacher can help each student generate a study plan and methods of monitoring progress. As self-direction is a quality that should be gradually developed in medical school, the degree of control can also be gradually reduced as the student matures in the school.

Surprisingly, Lockwood (1986) found that many adult distant learners had not received advice on how to prepare for self-study, read, take notes or prepare an essay. Those who had received advice on these activities, showed their willingness to heed the advice.

Developing students' creativity

The importance of creativity for the physician mandates that the teacher provides opportunities for students to develop this attribute. Assignments that force the student to solve problems for which they may not have the background knowledge are one way of encouraging creative thinking.

Another way is to encourage students to undertake creative writing through assignments which require them to compose original essays ('thought papers') without reference to published literature, a practice rarely used in medical education. They have the further advantage of developing students' skills in composition, an attribute which seems to be declining in the average medical student as multiple choice questions increasingly replace free-response questions in student assessment procedures.

Another way of developing creative thinking skills is through student research projects undertaken individually or in groups. The latter forces each student to think creatively. Such projects may be associated with field activities which students undertake during their community attachments. The added advantage of encouraging community orientation would accrue from such research projects.

Give students feedback on their accomplishments

Feedback can be generated internally (by students themselves while studying) and externally (by teachers and peers). When a learner realizes that a discrepancy exists between expected performance and achievement, external feedback is sought. Butler and Winne (1995) advise that feedback given by the teacher should relate not only to the content of learning, but also to the self study strategies adopted by the student. Schunk and Gunn (1986) are of the opinion that self-directed learners are more likely to attribute success or failure to feedback about effectiveness of strategies than about the student's ability or the effort put into study. Thus discussion with the student about methods of self-study is at least as important as pointing out the outcomes of study. Pressley et al. (1984) found, however, that feedback on strategy was more valuable in children than in adults, as the latter may have tried different strategies for learning and embarked on the strategy most effective for them.

Feedback is more useful for correcting errors of knowledge and understanding, and less useful for reinforcing correct knowledge, unless the student has some doubt about the correctness of knowledge (Kulhavy 1977). The nature of feedback determines its usefulness: for factual information, the correct answer is sufficient (Phye 1979); while for higher cognitive skills feedback should be more descriptive. Feedback on assignments should be descriptive, not merely quantitative scores or letter grades. The student should be informed of strengths and weaknesses, with suggestions for improvement.

Research generally shows that students are more effective when they attend to externally provided feedback than that generated internally (Bangert-Drowns et al. 1991). This may be related to the finding that students do not generally monitor their learning optimally. Pressley et al. (1990) found that university students show over-confidence about their ability to respond to questions and lack awareness of problems they have in understanding.

The feedback given to students should have the characteristics outlined in fig. 21.3.

Setting student assignments

Assignments are of two types: reading and written. The importance of reading assignments, which require critical thinking on the part of the student, has already been alluded to. If such reading assignments are given to a group of students, the teacher should assess each student's ability to criticize the assigned reading. One

- ◆ Realistic, on those aspects which the student can improve on and which are not beyond the student's scope
- ◆ Specific, pinpointing potential areas of improvement and avoiding generalizations and abstractions
- ◆ Sensitive to the student's personal goals
- ◆ Timely and prompt, as motivation to learn from the feedback may have diminished if postponed (Crooks 1988, p. 457)
- ◆ Clear, genuine, and accurate rather than manipulative
- ◆ Non-judgemental, avoiding value-laden statements, and without imposition of authority

Figure 21.3 Characteristics of good feedback.

method of assessment is through examining critiques written by each student, a time-consuming process in large student groups. Another strategy is to assign one or two students to lead (rather than present) a critique of the assigned reading, extracting contributions from each member of the group, in the teacher's presence. The teacher can then obtain a fair idea of each member's ability to criticize.

In many curricula student research projects are undertaken as a group activity. While this fosters pooling of ideas from each member of the group, it also provides opportunities for laggards to depend on enterprising students. Individual research projects may be more difficult to manage in a large batch of students. If group research projects are undertaken teachers should ensure that they appropriately reward the efforts of each group member's contribution to the task, even though Slavin (1983) concluded that group rewards based on individual contributions increased cooperation among group members. Assignments that involve cooperation among members of a group, but also competition among groups, seem to lead to higher average achievement than individual assignments (Johnson et al. 1981).

Students generally favour a strategic approach to learning in order to get the best grades possible. Assignments are undertaken depending on their perception of importance (Laurillard, 1979). It is up to the teachers to ensure and instil the belief in students that satisfactory completion of assignments is an important component of successful course completion.

Helping students prepare for examinations

A deep approach to learning should be encouraged when students prepare for impending examinations. The most potent factor which influences students' preparation is the nature of the questions they expect, based on previous examinations in the school. The aphorism 'assessment drives learning' is certainly true, especially in high stakes examinations. It is, therefore, of vital importance for the school to develop a culture of examining which requires students to display understanding, integration, application, critical thinking and problem-solving in answering questions. While testing recall is inevitable in many questions, the emphasis should be on these higher cognitive abilities.

Morgan (1993, p. 95) has stressed the importance of clearly communicating the teacher's demands to the students to help them improve their learning. Lucid learning objectives are a prerequisite to achieving clarity of expectations. If the content subsumed in some objectives has not been covered by the teacher, the objectives related to those 'uncovered' parts should be so clear that the

independent learner is aware of the teacher's expectations, even without attending the teacher's classes. In a critical review of the literature on the impact of classroom tests on student learning, Crooks (1988, p. 442) states that there is wide agreement that 'teacher-made tests tend to give greater emphasis to lower cognitive levels than the teacher's stated objectives would justify'. He presents evidence that the use of higher level questions in assessment enhances learning, retention, transfer, interest, and development of learning skills, unless such questions are too difficult or unclear for the students.

A second requirement for clarity relates to the taxonomic level of questions. In a school that has traditionally set recall-type questions, it is unfair to expect students to answer questions that test higher cognitive abilities in high stakes examinations, without having first given them practice in answering such questions. So-called 'mock examinations' before high stakes examinations are a good method of providing opportunities for practice. However, these examinations should always be followed by discussion of both content (answers to the questions) and process (issues related to the manner in which students should prepare for and answer such questions) with the students.

The third requirement is the nature of the grading system used. In high stakes examinations, in particular, where the consequences of pass/fail decisions are significant, students must be given every opportunity to maximize their grades. For this purpose, students should be aware of the relative weighting given to examination components, marking systems adopted by the examiners, methods of standard setting, and consequences of failure.

A truly integrated question tests students' ability to link content from different areas in a manner similar to the linking they would adopt in real life situations when called upon to manage patients. While many medical schools have replaced subject-based examinations with multidisciplinary ones, the latter often consist of a collection of questions from different subjects in a single question paper. Linking between subjects is not tested within each question. Consequently, students continue to undertake self-study subjectwise, and integrated learning is not encouraged (Bandaranayake 2011, p. 83). For this purpose question constructors must formulate questions which test links within and between subjects.

Conducting study skills courses

Study skills courses are not common in medical schools. An assumption is made that students know how to study at this level. While this may be true for students who have already undertaken undergraduate study before they enter medical school, in many countries they come directly from secondary school, bringing with them the practices they are accustomed to there. Though sometimes these practices are desirable ones, many students need to be oriented to effective ways of studying in medical school. Desirable study habits may not have been inculcated even in students who have already undertaken undergraduate study. Furthermore, as pointed out earlier, the study skills required for a medical student may differ in some aspects from those required for other students.

For the reasons stated already, a study skills course at the commencement of medical training is advantageous for all students. One suggestion for such a course would be a preliminary exposure to some of the principles of learning discussed earlier, followed by practice in each of the study skills that a medical student must acquire.

As lectures are a common method of teaching, students should develop skills in note taking. Many students are not skilled note takers, and the skills of effective note taking take time to learn. Aiken et al. (1975) found that information contained in notes is much more likely to be remembered later than that which is not. The act of taking notes, if done correctly, aids learning during a lecture, as the student is required to listen and process the information given by the lecturer before transcribing it into notes. The more common but less effective practice, however, is for the information to be transferred directly into notes without processing. Kiewra et al. (1991) suggest that study skills courses should address comprehension strategies in addition to note-taking skills.

A study by McGee (1991) demonstrated the positive outcomes of a brief course on study skills for premedical students. Ramsden et al. (1987) found, however, that a course to improve study skills of university students led to a greater use of surface than deep learning approaches. They attributed this finding to the course making students more aware of the nature of assessment procedures that favoured a surface approach. Study skills courses by themselves are unlikely, therefore, to improve students' study habits unless the assessment procedures also encourage desirable learning approaches.

In conducting a study skills course it would be best to use examples for demonstration and practice from the medical field to heighten students' interest and to provide them with a glimpse of the nature of studies which they are about to commence. Just as students see relevance in communication skills courses integrated with medical subject content, so also would study skills courses be seen as relevant when integrated with the same content.

Conclusions

◆ Increases in knowledge and technological developments, in costs of healthcare, and in public awareness have changed healthcare and education in ways that require the twenty-first century medical student to develop a set of study skills to effectively negotiate all phases of the continuum of medical education.

◆ In planning self-study students should be able to determine their priorities for learning, identify and access learning resources, retrieve and critically review information, and manage information in a manner that facilitates future use.

◆ In studying sourced material, students must adopt a deep approach to learning, reflecting on what they learn, integrating it with previous learning, and applying their learning to new situations.

◆ Creativity, self explanation, self assessment, and teaching peers are important skills to be developed in the physician of tomorrow.

References

Aiken, E.G., Thomas, G.S., and Shennum, W.A. (1975) Memory for a lecture: effects of notes, lecture rate and information density. *J Educ Psychol.* 67: 439–444

Bandaranayake, R.C. (2009) Study skills. In: J.A. Dent and R.M. Harden (eds) *A Practical Guide for Medical Teachers* (Chapter 50. p. 386). Edinburgh: Churchill Livingstone

Bandaranayake, R.C. (2010) The place of anatomy in medical education (Viewpoint: Throwing the baby out with the bath water!) AMEE Guide Supplement 41.3. *Med Teach.* 32: 607–609

Bandaranayake R.C. (2011) *The Integrated Medical Curriculum.* London: Radcliffe

Bandura, A. (1977) Self-efficacy: Toward a unifying theory of behavioral change. *Psychol Rev.* 84(2): 191–215

Bangert-Drowns, R.L., Kulik, C.C., Kulik, J.A., and Morgan, M.T. (1991) The instructional effect of feedback in test-like events. *Rev Educ Res.* 61: 213–238

Bielaczyc, K., Pirolli, P., and Brown, A.L. (1991) *The Effects of Training in Explanation Strategies on the Acquisition of Programming Skills.* Chicago: American Educational Research Association Annual Meeting, Chicago

Boud, D., Keogh, R. and Walker, D. (eds) (1985) *Reflection: Turning Experience into Learning.* London: Kogan Page

Bransford, J., Sherwood, R., Vye, N., and Reiser, J. (1986) Teaching thinking and problem solving. *Am Psychol.* 41: 1078–1089

Brown, A.L. and Campione, J.C. (1986) Psychological theory and the study of learning disabilities, *Am Psychol.* 41: 1059–1068

Buckley, S., Coleman, J., Davison, I., et al. (2009) The educational effects of portfolios on undergraduate student learning: a BEME systematic review. BEME Guide No. 11. *Med Teach.* 31(4): 282–298

Butler, D.L. and Winne, P.H. (1995) Feedback and self-regulated learning: a theoretical synthesis. *Rev Educ Res.* 65(3): 245–281

Candy, P.C. (1990) *Self-direction for Lifelong Learning: A Comprehensive Guide to Theory and Practice.* San Francisco: Jossey-Bass

Corno, I. and Mandinach, E.B. (1983) The role of cognitive engagement in classroom learning and motivation. *Educ Psychol.* 18: 88–108

Crooks, T.J. (1988) The impact of classroom evaluation practices on students. *Rev Educ Res* 58: 438–481

Entwistle, N.J. (1975) How students learn: information processing, intellectual development and confrontation. *Higher Educ Bull.* 3: 129–148

Entwistle, A. and Entwistle, N. (1992) Experiences of understanding in revising for degree examination. *Learn Instruct.* 2 (1): 1–22

Evans, T.D. and Nation, D. (1989) Dialogue in the theory, practice and research of distance education. *Open Learn.* 4(2): 37–46

Friere, P. (1982) *Pedagogy of the Oppressed.* Harmondsworth: Penguin

Gorsky, P., Caspi, A., and Trumper, R. (2004) Dialogue in a distance education physics course. *Open Learn.* 19(3): 265–277

Hattie, J., Biggs, J., and Purdie, N. (1996). Effects of learning skills interventions on student learning: a meta-analysis. *Rev Educ Res.* 66(2): 99–136

Holmberg, B. (1986) Improving study skills for distance students, *Open Learn.* 1(3): 29–33 and 52

Illich, I. (1984) *Deschooling Society.* Harmondsworth: Penguin Books

Inuwa, I.M., Taranikanti, V., Al-Rawahy, M., and Habbal, O. (2011) Perceptions and attitudes of medical students towards two methods of assessing practical anatomy knowledge. *Sultan Qaboos Univ Med J.* 11(3): 383–389

Johnson, D.W., Maruyama, G., Johnson, R., et al. (1981) Effects of cooperative, competitive and individualistic goal structures on achievement: A meta-analysis. *Psychol Bull.* 89: 47–62

Kear, K. (2004) Peer learning using asynchronous discussion systems in distance education. *Open Learn.* 19(2): 151–164

Kiewra, K.A. (1991) Aids to lecture learning. *Educ Psychol.* 26(1): 37–53

Knowles, M. (1980) *The Modern Practice of Adult Education: From Pedagogy to Andragogy,* New York: Cambridge

Knowles, M. (1990) *The Adult Learner: A Neglected Species.* 4th edn. Houston: Gulf Publishing, p. 174

Koestler, A. *The Act of Creation,* London: Penguin, 1964, p. 13.

Kulhavy, R.W. (1977) Feedback in written instruction. *Rev Educ Res.* 47: 211–232

Laurillard, D. (1979) The process of student learning. *Higher Educ.* 8: 395–409

Lockwood, F. (1986) Preparing students for distance learning. *Open Learn.* 1(1): 44–45

Marton, F. and Säljö, R. (1976a) On qualitative differences in learning. I. Outcome and process. *Br J Educ Psychol* 46: 4–11

Marton, F. and Säljö, R. (1976b) On qualitative differences in learning. II. Outcome as a function of the learner conception of the task. *Br J Educ Psychol.* 46: 115–127

Marton, F. and Säljö, R. (1984) Approaches to learning. In: F. Marton, D. Hounsell and N. Entwistle (eds) *The Experience of Learning* (pp. 36–45). Edinburgh: Scottish Academic Press.

McGee, H.M. (1991) Study skills instruction in medical school. *Irish Med J.* 84(3): 100–101

Morgan, A. (1993) *Improving your Students' Learning: Reflections on the Experience of Study.* Open and Distance Learning Series, London: Kogan Page.

Morgan, C.J., Dingsdaf, D., and Saenger, H. (1998) Learning strategies for distance learners: do they help? *Dist Educ.*19(1): 142–156

Musashi M. (1645) The Water Book. http://en.wikiquote.org/wiki/Miyamoto_Musashi#The_Water_Book. Accessed 26 February 2013

Novak, J.D. and Cañas, A.J. (2006) The theory underlying concept maps and how to construct and use them, Technical Report IHMC 2006-1 (Rev 01-2008) Florida Institute for Human and Machine Cognition [Online] http://cmap.ihmc.us/Publications/ResearchPapers/TheoryUnderlyingConceptMaps.pdf Accessed 21 March 2013

Pace, C.R. (1958) Educational objectives, In: N.B. Henry (ed.) *The Integration of Educational Experiences*, 57th Yearbook of the National Society for the Study of Education, Part III (Chapter IV, pp. 69–83). Chicago, IL: University of Chicago Press.

Paris, S.C. and Byrnes, J.P. (1989) The constructive approach to self-regulation and learning in the classroom. In: B.J. Zimmerman and D.H. Schunk (eds) *Self-regulated Learning and Academic Achievement: Theory, Research and Practice* (pp. 169–200). New York: Springer-Verlag

Phye, G.D. (1979) The processing of informative feedback about multiple-choice test performance. *Contemp Educ Psychol.* 4: 381–394

Prat-Sala, M. and Redford, P. (2010) The interplay between motivation, self-efficacy and approaches to studying. *Br J Educ Psychol.* 80: 283–305

Pratt, D.D. (1988) Andragogy as a relational construct. *Adult Educ Q.* 38(3): 160–172

Prawat, R.S. (1989) Promoting access to knowledge, strategy and disposition in students: a research synthesis. *Rev Educ Res.* 59(1): 1–41

Pressley, M., Ghatala, E.S., Woolshyn, V., et al. (1990) Sometimes adults miss the main idea and do not realize it: confidence in responses to short-answer and multiple-choice comprehension questions. *Reading Res Q.* 25: 232–249

Pressley, M., Levin, J.R., and Chatala, E.S. (1984) Memory strategy monitoring in adults and children. *J Verbal Learn Verbal Behav.* 23: 270–288

Pressley, M., Yokoi, L., van Meter, P., et al. (1997) Some of the reasons why preparing for exams is so hard: what can be done to make it easier? *Educ Psychol Rev.* 9(1): 1–38

Ramsden, P., Beswick, D., and Bowden, J. (1987) Learning processes and learning skills. In: J.T.E. Richardson, M.W. Eysenck and D.W. Piper (eds) *Student Learning: Research in Education and Cognitive Psychology* (pp. 168–176). Milton Keynes: Open University Press & Society for Research into Higher Education

Ramsden, P. and Entwistle, N.J. (1981) Effects of academic departments on students' approaches to studying. *Br J Educ Psychol.* 51: 368–383

Säljö R. (1979) Learning in the learner's perspective: 1. Some commonsense assumptions, Report No. 76, Goteberg, Sweden: University of Goteberg, Institute of Education

Saunders, K., Northup, D., and Mennin, S.P. (1985) The library in a problem-based curriculum. In: A. Kaufman (ed.) *Implementing Problem-Based Medical Education* (pp. 71–88). New York: Springer

Schunk, D.H. and Gunn, T.P. (1986) Self-efficacy and skill development: influence of task strategies and attributions. *J Educ Res.* 79(4): 238–244

Scouller, K. (1998) The influence of assessment method on students' learning approaches: MCQ examination vs assignment essay, *Higher Educ.* 35: 453–472

Slavin, R.E. (1983) When does cooperative learning increase student achievement? *Psychol Bull.* 94: 429–445

Steinberg, E.R. (1989) Cognition and learner control: a literature review, 1977–1988, *J Computer Based Instruct.* 16: 117–121

Thomas, P.R. and Bain, J.D. (1984) Contextual dependence of learning approaches: the effects of assessments. *Hum Learn.* 3: 227–240

Winne, P.H. (1995) Inherent details in self-regulated learning, *Educ Psychol.* 30: 173–187

World Health Organization (1978) *Primary Health Care*, Report of the International Conference on Primary Health Care, Alma Ata, USSR, 6–12 September, 1978. Geneva: World Health Organization

Supervision

CHAPTER 22

Educational supervision

Susan Kilminster and David Cottrell

Much teaching of supervision, and virtually all the literature on the subject, emphasises the importance of understanding supervision as a process of 'bringing forth' rather than 'holding forth'.

John Launer

Reproduced from Launer J, 'Reflective practice and clinical supervision: neutrality and honesty' Work Based Learning in Primary Care, 4, 4, pp. 384–386, © Radcliffe Publishing, 2006, with permission

Introduction

Doctors need to learn as they work and to do this they need to practise semi-autonomously. To enable safe patient care and an environment where doctors can learn, educational supervision is paramount. This chapter defines supervision and explains what it is for. It outlines different forms of supervision within medical education and the theoretical underpinnings of different supervision frameworks.

Supervision in practice: the evidence

Learning in the workplace is the basis of postgraduate medical education and training. Essentially, you learn to be a doctor by being one. Each training programme has formal educational activities, and doctors in training must undertake independent study, but the most important element of training is the opportunity to undertake medical practice under appropriate supervision. Although supervision has a vital role in medical education, it is still probably the least investigated and least developed aspect of clinical teaching. This chapter reviews current understandings about supervision; the evidence for supervision; why it matters to all doctors; and concludes by suggesting new directions for developing supervisory practice.

In the UK, educational and clinical supervision is required for both foundation and postgraduate trainees, as is the case in most countries. Although there has been a lack of clarity about supervision and the roles and responsibilities of supervisors, there are now explicit statements about what is expected at all levels of postgraduate training. The General Medical Council makes specific recommendations about supervision (GMC 2009, 2012): all trainees must have a named educational and clinical supervisor for each rotation; at times the same individual can fulfil both roles but their different roles and responsibilities must be clearly defined. At specialist trainee level, healthcare organizations are required to recognize supervised training as a core responsibility; the *Gold Guide* (MMC 2010) states that such supervision both ensures patient safety and promotes workforce

development (i.e. it has an educational function). The guidance for the Foundation programme (MMC 2012) explicitly recognizes that educational supervision, clinical supervision, and training more generally overlap, and that the same individual will move between a variety of supervisory roles at different times; for example a trainee may be both supervisor of a junior and receive supervision themselves.

The medical literature on supervision of doctors demonstrates general agreement that the two main purposes of supervision are to ensure patient safety and promote professional development. There seems to be consensus that supervision matters and is important for trainees. There is less agreement about what supervision actually means, what it is that supervisors and supervisees should actually do during supervision, when it should happen and how often. Supervision is commonly assumed to be something that supports the training and development of more junior doctors, and which takes place within a hierarchical relationship. There is thus virtually no discussion or investigation of peer supervision for consultants and GPs as part of a programme of continuing professional development. The next sections of this chapter will consider two main strands of the literature on supervision in medicine:

- ◆ guidance about effective supervision for trainees
- ◆ empirical evidence showing the relationship between supervision and patient safety.

We will then consider the theoretical frameworks for some models of supervision and explore the implications for these of recent developments in understanding workplace learning.

Effective supervision and postgraduate training

Supervision is often said to have three functions—educational, supportive, and managerial—although there are debates about the managerial function of supervision. In some of the literature about supervision there is a tendency for supervisory relationships to be idealized and for the realities of practice to be ignored. Some authors argue that because trust is important for the development of the supervisory relationship then there can be no managerial or hierarchical relationship and that the content of the supervisory relationship must be confidential. However, in medicine, and arguably, all healthcare professions, there is a managerial aspect to supervisory relationships and confidentiality is never absolute if there is a risk of harm. Indeed, the GMC guidance and the *Gold Guide* make it clear that supervision, assessment and performance review are linked.

Current UK guidance for postgraduate training states that educational supervisors are responsible for overseeing training—that is they must oversee a series of training posts that form part of a training programme; and clinical supervisors are responsible for overseeing day to day clinical practice. It also emphasizes that the purpose of supervision is to ensure patient safety and promote professional development or learning. Clearly, the content of what needs to be supervised and the level of supervision will vary according to the grade and relevant experience of the trainee, and also with the training context and the specialty. Supervisors must make judgements as to whether they should be present in the same room as the person being supervised, providing direct supervision; nearby and immediately available to come to the aid of the person being supervised; in the hospital or primary care premises and available at short notice able to offer immediate help by telephone and able to come to the aid of the person within a short time (local supervision); or on-call and available for advice and able to come to the trainee's assistance in an appropriate time (distant supervision). When Grant et al. (2003, pp. 140–149) asked supervisors and trainees about the type and frequency of activities that occur in supervision we found that supervision practices are variable; this finding has since been confirmed a number of times (Daelmans et al. 2004; Hore et al. 2009; Mourad et al. 2010; O'Brien et al. 2006; Wells et al. 2009).

A number of studies have investigated levels and types of supervision and there is some guidance about effective supervision which can help trainees and supervisors develop their practices (Anderson et al. 2011; Dwyer et al. 2011; Launer and Hogarth 2011; McKimm and Forrest 2010; Rudland et al. 2010; Swanwick et al. 2010). Overall, supervisors and trainees agree that discussing individual patients is the most frequent and the most effective supervisory activity and they agree on the importance of direct supervision (i.e. the supervisor being present and directly observing the clinical process) (Kilroy, 2006; Lewis et al 2009). A review of direct observation of practice in emergency medicine found a small number of studies which showed better outcomes for patients probably due to the consequent earlier involvement of senior doctors in patient care and improved decision making (Craig, 2011, pp. 60–67). There was some indication that more direct supervision may slow the speed at which patients are seen—longer waiting times may have negative effects on patients' conditions, although this may well be counterbalanced by the fact that over time, trainees who receive more direct supervision and feedback develop greater expertise.

The learning environment and the quality of the relationship are particularly valued (Busari et al. 2005; Van der Zwet et al. 2010; Wimmers et al. 2006). Other work has shown that it is possible to conduct supervision at a distance and that this is dependent on the relationship between the supervisor and trainee (Wearne 2005;

Hudson et al. 2011). However, supervisors and trainees can have different perceptions about the amount and type of supervision that trainees receive (trainees generally report receiving less supervision than supervisors report giving although Julyan (2009, p. 51) found approximately 70% agreement between psychiatry trainees and supervisors. Chur-Hansen and Maclean (2007, pp. 273–275) found that Australian psychiatry supervisors had different opinions to each other about what could be reasonably expected of trainees. Trainees often say that they do not receive sufficient supervision; they can be critical of aspects of supervision, particularly supervisors' commitment to supervision (Bruijn et al. 2006; Lloyd and Becker 2007).

There is general agreement that good supervision is dependent on the features outlined in fig. 22.1.

There is also general agreement that effective supervisors:

◆ involve trainees in patient care

◆ establish good relationships

◆ give direction and constructive feedback

◆ allow procedural opportunities

◆ offer chances to review patients

◆ give trainees responsibility.

Problems with supervision that have been identified are shown in fig. 22.2.

However, there is much less agreement about how to bring about these components of effective supervision. Previous work on supervision (Kilminster et al. 2007, Busari and Koot 2007; Bruijn et al. 2006) concluded that effective supervision for trainees is dependent on the quality of the supervisory relationship (see fig. 22.3).

In practice, supervision is much more complex than this literature suggests. There is often a tension in clinical education between enabling trainees to have opportunities for practice on the one hand and protecting patients on the other; supervisors have to make continual decisions about the activities they can entrust trainees to carry out and the level of supervision those trainees require (Sterkenburg et al. 2010; ten Cate and Scheele 2007). In addition, the supervisee can become the supervisor at different times in the same day and have to make those same decisions about others (Jelinek et al. 2010). A good supervisor may support a trainee in developing their own supervisory skills by making that trainee's supervision of a more junior trainee a component of supervision. Levels of responsibility and supervision also vary depending on time (e.g. out of hours), setting, speciality, local practices and culture, and previous experience. This is because the membership of clinical teams continually changes and lines of responsibility are not always clear; for instance, on some occasions, such as during

Good supervision is dependent on
◆ The attitudes and commitment of the trainee and supervisor
◆ The quality of the supervisory relationship
◆ Direct supervision
◆ Good practice in feedback
◆ Protected time for supervision meetings
◆ Regular meetings

Figure 22.1 Good supervision.

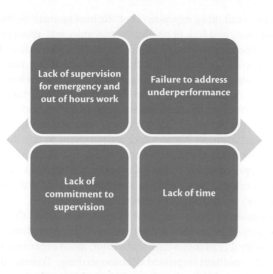

Figure 22.2 Problems with supervision.

Direct supervision—trainee and supervisor working together and observing each other—positively affects patients' outcomes and trainees' development.

Constructive feedback is essential and should be frequent.

Supervision should be structured and there should be regular timetabled meetings. The content of supervision meetings should be agreed and learning objectives determined at the beginning of the supervisory relationship. Continuity is important.

Supervision should include clinical management; teaching and research; management and administration; pastoral care; interpersonal skills; personal development; and reflection on practice, including reflection on the supervisory process.

The supervision process should be informed by a 360 degree perspective.

Figure 22.3 The supervisory relationship.

night-time emergencies, the most junior doctor in the team might be the most senior present, so that the daytime hierarchical and power relations are disrupted. The advent of more shift working and juniors working to teams of consultants means that older apprenticeship models are less common and trainees may find it harder to seek advice from seniors they know less well. More generally, trainees may be reluctant to ask for help or may try to hide specific gaps in their knowledge or experience—because they may be (justifiably) concerned about how they are perceived. This has obvious implications for patient safety.

Supervision and patient safety

There is convincing quantitative evidence that supervision has a positive effect on patient outcomes and that lack of supervision is harmful to patients and can be associated with increased morbidity and mortality (Kilminster et al. 2007). A recent systematic review of the effects of clinical supervision in North America found that it is associated with improved outcomes for both patients and trainees (Farnan et al. 2012). A specific case–control study of meningococcal disease in children (Ninis et al. 2005) found three factors which were associated with death: these included failures in supervision of junior doctors (the other two factors were not being seen by a paediatrician and failure to administer adequate inotropes). Overall, empirical evidence over the last 30 years shows that direct

supervision is important for patients as well as for trainees' development, especially when the supervisor gives the trainee focused feedback.

Over this period a number of studies have attempted to quantify the effects of supervision on patient outcomes. For example, 20 years ago a wide ranging review found evidence which suggests that increased deaths are associated with less supervision of junior doctors in surgery, anaesthesia, emergency care, obstetrics, and paediatrics (McKee andand Black 1992). The authors argued that the balance of evidence shows that patient care suffers when trainees are unsupervised—even though some trainees claim to benefit from the experience that lack of supervision gives them. McKee and Black (1992, pp. 549–558) also pointed out that trainees may not learn correct practice without appropriate supervision and that therefore unsupervised experience can lead to lower standards of care. Some recent studies have examined the effects of close supervision of trainees when performing more complex tasks—in cardiac surgery (Guo et al. 2008; Shi et al. 2011) and in gastrointestinal oncology (Yamamoto et al. 2009). These have shown that although such procedures may take trainees longer, the outcomes are acceptable and comparable to those of supervisors, when the trainees are closely supervised.

Other US studies have produced strong evidence for the importance of direct supervision. The effects of supervision on the quality of care were examined in five Harvard teaching hospitals (Sox et al. 1998). A range of measures was used—trainees' compliance with process of care guidelines (assessed by record review), patients' satisfaction, and patients' reported problems with care. Over a 7 month period all 3667 patients who presented at the study hospitals with abdominal pain, asthma or chronic obstructive pulmonary disease, chest pain, hand laceration, head trauma, and vaginal bleeding were included in the study; the trainees were unaware of the purpose of the study. All the patients were given a questionnaire to complete on site and some were randomly selected for a 10-day follow up interview. Analyses were adjusted for case mix, degree of urgency, and chief complaints. Using these measures the researchers found that the quality of care was higher when the resident was directly supervised (i.e. when the senior doctors also saw the patient). An earlier study compared senior doctors' findings in relation to patients with trainees' reports about those patients; they focused on history taking, assessment of severity of the patients' illness, diagnoses, treatment and follow-up plans (Genniss and Genniss 1993). When the senior doctors saw patients themselves, they rated the patients as more seriously ill than the trainees did and the senior doctors made frequent changes to the trainees' diagnosis and management plans. Once they had seen the patients the senior doctors made more critical assessments of the trainees. Although the authors acknowledge some weaknesses in their study design they conclude that, when supervisors see the patient themselves rather than relying on trainees' reports there is a significant difference in their assessments of residents' skills and patient management. Fallon et al. (1993, pp. 560–561) investigated each surgical procedure performed by the trauma service in one hospital over a year. The level of involvement of senior doctors was ranked and this data was matched to outcomes of death or complications. The results suggested that supervision had a greater impact where the trainee was less experienced. Griffiths et al. (1996, pp. 106–108) compared tests (X-rays, arterial blood gases (ABG) and electrolytes) ordered in the neonatal intensive care unit by staff with different levels of experience. They found that as workloads increased newly qualified doctors ordered more

ABGs, especially when they were less supervised. Furthermore, a recent study (Iwashyna et al. 2011) found that attending physicians (supervisors) had less impact on ordering of laboratory tests in one hospital; however, the authors note that the study was conducted in a setting where there is an existing emphasis on direct supervision. Therefore, the authors suggest that rates of ordering of laboratory tests might offer one way of measuring supervision.

Although the evidence shows that supervision affects patient outcomes and patient safety, trainees do not always ask for help. Kennedy et al. (2009, pp. S106–11) conducted an observational and interview study to investigate how and when medical trainees asked for clinical support. They showed clearly how trainees consider many factors besides clinical issues before asking for help from a supervisor. The trainees did consider the clinical situation and its importance but were reluctant to ask for help if they thought the problem was one that they ought to be able to deal with at their level of training. Their decisions were also affected by supervisor factors and trainee factors; trainees considered the availability and the approachability of their supervisors and were also concerned with their own desire to undertake independent practice and their wishes for positive assessments by their supervisors. Similarly, a questionnaire study that investigated perceived failures of supervision found that there were two main sources for such failures. These were supervisors failing to respond to trainees requests for guidance and support, and trainees' failing to ask for help. The authors suggest that the influence of the clinical environment was such that trainees put more weight on the way they appeared to their seniors than safe patient care (Stewart 2007; Ross et al. 2011). These findings, that trainees may perceive that asking for help presents a threat to their professional credibility, and sometimes, their professional progress, confirm those of earlier studies (Somers et al. 1994; Jolly and MacDonald 1986; Arluke 1980) as well as more recent questionnaire studies (Friedman et al. 2010). The findings have important practical implications. While it is incumbent on trainees to request help if they are uncertain, it is equally important for trainers to cultivate an atmosphere in which trainees feel supported in seeking help.

The studies just mentioned concentrate on procedural aspects of patient care; there is much less work on other aspects, including emotion. Iedema and colleagues (2009, pp. 1750–1756) argue that such procedural measurements dominate patient safety research, and that this ignores affective and narrative aspects of care. The affective and narrative aspects are, however, crucial to patient safety because they are the medium 'through which doctors' identity is nurtured, through which the intensely cohesive group memberships that are part and parcel of medical professionalism are sustained, and through which tactics for dealing with incidents and distress are negotiated' (p. 1750). Iedema et al. (2009) analysed young anaesthetists' 'horror' stories—that is stories about 'unexpected and unordinary' aspects of clinical practice, which evoke affective responses. They found three strands: identity, pedagogy and affectivity. In these stories, the strands unfolded as the doctors told their stories and began to talk more about their feelings and unresolved problems. At first the talk distanced horror, the stories were told in a way that objectified the situation, often with humour, and provided some narrative closure. This functioned to normalize horror and provided a way to accommodate it. The individual moral and pedagogic aspects of the stories were stressed; hence, such horror stories have a cautionary function in the trainees' experience of becoming an anaesthetist. As the discussions continued, the stories involved more expressions of the protagonists' feelings, the contradictions and lack of resolution and more talk about personal impacts. The authors describe how the doctors share their distress with their colleagues and argue that this 'is crucial for young doctors in coming to terms with failure, preparing themselves for any subsequent ones, and learning to "hear" similar uncertainties and concerns expressed by their own trainees' (p. 1755). Such talk actually promotes patient safety because it strengthens the fabric of clinical relationships. These issues are pertinent to any discussion of supervision. Engel et al. (2006, pp. 86–93) found that discussions with colleagues and supervisors were critical to trainees learning to cope with errors. They reinforce the importance of critical reflection as a key characteristic of effective supervision.

In summary, it seems clear that supervision has both immediate and long-term benefits for patient care. The immediate benefits are probably due to involvement of senior, more experienced clinicians, with resultant improved decision making. Trainees develop expertise through effective supervision—this results in medium- and long-term benefits to patients.

Theoretical perspectives

There are a number of discernible influences on the current understandings of and assumptions about supervision and supervisory practices. These include social learning and role modelling; reflective practice; cognitive apprenticeships; and behavioural models—see fig. 22.4. Each of these will now be briefly considered.

Ideas about role modelling are often present in the supervision literature. The basic assumption is that observing other people behaving in particular ways influences the individual who then behaves in similar ways. This derives from social learning theories originally developed by Bandura (1977, 1986); the emphasis is on individuals as models and the weakness with this approach is that the focus on individuals excludes relationships between individuals and the context in which the trainee is working.

Reflective practice is based on Donald Schon's (1983, 1987) work on reflection-in-action and reflection-on-action; these

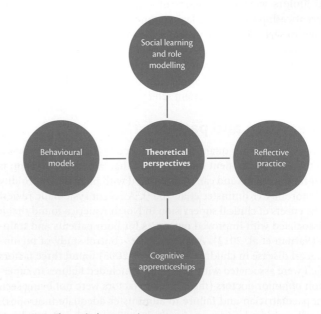

Figure 22.4 Theoretical perspectives.

were initially taken up strongly in nursing but have been increasingly adopted by other healthcare professions. They now frequently feature in reflective portfolios. They often encourage the trainee to consider how they are working with patients (and sometimes other members of the clinical team) and the consequences of their interventions and interactions. In some models of supervision reflective practice is seen as integral to the supervision process.

Cognitive apprenticeship approaches are concerned with the development of skills through *modelling* (the expert demonstrates the skill or tasks, sometimes providing verbal reasoning), *scaffolding* (where the task may be tried out in sections or learnt with particular supports in place), and *fading* (where the supports are gradually removed until the task can be performed independently). This approach focuses on coaching thorough observation, feedback and other interventions intended to promote expert performance. O'Neill et al. (2006, pp. 348–354) conducted an observational and questionnaire study to investigate supervisors' approaches to student and trainee doctors learning in clinical settings. They found that, in practice, supervisors predominantly used a modelling approach with students and an 'arms-length' supervision approach with trainees. Stalmeijer et al. (2009, pp. 535–546) investigated the cognitive apprenticeship model in student clerkships. They used an instructional model, which included modelling, coaching, scaffolding, articulation, reflection, and exploration. They found that modelling, coaching, and articulation were the most used and that scaffolding, reflection, and exploration were only used in longer placements. There was wide variation in the supervisors' use of the different methods—this was seen as a problem in this study. The authors conclude that this model is useful for evaluation, feedback, self-assessment, and faculty development.

Behavioural models rely on learning contracts and similar approaches to managing trainees' learning and performance. These are prevalent in medicine, although many problems with the

underpinning assumptions and actual practices have been identified in the literature (ten Cate and Scheele 2007).

Elements of all these approaches are often present in supervision practices; quite often in conjunction with managerial and audit approaches. Such approaches can limit independent action by trainees and there are some risks with this. Kennedy et al (2005, pp. S106–111) considered theoretical perspectives and empirical evidence relating to the role of progressive autonomy in clinical learning. They argued that although there was limited empirical support for the principle of progressive independence it is clear that different theoretical perspectives in psychology, sociology, education, and medical education suggest that progressive independence is critical to learning. While each of these theoretical approaches can have some positive effects on learning, they are limited. This is because they all tend to individualize learning and minimize or ignore the complexities of actual practice (fig. 22.5). Consequently, there has been increasing interest in notions of communities of practice and situated learning—these attempt to address some of these complexities. These perspectives emphasize practice as the basis for learning, which is understood through the metaphor of participation (Sfard 1998; Hager and Hodkinson 2009) Learning is often defined as a form of becoming. Learning involves engaging in legitimate peripheral practice under the guidance of experts. Knowledge, skills and values are learnt in practice and are not separate from practice (Lave and Wenger 1991; Wenger 1998; Bleakley 2005; Dornan 2005).

Models of supervision in medicine

A number of authors have tried to develop models to explain supervision in medicine. For example, Deketelaere et al (2006, pp. 908–915) suggested a conceptual framework to help understand learning in clinical placements. This framework was derived from a study of learning during internships in clinical placements. They identified

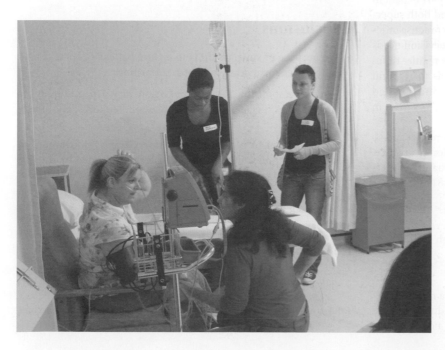

Figure 22.5 Supervision in action.

five components, which are in dynamic tension with each other in clinical learning experiences. The components are:

+ the agenda of the internship (working versus learning)

+ the attitude of the supervisor (evaluator versus coach)

+ the culture of the training setting (work-orientated versus training-orientated)

+ the intern's learning attitude (passive versus proactive) and

+ the nature of the learning process (informal versus formal).

Students have to continually '(re-) define and (re) position' themselves in relation to these components. Deketelaere et al. (2006) suggest that these components not only offer a way to conceptualize clinical learning but also provide a structure to help improve the quality of learning in clinical placements and the nature of supervision and support.

Kennedy et al. (2007, pp. 1080–1085) undertook an observational study on an emergency medicine department and a medical ward in a Canadian hospital. Their focus was to sample different clinical activities conducted under two different systems of supervision and their purpose was to develop a conceptual model of patterns of supervision. They distinguished between supervisory activities which relate specifically to patient care and other types of supervisory activities (they give the example of formal teaching). They use the term 'clinical oversight' to describe supervisors' participation in clinical activities where the purpose is to ensure quality of care. They elaborate three types of clinical oversight: routine oversight (preplanned monitoring of clinical work); responsive oversight (responding to the trainee's activity); and backstage oversight (of which the trainee is not directly aware). They argue that using these three categories to describe clinical oversight provides a framework to give concrete recommendations about clinical supervision and thus provides a potential way for clinical supervision to be measured.

Iedema et al. (2010, pp. 286–291) investigated junior doctors' experiences of supervision—the types and frequency of supervision they experienced and the nature of their supervisory relationships. They found that most supervision occurred as part of patient care and was rarely planned; the junior doctors valued both supervisory help when they needed it and opportunities to practise independently. Iedema and colleagues conclude that supervision needs to be both structured and dynamic: there needs to be regular times for discussion and reflection; and supervision needs to respond to individual doctors, to 'navigate between being hands-on and hands-off'. They consider that this will help junior doctors to be in a 'zone of safe learning'.

Other models seem overly reductionist and instrumental and so thereby neglect many of the complexities of supervision in practice. They include attempts to develop instruments to quantify supervision. For example Byrne et al. (2010, pp. 1171–1181) describe a survey tool which quantifies supervision in terms of

+ trainees' understanding of 'cases'

+ supervisors' contributions to patient care through feedback to the trainee and

+ supervisors' time.

There is sometimes an assumption that introducing a new requirement or assessment will have a direct effect and produce a desired change. However, things are rarely that simple. For example,

Daelmans et al. (2006, pp. 51–58) report on the effects of an in-training assessment programme on feedback and supervision for students .The effects of this programme were not those intended. In particular there was little follow-up on supervision and feedback given by the supervisors during the students' assessments. In addition, although the students said they wanted more supervision and feedback they rarely requested it.

While the models suggested by Deketelaere, Kennedy and Iedema do offer some explanatory value their focus is largely still on individuals and, to some extent, on the supervisory dyads—that is the supervisor–trainee (or student) pairs; these models still do not adequately account for details of practice nor do they show how learning is integral to practice. Fundamental to any model of supervision are understandings and assumptions about learning and knowledge. Many of the dominant perspectives in medical education assume that knowledge is individually acquired. However, more recent theories of workplace learning show that knowledge is situated and constructed. Clinical practice is the basis for learning and it is situated; supervision is part of practice and so it is also situated.

This analysis is derived from practice-based sociomaterial approaches that have three key features (Fenwick et al. 2011). The first is that whole systems, rather than a specific activity, are included in the analysis. Second, interactions and relationships among non-human as well as human parts of the system are considered. Third, knowledge and learning are understood as embedded in actions and interactions. So, for example, an inquiry into prescribing errors would need to include regulatory systems and prescribing practices and decisions at the specific sites along with the material processes of prescribing, rather than just the more usual focus on deficiencies in specific professional's knowledge and/or practice. The particular relevance of this for supervision is that supervision is both as situated and distributed as is practice. This means that the whole context, the specific local practices and the roles and participation of the clinical team need to be considered, not just the supervisor–trainee dyad. This recognition that practice and supervision are distributed can decrease the isolation that responsibility places on both junior doctors and their supervisors.

Conclusions

+ The purpose of supervision is to ensure patient safety and promote professional development and learning.

+ Levels of responsibility and supervision vary depending on the time, setting, speciality, local practices and cultures, and previous experience

+ It is important to recognize that supervision is not limited to supervisor–trainee dyads but is significantly affected by activity, practices, and cultures of each specific setting.

+ Supervision is an integral part of clinical activity, not separate from it—it is both situated and distributed.

References

Anderson, F., Cachia, P.G., Monie, R., and Connacher, A.A., (2011) Supporting trainees in difficulty: a new approach for Scotland. *Scottish Med J.* 56(2): 72–75

Arluke, A. (1980) Roundsmanship: inherent control on a medical teaching ward. *Social Sci Med* 14A: 297–302

Bandura, A. (1977) Self-efficacy: toward a unifying theory of behavioral change. *Psychol Rev.* 84: 191–215

Bandura, A. (1986) *Social Foundations of Thought and Action: A Social Cognitive Theory.* Englewood Cliffs, NJ: Prentice-Hall

Bleakley, A. (2005) Stories as data, data as stories: making sense of narrative inquiry in clinical education. *Med Educ.* 39(5): 534–540

Bruijn, M., Busari J.O., and Wolf, B.H. (2006) Quality of clinical supervision as perceived by specialist registrars in a university and district teaching hospital. *Med Educ.* 40(10):1002–1008

Byrne, J.M., Kashner, M., Gilman, S.C., et al. (2010) Measuring the intensity of resident supervision in the Department of Veterans Affairs: the Resident Supervision Index *Acad Med.* 85(7): 1171–1181

Busari, J.O. and Koot, B.G. (2007) Quality of clinical supervision as perceived by attending doctors in university and district teaching hospitals. *Med Educ.* 41(10): 957–964

Busari, J.O., Weggelaar, N.M., Knottnerus, A.C., Greidanus, P.M., and Scherpbier, A.J.J.A. (2005) How medical residents perceive the quality of supervision provided by attending doctors in the clinical setting. *Med Educ.* 39(7): 696–703

Chur-Hansen, A. and McLean, S. (2007) Supervisors' views about their trainees and supervision. *Aust Psychiatry.* 15(4): 273–275

Craig, S. (2011) Direct observation of clinical practice in emergency medicine education. *Acad Emerg Med.*18: 60–67

Daelmans, H.E.M., Hoogenboom, R.J.I., Donker, A.J.M., et al. (2004) Effectiveness of clinical rotations as a learning environment for achieving competences. *Med Teach.* 26(4): 305–312

Daelmans H.E., Overmeer R.M., van der Hem-Stokroos H.H., Scherpbier A.J., Stehouwer C.D., and van der Vleuten C.P. (2006) In-training assessment: qualitative study of effects on supervision and feedback in an undergraduate clinical rotation. *Med Educ.* 40(1): 51–58

Deketelaere A., Kelchtermans G., Struyf E., and De Leyn P. (2006) Disentangling clinical learning experiences: an exploratory study on the dynamic tensions in internship. *Med Educ.* 40(9): 908–915

Dornan, T., Scherpbier, A., King, N., and Boshuizen, H. (2005) Clinical teachers and problem-based learning: a phenomenological study. *Med Educ.* 39(2): 163–170

Dwyer, A.J., Morley, P., Reid, E., and Angelatos, C. (2011) Distressed doctors: a hospital-based support program for poorly performing and 'at-risk' junior medical staff. *Med J Aust.* 194(9): 466–469

Engel, K.G., Rosenthal, M. and Sutcliffe, K.M. (2006) Residents' responses to medical error: coping, learning and change. *Acad Med.* 81(1): 86–93

Fallon Jr, W.F., Wears, R.L., and Tepas III, J.J. (1993) Resident supervision in the operating room: does this impact on outcome? *J Trauma.* 35: 560–561

Farnan, J.M., Petty, L.A., Georgitis, E., et al. (2012) A systematic review: the effect of clinical supervision on patient and residency education outcomes. *Acad Med.* 87(4): 428–442

Fenwick, T., Edwards, R. and Sawchuk, P. (2011) *Emerging Approaches to Educational Research: Tracing the Socio-material.* London: Routledge

Friedman, S.M., Sowerby, R.J., Guo, R., and Bandiera, G. (2010) Perceptions of emergency medicine residents and fellows regarding competence, adverse events and reporting to supervisors: a national survey. *Can J Emerg Med Care.* 12(6): 491–499

General Medical Council (2009) *Good Medical Practice.* London: GMC

General Medical Council (2012) *Leadership and Management for All Doctors.* London: GMC

Genniss, V.M. and Genniss, M.A. (1993) Supervision in the outpatient clinic: effects on teaching and patient care. *J Gen Intern Med.* 8: 378–380

Grant, J. Kilminster, S.M., Jolly, B., and Cottrell, D. (2003) Clinical supervision of SpRs. Where does it happen, when does it happen and is it effective? *Med Educ.* 37(2): 140–149

Griffiths, C.H., Desai, N.S., Wilson, E.A., Powell, K.J., and Rich, EC. (1996) Housestaff experience, workload and test ordering in a neonatal intensive care unit. *Acad Med.*71: 106–110

Guo, L.R., Chu, M.W.A., Tong, M.Z.Y., et al. (2008) Does the trainee's level of experience impact on patient safety and clinical outcomes in coronary artery bypass surgery? *J Cardiac Surg.* 23(1): 1–5

Hager, P. and Hodkinson, P. (2009) Moving beyond the metaphor of transfer of learning. *Br Educ Res J.* 35(4): 619–638

Hore, C.T., Lancashire, W., and Fassett, R.G. (2009) Clinical supervision by consultants in teaching hospitals. *Med J Aust.* 191(4): 220–222

Hudson, J.N., Weston, K.M., and Farmer, E.A. (2011)Engaging rural preceptors in new longitudinal community clerkships during workforce shortage: a qualitative study. *BMC Fam Pract.* 12: 103

Iedema, R., Brownhill, S., Haines, M., Lancashire, B., Shaw, T., and Street, J. (2010) 'Hands on, Hands off': a model of clinical supervision that recognises trainees' need for support and independence. *Aust Health Rev.* 34(3): 286–291

Iedema, R. Jorris, C., and Lum, M. (2009) Affect is central to patient safety: the horror stories of young anaesthetists. *Soc Sci Med.* 69: 1750–1756

Iwashyna, T.J., Fuld, A., Asch, D.A., and Bellini LM. (2011)The impact of residents, interns, and attendings on inpatient laboratory ordering patterns: a report from one university's hospitalist service. *Acad Med.* 86(1): 139–145

Jelinek, G.A., Weiland, T.J., and Mackinlay, C. (2010) Supervision and feedback for junior medical staff in Australian emergency departments: findings from the emergency medicine capacity assessment study. *BMC Med Educ.* 10: 74.

Jolly, B.C. and Macdonald, M.M. (1986) Practical experience in the pre-registration year in relation to undergraduate preparation. *Proc Ann Conf Res Med Educ.* 25: 171–176

Julyan, T.E. (2009) Educational supervision and the impact of workplace-based assessments: a survey of psychiatry trainees and their supervisors. *BMC Med Educ.* 9: 51

Kennedy, T.J., Lingard, L., Baker, G.R., Kitchen, L., and Regehr, G. (2007) Clinical oversight: conceptualizing the relationship between supervision and safety. *J Gen Intern Med.* 22(8): 1080–1085

Kennedy, T.J.T., Regehr, G., Baker, G.R., and Lingard, L.A. (2005) Progressive independence in clinical training: A tradition worth defending? *Acad Med.* 80(10): S106–S111

Kennedy, T.J., Regehr, G., Baker, G.R., and Lingard, L. (2009) Preserving professional credibility: grounded theory study of medical trainee's requests for clinical support. *BMJ.* 338: 128

Kilminster, S.M., Jolly, B.C., Grant, J., and Cottrell, D. (2007) AMEE Guide No. 27: Effective educational and clinical supervision. *Med Teach.* 29(1): 2–19

Kilroy, D.A. (2006) Clinical supervision in the emergency department: a critical incident study. *Emerg Med J.* 23(2): 105–108

Launer, J. and Hogarth, S. (2011) What is good supervision? *Postgrad Med J* 87(1030): 573–574

Launer, J. (2006) Reflective practice and clinical supervision: neutrality and honesty. *Work Based Learning in Primary Care.* 4(4): 384–386

Lave, J. and Wenger, E. (1991) *Situated learning: Legitimate Peripheral Participation.* Cambridge: Cambridge University Press

Lewis, G,H., Sullivan, M,J., Tanner, R., et al. (2009) Exploring the perceptions of out-of-hours training for GP registrars in Wales. *Educ Prim Care.* 20(3): 152–158

Lloyd, B.W. and Becker, D. (2007)Paediatric specialist registrars' views of educational supervision and how it can be improved: a questionnaire study. *J Roy Soc Med.* 100(8): 375–378

McKee M. and Black N. (1992) Does the current use of junior doctors in the United Kingdom affect the quality of medical care. *Soc Sci Med.* 34: 549–558

McKimm, J. and Forrest, K. (2010) Using transactional analysis to improve clinical and educational supervision: the Drama and Winner's triangles. *Postgrad Med J.* 86(1015): 261–265

MMC (2010) *A Reference Guide for Postgraduate Specialty Training in the UK.* 4th edn. http://www.mmc.nhs.uk/pdf/Gold%20Guide%202010%20 Fourth%20Edition%20v08.pdf Accessed 29 March 2012

MMC (2012) *Foundation Programme Curriculum.* http://www. foundationprogramme.nhs.uk/pages/home/training-and-assessment Accessed 29 March 2012

Mourad, M., Kohlwes, J., Maselli, J., Auerbach, A.D., and MERN Group (2010) Supervising the supervisors—procedural training and supervision in internal medicine residency. *J Gen Intern Med.* 25(4): 351–356

Ninis, N., Phillips, C., Bailey, L., et al. (2005) The role of healthcare delivery in the outcome of meningococcal disease in children; case- control study of fatal and non-fatal cases. *BMJ.* 330: 1475

O'Brien, M., Brown, J., Ryland, I., et al. (2006) Exploring the views of second-year Foundation Programme doctors and their educational supervisors during a deanery-wide pilot Foundation Programme. *Postgrad Med J.* 82(974): 813–816

O'Neill, P.A., Owen, A.C., McArdle, P.J., and Duffy, K.A. (2006) Views, behaviours and perceived staff development needs of doctors and surgeons regarding learners in outpatient clinics. *Med Educ.* 40(4): 348–354

Ross, P.T., McMyler, E.T., Anderson, S.G., et al. (2011) Trainees' perceptions of patient safety practices: recounting failures of supervision. Joint Commission. *J Qual Patient Safety.* 37(2): 88–95

Rudland, J., Bagg, W., Child, S., et al. (2010) Maximising learning through effective supervision. *N Zeal Med J.* 123(1309): 117–126

Schon, D. (1983) *The Reflective Practitioner; How Professionals Think in Action.* London: Temple Smith

Schon, D.(1987) *Educating the Reflective Practitioner.* San Francisco,CA: Jossey-Bass

Sfard, A. (1998) On two metaphors for learning and the dangers of choosing just one. *Educ Res.* 27(2): 4–13

Shi, W.Y., Hayward, P.A., Yap, C.H., et al. (2011) Training in mitral valve surgery need not affect early outcomes and midterm survival: a multicentre analysis. *Eur J Cardio-Thorac Surg.* 40(4): 826–833

Shojania, K.G., Fletcher, K.E., and Saint, S. (2006) Graduate medical education and patient safety: a busy—and occasionally hazardous—intersection. *Ann Intern Med.* 145(8): 592–598

Somers, P.S., Muller, J.H., Saba, G.W., Draisin, J.A., and Shore, W.A. (1994) Reflections on action: medical students' accounts of their implicit beliefs and strategies in the context of one-to-one clinical teaching. *Acad Med.* 69: 584–587

Sox, C.M., Burstin, H.R., Orav, E.J., et al. (1998) The effect of supervision of residents on quality of care in five university-affiliated emergency departments. *Acad Med.* 73: 776–782

Stalmeijer, R.E., Dolmans, D.H.J.M., Wolfhagen, I.H.A.P., and Scherpbier, A.J.J.A. (2009) Cognitive apprenticeship in clinical practice: can it stimulate learning in the opinion of students? *Adv Health Sci Educ.* 14(4): 535–546

Sterkenburg, A., Barach, P., Kalkman, C., Gielen, M., and ten Cate, O. (2010) When do supervising physicians decide to entrust residents with unsupervised tasks? *Acad Med.* 85(9): 1408–1417

Stewart, J. (2007) Don't hesitate to call—the underlying assumptions. *Clin Teach.* 4: 6–9

Swanwick, T., McKimm, J., and Clarke, R. (2010) Introducing a professional development framework for postgraduate medical supervisors in secondary care: considerations, constraints and challenges. *Postgrad Med J.* 86(1014): 203–207

ten Cate, O. and Scheele, F. (2007) Competency-based postgraduate training: can we bridge the gap between theory and clinical practice? *Acad Med.* 82(6): 542–547

Van der Zwet, J., Hanssen, V.G.A., Zwietering, P.J., et al. (2010) Workplace learning in general practice: Supervision, patient mix and independence emerge from the black box once again. *Med Teach.* 32(7): 294–299

Wearne S. (2005) General practice supervision at a distance—is it remotely possible? *Aust Fam Phys.* 34(Suppl 1): 31–33

Wells, C.W., Inglis, S., and Barton, R. (2009) Trainees in gastroenterology views on teaching in clinical gastroenterology and endoscopy. *Med Teach.* 31(2): 138–144

Wenger, E. (1998) *Communities of Practice. Learning, Meaning and Identity.* Cambridge: Cambridge University Press

Wimmers, P.F., Schmidt, H.G., and Splinter, T.A.W. (2006) Influence of clerkship experiences on clinical competence. *Medl Educ.* 40(5): 450–458

Yamamoto, S., Uedo, N., Ishihara, R., et al. (2009) Endoscopic submucosal dissection for early gastric cancer performed by supervised residents: assessment of feasibility and learning curve. *Endoscopy.* 41(11): 923–928

CHAPTER 23

Mentoring

Erik Driessen and Karlijn Overeem

Mentoring encourages constructive reflection before exploring alternative courses of action.

Robert Alliott

Reproduced from *British Medical Journal*, Robert Alliot, 'Facilitatory mentoring in general practice', 313, pp. S2–7006, copyright 1996, with permission from BMJ Publishing Group Ltd.

Introduction

Studies have reported beneficial effects of mentoring in both medicine and medical education, with mentoring having positive effects on career success, productivity, job satisfaction, career preparation, and workplace-based learning (Driessen et al. 2011a). Mentoring thus appears to be a promising instrument to alleviate the burden of consultants, GPs and residents, who are expected to deliver excellent patient care, advance research and educate and train their future colleagues in an increasingly demanding and stressful environment. Not surprisingly, medical students, residents, and doctors appear to be increasingly vulnerable to burnout and stress, as evidenced by the growing prevalence of these complaints among members of the medical profession (Shanafelt and Habermann 2002). A nurturing workplace and a positive learning environment can go a long way to help students and professionals to successfully survive and grow in the complicated and competitive environment of today's healthcare by fostering learning and continuous professional development (Memon and Memon 2010). However, despite evidence that mentoring can alleviate the burden of physicians and trainees, the literature shows that mentoring has a long way to go before it is widely accepted and implemented, whether in medical practice or in medical education. A systematic review of the literature on mentoring by Sambunjak et al. (2006, p. 1113) reported that less than 50% of medical students and, in some specialties, less than 20% of faculty members had a mentor, while a recent Swiss study showed that since Sambunjak's review nothing much has changed, with only 37 to 50% of residents reporting that they had a mentor (Stamm and Buddeberg-Fischer 2011).

Like so many things that we are told are good for us, mentoring has remained underused, despite ample evidence of its beneficial effects. A probable explanation for this is that mentoring is surrounded by numerous unanswered questions, unknown opportunities, and uncertainties about pitfalls. In this chapter we aim to shed some informative light on mentoring and its potential role in undergraduate, postgraduate, and continuing medical education by discussing the literature on mentoring, the role and tasks of mentor and mentee, and the implementation of mentoring programmes.

First, we will take a closer look at how the terms mentor and mentoring are defined.

Since the mid-1970s, over 20, widely varying, definitions of mentoring and mentor have been proposed in the literature (Berk et al. 2005), suggesting persistent difficulties in reaching a professional consensus on a generally acceptable definition. In 2005, a Faculty Mentoring Committee at Johns Hopkins University proposed the following definition:

> A mentoring relationship is one that may vary along a continuum from informal/short-term to formal/long-term in which a faculty member with useful experience, knowledge, skills, and/or wisdom offers advice, information, guidance, support, or opportunity to another faculty member or student for that individual's professional development.
>
> Berk et al. (2005, p. 67).

A mentor has been defined as 'a person providing quality support, advice and counselling', 'a person who provides guidance and recommendations to a more junior person for courses of action and behaviour'—or even 'a person who shares experience, knowledge and wisdom about a particular occupation, their occupation or about the workplace in general' (Memon and Memon 2010).

In this chapter we use a broad interpretation of mentoring, defining it as situational, contextual, and dependent on institutional philosophy and the objectives pursued, which may range from guiding first-year students during the transition from secondary school to university, to optimizing workplace-based learning for undergraduate students, to career support for residents, and to guidance for healthcare practitioners who have run into problems. For situations where guidance and counselling are the salient aspects of mentoring, the terms coaching, supervision, and mentoring are often used almost interchangeably, which seems quite justified since the tasks of the mentor may indeed involve coaching and supervision. The term mentoring as used in this chapter encompasses all of the above-mentioned aspects (fig. 23.1). For those who are interested in the intricacies of the demarcation of these areas, we recommend the comprehensive discussion of the differences and similarities

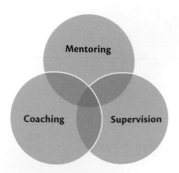

Figure 23.1 Mentoring, coaching and supervision.

between supervision, mentoring, and coaching by Launer (2006). We now turn our attention to the research evidence on mentoring.

Evidence on mentoring

We will consider the published research on mentoring from three perspectives: effects of mentoring on the mentee, on the mentor, and on the organization. Additionally, we will discuss different explanations that have been proposed for the persistent underuse of mentoring. We refer to the literature on health professions education, but we will also make some excursions into the management and organizational literature, which have a much longer tradition of research into mentoring.

The mentee

The 2006 review by Sambunjak et al. (2006), to which we referred earlier, focuses on the impact of mentoring on the career development of students and doctors. Of eight studies investigating the relationship between mentoring, career guidance, and personal development, five reported that mentoring was an important career-enhancing factor for students, fellows, and staff physicians in various disciplines. In another review, Sambunjak et al. (2010) found nine studies providing support for the conclusion that mentorship is an influential factor with regard to students' choice of specialty training and 21 studies in which mentees reported a marked effect of mentoring on research guidance, productivity, and success. Since many of these findings are based on cross-sectional self-report surveys without control groups, one might question whether the results qualify as convincing evidence. More convincing are results reported by Steiner et al. (2004), who, after controlling for other predictors, conclude that sustained mentorship is an important determinant of career development in research. Some of the studies that have been published since Sambunjak's review used methods with control groups and consequently provide more trustworthy results. Buddeberg-Fischer and Herta (2006) report short-term and long-term success of mentoring in improving mentees' professional development and social skills and in enhancing their interest in pursuing a scientific career. Other studies, too, report strong relationships between career success and having one or more mentors, although there is no correlation with career satisfaction (Stamm and Buddeberg-Fischer 2011). Ramanan et al. (2006) demonstrate that internal medicine residents who have a mentor are nearly twice as likely as their colleagues without mentors to report excellent career preparation. Feldman et al. (2010) find an association between mentoring and high scores on work satisfaction and self-efficacy. Other reported beneficial effects for medical mentees include: learning to

appreciate different or conflicting ideas, learning to overcome setbacks and obstacles, and acquiring an open and flexible attitude towards learning (Lingam and Gupta 1998). Later in this chapter we will consider the significance of the mentor as a non-judgemental advisor in workplace-based learning with one-to-one mentoring encompassing all the dimensions of creating learning opportunities in a safe environment (Lee et al. 2006). A similar comprehensive approach to mentoring has been introduced in many residency programmes as well as in formative assessments of the performance of qualified doctors using tools such as 360-degree feedback. Mentoring has been shown to be both effective in supporting workplace-based learning and a significant predictor of improvement following 360-degree feedback (Overeem et al. 2009). It was introduced in workplace-based learning in the UK in 2003 as an instrument for the appraisal of GP performance, aimed at stimulating GPs to plan and implement practice improvements and to equip them with skills for lifelong learning. The participating GPs took part in formative appraisal interviews with trained mentors (appraisers) aimed at supporting GPs' self-reflection. According to the GPs, the appraisal process actually resulted in practice improvement, and a majority of them said it had enhanced their continuous professional development (Bruce et al. 2004). Participants in another study mentioned that being appraised by a respected peer (mentor) was vital to the appraisal process; they also emphasized the importance of independent appraisers (Finlay and McLaren 2009). In business settings, participation in a mentoring programme has been shown to enhance professional growth, with mentees being more likely to have a degree, and to report greater job satisfaction. Hansford et al. (2002) conclude that mentoring programmes enhance job satisfaction, motivation, and promotion (Ehrich et al. 2002).

These positive findings may be offset, however, by detrimental effects when mentoring programmes are of poor quality or poorly implemented. Ehrich and Hansford (1999) call this the 'dark side of mentoring' and Sambunjak et al. (2010) speak of 'dysfunctional mentoring'. Problems can be caused by 'bossy mentoring', competitiveness, taking advantage of the mentee, or structural problems—such as conflicts of interest and lack of continuity. To this list might be added situations where mentors hold preconceived ideas about the choices to be made by mentees, demand that mentees meet only certain outcomes, or where clinician-mentors of students also decide on students' admission to residency programmes (Sambunjak et al. 2010).

Benefits to the mentor

It goes without saying that mentors are not primarily motivated by personal interests. It is equally indisputable, however, that mentors can reap benefits from undertaking this selfless task. These benefits are shown in fig. 23.2.

In a questionnaire survey among a network of senior physicians acting as mentors, the participants reported that they profited from being part of that network (Connor et al. 2000). In a recent study among senior medical specialists acting as mentors in a 360-degree feedback programme, 64% of the participants said they had learned a great deal from mentoring colleagues—specifically interview skills and ways of presenting feedback (Overeem et al. 2010a). Similarly, in a pilot study of a peer appraisal system for GPs in the UK, mentors (appraisers) reported more gains than did the mentees (appraisees) and regarded mentoring as a rewarding and educational experience (Lewis et al. 2003). They valued sharing the experiences of other GPs (mentees) facing problems that were

Learning from mentees' experiences

Learning from sharing one's experiences with mentees

Improved interviewing skills

Satisfaction on witnessing mentees making progress

Figure 23.2 Benefits to the mentor.

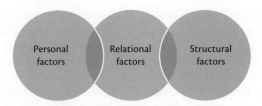

Figure 23.3 Barriers to mentoring.

similar to their own and gaining ideas about how to improve their own practice. Sackin et al. (1997) assume that mentoring reduces stress in GPs involved in peer mentoring as a result of the knowledge and skills they acquire in the process.

Mentors in an academic programme for promoting research careers mentioned the joy of empowering others and appreciated the opportunity to provide guidance and plant 'seeds' for the future (Ludwig and Stein 2008). Mentors can also experience personal satisfaction and increased professional recognition (Keyser et al. 2008), as well as a rekindled passion and enthusiasm for their specialty (Garmel 2004).

Benefits for the organization

For any organization in healthcare, whether this is a research department, hospital, or medical school, the satisfaction of its workforce is an invaluable asset. As mentoring can contribute to mentees' career satisfaction and make mentors feel valued, and as physicians' job satisfaction can lead to better care provision, it seems logical to conclude that mentoring can make an indirect contribution to the quality of healthcare. With regard to clinical governance, Young (1999) reports positive effects of a mentoring intervention to address the problems of doctors who have run into difficulties. Positive effects for hospitals, such as improved in-house relations, are reported from a peer-mentoring programme in the Netherlands (Overeem et al. 2010a). Mentors in this programme said that, because the mentor role made them look at situations objectively, their prejudices toward colleagues disappeared, and, because they were better informed about their colleagues' thoughts, solidarity, and mutual respect were increased. As mentors often have to provide feedback for formative assessment in workplace-based learning, however, potentially adverse effects of mentoring deserve serious consideration. Assessing the performance of colleagues and giving feedback to them may cause tensions, as was underlined in the study among mentors (appraisers) in the UK, who expressed enthusiasm for the programme but also pointed to the possibility of emotional difficulties and burden (Boylan et al. 2005). In a focus group study, mentors referred to tensions and discomfort caused by judging a colleague's work in the performance assessment procedure (Murie et al. 2009). One mentor said he felt like 'the messenger of bad news'.

Barriers to mentoring

The underuse of mentoring to support students, residents and practising physicians warrants a thorough investigation of the formal and informal barriers to participating in a mentoring programme, as mentor or as mentee (fig, 23.3). Sambunjak et al. (2010) distinguishes three main categories of barriers: personal factors, relational factors, and structural factors.

Personal factors relate to personality traits of mentors and mentees, such as mentees being unable or unwilling to engage in self-

reflection. In a case report on an eventually successful mentoring relationship between a 31-year-old internist and a 50-year-old professor, the mentor describes that the mentee initially 'struggled with the courage needed to face his inadequacies and to make effective changes', causing the mentee to cancel appointments with the mentor (Rabatin et al. 2004). This type of situation makes heavy demands on the skills of the mentor in stimulating reflection, asking probing questions, and monitoring progress. Unless the mentor has a strong commitment and excellent mentoring skills, mentoring in such cases is more likely than not bound for failure (Rabatin et al. 2004). Taherian and Shekarchian (2008) describe 'the tendency of mentors to adopt a patronising attitude towards the mentee' as an attribute of mentors that is associated with a strong risk of a dysfunctional mentor–mentee relationship, adding that mentors should be on the alert for this risk. An example is provided by UK students who remarked that mentoring was less useful when mentors have preconceived ideas about what choices students should make (Hauer et al. 2005). It is not the task of the mentor to advise mentees about the best course of action in a particular situation, but rather to help mentees reflect on their choices thereby enabling them to make their own decisions and arrive at their own solutions. Unfortunately, these are skills that physicians find particularly hard to master. In a qualitative study, doctors explained why this was such a challenge by pointing out that in their clinical work they are expected to intervene and offer concrete solutions, which runs counter to what a mentor is expected to do (Overeem et al. 2010a). A study by Memon and Menon (2010) conducted in surgical training reveals yet another barrier to mentoring, which seems to be particularly powerful in certain environments: the fact that seeking mentoring may be interpreted as a sign of weakness and of inability to cope with the challenges of training. In this type of environment showing weakness can be detrimental to a physician's career prospects.

The second category of barriers, relational factors, is concerned with aspects of the mentor–mentee relationship that may cause dysfunctional mentoring. There are two types of relationship barriers: an inadequate match of mentor and mentee and competition between mentor and mentee. The former barrier was identified in a qualitative study among faculty of an academic institution in the United States, where several mentees emphasized the importance of 'chemistry' in the mentoring relationship; mentoring is a relationship which '…can be as complex as the relationships we have with friends or family and be equally personal'. This complex relationship can be enhanced by shared interests and challenged by differences in race or gender (Jackson et al. 2003). The question whether differences in background should or should not be deliberately avoided in mentoring relationships has been the topic of numerous studies, but the results so far have remained inconclusive. Some studies emphasize the importance of concordance of background between mentors and mentees (Thomas 2001), but a recent study reports no effect of resident or faculty characteristics on satisfaction with mentoring (Ramanan et al. 2006). Similarly, a recent study among students of mathematics demonstrates that matching mentor and mentee on the basis of similarities in race and gender does not affect academic outcomes or satisfaction (Blake-Beard et al. 2011). However, other studies point out that, although mentors with different backgrounds can provide significant support, mentees from groups which due to gender and/or background are underrepresented in the environment of interest may find it important to have mentors matched on similar characteristics, and many studies report that such mentors can provide important psychosocial support and role modelling in how to succeed as a member of a minority group in work or academic environments (McAllister et al. 2009). Another relational cause of dysfunctional mentoring is associated with mentors accumulating a wealth of personal and work-related information about mentees during long-term mentoring relationships. This information may be shared with others, either deliberately or inadvertently, with consequences varying from a breach of confidence and disclosing confidential information to others (Garmel 2004) to mentors using their knowledge of mentees' ideas to compete with them for research grants (Taherian and Shekarchian 2008; Straus et al. 2009; Williams et al. 2004). A situation that involves a strong threat of relational problems arises when mentors are involved in assessing the performance of their mentees. This may force the mentor to disclose confidential information or put them in the position of a breaker of bad news (Overeem et al. 2010a).

Finally, structural factors that stand in the way of a satisfactory mentoring relationship include lack of time (Straus et al. 2009; Williams et al. 2004), lack of continuity, conflicts of interest (Hauer et al. 2005), and lack of (financial) support and recognition from management (Straus et al. 2009). In interviews with 21 mentees and seven mentors, Straus et al. (2009) identify lack of time as the single most important barrier to adequate mentoring. Medical students cited the organization of medical education, more specifically the disconnection between preclinical and clinical training, as an obstacle to a fruitful mentoring relationship (Hauer et al. 2005). In their first years as students they were not really paying much attention to their future careers, but once they started to do so, which typically happened in the clinical years, they were too busy to build a proper mentoring relationship. A second structural obstacle mentioned by the students is the short duration of courses and clerkship rotations, precluding the development of longitudinal relationships with faculty members (Hauer et al. 2005). And last but not least there is the problem of a shortage or even absence of mentors or the inability of mentees to find them. This is a multifactorial problem: faculty and staff are prevented from acting as mentors by time constraints and a lack of incentives; the organization does not have a dedicated mentoring programme; and students, residents, and physicians have no idea how or where they might find a mentor (Hauer et al. 2005; Straus et al. 2009; Williams et al. 2004). To clarify how organizations and institutions might advance the use of mentoring, we now describe some organizational mentoring models.

Mentoring models

At the beginning of this chapter, we expressed our misgivings at the contrast between the overwhelming evidence for the beneficial effects of mentoring with respect to career development, work satisfaction, learning, and performance and the scarcity of formal mentoring programmes, and learners' failure to take steps to establish mentorships. In our view, mentoring is too important to be left entirely to the initiative of learners (Driessen et al. 2011a) and we therefore strongly recommend that mentoring should be an integral component of medical education.

Despite many studies advocating mentoring, informal as well as formal mentoring programmes have remained rare. This gives cause for concern, for, unless mentoring is an integral component of an (educational) organization, it will reach only a small percentage of physicians, residents and students. Our concerns are supported by results of research emphasizing the need for organizational measures to deal with structural barriers to effective mentoring. One study underlines the impact of inequalities between mentees, showing that underrepresented minority residents are significantly less likely to establish a mentoring relationship than their peers (Ramanan et al. 2006). Another study reveals a remarkable gender effect, with female physicians being slower to make use of mentoring than their male colleagues (Stamm and Buddeberg-Fischer 2011). The authors speculate that this may be due to women being less assertive than men and consequently more hesitant to make a claim on the time of senior colleagues or to men being more career oriented, which induces them to seek support from a mentor. The latter explanation is supported by the finding that the mentors of the male physicians held positions higher in the organizational hierarchy than the mentors of the female physicians (Stamm and Buddeberg-Fischer 2011). To ensure that all students, residents and physicians are able to reap the benefits of proper mentoring, we recommend that formal mentoring programmes should be set up by organizations that are responsible for healthcare professionals' education and training.

We will discuss three models of formal mentoring programmes (Driessen et al. 2011a): the mentor-on-demand model, the mentor-is-appointed model, and the mentor network model (fig. 23.4).

In the first model, junior mentees (students, residents, and fellows) can select a mentor from a group of trained and respected senior staff members (researchers, consultants, or residents). For mentees, this model offers the advantage of being able to select a mentor with whom they expect to have a good rapport. However, this advantage has a downside in that it relies on mentees taking the initiative, which, as we explained earlier, will at best offer only a limited solution to the problem of the underutilization of mentoring.

With the mentor-is-appointed model, mentees are assigned a mentor without having any say in the choice of the mentor. Mentoring relationships may last for a certain period of time or even for the entire duration of a training programme, but mentees may also have different mentors in different periods depending on the objectives of mentoring in the different periods. The type of relationship-related problems we described earlier can be counteracted by offering an opt-out option to both mentors and mentees. This would go some way toward meeting the wishes of mentees, who in a recent study indicate a strong preference for selecting their own mentors over being assigned one, arguing that assigned

Mentor-on-demand model

Mentor-is-appointed model

Mentor network model

Figure 23.4 Models of mentoring programmes.

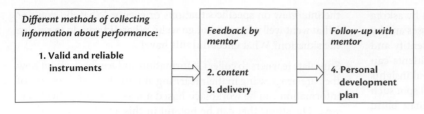

Figure 23.5 Elements and procedures of a formative assessment system.

mentors can lead to superficial or inadequate mentorship relations (Straus et al. 2009).

The mentor network model is in line with developmental network theory, which was first described by Higgins and Kram (2001) and posits that, due to organizational and societal changes, mentees nowadays should have more than one mentor, both from within and outside the organization. Mentees may have one of the clinical teachers in their department as a learning coach to help them reflect on their learning experiences and set learning goals, whereas for career advice they can turn to a mentor from a group of experienced doctors outside the department. For this type of model, some authors make a distinction between primary and secondary mentors. The primary mentor has an emotional bond with the mentee and provides a more profound experience. The strength of the primary mentor is that they spend a lot of time with the mentee and are able to empower mentees by providing acceptance and confirmation. As a role model, a primary mentor can show mentees alternative ways of responding to learning experiences (Freeman 1998). In contrast, the relationship with the secondary mentor is more businesslike and focused on career guidance. Secondary mentors may suggest projects, help mentees solve work-based problems, and coach them in certain skills (Lee 2007).

The literature presents several examples of ways in which a formal mentoring programme can be implemented (Buddeberg-Fischer and Herta 2006). In the next section we discuss in detail some examples of mentoring for continuous professional development.

Appraisal and formative assessment systems

Two examples of mentoring programmes aimed at enhancing professional development are the appraisal system introduced in the UK in 2001 for consultants and general practitioners employed by the National Health Service (NHS) and the performance assessment system with peer mentoring for consultants in the Netherlands (Conlon 2003; Overeem et al. 2010a). Physicians are invited to review their professional activities comprehensively, and to identify strengths and weaknesses in their performance. In this process three important steps can be distinguished (fig. 23.5). In the first step, physicians collect information about their performance from different sources on different occasions. Both in the UK and the Netherlands, multisource feedback (MSF) tools have been available since 2007 to collect information about various aspects of physician performance. Other sources of information are: medical audits, video consultations, or the results of patient satisfaction surveys. In the second step, the information gathered in step 1 is processed and communicated to the appraisee. The mentor plays a prominent role in this step. The effects of interactive delivery of feedback facilitated by a mentor have been established in quality improvement research (Winkens et al. 1995). In step 3, the follow up phase, the new insights gained from the previous steps are used to develop improvement goals and to follow up on them. The importance of follow-up is frequently highlighted in quality improvement research (Grol 2011). For feedback to achieve an optimal effect, it should ideally be integrated in a system of continuous monitoring, including systematic progress evaluation. Thus, follow-up is not limited to setting improvement goals and monitoring whether they are achieved, but covers the entire process following the provision of feedback. This can develop into an ongoing process of mentoring aimed at practice improvement.

Research findings show that the majority of physicians feel supported in their professional development by the mentoring and assessment systems and that, after the assessment, the majority intends to improve performance (Overeem et al. 2010b). The most significant benefit of the appraisals in the UK as perceived by the physicians who were appraised was the opportunity to reflect on their professional performance with a supportive colleague (Boylan et al. 2005). The Dutch appraisal programme comprises confidential conversations with a mentor about issues related to collaboration, communication, and management. Participating physicians reported that discussing feedback with a mentor helped them to accept the feedback and use it to make changes in their professional performance (Overeem et al. 2009). A study by psychology researchers confirms that interviews in which reflection is stimulated can enhance self-efficacy (Kluger and Van Dijk 2010). Studies in business settings report that managers who received MSF and were supported by a mentor showed significantly more improvement than managers receiving MSF without the support of a mentor (Smither et al. 2003).

The role of mentors in performance assessment and appraisals is as difficult as it is important. Mentors have to ensure that feedback recipients integrate the feedback into their self-concepts, as this is a crucial prerequisite for practice improvement and change. Since mentors are often inexperienced with regard to the required skills (Lewis et al. 2003; McKinstry et al. 2005), focused training of mentors is important.

We will now discuss how mentors can support mentees in learning from experience.

The role of the mentor with regard to learning from experience

How much someone learns from experience depends on how self analytical and critical they are (Driessen et al. 2008). According to Eva and Regehr (2008), reflection involves 'a conscious and deliberate reinvestment of mental energy aimed at exploring and elaborating one's understanding of the problem one has faced (or is facing) rather than aimed at simply trying to solve it'. Research provides clear evidence that learners tend to have difficulty reflecting on their experiences (Driessen et al. 2003). All too often it is shown that the support of a mentor is essential for learning from reflection. It is the mentor who can give the right push by asking the right questions to focus the learner's thinking processes and by giving feedback on performance to help the learner identify and develop learning goals (Driessen 2011b). Critical incidents can provide rich food for reflection, as they reveal also useful insights regarding existing concerns. An experienced mentor will spot such opportunities to open doors, reveal trends, and illuminate blind spots (Egan 2002). The effectiveness of mentoring aimed at steering learners' reflective processes depends on the mentor's communication skills, which are typically applied during progress interviews. We will now discuss the mentoring skills that are required for those interviews in more detail.

The mentoring strategies that we present here are based on the Guideline for Progress Interviews in postgraduate medical education developed by the Netherlands Association for Medical Education (Driessen et al. 2011c). According to the guideline, the main objectives of progress interviews are to coach learners and discuss how they are progressing in their professional development. The task of the mentor is thus primarily coaching, and the task of the mentor is to ask questions rather than give answers. Mentoring of professional development is especially effective when the mentor helps the learner to self-reflect on their performance and use the outcomes to develop new learning objectives. Learners should actively seek information and feedback about their performance to be able to self-direct their learning—so the mentor should stimulate learners to seek feedback and use the feedback to drive their learning. There are several strategies that mentors can use. Which strategies are used depends on the extent of the learner's experience. Mentor meetings with novice learners will be more structured and focus on concrete and practical learning objectives and topics. Meetings with more advanced learners will probably be of a more collegial nature and more holistic, with learner and mentor reflecting on standards of professional practice and the learner's performance and progress in relation to these.

A review of the literature on the quality of physicians' and residents' self-assessment reveals that this type of assessment is particularly vulnerable to bias (Davis et al. 2006). For this reason, Eva and Regehr (2008) stress the importance of confirmation of self-assessment by external assessment. It is important for mentors to stimulate learners to deliberately seek feedback and information from other sources that can guide them in directing their learning process. This can help learners to make a realistic assessment of their own performance and effectively direct their efforts to improve their performance. The following strategies can be used to stimulate learners to ask for feedback and improve self-reflection (Driessen 2011b):

- Create a safe learning environment. Learners who acknowledge their weaknesses should not be criticized but reassured that they are still learners and consequently not expected to show perfect performance.

- Open the mentor meeting by inquiring about the learner's general wellbeing to put learners at ease and make them feel the mentor is interested in how they are doing. Such questions have additional relevance, as general wellbeing can have a strong impact on learners' work and performance.

- Stimulate learners to present concrete observations. Most people tend to speak in general terms when they describe their own or other people's performance. The following questions can focus the interview on specific situations or events: What did you do? What went well what did not go well? What did you do to resolve the situation? What effect did this have?

- Stimulate learners to collect information and feedback about how they are progressing in their learning and work. Useful sources of information can be workplace-based assessments or patient surveys. Questions that can be helpful in this are: Which available information supports this? Which available information contradicts this?

- Stimulate learners to broaden their perspective. Relevant questions are: What did you want to achieve? What do you think the patient, colleague or nurse wanted? What did you think? What do you think the others were thinking? What did you do? What did the others do? Which emotions did you feel? Which emotions did the others feel?

Another important strategy is aimed at encouraging learners to reflect. By reflecting on their learning and performance learners can gain a new and improved understanding of situations and events. To achieve this mentor and learner can scrutinize the available feedback to detect patterns, and identify causes and consequences. The focus can be on the strategies the learner has used to achieve an objective and whether or not these strategies were appropriate and effective. The learner might also consider whether the objective was appropriate for the situation at hand. Learners can also be stimulated to reflect on moral and ethical aspects of their experiences and learning objectives.

As we observed earlier, it is the task of the mentor to stimulate learners to reflect on experiences in order to learn from them. To perform this task well it is not necessary for the mentor to have all the right answers. The main thing is to ask the right questions. Questions to stimulate reflection can relate to (Driessen 2011b):

- *Method or strategy*: Which methods or strategies did you use to achieve your objective? Why did you use these particular methods or strategies? Which methods or strategies were effective and which were not effective? Do you think that this method or strategy would work differently in another situation?

- *Objectives*: What were you trying to achieve? Were you successful? What do you consider successful? Why is this objective important?

- *Ethical reflection*: Do you think that others (patients, colleagues, nurses) were satisfied with the results? What are their primary concerns?

- *Confrontation with discrepancies*: It says in your portfolio that you are pleased with your development but when you are talking your face tells a different story. You assess your competence in this area higher or lower than your colleagues. Do you have an idea why this should be so? Your objectives are not consistent with the areas for improvement indicated in your portfolio. You did not work on the objectives you said you were going to pursue in the last interview.

- *Making connections*: Which similarities and dissimilarities do you notice between this particular situation and other situations? Does this situation occur more often? When does this happen? Do you see a pattern? Do you understand why this particular feedback is given and do you see similarities with your own analysis of the situation?

Analysing previous actions can initiate a search for alternative strategies or result in abandonment of the original objectives. New objectives and alternative strategies should be defined clearly and in detail. A recent study shows that setting objectives can stimulate learning and also that the mentor has an important contribution to make in this respect (Overeem et al. 2009). Learners who work with a mentor formulate more specific objectives and make better progress than learners who are not mentored (Smither et al. 2003). The objectives to be attained and the changes required to achieve them are often documented in a personal development plan (PDP) to ensure that they will be discussed in subsequent mentor meetings. Obviously, objectives will be pursued more effectively when both mentor and learner commit to them. PDPs tend to be rather vague, and mentors should ensure that learners formulate objectives as concretely as possible and describe a detailed strategy to pursue them. This can be done using the SMART approach: objectives should be Specific, Measurable, Achievable, Realistic and Time-scaled in order to enhance the chance of success.

So far we have looked at mentoring from the perspective of the mentor: which communication skills are important and which mentoring strategies should be used. We now move on to the perspective of the mentee: what can mentees do to promote successful mentoring and to receive optimal support for their development?

The mentee

A prerequisite for successful mentoring is mentees taking ownership of and directing the mentoring relationship, informing the mentor about their needs, and communicating the way they prefer (Zerzan et al. 2009). Mentees should be aware that mentoring relationships are not static and that each phase of the relationship requires a different approach. Ragins and Kram (2007) define four different phases: initiation, cultivation, separation, and redefinition. In the initiation phase mentor and mentee get to know each other and discuss what they expect from the mentoring process. When mentor and mentee have become acquainted, a proper start can be made with the actual mentoring process. At that point, the initiation phase becomes the cultivation phase, which turns into the separation phase when the needs of the participants change due to personal or organizational aspects.

Changes in individual needs usually relate to the growing independence of the mentee which moves the relationship in the

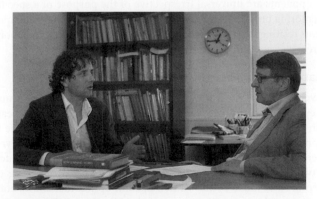

Figure 23.6 Mentoring in action.

direction of a peer relationship. Organizational change occurs when the mentee completes (a phase of) their training or when the mentor or the mentee moves to a different department or when there are changes in the organization. Many mentoring relationships end after the separation phase, but when the relationship has a strong psychosocial component it may continue into the redefinition phase, where the mentoring function fades and mentor and mentee become friends and/or colleagues, although this does not preclude occasional coaching or counselling.

We will discuss for each phase how mentees can contribute to a satisfactory mentoring relationship.

The initiation phase

Mentees should have a clear idea of their own goals and their expectations of the mentor. Also mentees should be open and honest about what they expect of mentoring and about their career plans (Detsky and Baerlocher 2007). Mentees may be inclined to say what they think the mentor wants to hear, but obviously this will not be conducive to a fruitful relationship. So when the mentee is not interested in a career in research, they should not pretend to be, just because the mentor is a renowned scientist. Before starting to look for a mentor or before the first encounter with an assigned mentor, mentees should carefully consider what their interests and ambitions are. Apart from their goals, mentees can think about which mentoring style would be most congenial to them. They might approach this question by recalling earlier mentoring experiences and considering which aspects determined whether the relationship with the mentor was fruitful. During the first interview with the mentor, the mentee should discuss their expectations concerning the nature of mentoring, the intensity, the responsibilities, and what and how the mentor and the mentee are expected to contribute to the relationship.

In some cases, mentors will be assigned by the educational institute or the employer, but in other cases mentees will have to find their own mentor. In selecting a mentor, mentees should give careful consideration to what is referred to in the literature as the mentor's willingness to mentor others and the mentor's experience of mentoring (Allen 2007). This means they should look at the prior experiences of potential mentors: how many mentees has the mentor guided? Were the mentees successful in their field? Additionally, they should consider characteristics like the mentor's gender, age, and position in the organization.

The cultivation phase

In the cultivation phase the mentoring relationship has become established. In this phase research shows that mentees who have a strong desire to learn and who seek advice and guidance from their mentor will have a more positive relationship (Turban 2007). This implies that mentees with a learning-directed orientation will benefit more from mentoring, because they tend to regard their mistakes, insecurities and problems as integral to the learning process and consequently share them easily with their mentor. Performance-oriented students, on the other hand, will be less likely to interpret mistakes as learning experiences and are therefore hesitant to bring them to the attention of the mentor. A safe and supportive learning climate in the cultivation phase can possibly stimulate movement to a learning orientation. Mentees can contribute to this by preparing carefully for meetings with the mentor by collecting information about their performance and learning, by giving serious thought to that information, and by self-reflection on their work and learning, which they should ideally put down in writing. Reflections of mentees about their performance, any problems they have experienced, and questions about their performance are a good starting point for conversations with the mentor. It is again important for mentees to reflect on issues and events that are important to them instead of focusing on what they assume the mentor considers important. It can be helpful if mentees prepare an agenda and send this to the mentor before the meeting. One of the threats to good mentoring is that mentor–mentee encounters are skipped because it is difficult to make time for them in busy schedules. Advance planning and a meeting schedule can prevent this. Mentees may take the initiative and monitor adherence to the schedule. Should the mentee discover, in the cultivation phase, that there is no chemistry with their mentor, the mentee may consider ending the relationship and may wish to look for another mentor (preferably one who uses a different mentoring style).

The separation phase

Generally, the mentoring relationship will find its natural endpoint when the course, training programme, or activity of which mentoring is a component, finishes or when the mentor or the mentee accepts another job. The relationship may also end, however, because the mentee is able to perform independently without guidance and moves on to the next stage of their career. At this point the mentoring relationship enters the redefinition phase and changes into a relationship on a more even footing. In this phase mentees should be confident about their ability to work as an independent professional. It is advisable for mentees not to just let the relationship peter out, but to talk with their mentor about the closure of the relationship.

At several places in this chapter, we have reiterated our concerns about the scarcity of mentoring programmes that are implemented effectively. Given the importance of such mentoring programmes, we will discuss this issue in considerable detail with reference to the relevant literature.

How to implement a mentoring programme

A recurring observation in articles on quality improvement in healthcare is that achieving change is fraught with difficulties. According to the literature, the majority of interventions are targeted at individual healthcare professionals, but the success of interventions may rely on other factors besides those relating to individuals (Grol et al. 2007). The successful implementation of mentoring programmes in medical schools, hospitals, or research institutes hinges on a number of conditions that have to be met. We will clarify each of these conditions.

Identification of barriers

The literature on interventions aimed at improving the quality of healthcare shows that potential barriers should be taken into account during the planning stage of interventions (Bosch et al. 2007). This applies equally to educational interventions and to interventions aimed at improving the performance and wellbeing of healthcare professionals, such as mentoring. Thus, ideally, before developing a new mentoring programme, programme designers should identify potential barriers and determine ways of dealing with them. Earlier, we described different barriers, such as ignorance of the benefits of mentoring, lack of time, lack of (financial)

incentives, and organizational problems. Barriers can be identified through focus groups or individual interviews with stakeholders (future mentors and mentees). Programme developers should take measures to prevent, counteract, or ameliorate the expected effects. All barriers that are identified deserve serious consideration. For example, when stakeholders do not see the value of mentoring, programme designers might first convince stakeholders of the benefits of mentoring by giving them relevant mentoring literature (Mahayosnand 2000).

Unrealistic expectations

According to Garmel et al. (2004), mentoring is inherently susceptible to the pitfall of unrealistic expectations on the part of both mentors and mentees. This pitfall can be circumvented by inviting members of different groups of stakeholders to sit on a committee charged with defining the objectives of the mentoring programme and explaining these to mentors and mentees (Keyser et al. 2008; Coates 2004). Such a committee could also develop a role description of the mentor with detailed descriptions of the mentor's tasks and job requirements.

Selection and training of mentors

As we noted earlier, mentoring is challenging but also enjoyable and rewarding. Mentors should have various communication skills—e.g. active listening, confronting, and encouraging reflection. These skills partly overlap with the interview techniques that physicians use during patient encounters. There is one crucial difference, however; physicians are expected to diagnose the patient's problem and determine what should be done about it, whereas mentoring conversations require a less directive, coaching approach. Not everybody is equally comfortable with or suited to this role, and it is advisable to select mentors that have excellent communication skills and are motivated to work with mentees. Keyser et al. (2008) propose the following two selection criteria for research mentoring: experience and contacts in the mentee's research interest. Although research mentoring obviously requires research experience, experience in the area of interest of the mentee is not necessarily required for all types of mentoring. Medical students for example can be mentored by behavioral and non-clinical scientists (Driessen et al. 2003).

Mentors should receive dedicated training in communication skills. Johnson et al. (2010) describe the following essential components of mentor training: defining the mentor team concept, the related roles and expectations, the rewards and challenges of mentoring, effective communication with mentees, work–life balance, and understanding the effects of diversity among mentees. These components are universal irrespective of the purpose of a specific mentoring programme. Additionally, training might cover components relating to specific mentoring goals, such as research support, career success, and performance improvement.

Matching mentors and mentees

Several authors have proposed a formal matching programme (Keyser et al. 2008; Overeem et al. 2010a), and the literature repeatedly contends that a good match between mentor and mentee is a prerequisite for a good mentor–mentee relationship. However, there are no hard and fast rules that guarantee a perfect match between mentor and mentee. We propose formal matching of mentors and mentees but with an opt-out option that allows both mentors and mentees to request another matching. With regard to matching, both mentors and mentees should be aware of diversity issues as 'many cross-race mentoring relationships' suffer from 'protective hesitation': both parties refrain from raising 'touchy issues' (Thomas 2001).

Peer feedback for mentors

Mentors may face many different challenges (e.g. having to identify with mentees from a variety of different backgrounds). Not all mentors will be aware of problems or realize that they can do better. Peer feedback sessions with other mentors can encourage mentors to reflect on their performance and share experiences with colleagues (which may help them to improve their performance).

Appoint a confidential advisor with whom mentors and mentees can discuss problems

Both mentors and mentees may encounter problematic situations (e.g. breaches of confidentiality on behalf of mentor or mentee). Mentors and mentees should have someone to turn to for help or advice about how to handle these situations. A confidential advisor can also compile a list of frequent problems that need addressing at the institutional level in the near future.

Incentives for mentors

A major obstacle to successful implementation of mentoring, which we mentioned earlier, is the lack of incentives in the form of time and money, and also academic recognition. To motivate people to become and remain a mentor, various incentives can be used: these include institutional recognition, career advancement, awards and protected time (Keyser et al. 2008; Straus et al. 2009; Sambunjak et al. 2010).

Evaluate the implementation process: look inside the black box of the intervention

Many quality improvement studies show that a crucial factor in designing successful interventions is to look inside the black box of the intervention, in other words process evaluation (Hulscher et al. 2003). Process evaluation is an important tool to gain insight into the intervention, the actual exposure to the intervention, and the experiences of those exposed to the intervention (participants). It is vital that mentoring programmes be subject to process evaluation.

Conclusions

- Mentoring can be beneficial for several important aspects of the professional development of physicians and trainees.

- Mentoring has remained underused, especially amongst professionals from underrepresented minorities and amongst females.

- The development and implementation of formal mentoring programmes could help to stimulate a wider use of mentoring in the medical profession.

- A mentor asks questions rather than gives answers.

- A prerequisite for successful mentoring is mentees taking ownership of and directing the mentoring relationship.

References

Allen, T.D. (2007) Mentoring relationships from the perspective of the mentor. In: B.R. Ragins, and K.E. Kram (eds) *The Handbook of Mentoring at Work: Theory, Research and Practice* (pp. 123–147). Los Angeles: Sage Publications

Berk, R.A., Berg, J., Mortimer, R., Walton-Moss, B., and Yeo, T.P. (2005) Measuring the effectiveness of faculty mentoring relationships. *Acad Med.* 80: 66–71

Blake-Beard, S., Bayne, M.L., Crosby, F.J., and Muller, C.B. (2011) Matching by race and gender in mentoring relationships: keeping our eyes on the prize. *J Soc Issues.* 67: 622–643

Bosch, M., Van Der Weijden, T., Wensing, M., and Grol, R. (2007) Tailoring quality improvement interventions to identified barriers: a multiple case analysis. *J Evaluation Clin Pract.* 13: 161–168

Boylan, O., Bradley, T., and McKnight, A. (2005) GP perceptions of appraisal: professional development, performance management, or both? *Br J Gen Pract.* 55: 544–545

Bruce, D., Phillips, K., Reid, R., Snadden, D., and Harden, R. (2004) Revalidation for general practitioners: randomised comparison of two revalidation models. *BMJ.* 328: 687–691

Buddeberg-Fischer, B. and Herta, K.D. (2006) Formal mentoring programmes for medical students and doctors—a review of the Medline literature. *Med Teach.* 28: 248–257

Coates, W.C. (2004) An educator's guide to teaching emergency medicine to medical students. *Acad Emerg Med.* 11: 300–306

Conlon, M. (2003) Appraisal: the catalyst of personal development. *BMJ.* 327: 389–391

Connor, M.P., Bynoe, A.G., Redfern, N., Pokora, J., and Clarke, J. (2000) Developing senior doctors as mentors: a form of continuing professional development. Report of an initiative to develop a network of senior doctors as mentors: 1994–99. *Med Educ.* 34: 747–753

Davis, D.A., Mazmanian, P.E., Fordis, M., Van Harrison, R., Thorpe, K.E., and Perrier, L. (2006) Accuracy of physician self-assessment compared with observed measures of competence: a systematic review. *JAMA.* 296: 1094–1102

Detsky, A.S. and Baerlocher, M.O. (2007) Academic mentoring—how to give it and how to get it. *JAMA.* 297: 2134–2136

Driessen, E., van Tartwijk, J., Vermunt, J., and van der Vleuten, C. (2003) Use of portfolios in early undergraduate medical training. *i.* 25: 18–23

Driessen, E., van Tartwijk, J., and Dornan, T. (2008) The self critical doctor: helping students become more reflective. *BMJ.* 336: 827–830

Driessen, E.W., Overeem, K., and van der Vleuten, C.P.M. (2011a) Get yourself a mentor. *Med Educ.* 45: 438–439

Driessen, E., Overeem, K., and van Tartwijk, J. (2011b) Learning from practice: mentoring, feedback and portfolios. In T. Dornan, K. Mann, A. Scherpbier, and J. Spencer (eds) *Medical Education Theory in Practice* (pp. 211–227). Edinburgh: Elsevier

Driessen, E., Kenter, G., de Leede, B., et al. (2011c) Richtlijn voortgangsgesprek in de medische vervolgopleiding (the Guideline for Progress Interviews in postgraduate medical education). *Tijdschrift voor Medisch Onderwijs.* 30(6 Suppl 3): 51–62

Egan, G. (2002) *The Skilled Helper.* Pacific Grove, CA: Thomson

Ehrich, L.C. and Hansford, B. (1999) Mentoring: pros and cons for HRM. *Asia Pacific J Hum Resources.* 37: 92–107

Ehrich, L., Tennent, L., and Hansford, B. (2002) A review of mentoring in education: some lessons for nursing. *Contemp Nurse.* 12: 253–264

Eva, K.W. and Regehr, G. (2008) 'I'll never play professional football' and other fallacies of self assessment. *J Contin Educ Health Prof.* 28: 14–19

Feldman, M.D., Arean, P.A., Marshall, S.J., Lovett, M., and O'Sullivan, P. (2010) Does mentoring matter: results from a survey of faculty mentees at a large health sciences university. *Med Educ Online.* 15: doi: 10.3402/meo.v15i0.5063

Finlay, K. and McLaren, S. (2009) Does appraisal enhance learning, improve practice and encourage continuing professional development? A survey of general practitioners' experiences of appraisal. *Qual Prim Care.* 17: 387–395

Freeman, R. (1998) *Mentoring in General Practice*. Oxford: Butterworth-Heinemann

Garmel, G.M. (2004) Mentoring medical students in academic emergency medicine. *Acad Emerg Med*. 11: 1351–1357

Grol, R.P.T.M., Bosch, M.C., Hulscher, M.E.J.L., Eccles, M.P., and Wensing, M. (2007) Planning and studying improvement in patient care: the use of theoretical perspectives. *Milbank Q*. 85: 93–138

Grol, R. and Wensing, M. (2011) *Implementatie: Effectieve verbetering van de patiëntenzorg*. Amsterdam: Reed Business

Hansford, B., Tennent, L., and Ehrich, L.C. (2002) Business mentoring: help or hindrance? *Mentoring & Tutoring: Partnership in Learning*. 10: 101–115

Hauer, K.E., Teherani, A., Dechet, A., and Aagaard, E.M. (2005) Medical students' perceptions of mentoring: a focus-group analysis. *Med Teach*. 27: 732–734

Higgins, M.C. and Kram, K.E. (2001) Reconceptualizing mentoring at work: a developmental network perspective. *Acad Manage Rev*. 26: 264–288

Hulscher, M.E.J.L., Laurant, M.G.H., and Grol, R.P.T.M. (2003) Process evaluation on quality improvement interventions. *Qual Saf Health Care*. 12: 40–46

Jackson, V.A., Palepu, A., Szalacha, L., Caswell, C., Carr, P.L., and Inui, T. (2003) 'Having the right chemistry': a qualitative study of mentoring in academic medicine. *Acad Med*. 78: 328–334

Johnson, M.O., Subak, L.L., Brown, J.S., Lee, K.A., and Feldman, M.D. (2010) An Innovative program to train health sciences researchers to be effective clinical and translational research mentors. *Acad Med*. 85: 484–489

Keyser, D.J., Lakoski, J.M., Lara-Cinisomo, S., et al. (2008) Advancing institutional efforts to support research mentorship: a conceptual framework and self-assessment tool. *Acad Med*. 83: 217–225

Kluger, A.N. and Van Dijk, D. (2010) Feedback, the various tasks of the doctor, and the feedforward alternative. *Med Educ*. 44: 1166–1174

Launer, J. (2006) Supervision, *Mentoring and Coaching: one-to-one learning encounters in medical education*. Edinburgh: ASME Understanding Medical Education

Lee, A. (2007) Special section: how can a mentor support experiential learning? *Clin Child Psychol Psychiatry*. 12: 333–340

Lee, J.M., Anzai, Y., and Langlotz, C.P. (2006) Mentoring the mentors: Aligning mentor and mentee expectations. *Acad Radiol*. 13: 556–561

Lewis, M., Elwyn, G., and Wood, F. (2003) Appraisal of family doctors: an evaluation study. *Br J Gen Pract*. 53: 454–460

Lingam, S. and Gupta, R. (1998) Mentoring for overseas doctors. *BMJ*. 317: S2-7151

Ludwig, S. and Stein, R.E.K. (2008) Anatomy of mentoring. *J Pediatr*. 152: 151–152

Mahayosnand, P.P. (2000) Public health E-mentoring: an investment for the next millennium. *Am J Public Health*. 90: 1317–1318

McAllister, C., Harold, R., Ahmedani, B., and Cramer, E. (2009) Targeted mentoring: evalution of a program. *J Soc Work Educ*. 45: 89–104

McKinstry, B., Peacock, H., and Shaw, J. (2005) GP experiences of partner and external peer appraisal: a qualitative study. *Br J Gen Pract*. 55: 539–543

Memon, B. and Memon, M.A. (2010) Mentoring and surgical training: a time for reflection! *Adv Health Sci Educ Theory Pract*. 15: 749–754

Murie, J., McCrae, J., and Bowie, P. (2009) The peer review pilot project: a potential system to support GP appraisal in NHS Scotland? *Educ Prim Care*. 20: 34–40

Overeem, K., Driessen, E.W., Arah, O.A., Lombarts, K.M., Wollersheim, H.C., and Grol, R.P. (2010a) Peer mentoring in doctor performance assessment: strategies, obstacles and benefits. *Med Educ*. 44: 140–147

Overeem, K., Wollersheim, H., Driessen, E., et al. (2009) Doctors' perceptions of why 360-degree feedback does (not) work: a qualitative study. *Med Educ*. 43: 874–882

Overeem, K., Lombarts, M.J., Arah, O.A., Klazinga, N.S., Grol, R.P., and Wollersheim, H.C. (2010b) Three methods of multi-source feedback compared: a plea for narrative comments and coworkers' perspectives. *Med Teach*. 32: 141–147

Rabatin, J.S., Lipkin, M., Rubin, A.S., Schachter, A., Nathan, M., and Kalet, A. (2004) A Year of mentoring in academic medicine. *J Gen Intern Med*. 19: 569–573

Ragins, B.R., and Kram, K.E. (2007) The roots and meaning of mentoring. In B.R. Ragins and K.E. Kram (eds) *The Handbook of Mentoring at Work: Theory, Research and Practice* (pp. 3–15). Los Angeles: Sage Publications

Ramanan, R.A., Taylor, W.C., Davis, R.B., and Phillips, R.S. (2006) Mentoring matters. Mentoring and career preparation in internal medicine residency training. *J Gen Intern Med*. 21: 340–345

Sackin, P., Barnett, M., Eastaugh, A., and Paxton, P. (1997) Peer-supported learning. *Br J Gen Pract*. 47: 67–68

Sambunjak, D., Straus, S.E., and Marusic, A. (2006) Mentoring in academic medicine: a systematic review. *JAMA*. 296: 1103–1115

Sambunjak, D., Straus, S., and Marusic, A. (2010) A systematic review of qualitative research on the meaning and characteristics of mentoring in academic medicine. *J Gen Intern Med*. 25: 72–78

Shanafelt, T. and Habermann, T. (2002) Medical residents' emotional well-being. *JAMA*. 288: 1846–1847; author reply 7

Smither, J.W., London, M., Flautt, R., Vargas, Y., and Kucine, I.V.Y. (2003) Can working with an executive coach improve multisource feedback ratings over time? A quasi-experimental field study. *Personnel Psychol*. 56: 23–44

Stamm, M. and Buddeberg-Fischer, B. (2011) The impact of mentoring during postgraduate training on doctors' career success. *Med Educ*. 45: 488–496

Steiner, J.F., Curtis, P., Lanphear, B.P., Vu, K.O., and Main, D.S. (2004) Assessing the role of influential mentors in the research development of primary care fellows. *Acad Med*. 79: 865–872

Straus, S.E., Chatur, F., and Taylor, M. (2009) Issues in the mentor-mentee relationship in academic medicine: a qualitative study. *Acad Med*. 84: 135–139

Taherian, K. and Shekarchian, M. (2008) Mentoring for doctors. Do its benefits outweigh its disadvantages? *Med Teach*. 30: e95–e99

Thomas, D.A. (2001) The truth about mentoring minorities. Race matters. *Harv Bus Rev*. 79: 98–107, 68

Turban, D.B. and Lee, F.K. (2007) The role of personality in mentoring relationships. In B.R. Ragins and K.E. Kram, (eds) *The Handbook of Mentoring at Work: Theory, Research and Practice* (pp. 21–50). Los Angeles: Sage Publications

Williams, L.L., Levine, J.B., Malhotra, S., and Holtzheimer, P. (2004) The good-enough mentoring relationship. *Acad Psychiatry*. 28: 111–115

Winkens, R.A.G., Pop, P., Bugter-Maessen, A.M.A., et al. (1995) Randomised controlled trial of routine individual feedback to improve rationality and reduce numbers of test requests. *Lancet*. 345: 498–502

Young, G. (1999) General practitioners' experiences of patients' complaints. Mentoring should be more widespread. *BMJ*. 319: 852–853

Zerzan, J.T., Hess, R., Schur, E., Phillips, R.S., and Rigotti, N. (2009) Making the most of mentors: a guide for mentees. *Acad Med*. 84: 140–144

CHAPTER 24

Professionalism

John Goldie, Al Dowie, Phil Cotton, and Jill Morrison

Example is contagious, and descends from teacher to pupil.

William Gull

Reproduced from *British Medical Journal*, William W. Gull, 'Introductory Address on the Study of Medicine', 2, p. 425, copyright 1874, with permission from BMJ Publishing Group Ltd.

Professionalism in medicine

Professionalism in Western medicine dates back to Hippocrates. It has traditionally encompassed a profession's public commitment to a set of values (Cruess et al. 2000), the word profession being derived from the Latin *profeteri*, to avow or confess. It was first used in a book of prescriptions written by Scribonius, a physician or pharmacist in the court of the Roman emperor Claudius, who linked humanism to virtues such as compassion and competence (Pellegrino and Pellegrino 1988). It is not an exclusive Western phenomenon and has played an important role in Hindu and Oriental medicine for a similar length of time (Sethuraman 2006; Nishigori 2007). Its meaning and definition are historically and culturally based (Hodges et al. 2011).

The archetypal Western professions, medicine, law and the clergy, were the offspring of the universities and medieval European craft guilds. By the middle of the 19th century the medical profession in most developed countries had come together to form national associations adopting codes of ethics to govern the behaviour of their members. They successfully lobbied governments to establish medical licensure, which granted a monopoly over practice to allopathic medicine (Krause 1996). The medical profession was delegated a 'market shelter' in the labour market, which enabled it to exclude potential competitors from outside the profession, thus creating sufficient economic security for members to make a long-term commitment to the profession as a career. It also allowed the profession to control its own work. Such protection, in theory, allowed members to concentrate on the integrity of their work and use it for the benefit of their patients and wider society (Friedson 1994).

Medicine has been a model for the conceptualization of professionalism as both an ethic and a process (Freidson 1970a). To help distinguish professions from other occupations early sociologists concentrated on their primary characteristics or traits (Jones 2003) (fig. 24.1). Most sociologists now view them as similar social forms with the differences being of degree not kind (Evetts 2006).

From the characteristics shown in fig. 24.1 three pillars of medical professionalism emerged in medical discourses (Irvine 1997; Arnold and Stern 2006): expertise, ethics, and service.

The profession's autonomy was granted by society on the basis that professionals will place individual and societal welfare before their own. This relationship is fiduciary rather than altruistic, as altruism's notion of self-denying service takes the ordinary virtue of assisting another person professionally to an extreme (Freidson 1994; O'Neill 2002). The autonomy of the medical profession is regulated by codes of ethics on one hand (Cruess and Cruess 1997), and laws and statutory frameworks outlining licensing, regulation, and guidelines on the other (Wynia et al. 1999; Pellegrino and Relman 1999). In Western medicine, like Western society, there has been a shift in the uses and forms of power from juridical, which uses the language of rights and obligations (e.g. codes of ethics), to forms of normalizing or regulatory power, which uses the language of normality (Foucault 1980). Regulatory power is dispersed throughout the social network rather than being concentrated in the hands of controlling bodies such as the General Medical Council (GMC). One way regulatory power works is by categorizing people in terms through which they come to understand themselves. Individuals become subjected to the rules and norms engendered by knowledge about what it means to be a professional. They adopt ways of being influenced by discourses from experts whose authority is based on rationality. These convey unofficial rules, implicit values, benefits, and attitudes, which are subsequently reproduced and reinforced in day-to-day interactions (de Montigny 1995). Individuals are encouraged to scrutinize themselves for signs of pathology through self-reflection shaped by institutional discourses (Foucault 1982; Hodges 2004; Hodgson 2005) such as the Royal College of Physicians' Medical Professionalism (2005).

The medical profession has thrived by existing in equilibrium with the forces of capitalism and the state (Krause 1996). The profession has maintained its 'market shelter' and sustained its status and privilege by adapting to changing political and economic environments. This requires maintaining sufficient cohesion of the

Discrete body of knowledge, under the control of its members, which is kept up to date

Monopoly over market for services

Autonomy over conditions of work and from state and capital

Is guided by codes of ethics

Altruism as a core motive, performance valued more than financial reward

Training, usually at tertiary education level, is lengthy and its content and standards are determined by the profession

Figure 24.1 Primary characteristics of a profession identified by early sociologists.

profession as a whole, protecting the profession's public face and deflecting efforts by employers and governments from exercising control over members' work. A number of factors contribute to this cohesion (Friedson 1994):

+ the members' distinct prestigious public identity, which provides the basis for solidarity and mutuality among members

+ the demanding entry standards and exacting training encourage long-term commitment to the profession as a career

+ the socialization experience of medical education

+ codes of ethics that promote solidarity between members.

There has been a disruption of the relationship between the medical profession and society in recent years in North America and Europe, although Gerstl and Jacobs (1976, p.1) suggest it could be part of a cycle of professionalization, deprofessionalization and reprofessionalization. Its autonomy has come under threat due to a loss of trust in the profession and its ability to self-regulate (Stevens 2000). This was due to a combination of factors that include the rise of consumerism and the emergence of the concept of profit in healthcare, which has compromised the fiduciary relationship (Cruess and Cruess 1997). Other societal and institutional factors influencing current reflection on professionalism and professional behaviour include (Irvine 1997; Castellani and Wear 2000):

+ the rapid expansion of medical knowledge and skills

+ the revolution in information technology

+ increased media attention, which has highlighted high-profile cases of negligence and malpractice, e.g. the Bristol paediatric heart surgery scandal

+ changes in philosophy of care, e.g. multidisciplinary teamwork, shared care

+ rapid changes in the management of care

+ changes in doctor's attitudes, e.g. work–life balance issues, enforced reduction of working hours

+ feminization of medicine.

As a result of these developments, professionalism has become one of the foremost issues for the medical profession. The profession's adaptive response has been to reaffirm its essential values and reestablish its commitment to the service nature of its work (Calman 1994; American Board of Internal Medicine 1995; Cruess and Cruess 1997; Irvine 1999; Accreditation Council for Graduate Medical Education 1999; Medical Professionalism Project 2000; CanMEDS 2000; Sox et al. 2002; GMC 1993, 2002, 2003; Hilton and Slotnick 2005; RCP London 2005; Project Team Consilium

Abeundi 2005). Critical scholars of professionalism and professionalization would argue that the profession's response is an attempt to assert its power and legitimize and maintain its monopoly in the healthcare market, in part by emphasizing the difference between medicine and other healthcare professions/occupations (Martimiankis et al. 2009). It may also reflect an attempt to retain its ability to define and control fundamental concepts such as what constitutes health, sickness, and treatment (Larson 1977). It is interesting to note that the drive to redefine professionalism has come from some of the most powerful, hierarchical, and male-dominated groups within the profession. It is an example of what Witz (1992, p. 61) described as 'professionalization projects of class-privileged male actors in a particular point in history and in particular societies'. Professionalism may represent a part of societal processes that construct and sustain social, gender and cultural inequalities (Martimiankis et al. 2009).

The profession has also imposed greater collegial authority—for example the publication in the UK of the GMC's standards of practice (GMC 2002) and the introduction of revalidation for all practising doctors (Jones 2003). Professionalism as a role played in society draws attention away from the traits and behaviours of individuals and towards the roles played by professionals in general. Unprofessional behaviour by an individual reflects on the profession as a whole. Socializing doctors to a lifetime commitment to high standards and obedience to a code of ethics and professional behaviour is seen as being in the interests of the public, the individual professional and the profession as a whole (Swick 2000).

What has been produced in these discourses is what Castellani and Hafferty (2006, p. 3) terms 'nostalgic professionalism', tradition-bound and hierarchically driven. We believe the term 'romantic professionalism' is more appropriate given its idealistic nature. Focusing on normative definitions of professionalism; trait-based, behaviour-based, or role-based, misses the influence of context, institutions and socioeconomic and political concerns in the creation of the definitions, and leads to an overemphasis on codes of behaviour (Martimiankis et al. 2009). Professionalism is a complex, multidimensional construct that varies across historical time periods and cultural contexts. It has elements at individual, interpersonal and societal–institutional levels, which interact. Freidson (1970b, 1986) showed that the culture and values of the institutions where doctors practice are more important determinants of their behaviour than their experiences at medical school.

An individual's behaviour arises not only from individual cognitive or personality dimensions, but in response to situational and contextual phenomena arising during learning and practice. The correlation between context and behaviour is stronger than between behaviour and underlying attitudes (Wallace et al. 2005; Rees and Knight 2007). They may look to institutionalized norms and conventions, which are influenced by the profession's wider economic and political concerns, to structure and give meaning to their behaviour. These are reproduced and reinforced in day-to-day interactions. By this process social structure is reproduced, culture transmitted and social control mechanisms applied (Giddens 1984). It is not necessarily a one-way process. The post-modern view is that coherence of an organization's culture derives from the partial and mutually dependent knowledge of each individual involved in the process and develops out of the work they do together. Meaning is created rather than transmitted and culture is constantly being recreated (Tierney 1997).

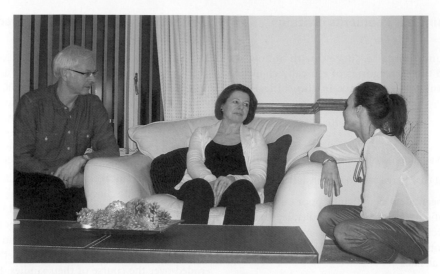

Figure 24.2 Professionalism in medical education.

Professionalism is not a stable construct that can be defined in isolation, taught and assessed. It is something that is socially constructed in interaction and sustained through institutional structures (Martimiankis et al. 2009). As such, it is a distributed attribute best understood in 'systemic considerations' rather than a reflection of individuals and their motives (Hafferty and Castellani 2009, p. 826). This position takes a wider view of professionalism than the lists of characteristics or behaviours favoured by the mainstream medical profession or the view of professionalism as the development of medical morality taken by moral philosophers such as Huddle (Huddle 2005). An acceptable, clearly articulated operational definition, which is regularly reviewed and refined, should be developed. It should be conceptualized at individual, institutional and interactional levels and developed through dialogue between the profession and the wider society (Cohen 2006). Initiatives like the International Ottawa Conference Working group on Professionalism (Hodges et al. 2011) point the profession in this direction. A complexity science approach, based on systems theory, which provides for analysis at multiple levels, could be useful (Hafferty and Levinson 2008). These theories encourage a non-reductionist, non-linear approach to studying complex phenomena and allow for multilevel analysis from the micro to the macro (Fogelberg and Frauwirth 2010).

Professionalism as an area for medical education

In tandem with the profession's re-evaluation of its ethical and professional responsibilities, professionalism has become an important issue for medical education (Swick et al. 1999; Ginsburg et al. 2000; Maudsley and Strivens 2000; Wear and Castellani 2000; Stevenson et al. 2001; Arnold 2002; Hilton and Slotnik 2005; Veloski et al. 2005; Stern 2006; Holtman 2008; Thistlethwaite and Spencer 2008; Cruess et al. 2009; Martimiankis et al. 2009; Hafferty and Castellani 2009; van Mook et al. 2009a; Wilkinson et al. 2009; Hodges et al. 2011), with medical education being viewed as the principal agent for remediation (Hafferty 2009) (fig. 24.2).

Medical education traditionally entrusted learning professionalism to the informal and hidden curricula. The informal curriculum has been conceptualized by Hafferty (1998, p. 404) as 'an

unscripted, predominantly ad hoc, and highly interpersonal form of teaching and learning that takes place among and between faculty and students'. The hidden curriculum is conceptualized as 'a set of influences that function at the level of organizational structure and culture'. What resulted was not always what was intended.

From an early stage, students interact with peers, teachers, scientists, laboratory staff, other doctors, nurses, other healthcare professionals, ancillary staff, and patients. These interactions occur in social institutions with established practices such as universities, hospitals, hospices, and community care organizations. Most of these interactions involve regular, routine, everyday aspects of professional practice. During these interactions students are exposed to role models who can have both positive and negative effects. Students may witness events and behaviours, particularly in the clinical years, which challenge their ethical and professional identities in both positive and negative ways. The literature on medical students' experiences is limited, focuses on dilemmas and relies mainly on the recollection of the frequency and severity rather than their nature (Ginsburg et al. 2002; Baldwin et al, 2006). van Mook et al (2009b) classified the most salient dilemmas encountered, and these are discussed next.

Mistreatment and abuse

This has been reported since the 1950s (Eron 1955). Baldwin et al. (1991; Baldwin and Daugherty 1997) reported a high prevalence of perceived unprofessional behaviour in US medical schools and residency programmes. Other authors reported similar findings in US and Finnish undergraduate and North American graduate medical education (Sheehan et al. 1990; Silver and Glicken 1990; Uhari et al. 1994; Cook et al. 1996). Monrouxe et al.'s (2011) UK wide survey found 16.2% of preclinical and 56.1% of clinical students had suffered verbal abuse; 16.2% of preclinical and 53.3% of clinical students reported experiencing sexual discrimination and harassment, with 14.9% preclinical and 39% of clinical students also reporting other forms of discrimination; 83.3% of clinical and 36.2% preclinical students had experienced indirect covert status abuse in the previous 12 months, for example feeling ignored or shunned by tutors, being excluded from learning opportunities or being humiliated in front of a patient by clinician; 70.9% of clinical and 22.4% preclinical students reported witnessing abuse of other students.

Unprofessional learning environments inviting conflicts

Hicks et al.'s (2001) questionnaire survey, with follow up focus groups, identified three categories of ethically challenging situations, which students experience in clinical learning environments:

1. Conflict between the priorities of medical education and patient care

2. Responsibility beyond a student's capacities

3. Involvement in patient care perceived to be substandard.

Other factors that have been identified include poor communication, objectification of patients, lack of accountability, lapses in the level of care, lack of respect for patients, failure to maintain professional norms, and students being caught in the crossfire between supervisors (Ginsburg et al. 2002).

Feudtner's (1994) study found 98% of students had heard physicians refer to patients using derogatory terms. Monrouxe et al. (2011) found 23.1% of preclinical and 59.8% of clinical students had reported compromising the safety or dignity of a patient—such as leaving a patient physically exposed for an unnecessary length of time, or acting beyond their level of competence without adequate supervision. Thirty-six point seven percent of preclinical and 81.4% of clinical students reported witnessing a clinician breach patient safety or dignity. Roberts et al (2004) compared medical students' and residents' perspectives. They found that ethical conflicts are perceived as common; 58% of respondents reporting a high frequency of ethical conflict encounters. Females and advanced trainees reported the highest levels of encounters.

Personal learning benefit resulting in patient harm

Professional conflict may arise when students and doctors in training take part in daily patient care. Patients may not benefit from the experience and may even be harmed by it (Hicks et al. 2001). The potential benefit for the individual student/trainee, and for the wider society in having appropriately trained doctors, has to be balanced against potential harm to the patient and respect for her/his autonomy (Jagsi and Lehman 2004). In a competitive healthcare market there is also a financial cost for the teaching hospital as the process of training inexperienced physicians may represent an important source of inefficiency (Rich et al. 1990).

Often the patient is willing to allow participation based on the altruistic belief that the balance of potential benefits to themselves and society outweighs the risks (Magrane et al. 1996). Teachers have to decide whether the balance of risks and benefits justifies requesting participation in patient care. Patients must be fully consented. However, Monrouxe et al. (2011) reported that 0.8% preclinical and 8.2% clinical students had instigated an intimate examination/procedure on a female patient without valid consent of their own accord in the previous 12 months. For male patients the figures were 0.9% and 8.2% respectively. Two percent of preclinical and 20.7% clinical students reported being asked by a clinician to perform an intimate examination/procedure on a female patient without valid consent. The figures for male patients were 2% of preclinical and 21% of clinical students.

Difficulty assessing newly observed behaviour as professional or unprofessional

Medical students are faced with behaviours often not previously observed. Knowing what is acceptable and what is morally questionable can be difficult (Robins et al. 2002), even for students who would otherwise naturally tend toward avowed professional virtues (Brainard and Brislen 2007). This has implications for the interpretation of the reporting of such behaviour.

Students who witness, or are victims of, mistreatment have been found to become increasingly cynical (Sheehan et al. 1990), which can lead to the ethical erosion reported in students as they progress through medical school (Sheehan et al. 1990; Wear et al. 2006). Feutender et al.'s (1994) study found 61% of clinical students had witnessed unethical behaviours, 58% reported behaving unethically, 67% felt guilty about something they had done as a student. Sixty-two percent of students believed their ethical principles had been eroded over the course of their studies. Satterwhite et al.'s (2000) survey found that the number of students who felt that derogatory comments made by doctors about patients were appropriate rose from 24% in year 1 to 55% in year 4. In the UK Cordingley et al. (2007) also found clinical students regularly experienced ethically challenging situations. Unethical conduct may be accompanied by acts that contribute to the 'moral exclusion' (Brass et al. 1998, p. 17) of patients such as the use of gallows humour (Fox and Lief 1963; Bosk 1979) or derogatory labels (Becker et al. 1961; Bosk 1979; Feudtner et al. 1994, Satterwhite et al. 2000) that dehumanize patients and create emotional distance from them (Holtman 2008).

However, what appears to be a steady loss of moral direction among medical students may reflect healthy coping strategies accompanying their growing orientation to a more practical set of working norms (Becker et al. 1961). Professional lapses can often be interpreted as manifestations of the normal social mechanisms that accompany all moral learning and their implications for the moral health of both the individual and the environment depend on their prevalence and context (Bandura 1986). Professional lapses form part of the social ecology of professionalism (Holtman 2008). Deviance theory suggests that deviance can serve as a positive social resource by drawing a boundary around normative expectations (Erikson 1962; Durkheim 1982). The problem arises where there is 'normative drift' (Holtman 2008, p. 236)—i.e. decoupling of local practice from global norms, which can be an important antecedent to high-technology accidents (Snook 2000). The ability to juggle conflicting normative expectations is part of any well-adjusted person's behavioural repertoire (Holtman 2008).

Integrating professionalism into modern medical curricula

Growing dissatisfaction with the limitations of traditional medical education and its ability to produce graduates who are 'fit for purpose' (Callahan 1999, p. 3), and influenced by the profession's wider political and economic concerns, led the Association of American Medical Colleges (AAMC) to produce the *General Professional Education of the Physician Report* (AAMC 1984) and the GMC to produce *Tomorrow's Doctors* (GMC 1993). Both the AAMC and the GMC stressed the importance of teaching professionalism and assessing professional behaviour. The GMC recommended professionalism is included as a curricular theme and that all medical schools establish 'fitness to practise' committees to identify medical students unsuited to the profession of medicine regardless of their academic standing (GMC 2003). Lapses in professional behaviour in medical school have been shown to be associated with subsequent problems during active practice as a doctor (Papadakis et al. 2005, 2008). Recognition and remediation of such behaviours provides possibilities for future prevention in some cases.

Implementation of teaching on professionalism has been slow. Barry et al.'s (2000) questionnaire survey of medical students, house officers and physicians found 73% of respondents reported receiving 10 hours or less formal curriculum teaching. Arnold (2002) found only half of US medical schools had identified between four and nine elements of professionalism and developed written criteria and methods for their assessment. Stevenson et al. (2006, p. 1075) found 23 of the 28 UK medical schools had written 'attitudinal objectives', but only 19 used some form of assessment to measure whether these objectives had been achieved. Formal inclusion of professionalism and ethics teaching in curricula has led to improved student awareness. Wagner et al. (2007) found students recognized the areas of patient relationship and communication with patients and colleagues as being of particular importance to them. However, while most students express enthusiasm for beneficence and being service-orientated (Brainard and Brislen 2007), they are not necessarily receptive of the notion that they are obliged to act accordingly in these respects (Hafferty 2002).

Curriculum planning

There is no clear consensus on how professionalism should be integrated into medical curricula (van de Camp 2004; Goldie 2008; Holtman 2008; van Mook et al. 2009a; Wilkinson et al. 2009; Passi et al. 2010). The outcome-based approach to curriculum planning has gained prominence in recent years. It is said to offer advantages over other approaches in helping 'prepare graduates to practice in an increasingly complex healthcare environment with changing patient and public expectations and increasing demands from employing authorities' (Harden et al. 1999, p. 7). In outcome-based education the educational outcomes are clearly specified and these determine the curriculum content and its organization, the teaching methods and strategies used; they also inform the assessment process and influence the educational environment.

Educational outcomes

Framing outcomes for professionalism has proved difficult. Medical education has focused on the teaching, learning, and assessment of elements of competency considered to be relatively stable and less context-dependent—e.g. the knowledge and technical skills required for clinical practice, and has found the operationalization of a dynamic, context-dependent construct, such as professionalism, difficult (van Mook et al. 2009c). For example, the latest edition of *Tomorrow's Doctors* (GMC 2009) frames outcomes relating to professionalism as lists of knowledge, skills, attitudes, and behaviours. Many definitions of modern professionalism, however, call for transformation at the level of values and self-identity, which has major pedagogical implications for educators. Outcomes, conceptualized at individual, institutional and interactional levels, and which call for deeper learning at the level of values and self-identity, need to be specified.

Content

Cruess et al. 2009 have suggested the following content areas for the formal professionalism curriculum:

- the nature of professionalism
- professionalism's historical roots
- the reasons society uses the professions
- the obligations necessary to sustain professional status
- professionalism's relationship to medicine's social contract with society.

Sociological perspectives also need to be embedded to raise awareness, and encourage reflection on the dynamics of professionalism and how individuals' actions relate to broader systemic considerations. Martimiankis et al. (2009) recommend that teaching around professionalism should make clear that:

- the construct of professionalism is central to the identity of a doctor
- the factors that constitute professionalism are not static
- professionalism is a nexus of power with dimensions of gender, race, and class
- the actions of professionals have far-reaching consequences.

Methods and strategies

Teaching on professionalism should be integrated horizontally and vertically in the medical curriculum (Goldie et al. 2007, 2008; Cruess et al. 2009; van Mook et al. 2009a, b, c). The purpose of integration is to demonstrate the ubiquitous nature of professionalism and to convey the message that being professional is central to being a doctor.

Theoretical considerations

Situating teaching and learning professionalism in a theoretical context promotes a more systematic approach (Steinert 2009). We have identified a number of relevant theories that underpin effective teaching and learning professionalism within medical curricula. These are outlined in the following sections.

Situated learning theory

Situated Learning Theory (Lave and Wenger 1991), an elaboration of the apprenticeship model, provides effective models to assist in the design of curricula where learning is 'situated' in practice allowing learners to develop their knowledge and skills in authentic contexts and absorb, and be absorbed into, the culture of the profession they desire to enter (Maudsley and Strivens 2000).

A key concept is legitimate peripheral participation. Learners enter the community of practice at the periphery and as they move towards fuller participation, they participate as a way of learning and both absorb and are absorbed into the culture of practice. A key element is having the opportunity to observe and participate in the framing of problems and understand how knowledge is structured. As a result learners' existing schemas, which guide their thinking and actions, are revised and over time become more elaborate, complex, and integrated (Kenny et al 2003). Learners' recognition of their learning needs and their desire to become full practitioners motivate learning and participation.

Legitimate peripheral participation provides role models who are the basis of, and also help motivate learners' activities. By observation of these role models students learn what to observe, what interpretations to link to observations, and what words and actions to use when conveying these to both patients and colleagues i.e. ways of being. It also demonstrates how these behaviours and knowledge are affected by the context in which they are applied (Johnson and Pratt 1998).

The peer pressure of respected role models is an enormously powerful tool. Negative role modelling, on the other hand, is pervasive and destructive as we have seen. Role models also have the potential to promote transformation at the level of self-identity (Kenny et al. 2003).

The characteristics of effective role models include (Steinert 2009):

* Clinical competence—technical knowledge and skills, interpersonal skills and sound clinical reasoning and decision making.

* Teaching skills—interpersonal skills, provision of feedback and opportunities for reflection that promotes student-centred learning.

* Personal qualities—e.g. compassion, honesty, integrity, enthusiasm for practice, and teaching.

Learning from role models occurs through observation and reflection. Active reflection, often expressing ideas in abstract terms, can result in unconscious thoughts and feelings being brought into the conscious where they can be actively translated into principles and action. An equally powerful process is where observed behaviours are unconsciously incorporated into the belief patterns and behaviours of students (Epstein et al. 1998).

Learning is viewed as more than achieving competence in specific practices, but also involves identity negotiation and formation. Learners develop identity by participating in the practices of the relevant community. Identities are constituted by narratives during interactions. These help students make sense of their experiences and interpret their emerging identity in light of cultural and social expectations (Lawler 2008). Identities are, therefore, moulded to provide meaning, a sense of coherence (McAdams 1993), and a guide to their actions (Ricoeur 1992). Narratives influencing identity formation are often seen in ordinary conversations as well as the 'big stories' students tell of their lives (Monrouxe 2009, p.44). Students need to be provided with the pedagogical space (to understand and synergize their developing identities (Atkinson 1995). It is important to provide this space from the start of the curriculum. While reflective journals can be useful tools, it requires a more interactional context to examine multiple perspectives and develop students' understanding of their developing professional identity (Monrouxe 2009).

The provision of feedback is important. Pratt et al. (2006) found doctors in training used performance feedback and role models in validating their professional identities. Identity theory proposes that individuals develop meaning about themselves through feedback from others (Stryker and Stratham 1985). This feedback, termed reflected appraisals, can be congruent or incongruent with a person's self-perception (Kiecolt 1994). Burke (1991) proposed that, where reflected appraisals are incongruent with an individual's self-perception, behaviour is changed to conform to the appraisal. Swann (1987) however, found that individuals do not change their behaviour if it means changing their self-perception. Alternatively

they associate with, and search out feedback from, individuals who confirm their self-perceptions.

Learning is seen as a dynamic process. While learners are building and revising their schemas the community of practice is simultaneously changing. Each learner adds to the community and learning extends beyond the development of cognitive structures to reflect the larger changes in society and the work of the community.

A major criticism of the Situated Learning perspective has been the underestimation of the role of reflection on experience. Maudsley and Strivens (2000) advise that for situated learning models to be useful to medical educators they should be supplemented by consideration of models which build-in reflection. Undergraduate curricula should aim to provide stage-appropriate opportunities for gaining experience and reflecting on it (Dreyfus and Dreyfus 1980; Leach 2002). There should be structured opportunities which allow students to discuss professional issues in a safe environment (Wear and Castellani 2000; Maudsley and Strivens 2000; Inui 2003; Goldie et al. 2007).

Reflective practice

The concept of the reflective practitioner proposes that theory and practice inform each other. Schon's (1983, 1987) theories are the most widely recognized in this area. Experienced professionals, he advocates, develop zones of mastery around areas of competence. They practice within these zones as if automatic. Schon terms this 'knowing-in-action' (1987, p. 25). Occasionally professionals encounter an unexpected outcome or surprise. Two types of reflection are triggered at this time, 'reflection-in-action' and 'reflection-on-action' (1987, p. ix). Reflection-in-action occurs during the activity and consists of three components:

1. Reframing and reworking the problem from different perspectives

2. Establishing where the problem fits into existing schemas

3. Understanding the elements and implications present in the problem, its solution and consequences.

Reflection-on-action follows the experience and involves revisiting the event to consider what occurred, what was learned and how to incorporate new learning into 'knowing-in-action'. Reflective practice is more than thoughtful practice; it is the process of intentionally turning thoughtful practice into a potential learning situation. Moreover, reflective practice also goes beyond examining knowledge components to include the affective aspects of a situation. However, it does not account for circumstances where decisions have to be rapid and the scope for reflection is extremely limited. In this case reflection is best seen as an intuitive, metacognitive process drawing on previous experience with little deliberation.

In order for students to develop the necessary skills for reflective practice they must have opportunities to acquire them. Teachers must initially model, share and demonstrate the skills. They facilitate the students' abilities to perceive options and alternatives, to 'frame and re-frame problems' (1987, p. 250). They also assist students to reflect on actions and the options they choose, and on what values may have influenced their choice. Finally, they help students to consider critically what they have learned and to integrate it into their existing knowledge. Once the student has achieved sufficient experience and insight, the teacher's role becomes facilitative, observing and commenting constructively on situations in which students' 're-framing' has occurred, which helps them become consciously aware of the process of reflection (Kaufman et al. 2000).

Critical thinking is a prerequisite for critical reflection. Group learning has been shown to be particularly effective in fostering critical thinking (Maudsley and Strivens 2000). Monrouxe and Rees (2011) found physician led small-group teaching, encouraging reflection on professionalism resulted in complex, embodied understandings of professionalism. In contrast students who learned predominantly through lectures had a simpler, more superficial understanding.

Brookfield (1987) maintains that the critical thinking process is person-specific, emotion-centred and both intrinsically and extrinsically motivated. He warns against forcing critical thinking on learners without their consent. In his rules of thumb for facilitating critical thinking he emphasizes there is no standard approach. Diversity is seen as essential, perfection impossible, learner satisfaction is seen as only one aim and risk-taking, for example recognizing opportunistic teaching moments, is considered important. He makes a number of recommendations for facilitators of critical thinking:

- affirm the learner's self-worth
- listen attentively
- show support
- reflect and mirror learner's ideas and actions
- motivate learners
- regularly evaluate the process
- help learners create social networks with like-minded networks
- be critical educators
- raise awareness of how to learn to be critical thinkers
- be role models for critical thinking.

Critical thinking needs be extended beyond the cognitive, rational, and intellectual dimensions to also be concerned with bringing into the learner's consciousness those assumptions, beliefs and values which have been uncritically assimilated and internalized during childhood and adolescence and during their time at medical school. Critical awareness can help learners become aware of, and liberate themselves from the social and cultural restraints on their behaviour, Berger's (1965, p. 25) sociologic consciousness. Some critical theorists go further suggesting that such awareness should lead to social action (Carr and Kemmis 1983; Freire 1985). One of the commonly stated aims of professionalism teaching is to increase students' awareness of their social responsibilities as doctors in terms of social justice, which potentially could include taking action, although this has been the subject of a great deal of recent debate among US medical educators (Kanter 2011).

However, in helping students explore their personal attitudes, issues relating to students' unconscious may affect the interpersonal dynamics. This requires teachers who are able to recognize these conflicts and are clear on their boundaries. In many cases teachers will require appropriate training, which has resource implications for medical schools.

Experiential learning

The definition of experiential learning is important as all learning can be viewed as experiential to some extent. Eraut (2006, p. 107) restricts the term 'experiential learning' to situations where experience is initially apprehended at the level of impressions, thus requiring a further period of reflective thinking. Most models of experiential learning assume further reflection will occur, depending on the learner's disposition. The best known model is Kolb's (1984). Kolb (1984) describes four main environments: Affectively orientated (feeling), symbolically orientated (thinking), perceptually orientated (watching) or behaviourally orientated (doing). He conceives learning tasks within these environments as being composed of grasping and transforming experiences. Grasping experiences have two components, concrete experience, which filters through the senses, and abstract conceptualization, which is indirect and symbolic. Transforming experiences consist of two processes, reflection and action. Learning is enhanced if learners are encouraged to use all four components.

Experiential learning helps learners connect their previous knowledge, abilities, values, and beliefs with their current experiences promoting new learning. It also allows them to assume responsibility for their learning, and transfers learning from an academic mode to the environments where students will ultimately operate. The role of the teacher will depend on the orientation of the learning environment. For example, in the affectively-orientated environment, where activities are directed towards the learner experiencing what it would be like to be a practising doctor, they act as role models. In the behaviourally orientated environment, where activities are focused on learners applying their competencies to practical problems or practices, they act as mentors.

Professional identity arises from a long-term combination of experience and reflection on experience (Hilton and Slotnik 2005). As mentioned previously, medical education should aim to provide stage-appropriate opportunities for gaining experience and reflecting on it. There should structured opportunities, which allow students to discuss professional issues in a safe environment.

Self-directed learning

Self-directed learning is one of the foundation concepts in adult education. Being self-directed enables learners to achieve more autonomy, which is particularly important as learners move towards fuller participation in the community of practice. It is a quality which promotes successful reflective practice and experiential learning. It is also an essential quality for portfolio-based learning.

Self-directed learning occurs when learners determine goals and objectives, locate appropriate resources, plan their learning strategies and evaluate the outcomes. It is seen as the appropriate way for mature adults to learn. It is said to promote freedom, autonomy, independence, learner-centeredness and relevance. Learning is the responsibility of the learner. The teacher's role is that of learning facilitator (Tennant 1997).

Learners must have the opportunity to develop and practise the skills required to be self-directed learners. These include competency at asking questions and critical appraisal of new information. A fundamental skill in self-direction is that of critical reflection on one's own learning and experience. Learners must practise and develop skills at reflecting on all aspects of their learning to determine additional learning needs. Self-directed learning is facilitated by the creation of a supportive learning environment where learners feel safe to ask questions and admit to not understanding (Tennant 1997; Kaufman et al. 2000). It has been embraced by many medical educators in both undergraduate and continuing professional development programmes as a prerequisite for life-long learning (Tennant 1997; Kaufman et al. 2000). However, the ability and motivation to be self-directed varies with the context of learning (Candy 1991; Merriam and Caffarella 1999). The extent to which self-directedness is possible or likely to happen depends on the subject matter, the social, cultural and educational setting, past experiences, self-concept and relevant study skills (Greveson and Spencer 2005).

Socialization theory

Socialization in essence is about learning to be an insider. There is no single theory of socialization. It has evolved over time and across various disciplines. There are many types of socialization along a number of dimensions e.g. primary/secondary, child/adult, gender or religious. Professional socialization is a form of adult or secondary socialization. A number of basic principles of socialization theory can be drawn upon when exploring teaching and learning professionalism (Hafferty 2009):

The recognition of medical education as a site of occupational culture links it directly to the concept of socialization (Hafferty 2009). Socialization is different from occupational training. Occupational training involves learning role-specific knowledge, skills, and behaviours. While socialization theory addresses these issues it also involves training for self-image and identity. Socialization is fundamentally both a process and an outcome of personal transformation.

Culture is viewed by modernists as the sum of activities, symbolic and instrumental, which exist in the organization and create shared meaning. Socialization is viewed as the process through which individuals acquire and incorporate an understanding of these activities. Culture is seen as relatively constant and can be understood through reason. An organization's culture, therefore, teaches individuals how to behave, what to hope for, and what it means to succeed or fail. Some individuals become competent; some do not (Tierney 1997).

The post-modernist view, however, rejects the rationalist view of the world in which reality is fixed and understandable and culture discovered. It also rejects the idea of the individual having an immutable identity awaiting organizational imprinting. Culture is seen as the interpretation by participants of the organization's activities rather than simply the sum of activities. It is less a definition of the world as it is, but more a conglomeration of the aspirations of what the organizational world might be. Culture is open to challenge and change, although historical and social forces may limit change. Socialization, in this perspective, involves an interpretive process where new recruits make sense of an organization through the lens of their own unique backgrounds and in the organization's current context. It is not simply a planned sequence of learning activities occurring in unchanging contexts irrespective of individual and group identity, where individuals acquire static facts one after another. Instead these facts are open to multiple interpretations, meaning is created rather than transmitted, and culture is constantly being recreated (Tierney 1997).

The hidden curriculum is closely aligned with Schein's (1992) model of occupational culture. Schein proposes that cultures can be interpreted and understood by examining their core values and assumptions. The model proposes culture exists simultaneously on three levels which interact:

- Artefacts—these are the visible elements in a culture e.g. dress codes, use of instruments such as stethoscopes or organizational structures. They can be recognized by people who are not part of the culture, but not fully understood by them. To understand their origin they must look to the espoused values in the culture.

- Espoused values—these are values normally espoused by leading figures of the culture, e.g. the GMC. These are also prominent in the formal curriculum. They are represented in the attempts to define modern professionalism by influential bodies. Espoused values must be rooted in shared assumptions of the members otherwise problems can arise.

- Assumptions—these reflect the shared values within a culture. These are often tacit, taken-for-granted and not especially visible to members. Core assumptions can be assumptions about the importance of work life balance or the importance of maximizing income. Where these conflict with espoused values it can lead to problems such as low morale and disillusionment.

Much of what takes place during socialization is at tacit level. It is a process where what is seen as unusual, non-routine or incongruous to the outsider becomes as commonplace and taken-for-granted as for those within the group they seek to join. It works best when it unfolds in a subtle and incremental manner. While there is value in formalized organizational rituals to promote transmission of group values and norms, e.g. 'White Coat' ceremonies, it is the less dramatic taken-for-granted routine day-to-day activities that have most impact (van Maanen and Barley 1984). The informal curriculum is awash with these activities.

Medical education is challenging and stressful and, as has been illustrated, students can be subjected to bullying and abuse. Independent of environmental pressures students are high achievers who are anxious to do well and become members of the medical profession. As such they are the 'perfect objects' for socialization. This is heightened by a culture in medicine which, until recently, devalued introspection and reflection (Hafferty 2009). Some forms of socialization are less visible. Medical education has the potential to be a form of re-socialization due to:

- Its structure: hierarchical and extended

- Its institutional setting (often linked to Goffman's (1961, p. 4) concept of the 'total institution', one in which virtually every aspect of members' lives is controlled by the institution and calculated to serve its goals and

- Its cognitive and emotional demands (Hafferty 2009).

Resocialization is an active social process in which new ways of thinking, acting and valuing can result from manipulation of the environment (Hafferty 1991). This process is most likely to occur when individuals are repeatedly and purposively stressed. The potential dangers of resocialization must be countered.

Teaching and learning methods

Passi et al.'s (2010) review of teaching and learning methods for professionalism identified three main themes which have emerged:

1. The development of patient-centred approaches

Experiential: reflective practice
Clinical contact including tutor feedback
Undergraduate ethics teaching
Problem based learning
Role play exercises
Bedside teaching
Educational portfolios
Videotaped consultation analysis
Significant event analysis
Workshops: interactive lectures
Humanities writing: reading literature related to patients and doctors
Mentoring programmes

Figure 24.3 Teaching and learning methods used for professionalism.

2. The focus on encouraging the development of reflective practice

3. The development of ethical approaches to practice.

The teaching and learning methods described in the literature are shown in fig. 24.3. However, there has been little evaluation of individual methods or comparison between them (Passi et al. 2010).

We would suggest that undergraduate ethics teaching should not be classified as a teaching and learning method for professionalism. Ethical practice is integral to professional practice and needs to be developed along similar lines. We would direct those wishing a more in depth examination of ethics and law in medical curricula to Dowie and Martin (2011).

Educational environment

The institutional culture can promote professional behaviour or subvert it. Medical education takes place in a milieu heavily influenced by the atmosphere created within medicine's institutions and by the healthcare system (Cruess and Cruess 2009).

While formal teaching is important it is in the informal and hidden curricula that professionalism is operationalized and where most learning takes place. The informal and hidden curricula are more powerful than the formal curriculum in transmitting the values of the profession (Stern 1998). Optimizing the effectiveness of the formal curriculum must be combined with maximizing the potential for learning in informal and hidden curricula and controlling for its negative effects.

Tackling the informal and hidden curricula involves active recognition of the importance of professionalism by heads of medical schools and healthcare organizations. This sends a message of its importance. Their support must be manifested by decisions taken on pedagogical approaches and the allocation of space, teaching time and financial resources (Cruess and Cruess 2009). Appointing a leader or champion to establish and direct the implementation of a programme for teaching and learning professionalism is recommended. They should be supported by a working group or committee consisting of academics and teachers as well as local experts on professionalism and its evaluation. Students and doctors from different generations working in clinical teaching units are important stakeholders who should be involved in the process. This may also help counter their potential scepticism about professionalism (Hafferty 2002).

Students can offer the potential for reflection and challenge to institutional habitas—the behaviours and practices of institutions such as medical schools that are often strongly influenced by tradition (Monrouxe 2009). To promote this challenge institutions and individual members need to be aware of existing power relations and develop strategies to empower students' contributions both as peripheral members of communities of practice and at institutional level. These need to be reflected in the discourses of the medical profession.

Faculty development programmes should be directed at both individual and organizational levels (Wilkerson and Irby 1998). At individual level they can:

◆ address attitudes and beliefs that can impede the teaching and learning of professionalism

◆ transmit knowledge about the core content of professionalism as well as effective teaching and assessment practices

◆ develop skills in teaching and evaluating behaviours that exemplify professionalism.

Individuals involved in learning environments need to reflect on how they learn and facilitate the learning of others. This may involve the identification of values-relevant experiences for individual and group reflection. At the level of 'community of practice' the larger academic community should reflect on professionalism and professional values. Medical educators should look outward and learn from other helping professions that combine experience and reflection to foster moral growth and deepening of values (Inui et al. 2009).

At organizational level faculty development may help:

◆ define a shared vision of professionalism and how it should be taught and evaluated

◆ create opportunities for teaching and learning professionalism

◆ address system issues that can impeded the teaching and learning of professionalism in the formal, informal and hidden curricula.

Kotter (1996) has outlined the following steps to promote change at organizational level:

◆ establish a sense of urgency

◆ form a powerful guiding coalition

◆ create a vision

◆ communicate the vision

◆ empower others to act on the vision

◆ generate short-term wins

◆ consolidate gains and produce more change

◆ anchor new approaches in the culture.

The social and physical environments where students are educated have been intentionally constructed. These have often been organized to meet the needs of teaching staff or the efficiency of the medical care system without explicit attention being paid to the moral values they express. There needs to be reflection on the institutionalized norms and conventions that influence student's behaviours (Du Gay et al. 2000). Schein's model can be used to examine an organization's culture, understand cultural elements and analyse the relationship between deep-rooted assumptions and common practices. Attempts can then be made to change the culture by changing basic assumptions to fit the desired espoused values and artefacts of the organization. Another potential approach, based on third-generation activity theory (Engestrom, 2007), is to introduce 'change laboratory' interventions designed to bring about change in the day-to-day practices and social structures of organizations.

Conclusions

- Definitions of professionalism are historically and culturally based.

- There has been a disruption of the relationship between the medical profession and society in recent years in North America and Europe. In response the Western medical community has started to redefine professionalism.

- What has been produced can be described as 'romantic professionalism'. It focuses on normative definitions and misses the influence of context, institutions and socioeconomic and political concerns in the creation of the definitions. Professionalism is a nexus of power with dimensions of gender, race and class. It is a distributed attribute best understood in 'systemic considerations', rather than as a reflection of individuals and their motives.

- There is no clear consensus on how medical education should teach and promote learning on professionalism.

- While formal teaching is important, it is in the informal and hidden curricula that professionalism is operationalized and where most learning takes place. Optimizing the effectiveness of the formal curriculum must be combined with maximizing the potential for learning in informal and hidden curricula and controlling for their sometimes negative effects.

- Teaching and learning professionalism is the collective responsibility of educators, students, medical and other healthcare professionals with whom students come into contact, and the institutions associated with medical education. This must take place in partnership with wider society.

- Medical education is not a panacea for remediation.

References

Accreditation Council for Graduate Medical Education (1999) Enhancing residency education through outcomes assessment: General competencies. *ACGME Outcome Project*. [Online] http://www.acgme.org/outcome/comp/compFull.asp Accessed March 2013

American Association of Internal Medicine Committee on Evaluation of Clinical Competence (1995) *Project Professionalism*. Philadelphia: ABIM

Arnold, L. (2002) Assessing professional behaviour: yesterday, today and tomorrow. *Acad Med.* 77(6): 502–515

Arnold, L. and Stern, DT. (2006) What is medical professionalism? In: D.T. Stern (ed) *Measuring Medical Professionalism* (pp. 15–39). New York: Oxford University Press

Association of American Medical Colleges (1984) Physicians for the twenty-first century. Report on the General Professional Education of the Physician. Washington, DC: AAMC

Atkinson, P. (1995) *Medical Talk and Medical Work*. London: Sage

Baldwin, D.C. and Daugherty, S.R. (1997) Do residents feel 'abused'? Perceived mistreatment during internship. *Acad Med.* 72: S51–S53

Baldwin, D.C. and Daugherty, S.R. (2006) Using surveys to assess professionalism in individuals and institutions. In: D.T. Stern (ed) *Measuring Medical Professionalism* (pp. 95–117). New York: Oxford University Press

Baldwin, D.C., Daugherty, S.R., and Eckenfels, E.J. (1991) Student perceptions of mistreatment and harassment during medical school. A survey of ten United States schools. *W J Med.* 155(2): 140–145

Bandura, A. (1986) *Social Foundations of Thought and Action: A Social Cognitive Theory*. Englewood Cliffs, NJ: Prentice-Hall

Barry, D., Cyran, E., and Anderson, RJ. (2000) Common issues in medical professionalism: room to grow. *Am J Med.* 108(2): 136–142

Becker, H.S., Geer, B., Hughes, E.C., and Strauss, A.L. (1961) *Boys in White: Student Culture in Medical School*. Chicago IL: University of Chicago Press

Berger, P. (1965) *Invitation to Sociology*. New York: Anchor Books

Bosk, C. (1979) *Forgive and remember: Managing medical failure*. Chicago: University of Chicago Press

Brainard, A.H. and Brislen, H.C. (2007) Viewpoint: learning professionalism: a view from the trenches. *Acad Med.* 82(11): 1010–1014

Brass, D.J., Butterfield, K.D., and Skaggs, B.C. (1998) Relationships and unethical behaviour; A social network perspective. *Acad Manage Rev.* 23: 14–31

Brookfield, S.D. (1987) *Developing Critical Thinkers: Challenging Adults to Explore Alternative Ways of Thinking and Acting*. Milton Keynes: Open University Press

Burke, P.J. (1991) Identity processes and social stress. *Am Sociol Rev.* 56: 836–849

Callahan, D. (1999) Medical education and the goals of medicine. *AMEE Medical Education Guide No 14*, 3–4

Calman, K. (1994) The profession of medicine. *BMJ.* 309: 1140–1143

Candy, P.C. (1991) *Self-Direction for Lifelong Learning: A Comprehensive Guide to Theory and Practice*. San Francisco: Jossey-Bass

CanMEDS. (2000) Extract from the CanMEDS 2000 Project Societal Needs Working Group Report. *Med Teach.* 22(6): 549–554

Carr, W. and Kemmis, S. (1983) *Becoming Critical: Knowing Through Action Research*, Waure Ponds: Deakin University Press

Castellani, B. and Hafferty, F. (2006) The complexities of professionalism: a preliminary investigation. In: A. Wear, J.M. Aultman (eds) *Professionalism in Medicine: Critical Perspectives* (pp. 3–23). New York: Springer.

Castelani, B. and Wear, D. (2000) Physicians views on practicing professionalism in the corporate age. *Qual Health Res.* 10(4): 490–506

Cohen, J.J. (2006) Professionalism in medical education, an American perspective: from evidence to accountability. *Med Educ.* 40: 607–617

Cook, D.J., Liukus J.F., Risdon, C.L., Griffith, L.E., Guyatt, G.H., and Walter, S.D. (1996) Residents' experiences of abuse, discrimination and sexual harassment during residency training. *CMAJ.* 154(11): 1657–1665

Cordingley, L., Hyde, C., Peters, S., Vernon, B., and Bundy, C. (2007) Undergraduate medical students' exposure to clinical ethics: a challenge to the development of professional behaviours? *Med Educ.* 41(12): 1202–1209

Cruess, S. R. and Cruess, R.L. (1997) Professionalism must be taught. *BMJ.* 315: 1674–1677

Cruess, R.L., and Cruess S.R., (2009) Principles for designing a program for the teaching and learning of professionalism at the undergraduate level. In: R.L. Cruess, S.R. Cruess, and Y. Steinert (eds) *Teaching Medical Professionalism*. New York: Cambridge University Press, pp. 73–93.

Cruess, R.L., Cruess, S.R., and Johnston, S.E. (2000) Professionalism: an ideal to be sustained. *Lancet.* 356(9224): 156–159

Cruess, R.L., Cruess, S.R., and Steinert, Y. (eds) (2009) *Teaching Medical Professionalism*. New York: Cambridge University Press, pp. 31–53

de Montigny, G. (1995) The power of being professional. In: A. Manicom, M. Campbell (eds) *Knowledge, Experience and Ruling Relations* (pp. 209–220). Toronto, ON: University of Toronto Press

Dowie, A., and Martin, A. (2011) Ethics and law in the medical curriculum. *AMEE Curriculum Guide. No 53*. Dundee, UK: Association for Medical Education in Europe

Dreyfus, H.L., and Dreyfus, S.E. (1980) *A Five Stage Model of the Mental Activities Involved in Directed Skill Acquisition*. Berkeley, CA: University of California Press

Durkheim, E. (1982) Rules for the distinction of the normal from the pathological. In: S. Lukes (ed.) *The Rules of Sociological Methods and Selected Texts on Sociology and its Method* (pp. 85–108). New York: Free Press

Du Gay, P., Evans, J., and Redman, P. (2000) *Identity: a Reader*. London: Sage

Engestrom, Y. (2007) Putting Vygotsky to work. The change laboratory as an application of double stimulation. In: H. Daniels, M. Cole, and J.V. Wertsch (eds) *The Cambridge Companion to* Vygotsky (pp. 362–382). Cambridge: Cambridge University Press

Epstein, R.M., Cole, D.R., Gawinski, B.A., Pitrowski-Lee, S., and Ruddy N.B. (1998) How students learn from community-based preceptors. *Arch Fam Med*. 7: 149–154

Eraut, M. (2006) *Developing Professional Knowledge and Competence*. 3rd edn. Oxford: Routledge Falmer

Erikson, K.T. (1962) Notes on the sociology of deviance. *Social Problems*. 9: 307–314

Eron, L.D. (1955) Effect of medical education on medical students' attitudes. *J Med Educ*. 30(10): 559–566

Evetts, J. (2006) Short note: the sociology of professional groups: new directions. *Curr Sociol*. 54: 133–143

Feudtner, C., Christakis, D.A., and Christakis, N.A. (1994) Do clinical clerks suffer ethical erosion? Students' perceptions of their ethical and personal development. *Acad Med*. 69: 670–679

Fogelberg, D., and Frauwirth, S. (2010) A complexity science approach to occupation: moving beyond the individual. *J Occup Sci*. 17(3): 131–139

Foucault, M. (1980) Truth and power. In: C. Gordon (ed), trans C. Gordon, L Marshall, J, Mepham, and K. Soper. *Power/Knowledge* (pp. 109–133) Hemel Hempstead: Harvester Wheatsheaf

Foucault, M. (1982) The subject and power. In: H. Dreyfus and P. Rabinow (eds) *Michael Foucault: Beyond Structuralism and Hermeneutics* (pp. 208–226). Chicago: Chicago University Press

Fox, R.C. and Lief, H. (1963) Training for 'detached concern'. In: H.I. Lief(ed) *The Psychological Basis of Medical Practice* (pp. 12–35). New York: Harper and Row

Freire, P. (1985) *The Politics of Education: Culture, Power and Liberation*. London: Macmillan

Freidson, E. (1970a) *Professional Dominance: the Social Structure of Medical Care*. New York, NY: Atherton Press

Freidson, E. (1970b) *Profession of Medicine: a Study of the Sociology of Applied Knowledge*. New York: Harper & Row

Freidson, E. (1986) *Professional Powers: a Study of Institutionalization of Formal Knowledge*. Chicago, IL: University of Chicago Press

Freidson, E. (1994) *Professionalism Reborn: Theory, Prophecy, and Policy*. Cambridge: Polity Press

General Medical Council (1993) *Tomorrow's Doctors*. London: GMC

General Medical Council (2002) *Good Medical Practice*. London: GMC

General Medical Council (2003) *Tomorrow's Doctors: Recommendations on undergraduate medical education*. London: GMC

General Medical Council (2009) *Tomorrow's Doctors*. London: GMC

Gerstl, J. and Jacobs, G. (1976) *Professions for the People. The Politics of Skills*. New York: New Schenkman Publishing Company

Giddens, A. (1984) *The Constitution of society: Outline of the Theory of Structuration*. Cambridge: Polity Press

Ginsburg, S., Regehr, G., Hatala, R. et al. (2000) Context, conflict and resolution: a new conceptual framework for evaluating professionalism. *Acad Med*. 75(10): S6–S11

Ginsburg, S., Regehr, G., Stern, D., and Lingard, L. (2002) The anatomy of the professional lapse: bridging the gap between traditional frameworks and students' perceptions. *Acad Med*. 77(6): 516–522

Goffman, E. (1961) *Asylums: Essays On The Social Situation Of Mental Patients And Other Inmates*. Garden City NY: Doubleday

Goldie, J., Cotton, P., Dowie, A., and Morrison, J. (2007) Teaching professionalism in the early years of a medical curriculum: A qualitative study. *Med Educ*. 41: 610–617

Goldie, J. (2008) Integrating professionalism teaching into undergraduate medical education in the UK setting. *Med Teach*. 30(5): 513–527

Greveson, G.C. and Spencer, J.A. (2005) Self-directed learning—the importance of concepts and contexts. *Med Educ*. 39: 348–349

Gull, W.W. (1874) Introductory address on the study of medicine. *BMJ*. 2: 425

Hafferty, F.W. (1991) *Into the Valley: Death and the Socialization of Medical Students*. New Haven, CT: Yale University Press

Hafferty, F.W. (1998) Beyond curriculum reform: Confronting medicine's hidden curriculum. *Acad Med*. 73(4): 403–407

Hafferty, F.W. (2002) What medical students know about professionalism. *Mount Sinai Med J*. 69(6): 385–397

Hafferty, F.W. (2009) Professionalism and the socialization of medical students. In: R.L. Cruess, S.R. Cruess, Y. Steinert (eds) *Teaching Medical Professionalism* (pp. 53–73). New York: Cambridge University Press

Hafferty, F.W. and Castellani, B. (2009) A sociological framing of medicine's modern-day professionalism movement. *Med Educ*. 43: 826–828

Hafferty, F.W. and Levinson, D. (2008) Moving beyond nostalgia and motives: toward a complexity science view of medical professionalism. *Perspectives Biol Med*. 51(4): 599–615

Harden, R.M., Crosby, J.R., and Davis M.H. (1999) An introduction to outcome-based education. *Med Teach*. 21(2): 7–14

Hicks, L.K., Lin, Y., Robertson, D.W., Robinson, D.L., and Woodrow, S.I. (2001) Understanding the clinical dilemmas that shape medical students' ethical development: questionnaire survey and focus group study. *BMJ*. 332(7288): 709–710

Hilton, S.R. and Slotnik, H.B. (2005) Proto-professionalism: how professionalisation occurs across the continuum of medical education. *Med Educ*. 39: 58–66

Hodges, D. (2004) Medical student bodies and the pedagogy of self-reflection, self-assessment, and self-regulation. *J Curriculum Theorizing*. 20: 41–51

Hodges, B.D., Ginsburg, S., Cruess, R. et al. (2011) Assessment of professionalism: recommendations from the Ottawa 2010 Conference. *Med Teach*. 33(5): 354–363

Hodgson, D. (2005) 'Putting on a professional performance': performativity, subversion and project management. *Organization*. 12: 51–68

Holtman, M.C. (2008) A theoretical sketch of medical professionalism as a normative complex. *Adv Health Sci Educ*. 13: 233–245

Huddle, T.S. (2005) Teaching professionalism: is medical morality a competency? *Acad Med*. 80(10): 885–891

Inui, T.S. (2003) *A flag in the Wind: Educating for Professionalism in Medicine*. Washington DC: Association of American Medical Colleges

Inui, T.S., Cottingham, A.H., Frankel, R.M., Litzelman, M.D., Suchman, A.L., and Williamson, P.R. (2009) Supporting teaching and learning of professionalism—changing the educational environment and students' 'navigational skills'. In: R.L. Cruess, S.R. Cruess, Y. Steinert (eds) *Teaching Medical Professionalism* (pp. 108–125). New York: Cambridge University Press

Irvine, D. (1997) The performance of doctors: Professionalism and self regulation in a changing world. *BMJ*. 314: 1540–1542

Irvine, D. (1999) The performance of doctors: the new professionalism. *Lancet*. 353: 1174–1177

Jagsi, R. and Lehmann, L.S. (2004) The ethics of medical education. *BMJ*. 329(7461): 332–334

Johnson, J. and Pratt, D.D. (1998) The apprenticeship perspective: modelling ways of being. In: D.D. Pratt et al. (eds) *Five Perspectives of Teaching in Adult and High Education* (pp. 83–104). Malabar, FL: Kreiger Publishing

Jones, I.M. (2003) Health professions. In: G. Scambler. (ed) *Sociology as Applied to Medicine* (pp. 235–248). London: Saunders

Kanter, S.L. (2011) On physician advocacy. *Acad Med*. 86(9): 1059–1060

Kaufman, D.M., Mann, K.V., and Jennett, P.A. (2000) *Teaching and Learning in Medical Education: How theory can inform practice*. Edinburgh: ASME

Kenny, N.P., Mann, K.V., and MacLeod, H. (2003) Role modelling in physicians' professional formation: reconsidering an essential but untapped educational strategy. *Acad Med*. 78: 1203–1210

Kiecolt, K.J. (1994) Stress and the decision to change oneself: A theoretical model. *Soc Psychol Q*. 57: 49–63

Kotter, J.P. (1996) *Leading Change*. Boston (MA): Harvard Business School Press

Kolb, D.A. (1984) *Experiential learning: Experience as the Source of Learning and Development*. Englewood Cliffs (NJ): Prentice Hall

Krause, E.A. (1996) *Death of the Guilds*. New Haven, CT: Yale University Press

Larson, M.S. (1977) *The Rise of Professionalism: A Sociological Analysis*. Berkeley, CA: University of California Press

Lawler, S. (2008) *Identity: Sociological Perspectives*. Cambridge: Polity Press

Lave, J. and Wenger, E. (1991) *Situated Learning. Legitimate Peripheral Participation*. Cambridge: Cambridge University Press

Leach, D.C. (2002) Competence is a habit. *JAMA*. 287:243–244

Magrane, D., Gannon, J., and Miller, C.T. (1996) Student doctors and women in labour: attitudes and expectations. *Obstet Gynaecol*. 88(2): 298–302

Martimiankis, M.A., Maniate, J.M., and Hodges, B.D. (2009) Sociological interpretations of professionalism. *Med Educ*. 43: 829–837

Maudsley, G. and Strivens, J. (2000) Promoting professional knowledge, experiential learning and critical thinking for medical students. *Med Educ*. 34: 535–544

Medical Professionalism Project (2000) Medical professionalism in the new millennium: a physician's charter. *Lancet*. 359: 520–522

Merriam, S.B. and Caffarella, R.S. (1999) *Learning in Adulthood*. San Francisco: Jossey-Bass

Monrouxe, L. (2009) Identity, identification and medical education: why should we care? *Med Educ*. 44: 40–49

Monrouxe, L. and Rees, C. (2011) Differences in medical students' explicit discourses of professionalism: acting, representing, becoming. *Med Educ*. 45(6): 585–602

Monrouxe, L., Rees, C., Wells, S., and Linford, H. (2011) Medical Students' Professional Dilemmas UK Questionnaire: Report to Head of Schools. ASME Annual Scientific Meeting. Edinburgh, July 2011

McAdams, D. (1993) *The Stories We Live By*. New York, NY: Guilford Press

Nishigori, H. (2007) Professionalism learned from BUSHIDO. 39th Annual Meeting Japanese Society for Medical Education. Iwate, Japan

O'Neill, O. (2002) *A Question of Trust*: The BBC Reith Lectures 2002. Cambridge: Cambridge University Press

Papadakis, M.A., Arnold, G.K., Blank L.L., Holmboe, E.S., and Lipner, R.S. (2008) Performance during internal medicine training and subsequent disciplinary action by state licensing boards. *Ann Intern Med*. 148(11): 869–876

Papadakis, M.A., Teherani, A., Banach, M.A., et al. (2005) Disciplinary action by medical boards and prior behaviour in medical school. *N Engl J Med*. 353(25): 2673–2682

Passi, V., Manjo, D., Peile, E., Thistlethwaite, J., and Johnson, N. (2010) Developing medical professionalism in future doctors: a systematic review. *Int J Med Educ*. 1: 19–29

Pellegrino, E.D. and Pellegrino, AA. (1988) Humanism and ethics in Roman medicine: translation and commentary on a text of Scribonius Largus. *Literature and Medicine*. 7: 22–38

Pellegrino, E.D. and Relman, A.S. (1999) Professional medical associations: ethical and practical guideline. *JAMA*. 282(10): 984–986

Pratt, M.G., Rockmann, K.W., and Kaufmann, J.B. (2006) Constructing professional identity; The role of work and identity learning cycles in the customization of identity among medical residents. *Acad Manage J*. 49(2): 235–252

Projectteam Consilium Abeundi (2005) In: Luijk, S.J. (ed) *Professional Behaviour: teaching, assessing and coaching students*. ISBN 90-5278-442-6

Rees, C.E. and Knight, L. V. (2007) The trouble with assessing students' professionalism: Theoretical insights from sociocognitive psychology. *Acad Med*. 82: 46–50

Rich, E.C., Gifford, G., Luxenberg, M., and Dowd, B. (1990) The relationship of house staff experience to the cost and quality of inpatient care. *JAMA*. 263(7): 953–957

Ricoeur, P. (1992) *Oneself as Another*. Chicago, IL: University of Chicago Press

Roberts, L.W., Green Hammond, K.A., Geppert, C.M., and Warner, T.D. (2004) The positive role of professionalism and ethics training in medical education: a comparison of medical student and resident perspectives. *Acad Psychiatry*. 28(3): 170–182

Robins, L.S., Braddock, C.H., and Fryer-Edwards, K.A. (2002) Using the American Board of Internal Medicine's 'Elements of Professionalism' for undergraduate ethics education. *Acad Med*. 77(6): 523–531

Royal College of Physicians (2005) *Medical Professionalism in a Changing World*. RCP. London

Satterwhite, R.C., Satterwhite, W.M., and Enarson, C. (2000) An ethical paradox: the effect of unethical conduct on medical students' values. *J Med Ethics*. 26(6): 462–465

Schein, E.H. (1992) *Organizational Culture and Leadership*. Hoboken NJ: John Wiley & Sons Inc.

Schon, D.A. (1983) *The Reflective Practitioner: How Professionals Think in Action*. New York: Basic Books, Inc.

Schon, D.A. (1987) *Educating the Reflective Practitioner: Toward a New Design for Teaching and Learning in the Professions*. San Francisco, CA: Jossey-Bass

Sethuraman, K.R. (2006) Professionalism in medicine. *Regional Health Forum*. 10(1): 1–10

Sheehan, K.H., Sheehan, D.V., White, K., Leibowitz, A., and Baldwin, D.C. (1990) A pilot study of medical student 'abuse'. Student perceptions of mistreatment and misconduct in medical school. *JAMA*. 263(4): 533–537

Silver, H.K. and Glicken. A.D. (1990) Medical student abuse. Incidence, severity, and significance. *JAMA*. 263(4): 527–532

Sox, H. (2002) Medical professionalism in the new millennium: a physician charter. *Ann Intern Med*. 136(3): 243–246

Snook, S.A. (2000) *Friendly Fire: The Accidental Shoot Down of US Blackhawks over Northern Iraq*. Princeton: Princeton University Press

Steinert, Y. (2009) Strategies for teaching and learning professionalism. In: R.L. Cruess, S.R. Cruess, and Y. Steinert (eds) *Teaching Medical Professionalism* (pp. 31–53). New York: Cambridge University Press

Stern, D.T. (1998) In search of the informal curriculum: when and where professional values are taught. *Acad Med*. 73: S28–S30

Stern, D.T. (ed) (2006) *Measuring Medical Professionalism*. New York: Oxford University Press, pp. 3–15

Stevenson, A., Adshead, L., and Higgs, R. (2006) The teaching of professional attitudes within UK medical schools: reported difficulties and good practice. *Med Educ*. 11: 1072–1080

Stevenson, A., Higgs, R., and Sugarman, J. (2001) Teaching professional development in medical schools. *Lancet*. 357: 867–887

Stevens, R.A. (2000) Themes in the history of medical professionalism. *Mount Sinai J Med*. 69(6): 357–362

Stryker, S. and Stratham A. (1985) Symbolic interaction role theory. In: E. Aronson and G. Lindzey (eds) *Handbook of Social Psychology* (pp. 311–378). New York: Random House

Swann, W.B. (1987) Identity negotiation: Where two roads meet. *J Personality Soc Psychol*. 53: 1038–1051

Swick, H.M., Szenas, P., Danoff, D., and Whitcomb, M.E. (1999) Teaching professionalism in undergraduate medical education. *JAMA*. 282(9): 830–832

Swick, H.M. (2000) Toward a normative definition of medical professionalism. *Acad Med*. 75: 612–616

Tennant, M. (1997) *Psychology and Adult Learning*. 2nd edn. Routledge: London

Thistlethwaite, J.E. and Spencer, J.A. (2008) *Professionalism in Medicine*. Abingdon, UK: Radcliffe Publishing Ltd

Tierney, W.G. (1997) Organizational socialization in higher education. *J Higher Educ*. 68: 1–16

Uhari, M., Kokkonen, J., Nuutinen, M. et al. (1994) Medical student abuse: an international phenomenon. *JAMA*. 271(13): 1049–1051

van de Camp, K., Vernooij-Dassen, M.J.F.J., Grol, R.P.T.M., and Bottema, B.J.A.M. (2004) How to conceptualize professionalism. *Med Teach*. 26(8): 696–702 van Maanen, J. and Barley, S.R. (1984) Occupational communities: culture and control in organizations. In: B.M. Staw, L.L. Cummings (eds) *Research in Organizational Behavior* (Vol 6 pp. 287–365). Greenwich, CT: JAI Press

van Mook, W.N., van Luijk, S.J., O'Sullivan, H., et al. (2009a) The concepts of professionalism and professional behaviour; Conflicts in both definition and learning outcome. *Eur J Intern Med.* 20(8): e85–e89

van Mook, W.N., de Grave, W.S., van Luijk, S.J., et al. (2009b) Training and learning professionalism in the medical school curriculum: Current consideration. *Eur J Intern Med.* 20(8): e96–e100

van Mook, W.N., de Grave, W.S., Wass, V., et al. (2009c) Professionalism: evolution of the concept. *Eur J Intern Med.* 20(8): e81–e84

Veloski, J.J., Fields, S.K., Boex, J.R., and Blank, L.L. (2005) Measuring professionalism: a review of studies with instruments reported in the literature between 1982 and 2002. *Acad Med.* 80: 366–370

Wagner, P., Hendrich, J., Moseley, G., and Hudson, V. (2007) Defining medical professionalism: a qualitative study. *Med Educ.* 41(3): 288–294

Wallace, D., Paulson, R., Lord, C., and Bond, CJ. (2005) Which behaviours do attitudes predict? Meta-analysing the effects of social pressure and perceived difficulty. *RevGen Psychol.* 9: 214–227

Wear, D., Aultman, J.M., Varley, J.D., and Zarconi, J. (2006) Making fun of patients: medical students' perceptions and use of derogatory and cynical humour in clinical settings. *Acad Med.* 81(5): 454–462

Wear, D. and Castellani, B. (2000) The development of professionalism: curriculum matters. *Acad Med.* 75: 602–611

Wilkerson, L. and Irby, D.M. (1998) Strategies for improving teaching practices: a comprehensive approach to faculty development. *Acad Med.* 73(4): 387–396

Wilkinson, T.J., Wade, W.B., and Knock, L.D. (2009) A blueprint to assess professionalism—results of a systematic review. *Acad Med.* 84: 551–558

Witz, A. (1992) *Professions and Patriarchy.* London: Routledge

Wynia, M.K., Latham, S.R., Kao, A.C., Berg, J.W., and Emanuel, L.L. (1999) Medical professionalism in society. *N Engl J Med.* 314(21): 1612–1616

CHAPTER 25

The resident as teacher

Tzu-Chieh Yu, Susan E. Farrell, and Andrew G. Hill

Therefore, the essential question is not, 'Do house officers function as teachers?' but rather, 'How can house officers be good teachers?'

Mark Barrow

Introduction

Residents are unique in their role as physician teachers and deserve encouragement, support and formal training on how to become effective and efficient clinical supervisors and teachers. This chapter begins with a primer on the vital role of resident teachers as well as the challenges they might face and the qualities they need in order to be successful. It also provides an up to date review of resident as teacher training programmes and their effectiveness at improving teaching knowledge, skills, and behaviours. Lastly, the chapter provides practical tips to guide readers through the essential steps involved in designing and implementing resident as teacher programmes.

Resident as teacher: roles, motivators, and challenges

The role of the resident teacher has taken on significant meaning in the last 40 years (Hill et al. 2009) and expanded to include a number of different functions and responsibilities. Residents are driven by a number of different motivating factors to participate in teaching but also face challenges as clinical teachers and supervisors including how best to achieve a balance with their clinical responsibilities. Understanding these aspects of the resident as teacher allows for planning and implementation of educational training programmes and organizational policies to better support resident teachers and to meet their professional development and learning needs.

It is widely recognized that residents fulfil crucial roles in undergraduate medical education. As clinical teachers and supervisors for medical students, residents are advantaged by the large amount of clinical time they spend with their learners, the directness of their supervision, and their closeness in age and professional development to students (Bordley and Litzelman 2000). Medical students identify residents as their most important clinical trainers (Remmen et al. 2000) and attribute up to one-third of their clinical education to teaching by interns and residents (Barrow 1966; Lowery 1976; Bing-You and Sproul 1992). Correspondingly, residents spend up to 25% of their time supervising, teaching and evaluating students and junior colleagues (Bing-You and Sproul 1992; Brown 1970; Hafler 2003).

Professional development of residents as teachers grew in popularity during the 1990s with an expansion of resident teacher-training interventions (Brown 1971) and a number of medical accreditation agencies coming to recognize that residents are a unique and essential group of clinical teachers deserving of acknowledgement and support. These included the Accreditation Council for Graduate Medical Education (ACGME) (2011), the Liaison Committee on Medical Education (LCME) (2011), The Royal College of Physicians and Surgeons of Canada (2005), and the General Medical Council (2006). Besides being a significant individual responsibility within the modern day multifaceted definition of 'professional practice', teaching also ties in with several other competencies including medical and technical knowledge, practice-based learning, and interpersonal and communication skills.

Teaching and supervision provided by residents has a number of distinguishing features. Most evidently, the resident teacher's role is predominantly practical, whereas teaching by faculty and attending clinicians is often dominated by theory (Stark 2003). Resident teaching focuses on the day-to-day management of patients and rarely involves the in-depth discussion and problem-solving teaching style typical of senior clinicians (Tremonti and Biddle 1982). A study of obstetrics and gynaecology clerkships found that medical students performed significantly more physical examinations and bedside investigative procedures during sessions with residents than with faculty (Johnson and Chen 2006). In this way, teaching contributions of residents complements, rather than duplicates, the teaching carried by senior clinicians (Bordage 1994; Bordage and Lemieux 1991; Wilkerson et al. 1986).

The approachability of residents also distinguishes them from senior attending clinicians (Kaji and Moorehead 2002) who can be perceived by medical students and allied healthcare staff to be distant figures of leadership and authority. It is often the resident who takes the time to direct patient management and explain the scientific reasoning behind clinical decisions to patients, medical students, junior colleagues, and members of the multidisciplinary healthcare team so that all efforts are coordinated.

Residents also 'teach on the run' and are seldom focused solely on teaching. In fact, they are constantly interchanging and combining their 'physician', 'learner', and 'teacher' roles in response to shifting expectations arising from the clinical environment (Busari and Scherpbier 2004). For example, grand rounds conducted in the presence of attending clinicians require residents to play the role of the 'physician-learner' who demonstrates clinical competency and an enthusiasm for acquiring new knowledge and skills. In comparison, during working ward rounds the same resident becomes the 'physician–teacher' at the patient's bedside who is striving to deliver efficient patient care whilst supervising and teaching interns and promoting medical student engagement and education. This ability to multitask makes residents effective role models of time-management and clinical prioritization. The nature of their clinical role constrains the time they have for teaching and self-learning and effective residents are adept at integrating learning and teaching within the fast-paced environment of inpatient clinical practice (Vu et al. 1997).

Residents are also credited with conveying the 'informal' or 'hidden' curriculum to medical students and junior colleagues, largely during contact outside of normal working hours when attending physicians are not present (Stern 1998). Taught alongside the formal structured curriculum, this parallel set of knowledge and skills is founded on the values, norms, and expectations of the clinical working and learning environment. Student development of medical professionalism is thought to partly develop from impromptu resident teaching of this unofficial and implicit curriculum (Stern 1998): as residents and students chat over meals, work together in emergency rooms, and walk the wards, they take the opportunity to reflect on and discuss the nature of their work and significance of values such as compassion, honesty, and accountability.

Even without outwardly discussing these issues, residents still impart them through role modelling and mentoring of medical students and interns (Remmen et al. 2000; De et al. 2004; Whittaker et al. 2006). This unscheduled 'real-life' demonstration and coaching of functional skills has been found to significantly impact self-evaluated 'preparedness to practise' of final-year medical students (Gome et al. 2008; Cave et al. 2009; Sheehan et al. 2005). Furthermore, mentoring by residents influences future career choices of medical students (Schwartz et al. 1991). This is particularly evident in the promotion of surgical specialties (Ek et al. 2005; McCord et al. 2009; Musunuru et al. 2007; Nguyen and Divino 2007; Ehrlich and Seidman 2006).

As well as influencing their learners' acquisition of knowledge and skills, residents help to create a positive and relaxed learning environment around students and interns, communicate a sense of enthusiasm, and demonstrate commitment to keeping abreast of research advances (Miller 1980). It is understood that residents influence the learning environment of students by adjusting their teaching style, demonstrating concern and interest in learner progress and welfare, and role-modelling (Hutchinson 2003). In these ways, residents contribute to learner satisfaction, engagement, and enjoyment (Whittle et al. 2007; Bassaw et al. 2003). After implementing a teacher-training workshop for obstetrics and gynaecology residents at the University of Michigan Hospital, Hammoud et al. (2004) found that medical students perceived an improvement in overall clerkship quality at this hospital. Similarly, a study of general surgery clerkships over 5 consecutive years at Jefferson

Medical College found that overall clerkship assessment by third-year medical students was influenced by three specific aspects of resident teaching: residents respecting students, providing teaching experiences, and serving as role models (Xu et al. 1998).

Residents are motivated to teach by a number of factors including a strong sense of intrinsic responsibility (Busari et al. 2002; Wilkerson et al. 1986). Residents also report that clinical teaching is enjoyable and consider it an important component of their own experience and education, presenting them with opportunities to revise prior clinical knowledge and skills and initiate self-directed learning (Apter et al. 1988; Sheets et al. 1991; Greenberg et al. 1984; Busari et al. 2000; Seely et al. 1999). This positivity is imperative because the resident teacher's enjoyment of and sense of responsibility towards clinical teaching ultimately influences its effectiveness (Wilkerson et al. 1986; Bing-You and Harvey 1991). A survey of 83 medical students from the University of Vermont College of Medicine has suggested that most residents develop an interest in clinical teaching prior to residency (Bing-You and Sproul 1992). The survey found that 80% of respondents had aspirations to teach peers during medical school and 93% had plans to resume this teaching responsibility during residency. Furthermore, 90% of the students surveyed indicated an interest in participating in formal teacher-training to improve their teaching skills prior to residency.

A common incentive for participating in teaching is the belief by residents that teaching benefits their personal learning (Apter et al. 1988; Greenberg et al. 1984). In theory, teaching allows clinical teachers to understand the medical educational process and this reinforces and improves their own didactic, cognitive, and clinical skills (Irby 1994). In practice, there is evidence to confirm that clinical teaching indeed allows for development of residents' own ability for self-directed learning, giving them a chance to review, reorganize and solidify knowledge and skills they already possess. Formal teaching by surgical residents has been found to enhance their knowledge acquisition independent of lecture attendance and self-study (Pelletier and Belliveau 1999) and their performance in formal examinations positively correlates with their rated teaching skills and abilities (Seely et al. 1999).

Despite indicating an enthusiasm for teaching and believing that teaching benefits not only the students but also themselves, a number of challenges stand in the way of residents participating in clinical teaching. Residents report that the presence of medical students can make their clinical responsibilities more difficult to carry out (Greenberg et al. 1984). One of the main challenges faced by residents is the conflict arising from efforts to prioritize multiple roles and duties bestowed upon them (Yedidia et al. 1995). Together with a lack of confidence as teachers, insufficient preparation prior to becoming clinical teachers, and a lack of support from senior clinicians, these represent the main barriers preventing residents from participating in clinical teaching (Apter et al. 1988; Busari et al. 2002). Residents are therefore likely to need significant encouragement, support, and recognition as clinical teachers because residency is a time when residents have a need for emotional support themselves yet they are relied on and feel obligated to nurture and give support to others (Yedidia et al. 1995).

Resident as teacher attributes

Effective and memorable resident teachers possess a number of different attributes and a diverse range of methods have been used to ascertain what these are in the hope that they can be engendered in all residents. Most studies have involved major stakeholders—residents, medical students, senior clinicians, medical educationists, and residency programme directors and used questionnaires, interviews, and focus groups (Dunnington and DaRosa 1998; Katzelnick et al. 1991; Susman and Gilbert 1995; White et al. 1997). A smaller number of studies have been predominantly grounded in theories and observations.

As a way of assessing the needs of resident teachers, Wilkerson et al. (1986) observed 14 first- and second-year residents during working ward rounds and found that the most frequent teaching behaviours demonstrated by residents were those associated with patient care at the bedside: providing a model of appropriate interaction with patients and verifying clinical findings. They also found that, away from the bedside, residents frequently required lecturing skills but did not habitually demonstrate skills in giving feedback, asking stimulating questions, or referring to the literature. With this information, the investigators initiated a course on clinical teaching for residents. In pursuit of the same objective, Katz et al. (2003) performed a needs assessment of resident teaching skills by observing their teaching encounters with medical students in obstetrics and gynaecology outpatient clinics and recording behaviours with an 18-item checklist. Residents were found to be efficient managers of time, enthusiastic teachers, and role-models of professional behaviour but deficient in giving feedback, planning future learning, and orientating learners to their surroundings.

Busari et al. have also made significant contributions in this area by exploring the perceptions of residents (Busari et al. 2002) and attending clinicians (Busari et al. 2003) towards the skills and cognitions thought necessary to be effective resident teachers (table 25.1). Other authors who have contributed in similar ways include Brown (1970) who found that resident teachers asked for training in instructional methods, public speaking, and student evaluation, and Rotenberg et al. (2000) who found that surgical residents need time management skills, an understanding of the students' formal learning objectives, appreciation for the appropriate times and locations to teach, and the ability to foster good team relationships. Resident participants also reported that having the right attitude towards clinical teaching is an important resident teacher attribute.

Ultimately, as the harshest critic of resident teachers, the perceptions and insights of medical students are important in defining the attributes of good resident teachers (Tonesk 1979). Most frequently in a position to receive teaching by residents, medical students and residents have been shown to agree on the levels of competence, confidence, and motivation required by resident teachers (Henry et al. 2006). Elnicki and Cooper (2005) surveyed 72 third-year medical students at the completion of their 4-week general internal medicine rotation and found that the perceived effectiveness of resident teaching correlated most with the resident teachers' role-modelling, availability to students, demonstration of effective patient education, confidence in clinical knowledge and skills, and enthusiasm for teaching.

Based on current understanding of resident roles and responsibilities, several other teacher attributes come to mind including the ability to integrate teaching and learner supervision into patient care. This was recognized by Irby who found that attending physicians who were successful at combining clinical and teaching responsibilities accomplished this by completing three tasks: 'diagnose the patient', 'diagnose the learner', and 'teach the learner' (Irby 1992). Residents need practical and realistic teaching strategies that allow them to simultaneously

Table 25.1 The skills of effective resident teachers

Residents' suggestions (Busari et al. 2002)	Attending clinicians' suggestions (Busari et al. 2003)
Ability to present information Ability to transfer knowledge Ability to explain concepts	1. Teaching skills ◆ Set teaching objectives ◆ Problem-solve ◆ Stimulate learners to learn
Ability to give feedback to learners	2. Communication ◆ Ability to interact with medical students ◆ Ability to give feedback
	3. Clinical skills ◆ Perform and teach clinical skills effectively ◆ Conduct literature searches to answer clinical questions and teach this skill
	4. Attitude ◆ Appropriate professional conduct towards students, patients, and nursing staff ◆ Professional responsibility
	5. Self-assessment ◆ Rate own ability as a doctor ◆ Rate own ability as a clinical teacher
	6. Time management skills
	7. Assessment of peers and students

teach and delivery patient care. Bordley and Litzelman (2000) argue that having a student on their team should not require residents to change daily routines or reduce clinical activities.

An organized and structured method of defining resident attributes for precepting medical students is to breakdown the clinical clerkship into stages where each stage requires a specific set of teaching and supervision skills. Kates and Lesser (1985) proposed that specific tasks can be systematically assigned to four different stages of student supervision (table 25.2). Alseidi (2007) proposed a similar structure that also divided student clerkships into four phases. To produce mutually beneficial and enjoyable teaching and learning experiences, residents and medical students should aim to fulfil the conditions within each phase.

Different clinical environments within medical specialties also play a part in shaping the combination of teaching attributes required by residents. For example, residents in surgical specialties may teach under tremendous time constraints as a consequence of responsibilities in the operating theatre, outpatient clinic, ward, and emergency room. If they are to be successful teachers, their teaching repertoire needs to overcome this obstacle and a set of practical teaching concepts, skills, and techniques have been suggested by Jamshidi and Ozgediz (2008) for the time-constrained surgical resident. These include the ability to recognize teachable moments, demonstrate model behaviour, think aloud to provide learners with the clinician's train of thought, make the student the teacher, prearrange teaching times, and provide orientation to learning expectations.

Table 25.2 The resident teacher's roles and responsibilities during different phases of the student clerkship

Clerkship phase	Description	Resident teacher responsibilities
Preparation	Prior to commencement of student clerkship	Residents should familiarize themselves with clerkship learning objectives and negotiate their own clinical responsibilities to make time for teaching.
Negotiation and planning	Resident and students meet to clarify roles and expectations	Residents should be able to clearly specify what is expected of students and also gauge their prior knowledge and experience.
Working	Resident and student work together on the job, sticking to previously negotiated expectations and learning outcomes	Residents need a range of teaching skills during this stage—these include being able to adjust teaching to diverse clinical settings, coach students on clinical and technical skills, offer regular feedback, stimulate independent learning, and role-model professionalism.
Closing	Resident performs student assessment, debrief, and send-off	Residents should perform student assessment and debriefing

Residents and interns are exposed to medical students at a time when their own knowledge has not yet solidified and they may feel uncomfortable teaching because attempts to meet the needs of student learners might undermine their self-confidence (Yedidia et al. 1995). With the emphasis placed on residents 'knowing' and 'comprehending', successful resident teachers also need assurance that occasionally admitting to 'not knowing' is part of the teaching experience.

Interventions to develop effective resident teachers

One of the most recent notable advances in medical education is the realization that clinical teachers should be and can be trained to teach more effectively. Resident as teacher programmes were first described in the 1960s and 1970s and became widely recognized in the 1990s (Brown 1971) as a means of improving resident teaching skills. In 2001, a survey conducted by Morrison et al. (2001) found that 55% of residency programmes in the US included a formal component of teacher-training.

Resident as teacher programmes can vary significantly in curricula and delivery methods and also in how they have been evaluated. Current understanding of how they should be developed, implemented, and evaluated, and what impact they deliver arises from a combination of teaching and learning theories, methodical research, and practical experience and expertise.

Curriculum content, structure, and delivery

With so many recognized competencies and teaching skills required by resident teachers and no consensus as to which ones should be prioritized, it follows that resident as teacher programmes vary significantly in their interventional focus and curriculum content. On examining the course structures and delivery methods, significant discrepancy is also found. One further distinguishing factor of resident as teacher programmes is whether they are focused on resident teachers of specific professional disciplines or whether a generic interdisciplinary model is used.

Resident as teacher programmes have included theoretical concepts and practical skill sets. Principles and philosophies of instructing and the theories of adult learning are found alongside the distinguishing features of individual learning and teaching styles and various learner-centred and teacher-centred approaches to knowledge transfer. Practical teaching skills and techniques that have been utilized include learner orientation, micro-skills of teaching, bedside teaching, teaching psychomotor skills, teaching in the operating theatre, structuring a teaching lesson, and giving lectures. Giving effective feedback and learner evaluation also feature in many courses. While the majority of resident as teacher programmes are a combination of theory and practice structured into multiple training modules, a small number of programmes have focused on improving a specific teaching proficiency. For example, Furney et al. (2001) implemented a brief 1-hour course for resident teachers focused on Neher's 'One-minute Preceptor' model of microskills teaching and Frattarelli and Kasuya (2003) developed a 4.5 hour programme aimed at instructing residents on the microskills of facilitating problem-based learning.

Concepts of the 'professionalism of teaching' can also be found in the curricula of a number of resident as teacher programmes, summed up under headings such as 'improving the learning climate' (Rubak et al. 2008) and 'what makes a good teacher' (Hammoud et al. 2004). These modules recognize that residents need to be prepared for their role in covering the 'informal' curriculum and demonstrate caring teacher attitudes and professional conduct towards students, patients, and colleagues. Moving beyond the resident as educator, resident as teacher curricula have also been combined with other professional development courses. Subject matter has included leadership, planning and time management skills, mentoring, and career counselling (Wipf et al. 1999; Susman and Gilbert 1995; Rubak et al. 2008; Busari et al. 2006b).

Significant variations in programme participants, delivery settings, and methods used to evaluate educational value and effectiveness exist among resident as teacher programmes that have been evaluated. While some recruit only residents, others have involved faculty members participating alongside residents (Pandachuck et al. 2004; Rubak et al. 2008). Programme structures of programmes have consisted of singular to multiple sessions or workshops of varying duration and frequency over the span of several weeks or months. They have also included intensive multiday retreats (Litzelman et al. 1994), month-long fellowships (Troupin 1990) and electives (Weissman et al. 2006). 'Refresher' courses have also featured in the delivery of a number of resident as teacher interventions, providing revision and feedback after the predominant initial session. For example, Roberts et al. (1994) implemented a 1-hour refresher session for paediatric resident teachers 6 months after they had attended a 2-day training retreat.

Programme instructional methods have included lectures and small-group discussions, as well as more interactive role-play and simulation training activities. Teaching scenarios are set up involving standardized students and revolve around common challenges faced by resident teachers. Many involve the use of audiovisual recording of simulated teaching sessions before, during, and after actual training interventions for the purposes of resident self-reflection and examination of improvements. Table 25.3 outlines the structure and instructional methods of well-described resident as teacher programmes that have had significant effects on participant teaching knowledge, skills, and behaviour.

Evaluation and evidence of effectiveness

The evaluation of resident as teacher programmes has progressed alongside their development—evaluations have featured a range of different measurement tools and endpoints. Attempts have been made to systematically review and summarize a growing body of evidence conveying the educational impact of resident as teacher programmes (Busari and Scherpbier 2004; Dewey et al. 2008; Wamsley et al. 2004; Morrison and Hafler 2000), but efforts have been hampered by marked heterogeneity amongst described programmes and evaluation strategies, and a general lack of research rigour (Hill et al. 2009). As a consequence, no conclusions have been drawn in regards to the common features of successful programmes and the true total impact of resident as teacher programmes. There is also limited research on how resident as teacher programmes affect the learning outcomes of those who are taught and supervised by resident participants. These issues remain the focus for future research efforts.

Medical educationalists commonly conceptualize education outcomes as a series of levels through which the learner progresses. Such outcomes-focused models provide programme coordinators and designers with a summative knowledge of the intervention's rationale, goal, and intended outcomes as well as the inputs and processes require to arrive at those outcomes. A frequently used framework to define evaluation endpoints and measure impact 'size' from educational interventions is the Kirkpatrick's 'Model of Learning'. Its basic structure provides an appropriate basis for evaluation of medical education interventions and modifications can be made so that levels match learning outcomes and competencies specific to residents as teachers (table 25.4). Assembled from four levels, with defined achievement criteria at each level, it provides educationists, programme co-ordinators, and researchers with a basic organised structure to explore the impact of resident as teacher interventions.

At the basic levels of the Kirkpatrick's model, an intervention should bring about a subjective response and a change in perceptions and attitudes in participants. A number of resident as teacher programmes have been shown to increase resident enthusiasm for teaching and to improve their confidence as teachers over a sustained period of time (Litzelman et al. 1998; Lawson and Harvill 1980; Edwards et al. 1986, 1988; Dunnington and DaRosa 1998; Jewett et al. 1982). Although not often valued in the same way as objective outcomes, subjective and qualitative outcome measures often reveal important details that can otherwise be missed (Johnson et al. 1996). Success of resident as teacher programmes can lie in the residents' acceptance of the curricula and delivery methods and the value they place on the training provided. In fact, the attitudes and self-perceived capabilities of newly trained residents may go on to influence their future plans to participate in teaching (Janicik et al. 2001).

Preparation of residents for teaching also influences their enjoyment of and enthusiasm for teaching. A year after implementing a resident as teacher workshop, Morrison et al. (2005) found that resident participants expressed greater enthusiasm for teaching, more learner-centred and empathic approaches, and a richer understanding of teaching principles and skills. In comparison, those who did not receive the formal teacher training did not enjoy teaching, had few plans to teach in the future, became frustrated by clinical time constraints, and demonstrated cynicism and blame toward learners (Morrison et al. 2005). This suggests that one main goal of resident as teacher interventions is not to transform residents into fully fledged clinical teachers but to arm them with basic teaching knowledge and skills so that they can participate with confidence, enjoy teacher-learner interactions, and eventually develop their own individual teaching styles.

To advance to middle-ranking levels of the Kirkpatrick's model, educational interventions should bring about measurable improvements in participant knowledge, skills, and behaviour and there is a substantial body of evidence to show that resident as teacher programmes achieve these criteria (Hill et al. 2009). A wide variety of evaluation methods have been used to show this and involve including self-assessment by participating residents or assessment by course facilitators, independent 'experts', standardized students, peers, and actual students and interns. Post-, pre-post-, and retrospective pre-post study designs are common but comparison studies can also be found including several randomized controlled trials (Jewett et al. 1982; Morrison et al. 2004; D'Eon 2004; Dunnington and DaRosa 1998). Iinvestigators have sought to use validated evaluation tools and checklists and the direct observation of residents has occurred during actual and videotaped teaching sessions. Written examinations and objective structured teaching examinations also feature prominently as standardized quantitative methods of assessing improvements in teaching ability brought about by resident as teacher interventions.

The objective structured teaching examination is modelled after the objective structured clinical examination (OSCE) but concentrates on demonstration and application of teaching knowledge and skills (Zabar et al. 2004). Developed to provide standard evaluation of faculty and resident teaching skills, it is widely believed to be the most objective tool available and has contributed significantly to outcome-based research. The objective structured teaching examination has been used to evaluate the effectiveness of several programmes (Dunnington and DaRosa 1998; Gaba et al. 2007; Morrison et al. 2004; Zabar et al. 2004) and there have been efforts to improve its reliability and validity (Morrison et al. 2002; Prislin et al. 1998). Standardized learners, like standardized patients, are trained to portray challenging learners and can also be called upon to rate resident teachers and provide feedback. When not used in an assessment capacity, objective structured teaching examinations double as structured teaching encounters that have been used to improve teaching performance of residents and faculty. Their qualitative evaluation has generally been positive (Trowbridge et al. 2011). The drawbacks of using objective structured teaching

Table 25.3 Curriculum and delivery methods of sample resident as teacher interventions that have been evaluated

Reference	Specialty	Structure	Curriculum
(Lawson and Harvill 1980)	Family practice, internal medicine	13 × 1-hour weekly sessions (= 13 hours)	5 instructional packages: *objectives and planning; delivery methods; discussion questioning; demonstration techniques audiovisuals; lecturing*
(Snell 1989)	Internal medicine	5 × 3-hour seminars (= 15 hours)	6 resident teaching skills: *large-group teaching (the lecture); small-group teaching (leading a discussion); one-on-one teaching (tutorials); bedside and clinical teaching; the art of feedback; teaching and learning styles*
(Katzelnick et al. 1991)	Psychiatry	1-day workshop	Multiple topics including: *'importance of residents as teachers'; 'basic concepts of learning'; 'roles of teaching in psychiatry'; 'organizing and presenting effective lectures'; 'task-oriented small-group learning'; 'principles of problem-based learning'; 'bedside clinical teaching and supervision'; 'evaluation of medical students in psychiatry'; 'problematic student encounters'*
(Litzelman et al. 1994)	Internal medicine	2-day retreat	Stanford Faculty Development Program (SFDP) Clinical Teaching Component
(Spickard et al. 1996)	Internal medicine	3-hour workshop	2 core teaching topics: 1. Learning climate: *stimulate learner participation in discussions and decisions; identify the learner's understanding of the patient case* 2. Giving feedback: *communicate teacher's assessment of learner performance*
(Dunnington and DaRosa, 1998)	General surgery	3 × sessions, over 2 days (= 10.5 hours)	7 × instructional modules: *adult learning principles or microskills of teaching; teaching at the bedside; feedback skills; teaching psychomotor skills; teaching in the clinic; teaching in the operating room; senior resident as manager*
(Wipf et al. 1999)	Internal medicine	3 × 2-hour sessions (= 6 hours)	Multiple topics including: *developing team leadership skills; conducting effective work rounds; interacting with attending physicians; practising teaching skills; teaching medical students; using feedback and evaluation; dealing with problem behaviour*
(Furney et al. 2001)	Internal medicine	1-hour session	One-Minute Preceptor teaching model – '5 micro-skills'
(Morrison et al. 2004)	Family practice, internal medicine, paediatrics	1 × 3-hour mini-retreat + 10 × 1-hour sessions (= 13 hours)	– Bringing Education & Service Together (BEST): 8 × modules (*leadership/role modelling; orienting learners; giving feedback; bedside teaching; teaching procedures; inpatient teaching; teaching charting; giving lectures*) – Exploring *'teachable moments'* – '5-step microskills' model
(Busari et al. 2006a)	Paediatrics, O&G	2-day workshop	6 educational modules: *effective teaching; self-knowledge and teaching ability; feedback skills; assessing prior knowledge; trouble shooing; time management*
(Gaba et al. 2007)	O&G	6 × 1.5 hour workshops (= 10.5 hours)	3-Function model of clinical teaching (*prepare for the learning exercise; perform the exercise; process what happened*)
(Moser 2008)	Internal medicine, paediatrics, O&G	8-hour programme + 7 × 1-hour sessions, over 6 months (= 15 hours)	– 'Train-the-trainer' teaching skills program: *'why residents can be excellent teachers'; 'one-minute preceptor'; 'how do we learn best?'; 'five-minute teaching strategies'; 'how to give effective feedback'; 'orienting your students to goals and expectations'; 'what's in a great question?'* – Facilitation skills developed through role-play, brainstorming, reflection, and small-group discussions
(Hill et al. 2012)	Not applicable	1.5 day workshop	4 learning modules: *General principles of clinical teaching; bedside teaching; giving effective feedback; teaching effective discussion; leading and lecturing*

Table 25.4 Modified Kirkpatrick's 'Model of Learning' Framework

Level 1	Reaction	Participants' views of the learning experience, its organization, presentation, content, teaching methods, and quality of instruction.
Level 2	Learning Change in attitudes; modification of knowledge or skills	Changes in the attitudes or perceptions among participants towards teaching and learning Modified knowledge: acquisition of concepts, procedures and principles Modified skills: acquisition of thinking/problem-solving, psychomotor and social skills.
Level 3	Behaviour Change in behaviour	Documents the transfer of learning to the workplace. Willingness of learners to apply new knowledge and skills.
Level 4A	Results Change in system/organizational practice	Refers to wider changes in the organization, attributable to the educational programme
Level 4B	Results Change among participants' learners, students, peers	Refers to improvement in medical student or resident peer learning or performance as a direct result of the educational intervention.

Reproduced from Hill, A. G., Yu, T. C., Barrow, M. & Hattie, J., 'A systematic review of resident-as-teacher programmes', *Medical Education*, 43, pp. 1129–1140, 2009, with permission from Association for the Study of Medical Education and Wiley.

examinations outside of research settings are the time and expense requirements (Morrison and Hafler 2000).

While the objective structured teaching examination remains an artificial environment, a number of studies have found that teaching skills obtained during resident as teacher interventions can be transferred to real-life clinical environments. By recruiting medical students and interns as learner-observers, the effectiveness of resident as teacher programmes has been rated in pre-post intervention and comparison–control studies. For example, resident teaching skills after a half-day workshop were rated by third-year medical students (Edwards et al. 1988) using the Clinical Teaching Assessment developed by Irby and Rakestraw (1981). In comparison to controls, residents who had attended the workshop received significantly higher scores for four of the nine assessment items ('knowledge', 'organizational skills', 'demonstration of clinical skills', and 'overall teaching effectiveness'). Several similar studies have also demonstrated improvements in resident teacher ratings after programme attendance (Moser 2008; Wipf et al. 1999; Pandachuck et al. 2004). Potential challenges with using rating scales include deciding which instrument to use and how best to have the raters complete it an objective and independent manner.

The most convincing measure of resident teaching effectiveness maybe the achievement of learning objectives by their students. Without a good understanding of how residents' teaching abilities affect the performance of their learners, it has been difficult to determine whether improving residents' teaching skills improves their learners' clinical performance (Morrison and Hafler 2000). Thomas et al. (2002) demonstrated that a brief resident as teacher tutorial outlining the principles of teaching clinical skills coupled with an expert demonstration of common physical examination skills led to significantly improved OSCE performances by medical students under the supervision of resident participants. The study however was small and did not provide a full description of the resident as teacher intervention.

Most recently, Hill et al. (2012) attempted to demonstrate the same link between improved resident teaching skills and enhanced student performance by implementing a 1.5-day residents as teacher workshop for interns. They found improved intern attitudes and perceptions towards clinical teaching (Yu et al. 2010)

and observable advances in their teaching behaviour (Hill et al. 2012). Disappointingly, medical student OSCE grades did not show obvious improvements in achievement of surgical clerkship learning objectives (Hill et al. 2012). Thus, at the highest level of Kirkpatrick's model, evidence supporting residents as teacher interventions is limited (Hill et al. 2009). It is important to remember that outcomes-focused models such as Kirkpatrick's model provide little insight into the processes by which an educational programme yields its desired outcomes and the underlying mechanisms that hinder or enable the achievement of such outcomes. These models also have no way of capturing any unintended effects and outcomes that provide investigators with a richer and more comprehensive understanding of the programme's value. Consequently, the following points are speculation at this stage.

To dissect out some of the possible reasons for their findings, Hill et al. (2012) raised several important considerations aside from the suitability of the resident as teacher intervention. First, they question whether resident as teacher programmes actually have the potential to immediately improve formal learning outcomes of medical students. They refer to faculty development programmes that have been developed to improve the teaching skills of senior clinicians. Like resident as teacher programmes, these parallel interventions improve the pedagogic skills of faculty and attending clinicians but there is little evidence to suggest that they positively impact student performance and learning outcomes (Steinert et al. 2006). Medical students are individuals with profound capacity to adapt and self-motivate, likely possessing the ability to achieve assessed learning outcomes regardless of the teaching they receive. Perhaps even the best clinical teachers only play a minor part in their learning.

Secondly, as pointed out by Hill et al. (2012), the clinical skills and knowledge taught to students by residents are not necessarily those examined by formal curriculum-based assessments. It is widely accepted that residents teach a significant proportion of the 'informal' curriculum where skills and knowledge are focused on the day-to-day aspects of patient management (procedural skills, patient communication, task prioritization) (Tremonti and Biddle 1982). Without detailed descriptions of how residents of different disciplines contribute to the learning environment of medical students and interns, researchers cannot conclusively evaluate the effectiveness of their teaching contributions.

Practical tips for design and implementation

The wealth of literature about programmes to develop residents as teachers makes this educational endeavour an appealing project for post-graduate programme directors and academic faculty. Furthermore, they have a responsibility to help residents achieve all the skills and behaviours which will make them the best physicians that they can be. It follows that having skills as a teacher should enhance a trainee's abilities to communicate with both learners and patients. Therefore, investment in residents as teachers is a logical choice for promoting, improving, and sustaining the medical profession. However, because the evidence for the long-term impact of resident as teacher programmes is scant, designing and implementing these resource-intensive programmes should be undertaken with much planning and a realistic assessment of residents' needs and the intended institutional outcomes.

Several issues and challenges need to be considered when designing a resident as teacher programme. These include decisions about programme content and methods of implementation and evaluation such as:

♦ What educational content will be focused on, and how will it be defined and operationalized?

♦ What teaching skills and behaviours will be taught to residents?

♦ What are the contexts in which residents will apply these skills?

♦ How will the programme be implemented?

♦ How will the impact of the programme be evaluated, relative to intended goals and outcomes?

The answers to these questions will depend on the intended goals of the programme and the resources available to implement and evaluate it.

One of the first decisions to be made in designing a programme is the focus of the content. Should the content consist of specialty-specific knowledge, skills, or behaviours that are part of the residents' daily interactions with learners? Or should the programme focus on general professional behaviours that are part of the teaching–learning encounter and the doctor–patient relationship? Examples of these behaviours may include residents' role-modelling of professional behaviours that reflect interpersonal communications skills, ethical interactions with patients and families, the development of practice-based learning and improvement plans, interprofessional systems-based practice, and the importance of giving effective feedback. It is also plausible to construct a balanced programme covering both general and specialty-specific teaching skills and behaviours.

The breadth of content for a programme can be expansive and this initial decision should be based on a needs assessment of the teaching behaviours and skills that are felt to be important for the residents' personal improvement, the educational needs of the learners with whom the residents have frequent contact, and the educational goals of the institution. The expertise and availability of programme faculty and the availability of necessary resources (programme funding, programme time within the residents' training curriculum, physical teaching space, and course materials) will also impact decisions about course content.

The context in which residents are expected to teach should be considered when defining the programme content as well as the programme's pedagogical methods. Residents, who are being asked to learn and practise new teaching skills within their existing responsibilities, need to understand why teaching skills are pertinent and beneficial to their personal development. They need to feel confident that they will acquire education-related knowledge and skills that will be feasible and gratifying for them to use in their daily work.

Alternatively, the decision about teaching context may be influenced by the clinical areas in which residents are the primary patient care providers, where residents can make the greatest educational impact for learners, or in which there is a specific need for enhanced teaching. For example, is there a need to enhance residents' teaching in the outpatient clinic, on inpatient ward rounds, or in specific physical spaces in the clinical setting, such as the operating theatre, emergency department, or procedural suite? Defining the teaching context will inform subsequent decisions about the teaching skills and methods to be imparted and practised in the programme.

Finally, careful consideration should be given to the teaching knowledge and skills most compatible with the daily work and patient care responsibilities of residents. An educational 'toolbox' that consists of teaching skills that are adaptable and can be efficiently employed are the best skills on which to focus during the programme. Teaching skills that most commonly align with the resident role are often patient-centred, and include bedside teaching (or teaching with the patient present during the encounter), clinical case-based discussions, and procedural teaching. Many residency programmes also expect residents to be able to lead small group teaching discussions and to lecture to larger groups of learners. The majority of these clinical teaching responsibilities and patient-centred teaching behaviours are opportunities for the explicit training of residents in the educational importance of professional role-modelling and providing effective feedback to learners.

Once the programme content has been prioritized, the programme director should assess the available resources for implementing the programme. These resources include programme funding, personnel, programme time within the residents' training curriculum, physical teaching space, and programme equipment and materials. In terms of personnel, it may be desirable to bring a team of additional faculty and educators into the programme as content and pedagogical experts. It may be necessary to recruit and train faculty to facilitate small groups of residents in practising new teaching skills, fostering individual reflection on the challenges of applying newly learned skills, and providing individualized feedback and ideas for adapting new teaching skills in the clinical workplace. Recently appointed specialists who practise in academic clinical environments are potential faculty who can reinforce the importance of having a solid teaching background, and provide real-world context to future teaching requirements.

Time is a significant resource in any postgraduate training curriculum and the intentions of the resident as teacher programme and its expected outcomes need to be realistic (considering the time allowed). Obviously, the more expansive the resident as teacher programme, the longer the required programme time. It is important to note that the literature indicates that once-off intensive resident as teacher sessions can have an immediate impact on residents' confidence in and application of new teaching behaviours, but that many teaching behaviours will not be sustainable

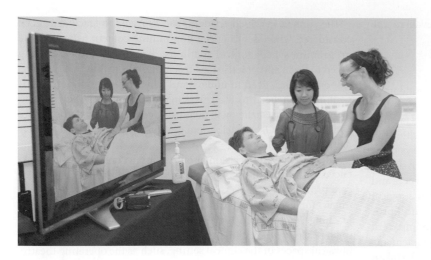

Figure 25.1 A resident as teacher course participant is captured on video while she directly observes her student learner demonstrate clinical skills during a simulated bedside teaching scenario.
Courtesy of Dr Susan Hawken, University of Auckland

over a prolonged period of time (greater than 6 to 10 months) if there is no opportunity for support through refresher sessions and on-going feedback. Ideally, the resident as teacher curriculum is one that is integrated longitudinally across the residency programme curriculum. This longitudinal approach to resident teacher training allows for ongoing skills building and reinforcement, and recurrent opportunities for review, discussion, and problem-solving about real-life teaching challenges. Although time-intensive, a longitudinal resident as teacher curriculum, integrated into the formal programme curriculum, signifies to the residents the importance and value of teaching in their programme's academic environment.

The implementation of a resident as teacher programme should model principles of experiential learning as they apply to the programme content and the intended outcomes. Residents learn much of their medicine as apprentices in the clinical environment. They are used to active learning that is based on their need to understand medicine in order to care for their patients and they use recurrent clinical experiences to improve their clinical skills. A resident as teacher programme should follow similar principles.

Consider using clinical teaching case vignettes that are realistic to residents' work experiences in order to prompt an interest and desire to know more about teaching skills. Activate residents' prior knowledge about clinical teaching experiences, as both teachers and learners in the clinical environment. The challenge of teaching in the context of clinical work is real for both residents and faculty, but programme faculty should role-model the fact that clinical teaching is not an insurmountable task. Help residents to share their successes, challenges, or concerns about their teaching role. Provide a safe, non-judgemental environment in which residents can openly contribute, and develop mutual respect for common challenges related to resident teaching. Address challenges in collaborative, problem-solving discussions that focus on the feasibility of acquiring and practising new skills together.

Give residents evidence-based information about educational principles and teaching skills that are realistic to the residents' work life. Allow for questions and then create opportunities for practice. Devote time to residents' active teaching skills practice in facilitated small groups that foster shared learning and allow time for

individual reflection and feedback. Depending on the skill being taught, practice may include the use of volunteer students, standardized patients, and videotaped practice with time for individual review (fig. 25.1). Videotape review and cooperative peer and faculty feedback, focused on positive teaching behaviours and problem-solving ideas to approach challenges should further residents' reflection on their new learning, and thoughts about ways to adapt and improve their teaching skills. Finally, individual and group brainstorming about how to adapt new teaching skills in realistic environments should help resident participants to visualize and plan teaching and learning encounters with clinical learners.

It cannot be stressed too much how important it is to provide ongoing supervision, one-on-one observation and consultation, and feedback to residents who are becoming teachers for the first time in their clinical workplace. Resident as teacher programme faculty need to support the programme outcomes through their willingness to continue to advise on difficult teaching encounters after the formal programme ends.

Conclusions

◆ Helping residents carry out the important mission of teaching perpetuates medical education as the basis for promoting and imparting clinical knowledge as well as the values of communication, self-reflection, and nurturing that are core characteristics of medical professionals.

◆ The role of the resident teacher is complex and challenging. They have to possess clinical competence and also the ability to convey their clinical knowledge and skills to learners while at the same time ensuring patient care and safety.

◆ Resident as teacher training programmes have become a key feature in the development of new teachers and have a number of positive effects, including improved resident attitudes and perceptions towards clinical teaching, as well as enhanced teacher confidence, knowledge, skills, and behaviours

◆ Effective resident as teacher programmes require advanced planning and preparation, careful assessment of resident needs, dedicated co-ordinators and facilitators with adequate expertise, and a comprehensive evaluation plan.

References

Accreditation Council for Graduate Medical Education (2011) *Accreditation Council for Graduate Medical Education. Common Program Requirements, Effective July 2011* [Online]. http://www.acgme.org/acWebsite/dutyHours/dh_dutyhoursCommonPR07012007.pdf Accessed 12 September 2011

Alseidi, A. (2007) The resident-student teaching encounter: a structured method. *Am J Surg.* 193: 784–785

Apter, A., Metzger, R., and Glassroth, J. (1988) Residents' perceptions of their roles as teachers. *J Med Educ.* 63: 900–905

Barrow, M.V. (1965) The house officer as a medical educator. *J Med Educ.* 40: 712–714.

Barrow, M. (1966) Medical students' opinions of the house officer as teacher. *J Med Educ.* 41: 807–810

Bassaw, B., Roff, S., Mcaleer, S., et al. (2003) Students' perspectives on the educational environment, Faculty of Medical Sciences, Trinidad. *Med Teach.* 25: 522–526

Bing-You, R.G. and Harvey, B.J. (1991) Factors related to residents' desire and ability to teach in the clinical setting. *Teach Learn Med.* 3: 95–100

Bing-You, R.G. and Sproul, M.S. (1992) Medical students' perceptions of themselves and residents as teachers. *Med Teach.* 14: 133–138

Bordage, G. (1994) Elaborated knowledge: a key to successful diagnostic thinking. *Acad Med.* 69: 883–885

Bordage, G. and Lemieux, M. (1991) Semantic structures and diagnostic thinking of experts and novices. *Acad Med.* 66: S70–S72

Bordley, D.R. and Litzelman, D.K. (2000) Preparing residents to become more effective teachers: a priority for internal medicine. *Am J Med.* 109: 693–696

Brown, R.S. (1970) House staff attitudes towards teaching. *J Med Educ.* 45: 156–159

Brown, R S. (1971) Pedagogy for surgical house staff. *J Med Educ.* 46: 93–95

Busari, J.O. and Scherpbier, A.J. (2004) Why residents should teach: a literature review. *J Postgrad Med.* 50: 205–210

Busari, J.O., Prince, K.J., Scherpbier, A.J., van der Vleuten, C.P., and Essed, G.G. (2002) How residents perceive their teaching role in the clinical setting: a qualitative study. *Med Teach.* 24: 57–61

Busari, J.O., Scherpbier, A.J.J.A., van der Vleuten, C.P.M., and Essed, G.E. (2000) Residents' perception of their role in teaching undergraduate students in the clinical setting. *Med Teach.* 22: 348–353

Busari, J.O., Scherpbier, A.J., van der Vleuten, C.P, and Essed, G.G. (2003) The perceptions of attending doctors of the role of residents as teachers of undergraduate clinical students. *Med Educ.* 37: 241–247

Busari, J.O., Scherpbier, A., van der Vleuten, C.P.M. and Essed, G.G.M. (2006a) A Two-day Teacher-Training Programme for Medical Residents: Investigating the Impact on Teaching Ability. *Adv Health Sci Educ.* 11: 133–144

Busari, J.O., Scherpbier, A.J.J.A., van der Vleuten, C.P.M., Essed, G.G.M., and Rojer, R. (2006b) A description of a validated effective teacher-training workshop for medical residents. *Med Educ Online.* 11: 1–8

Cave, J., Woolf, K., Jones, A., and Dacre, J. (2009) Easing the transition from student to doctor: how can medical schools help prepare their graduates for starting work? *Med Teach.* 31: 403–408

D'eon, M.F. (2004) Evaluation of a teaching workshop for residents at the University of Saskatchewan: a pilot study. *Acad Med.* 79: 791–797

De, S.K., Henke, P.K., Ailawadi, G., Dimick, J.B., and Colletti, L.M. (2004) Attending, house officer, and medical student perceptions about teaching in the third-year medical school general surgery clerkship. *J Am Coll Surg.* 199: 932–942

Dewey, C.M., Coverdale, J.H., Ismail, N.J., et al. (2008) Residents-as-teachers programs in psychiatry: a systematic review. *Can J Psychiatry.* 53: 77–84.

Dunnington, G.L. and Darosa, D. (1998) A prospective randomized trial of a residents-as-teachers training program. *Acad Med.* 73: 696–700

Edwards, J.C., Kissling, G.E., Plauche, W C. and Marier, R.L. (1986) Long-term evaluation of training residents in clinical teaching skills. *J Med Educ.* 61: 967–970

Edwards, J.C., Kissling, G.E., Plauche, W.C., and Marier, R.L. (1988) Evaluation of a teaching skills improvement programme for residents. *Med Educ.* 22: 514–517

Ehrlich, P.F. and Seidman, P.A. (2006) Deconstructing surgical education-teacher quality really matters: implications for attracting medical students to surgical careers. *Am Surg.* 72: 430–434

Ek, E.W., Ek, E.T., and Mackay, S.D. (2005) Undergraduate experience of surgical teaching and its influence on career choice. *ANZ J Surg.* 75: 713–718

Elnicki, D.M. and Cooper, A. (2005) Medical students' perceptions of the elements of effective inpatient teaching by attending physicians and housestaff. *J Gen Intern Med.* 20: 635–639

Frattarelli, L.C. and Kasuya, R. (2003) Implementation and evaluation of a training program to improve resident teaching skills. *Am J Obstet Gynecol.* 189: 670–673

Furney, S.L., Orsini, A.N., Orsetti, K.E., Stern, D.T., Gruppen, L.D., and Irby, D.M. (2001) Teaching the one-minute preceptor. A randomized controlled trial. *J Gen Intern Med.* 16: 620–624

Gaba, N.D., Blatt, B., Macri, C.J., and Greenberg, L. (2007) Improving teaching skills in obstetrics and gynecology residents: evaluation of a residents-as-teachers program. *Am J Obstet Gynecol.* 196(87): e1–e7

General Medical Council (2006) *Good medical practice* [Online]. http://www.gmc-uk.org/guidance/good_medical_practice/index.asp Accessed 4 September 2011

Gome, J.J., Paltridge, D., and Inder, W.J. (2008) Review of intern preparedness and education experiences in General Medicine. *Intern Med J.* 38: 249–253

Greenberg, L.W., Goldberg, R.M., and Jewett, L.S. (1984) Teaching in the clinical setting: factors influencing residents' perceptions, confidence and behaviour. *Med Educ.* 18, 360–365.

Hafler, J.P. (2003) Residents as teachers: a process for training and development. *J Nutr.* 133: 544S–546S

Hammoud, M.M., Haefner, H.K., Schigelone, A., and Gruppen, L.D. (2004) Teaching residents how to teach improves quality of clerkship. In: CREOG/APGO 2004 Annual Meeting, 3–6 March 2004 Lake Buena Vista, FL

Henry, B.W., Haworth, J.G., and Hering, P. (2006) Perceptions of medical school graduates and students regarding their academic preparation to teach. *Postgrad Med J.* 82: 607–612

Hill, A.G., Yu, T.C., Barrow, M., and Hattie, J. (2009) A systematic review of resident-as-teacher programmes. *Med Educ.* 43: 1129–1140

Hill, A.G., Srinivasa, S., Hawken, S., et al. (2012) Impact of a resident-as-teacher workshop on teaching behavior of interns and learning outcomes of medical students. *J Grad Med Educ.* 4(1): 34–41

Hutchinson, L. (2003) Educational environment. *BMJ.* 326: 810–812

Irby, D.M. (1992) How attending physicians make instructional decisions when conducting teaching rounds. *Acad Med.* 67: 630–638

Irby, D. (1994) What clinical teachers in medicine need to know. *Acad Med.* 69: 333–342

Irby, D. and Rakestraw, P. (1981) Evaluating clinical teaching in medicine. *J Med Educ.* 56: 181–186

Jamshidi, R. and Ozgediz, D. (2008) Medical student teaching: a peer-to-peer toolbox for time-constrained resident educators. *J Surg Educ* 65: 95–98

Janicik, R.W., Schwartz, M.D., Kalet, A., and Zabar, S. (2001) Residents as teachers. *J Gen Intern Med.* 16(suppl): 101

Jewett, L.S., Greenberg, L.W., and Goldberg, R.M. (1982) Teaching residents how to teach—a one-year study. *J Med Educ.* 57: 361–366

Johnson, C.E., Bachur, R., Priebe, C., Barnes-Ruth, A., Lovejoy, F.H., and Hafler, J.P. (1996) Developing residents as teachers: process and content. *Pediatrics.* 97: 907–915

Johnson, N.R. and Chen, J. (2006) Medical student evaluation of teaching quality between obstetrics and gynecology residents and faculty as clinical preceptors in ambulatory gynecology. *Am J Obstet Gynecol.* 195: 1479–1483

Kaji, A. and Moorehead, J.C. (2002) Residents' perspective. Residents as teachers in the emergency department. *Ann Emerg Med.* 39: 316–318

Kates, N.S. and Lesser, A.L. (1985) The resident as a teacher: a neglected role. *Can J Psychiatry*. 30: 418–421

Katz, N.T., Mccarty-Gillespie, L., and Magrane, D. M. (2003) Direct observation as a tool for needs assessment of resident teaching skills in the ambulatory setting. *Am J Obstet Gynecol*. 189: 684–687

Katzelnick, D.J., Gonzales, J.J., Conley, M.C., Shuster, J.L., and Borus, J.F. (1991) Teaching psychiatric residents to teach. *Acad Psychiatry*. 15: 153–159

Lawson, B.K. and Harvill, L.M. (1980) The evaluation of a training program for improving residents' teaching skills. *J Med Educ*. 55: 1000–1005

Liaison Committee on Medical Education (2011) *Functions and Structure of a Medical School* [Online]. http://www.lcme.org/functions2011may.pdf Accessed 9 September 2011

Litzelman, D.K., Stratos, G.A., Marriott, D.J., Lazaridis, E.N., and Skeff, K.M. (1998) Beneficial and harmful effects of augmented feedback on physicians' clinical-teaching performances. *Acad Med*. 73: 324–332

Litzelman, D.K., Stratos, G.A., and Skeff, K.M. (1994) The effect of a clinical teaching retreat on residents' teaching skills. *Acad Med*. 69: 433–434

Lowery, S.F. (1976) The role of house staff in undergraduate surgical education. *Surgery*. 80: 624–628

Mccord, J.H., Mcdonald, R., Sippel, R.S., Leverson, G., Mahvi, D.M., and Weber, S.M. (2009) Surgical career choices: the vital impact of mentoring. *J Surg Res*. 155: 136–141

Miller, G.E. (1980) *Educating Medical Teachers*. Cambridge, MA: Harvard University Press

Morrison, E.H. and Hafler, J.P. (2000) Yesterday a learner, today a teacher too: residents as teachers in 2000. *Pediatrics*. 105: 238–241

Morrison, E.H., Friedland, J.A., Boker, J., Rucker, L., Hollingshead, J., and Murata, P. (2001) Residents-as-teachers training in the US residency programs and offices of graduate medical education. *Acad Med*. 76: S1–S4

Morrison, E.H., Boker, J.R., Hollingshead, J., Prislin, M.D., Hitchcock, M.A., and Litzelman, D. K. (2002) Reliability and validity of an objective structured teaching examination for generalist resident teachers. *Acad Med*. 77: S29–S32

Morrison, E.H., Rucker, L., Boker, J.R., et al. (2004) The effect of a 13-hour curriculum to improve residents' teaching skills: a randomized trial. *Ann Intern Med*. 141: 257–263.

Morrison, E.H., Shapiro, J.F., and Harthill, M. (2005) Resident doctors' understanding of their roles as clinical teachers. *Med Educ*. 39: 137–144

Moser, E.M. (2008) Chief Residents as educators: an effective method of resident development. *Teach Learn Med*. 20: 323–328

Musunuru, S., Lewis, B., Rikkers, L.F., and Chen, H. (2007) Effective surgical residents strongly influence medical students to pursue surgical careers. *J Am Coll Surg*. 204: 164–167

Nguyen, S.Q. and Divino, C.M. (2007) Surgical residents as medical student mentors. *Am J Surg*. 193: 90–93

Pandachuck, K., Harley, D., and Cook, D. (2004) Effectiveness of a brief workshop designed to improve teaching performance at the University of Alberta. *Acad Med*. 79: 798–804

Pelletier, M. and Belliveau, P. (1999) Role of surgical residents in undergraduate surgical education. *Can J Surg*. 42: 451–456

Prislin, M.D., Fitzpatrick, C., Giglio, M., Lie, D., and Radecki, S. (1998) Initial experience with a multi-station objective structured teaching skills evaluation. *Acad Med*. 73: 1116–1118

Remmen, R., Denekens, J., Scherpbier, A., et al. (2000) An evaluation study of the didactic quality of clerkships. *Med Educ*. 34: 460–464

Roberts, K.B., Dewitt, T.G., Goldberg, R.L., and Scheiner, A.P. (1994) A program to develop residents as teachers. *Arch Pediatr Adolesc Med*. 148: 405–410

Rotenberg, B.W., Woodhouse, R.A., Gilbart, M., and Hutchison, C. R. (2000) A needs assessment of surgical residents as teachers. *Can J Surg*. 43: 295–300

Royal College of Physicians and Surgeons of Canada (2005) *The CanMEDS 2005 physician competency framework* [Online]. http://www.royalcollege.ca/portal/page/portal/rc/common/documents/canmeds/resources/publications/framework_full_e.pdf Accessed 22 March 2013

Rubak, S., Mortensen, L., Ringsted, C., and Malling, B. (2008) A controlled study of the short- and long-term effects of a Train the Trainers course. *Med Educ*. 42: 693–702

Schwartz, M., Linzer, M., Babbott, D., Divine, G.W., and Broadhead, E. (1991) Medical student interest in internal medicine. Initial report of the Society of General Internal Medicine Interest Group Survey on Factors Influencing Career Choice in Internal Medicine. *Ann Intern Med*. 114: 6–15

Seely, A.J., Pelletier, M.P., Snell, L.S. and Trudel, J.L. (1999) Do surgical residents rated as better teachers perform better on in-training examinations? *Am J Surg*. 177: 33–37

Sheehan, D., Wilkinson, T.J., and Billett, S. (2005) Interns' participation and learning in clinical environments in a New Zealand hospital. *Acad Med*. 80: 302–308

Sheets, K.J., Hankin, F.M. and Schwenk, T.L. (1991) Preparing surgery house officers for their teaching role. *Am J Surg*. 161: 443–449

Snell, L. (1989) Improving medical residents' teaching skills. *Ann Roy Coll Phys Surg Can*. 22: 125–128

Spickard, A., 3rd, Corbett, E.C., Jr., and Schorling, J.B. (1996) Improving residents' teaching skills and attitudes toward teaching. *J Gen Intern Med*. 11: 475–480

Stark, P. (2003) Teaching and learning in the clinical setting: a qualitative study of the perceptions of students and teachers. *Med Educ*. 37: 975–982

Steinert, Y., Mann, K., Centeno, A., et al. (2006) A systematic review of faculty development initiatives designed to improve teaching effectiveness in medical education: BEME Guide No. 8. *Med Teach*. 28: 497–526

Stern, D.T. (1998) In search of the informal curriculum: when and where professional values are taught. *Acad Med*. 73: S28–S30

Susman, J.L. and Gilbert, C.S. (1995) A brief faculty development program for family medicine chief residents. *Teach Learn Med*. 7: 111–114

Thomas, P. S., Harris, P., Rendina, N., and Keogh, G. (2002) Residents as teachers: outcomes of a brief training programme. *Educ Health*. 15: 71–78

Tonesk, X. (1979) The house officer as a teacher: what schools expect and measure. *J Med Educ*. 54: 613–616

Tremonti, L.P. and Biddle, W.B. (1982) Teaching behaviors of residents and faculty members. *J Med Educ*. 57: 854–859

Troupin, R.H. (1990) The mini-fellowship in teaching. A senior resident elective. *Invest Radiol*. 25: 751–753

Trowbridge, R.L., Snydman, L.K., Skolfield, J., Hafler, J., and Bing-You, R.G. (2011) A systematic review of the use and effectiveness of the Objective Structured Teaching Encounter. *Med Teach*. 33: 893–903

Vu, T.R., Marriott, D.J., Skeff, K.M., Stratos, G.A., and Litzelman, D.K. (1997) Prioritizing areas for faculty development of clinical teachers by using student evaluations for evidence-based decisions. *Acad Med*. 72: S7–S9

Wamsley, M.A., Julian, K.A., and Wipf, J.E. (2004) A literature review of 'resident-as-teacher' curricula: do teaching courses make a difference? *J Gen Intern Med*. 19: 574–581

Weissman, M.A., Bensinger, L., and Koestler, J.L. (2006) Resident as teacher: educating the educators. *Mt Sinai J Med*. 73: 1165–1169

White, C.B., Bassali, R.W. and Heery, L.B. (1997) Teaching residents to teach. An instructional program for training pediatric residents to precept third-year medical students in the ambulatory clinic. *Arch Pediatr Adolesc Med*. 151: 730–735

Whittaker, L.D., Jr., Estes, N.C., Ash, J., and Meyer, L.E. (2006) The value of resident teaching to improve student perceptions of surgery clerkships and surgical career choices. *Am J Surg*. 191: 320–324

Whittle, S.R., Whelan, B., and Murdoch-Eaton, D.G. (2007) DREEM and beyond; studies of the educational environment as a means for its enhancement. *Educ Health*. 20: 7.

Wilkerson, L., Lesky, L., and Medio, F.J. (1986) The resident as teacher during work rounds. *J Med Educ*. 61: 823–829

Wipf, J.E., Orlander, J.D., and Anderson, J.J. (1999) The effect of a teaching skills course on interns' and students' evaluations of their resident-teachers. *Acad Med*. 74: 938–942

Xu, G., Wolfson, P., Robeson, M., Rodgers, J.F., Veloski, J.J., and Brigham, T.P. (1998) Students' satisfaction and perceptions of attending physicians' and residents' teaching role. *Am J Surg.* 176: 46–48

Yedidia, M.J., Schwartz, M.D., Hirschkorn, C., and Lipkin, M., Jr. (1995) Learners as teachers: the conflicting roles of medical residents. *J Gen Intern Med.* 10: 615–623

Yu, T.C., Srinivasa, S., Steff, K., et al. (2010) Attending a house officer-as-teacher (HOT) workshop changes attitudes and perceptions towards clinical teaching. *Focus on Health Professional Education: A Multi-Disciplinary Journal.* 12: 86–96

Zabar, S., Hanley, K., Stevens, D.L., et al. (2004) Measuring the competence of residents as teachers. *J Gen Intern Med.* 19: 530–533

CHAPTER 26

Students learning to teach

Michael T. Ross and Terese Stenfors-Hayes

The safest thing for a patient is to be in the hands of a man engaged in teaching medicine. In order to be a teacher of medicine the doctor must always be a student.

Charles Mayo

This quotation was published in Mayo Clinic Proceedings, 2, Charles Mayo, 'Proceedings of the Staff Meetings of the Mayo Clinic', p. 233, Copyright Elsevier, 1927

Why are students learning to teach?

Many reasons are given in the literature for medical students learning to teach. Most ultimately relate to the enhancement of patient care. If clinicians are trained and motivated to teach, students and trainees are more likely to experience high quality teaching, and in turn are more likely to deliver high quality patient care. A good teacher can also help equip patients and colleagues with what they need to help themselves, not only in terms of information but also in terms of confidence in their own abilities and self-efficacy (Roter 2000; Dandavino et al. 2007). Increased clinical teaching may also directly enhance patient care by giving patients extra time to talk with doctors and students and to ask questions, and by making patients feel valued.

Recent medical graduates are also increasingly learning to teach, both in relation to specific teaching roles and in relation to more generic principles of teaching (e.g. Bharel and Jain 2005; James et al. 2006; Mann et al. 2007; Rodrigues et al. 2008; Hill et al. 2009; Ostapchuk et al. 2010; Qureshi et al. 2013). Graduate teaching is explored further in Chapter 25. Such initiatives raise the question of whether medical students really need to learn to teach during their undergraduate studies at all, or if they could instead learn to teach after graduation. If recent graduates are expected to be able to teach effectively from their first day of work, however, it is not sufficient to wait until they have graduated to begin their training in teaching. Also teaching is a complex activity requiring considerable skill to undertake effectively, so they need to start learning and gaining experience through deliberate practice as early as possible (Ericsson 2004). There are therefore many reasons why institutions and health services may want medical students to learn to teach, and students themselves may also want to learn to teach—to address their own learning needs, for career intentions or interests, or simply because they enjoy teaching and find it rewarding. Some of these reasons for learning to teach are explored further in fig. 26.1 and the following text.

Because medical graduates are expected to be able to teach patients

Good patient education and patient-centred care has been shown to lead to better health outcomes (Stewart 1995; Stewart et al. 2000; Adams 2010). Medical students are typically expected to learn how to teach patients, and in many countries have explicitly been taught and assessed on this for years. Typically, this is incorporated into the undergraduate curriculum as part of communication or consultation skills and not explicitly referred to as teaching. All new UK medical graduates, for example, are required by the General Medical Council (GMC) to be able to 'provide explanation, advice, reassurance, and support' to patients (GMC 2009, p. 19). Similarly, all Canadian medical graduates are required by the Medical Council of Canada to be able to 'facilitate the learning of others as part of professional responsibility (patients, health professionals, society' (Medical Council of Canada 2009, Physician as Scholar, Objective 3).

Because medical graduates are expected to be able to teach colleagues

All students may be required to learn to teach by national regulatory bodies or healthcare systems or by their local institution. All new UK medical graduates, for example, are now also required by the GMC to be able to:

> function effectively as a mentor and teacher including contributing to the appraisal, assessment and review of colleagues, giving effective feedback, and taking advantage of opportunities to develop these skills

GMC (2009, p. 27)

Even where there is no statutory requirement for all students to learn to teach, there may be an expectation that they will do so. A recent European project identified strong consensus between medical academics, graduates and students that all European medical graduates should have the 'ability to teach others' (Cumming and Ross 2008, p. 17). Teaching was also one of nine domains in

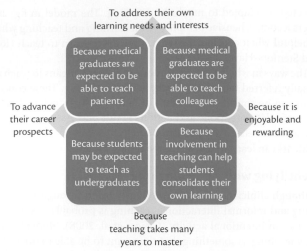

Figure 26.1 Reasons undergraduates should learn to teach.

the European Core Curriculum for undergraduate medicine proposed by a collaboration of European medical student organizations (Hilgers and De Roos 2007; Rigby 2007), and teaching programmes have been proposed by many other authors in the literature (e.g. Pasquale and Pugnaire 2002; Dandavino et al. 2007; Zijdenbos et al. 2011). Recent research in Scotland identified a wide range of teaching undertaken by doctors in their first year after graduation (Ross 2012). These were grouped into three broad domains as follows:

- Informal opportunistic teaching
  - Involving medical students in day to day practice
    - Encouraging medical students to follow and observe practice
    - Providing a commentary and explanation of practice
    - Responding to student questions
    - Supporting students in difficult or stressful situations
    - Delegating tasks or responsibilities to students
  - Getting medical students to see patients on their own
    - Finding patients for students to see
    - Getting students to clerk and present patients
  - Observing or testing medical students and giving feedback
    - Bedside teaching
    - Supervising students doing clinical procedures
    - Testing knowledge and clinical reasoning
  - Giving medical students opportunistic mini-tutorials
  - Teaching doctors at the same or higher level
  - Teaching nurses, nursing students and allied health professionals.
- Semiformal prearranged teaching
  - Having students on shadowing placements
  - Pre-arranged topic or case based tutorials
  - Hosting school pupils for work experience

- Teaching for societies and friends outside work
- Prearranged formative assessments (e.g. mock objective structured clinical examinations (OSCEs))
- Formal organized teaching
  - Teaching as part of a formalized teaching scheme
  - Covering timetabled tutorials if seniors unavailable
  - Formal timetabled teaching of clinical procedures
  - Giving presentations or lectures
  - Organizing teaching
  - Identifying or creating learning resources.

As doctors become more senior, they often take on further teaching responsibilities and roles in addition to those more general teaching activities they will be expected to undertake immediately after graduation. Examples of these special roles include lecturer, tutor, clinical supervisor, preceptor, mentor, and examiner. The teaching activities undertaken, title given to the role, and any training required can vary considerably. Some of these roles may be well-defined and doctors may compartmentalize them from other clinical and teaching roles, but others may be more difficult to define and differentiate (Stenfors-Hayes et al. 2010, 2011; Stenfors-Hayes 2011).

Because students may be expected to teach as undergraduates

Many medical students teach while undergraduates (Soriano et al. 2010), particularly in relation to different types of peer-assisted learning (PAL) activities (Ross and Cameron 2007). For the majority, participation such PAL activities and associated training will be voluntary. In a few institutions PAL has become so embedded in the curriculum that all medical students are expected to undertake training and to teach as undergraduates (Ten Cate 2007; Zijdenbos et al. 2011). Medical students may also be expected to teach patients as undergraduates, although often this is in simulations or under supervision rather than independently.

Because involvement in teaching can help students consolidate their own learning

Learning content with the intention to teach it can result in significantly better retention than learning it for an exam (Bargh and Schul 1980). Actually teaching that content seems to consolidate students' learning further, and can lead to measurable improvements in theoretical and practical tests (Knobe et al. 2010). PAL tutors frequently state that one reason for volunteering as tutors was to help them revise or consolidate their own learning. Medical students and trainees who learn to teach are also likely to think differently, and to approach their clinical practice differently (Weiss and Needlman 1998).

What does it mean to learn to teach?

Asking what it means to learn to teach can be compared to asking what it means to learn to do research or to undertake clinical care. There is no one simple answer. Adequate content knowledge, for example, seems to be an important prerequisite for teaching, but is not sufficient. As Miller (1990) and many other researchers since have highlighted, there is a great difference between knowing about a skill or how to do it and actually being able to demonstrate it or to do it in real practice. Shulman (1987) argues that teachers require knowledge in the following seven domains:

- content knowledge (in this case about medicine)
- general pedagogical knowledge (e.g. principles and strategies of organization and management of teaching)
- curriculum knowledge
- pedagogical content knowledge (the amalgam of content and pedagogy)
- knowledge of learners
- knowledge of educational contexts (e.g. classroom or hospital department, community and culture)
- knowledge of educational ends, purposes and values.

This can be helpful when trying to determine the content of any teacher training for students. Many authors would add an eighth domain of 'knowledge of self'. This would highlight the need for teachers to be self-aware, and to be reflexive about how their values, beliefs, experiences and preferences may influence their teaching.

Teaching is often conceptualized as what teachers and students do together in the lecture theatre, classroom or at the bedside—indicated as shared activities in fig. 26.2. From that perspective, one might expect learning to do this is simply a matter of learning how to deliver a lecture, lead a small group or talk with students about a patient. This represents only one particular aspect of what it means to learn to teach, however, and ignores the prior learning, expectations, and concerns of the learner and the independent learning activities they can undertake. It also ignores the personality, experience, and skills of the individual teacher, other teaching activities they undertake such as preparation, resource production and evaluation which may not involve learners, the content to be learned, and aspects of the learning and teaching situation which can be selected or adapted to maximize learning. The model in fig. 26.2 offers a comprehensive perspective on learning and teaching which is helpful when considering what it means to learn to teach (Ross and Stenfors-Hayes 2008a, b).

The ways in which teachers understand what it means to teach are usually referred to as their conceptions of teaching. These conceptions can be considered in terms of beliefs (which include knowledge of self), intentions and actions (Pratt and Associates 1998). These three related aspects can be helpful when considering how students can learn to teach and are expanded upon in table 26.1.

Identifying with a teaching role

Although clinicians may subconsciously teach through role modelling and informal interactions, teaching is probably best considered as an intentional activity (Cruess et al. 2008). Students must view teaching as something that they want to be able to do, so that they can deliberately practise and develop their teaching skills (Ericsson et al. 1993; Ericsson 2004). A prerequisite for learning to teach, therefore, is to believe it is possible, and to identify oneself with a current or future teaching role. Recent research, however, identified that many junior doctors and students do not consider teaching to be part of their role (Ross 2012), and even many senior doctors involved in teaching consider themselves to be 'doctors who teach' rather than 'teachers' (Stone et al. 2002; Higgs and McAllister 2007; Taylor et al. 2007). Most doctors do seem to have teaching roles however, and in some circumstances these may be in direct competition with their patient care and other roles (Rotem and Bandaranayake 1981; McInnins 2000; Stark 2003; MacDougall and Drummond 2005; Young 2006; Taylor et al. 2007; Schofield et al. 2010). Clinicians may at the same time be responsible for patients as well as students, for example, and may need to adopt different roles simultaneously or prioritize between them if they conflict (Higgs and McAllister 2005). Those helping students learn to teach need to be aware of the potential conflict generated from

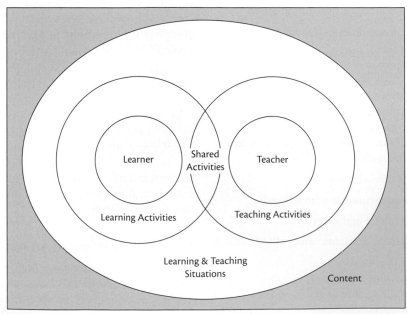

Figure 26.2 Learning and teaching model.
Reproduced from Michael T. Ross, Terese Stenfors-Hayes, 'Development of a framework of medical undergraduate teaching activities', Medical Education, 42, 9, pp. 915–922, 2008, with permission from Wiley.

Table 26.1 Developing student conceptions of teaching

Beliefs	Students need to believe that teaching can be learned, and they must begin to identify with a teaching role
Intentions	Students need to be able to define their intentions both in broad terms and more specifically with the intended outcomes of any teaching session
Actions	Students need to be able to undertake certain actions and teaching techniques

their emerging identities in relation to teaching, and provide support to help them recognize and manage the tensions inherent in such multiple roles (Lieff et al. 2012).

The issue of the teacher role not being sufficiently recognized is not new, having already been noted in the 1890s (Calman 2007). Today, teaching is still often not discussed and is just something that doctors do (Rotem and Bandaranayake 1981; Handal 1999; Young 2006). Learning to teach is as much about the development of a professional identity as it is about content learning. Clinicians who think of themselves as teachers may be more likely to enjoy teaching, to teach more, and to be recognized by students and other faculty as good teachers (Starr et al. 2003), which suggests that early identification of this role is important. The ways in which students develop their professional identity and conceptualize their multiple roles has important implications for their own wellbeing and for the relationships they form with colleagues and patients (Monrouxe 2010). Learning to teach as part of the undergraduate curriculum may help strengthen the teacher identity for future graduates and thereby also improve teaching.

Reflecting on the intention(s) of teaching

In order to learn about teaching, students need to gain some understanding of what teaching is and what it is for. This is not as straightforward as it may sound because the nature and purpose of teaching can be understood in many different ways. Such differences in understanding will influence the way in which teachers see the world and interpret and act on what they see (Pratt and Associates 1998; Entwistle et al. 2000). The way teachers understand being a teacher provides direction and justification for what they do. It also informs their roles and expectations regarding acceptable forms of teaching. Teachers' values, beliefs and conceptions of teaching may be affected by their current discipline (Knight and Trowler 2000), and their disciplinary background (Jarvis-Selinger et al. 2006). There is evidence that teacher's conceptions of teaching impact on the way they approach their teaching (Prebble et al. 2004), and that this in turn impacts on the learning of those they teach (Trigwell et al. 1999; Martin et al. 2000). For this reason faculty development strategies often deliberately seek to influence participant conceptions of teaching (Trigwell and Prosser 1996; Kember and Kwan 2000; Ho et al. 2001; Richardson 2005; Knight and Bligh 2006; Bulik and Shokar 2007; Åkerlind 2008). Some even argue that 'fundamental changes to the quality of teaching and learning are unlikely to happen without changes to lecturers' conception of teaching' (Kember and Kwan 2000, p. 469).

A number of studies in higher education highlight the differences between teacher-centred approaches to teaching, in which the focus is on what teachers do in order to present content clearly and accurately to students, and learner-centred approaches, in which the focus is on the learners' experience of learning and on adapting teaching to enhance student learning and development (Kember 1997; Kember and Kwan 2000; Wood 2000; Samuelovicz and Bain 2001; Åkerlind 2004; Postareff and Lindblom-Ylänne 2008; Weurlander and Stenfors-Hayes 2008). The teacher's intention in each case is quite different, and most studies suggest learner centred approaches are better than teacher centred ones. Pratt et al. (1998), however, do not support this polarized dichotomy and instead suggest five perspectives on good teaching, which can be summarized as:

- The *transmission* perspective, characterized by the notion that good teaching involves presenting content to students clearly and accurately in a structured manner. The focus is on the teacher and the content, and how content can be delivered and goals achieved most efficiently.

- The *apprenticeship* perspective, in which learners interact with teachers and are gradually enculturated to think and act in a similar way, with similar social norms and ways of working, through modelling, questioning and feedback. The teacher is perceived as inseparable from content as they exemplify the values and knowledge to be learned.

- The *developmental* perspective, which involves planning and delivering teaching appropriate to students' current knowledge and experience, focusing on helping learners develop their abilities in critical thinking and their personal autonomy. This requires that the teacher appreciates how learners think in relation to the content. Knowledge is interrogated, and the teacher's authority is open to discussion.

- The *nurturing* perspective, which emphasizes the importance of creating a safe and supportive environment for learners which minimizes feelings of failure among learners. It emphasizes the need for emotional support, personal relationships, mutual trust, and respect.

- The *social reform* perspective, which adopts a broader critical stance in which the function of teaching is to reform practice and/or society. The focus is therefore on the collective rather than the individual. Students are encouraged and empowered to take a critical stance themselves, and to be agents for social change.

Pratt et al. (1998) argue that none of the five perspectives are inherently better or worse than the others, and that each may be more or less appropriate depending on the context, culture and discipline. This relates to the model in fig. 26.2 in terms of the interdependent relationship between learner, teacher, content, and situation, and the need to consider all of them when selecting teaching activities. Each perspective is presented with sound epistemological and philosophical underpinnings, and will be appropriate for certain learners, contexts, and purposes. Teachers typically describe multiple perspectives of teaching, although there is often one that dominates at particular times.

A number of resources and tools have been developed to help novice teachers reflect broadly on what they think is the purpose of teaching. Probably the best-known example is the Approaches to Teaching Inventory by Trigwell and Prosser (2004), which distinguishes more teacher-centered and learner-centered approaches. Another example is the Teaching Perspectives Inventory (TPI), which is based on Pratt's research, and distinguishes the five non-hierarchical conceptions of teaching listed earlier (Collins and Pratt 2011; Pratt and Collins 2012). Both instruments have been widely used in different contexts with large numbers of teachers, and offer an accessible introduction to different conceptions of teaching.

Aligning with the intended outcomes of any teaching session or course

The intention of teaching can also be considered more specifically in terms of what the teacher is trying to achieve in a particular activity, session, course, or programme. Although conceptually such purposes may be diverse, when practically planning a session or course teachers typically try to identify specifically what they want learners to learn. In medical education this content is most commonly defined as either the intended learning outcomes of a programme of study, or as the competencies that learners will develop and be able to demonstrate on completion of a programme. Students learning to teach therefore need to be aware of the intended learning outcomes or competencies of any teaching they are involved in, and the importance of constructively aligning any teaching, learning, assessment, and evaluation with these (Biggs 1996). They also need to be aware of the level of proficiency, depth and application to practice that learners are expected to achieve (Harden 2007).

In most teaching situations, with the notable exception of non-expert problem-based learning tutors, students and more senior medical teachers are likely to have already achieved the outcomes or competencies themselves before teaching them. In some cases they have only learned these a short time before, and so are likely to remember any difficulties they had in learning them and what best helped them to learn, and may also be able to reflect on the experiences of their colleagues. Understanding the concept of constructive alignment can empower novice teachers to think about what activities are most likely to help their learners achieve the intended outcomes, rather than uncritically modelling their teaching on formats they have been exposed to in the past themselves, or trying to deliver comprehensive textbook-style details of the topic.

Learning specific teaching techniques and approaches

Teaching can also be thought of as a number of different activities, each of which can be described, learned and practised. When asked, undergraduate medical teachers often initially describe what they do in relation to hands-on teaching activities such as providing information, demonstrating, facilitating learning, assessing, and giving feedback (Ross and Stenfors-Hayes 2008b). Many will also describe background or management teaching activities, which may not be so visible to students, such as leading a course, curriculum development, and the recruitment of students and teachers. Most teachers also take part in personal learning and community building activities, including formal training, networking, and educational research, although they may not initially describe this as teaching (Ross and Stenfors-Hayes 2008b). Such activities, especially the formal training, are often undertaken to support or prepare teachers for their hands-on teaching.

How can students learn to teach?

There are many ways in which students can learn to teach, and many ways in which different undergraduate curricula could ensure all students achieve this. These include learning to teach patients, making explicit links with content learned elsewhere in the curriculum, learning from role models, and the experience of being taught, gaining practical experience of teaching—most commonly as some form of PAL initiative, and specific training in teaching (see fig. 26.3).

Learning to teach patients

Medical students already explicitly learn how to deliver patient education and are typically assessed on their ability to do this. There are many similarities between teaching patients and teaching colleagues, which makes some of the skills learnt in these courses transferable to other teaching contexts (Cohen and Dennick 2009; O'Sullivan and Irby 2011). The clinical concept of patient-centredness, for example, relates closely to the educational concept of learner-centredness (Smith et al. 2007). Similarly, relationships between experienced doctors and students or trainees, and between doctors and patients, are both complicated by a power differential (Ong et al. 1995), which the doctor and teacher need to consider. Also, to earn a patient's trust and deliver effective healthcare, doctors must be able to establish a rapport with patients (Tate 2009). Likewise, with the relationship between medical teachers and students or trainees, effective teaching requires the establishment of rapport and trust (Neighbour 2004). Principles describing good communication skills such as promoting dialogue rather than one-way transmission, planning and thinking in terms of outcomes, and following an iterative and contingent rather than linear plan, can be equally applied to teaching colleagues as to consulting with patients (Dandavino et al. 2007). The experiences students gain in their clinical training and interaction with patients can easily be used and reflected upon from a teaching and learning perspective to facilitate students learning to teach. In both situations, the aim is to help the individual patient or student to learn, promote self-efficacy, and avoid the development of dependence or other unhelpful and unprofessional relationships (Roter 2000).

Making links with content learned elsewhere in the curriculum

Medical students already learn a diverse range of content during their undergraduate education which seems to be relevant to learning to teach, but is typically not labelled as such. Aspects of clinical communication related to teaching patients have already been described, but other aspects such as the principles of breaking bad news to a patient can also be applied to giving difficult feedback to a student or trainee (Tate 2009). Similarly, ethical principles of consent, confidentiality, beneficence, non-maleficence, autonomy, and social justice, are as important for educational as for clinical practice (Campbell et al. 2005). Other aspects of the undergraduate medical curriculum such as team-working, literature searching, and critique, writing reports and essays, preparing presentations, time management, reflective practice, peer assessment, peer feedback,

Learning to teach patients
Making explicit links with content learned elsewhere in the curriculum
Learning from role models and the experience of being taught
Gaining practical experience of teaching
Specific training in teaching

Figure 26.3 How students can learn to teach.

and continuing professional development, are also all relevant to learning about teaching.

Learning from role models and the experience of being taught

Medical students are also typically exposed to a large and diverse range of teachers from whom they will inevitably learn through role modelling and the experience of being taught (MacDougall and Drummond 2005; Knight et al. 2006). These may include positive role models and examples of good teaching they would like to emulate, but are also likely to include negative role models and examples of poor teaching that they would want to carefully avoid emulating. There is some evidence that influencing student experiences through 'deliberate role modelling' and exposing them to examples good teaching can have a positive impact on student learning (Cruess et al. 2008). Such teaching role models, of course, are not limited to medical teachers, and may also include previous school teachers, sports instructors, family members, and even the medical students' own doctors.

Gaining practical experience of teaching

Teaching is a complex activity, and there is an extensive body of literature which supports the value of learning complex activities through experience and deliberate practice (Schön 1983; Kolb 1984; Ericsson et al. 1993; Ericsson 2004; Van de Wiel et al. 2011). Some may even argue that it is impossible to learn how to teach without practical experience of teaching. Without practical experience, students will have less to reflect upon, and so are likely to derive less benefit from any more formal training in teaching. As well as offering opportunities to learn and practise skills and techniques, practical experience of teaching can influence an individual's developing professionalism, their attitudes towards teaching and learning, and can also lead to the development of so-called 'practical wisdom' (Carr 2000; Korthagen et al. 2001; Shulman 2007). Such practical wisdom (Greek: *phronesis*) is based on experience and is situation-specific, concrete, and subjective. It is quite different to the more general and abstract scientific knowledge (Greek: *episteme*), which can be presented in a lecture or read in a book (Korthagen et al. 2001). Ideally students learning to teach patients and colleagues should therefore gain practical experience of actually teaching. Such practical experience can also help students develop their sense of identity as a teacher (Stone et al. 2002). Undergraduate medical teaching experiences may take different forms, but most commonly involve various types of PAL initiatives (see fig. 26.4). Students, who have not yet had PAL experiences particularly in the early years, may instead reflect on any teaching experiences they have had in other contexts such as teaching siblings, coaching sports or leading youth groups. All students, even those who do not remember ever being involved in teaching, can also reflect on their varied experiences of being taught.

Specific training in teaching

Motivation to participate in teacher training, and what students aim to achieve through such training, will vary depending on their conceptions of teaching. Students with a transmission focus of teaching are more likely to be interested in presentation techniques, while students with a developmental perspective are likely to be more interested in learning how to engage learners in critical thinking

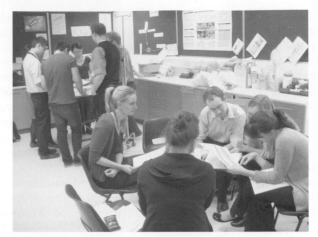

Figure 26.4 Students in a PAL session on fluid balance.

or reflection (Åkerlind 2003). The focus in faculty development for medical teachers has shifted over time from skills practice, teaching aids and communication techniques, towards encouraging student-centredness, self-directed learning, collaborative learning, and more conducive learning environments (Wilkerson and Irby 1998; McClean et al. 2008). Activities used today include workshops, consultations, mentoring, reflective diaries, self-assessment, student and peer feedback, role play, critical incident analysis, observation of teaching, and scholarship activities (Knight 2002; Prebble et al. 2004; Steinert et al. 2006; McClean et al. 2008; McLeod and Steinert 2010). All of these activities can also be used with students learning to teach. Other potential activities might include analysing video recordings of student teaching, teaching in teams with the opportunity to give feedback and reflect, and participating in reading groups or journal clubs on educational literature. For in-depth understanding of teaching, however, reflection is generally considered a prerequisite (Tigelaar et al. 2008). This needs to be framed within the learning context in which it takes place (Boud and Walker 1998), and is considered more effective when related to personal experience (Sharpe 2004). This again reinforces the view that students should ideally have some teaching experiences themselves before participating in more formal teacher training.

Peer-assisted learning

PAL can be defined as 'people from similar social groupings who are not professional teachers helping each other to learn and learning themselves by teaching' (Topping 1996, p. 322). Thus defined, PAL always involves non-professional teachers undertaking some form of teaching, but excludes other learning activities in groups or pairs which do not involve teaching. Medical students in the same or different years, and students from different healthcare disciplines, are generally considered to be peers because they are in similar social groupings in terms of their professional activities and career stage (Ross and Cameron 2007). PAL terminology in medical education is not standardized, and alternative terms include 'peer teaching', 'student tutoring', or 'supplemental instruction'. Various terms have also been used to describe PAL participants, activities and situations, but in this chapter we refer to discrete PAL initiatives or projects in which tutors assist the learning of tutees in one or more interactions or sessions. However, it is recognized that in some PAL projects tutors will only interact with tutees indirectly online or through the production of learning resources, and, in reciprocal forms of PAL, each participant may at different times be tutor and tutee.

PAL initiatives are widespread in undergraduate medical education, and examples of PAL can be traced back as far as Aristotle in 340 BCE (Wagner 1982). PAL initiatives have not always been formalized or reported, but over the past few decades a considerable volume of PAL-related studies have appeared in the literature. These have related to most subject areas and stages of training, and to many different teaching approaches and strategies including revision tutorials, problem-based learning facilitation, student support, formative assessment and feedback, summative assessment, lectures, and the production of learning resources.

The literature suggests that teaching from peers is qualitatively different to that delivered by more experienced medical teachers. While studies directly comparing peer tutors to faculty have shown that students can, in certain circumstances, achieve similar or even better outcomes in terms of tutee evaluation and examination scores (e.g. Perkins et al. 2002; Knobe et al. 2010), they have also been shown to be less effective in other situations (Rogers et al. 2000). PAL teaching, like any other approach to teaching and learning, will have advantages and disadvantages in any given situation. All new PAL initiatives therefore should be carefully monitored and evaluated to ensure that they are achieving the desired outcomes. Those considering developing their own PAL initiatives are therefore encouraged to identify examples of PAL in the literature relating to their own discipline, and to follow a template or framework for planning and implementing the project, such as that described by Ross and Cameron (2007).

Reported benefits of PAL

Most examples of PAL in the literature report that both tutors and tutees enjoyed participating and felt they benefited in various ways. Topping and Ehly (2001) suggest that the perceived success and effectiveness of PAL is due to cognitive, communication, organizational, affective, and social factors. Cognitive factors include Piagetian 'cognitive conflict' resulting from tutors and tutees being challenged in their understanding, beliefs and assumptions (Piaget 1973); Vygotskian 'scaffolded learning', with slightly more experienced tutors helping peers in their 'zone of proximal development' (Vygotsky 1978); 'cognitive congruence' with tutors being better able to understand the difficulties of tutees than faculty (Ten Cate and Durning 2007); and the advantage to tutors of learning and structuring knowledge with the purpose of teaching it (Bargh and Schul 1980; Ten Cate and Durning 2007). Communication factors relate to tutees and particularly tutors having to recall, structure and verbalize their understanding of content, perhaps for the first time, and the related tasks of listening, explaining, questioning, clarifying, simplifying, summarizing and hypothesizing about content with their peers (Topping 1996). Organizational factors typically relate to students spending increased time engaging with content, in many cases receiving additional teaching either from faculty in tutor-training or from PAL tutors if the sessions are offered in addition to the core curriculum; smaller group sizes with increased immediate feedback from peers; and also various rewards, which may be intrinsic (interest, variety, enjoyment, sense of purpose) or extrinsic (PAL sometimes results in additional privilege, certification of participation or even payment for tutors). Affective and social factors for tutees include the relaxed and often informal learning environment which allows tutees to speak freely and ask even 'silly' questions; enhanced role-modelling and motivation due to tutors being only slightly ahead of them in stage; and increased transmission of a positive hidden curriculum (Snyder 1970; Lockspeiser et al. 2008). For tutors, PAL also seems to resonate with a perceived human need for esteem with aspects of role theory and self-determination theory, which suggest that by acting as a relative expert, PAL tutors will increasingly feel and then become more like an expert in terms of competency, autonomy, esteem, and motivation (Ten Cate and Durning 2007). From the institutional perspective, PAL can help students learn about and gain practical experience in teaching; can address content gaps in the core curriculum; can give students practical experience of team-working, leadership, and increased responsibility; and can help students develop empathy and professionalism, as well as a greater sense of engagement with the core curriculum. It has also been reported that using PAL tutors instead of faculty in certain situations can result in cost-savings, although this is also a potential concern.

Potential concerns and disadvantages of PAL

Potential disadvantages of PAL most commonly relate to concerns that tutors will have inadequate depth of knowledge and so may give inappropriate or incomplete information to tutees: that they may not be experienced enough in teaching to maintain discipline or to present content clearly; and that they may not appreciate what is core and so overload tutees with too much information or confuse tutees with regard to what they need to learn (Topping 1996; Rogers et al. 2000). Although many PAL initiatives result in additional cost and faculty time commitments, concerns have also been expressed that in some circumstances PAL tutors have been used as cheap labour to teach on established courses instead of faculty—to the detriment of both PAL tutors and tutees. Another controversial issue discussed in the medical education literature in relation to PAL is peer physical examination. While clear benefits have been reported for many students who undertake peer physical examination, not all students want to examine or be examined by their peers, and there seems to be some potential for peer pressure, coercion, embarrassment, and even inappropriate behaviour (Chang and Power 2000; Rees et al. 2005; Wearn et al. 2008; Rees et al. 2009). When developing new PAL initiatives it is worth considering these potential concerns and disadvantages early so they can be avoided or minimized.

Planning and implementing a PAL initiative

Ross and Cameron (2007) developed a framework of questions to guide curriculum developers and PAL organizers seeking to develop new PAL initiatives, the responses to which constitute the basis of a comprehensive project plan or proposal. These relate to the background, leadership, and aims of the PAL, recruitment and training of participants, format and arrangement of proposed PAL sessions, approaches to evaluation and research, resource implications, potential pitfalls, and a timeline with action points for implementation. Details of these questions and a worked example can be found elsewhere (Ross and Cameron 2007).

Assessing and evaluating student teaching abilities

How can faculty determine whether students have learned to teach? To date little attention has been given in the literature to the formal assessment of student teaching abilities, although this is likely to change as schools respond to external requirements to demonstrate that all of their graduates are able to teach. The most common approach described in the literature is to review feedback from PAL tutees, although observations by peers and faculty, scrutiny of the assessment results attained by participants, and reflective diaries have also been reported. Teaching can also be assessed using an OSCE format, either as solitary stations in a traditional OSCE (Zabar et al. 2004), or as an objective structured teaching examination (OSTE) with multiple teaching-related stations (Morrison et al. 2002; Wamsley et al. 2005). University faculty are often assessed on their teaching by means of a teaching portfolio (Centra 2000; Seldin et al. 2010), following the general principles of portfolio based learning applied to teaching practice (see for example Snadden and Thomas 1998; Ben-David et al. 2001). The teacher gradually adds evidence, feedback, and personal reflections about their teaching to their portfolio, which can be a useful focus to help teachers develop reflective practices, and can also be a way for their development as a teacher to be followed and assessed. Students could also be assessed in this way and, for example, start a teaching portfolio in the early years of the undergraduate curriculum and carry it on into postgraduate training and beyond.

Embedding learning to teach in the curriculum

Although now a statutory requirement for many medical schools, there are few examples in the literature of focused curriculum development to ensure that all graduates are able to teach. The University Medical Centre Utrecht in the Netherlands, for example, has instituted a compulsory week-long teacher training course for all of their senior medical students (Ten Cate 2007; Zijdenbos et al. 2011). Barts and the London School of Medicine and Dentistry have introduced a 2-day programme of practical and theoretical training in teaching (Cook et al. 2010). The University of Edinburgh have developed a core introductory session on teaching for all medical students in their fourth year, and a broad range of PAL projects in which students can volunteer to participate as tutors or co-organizers, each with bespoke PAL tutor training and support. This core introductory session presents some basic educational theory structured around the model in fig. 26.2, makes explicit links with relevant teaching content learned elsewhere in the curriculum, introduces the various PAL opportunities, and encourages students to volunteer for projects. Teaching undertaken by students in the different PAL projects includes demonstrating in practical anatomy classes, teaching a range of clinical procedures and skills, teaching electrocardiogram and X-ray interpretation, offering advice and support to students in junior years, designing and delivering practice OSCE assessments, and helping to develop teaching resources and revision aids. The Edinburgh PAL programme has in many ways been successful since its inception in 2003, but there has been variable uptake of tutoring opportunities, few assessment of students on their teaching abilities, and considerable variation in training, evaluation and student experience depending upon the project undertaken and individual student engagement. For example, although there were more than enough places for all 260 fourth year students to teach in a PAL project in 2009-10, evaluation revealed that only two-thirds of the year had taken up this opportunity. Many of those who did tutor or organize PAL had also participated in more than one project. It is often said that assessment drives learning, and the evaluation found that many students did not participate because they knew their participation was not assessed nor compulsory. These issues are now being addressed.

Conclusions

◆ The importance of medical students learning to teach is increasingly highlighted in the literature, and doctors are often expected to teach patients and colleagues from graduation or before.

◆ Learning to teach is much more than just learning content and specific teaching techniques and skills. It includes developing a sense of an identity as a teacher, greater understanding of the purpose and nature of teaching, consideration of the learner, and appreciation of the importance of context.

◆ Ensuring that all medical students learn to teach does not imply that schools will necessarily have to introduce a compulsory course on teaching into their core curriculum. In this chapter we presented an alternative pragmatic approach which makes best use of prior learning and existing programme content. Medical students already learn to teach patients, learn to communicate well, and behave professionally and ethically, and are surrounded by role-models they can learn from. Many also have opportunities to teach and gain practical experience of teaching through PAL.

◆ If medical students are to be expected to learn to teach, they need to know this early in the undergraduate curriculum and need to have some opportunities to gain practical experience of teaching, in addition to any specific training in teaching.

References

Adams, R.J. (2010) Improving health outcomes with better patient understanding and education. *Risk Manage Healthcare Policy.* 2010(3): 61–72

Åkerlind, G.S. (2003) Growing and developing as a university teacher—variation in meaning. *Studies Higher Educ.* 28: 375–390

Åkerlind, G.S. (2004) A new dimension to understanding university teaching. *Teach Higher Educ.* 9(3): 363–375

Åkerlind, G.S. (2008) A phenomenographic approach to developing academics' understanding of the nature of teaching and learning. *Teach Higher Educ.* 13(6): 633–644

Aspegren, K. (1999) BEME Guide No.2: Teaching and learning communication skills in medicine—a review with quality grading of articles. *Med Teach.* 21(6): 563–570

Bargh, J.A. and Schul, Y. (1980) On the cognitive benefits of teaching. *J Educ Psychol.* 72(5): 593–604

Ben-David, M.F., Davis, M.H., Harden, R.M., Howie, P.W., Ker, J., and Pippard, M.J. (2001) AMEE Guilde No. 24: Portfolios as a method of student assessment. *Med Teach.* 23(6): 535–551

Bharel, M. and Jain, S. (2005) A longitudinal curriculum to improve resident teaching skills. *Med Teach.* 27(6): 564–566

Biggs, J.B. (1996) Enhancing teaching through constructive alignment. *Higher Educ.* 32: 347–364

Boud, D. and Walker, D. (1998) Promoting reflection in professional courses: the challenge of context. *Studies Higher Educ.* 23(2): 191–206

Bulik, R.J. and Shokar, G.S. (2007) 'Coming about!'—a faculty workshop on teaching beliefs. *Teach Learn Med.* 19(2): 168–173

Busari, J.O., Scherpbier, A.J.J.A., van der Vleuten, C.P.M., and Essed, G.E. (2000) Residents' perception of their role in teaching undergraduate students in the clinical setting. *Med Teach.* 22(4): 348–353

Calman, K.C. (2007) *Medical Education: Past, Present and Future.* Edinburgh: Elsevier

Campbell, A., Gillet, G., Jones, G. (2005) *Medical Ethics.* 4th edn. Oxford: Oxford University Press

Carr, D. (2000) *Professionalism and Ethics in Teaching.*. London: Routledge

Centra, J.A. (2000) Evaluating the teaching portfolio: a role for colleagues. *New Directions Teach Learn.* 83: 87–93

Chang, E.H. and Power, D.V. (2000) Are medical students comfortable with practicing physical examinations on each other? *Acad Med.* 75(4): 384–389

Cohen, S. and Dennick, R. (2009) Applying learning theory in the consultation. *The Clin Teach.* 6: 117–121

Collins, J.B. and Pratt, D.D. (2011) The Teaching Perspectives Inventory at ten years and 100 000 respondents: reliability and validity of a teacher self-report inventory. *Adult Educ Q.* 61(4): 358–375

Cook, V., Fuller, J.H., and Evans, D.E. (2010) Helping students become the medical teachers of the future—the doctors as teachers and educators (DATE) programme of Barts and the London School of Medicine and Dentistry, London. *Educ Health.* 23(2): 1–6

Cruess, S.R., Cruess, R.L., and Steinert, Y. (2008) Role modeling—making the most of a powerful teaching strategy. *BMJ.* 336: 718–721

Cumming, A.D. and Ross, M.T. (2008) *The Tuning Project (medicine)—learning outcomes/competences for undergraduate medical education in Europe.* Edinburgh: The University of Edinburgh. http://www.tuning-medicine.com Accessed 23 April 2012

Dandavino, M., Snell, L., Wiseman, J. (2007) Why medical students should learn how to teach. *Med Teach.* 29: 558–565.

Entwistle, N., Skinner, D., Entwistle, D., and Orr, S. (2000) Conceptions and beliefs about 'good teaching': an integration of contrasting research areas. *Higher Educ Res Dev.* 19(1): 5–26

Ericsson, K.A. (2004) Deliberate practice and the acquisition and maintenance of expert performance in medicine and related domains. *Acad Med.* 79(10 Supplement): S70–S81

Ericsson, K.A., Krampe, R.T., and Tesch-Römer, C. (1993) The role of deliberate practice in the acquisition of expert performance. *Psychol Rev.* 100(3): 363–406

GMC (2009) *Tomorrow's Doctors: outcomes and standards for undergraduate medical education.* London: The General Medical Council

GMC (2011) *Developing teachers and trainers in undergraduate medical education: advice supplementary to Tomorrow's Doctors (2009).* London: The General Medical Council

Handal, G. (1999) Consultation using critical friends. *New Directions Teach Learn.* 79: 59–70

Harden, R.M. (2007) Learning outcomes as a tool to assess progression. *Med Teach.* 29: 678–682

Higgs, J. and McAllister, L. (2005) The lived experiences of clinical educators with implications for their preparation, support and professional development. *Learn Health Soc Care.* 4(3): 156–171

Higgs, J. and McAllister, L. (2007) Being a clinical educator. *Adv Health Sci Educ.* 12: 187–199

Hilgers, J. and De Roos, P. (2007) European Core Curriculum-the Students' Perspective, Bristol, UK, 10 July 2006. *Med Teach.* 29: 270–275

Hill, A.G., Yu, T.C., Barrow, M., and Hattie, J. (2009) A systematic review of resident-as-teacher programmes. *Med. Educ.* 43: 1129–1140

Ho, A., Watkins, D., and Kelly, M. (2001) The conceptual change approach to improving teaching and learning: an evaluation of a Hong Kong staff development programme. *Higher Educ.* 42: 143–169

James, M.T., Mintz, M.J., and McLaughlin, K. (2006) Evaluation of a multifaceted 'resident-as-teacher' educational intervention to improve morning report. *BMC Med Educ.* 6: 20

Jarvis-Selinger, S., Collins, J.B., and Pratt, D.D. (2006) Do academic origins influence perspectives on teaching? *Teach Educ Q.* 34(3): 67–82

Kember, D. (1997) A reconceptualisation of the research into university academics' conceptions of teaching. *Learn Instruct.* 7(3): 255–275

Kember, D. and Kwan, K.P. (2000) Lecturers' approaches to teaching and their relationship to conceptions of good teaching. *Instruct Sci.* 28: 469–490

Knight, P. (2002) *Being a Teacher in Higher Education.* Maidenhead, UK: Society for Research in Higher Education and the Open University Press

Knight, L.V. and Bligh, J. (2006) Physicians' perceptions of clinical teaching: a qualitative analysis in the context of change. *Adv Health Sci Educ.* 11(3): 221–234

Knight, P., Tait, J., and Yorke, M. (2006) The professional learning of teachers in higher education. *Studies Higher Educ.* 31(3): 319–339

Knight, P.T. and Trowler, P.R. (2000) Department-level cultures and the improvement of learning and teaching. *Studies Higher Educ.* 25(1): 69–83

Knobe, M., Münker, R., Sellei, R.M., et al. (2010) Peer teaching: a randomised controlled trial using student teachers to teach musculoskeletal ultrasound. *Med Educ.* 44: 148–155

Kolb, D.A. (1984) *Experiential Learning. Experience as the source of learning and development.* New Jersey: Prentice-Hall

Korthagen, F.A.J., Kessels, J., Koster, B., Lagerwerf, B., and Wubbels, T. (2001) *Linking Practice and Theory: the pedagogy of realistic teacher education.* Mahwah, New Jersey: Lawrence Erlbaum Associates Inc. Reprinted 2008, New York: Routledge

Lieff, S., Baker, L., Mori, B., Egan-Lee, E., Chin, K., and Reeves, S. (2012) Who am I? Key influences on the formation of academic identity within a faculty development program. *Med Teach.* 34(3): e208–e215

Lockspeiser, T.M., O'Sullivan, P., Teherani, A., and Muller, J. (2008) Understanding the experience of being taught by peers: the value of social and cognitive congruence. *Adv Health Sci Educ.* 13: 361–372

MacDougall, J. and Drummond, M.J. (2005) The development of medical teachers: an enquiry into the learning histories of 10 experienced medical teachers. *Med Educ.* 39(12): 1213–1220

Mann, K.V., Sutton, E., and Frank, B. (2007) Twelve tips for preparing residents as teachers. *Med Teach.* 29: 301–306

Martin, E., Prosser, M., Trigwell, K., Ramsden, P., and Benjamin, J. (2000) What university teachers teach and how they teach it. *Instruct Sci.* 28: 387–412

Mayo, C.H. (1927). Proceedings of the Staff Meetings of the Mayo Clinic 2: 233

McClean, M., Cilliers, F., and van Wyk, J.M. (2008) Faculty development: yesterday, today and tomorrow. *Med Teach.* 30(6): 555–584

McInnins, C. (2000) Changing academic work roles: the everyday realities challenging quality in teaching. *Qual Higher Educ.* 6(2): 143–152

McLeod, P. and Steinert, Y. (2010) The evolution of faculty development in Canada since the 1980s: coming of age or time for a change? *Med Teach.* 32: e31–e35

Medical Council of Canada (2009) *Objectives for the qualifying examination.* https://apps.mcc.ca/objectives_online/objectives.pl?lang=english&role=scholar Accessed 23 April 2012

Miller, G.E. (1990) The assessment of clinical skills / competence / performance. *Acad Med.* 65(9 Supplement): S63–S67

Monrouxe, L.V. (2010) Identity, identification and medical education: why should we care? *Med. Educ.* 44(1): 40–49

Morrison, E.H., Boker, J.R., Hollingshead, J., Prislin, M.D., Hitchcock, M.A., and Litzelman, D.K. (2002) Reliability and validity of an objective structured teaching examination for general resident teachers. *Acad Med.* 77(10): S29–S32

Neighbour, R. (2004) *The Inner Apprentice: an awareness-centred approach to vocational training for general practice.* 2nd edn. Abingdon: Radcliffe Medical Press

O'Sullivan, P.S. and Irby, D.M. (2011) Reframing research on faculty development. *Acad Med.* 86 (4): 421–428

Ong, L.M.L., de Haes, J.C.J.M., Hoos, A.M., and Lammes, F.B. (1995) Doctor-patient communication: a review of the literature. *Soc Sci Med.* 40 (7): 903–918

Ostapchuk, M., Patel, P.D., Hughes Miller, K., Ziegler, C.H., Greenberg, R.B., and Haynes, G. (2010) Improving residents' teaching skills: a program evaluation of residents as teachers course. *Med Teach.* 32: e49–e56

Pasquale, S.J. and Pugnaire, M.P. (2002) Preparing medical students to teach. *Acad Med.* 77(11): 1175

Perkins, G.D., Hulme, J., and Bion, J.F. (2002) Peer-led resuscitation training for healthcare students: a randomised controlled study. *Intens Care Med.* 28: 698–700

Piaget, J. (1973) *Memory and Intelligence* (English translation). London: Routledge and Kegan Paul

Postareff, L. and Lindblom-Ylänne, S. (2008) Variation in teachers' descriptions of teaching: broadening the understanding of teaching in higher education. *Learn Instruct.* 18: 109–120

Pratt, D., Associates (1998) *Five Perspectives on Teaching in Adult and Higher Education.* Malabar, Florida: Krieger Publishing

Pratt, D. and Collins, J.B. (2012) *Teaching Perspectives Inventory.* http://www.teachingperspectives.com Accessed 5 May 2012

Prebble, T., Hargraves, H., Leach, L., Naidoo, K., Suddaby, G., and Zepke, N. (2004) Impact of student support services and academic development programmes on student outcomes in undergraduate tertiary study: a synthesis of the research. Wellington, New Zealand: Ministry of Education. Online: http://www.educationcounts.govt.nz/__data/assets/pdf_file/0013/7321/ugradstudentoutcomes.pdf Accessed 23 April 2012

Qureshi, Z., Ross, M.T., Maxwell, S., Rodrigues, M., Parisinos, C., and Hall, H.N. (2013) Developing junior doctor-delivered teaching. *Clin Teach.* 10(2): 118–123

Rees, C.E., Bradley, P., Collett, T., and McLachlan, J.C. (2005) 'Over my dead body?': the influence of demographics on students' willingness to participate in peer physical examination. *Med Teach.* 27(7): 599–605

Rees, C.E., Wearn, A.M., Vnuk, A.K., and Bradley, P. (2009) Don't want to show fellow students my naughty bits: medical students' anxieties about peer examination of intimate body regions at six schools across UK, Australasia and Far-East Asia. *Med Teach.* 31: 921–927

Richardson, J.T.E. (2005) Students' approaches to learning and teachers' approaches to teaching in higher education. *Educ Psychol.* 25(6): 673–680

Rigby, E. (2007) Taking forward aims of the Bologna Declaration: European core curriculum—the students' perspective. *Med Teach.* 29: 83–84

Rodrigues, J., Sengupta, A., Mitchell, A., et al. (2008) The South-East Scotland foundation doctor training programme—is 'near-peer' teaching feasible, efficacious and sustainable on a regional scale? *Med Teach.* 31(2): 51–57

Rogers, D.A., Regehr, G., Gelula, M., Yeh, K.A., Howdieshell, T.R., and Webb, W. (2000) Peer teaching and computer-assisted learning: An effective combination for surgical skill training? *J Surg Res.* 92(1): 53–55

Ross, M.T. (2012) Learning about teaching as part of the undergraduate medical curriculum: perspectives and learning outcomes. Doctor of Education Thesis. Edinburgh: The University of Edinburgh

Ross, M.T. and Cameron, H.S.C. (2007) AMEE Guide 30: Peer assisted learning: a planning and implementation framework. *Med Teach.* 29: 527–545

Ross, M.T. and Stenfors-Hayes, T. (2008a) What do Medical Teachers do? *Clin Teach.* 5(3): 159–162

Ross, M.T. and Stenfors-Hayes, T. (2008b) Development of a framework of medical undergraduate teaching activities. *Med. Educ.* 42(9): 915–922

Rotem, A. and Bandaranayake, R. (1981) Difficulties in improving medical education: a framework for analysis. *Higher Educ.* 10(5): 597–603

Roter, D. (2000) The enduring and evolving nature of the patient-physician relationship. *Patient Educ Counsell.* 39: 5–15

Samuelovicz, K. and Bain, J.D. (2001) Revisiting academics' beliefs about teaching and learning. *Higher Educ.* 41: 299–325

Schofield, S.J., Bradley, S., MacRae, C., Nathwani, D., and Dent, J.A. (2010) How we encourage faculty development. *Med Teach.* 32(11): 883–886

Schön, D.A. (1983) *The Reflective Practitioner: How Professionals Think in Action.* London: Temple Smith

Seldin, P., Miller, J.E., and Seldin, C.A. (2010) *The teaching portfolio: a practical guide to improved performance and promotion / tenure decisions,* 4th edition. San Francisco: Jossey-Bass

Sharpe, R. (2004) How do professionals learn and develop? Implications for staff and educational developers. In Baume D, Kahn P (eds) *Enhancing Staff and Educational Development* (pp. 132–153). London: Routledge Falmer

Shulman, L. (1987) Knowledge and teaching: foundations of a new reform. *Harv Educ Rev* 57(1): 1–22

Shulman, L. (2007) Practical wisdom in the service of professional practice. *Educ Res* 36(9): 560–563

Simpson, J. and Weiner, E. (1989) *The Oxford English Dictionary,* 2nd edn. Oxford: Clarendon Press

Smith, S., Mitchell, C., andBowler, S. (2007) Patient-centered education: applying learner-centered concepts to asthma education. *J Asthma* 44(10): 799–804

Snadden, D. and Thomas, M. (1998) The use of portfolio learning in medical education. *Med Teach.* 20(3): 192–199

Snyder, B.R. (1970) *The Hidden Curriculum.* New York: Alfred A. Knopf, Inc

Soriano, R.P., Blatt, B., Coplit, L., et al. (2010) Teaching medical students how to teach: a national survey of students-as-teachers programs in US medical schools. *Acad Med.* 85(11): 1725–1731

Stark, P. (2003) Teaching and learning in the clinical setting: a qualitative study of the perceptions of students and teachers. *Med Educ.* 37: 975–982

Starr, S., Ferguson, W.J., Haley, H.-L., and Quirk, M. (2003) Community preceptors' views of their identities as teachers. *Acad Med.* 78(8): 820–825

Steinert, Y., Mann, K., Centeno, A., et al. (2006) A systematic review of faculty development initiatives designed to improve teaching effectiveness in medical education: BEME Guide No. 8. *Med Teach.* 28(6): 497–526

Stenfors-Hayes, T., Hult, H., and Dahlgren, L.O. (2010) What does it mean to be a good teacher and clinical supervisor in medical education? *Adv Health Sci Educ.* 16(2): 197–210

Stenfors-Hayes, T., Hult, H., and Dahlgren, L.O. (2011) What does it mean to be a mentor in medical education? *Med Teach.* 33(8): e423–e428

Stenfors-Hayes, T. (2011) Being and becoming a teacher in medical education. PhD thesis. Stockholm: Karolinska Institutet

Stewart, M.A. (1995) Effective physician-patient communication and health outcomes: a review. *Can Med Ass J.* 152(9): 1423–1433

Stewart, M.A., Brown, J.B., Donner, A., et al. (2000) The impact of patient-centered care on outcomes. *J Fam Pract.* 49(9): 805–807

Stone, S., Ellers, B., Holmes, D., Orgren, R., Qualters, D., and Thompson, J. (2002) Identifying oneself as a teacher: the perceptions of preceptors. *Med Educ.* 36: 180–185

Tate, P. (2009) *The Doctor's Communication Handbook,* 6th edn. Abingdon: Radcliffe Publishing Ltd

Taylor, E.W., Tisdell, E.J., and Gusic, M.E. (2007) Teaching beliefs of medical educators: perspectives on clinical teaching in paediatrics. *Med Teach.* 29(4): 371–376

ten Cate, O. (2007) A teaching rotation and a student teaching qualification for senior medical students. *Med Teach.* 29: 566–571

ten Cate, O. and Durning, S. (2007) Dimensions and psychology of peer teaching in medical education. *Med Teach.* 29: 546–552

Tigelaar, D.E.H., Dolmans, D.H.J.M., Meijer, P.C., de Grave, W.S., and van der Vleuten, C.P.M. (2008) Teachers' interactions and their collaborative reflection processes during peer meetings. *Adv Health Sci Educ.* 13(3): 289–308

Topping, K.J. (1996) The effectiveness of peer tutoring in further and higher education: A typology and review of the literature. *Higher Educ.* 32(3): 321–345

Topping, K.J. and Ehly, S.W. (2001) Peer assisted learning: a framework for consultation. *J Educ Psychol Consult.* 12(2): 113–132

Trigwell, K. and Prosser, M. (1996) Changing approaches to teaching: a relational perspective. *Studies Higher Educ.* 21(3): 275–284

Trigwell, K. and Prosser, M. (2004) Development and use of the approaches to teaching inventory. *Educ. Psychol Rev.* 16(4): 409–424

Trigwell, K., Prosser, M., and Waterhouse, F. (1999) Relations between teachers' approaches to teaching and students' approaches to learning. *Higher Educ Res Devel.* 27(2): 143–153

Van de Wiel, M.W.J., Van de Bossche, P., Janssen, S., and Jossberger, H. (2011) Exploring deliberate practice in medicine: how do physicians learn in the workplace? *Adv Health Sci Educ.* 16: 81–95

von Fragstein, M., Silverman, J., Cushing, A., Quilligan, S., Salisbury, H., and Wiskin, C. (2008) UK consensus statement on the content of communication curricula in undergraduate medical education. *Med Educ.* 42: 1100–1107

Vygotsky, L.S. (1978) *Mind in society: the development of higher psychological processes.* Cambridge, MA: Harvard University Press

Wagner, L. (1982) *Peer Teaching: Historical Perspectives.* Westport, CT: Greenwood Press

Wamsley, M.A., Julian, K.A., Vener, M.H., and Morrison, E.H. (2005) Using an objective structured teaching evaluation for faculty development. *Med Educ.* 39: 1143–1172

Wearn, A.M., Rees, C.E., Bradley, P., and Vnuk, A.K. (2008) Understanding student concerns about peer physical examination using an activity theory framework. *Med Educ.* 42: 1218–1226

Weiss, V. and Needlman, R. (1998) To teach is to learn twice. Resident teachers learn more. *Arch Pediatr Adolesc Med.* 152(2): 190–192

Weurlander, M., Stenfors-Hayes, T. (2008) Developing medical teachers' thinking and practice: impact of a staff development course. *Higher Educ Res Devel.* 27(2): 143–153

Wilkerson, L. and Irby, D.M. (1998) Strategies for improving teaching practices: a comprehensive approach to faculty development. *Acad Med.* 73(4): 387–396

Wood, K. (2000) The experience of learning to teach: changing student teachers' ways of understanding teaching. *J Curriculum Studies.* 32(1): 75–93

Young, P. (2006) Out of balance: lecturers' perceptions of differential status and rewards in relation to teaching and research. *Teach Higher Educ.* 11(2): 191–202

Zabar, S., Hanley, K., Stevens, D.L., et al. (2004) Measuring the competency of residents as teachers. *J Gen Intern Med.* 19: 530–533

Zijdenbos, I., Fick, T., and ten Cate, O. (2011) How we offer all medical students training in basic teaching skills. *Med Teach.* 33: 24–26

CHAPTER 27

Patient involvement in medical education

Angela Towle and William Godolphin

I'm unique; not merely a diagnosis. Don't assume! Take time to listen, understand & give options. I hope you'll guide me on my journey.

Reproduced from a Tweet from a group of interprofessional students and mentor with a chronic condition, in a Health Mentors Program summarizing their key message as a group for a symposium to share their learning. With kind permission from Diane Desjardins (patient teacher), Milena Semproni, Jennifer Lukomskyj, Amy Le, and Lindsey McCloy (students)

Introduction

Patients have always been involved in medical education but too often in the past they have been used as convenient and passive tools for learning and practice. The first major review of the contribution that patients can make in the education of medical students, beyond their traditional role as 'clinical material' and teaching aids, was by Spencer et al. (2000). Since then, several reviews have explored both theoretical and practical aspects of patient involvement (Wykurz and Kelly 2002; Repper and Breeze 2007; Morgan and Jones 2009; Jha et al. 2009a; Towle et al. 2010; Spencer et al. 2011). We have assembled a comprehensive bibliography comprising over 400 papers published in English between 1970 and 2011 covering healthcare professional education (Towle and Godolphin 2012).

The focus of this chapter is the *active* involvement of patients, a term we use to describe the involvement of people who are engaged in teaching, assessment or curriculum development because of their expertise or experiences of health, illness or disability and who are aware that they have designated teaching roles. We exclude involvement of people who role-play patients to express symptoms, conditions or life stories they do not actually have (simulated patients). We include examples of standardized patients where they are being themselves (such as women who teach intimate examinations), though we admit this is a grey area. We exclude examples of patient stories (narratives) considered as learning resources; we also exclude indirect assessment of learning through anonymized feedback forms. Finally, we exclude informal learning in clinical settings where the patient's role is still essentially passive and their priority is to receive care.

Active patient involvement occurs throughout the continuum from undergraduate education, postgraduate education, continuing professional development (CPD), and in-service training, although the majority of reported initiatives occur in undergraduate courses or in postgraduate training of mental health professionals. In theory, patients can contribute to many different aspects of the educational process, including direct delivery of teaching and learning, curriculum and course planning, programme management,

recruitment and selection of students, student assessment, and course evaluation (Tew et al. 2004). In medical education, patients are mainly involved in curriculum delivery and, to a much lesser extent, curriculum development and student assessment (Jha et al. 2009a); few other roles are currently represented. A greater range of patient involvement is found in nursing and social work education (Repper and Breeze 2007).

The earliest examples of active patient involvement in teaching are interventions in which the patient was an instructor of clinical skills. The longest-lasting programmes are those in which patient instructors teach intimate examinations or musculoskeletal examination (Towle et al. 2010). Over the last two decades, professional educators have made use of the expertise of patients in order to enrich the education of students in a variety of ways, providing learning experiences that could not otherwise occur and broadening the curriculum from the biomedical model. There is a wide variety in the range of patients who have shared their experiences of living with illness or disability, although most medical schools only focus on one patient population or a limited selection. Typically, one or more patients are invited into the classroom or a small group tutorial to tell their stories and answer questions from students. The range includes people with human immunodeficiency virus (HIV) infection, cancer, disability and mental illness, and caregivers (Anderson et al. 2011; Wittenberg-Lyles et al. 2011). Patients may co-tutor sessions with faculty (Solomon et al. 2005). Home or family attachment schemes permit students to interact with patients over a period of time to learn about a variety of conditions in the wider community context (Shapiro et al. 2009). The aim may be to promote humanism and patient-centred care (Kumagai 2008), or foster more positive student attitudes towards certain stigmatized or underserved groups. Examples include workshops run by professional actors with learning disabilities or teaching by parents of children with chronic illness (e.g. Hall and Hollins 1996; Blaylock 2000). Community-based programmes include senior mentor programmes in which students are partnered with an elderly person who is 'ageing well' (Stewart and Alford 2006), health mentor programmes in which interprofessional groups of students learn from someone with a chronic condition (Collins et al. 2011), and placements in which students or residents learn from people living in deprived inner city areas and workers in the agencies that provide them with services (Anderson and Lennox 2009; Sturm et al. 2011). Patient organizations may contribute to, or lead, CPD activities on specialized topics such as fetal alcohol syndrome and there may be public members on committees that plan CPD (British Medical Association 2008).

In this chapter we explain why it is helpful to involve patients as active partners in education; we describe examples of some of the most well developed patient-as-teacher approaches, and examine the evidence that involving patients can improve outcomes. We conclude by giving a practical guide to involving patients.

Language: words, meanings, terminology

We use the term patient, for the sake of brevity, to include people with health problems (service user, client, or consumer), their caregivers (including carers, parents, and families), and healthy people (community member, citizen, or lay person). We chose to use 'patient' as our umbrella term—it being the most commonly recognized word; however, the language of 'patient involvement' is confusing and controversial.

Language not only transmits values and beliefs, but also reflects existing power relations. The use of the word patient is emotive, because in many people's minds it is associated with passivity, the sick role and disempowerment. As such it sits oddly with recent rhetoric about the importance of patient empowerment and activated patients. In the UK the term user or service user has increasingly replaced patient in relation to involvement in health and social care service delivery. However, in other parts of the world, including North America, 'user' is associated with illicit drug use. Even in the UK there are those who consider the term service user as passive and not inclusive of those who cannot or do not access services (McLaughlin 2009), or as implying provision of a technical service rather than holistic, relationship-centred care.

In some health professions, client is the preferred term—and preferred relationship. But there are also 'consumers', 'mental consumers', 'people with…' [a condition, disability], such as 'people with HIV infection', 'survivors', 'activists', 'people in recovery', 'experts by experience', and so on. The words people use to think of themselves in relation to the healthcare system vary according to the practitioner they are consulting, their condition and the stage of their illness, and can therefore have personal and emotional significance (Speed 2006). For example, some people who have battled with cancer or mental illness regard themselves as survivors, and this is how they prefer to be known, leading to a proliferation of literature on survivorship. The lack of agreed terminology is important for educators for several reasons. Strong emotions generated by language and labels create barriers to communication and partnerships. Whichever discourse we use identifies a power dimension and hierarchy of control (McLaughlin 2009) and is descriptive not of a person but of a relationship. Each of these words carries different meaning and none is acceptable by everyone as an alternative to patient. The inevitable multiplicity of terms complicates scholarly activity: it makes searching the literature difficult, and writing and talking about the topic cumbersome.

Furthermore, not all patients involved in health professional education are ill or are currently receiving care. There are many well people who have perspectives or experiences of value to health professional learning. These include older people, caregivers of people with chronic illness or disability, parents of normal children, people from specific ethnic groups, refugees, people who are marginalized or disadvantaged (for example the homeless or recent immigrants). The term 'lay' may be more inclusive but it defines people in terms of what they are *not* (a professional) and implies a lack of expertise and in our experience is universally disliked even by people who cannot agree on any other term. Other terms found are 'citizens', 'community members' and 'the public', but these do not clearly differentiate health professionals from non-professionals.

Complications of terminology extend to the many names used for patients actively involved in medical or other health professions education. For example, patients may be teachers, educators, instructors, teaching associates, professional patients, mentors, partners or consultants. Many patient involvement initiatives have coined their own local terminology and the meaning of terms is not always consistent. This makes literature searches difficult and may be one reason why reviews of the literature using similar but not identical inclusion criteria miss many relevant papers.

Classification schemes

The diversity of educational initiatives in which patients are involved requires a classification scheme. Without such a framework there is no agreed way that authors can characterize the role of patients in their initiatives, making scholarly communication difficult. It is often difficult to find out from published work exactly what the patient's role was in the educational programme described, especially the degree to which patients were actively involved, whether their role was explicitly identified as teacher and the degree to which they participated in decision making. For example, early patient or community contact in medical school frequently consists of an attachment to a patient with a chronic illness, a pregnant woman, a family, or a community agency; in some cases the patient, family, or community agency may be explicitly identified as a teacher or mentor, whereas in other cases their role is to be interviewed. The expected learning outcomes would be quite different for those different roles. Several schemes have been developed to classify the variables so that initiatives can be consistently described and compared, for example with respect to outcomes. They can also be used to track changes over time to answer questions about how and why the role or degree of involvement changes.

The Cambridge Framework (Spencer et al. 2000) was developed to facilitate discussion about involvement of patients in clinical education. It is based on four sets of attributes of situations and environments in which patients, students, and teachers interact:

Who: the individual background, culture and experience of each patient, their family and carers.

How: including patient role (passive or active), nature of encounter, length of contact, degree of supervision.

What: the educational content, including type of problem (general versus specific) and the knowledge, skills and values to be learned.

Where: location of interaction, e.g. community, hospital ward, clinic.

The Cambridge Framework is a tool that could be used by curriculum planners and educators to review and monitor the extent to which patients are actively involved. It has not been validated.

A different approach to classification is based on the degree of engagement, from minimal involvement to full partnership. Tew et al. (2004) described a 'Ladder of Involvement' in curricular development and delivery ranging from Level 1 'No involvement' to Level 5 'Partnership'. Their tool, developed in the context of mental health education and training, can be applied to other educational programmes and across the educational continuum.

Level 1: Little involvement—curriculum is planned and delivered with no consultation or involvement.

Level 2: Emerging involvement—outreach and liaison with local user and carer groups; they are invited to tell their story and are occasionally consulted in relation to planning, but have no opportunity for shaping as a whole.

Level 3: Growing involvement—users and carers contribute regularly in more than one aspect of education and training. They are reimbursed and there is some support. Key decisions on education may be made in forums, in which users or carers are excluded.

Level 4: Collaboration—users and carers may contribute to key discussions and decisions; the value of this is acknowledged by all concerned. A coordinated programme of involvement and support is developing.

Level 5: Partnership—all partner groups work together systematically and strategically, underpinned by explicit statement of partnership values. All key decisions are made jointly. Infrastructure is funded and in place for support and training.

We have developed and field-tested a taxonomy with elements of both these models that identifies six main educational roles and for each role identifies six attributes associated with the degree of involvement (Spencer et al. 2011).

Rationale for involvement of patients in medical education

There are many reasons for patient involvement in health professional education, which differ by profession, country, and over time

(fig. 27.1). In general, decisions to involve patients have originated from socio-cultural change and associated policy responses. We discuss three clusters of reasons that are not mutually exclusive but are each rooted in a different discourse. It is important to recognize that, at the time of writing, the movement to involve patients actively in the education of health professionals is based more on the power of these rationales than on educational theory or robust evidence of beneficial educational or health outcomes.

Public and patient involvement in healthcare: government and professional policy directives

The importance of public and patient involvement in healthcare is recognized in many countries. Members of the public are frequently consulted about services, policy and research as part of a growing consumerist model of healthcare. In the UK, government policy has placed the public and individual patients at the centre of healthcare over the past 20 years and successive policy documents have emphasized a patient-led service based on choice, participation, and partnership. Within this context the UK government has recently made clear its expectations that service users and carers should be involved in the education and training of health professionals, a policy directive that has been taken up by accrediting bodies. Although medical education lags behind nursing and social work in its requirements for extensive patient–public involvement, the General Medical Council does require data on the quality of medical education programmes to include feedback from patients. The most significant activity has been in the field of mental health; originally in mental health nursing, extended more recently to social work, psychiatry, and clinical psychology. These policy directives have resulted in a large number of initiatives such that the UK leads in institutionalizing patient involvement in education.

Irrespective of national government policy, however, almost all health professions espouse a version of patient-centred care in their good practice model, which involves patients in decision-making, with a focus on individual people's preferences, life circumstances, and experience of illness. There is at least a conceptual link between patient involvement in education, patient involvement in care, and improved health outcomes. However, patient-centredness is typically framed as a set of values and virtues learned from doctors as role models, reinforced through structured educational input from

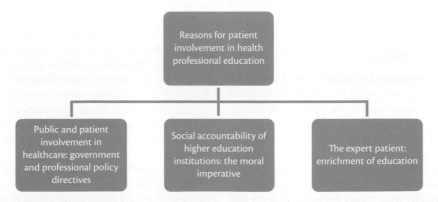

Figure 27.1 Reasons for patient involvement in health professional education.

medical educators, and, paradoxically, not from patients (Bleakley and Bligh 2008).

Social accountability of higher education institutions: the moral imperative

Universities and medical schools are being increasingly scrutinized with regard to the gap between societal needs and the educational system (Towle and Godolphin 2011a). Community engagement initiatives signal recognition by academic institutions that they need to respond effectively to society's evolving health needs. Involving patients in medical education is one way to bring the voice of the community into the medical school. Initiatives such as community-based service learning, especially in the USA, come from the moral imperative to address health disparities. Although active patient or community involvement are not in themselves prerequisites for service learning activities, people in the community play a variety of roles along the spectrum of involvement from passive recipients of care (the classic provider–patient relationship), to facilitators of reflection seminars, mentors, and assessors of students. The provision of opportunities for service learning has recently been adopted as an accreditation standard for North American medical schools. However, there remains a wide gap between service or outreach and collaborative partnerships with the community, leading to the integration of community members into academic medicine as mentors and teachers (Hunt et al. 2011). Other patient involvement initiatives in the USA (e.g. the senior mentor programmes) have their origin in the need to improve healthcare for the underserved.

The expert patient: enrichment of education

Patients bring a diversity of expertise to their teaching role (Wykurz and Kelly 2002). The recognition of patients as experts comes in part from the concept of encounters between professionals and patients as 'meetings of experts', first elaborated by Tuckett et al. (1985). Health professionals bring biomedical expertise and patients bring expertise of their personal and cultural background and their experience of living with illness or disability. Broadening curricula to include the psychosocial is especially necessary when educating professionals to deal with the increasing burden of chronic disease, where patient and family are the chief providers of care and where day-to-day management involves much more than attention to biomedical concerns (Towle and Godolphin 2011b). In some disciplines, the expertise of patients has been used to augment a scarce pool of clinical teachers or to create safe learning environments in which students can practise clinical skills.

Theoretical perspectives

The impetus for patient involvement has largely come from social change and policy directives. Not much of the literature about patient involvement in education is informed by learning theory. Patients as educators challenge the nature of expertise and power, yet so far there has been a failure to explore social issues surrounding patient involvement such as how students learn *with* rather than just *about* patients (Rees et al. 2007). Such learning not only implies a greater level of activity on the part of patients but also reflects the dynamic mutuality that occurs between students and patients. An example of the kind of work that would advance

understanding of learning from patients is the study by Henriksen and Ringsted (2011) who interviewed occupational therapy and physical therapy students about their experience of learning from patient instructors with arthritis (in the absence of faculty); in this context the added value derived from the combination of content matter, pedagogical format and patient–student power relations. The content matter was complemented by the provision of realism and individual perspectives on rheumatism; the pedagogical format was authentic and intimate in the style of instruction and feedback; and the patient instructor-student relationship was characterized by balanced power relations that supported the legitimacy of learning and allowed mistakes and questions (Henriksen and Ringsted 2011).

Socio-cultural learning theory in which learning is conceptualized as participation in a social process provides a useful way to contrast learning with patients to the usual concept of individual knowledge acquisition. Learning by participation also appears to be consistent with the ways in which community-based organizations conceptualize learning as compared to faculty in higher education (Bacon 2002): for example, faculty identify themselves as 'knowers' and 'individuals'; community members identify themselves as 'learners' and 'collective'. Theories such as situated learning (Lave and Wenger 1991) offer insights into issues such as power relationships, identity, roles and discourse that are pertinent to considerations about patient or user involvement. The work of Katz et al. (2000) provides an example of how a sociocultural perspective can be used to explore how students learn *with* rather than simply *about* patients in the context of a conversational forum that permits appreciation of the different points of view that participants bring to bear on an ethical dilemma. Rees et al. (2007) used sociocultural learning theory to show that both students and patients are legitimate peripheral participants in the community of medical practice, and generated recommendations that would lead to active collaboration between qualified health professionals and patients. They hypothesized that, as a consequence, a new level of knowledge 'production' rather than 'reproduction' may emerge within the medical education community. Similarly, Bleakley and Bligh (2008) propose a theoretical model of collaborative knowledge production based on theories of text, identity construction and work-based learning in which the prime locus for knowledge production is the student's reading of the patient's condition in collaboration with the patient. In this radical model, the teacher's task shifts from that of knowledge transfer to genuine facilitation, and the process of education becomes a 'mutually beneficial dialogue supported by experts'.

Another area ripe for theoretical exploration is that of patient expertise within the context of health professional education, i.e. what knowledge can patients contribute? Theories of development of professional expertise and the literature on the expert patient or lay expertise are difficult to apply in this context. Exploration of patient expertise is located within the broader theoretical debate about the status of medical and scientific expertise in late modern society and the value and distinctiveness of ordinary people's knowledge, and whether these are two distinctly different types of knowledge or a continuum (McClean and Shaw 2005). The most relevant analysis we have found is in relation to the added value of patient participation in biomedical research by Caron-Flinterman et al. (2005). They use the term 'experiential knowledge' to refer to the ultimate source of patient-specific knowledge, the often implicit lived experiences of individual patients with their bodies and their illnesses as well as with care and cure. It arises when these experiences are converted, consciously or unconsciously, into personal insight that helps someone to manage their condition. Experiential expertise arises when patients share this knowledge so that the communal body of knowledge exceeds the boundaries of individual experiences. The theories of expertise and the validity of knowledge outlined by Caron-Flinterman et al. (2005) are as applicable to education as to research and have important implications. For example, they may determine criteria for selection of patient educators (stage of development of experiential knowledge; extent to which patients have shared experiences with peer groups) and attitudes of faculty towards patients as educators (perceptions about the validity of their knowledge).

Examples of patient involvement in medical education

We give four examples that illustrate a range of ways in which patients have been involved as teachers. We chose these because there is a unifying theme that permits different initiatives to be clustered together and some conclusions to be drawn: patients as teachers of clinical skills; senior mentor programmes; involvement of people with mental health problems; and parents as teachers (see fig. 27.2). Other examples can be found in reviews by Wykurz and Kelly (2002), Repper and Breeze (2007), Morgan and Jones (2009), Jha et al. (2009a), Towle et al. (2010), Spencer et al. (2011), and Towle and Godolphin (2012).

Patients as teachers of clinical skills

There is cross-over between standardized patients (SPs), simulated patients, and patients who teach clinical and communication skills. We deal here only with cases where patients are being themselves, teaching on their own bodies and using their own lived experiences (although they may have been trained to teach in a standardized way).

Physical examination skills

Patient Instructor (PI) programmes, in which patients teach physical examination and communication skills, were developed in the early 1970s as a response by professional educators to perceived problems with the teaching of basic clinical skills by clinicians,

notably that students were rarely observed or given feedback on their performance (Towle et al. 2010). Early studies provided evidence of acceptability, short-term effectiveness and cost efficiency. PIs provided a safe learning environment in which students felt less pressure to perform because of the reduced power differential between student and patient compared with student and clinician. The first programmes used PIs who were themselves (either normal or with defined signs and symptoms); however, by the late 1970s Barrows and colleagues had developed sophisticated simulation techniques, the foundation for the wide and varied use of SPs today (Wallace 1997). The PI concept went into decline apart from female and male intimate examinations and musculoskeletal examinations, although it has witnessed a renaissance in recent years, in part because of its perceived cost effectiveness (teaching basic physical examination skills is expensive).

Intimate examinations

Intimate examinations include pelvic, breast, testicular and rectal examinations, although most examples in the literature describe patients teaching the female examination. The first Gynecology Teaching Associate (GTA) programme in the late 1960s was inspired by Barrows' early work (Kretzschmar 1978). By the early 1980s the use of GTAs had become widespread in North American medical schools; male TAs were introduced to teach the genitorectal examination, but these programmes did not become as well established. The Netherlands, Sweden, Belgium, Australia, and the UK have adopted GTA programmes more recently. Reasons for the success and longevity of the programmes include the anxiety faced by students in learning these skills, and the inherent difficulty in teaching and assessing intimate examinations in an ethical manner, although the fact that students continue to report learning on unconsenting anaesthetized women suggests that patients are still inappropriately used as teaching material (Rees and Monrouxe 2011). The objectives of GTA programmes may include not only technical and communication skills, but attitudes towards women and women's health issues, including well-women checks and contraception. Another common objective is to reduce anxiety for students and patients. In general, students report high satisfaction with the experience: learning is non-stressful and they receive immediate and constructive feedback on their performance; improvements in clinical skills have been convincingly demonstrated (Jha et al. 2010).

Musculoskeletal examination

One of the most developed, institutionalized and widespread PI programmes is the arthritis educator programme in which arthritis patients teach and assess the musculoskeletal examination (total or specific joints). Since the 1980s, it has spread to other schools in the USA, Canada, and Australia, and thence to several other countries, more recently appearing, apparently independently, in Switzerland and the UK. Long-term stable funding has come largely from pharmaceutical companies. The patients (Patient Instructors, Patient Partners, Patient Educators, or Arthritis Educators) receive intense structured and standardized training from physicians within the biomedical model; there is a strong emphasis on anatomy and the reliable assessment of the performance of the joint examination using a standardized checklist (Gruppen et al. 1996). The autonomy of the patient as educator is limited, but in some programmes patients also teach about psychosocial issues and the experience of living with arthritis. Learners are generally preclinical medical students, but some involve clinical level students, postgraduates, and

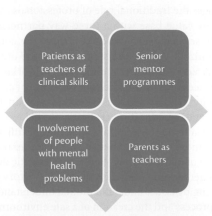

Figure 27.2 Examples of patient involvement in medical education.

physical therapy students. In general, arthritis educators are used in addition to interactive small group discussion and computer-assisted learning. Because of differences in programme design and evaluation methods, it is difficult to draw strong conclusions about outcomes. Student satisfaction is high although in comparative studies students tend to prefer being taught by specialists. Some programmes employ arthritis educators because of a shortage of specialists. Students taught by patients generally have equivalent examination skills to those taught by specialist physicians (Oswald et al. 2011a) although the teaching style is qualitatively different (Oswald et al. 2011b). Patient satisfaction is high and no adverse effects of being a patient teacher have been noted.

Senior mentor programmes

Senior Mentor Programmes (SMPs) emerged in US medical schools in 2000 to improve attitudes of students towards older people and reduce ageism as part of the evolution of geriatrics curricula in the face of a rapidly aging population. At least 20 programmes have been developed, all with a primary goal: to provide students an experience with older, well adults. The first wave of programmes that developed between 2000 and 2005 with John A Hartford Foundation and Association of American Medical Colleges support had such promising results that other medical schools subsequently adopted or adapted their own SMP. Detailed descriptions of eight of the original programmes were published in a special issue of *Gerontology and Geriatrics Education* (Stewart and Alford 2006). The SMPs vary greatly in format, including length (from one day to 4 years), whether required or elective, and extent of integration into medical school curricula. Most have a mixture of social activities and formal assignments that students and mentors complete together through interviews or standard assessment instruments (e.g. medication review), but differ in the extent to which the relationship between students and mentors is viewed as a defining aspect of the programme. Students and mentors need to respond to role changes as the relationship and the nature of academic activities evolve. In programmes that last 3 or 4 years, students find it challenging to sustain the relationship and to fulfil SMP obligations during the clinical years.

SMPs use older adults who are basically well and living in the community with no cognitive problems. Most programmes appear to have no difficulty recruiting mentors and some have waiting lists, though all struggle to recruit an ethnically and socioeconomically diverse pool of mentors, an issue raised frequently in descriptions of other patient-as-teacher programmes. Student and mentor acceptance is high, there is a positive effect on student attitudes towards older adults and there is some indication that the experience promotes student empathy and patient-centredness (Eleazer et al. 2009). For example, Breytspraak et al. (2008) found that an intergenerational relationship developed between medical student and senior mentor, characterized by affective reciprocity (empathy, intimacy), instrumental reciprocity (such as advice, role modeling, support), and the discovery of similarities and differences. SMPs appear to be sustained by the medical school because they increase the visibility and acceptance of gerontology, and are economical and easy to operate (Eleazer et al. 2009).

A different model that addressed some of the same concerns about helping physicians to provide better care for the elderly is the 'Council of Elders' (Katz et al. 2000) in which community elders were invited to function as 'Senior Faculty' to whom medical

residents in a geriatrics rotation presented their challenging and heartfelt dilemmas in caring for elderly patients. Particular attention was paid to the preparation felt necessary to build a dialogue relationship between participants from two very different worlds—i.e. different generations and cultures. Unfortunately it is also an example of how patient-as-educator initiatives are often short-lived—this can be for various reasons: for example the amount of work required may not be sustainable, champions leave, institutional support (including funding) is lacking, or because the initiative was only ever intended as a time-limited research project and not an ongoing programme.

Mental health

People with mental health problems are involved in the education of medical students and trainee psychiatrists as well as mental health nurses, clinical psychologists, social workers and interprofessional mental health teams. A general review is provided by Livingston and Cooper (2004) and a detailed practical guide by Tew et al. (2004). Most of the extensive literature relates to involvement in non-physician training, and most comes from the UK. In 2005 the UK Royal College of Psychiatrists made service user and carer involvement an accreditation requirement of postgraduate training programmes in psychiatry through, for example, selection of trainees, planning of training, sharing experiences, interview skills training and giving feedback on performance (Fadden et al. 2005). Patients have identified that they can contextualize the part mental health plays in people's lives, dispel myths and fantasies; offer positive aspects of mental health to counterbalance negative media portrayals, and illustrate diversity, hope and recovery (Dogra et al. 2008).

Although most psychiatry trainees see benefit to learning about patient perspectives, they have concerns about the representativeness of views expressed and the potential undermining of physician authority; few support patients being assessors because of concerns about objectivity. Indeed, the involvement of people with mental health problems raises some of the thorniest issues in the patient-as-teacher movement. For example, the widespread stereotypes of mental illness, including irrationality and irresponsibility, make the credibility of mental health patients as educators suspect. In the pervasive medical model professionals have the power and legitimized expertise to define the mentally ill as lacking in competence, and contact in a psychiatric hospital setting does not reinforce the view of a patient as an equal partner or member of the community (Scheyett and Kim 2004). On the other hand, patient involvement challenges the traditional role of professionals as experts and requires a new value base with a three-way partnership between professionals, service users and carers where the contribution of each is recognized, valued and respected by the others (Fadden et al. 2005). Academics perceive difficulties in working with mental health service users in the classroom because of assumptions of unpredictability, need for supervision and possible inability to cope with the demands of education (Felton and Stickley 2004). Those who genuinely attempt to work in collaboration with a patient find they become more aware of their own biases, assumptions and understanding of mental illness (Bennett and Baikie 2003).

Bringing together members of groups with a history of tension to discuss challenging issues and build mutual understanding requires attention to process and the creation of a safe environment for sharing. Techniques such as facilitated dialogue have been used when the aim is to change attitudes (Scheyett and Kim 2004). A number of approaches have been developed to legitimize the involvement of mental health patients through training, co-teaching and accreditation of patient teachers (e.g. consumer tutors) and academic appointments such as 'Service User Academic' (Simons et al. 2007). However, this transition from user to academic has led to charges that service users who become part of the educational culture are of limited value as they have become distanced from their experiences and so are not representative of other individuals with mental health problems. In this respect service users are in a no-win situation because as patients they are perceived as incompetent and irrational but neither are they accepted as professionals in the education system (Felton and Stickley 2004).

Parents as teachers

Parents as teacher programmes present learners with a holistic understanding of life with a chronically ill or disabled child—in order to promote family-centred care. They may also aim to prepare professionals for work in an interagency, interprofessional environment in collaboration with families. The most common models are the single home visit to a parent and child with a chronic condition and the family attachment programme in which preclinical students follow a family for a period of time, e.g. through pregnancy. US medical schools provide some of the best developed and long lasting examples in which parents are explicitly recognized as teachers and have been integrated into the curriculum, for example in paediatric residency training (Blasco et al. 1999), paediatric clerkships (Johnson et al. 2006), or throughout the undergraduate curriculum in multiple courses (Hanson and Randall 2007). Each programme involves parents in multiple roles—typically participation in curriculum development, panel discussions, interviews and home visits. A usual feature is involvement of a core group of activated parents, either a pre-existing community advocacy group (such as Parent to Parent Vermont), or a group created especially for purpose. These groups partner with faculty to make decisions about the curriculum, as well as provide a pool of parents for teaching purposes, and are often responsible for recruitment, training and support of new parent teachers. Reports of these programmes emphasize the inclusive developmental process and describe educational activities but have little information on student perspectives beyond acceptability. Other roles that parents may play include fostering interviewing skills, acting and role playing, sharing experiences of being a patient (e.g. students accompanying parents on a clinic visit), and collaborating in mutually beneficial service-learning activities (e.g. students providing respite care) (Blaylock 2000).

Patient involvement in other health professional programmes

Patient (service user and carer) involvement in the education of health and social care professionals has become expected practice in many countries, especially in the training of mental health professionals, although only in the UK and, to a lesser extent, Australia, has it become mandatory. In the UK involvement of service users or patients is a requirement at preregistration level for nurses, midwives and health visitors, and involvement in social work education was formalized with the introduction of the new social work degree in 2003. The British experience therefore provides the most complete understanding of the obstacles and opportunities that occur with systemic involvement. Although nursing, social work, and mental health workers are the major professions that involve patients in education; an international conference on patient involvement in health professional education in 2005 was also attended by representatives from pharmacy, occupational therapy, physical therapy, chiropractic, and psychology (Farrell et al. 2006). The intent of involvement is to promote the social model that puts service users at the centre of their care. Major goals are to remove attitudinal barriers, challenge stereotypes, tackle social exclusion, and redress historic power imbalances, especially in the case of people who use mental health and social services. In social work education, for example, underpinning values include respect, equality, genuine partnership, social inclusion and empowerment, and involvement is designed to change the power dynamics between clients and social workers (or between students and clients within practice placements) that make it difficult for clients to share experiential knowledge and contribute to the knowledge base of social work (Anghel and Ramon 2009).

Benefits have been shown in a few studies (Barnes et al. 2006) but there is little evidence of sustained impact on student learning. Making patient involvement a mandatory requirement has resulted in tokenistic involvement in many cases with a failure to fundamentally challenge existing power structures in educational relationships (Felton and Stickley 2004). It has also highlighted the barriers that exist in higher education to the development of authentic partnerships: requirements at the institutional level include strategic leadership and direction, access to local links and networks, and attention to those organizational and cultural issues that require creative solutions and infrastructure to support involvement (Gutteridge and Dobbins 2010). One of the most developed examples of sustained and authentic involvement at an institutional level is Comensus at the University of Central Lancashire, a faculty-wide initiative to involve service users and carers in the education of health and social care professionals across all schools and departments in the Faculty of Health (McKeown et al. 2010).

Outcomes of patient involvement

A consistent theme in reviews on patient involvement is lack of clear and measurable educational outcomes. The quality of the literature is generally low, as assessed by accepted criteria for quantitative and qualitative studies (Towle et al. 2010). Most studies are descriptive; some evaluation of short-term outcomes is reported for a subset of initiatives (primarily in the teaching of clinical skills), but few studies have rigorous experimental designs. Interventions are usually described only once, soon after implementation (often of a pilot project) along with preliminary evaluation data, usually student satisfaction and patient views. Reviews by Morgan and Jones (2009) and Jha et al. (2009a) provide summaries of the state of the art and note some evidence of short-term benefits to students and the patient teachers, and lack of evidence of long-term impact on students or the healthcare system. Methodological weaknesses, and the lack of specificity of objectives or intended outcomes, as well as their diversity, make it difficult to draw strong general conclusions about the effectiveness of patient involvement. However, some of the recurring themes and more notable studies are identified in the following sections.

Learners' perspectives

Most studies report high learner satisfaction with patient involvement. Students identify benefits such as perceived relevance, enhanced understanding of patient perspectives, enhanced communication skills, increased confidence talking to patients and learning in a non-threatening environment, especially for intimate examinations (Jha et al. 2009a, 2010). Comparisons of student perceptions as reported in pre/post-programme questionnaires indicate that students become more sensitive to the needs of vulnerable populations; and their assumptions and attitudes improve significantly in relation to chronic illness, disabled children, family involvement, mental illness, and senior care (Towle et al. 2010). Independent verification of these perceptions is lacking. Students learn physical examination skills equally well from patient teachers as from physicians (Oswald et al. 2011a).

Although few papers report student learning beyond post-encounter evaluation there is evidence that teaching by patients has a lasting impact in the areas of technical skills (Coleman et al. 2003), interpersonal skills, empathic understanding and an individualized approach to the patient (Klein et al. 2000). Studies of effects on subsequent practice are rare. In one follow up study of health professionals in a Masters level Community Mental Health course, all participants described how their practice had developed to enhance user involvement, and a higher proportion of their service users reported good user-centred assessment and care planning compared to a control group (Barnes et al. 2006).

The few negative experiences documented are almost always following sessions with people with mental health problems, and are associated with perceived antagonistic attitudes, unbalanced views, lack of representativeness and mixed views on the usefulness of feedback received (Morgan and Jones 2009). Other studies report that students are sometimes concerned about becoming a burden to patients. Patient attachment and mentorship programmes may provide the first real, long-term exposure that students have to patients and can be emotionally testing, especially if the patient's health deteriorates. Faculty support for students and having formal closure of the student–patient relationship are helpful (Towle et al. 2010).

Patients' perspectives

Benefits to patients occur because they feel their experiential knowledge of illness and the healthcare system should be included in medical education; they like to give something back to the community and feel their experiences can benefit future health professionals and patients (Stacy and Spencer 1999). Patients report specific therapeutic benefits such as raised self-esteem and empowerment, development of a coherent illness narrative, new insights into their problems and deeper understanding of the doctor-patient relationship (Walters et al. 2003). Senior mentors enjoy the companionship of students. Patients generally feel well treated by students.

Problems reported by patients starting their new role include concerns about revisiting negative experiences, about being judged by students and about how truthfully their experiences will be represented when students write up assignments (Towle et al. 2010). Consent and confidentiality are major concerns for patients and carers, but the ethics of patient involvement are not well addressed (Jha et al. 2009a). Concerns can be addressed by appropriate preparation and orientation: clearly explaining the purpose and importance of their involvement, obtaining informed consent, limiting medical information provided to students to that necessary to their learning, and providing strict guidelines about confidentiality (Towle et al. 2010). The potential for exploitation of people's goodwill has been raised (Stacy and Spencer 1999) and occasional evidence of negative consequences has been documented, for example in relation to mental health (Livingston and Cooper 2004) and intimate examinations (Jha et al. 2010).

Professionals' perspectives

Few studies have examined the views of health professionals involved in patient-as-teacher programmes. Most feel that students have valuable learning experiences, are exposed to important patient issues, are enabled to see the patient's perspective, and gain valuable patient interaction skills (fig. 27.3). Although they support teaching by patients, time to devote to these programmes is a concern (Towle et al. 2010). There is generally less support for expanding the role of patients to curriculum development or formal assessment of students (Jha et al. 2009b).

No specific negative impact on health professional educators has been documented. Some professionals have negative attitudes about involving patients, most frequently related to patients with mental health problems (Livingston and Cooper 2004). Some express concern about possible deleterious effects on patients such as psychological stress, emotional wellbeing, and physical fatigue but the little research on this is inconclusive (Gecht 2000). Some perceive that patients chosen by their doctors to be involved may either feel obligated to the commitment or conversely feel the commitment entitles them to preferential treatment, thus blurring professional boundaries (Walters et al. 2003) or that patients who repeat their stories frequently are in danger of becoming professionalized (Jha et al. 2009b). Research is needed to confirm whether these concerns are justified.

Practical considerations

Good practice guides that provide useful information have been produced in the UK for education in mental healthcare (Tew et al. 2004) and social work (Levin 2004). The INVOLVE guides, designed to promote patient involvement in health research, have information relevant to higher education (http://www.invo.org.uk). No such 'how to' resources yet exist for medical education but the British Medical Association (2008) published some useful

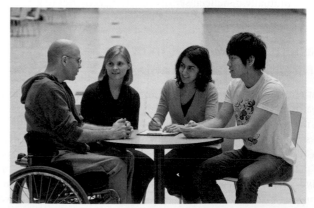

Figure 27.3 Patient involvement in action.

guidelines, especially on the important topic of ethics, including confidentiality and consent.

Each of these guides organizes the key tasks differently, but all identify a core set of issues as critical. These include: leadership (requires a champion); dedicated funding; recruitment of patients (diversity and representativeness); infrastructure for support, training, and supervision of patients; employment and contracting; payment and expenses; capacity building; and evaluation. They are good resources for those needing advice about initiating and sustaining involvement. However, these activities may be more effectively facilitated by designated support and development workers. A network of development workers has been established in the UK which has published guidelines for higher education institutions (Developers of User and Carers in Education 2009). This liaison role, also referred to as being a culture broker or boundary spanner, is one that many academic institutions have found essential to facilitate partnerships with community-based organizations and overcome the large power imbalance.

A guide produced by the Social Care Institute for Excellence (Levin 2004) articulates key practical considerations in 'preparing for participation':

+ Everyone benefits from working on and agreeing the values and principles of involvement as early as possible in the process of developing partnerships.

+ A comprehensive strategy for involvement makes it easier to include later new roles where progress may be slower or more complicated.

+ Effective participation requires patients, academic staff, administrators, students, and others working together in new ways—an opportunity for development.

+ Resources (people, time, money and support) are needed to make it work.

+ Actively promoting and sustaining participation is a process not a one-off event. It takes time to build respectful and purposeful relationships and to give attention to practicalities.

+ Enthusiasm and goodwill are required; initially only a small number of participants may be available and willing; widening participation is a key task.

Often the words involvement, collaboration, and partnership are used interchangeably. However, working in true partnership with people from the community brings challenges for academics. There are major institutional barriers to the authentic involvement of community members in higher education, including the hierarchical nature of academia, stigma and discrimination, validation and accreditation processes, academic jargon, definitions of knowledge, and inappropriate payment and support systems (Basset et al. 2006). The university, while paying lip service to community engagement and partnership, still views the benefits to the community to be the consequence of its expertise being given out (Towle and Godolphin 2011a). There is little scholarly debate about the benefits to academia of in-reach from the community, or the changes that may occur to the university as a consequence—that is, 'the reciprocal sharing of resources between the university and its community, each having different forms of assets and social capital' (McKeown et al. 2010, p. 52). Recognizing the difficulty of achieving authentic partnerships between academia and the community, the North American organization Community-Campus Partnerships for Health has developed a set of partnership principles that have been recognized and applied internationally (see http://www.ccph.info).

Based on our experience of developing several patient-as-teacher initiatives, we propose a framework that includes examples of the questions to be considered when planning (see table 27.1).

Some of the most important practical issues related to involving patients are now discussed in more detail.

Recruitment

Patients can be recruited through diverse means such as patient advocacy or support groups, community agencies or newspapers, through family practitioner offices or clinics. In our experience, recruitment works best through organizations such as patient support groups, especially those whose mandate includes educational activities such as peer support, and we recommend that academics take time to develop good working relationships with their local organizations. Most not-for-profit organizations have considerable expertise in the recruitment of volunteers for a variety of roles; we have found them to be of great assistance with recruitment of patient teachers. Two important considerations are diversity and representativeness. Recruitment of culturally or ethnically diverse groups is notoriously problematic. Identified barriers include language, the demographic profile of most patient support groups, the deference to doctors found in some cultures, concerns from families about losing face in the community if illness (especially mental illness) is disclosed, and the major power imbalance between academia and people who are already marginalized in society (Warren and Boxall 2009; Yeung and Ng 2011). Representativeness is a concern given the individual nature of the patient experience and that some patients will have a specific issue or agenda. Although some programmes recruit patients who meet specific criteria, such as good communication skills, in general there has been little substantive discussion in the literature about selection, or application of the ideas found in the work of Williamson (2007) about selection of patient representatives for consultation about healthcare services.

Preparation and training

Preparation of patients for their involvement in education is generally agreed to be important but varies widely in method, duration and intensity. Sometimes patients are given learning objectives to be covered with their student partners and there may be some form of training by the medical faculty. Intensive training is most often associated with teaching physical examination skills. Training appears to reduce patients' anxiety about their teaching role and makes their involvement seem more official and important. However, little attention has been paid to how training might occur within a partnership model rather than as an activity that is 'done to' patients by well-meaning experts. Moss et al. (2009) offer one model in which service users and carers played a leading role in identifying their training needs and developing a course to be taken jointly by service users and academic staff. We have found that by working with patient groups that have a mandate for education we are able to recruit many people who already have skills in facilitation, peer support or making presentations that are directly transferable to their role as teachers of health professionals.

Table 27.1 Example of a planning framework for a patient as educator programme

Issue	Questions to consider
Rationale, theory	What are the reasons for involving patients as educators? Does it fit with institutional philosophy? Has the community expressed an interest need? What are the expected outcomes/benefits?
Institutional/organizational context	Who are the leaders/champions? Are there existing collaborations with community volunteers/organizations? Where does the programme fit within existing curriculum? Is it a research project or curriculum development initiative?
Planning	What is the organizational structure for planning (planning committee mandate, leadership, membership of faculty, patients, students, decision making)? What resources are available (for start up, continuation)? Is it a pilot project? Who are the learners and how many? Is it required or voluntary (if voluntary, how are learners selected)?
Recruitment of patient educators	What are the roles (job description)? How are patients recruited (through community organisations, health professionals, brochures, word of mouth, websites)? How are patients screened and by whom (selection criteria, recruitment process)? How are representativeness and diversity managed?
Curriculum and assessment	What are the objectives (and who decides)? What are the roles of patients in teaching? Design and number of teaching sessions? Learning activities? How will students be assessed and by whom (role of patient)? Where does learning take place (classroom, clinic, community setting)?
Preparation and support of patient educators	Orientation (written and verbal information), individual or group? Training (what additional skills do patient educators require, initial and ongoing)? Support (support meetings, contact person for problem solving, updates on programme and student progress)? Recognition (honorary titles, payment, letters, certificates, appreciation events)?
Operational	Staffing requirements, e.g. coordination, administration (job description, new hire, existing position, secondment), qualifications—professional or administrative?
Programme evaluation and research	Evaluation/ research questions? Methods (surveys, interviews, focus groups, reflective journals)? Ethics, confidentiality and consent for use of data? Knowledge ownership and dissemination?
Sustainability	Moving from project to programme? Embedding in the institution? Institutional support through funding, staffing, space?

Remuneration and status

Payment models range from nothing, to expenses only, to expenses plus honorarium, to an hourly rate. Some patients do not wish to be paid and feel that the satisfaction of making a contribution to learning is sufficient reward; others feel that this is exploitative. Payment is associated with increased formal recognition and status, and academic leaders must be upfront about policies and practices. Payment for involvement may have repercussions for welfare benefit claims and needs to be negotiated locally and reviewed periodically. Traditional institutional policies and practices may create barriers, for example being slow to reimburse expenses, especially to those who are socially disadvantaged (Gutteridge and Dobbins 2010). Recognition by the institution may be demonstrated in the currency of academia, for example, by funding a formal academic position for a service user, or invitation to coauthor articles (Simons et al. 2007). However, the appropriate recognition of patients who teach contains a fundamental tension; do we provide recognition in a form that the academy values or does this turn people into 'professors' making them 'one of us' rather than marking and valuing their difference?

Retention and sustainability

Most programs have positive feedback from patients—who want to be repeatedly involved. Retention is best in programmes that involve patients in planning, acknowledge their involvement and regularly update them on the programme and student progress. Resources to train patients and maintain their skills, and faculty who are committed to working in partnership are essential for sustainable programmes. In an unpublished study of 59 patient-as-teacher initiatives we found that the most important factors for sustainability were leadership, institutional support, and funding. Descriptions of how initiatives representing a range of patient roles have been sustained over time may be found in the case studies developed by Spencer et al. (2011).

Future directions

The ongoing publication of new initiatives in the literature indicates that active patient involvement in medical education is increasing. The experience and expertise that patients have to offer continues to be explored, as do issues of working in authentic partnerships with patients and the community. For example, at the University of British Columbia we have worked with people with mental health problems, aphasia, arthritis, epilepsy, and HIV infection to develop patient-led workshops for interprofessional groups of students in which faculty play a supportive, not directive, role (Towle and Godolphin 2013). The patient educators not only run the workshops but identify the topics that they think are important for them to teach. The result is a wider diversity of topics than is usually taught by patients; topics include living with chronic disease, both day-to-day and the journey over time; the diversity of the illness experience; effects on partners and families; physical examination skills; diagnostic challenges; stigma and stereotyping; peer support; recovery; practical aids to daily living; advice about what health professionals can do; and information about support groups in the community.

However, most initiatives described in the medical education literature are single educational experiences the impact of which is limited. If education is to promote partnerships with patients as the basis for healthcare, then we must move from isolated initiatives to coordinated and sustained programmes: a patient involvement curriculum. This will require academic institutions to move from their ivory towers and engage with community organizations in a non-tokenistic way and to develop authentic partnerships at an institutional level. We recommend that medical educators learn from the experience of other health professions about the opportunities and the challenges of systemic involvement. An important consequence will be the way that the academy recognizes the contribution of people from the community who have a distinctive and unique expertise. Patient involvement will force the university to think and talk differently about intellectual authority, the nature of expertise and the role of the teacher, and will impact the current discourse of teaching in higher education as a scholarly activity, and teaching as a research-based profession (Towle and Godolphin 2011a).

Through scholarly thought and activity, patient involvement in medical education can not only grow as a movement in its own right but can contribute to other contemporary debates in the field such as professionalism, humanism, narrative competence, relationship-centred care, identity formation, moral development, and reflective capacity.

Conclusions

◆ Active patient involvement in medical education is widespread and increasing.

◆ Decisions to involve patients have originated from sociocultural changes and associated policy responses.

◆ Development of applicable learning theory and examination of long-term benefits are needed.

◆ Involvement of patients as teachers requires attention to practical matters not commonly encountered in medical education.

◆ Involvement of patients in an authentic and non-tokenistic way has implications for medical educators and academic institutions.

References

Anderson, E.S., Ford, J., and Thorpe, L. (2011) Learning to listen: improving students' communication with disabled people. *Med Teach.* 33: 44–52

Anderson, E.S. and Lennox, A. (2009) The Leicester model of interprofessional education: developing, delivering and learning from student voices for 10 years. *J Interprof Care.* 23: 557–573

Anghel, R. and Ramon, S. (2009) Service users and carers' involvement in social work education: lessons from an English case study. *Eur J Soc Work.* 12: 185–199

Bacon, N. (2002) Differences in faculty and community partners' theories of learning. *Michigan J Comm Service Learn.* 9: 34–44

Barnes, D., Carpenter, J., and Dickinson, C. (2006) The outcomes of partnerships with mental health service users in interprofessional education: a case study. *Health Soc Care Comm.* 14: 426–435

Basset, T., Campbell, P., and Anderson, J. (2006) Service user / survivor involvement in mental health training and education: overcoming the barriers. *Soc Work Educ.* 25: 393–402

Bennett, L. and Baikie, K. (2003) The client as educator: learning about mental illness through the eyes of the expert. *Nurse Educ Today.* 23: 104–111

Blasco, P.A., Kohen, H., and Shapland, C. (1999) Parents-as-teachers: design and establishment of a training programme for paediatric residents. *Med Educ.* 33: 695–701

Blaylock, B.L. (2000) Patients and families as teachers: inspiring an empathic connection. *Families, Systems and Health.* 18: 161–176

Bleakley, A. and Bligh, J. (2008) Students learning from patients: let's get real in medical education. *Adv Health Sci Educ: Theory Pract.* 13: 89–107

Breytspraak, L.M., Arnold, L., and Hogan, K. (2008) Dimensions of an intergenerational relationship between medical students and mentors-on-aging. *J Intergen Relat.* 6: 131–153

British Medical Association, Medical Education Subcommittee (2008) *Role of the Patient in Medical Education.* http://bma.org.uk/-/media/Files/PDFs/Developing%20your%20career/Becoming%20a%20doctor/Role%20of%20patient.pdf Accessed 14 March 2013

Caron-Flinterman, J.F., Broerse, J.E.W., and Bunders, J.F.G. (2005) The experiential knowledge of patients: a new resource for biomedical research? *So Sci Med.* 60: 2575–2584

Coleman, E.A., Lord, J.E., Heard, J.K., et al. (2003) The Delta project: increasing breast cancer screening among rural minority and older women by targeting rural healthcare providers. *Oncol Nursing Forum.* 30: 669–677

Collins, L., Arenson, C., Jerpbak, C., Kane, P., Dressel, R., and Antony, R. (2011) Transforming chronic illness care education: a longitudinal interprofessional mentorship curriculum. *J Interprof Care.* 25: 228–230

Developers of User and Carer Involvement in Education (2009) Involving service users and carers in education: the development worker role. Guidelines for higher education institutions. http://www.mhhe.heacademy.ac.uk/silo/files/ducie-guidelines.pdf Accessed 19 March 2012

Dogra, N., Anderson, J., Edwards, R., and Cavendish, S. (2008) Service user perspectives about their roles in undergraduate medical training about mental health. *Med Teach.* 30: 152–156

Eleazer, G.P., Stewart, T.J., Wieland, G.D., Anderson, M.B., and Simpson, D. (2009) The national evaluation of senior mentor programs: older adults in medical education. *J Am Geriatr Soc.* 57: 321–326

Fadden, G., Shooter, M., and Holsgrove, G. (2005) Involving carers and service users in the training of psychiatrists. *Psychiatr Bull.* 29: 270–274

Farrell, C., Towle, A., and Godolphin, W. (2006) *Where's the Patient's Voice in Health Professional Education?* Vancouver: Division of Health Care Communication, University of British Columbia

Felton, A. and Stickley, T. (2004) Pedagogy, power and service user involvement. *J Psychiatr Mental Health Nurs.* 11: 89–98

Gecht, M.R. (2000) What happens to patients who teach? *Teach Learn Med.* 12: 171–175

Gruppen, L.D., Branch, V.K., and Laing, T.J. (1996) The use of trained patient educators with rheumatoid arthritis to teach medical students. *Arthritis Care Res.* 9: 302–308

Gutteridge, R. and Dobbins, K. (2010) Service user and carer involvement in learning and teaching: a faculty of health staff perspective. *Nurse Educ Today.* 30: 509–514

Hanson, J.L. and Randall, V.F. (2007) Advancing a partnership: patients, families, and medical educators. *Teach Learn Med.* 19: 191–197

Hall, I.S. and Hollins S. (1996) The Strathcona Theatre Company: changing medical students' attitudes to learning disability (mental handicap) *Psychiatr Bull* 20: 429–430

Henriksen, A.-.H. and Ringsted, C. (2011) Learning from patients: students' perceptions of patient-instructors. *Med Educ.* 45: 913–919

Hunt, J.B., Bonham, C., and Jones, L. (2011) Understanding the goals of service learning and community-based medical education: a systematic review. *Acad Med.* 86: 246–251

Jha, V., Quinton, N.D., Bekker, H.L., and Roberts, T.E. (2009a) Strategies and interventions for the involvement of real patients in medical education: a systematic review. *Med Educ.* 43: 10–20

Jha, V., Quinton, N.D., Bekker, H.L., and Roberts, T.E. (2009b) What educators and students really think about using patients as teachers in medical education: a qualitative study. *Med Educ.* 43: 449–456

Jha, V., Setna, Z., Al-Hity, A., Quinton, N.D., and Roberts, T.E. (2010) Patient involvement in teaching and assessing intimate examination skills: a systematic review. *Med Educ.* 44: 347–357

Johnson, A.M., Yoder, J., and Richardson-Nassif, K. (2006) Using families as faculty in teaching medical students family-centered care: what are students learning? *Teach Learn Med.* 18: 222–225

Katz, A.M., Conant, J.L., Inui, T.S., Baron, D., and Bor, D. (2000) A council of elders: creating a multi-voiced dialogue in a community of care. *Soc Sci Med.* 50: 851–860

Klein, S., Tracy, D., Kitchener, H.C., and Walker, L.G. (2000) The effects of the participation of patients with cancer in teaching communication skills to medical undergraduates: a randomised study with follow-up after 2 years. *Eur J Cancer.* 36: 273–281

Kretzschmar, R.M. (1978) Evolution of the Gynecology Teaching Associate: an education specialist. *Am J Obstet Gynecol.* 131: 367–373

Kumagai, A.K. (2008) A conceptual framework for the use of illness narratives in medical education. *Acad Med.* 83: 653–658

Lave, J. and Wenger, E. (1991) *Situated Learning: Legitimate Peripheral Participation.* Cambridge, UK: Cambridge University Press

Levin, E. (2004) *Involving Service Users and Carers in Social Work Education.* London, UK: Social Care Institute for Excellence, Resource Guide No 4. http://www.scie.org.uk/publications/guides/guide04/files/guide04.pdf Accessed 19 March 2012

Livingston, G. and Cooper, C. (2004) User and carer involvement in mental health training. *Adv Psychiatr Treat.* 10: 85–92

McClean, S. and Shaw, A. (2005) From schism to continuum? The problematic relationship between expert and lay knowledge—an exploratory conceptual synthesis of two qualitative studies. *Qual Health Res.* 15: 729–748

McKeown, M., Malihi-Shoja, L., and Downe, S., supporting the Comensus Writing Collective. (2010) *Service User and Carer Involvement in Education for Health and Social Care.* Oxford, UK: Wiley Blackwell

McLaughlin, H. (2009) What's in a name: 'client', 'patient', 'customer', 'consumer', 'expert by experience', 'service user'—what's next? *Br J Soc Work.* 39: 1101–1117

Morgan, A. and Jones, D. (2009) Perceptions of service user and carer involvement in healthcare education and impact on students' knowledge and practice: a literature review. *Med Teach.* 31: 82–95

Moss, B., Boath, L., Buckley, S., and Colgan, A. (2009) The fount of all knowledge: training required to involve service users and carers in health and social care education and training. *Soc Work Educ.* 28: 562–572

Oswald, A.E., Bell, M.J., Wiseman, J., and Snell, L. (2011a) The impact of trained patient educators on musculoskeletal clinical skills attainment in pre-clerkship medical students. *BMC Med Educ.* 11: 65

Oswald, A.E., Wiseman, J., Bell, M.J., and Snell, L. (2011b) Musculoskeletal examination teaching by patients versus physicians: how are they different? Neither better nor worse, but complementary. *Med Teach.* 33: e227–e235

Rees, C.E., Knight, L.V., and Wilkinson, C.E. (2007) 'User involvement is a *sine qua non*, almost, in medical education': learning with rather than just about health and social care service users. *Adv Health Sci Educ: Theory Pract.* 12: 359–390

Rees, C.E. and Monrouxe, L. (2011) Medical students learning intimate examinations without valid consent: a multicentre study. *Med Educ.* 45: 261–272

Repper, J. and Breeze, J. (2007) User and carer involvement in the training and education of health professionals: a review of the literature. *Int J Nursing Studies.* 44: 511–519

Scheyett, A. and Kim, M. (2004) 'Can we talk?': using facilitated dialogue to positively change student attitudes towards persons with mental illness. *J Teach Soc Work.* 24: 39–53

Shapiro, D., Tomasa, L., and Koff, N.A. (2009) Patients as teachers, medical students as filmmakers: the video slam, a pilot study. *Acad Med.* 84: 1235–1244

Simons, L., Tee, S., Lathlean, J., Burgess, A., Herbert, L., and Gibson, C. (2007) A socially inclusive approach to user participation in higher education. *J Adv Nurs.* 58: 246–255

Solomon, P., Guenter, D., and Stinson, D. (2005) People with HIV as educators of health professionals. *AIDS Patient Care and STDs.* 19: 840–847

Speed, E. (2006) Patients, consumers and survivors: a case study of mental health service user discourses. *Soc Sci Med.* 62: 28–38

Spencer, J., Blackmore, D., Heard, S., et al. (2000) Patient-oriented learning: a review of the role of the patient in the education of medical students. *Med Educ.* 34: 851–857

Spencer, J., Godolphin, W., Karpenko, N., and Towle, A. (2011) *Can patients be teachers? Involving patients and service users in healthcare professionals' education.* London UK: The Health Foundation, www.health.org.uk Accessed 19 March 2012

Stacy, R. and Spencer, J. (1999) Patients as teachers: a qualitative study of patients' views on their role in a community-based undergraduate project. *Med Educ.* 33: 688–694

Stewart, T. and Alford, C.L. (2006) Older adults in medical education—senior mentor programs in U.S. medical schools. *Gerontol Geriatr Educ.* 27: 3–10

Sturm, L.A., Shultz, J., Kirby, R., and Stelzner, S.M. (2011) Community partners as co-teachers in resident continuity clinics. *Acad Med.* 86: 1532–1538

Tew, J., Gell, C., and Foster, S. (2004) *Learning from Experience. Involving Service Users and Carers in Mental Health Education and Training.* UK: Higher Education Academy/National Institute for Mental Health in England/Trent Workforce Development Confederation. http://www.mhhe.heacademy.ac.uk/resources/learning-from-experience-guide-and-updates/ Accessed 19 March 2012

Towle, A., Bainbridge, L., Godolphin, W., et al. (2010) Active patient involvement in the education of health professionals. *Med Educ.* 44: 64–74

Towle, A. and Godolphin, W. (2011a) A meeting of experts: the emerging roles of non-professionals in the education of health professionals. *Teach Higher Educ.* 16: 495–504

Towle, A. and Godolphin, W. (2011b) The neglect of chronic disease self-management in medical education: involving patients as educators. *Acad Med.* 86: 1350

Towle, A. and Godolphin, W. (2012) Patient involvement in health professional education: a bibliography 1975–2012. Division of Health Care Communication, University of British Columbia. http://www.chd.ubc.ca/dhcc/node/207 Accessed 28 February 2013

Towle, Aand, Godolphin, W. (2013) Patients as educators: Interprofessional learning for patient-centred care. *Med Teach.* T35: 219–223

Tuckett, D.M., Boulton, M., Olson, C., and Williams, A. (1985) *Meetings between Experts. An Approach to Sharing Ideas in Medical Consultations.* London, UK: Tavistock Publications Ltd

Wallace, P. (1997) Following the threads of an innovation: the history of standardized patients in medical education. *Caduceus (Springfield, Ill.,* 13: 5–28

Walters, K., Buszewicz, M., Russell, J., and Humphrey, C. (2003) Teaching as therapy: cross sectional and qualitative evaluation of patients' experiences of undergraduate psychiatry teaching in the community. *BMJ.* 326: 740–745

Warren, L. and Boxall, K. (2009) Service users in and out of the academy: collusion in exclusion? *Soc Work Educ.* 28: 281–297

Williamson, C. (2007) 'How do we find the right patients to consult?' *Qual Prim Care.* 15: 195–199

Wittenberg-Lyles, E., Shaunfield, S., Goldsmith, J., and Sanchez-Reilly, S. (2011) How we involved bereaved family caregivers in palliative care education. *Med Teach.* 33: 351–353

Wykurz, G. and Kelly, D. (2002) Developing the role of patients as teachers: literature review. *BMJ.* 325: 818–821

Yeung, E.Y.W. and Ng, S.M. (2011) Engaging service users and carers in health and social care education: challenges and opportunities in the Chinese community. *Soc Work Educ.* 30: 281–298

PART 6

Stages

CHAPTER 28

Undergraduate medical education

H. Thomas Aretz and Elizabeth G. Armstrong

By the age of 17, a youth would have had time to procure a good preliminary education, and the subsequent six years would admit of a good medical education, including a period—not of five years, but of some months—occupied in something analogous to the apprenticeship of the present day.

Charles Carter (Carter 1844 p593)

Introduction

Undergraduate medical education (UGME) continues to undergo significant change and reform (Aretz 2011; Frenk et al. 2010; Putnam 2006). Since many aspects of undergraduate education have been covered elsewhere in this textbook, this chapter will focus on two aspects of undergraduate medical education:

- A review of some of the major reforms since the 1970s categorized by their relationship to the demands of healthcare delivery. To provide historical context, there will be a brief overview of the history of Western medical education

- An evolving three-phase model for undergraduate curriculum planning that combines values and outcomes-based planning with resource and quality management guided implementation.

The context of UGME

As pointed out by Frenk et al. (2010 pp. 1929–33), medical education in the last 100 years has seen a shift from being science-based to patient- or problem-based to system-based. They make the argument that the instructional, institutional, and societal contexts have changed in parallel: while the institutional centre was once the university, it moved to the academic medical centre, and now spans the entire healthcare system. In parallel, instructional emphasis moved from a mostly scientific focus, to applied patient and problem-based models, and more recently competency and outcomes-based approaches responsive to societal requirements. All these changes have been made in response to significant changes in the healthcare and its delivery in many parts of the world.

The major drivers and trends in healthcare that are influencing medical education include (Irby and Wilkerson 2003; Bligh 1999; Frenk et al. 2010):

1. Changes in demographics and the epidemiology of diseases, especially a shift from acute to chronic conditions

2. Changes in medical knowledge, therapies and technologies

3. Changes in the delivery of healthcare, especially a shift from inpatient to outpatient therapy

4. Changes in the roles of healthcare professions, the composition of healthcare teams and the role of clinical and basic sciences faculty

5. Changes in societal and consumer expectations and requirements, including healthcare outcomes, quality and safety, and cost.

We will explore how these various drivers have influenced educational interventions and innovations, and how future trends will continue to influence the evolution of undergraduate medical education. In addition, there have been significant changes in our understanding of pedagogy and the evolution of pedagogical technology. The major changes in this regard include:

- better understanding of the neurobiology and psychology of learning

- the use of learning management systems

- the use of digital instruction materials, including distance learning

- the use of simulation and standardized patients.

Medical education prior to 1970

The major model of UGME in the world has its origin in the medieval European university model, which in turn has its roots in the classic teachings of medicine in ancient Greece, Rome, and the Middle East. In classical antiquity (Kudlien 1970a), medicine moved from being a 'family business' to being a subject taught to strangers. As medicine was identified as a field separate from philosophy, the struggle between theory and practice became evident almost immediately. Throughout antiquity medicine was considered not only a science but also a craft, embodied in the Latin words *physicus*, the learned physician trained in philosophy and theory, versus the *medicus*, the mere provider of care. The writings of the main authors of the day, Aristotle, Galen and Hippocrates, became the core of medical teachings for centuries (Talbot 1970). It is worth noting that medical education in medieval Islam (Hamarneh 1970) allowed more of a balance between theory and practice and saw the establishment of the first fully functioning academic medical centres (including community outreach to less fortunate sectors of society). The writings of Abu Bakr Muhammad ibn Zakariya al-Razi defined patient–doctor relationships and the essence of professionalism for physicians. This was built upon by Ibn Sina (Avicenna) in *Canons of Medicine*, which became an important textbook throughout the Middle Ages—the contents of which included such modern topics as exercise, environmental influences, and criteria for drug testing (Jacquart 2008).

With the advent of the Renaissance, medicine developed a more scientific approach (O'Malley 1970). The scientific basis of medicine and its education became firmly established in the 19th century, and standardized curricula began to emerge to assure relevance to the public mission (Coury 1970). The notions of 'academic freedom' (absence of influence over science and teaching by the state and the church) and the definition of requirements for entry into medical education were other trends that have their origins in that period. The ground-breaking Flexner report (Flexner 1910) introduced a systematic and scientific approach as the basis of medical education into the USA replacing the prevailing apprenticeship model (Flexner published a report on European schools two years later (Flexner 1912)). It should be noted, however, that Flexner did not intend to create a solely scientific model and eliminate any form of apprenticeship; in fact he explicitly warned against this (Flexner 1925).

This abbreviated history of medical education highlights some essential themes that are still being discussed today:

- What is the role of theory and how should it be balanced with practice?
- Who determines the curriculum—the university or society?
- What is the importance of 'soft skills', or more generally, what is the domain of medicine and its education?
- Who determines the prerequisites, and who certifies the graduate?
- Where in the healthcare system should students learn their craft?
- Is medical education an academic pursuit or a preparation for a profession?

Major changes in UGME since 1970

Multiple reports and position papers have made strong cases for the reform of medical education over the last 30 years—pointing out needed changes to make medical education more relevant to healthcare practice and health promotion (Muller 1984; General Medical Council 1993, 2003, 2009; Neufeld et al. 1998; Association of American Medical Colleges 1998; Maudsley et al. 2000; Josiah

Macy Jr. Foundation 2009; The Association of Faculties of Medicine of Canada 2010). The journal *Medical Teacher* (Gibbs 2011) dedicated an entire issue to the social accountability of medical education—enforcing the need for medial education's responsibility towards its stakeholders. There is also agreement throughout many parts of the world that UGME, which in many countries still includes a 1-year internship, is not sufficient to assure readiness for independent practice, but is the basis for medical practice under supervision (i.e. postgraduate education). This realization has provided additional focus on the purpose, scope and desired outcomes of UGME.

Rather than listing the various innovations and interventions in isolation, the following discussion uses the major healthcare trends mentioned earlier and the changes in the understanding of learning as contexts for the educational interventions along with their desired outcomes and impacts (table 28.1). It would be impossible in the space provided to review and analyse all the interventions and innovations listed in table 28.1. The following discussion will focus on those innovations that have tried to address multiple healthcare challenges, and those that have impacted medical education most significantly.

Trend 1: Changes in demographics and the epidemiology of diseases, especially a shift from acute to chronic conditions (also the ageing population)

The epidemiology of disease is changing dramatically across the world and life expectancy is increasing virtually everywhere. While acute diseases are not extinct, the efficient and effective management of chronic conditions has become a major goal of healthcare systems and modern medical education (Maeshiro 2010). Identifying experiences to train medical students in chronic care (Holman 2004), defining minimal competencies for the care of the elderly (Leipzig 2009), and using curricular themes have all been employed to address this issue. Rather than being taught as a separate subject, geriatrics is often woven into multiple courses taught by a variety of disciplines. Despite agreeing on many objectives in this area, there is still significant disagreement as to priorities and educational approaches (Pham 2004). The thematic approach to curricular planning is challenged by the predominant departmental organizational structures more traditionally supporting discipline based courses, leaving the theme without a strong institutional advocate.

Longitudinal clinical experiences and clerkships are becoming more frequent (Norris 2009), either as supplementary experiences in addition to traditional block clerkships (Peters 2001) or as outright replacements of those clerkships (Ogur 2007). A recent survey, however, showed that only 22% of US schools offered longitudinal clerkships (LCME 2011). Preliminary results reported by the three initial papers cited in this paragraph indicate that there was good longitudinal patient contact, that there was good student acceptance, that students felt more competent in chronic patient care, and that they were more likely to choose primary care careers; scores in standardized tests, however, showed no difference. A review of the literature (Ogrinc 2002) showed that there was sparse evidence of the effectiveness of ambulatory longitudinal clerkships and that more rigorous research was needed.

Table 28.1 Major trends in healthcare and pedagogy affecting undergraduate medical education relative to the desired outcomes and impacts

Trend	Interventions	Desired outcome	Desired impact
Changes in demographics and the epidemiology of diseases, especially a shift from acute to chronic conditions and the ageing population	◆ Curricular themes (e.g. geriatrics) ◆ Increased outpatient and community-based instruction ◆ Longitudinal clerkships/postings ◆ New community-based medical schools	◆ Ability to manage chronic conditions ◆ Better understanding of needs of geriatric population, including rehabilitation ◆ Better understanding of health system interactions	◆ Better management of chronic conditions and 'lifestyle' diseases ◆ Better care of the elderly ◆ Better utilization of healthcare resources
Changes in medical knowledge, therapies and technologies, and their impact on patient care, healthcare professionals and society	◆ Integrated and interdisciplinary curricula ◆ Professionalism courses ◆ Humanities and ethics ◆ Community education and projects ◆ Linkages to engineering schools and technology colleges	◆ Better use of relevant science for clinical care ◆ Improved clinical reasoning ◆ Greater breadth and depth of knowledge ◆ Professional and ethical behaviour including communication skills ◆ Understanding of holistic patient and community care ◆ Understanding of role of technology	◆ Patient-centred (relationship-centred) and community- centred care ◆ Evidence-based medicine ◆ Improved professional and ethical behaviour by physicians ◆ Reflective practice ◆ Expert systems in patient care, and care management
Changes in the delivery of healthcare, especially a shift from inpatient to outpatient therapy	◆ Longitudinal clerkships/postings ◆ Ambulatory and community clerkships/postings ◆ Rural clerkships/postings ◆ Community-based and hospital-based medical schools	◆ Better understanding of longitudinal care and healthcare systems ◆ Ability to function in community and rural environments ◆ Appropriate learning environments and educational focus	◆ Appropriate delivery and coordination of care in multiple settings and services ◆ Appropriate care to rural and urban populations ◆ Improvement of care across the entire healthcare system
Changes in the roles of healthcare professions, the composition of healthcare teams and the role of clinical and basic sciences faculty	◆ Team-based learning ◆ Interdisciplinary courses ◆ Curricular integration ◆ Interprofessional education ◆ Faculty development ◆ Enhanced promotion criteria ◆ Mission-based management ◆ Academies of medical educators ◆ Medical education programmes ◆ Combined MD-MBA/MPH programmes	◆ Teamwork ◆ Interprofessional understanding and collaborative practice ◆ Improved teaching and learning ◆ Recapture of educational mission ◆ Educational scholarship ◆ Educational mentorship ◆ Competence in management skills and systems approaches	◆ Interdisciplinary and interprofessional patient care ◆ Healthcare teams designed for specific needs ◆ Redefinition of role of academic medicine in the healthcare system ◆ Appropriate incentives for faculty and resource allocations ◆ Educational research ◆ Cost reductions and social accountability
Changes in societal and consumer expectations and requirements, including healthcare outcomes, quality and patient safety	◆ Focus on health promotion ◆ Curricular themes addressing this content ◆ Combined degree programmes ◆ Focus on assessment and new assessment modalities ◆ Competency based curricula ◆ Social accountability of medical education ◆ Simulation	◆ Able to promote health and not only cure disease ◆ Defined set of competencies and greater ability to better 'certify' graduates ◆ Understanding of principles of quality management and patient safety ◆ Understanding of principles of healthcare economics ◆ New professional careers	◆ Socially appropriate care ◆ Improved population health ◆ Improved healthcare quality and patient safety ◆ Decreased healthcare costs ◆ Professionals competent in multiple domains important to improving and managing healthcare systems
Changes in the science and technology of learning	◆ PBL and case-based learning ◆ Individualized and developmental approach ◆ Remediation programmes ◆ Learning communities ◆ Learning management systems ◆ Online interactive instructions ◆ Simulation	◆ Learner-centred educational environment ◆ More effective and efficient learning ◆ Critical thinking and clinical reasoning ◆ Increased motivation ◆ Active learning ◆ Practise in safe setting ◆ Improved mentoring and coaching ◆ Effective data and knowledge management	◆ Lifelong learning ◆ Adaptability to change ◆ Greater ability to solve problems and innovate ◆ Communities of practice

Trend 2: Changes in medical knowledge, therapies and technologies, and their impact on patient care, healthcare professionals, and society

Medical knowledge and technological advancement have grown exponentially in recent years. How to teach this vast specialized knowledge in a meaningful fashion that is relevant to clinical practice and how to assure that professionals behave ethically and do not overuse these therapies and technologies for personal gain have been major issues in UGME in recent years. This section will focus on two major UGME trends in response to this trend—curricular integration to assure an understanding of the core, and professionalism courses to produce ethical physicians.

The fact that 'nobody [is] able to master medicine as a whole' is a statement that goes back at least 1800 years (Kudlien 1970a, b, p. 25). Curricular integration has attempted to move UGME from being discipline-based to interdisciplinary-based (Harden et al. 1984; Bligh 1999)—with the degree of integration being varied (Harden 2000). The intent of integration was to define the core knowledge (Bligh 1995), essential skills and appropriate attitudes and experiences for all graduates (Harden et al. 1997, McNeil et al. 2006), while reducing redundancies and emphasizing connections and interrelationships as they apply to patient care.

Early attempts focused on interdisciplinary teaching of the basic sciences, as exemplified by the organ-based basic science curriculum at Case Western Reserve University (Wile and Smith 2000). This was however for the most part a 'horizontal' integration effort. The biopsychosocial model (Engel 1977) aimed to integrate the psychological and social aspects of patient care and took a more 'vertical' view of integration. Not only did it try to address the shortcomings of the pure biomedical model of care by integrating new aspects into the scientific curriculum, it also introduced a unifying longitudinal theme, a curricular design effort that has been expanded upon since. An early review of curricular innovations (Siu et al. 1985) showed disappointing results and could not demonstrate any definite improved outcomes. Nonetheless, modern curriculum models and planning all aim at integration, especially between theory and practice. The basic aim was to create 'a whole that is greater than the sum of the parts' (Harden et al. 1997, p. 264) by vertically integrating the content (e.g. spiral curricula), having longitudinal themes and providing a problem-based or clinical presentation-based focus across the continuum, while exposing students to the clinical environment from the beginning. Research has shown that integrated curricula have led to superior diagnostic skills (Papa and Harasym 1999).

A US study (Papadakis et al. 2004) correlated disciplinary action during physicians' professional lives with concerns raised during their clinical clerkships while in medical school. Authors have warned for some time now that there is an 'informal' or 'hidden curriculum' in medical schools (Hafferty 1998, p. 403) (i.e. an incongruence between what was formally taught and the way things were actually done, and the values as experienced by students each day (Gaufberg et al. 2010)). Coulehan (2005, pp. 892–898) warned that formal instruction in professionalism alone will not have the desired results if the clinical and educational environments do not demonstrate the desirable attributes.

Remedies proposed (Coulehan 2005; Stern and Papadakis 2006) suggest changes in student admissions and new education and assessment methods, with an emphasis on role modelling, community service, and a focus on self-awareness. The latter has been subject to extensive research, which has shown that novices in particular have poor metacognitive skills, making it difficult for them to judge their own abilities (Kruger and Dunning 1999), but that improving those skills will remedy the situation. Community service has been shown to help in the socialization of students into the profession (Dornan et al. 2006). Assessment methods have been developed that have been shown to be accurate in detecting unprofessional behaviour (Hemmer et al. 2000). For UGME design, this means that the entire educational environment needs to be taken into account when planning educational programmes and experiences. Attention will need to be paid to institutional culture, faculty development, and engagement, and moving from patient-centred care to 'relationship-centred care' which recognizes the emotional aspects of care for patients and physicians (Dobie 2007, pp. 423–424).

The recent proliferation of non-diagnostic and non-therapeutic technologies in healthcare, such as information technology, data banks, telehealth, mobile health, and communication technology in general, will all present continued challenges for future strategies in medical education. Studies have shown that students feel inadequately prepared in these areas (Jamshidi and Cook 2003). The Institute of Medicine (Committee on the Health Professions Education Summit 2003) and the World Health Organization (WHO) (Pruitt and Epping-Jordan 2005) have declared information and communication technology as core competencies for future healthcare professionals.

Trend 3: Changes in the delivery of healthcare, especially a shift from inpatient to outpatient therapy

With advances in medical technology, the epidemiological shift from acute to chronic diseases and the need to control healthcare costs, patient care continues to shift from inpatient to outpatient settings. The average length of stay across all Organization for Economic Cooperation and Development (OECD) countries continues to fall every year, despite significant variations between the countries (OECD 2011) resulting in heightened acuity of disease in hospitals, an increase in patients being treated outside the hospital and an inability of students to experience the continuum of care. Less than 0.1% of the population at risk over the period of one month is hospitalized in an academic medical centre (Green 2001). This means that the vast majority of healthcare delivery takes place outside academic medical centres, where most of UGME still takes place. Ambulatory and community-based medical education initiatives are some of the recent interventions to address this trend.

Community-based medical education tries to address several needs: it should make theoretical knowledge relevant, provide primary care experiences, instill professional values and move the understanding and practice of patient care beyond the individual level. A Best Evidence Medical Education (BEME) systematic review (Dornan et al. 2006) of early community experiences confirms that these aims are being at least partially accomplished. Students did gain a better understanding of the role of their profession, and gained better self-reflection skills, while learning about the healthcare system in action, especially the role of primary care. These experiences also helped recruitment into primary care. Since primary and community-based care may not be present in many teaching hospitals, its teaching required the integration of new and traditionally non-academic teaching sites, such as primary care physician practices, managed healthcare organizations (Moore et al. 1994) and public community clinics. Inclusion of community or ambulatory experience has been part of modern curricular models for a while (Harden et al. 1984) and it is required by many accrediting bodies for UGME.

More substantial and radical solutions to the training in community-based medicine have been the founding of new community-based, often rural schools, either independently or as part of established universities (Hurt and Harris 2005; Rabinowitz et al. 2008; Strasser et al. 2009; Worley and Murray 2011). The clinical teaching in these schools and programmes takes place in a dispersed community environment often necessitating significant information and telecommunications support to assure common curricular experiences and quality control (Hurt and Harris 2005; Rourke 2002). An analysis of rural programmes in the USA (Rabinowitz et al. 2008) showed that rural programmes increased the number of physicians practicing in rural settings, a finding reproduced in Australia. In the latter setting, student satisfaction with the experience did not translate directly into career choice, as the conditions in the rural workplace were deemed unattractive (Eley and Baker 2006). Targeted recruitment of students from rural and underserved populations is another strategy to address community care needs (Biggs and Wells 2011). There is no question that medical education will increasingly involve extra-hospital and non-traditional training sites, as more of medical care moves into the community. This will require not only new content and methods, but also new organizational structures (Hurt and Harris 2005), more use of information technology and better faculty development.

Trend 4: Changes in the roles of healthcare professions, the composition of healthcare teams and the role of clinical and basic sciences faculty

Medicine and medical education traditionally focused on the one-on-one relationship between the doctor and the patient, but the increasing complexity of modern medical care requires teamwork between the disciplines and across professions. Studies looking at overall hospital care (O'Leary et al. 2011), operating rooms (Hull et al. 2012), intensive care units (Mayer et al. 2011), geriatric and long-term care (Rand Europe and Ernst & Young 2012), and primary care (Gumbach and Bodenheimer 2004) have all shown superior patient outcomes as a result of integrated and interdisciplinary team approaches. In addition, the roles of non-physician healthcare professionals have evolved and proliferated. New technologies, healthcare system demands and shifts in care have created new professions (e.g. case managers), while some of the traditional roles of physicians are being supplemented or taken over by nurse practitioners and physician extenders, such as physician assistants. Community health workers and trained lay personnel are becoming integral parts of healthcare teams in many underserved environments (Frenk et al. 2010). These developments have heightened the need for teamwork and interprofessional education.

In parallel with shifting professional roles, the non-teaching responsibilities of clinical and basic science faculty have been dramatically impacted by clinical duty requirements and increasing time spent doing research, respectively. These developments have led to a re-examination of and re-emphasis on the mission of academic medical centres and on the scholarship of medical education (Irby and Wilkerson 2003).

Learning and teaching in small groups, whether as part of problem-based learning (PBL), team-based learning (TBL), group projects, simulator-based training, or ward teams has become a staple of UGME. Small group learning is meant to foster teamwork—in preparation for medical practice. While learning in groups has shown to improve individual learning (if groups have to solve problems and teach one another in the process), teamwork itself has not been a strong educational goal for UGME (Morrison et al. 2010). Teamwork itself requires specific knowledge, skills and attitudes as well as enabling conditions (Hackman 1990) that are typically not emphasized in UGME curricula. Turning 'a team of experts into an expert team' is a difficult task requiring the adoption of techniques and experiences from other fields (Burke et al. 2004, p. 96). It is rare to see teams in UGME that fulfil the conditions of the definition of a 'real' team—one that 'consists of two or more individuals, with complementary skills, that have a common commitment and purpose and that have a set of performance goals for which they hold themselves accountable' (Morrison et al. 2010, p. 255).

TBL tries to address some of these shortcomings. Multiple studies have shown that if the method is used as intended it leads to positive learning outcomes, more engaged and prepared learners, and improved problem-solving and teamwork skills (Parmelee 2010). TBL, like all other pedagogical methods, needs to be used as part of a well-thought-out educational strategy to help learners reach desired outcomes (Parmelee and Michaelsen 2010). Additional research is needed to evaluate the effectiveness of TBL, and certain conventions for reporting results will need to be followed (Haidet et al. 2012), since meaningful conclusions will otherwise not be possible.

There is an increasing interest in interprofessional education (IPE) in order to support collaborative healthcare environments (Hean et al 2012). Recent publications (Frenk et al. 2010; Health Professions Network Nursing and Midwifery in Human Resources for Health, World Health Organization 2010) have made a clear case for IPE being an important step towards better patient care. A review of the attitudes towards adopting IPE in medical clerkships across the USA showed that almost half of clerkship directors were skeptical and 81% of clerkships had no formal IPE curriculum (Liston et al. 2011). A study looking at changes in attitudes based on a longitudinal IPE curriculum as part of UGME showed positive results initially, but no significant long term effect could be demonstrated (Curran et al. 2010). In some countries, such as Sweden, interprofessional wards have shown great promise and early positive results—in terms of better acceptance by students, better understanding of roles and the development of positive attitudes (Hylin et al. 2007; Pelling et al. 2011;). Despite clear demonstration of the effectiveness of interprofessional team training in the specific areas mentioned in the beginning of this section, recent systematic reviews of the IPE literature looking at outcomes in the UGME setting have shown mixed results (Reeves et al. 2010; Hammick, et al. 2007), and others have pointed towards the need for more rigorous studies (Thistlethwaite 2012). In the meantime, the Interprofessional Education Collaborative (2011) has published a white paper outlining the four domains and specific competencies for interprofessional practice (values and ethics, communication, roles and responsibilities, and teamwork). The paper makes a clear distinction between profession-specific, common, and interprofessional competencies, which may be helpful for the planning and implementation of UGME curricula in the future.

The classical model for a medical school faculty member, sometimes called the 'triple-threat' or 'three-legged stool' of academia (research, teaching, and clinical practice) is becoming increasingly unattainable. Increased clinical responsibilities and the competitive environment and time commitments in research have forced faculty members to make choices. Teaching often 'drew the short straw', since clinical income and research publications were the recognized coin of the realm, and Ludmerer (2004, pp. 1163–1164) argued that the lack of 'learner-centered medical education' was not a matter of resources, but one of values and attitudes. The last 20 to 30 years has seen a redefinition of scholarship in general (Boyer 1990) and the scholarship of medical teaching in particular (Fincher et al 2000). Several publications have begun to clearly define competencies and scholarly activities for medical educators that provide a basis for the professionalization of teaching and the necessary academic recognition for promotion of teachers (Simpson, et al. 2007; Srinivasan et al. 2011; Milner et al. 2011).

These publications provide valuable frameworks for the design and implementation of competency-based faculty development programmes, targeted to the needs of the faculty as well as the medical school itself. A BEME review (Steinert et al. 2006) identified certain programmatic features that correlated with successful programmes, such as experiential learning, peer relationship building and the use of diverse teaching and learning methods.

Trend 5: Changes in societal and consumer expectations and requirements, including healthcare outcomes, quality and patient safety

Society is redefining the role of physicians in the healthcare system. This includes their role in health promotion and advocacy, in line with the WHO definition of health as 'a state of complete physical, mental and social well-being and not merely the absence of disease or infirmity' (WHO 1948). Patients are becoming much more informed about their healthcare options, and they have increasing access to health information and outcomes data, allowing them to make comparisons between selected institutions and individual providers. The reports by the Institute of Medicine (Kohn et al. 1999) in the USA about medical errors and the emphasis on patient safety and quality have all created a need for better quality control of professional education, and have given rise to the outcomes and competency movement (Harden 2002). Secondary efforts have

focused on competency assessment and practice in safe environments, such as simulation and the use of standardized patients.

Robyn Tamblyn (1999, pp. 9–25) defined clinical competence as a primary outcome of medical education, and—along with other determinants—as a prerequisite for good medical practice and positive health outcomes. It is this argument that has led to the development of outcomes and competency based curricula. Frank and colleagues (2010, p. 636) proposed the following definition: 'competency-based education (CBE) is an approach to preparing physicians for practice that is fundamentally oriented to graduate outcome abilities and organized around competencies derived from an analysis of societal and patient needs. It de-emphasizes time-based training and promises greater accountability, flexibility, and learner-centeredness'. The major aspects of such educational programmes are outlined in fig. 28.1.

Assessment in UGME has changed significantly and there is an enormous amount of literature on assessment methods for various competencies. Papers have outlined approaches to assessment in general (Crossley et al. 2002; Epstein and Hundert 2002; Epstein 2007) and competencies in particular (Holmboe et al. 2010). Manuals have been published to guide the assessment of specific sets of competencies (Rider et al. 2007). It can be safely stated that Miller's pyramid (i.e. 'knows' > 'knows how' > 'shows how' > 'does') has emerged as the basis of assessment for medical students and professionals (Miller 1990). However, schools are still struggling in the assessment of performance—the 'does' part of Miller's pyramid (Wass et al 2001). As assessment is becoming an increasingly prominent part of medical education, concerns are beginning to be raised about its extent and meaningfulness (Huddle and Heudebert 2007; Brooks 2009), as well as its practicality (Schuwirth et al 2002). Although most desirable competencies such as those required by the ACGME are felt to be 'linked to health care quality aims' (Swing 2007, p. 652), hard data concerning health outcomes are not available. Surveys of residency directors are serving as surrogate markers (Paolo and Bonaminio 2003; Wilkinson and Frampton 2004), showing some correlation between assessment methods and clinical performance.

Standardized patients and simulation are increasingly used for assessment, e.g. the Objective Structured Clinical Examination (OSCE). One of the main goals of this approach, besides providing a standardized and controlled testing environment, is to allow students to practise and be observed in a safe practice environment. The use of standardized patients in OSCEs has been reviewed on multiple occasions (Barrows 1993; Whelan et al. 2005) and the limitations and benefits have been described. The use of feedback by standardized patients has not yet been fully optimized or implemented (Bokken et al. 2009), despite the fact that such feedback has been shown to improve clinical skills and create a positive learning environment (Park et al. 2011).

> Outcomes are clearly defined and transparent to learners and teachers
>
> The design of the curriculum assures that these outcomes are achieved
>
> Developmental milestones for those competencies are clearly defined in order to allow for a less time-based approach to training
>
> The assessment process assures attainment and demonstration of competencies

Figure 28.1 Features of competency-based outcomes curricula.

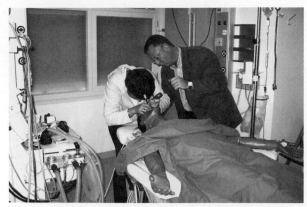

Figure 28.2 Becoming competent and advancing patient safety by learning how to intubate using a simulator.

The use of simulation (fig. 28.2) in medical training is increasing, as more sophisticated, cost-effective and task-specific simulators become available. A BEME review (Issenberg et al. 2005) concluded that simulation was useful and its utility has become increasingly evident, although direct correlation with clinical outcomes can rarely be demonstrated in UGME (Okuda et al. 2009). Simulation will definitely be an integral element in UGME in the future, but its optimal utilization and its relationship to clinical outcomes remain to be studied further.

Trend 6: Changes in the science and technology of learning

Enormous strides are being made in the understanding of the relationship between neurosciences, learning theories and educational interventions (Friedlander et al. 2011). Tools such as concept maps to aid critical thinking and clinical reasoning (Charlin et al. 2012), and experiential learning theory to form the basis of educational programme design (Armstrong and Parsa Parsi 2005) are but two examples. Special attention has been paid to the application of cognitive psychological principles to the development of expertise, a crucial goal in professional education (Regehr and Norman 1996). The use of information technology in education and the design of learning management systems (LMS) also require a deep understanding of learning theory and its application to online or virtual learning experiences.

A detailed treatise of these topics is beyond the scope of this chapter. This section will focus on two illustrative, but important examples in UGME in recent years: PBL, one of the more radical and pervasive medical education reforms in the last 50 years, as an example of an educational intervention based on learning theory; and online education in medical education, which is poised to revolutionize traditional education.

In 1969, McMaster University, a new Canadian medical school, introduced PBL as the basis of its 3-year curriculum (Neville and Norman 2007). Initially, three basic principles were identified as being the pedagogical basis for PBL (Schmidt 1989): activation of prior learning, learning in context, and elaboration through further experiences (O'Neill et al. 2002). With increasing experience of PBL, additional aspects became evident, such as the structuring of knowledge, motivation to learn, and effects of the group process itself (Schmidt 1993). These were in line with Barrows' (1986, pp. 481–486) original objectives for PBL. Much has been written about the effectiveness of PBL or lack thereof (Albanese and Mitchell 1993; Vernon and Blake 1993; Albanese 2000; Colliver 2000; Antepohl et al. 2003) and the results of these meta-analyses are still somewhat controversial. Over the years it became clear that everything that was called PBL was not always comparable—contributing to confusion in the literature and sometimes contradictory results. Two more recent reviews of the literature (Neville 2009; Koh et al. 2008) using an agreed upon definition of PBL (Maudsley 1999) have identified some distinct outcomes for PBL. There seems to be no difference in knowledge acquisition as measured by standardized tests amongst graduates of PBL schools, although there may be a trend towards better results on the clinical examination (Blake et al. 2000). Knowledge recall may be weaker in students from a PBL curriculum, while knowledge application may be superior (Neville 2009). Students in PBL programmes seemed to be better at 'coping with uncertainty', 'appreciation of legal and ethical aspects of healthcare', 'communication skills', and 'self-directed continuing learning' (Koh et al. 2008, p. 39). It is interesting in this context to look at the evolution of McMaster University's curriculum, since it was the original site of PBL in UGME. McMaster has undergone two curriculum reforms since 1969, in 1983 and in 2004 (Neville and Norman 2007). McMaster recognized that although concepts were embedded in the cases, the rich clinical context shifted discussions to clinical aspects rather than fundamental concepts. Without deviating from the basic initial educational philosophy, the curriculum, the cases and PBL sessions were significantly revised based on a solid understanding of the data and needed outcomes. It is clear from this example that data will need to be collected locally all the time to allow for evidence based revisions and improvement.

Online learning is gaining increasingly wide acceptance in medical education. Chumley-Jones and colleagues (2002, pp. S86–S93) and Ruiz and colleagues (2006, p. 209) found in their reviews of the literature that e-learning is at least equivalent to traditional methods in enabling the acquisition of knowledge, and sometimes better in enabling its retention. What has become clear from multiple studies, is that the design of online sessions, courses and programmes needs to be pedagogically sound and to utilize the special capabilities of the medium. It must: take advantage of being able to address audiences asynchronously and in various locations (Ruiz et al. 2006); use interactive multimedia (Issa et al. 2011); provide information online and focus on interaction and application in face-to-face environments, using a blended approach (Masie 2002); make resources available to wider, especially less resource-rich environments (MedEdPortal® (2012)); support online collaboration (Quattrochi et al. 2002); and use learning management systems to collect data about knowledge acquisition and learning activities (Johnson et al. 2004). Suffice to say that educational and other technologies will play an increasing role in UGME and research into their optimal use will be crucial.

Summary

UGME, not too long ago an academic endeavor under the sole control of universities needs to change in order to serve societies' evolving needs. Many innovations and educational developments have been introduced to address the increasingly complex and ever changing world of healthcare—into which our graduates venture. The previous sections have attempted to highlight some of the more significant changes and innovations as they try to achieve outcomes that will impact healthcare in the future. This process has become increasingly global, and local UGME is expanding its borders through student and faculty exchanges, global partnering with international schools, inclusion of global health curricula, and training of physicians as global citizens. It is hoped that this will lead to increasing exchange of ideas across the globe, as experimentation, new models and continued innovation will be crucial to arrive at the most effective ways to train physicians, while preserving the values important and intrinsic to the profession.

The next section will describe an approach to the planning and implementation of UGME curricula that combines an outcomes-based approach and the translation of institutional and professional values into reality. Kern and colleagues (2009, pp. 5–9) have publicized a widely adopted six-step approach to curriculum planning that outlines the various steps from needs assessment to maintenance and quality assurance; it is hoped that the concepts in the next section will help provide further guidance for conscientious and responsible curriculum planning and maintenance.

A model for UGME curriculum planning and implementation

Curriculum development can be viewed with several aspects in mind:

♦ *Curriculum development as an evolutionary process.* In order to plan and understand curricula, the historical background, and social, cultural and regulatory context need to be understood. Medical education is never designed in a vacuum, but it is firmly rooted in the locale and circumstance, in which it takes place.

♦ *Curriculum as the 'tangible expression of the soul of an educational institution'.* This anonymous quote emphasizes the fact that the curriculum of an institution needs to reflect that institution's values and principles. Paying attention to this aspect will alleviate many of the contradictions between the formal and informal curriculum, while providing a solid foundation for consensus among all stakeholders.

♦ *The curriculum as a product and a mirror of the organization that produces it.* Curriculum is not merely content and methods—it includes planning, implementation, operation and constant improvement.

♦ *The product of the curriculum, i.e. the competencies and characteristics of the graduates.* Stakeholder needs have to be met by what the curriculum produces. This means, that we have to understand those needs from the beginning and be able to measure whether we have accomplished our goals through a systems approach to educational planning and evaluation.

♦ *Curriculum as a record of resource allocation and resource management.* Resource allocation for academic activities and programmes need to be aligned with values, incentives and priorities, and should be part of the planning process from the beginning.

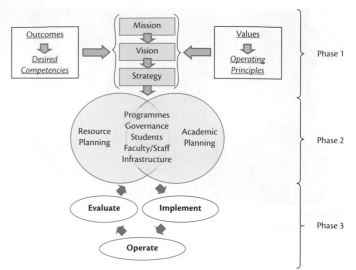

Figure 28.3 Model of a systematic approach to medical education planning.

On the other hand, if resource allocations do not support the espoused values, the values become worthless.

The following sections will touch upon these aspects as they describe three phases of curriculum planning, within a systems design framework (fig. 28.3).

Phase 1: Align values and outcomes

Phase 2: Plan with implementation in mind

Phase 3: Implement and operate for constant improvement.

Phase 1: Align values and outcomes

When Ludwig Mies van der Rohe became the director of the Armour Institute in Chicago in 1938, he stated in his inaugural speech to students that 'true education is concerned not only with practical goals but also with values...Our aims assure us of our material life, our values make possible our spiritual life' (Mies van der Rohe 1938). Curriculum planning needs to ensure that both goals of education are attained. Values need to be translated into operating principles and aims into desired competencies of the graduates. The desired outcomes and competencies must be informed by and must address society's needs. A needs assessment is important before defining a vision and mission for the institution or the programme (while keeping in mind regulatory constraints and requirements). As part of the competency movement, many countries and their accreditation agencies have defined minimum competencies for UGME, but these do not include everything that needs to be accomplished. All societal needs may not be able to be addressed by all schools, and as the development of niche schools has demonstrated in recent years, specific needs and fields can and should be addressed.

Let us use Mercer University School of Medicine (MUSM) (2002) in the USA as an example. MUSM describes its vision as 'to improve access to quality health care and enhance the health status of Georgia residents and to be a recognized leader in educating primary care, rural and community-based health professionals'. This statement clearly and succinctly describes what MUSM wants to accomplish and what it wants to be as an institution in the future. Its mission statement 'to educate physicians and health professionals to meet the primary care and health care needs of rural and medically underserved areas of Georgia' (Mercer University School of Medicine 2002) defines what it is going to do to attain the vision. Mission statements may also provide some detail about what graduates will look like, how they will be different or unique, and how the institution will foster those qualities. They should however, be brief. Like many other institutions, MUSM then defines its core values that are intended to support its vision and mission (Mercer University School of Medicine 2002). Values and broad goals (outcomes) in this example have thus been defined. What remains is to translate the outcomes into competencies, and the values into operating principles.

The competencies of graduates need to support the desired outcomes based on society's needs at a level expected at a particular stage of education and professional development. The competencies can be custom-designed *de novo* by the institution (G2010 Project Group 2010). Alternatively established sets of competencies germane to the regulatory environment can be adopted and adapted. MUSM chose the second route, and adopted the ACGME competencies in 2005 (Mercer University School of Medicine 2011), but modified them to align them with its own institutional goals so that they would 'reflect the knowledge, skills, behaviors, and attitudes expected of MUSM graduates'. (Mercer University School of Medicine 2011, p. 52) In light of an emerging list of global competencies applicable to healthcare professionals anywhere, such an approach uses an established framework of accepted benchmarks and standards, while allowing customization based on mission and local circumstances. If certain competencies are felt to be missing, they can be added.

The translation of values into operating principles further strengthens the cohesiveness of curriculum planning, as these operating principles provide guideposts and operational guidelines for everyone involved in curriculum development. The process can be described in three steps:

1. The first step is to agree on common values. Schools have multiple stakeholders (basic scientists, clinicians, non-physician healthcare professionals, students, residency directors, patients, donors, and alumni), all of whom may value different things. Holistic care may be of paramount important to primary care physicians, while the scientific basis of medicine may be the most important value for researchers. The initial process should create a common set of organizational values that are supported by all stakeholders.

2. The second step is to define operating principles based on these values, such that they can become an integral part of curriculum planning. For instance, if 'collaboration' is one of the values, corresponding operating principles could be: 'the curriculum needs to be integrated on multiple levels: basic science–clinical; biopsychosocial; school–community; primary care–specialties'; and 'the curriculum must foster collegiality, cooperation and respect among the professions'. While the first principle focuses on the curriculum content itself, and the integration and collaboration among the various fields, the second principle emphasizes the creation of a culture that will support not only the curriculum process, but also the development of professional attitudes and collaborative practice. Sets of operating principles should be developed to govern not only the content and methods of the academic programmes, but also the related aspects of

student admissions and student life; faculty development, and promotion; organizational structure; infrastructure and systems; and resource allocation.

3. The third step is to define pedagogical principles that support the attainment of the competencies and reflect the values of the organization. If 'collaboration' is an important value, a curriculum without team-based pedagogy would not be credible. The pedagogical principles may ask for 'methods to support collaborative learning' at this stage, but this principle does not specify pedagogical strategies. The specific strategies need to be defined as a next step for the various phases of the curriculum and its activities, keeping desired outcomes, available resources and local constraints in mind.

Phase 2: Plan with implementation in mind

Needs have to be paired with institutional capabilities and resources to ensure that the institution can actually deliver on its promises. This second phase can be seen as the translation of the values and principles underlying the mission into implementation. It is no accident that Phase 2 in fig. 28.3 is depicted as two partially overlapping circles of academic and resource planning. As planning goes through its multiple iterations, resource needs should be examined at every step to assure that what is desirable is also feasible.

The first step involves the creation of a curriculum blueprint that defines:

- the basic model (e.g. spiral, organ-system based, disease-based, or clinical-presentation based) (Papa and Harasym 1999; Bligh 1999)

- curriculum phases and

- longitudinal threads.

For instance, a spiral curriculum may have three classical phases: basic sciences (e.g. anatomy, biochemistry, and physiology), preclinical sciences (e.g. pathology, pathophysiology, and pharmacology), and clinical sciences (e.g. medicine, surgery, and paediatrics). Longitudinal threads may include scholarship, community medicine, and professional development. The blueprint will show courses, their sequence, lengths, and proportional time requirements over the various phases of the curriculum. Once this is done, the desired levels of attainment for the various competencies are now defined for each phase, thereby determining the desired outcomes at various curricular milestones (G2010 Project Group 2010). This allows for the determination of educational strategies, including assessment strategies. Developing schedules for 'prototypical weeks' can be helpful at this time as they illustrate the desired allocation for the various educational strategies in the various phases and threads in the curriculum (Armstrong 1997, p. 141), while also defining dedicated times in the curriculum for extracurricular activities, studying, reflection and institutional or community service. This information allows for an initial assessment of the required resources.

The types of resources that need to be kept in mind include:

- Human resources:
  - *Faculty*: What is the number of faculty needed? For what time? How do they need to be trained? Are they full-time or part-time? How will they be promoted or incentivized? Are there new career opportunities?

- *Staff*: What is the administrative and support staff needed? What other professionals (e.g. biometricians, education specialists, and psychologists) need to be brought on board?

  - *Patients*: What types of patients will be needed for the educational programmes and options? What is the need for standardized patients?

- Organizational structures: Will new structures be needed in the future? What are the structures needed for planning, implementation and operation? Are new policies and procedures required?

- Facilities: Do the facilities support the planned educational strategies? Are the clinical facilities adequate for teaching students? Are special facilities (e.g. simulation or clinical skills labs) required? What are the equipment requirements?

- Systems: What are the IT and technology requirements for the various strategic options? Do they need to be developed in-house?

- Funding: Is there adequate funding for planning and operations? What are the costs for the various options?

Reforming an existing and creating a new curriculum require initial and ongoing negotiations. The people planning and implementing the curriculum need to understand the political landscape, internal, as well as external. Who are the allies, opponents, and neutrals that need to be convinced, brought on board, or negotiated with? Bland and colleagues (2000, pp. 575–594) studied success factors for curriculum change in medical schools and emphasized the importance of the 'soft factors' in curriculum development, planning and implementation, i.e. mission, goals, leadership, politics, and participation by organizational members. Since almost all members of the school will be touched by the curriculum in one way or another, communication is crucial to inform the stakeholders and get feedback in a timely manner.

The project management literature has stressed for years that leadership involvement and organizational consensus early in a project are crucial for success and efficiency (Hayes et al. 1988). The same is true for curriculum planning. It is important to spend time talking through issues before moving to concrete solutions (however this does not mean that there should not be clear timelines). This important phase sets the stage for the implementation and operations phase of the curriculum.

Phase 3: Implement and operate for constant improvement

Phase 3 in fig. 28.3 is drawn as a cycle (like the quality improvement cycle). The success of any curriculum effort is measured against the attainment of its goals and outcomes. Curriculum implementation, dissemination, maintenance and evaluation have been described by Kern et al. (2009, pp. 84–182). The following section will emphasize three aspects of this phase

- an organizational design addressing integration

- setting teams up for success and

- creating a quality system.

Modern curricula are supposed to be integrated and developmental, requiring close collaboration among the various groups involved in planning, implementing, and operating the various courses and activities. Horizontal and vertical integration are the words used to describe coordination of activities happening in a course during a particular year. Groups need to be established that 'own' the various themes or courses, from now on called 'teams'. Coordinating mechanisms are required to assure adherence to guidelines, clear goal setting, lack of redundancies and gaps, and a progression of knowledge, skills, attitudes, and experiences that logically build on what went before. Here is one example that illustrates an approach to content integration in one curriculum.

The authors of this chapter were asked to participate in the early stages of curriculum planning for a new medical school, which had chosen to teach its first two preclinical years in organ-based modules—teaching normal structure and function in the first year and abnormal structure and function in the second year. There were eight longitudinal themes (including anatomy, physiology, pharmacology, and biochemistry) and eight organ systems (including pulmonary, cardiovascular, and gastrointestinal). Faculty for each organ system and theme was asked to define the most important concepts, termed 'buckets' that were felt to be germane to the field. In the pulmonary field these buckets might be normal and abnormal function in inspiration, expiration, and gas exchange. Once this was done, concepts were 'matched' to assure 'best fit'. This approach assured 'coverage without gaps', while minimizing redundancies. At the same time, while being organized as organ-based courses, the longitudinal themes (e.g. anatomy, physiology) need to also constitute cohesive and comprehensive courses across the organ systems. Integration is often harder in the clinical years, but developmental models such as the reporter–interpreter–manager–educator (RIME) system (Pangaro 2006) have tried to address this issue. Developmental approaches to learning (ten Cate et al. 2004) and assessment need to be similarly managed proactively.

The organizational framework suggested allows the teams responsible for implementation and operation of the curriculum to function effectively. Understanding clearly what has come before, what is happening in parallel, and most importantly, what is expected next, is of paramount importance for the implementation of successful educational programmes by the faculty that face the students every day. 'Team leaders' such as directors of courses, clerkships, postings and other educational activities need

- clearly defined goals in line with the operating principles

- team members who are appropriately incentivized to do the work and

- adequate material resources, not the least of which is time (Hackman and Walton 1986).

Lack of any of these conditions may lead to frustration for the faculty and staff, and suboptimal educational experiences for students. This framework should by no means prevent experimentation and innovation. On the contrary, a clear understanding of the team's task, and appropriate guidelines rather than rigid dictates should foster and encourage experiments to arrive at the best solutions.

Finally, how does the school know that the curriculum and its associated endeavours are working? Is the curriculum truly coordinated and efficient? Are the teams and the faculty achieving their goals? Is the institution thriving in its educational mission? Are the outcomes creating the desired impact? These are all questions that a quality improvement system tries to address.

As quality improvement efforts in industry and elsewhere have become increasingly pervasive and necessary, medical schools have been similarly pressured to apply quality management principles to their efforts. Authors have suggested using models from industry (Armstrong et al. 2004) to guide the planning and conduct of medical education, while others have reported the adoption and adaptation of industrial quality management processes to curriculum (Stratton et al. 2007; Dalt et al. 2010) and course (Goldman et al. 2012) management. It has become clear that a more comprehensive approach to quality management in education on a system-wide basis is necessary (McOwen et al. 2009).

Most medical schools collect a lot of evaluation data but this is often used for narrow purposes (such as faculty promotion) and is rarely part of an overall systematic approach to quality management. Comprehensive systems are needed that supply data and information about

* students' professional success, conduct and contentment and not just their academic success

* future employer satisfaction and patient outcomes, and not just graduate placements

* faculty engagement and growth, and not just student feedback

* curriculum innovation and responsiveness, and not just content covered

* corporate culture and institutional growth, and not just research grants obtained

* meeting society's needs and fulfilling its mission, and not just national rankings (see fig. 28.4).

In summary, curriculum planning and implementation is a complex process that requires a concerted organizational approach, and in most cases significant changes in organizational culture, structure and function. Curriculum planning that merely addresses changes in content will not be enough. Societal needs, mission and values set the stage; realistic and evidence-based planning translates the mission into a detailed strategy; and careful implementation based on quality improvement principles makes the curriculum dynamic, responsive to needs and data, and constantly changing.

Conclusions

* Significant changes in healthcare, biomedical sciences, and pedagogy required undergraduate medical education to change dramatically in the last 40 years.

* These changes have led to many innovations.

* The impact and outcomes in patient and population health are yet to be determined.

* Significant efforts will need to be made in educational research to address these issues in a context of social accountability.

* Educational planning in the future will need to assure desired outcomes, socially appropriate values, prudent use of resources, and a robust quality improvement system.

References

Albanese, M. (2000) Problem-based learning: why curricula are likely to show little effect on knowledge and clinical skills. *Med Educ.* 24: 729–738

Albanese, M.A. and Mitchell, S. (1993) Problem-based learning: a review of literature on its outcomes and implementation issues. *Acad Med.* 68: 52–81

Antepohl, W., Domeij, E., Forsberg, P., and Ludvigsson, J. (2003) A follow-up of medical graduates of a problem-based learning curriculum. *Med Educ.* 37: 155–162

Aretz, H.T. (2011) Some thoughts about creating healthcare professionals that match what societies need. *Med Teach.* 33: 608–613

Armstrong, E.G. (1997) A hybrid model of problem-based learning. In D. Boud and G. Feletti. (eds.) *The Challenge of Problem-based Learning* (pp. 137–150). 2nd ed. London: Kogan Press

Armstrong, E.G., Mackey, M., and Spear, S. (2004) Medical education as a process management problem. *Acad Med.* 79: 721–728

Armstrong, E.G. and Parsa Parsi, R. (2005) How can physicians' learning styles drive educational planning. *Acad Med.* 80: 680–684

Association of American Medical Colleges (1998) *Learning Objectives for Medical Student Education. Report I. Guidelines for Medical Schools.* Washington, DC: AAMC

Barrows, H.S. (1986) A taxonomy of problem-based learning methods. *Med Educ.* 20: 481–486

Barrows, H.S. (1993) An overview of the uses of standardized patients for teaching and evaluating clinical skills. *Acad Med.* 68: 443–451

Biggs, J.S. and Wells, R.W. (2011) The social mission of Australian medical schools in a time of expansion. *Aust Health Rev.* 35: 424–429.

Bland, C.J., Starnaman, S., Wersal, L., Moorhead-Rosenberg, L., Zonia, S., and Henry, R. (2000) Curricular change in medical schools: how to succeed. *Acad Med.* 75: 575–594

Bligh, J. (1995) Identifying the core curriculum: the Liverpool approach. *Med Teach.* 17: 383–390

Bligh, J. (1999) Curriculum design revisited. *Med Educ.* 33: 82–85

Blake, R.L., Hosokawa, M.C., and Riley, S.L. (2000) Student performances on step 1 and step 2 of the United States Medical Licensing Examination following implementation of a problem-based learning curriculum. *Acad Med.* 75: 66–70

Bokken, L., Linssen, T., Scherpbier, A., van der Vleuten, C., and Rethans, J.J. (2009) Feedback by simulated patients in undergraduate medical education: a systematic review of the literature. *Med Educ.* 43: 202–210.

Boyer, E.L. (1990) *Scholarship Revisited. Priorities of the Professoriate.* The Carnegie Foundation for the Advancement of Teaching. New York, NY: John Wiley & Sons Inc.

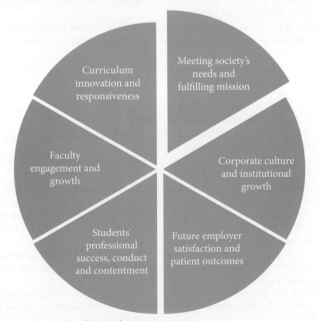

Figure 28.4 New goals to evaluate.

Brooks, M.A. (2009). Medical education and the tyranny of competency. *Persp Biol Med*. 52: 90–102

Burke, C.S., Salas, E., Wilson-Donnelly, K., and Priest, H. (2004) How to turn a team of experts into an expert medical team: guidance from the aviation and military communities. *Qual Saf Health Care*. 13: 96–104

Carter, C.T. (1844) Observations on the clauses and provisions of Sir James Graham's Medical Bill *Prov Med Surg J*. s1–8: 593

Charlin, B., Lubarsky, S., Millette, B., et al. (2012) Clinical reasoning processes: unravelling complexity through graphical representation. *Med Educ*. 46: 454–463

Chumley-Jones, H.S., Dobbie, A., and Alford, C.L. (2002) Web-based learning: sound educational method or hype? A review of the evaluation literature. *Acad Med*. 77(10 suppl): S86–S93

Colliver, J.A. (2000) Effectiveness of problem-based learning curricula: research and theory. *Acad Med*. 75: 259–266

Committee on the Health Professions Education Summit (2003) A.C. Greiner, and E. Knebel, (eds) Institute of Medicine of the National Academies. Health Profession Education: A Bridge to Quality. Washington, DC: The National Academies Press

Coulehan, J. (2005) Viewpoint: Today's professionalism: engaging the mind but not the heart. *Acad Med*. 8: 892–898

Coury, C. (1970) The teaching of medicine in France from the beginning of the seventeenth century. In C.D. O'Malley (ed.) *The History of Medical Education* (p. 123). UCLA Forum in Medical Sciences, Number 12. Berkeley: University of California Press

Crossley, J., Humphris, G., and Jolly, B. (2002) Assessing health professionals. *Med Educ*. 36: 800–804

Curran, V.R., Sharpe, D., Flynn, K., and Button, P. (2010) A longitudinal study of the effect of an interprofessional education curriculum on student satisfaction and attitudes towards interprofessional teamwork and education. *J Interprof Care*. 24: 41–52.

Dalt, L.D., Callegaro, S., Mazzi, A., et al. (2010) A model of quality assurance and quality improvement for post-graduate medical education in Europe. *Med Teach*. 32: e57–e64

Dobie, S. (2007) Reflections on a well-traveled path: self-awareness, mindful practice, and relationship-centered care as foundation for medical education. *Acad Med*. 82: 422–427

Dornan, T., Littlewood, S., Margolis, S.A., Scherpbier, A., Spencer, J., and Ypinazar, V. (2006) How can experience in clinical and community settings contribute to early medical education? A BEME systematic review. *Med Teach*. 28: 3–18

Eley, D. and Baker, P. (2006) Does recruitment lead to retention? Rural clinical school training experiences and subsequent intern choices. *Rural Remote Health*. 3 February, 6: 511

Engel, G.L. (1977) The need for a new medical model: a challenge for biomedicine. *Science*. 196: 129–136

Epstein, R.M. (2007) Assessment in medical education. *N Engl J Med*. 356: 387–396

Epstein, R.M. and Hundert, E.M. (2002) Defining and assessing professional competence. *JAMA*. 287: 226–235

Fincher, R.M., Simpson, D.E., Mennin, S.P, et al. (2000) Scholarship in teaching: an imperative for the 21st century. *Acad Med*. 75: 887–894

Flexner, A. (1910) Medical education in the United States and Canada: a report to the Carnegie Foundation for the Advancement of Teaching. New York: Carnegie Foundation for the Advancement of Teaching; Bulletin No. 4

Flexner, A. (1912) Medical Education in Europe: A Report to the Carnegie Foundation for the Advancement of Teaching. New York, NY: The Carnegie Foundation for the Advancement of Teaching; Bulletin No. 6

Flexner, A. (1925) *Medical Education: a Comparative Study*. New York: MacMillan

Frank, J.R., Mungroo, R., Ahmad, Y., Wang, M., de Rossi, S., and Horsley, T. (2010) Toward a definition of competency-based education in medicine: a systematic review of published definitions. *Med Teach*. 32: 631–637

Frenk, J., Chen, L., Bhutta, Z.A., et al. (2010) Health professionals for a new century: transforming education to strengthen health systems in an interdependent world. *Lancet*. 376: 1923–1958

Friedlander, M.J., Andrews, L., Armstrong, E.G., et al. (2011). What can medical education learn from the neurobiology of learning? *Acad Med*. 86: 415–420.

G2010 Project Group (2010) *Blueprint G2010. Revised Medical Curriculum RuG. The Groningen University*. [Online] http://www.rug.nl/umcg/onderwijs/g2010/blueprintg2010.pdf Accessed 12 March 2012

Gaufberg, E., Batalden, M., Sands, R., and Bell, S. (2010) The hidden curriculum: what can we learn from third year medical student narratives reflections? *Acad Med*. 85: 1709–1716

General Medical Council (1993) *Tomorrow's Doctors. Recommendations on Undergraduate Medical Education*. London: Education Committee of the General Medical Council

General Medical Council (2003) *Tomorrow's Doctors*. London: General Medical Council

General Medical Council (2009) *Tomorrow's Doctors. Outcomes and Standards for Undergraduate Medical Education*. London: General Medical Council

Gibbs, T. (2011) Medical Teacher. Social Accountability Special Issue. *Med Teach*. 33, Vol. 8, pp. 605–679

Goldman, E.F., Swayze, S.S., Swinehart, S.E., and Schroth, W.S. (2012) Effecting curricular change through comprehensive course assessment: using structure and process to change outcomes. *Acad Med*. 87: 300–307

Green, L.A., Fryer Jr., G.E., Yawn, B.P., Lanier, D., and Dovey, S.M. (2001) The ecology of medical care revisited. *N Engl J Med*. 344: 2021–2025

Gumbach, K., and Bodenheimer, T. (2004) Can health care teams improve primary care practice? *JAMA*. 291: 1246–1251

Hackman, J. R. and Walton, R. E. (1986). Leading groups in organizations. In P.S. Goodman (ed.), *Designing Effective Work Groups* (pp. 72–119). San Francisco: Jossey-Bass.

Hackman, J.R. (ed.) (1990) *Groups That Work (and Those That Don't). Creating Conditions for Effective Teamwork*. San Francisco: Jossey-Bass

Hafferty, F.W. (1998) Beyond curriculum reform: confronting medicine's hidden curriculum. *Acad Med*. 73: 403–407

Haidet, P., Levine, R.E., Parmelee, D.X., et al. (2012) Perspective: Guidelines for reporting team-based learning activities in the medical and health sciences literature. *Acad Med*. 87: 292–299

Hamarneh, S. (1970) Medical education and practice in medieval Islam. In C.D. O'Malley (ed.) *The History of Medical Education* (pp. 39–72). UCLA Forum in Medical Sciences, Number 12. Berkeley: University of California Press

Hammick, M., Freeth, D., Koppel, I., Reeves, S., and Barr, H. (2007) A best evidence systematic review of interprofessional education: BEME guide no. 9. *Med Teach*. 29: 735–751

Harden, R.M., Davis, M.H., and Crosby, J.R. (1997) The new Dundee medical curriculum: a whole that is greater than the sum of its parts. *Med Educ*. 31: 264–271

Harden, R.M., Sowden, S., and Dunn, R.W. (1984) Educational strategies in curriculum development: the SPICES model. *Med Educ*. 18: 284–297

Harden, R.M. (2000) The integration ladder: a tool for curriculum planning and evaluation. *Med Educ*. 34, 551–557

Harden, R.M. (2002) Developments in outcomes-based education. *Med Teach*. 24: 117–120

Hayes, R.H., Wheelwright, S.C., and Clark, K.B. (1988) *Dynamic Manufacturing* (p. 279). New York: The Free Press

Health Professions Network Nursing and Midwifery in Human Resources for Health, World Health Organization. (2010) *Framework for action on interprofessional education and collaborative practice*. WHO, Geneva. [Online] http://whqlibdoc.who.int/hq/2010/WHO_HRH_HPN_10.3_eng.pdf Accessed December 2010

Hean, S., Craddock, D., Hammick, M., and Hammick M. (2012) Theoretical insights into interprofessional education: AMEE Guide No. 62. *Med Teach*. 34: e78–e101

Hemmer, P.A., Hawkins, R., Jackson, J.L., and Pangaro, L.N. (2000) Assessing how well three evaluation methods detect deficiencies in medical students' professionalism in two settings of an internal medicine clerkship. *Acad Med.* 75: 167–173

Holman, H. (2004) Chronic disease—the need for a new clinical education. *JAMA.* 292, 1057–1059

Holmboe, E.S., Sherbino, J., Long, D.M., Swing, S.R., and Frank, J.R. for the International CBME Collaborators. (2010) The role of assessment in competency-based medical education. *Med Teach.* 32: 676–682

Huddle, T.S. and Heudebert, G.R. (2007). Taking apart the art: the risk of anatomizing clinical competence. *Acad Med.* 82: 536–541

Hurt, M.M. and Harris, J.O. (2005) Founding a new college of medicine at Florida State University. *Acad Med.* 80, 973–979

Hull, L., Arora, S., Aggarwal, R., Darzi, A., Vincent, C., and Sevdalis, N. (2012) The impact of nontechnical skills on technical performance in surgery: a systematic review. *J Am Coll Surg.* 214: 214–230

Hylin, U., Nyholm, H., Mattiasson, A.C., and Ponzer, S. (2007) Interprofessional training in clinical practice on a training ward for healthcare students: a two-year follow-up. *J Interprof Care.* 21: 277–288

Interprofessional Education Collaborative Expert Panel (2011) *Core Competencies for Interprofessional Collaborative Practice: Report of an Expert Panel.* Washington, DC: Interprofessional Education Collaborative

Irby, D.M. and Wilkerson, L. (2003). Educational innovations in academic medicine and environmental trends. *J Gen Intern Med.* 18: 370–376

Issa, N., Schuller, M., Santacaterina, S., et al. (2011) Applying multimedia design principles enhances learning in medical education. *Med Educ.* 45: 818–826

Issenberg, S.B., McGaghie, W.C., Petrusa, E.R., Lee Gordon, D., and Scalese, R.J. (2005) Features and uses of high-fidelity medical simulations that lead to effective learning: a BEME systematic review. *Med Teach.* 27: 10–28

Jacquart, D. (2008) Islamic pharmacology in the middle ages: theories and substances, *Eur Rev.* 16: 219–227

Jamshidi, H.R. and Cook, D.A. (2003) Some thoughts about medical education in the twenty-first century. *Med Teach.* 25: 229–238

Johnson, C.E., Hurtubise, L.C., Castrop, J., et al. (2004) Learning management systems: technology to measure the medical knowledge competency of the ACGME. *Med Educ.* 38: 599–608

Josiah Macy Jr. Foundation (2009) *Revisiting the Medical School Educational Mission at a Time of Expansion.* New York: Josiah Macy Jr. Foundation

Kern, D.E., Thomas, P.A., and Hughes, M.T. (eds). (2009) *Curriculum Development for Medical Education. A Six-Step Approach.* 2nd edn. Baltimore: The Johns Hopkins University Press

Koh, G.C.-H., Khoo, H.E., Wong, M.L., and Koh, D. (2008) The effects of problem-based learning during medical school on physician competency: a systematic review. *CMAJ.* 178: 34–41

Kohn, L.Y., Corrigan, J.M., and Donaldson, M.S. (eds) (1999) *To Err Is Human: Building a Safer Health System.* Institute of Medicine, Washington, DC: National Academy Press

Kruger, J. and Dunning, D. (1999) Unskilled and unaware of it: how difficulties in recognizing one's own incompetence lead to inflated self-assessments. *J Personality Soc Psychol.* 77: 1121–1134

Kudlien, F. (1970a) Medical education in classical antiquity. In C.D. O'Malley (ed.) *The History of Medical Education* (pp. 3–37). UCLA Forum in Medical Sciences, Number 12. Berkeley: University of California Press

Kudlien F. (1970b) Medical education in classical antiquity. In C.D. O'Malley (ed.) *The History of Medical Education* (p. 25). UCLA Forum in Medical Sciences, Number 12. Berkeley: University of California Press

LCME Annual Questionnaire, Part II (2011) *U.S. Medical Schools Offering One or More Longitudinal Clerkships. AAMC Curriculum Reports.* [Online] https://www.aamc.org/download/271138/data/longitudinalclerkships.pdf Accessed 27 March 2012

Leipzig, R.M., Granville, L., Simpson, D, et al. (2009). Keeping granny safe on July 1: Consensus on minimum geriatric competencies for graduating medical students. *Acad Med.* 84: 604–610

Liston, B.W., Fischer, M.A., Way, D.P., Torre, D., and Papp, K.K. (2011) Interprofessional education in the internal medicine clerkship: results from a national survey. *Acad Med.* 86: 872–876.

Ludmerer, K.M. (2004) Perspective: Learner-centered medical education. *N Engl J Med.* 351: 1163–1164

Maeshiro, R., Johnson, I., Koo D, et al. (2010) Medical Education for a Healthier Population: Reflections on the Flexner Report from a public health perspective. *Acad Med.* 85: 211–219

Masie, E. (2002). Blended learning: the magic is in the mix. In: Rossett A (ed.). *The ASTD E-Learning Handbook* (pp. 58–63). New York: McGraw-Hill

Maudsley, G. (1999) Do we all mean the same thing by 'problem-based learning'? A review of the concepts and a formulation of the ground rules. *Acad Med.* 74: 178–185

Maudsley, R.F., Wilson, D.R., Neufeld, V.R., et al. (2000) Educating future physicians for Ontario: Phase II. *Acad Med.* 75: 113–126

Mayer, C.M., Cluff, L., Lin, W.T., et al. (2011) Evaluating efforts to optimize TeamSTEPPS implementation in surgical and pediatric intensive care units. *The Joint Commission Journal on Quality and Patient Safety.* 37: 365–374.

McNeil, H.P., Hughes, C.S., Toohey, S.M., and Dowton, S.B. (2006) An innovative outcomes-based medical education program built on adult learning principles. *Med Teach.* 28: 527–534

McOwen, K.S., Bellini, L.M., Morison, G., and Shea, J.A. (2009) The development and implementation of a health-system-wide evaluation system for education activities: build it and they will come. *Acad Med.* 84: 1352–1359

MedEdPortal (2012) Association of American Medical Colleges, Washington, DC [Online] https://www.mededportal.org/ Accessed 10 May 2012

Mercer University School of Medicine (2002) [Online] http://medicine.mercer.edu/about/mission/ Accessed 17 May 2012

Mercer University School of Medicine (2011) *Medical Student handbook 2011–2012*, pp. 52–55. [Online] http://medicine.mercer.edu/mu-medicine/academics/catalogs/upload/studenthandbook.pdf Accessed 17 May 2012

Mies van der Rohe, L (1938) Speech to architecture students. Armour Institute, Chicago 1938. [Online] http://www.scribd.com/doc/91739267/Mies-speech-to-architecture-students-IIT-1938 Accessed 27 June 2012

Miller, G.E. (1990) The assessment of clinical skills/competence/performance. *Acad Med.* 65: 563–567

Milner R.J., Gusic, M.E., and Thorndyke, L.E. (2011) Perspective: Toward a competency framework for faculty. *Acad Med.* 86: 1204–1210

Moore, G.T., Inui, T.S., Ludden, J.M., and Schoenbaum, S.C. (1994) The 'teaching HMO': a new academic partner. *Acad Med.* 69: 595–600

Morrison, G., Goldfarb, S., and Lanken, P.N. (2010) Team training of medical students in the 21st century: would Flexner approve? *Acad Med.* 85: 254–259

Muller, S. (chair) (1984). Physicians for the twenty-first century: report of the project panel on the general professional education of the physician and college preparation for medicine (GPEP). *Journal of Med Educ.* 59 (11 Pt 2): 1–208

Neufeld, V.R., Maudsley, R.F., Pickering, R.J., et al. (1998) Educating future physicians for Ontario. *Acad Med.* 73: 1133–1148

Neville, A.J., and Norman, G.R. (2007) PBL in the undergraduate MD program at McMaster University: three iterations in three decades. *Acad Med.* 82: 370–374.

Neville, A.J. (2009) Problem-based learning and medical education forty years on. A review of its effects on knowledge and clinical performance. *Med Principles Pract.* 18: 1–9

Norris, T.E., Schaad, D.C., DeWitt, D., Ogur, B., and Hunt D.D. (2009) Consortium of Longitudinal Integrated Clerkships. Longitudinal integrated clerkships for medical students: an innovation adopted by medical schools in Australia, Canada, South Africa, and the United States. *Acad Med.* 84: 902–907

O'Leary, K.J., Buck, R., Fligiel, H.M., et al. (2011) Structured interdisciplinary rounds in a medical teaching unit: improving patient safety. *Arch Intern Med.* 171: 678–684

O'Malley, C.D. (1970) Medical education during the Renaissance. In C. D. O'Malley (ed.) *The History of Medical Education* (pp. 89–102). UCLA Forum in Medical Sciences, Number 12. Berkeley: University of California Press

O'Neill, P.A., Willis, S.C., and Jones, A. (2002) A model of how students link problem-based learning with clinical experience through 'elaboration'. *Acad Med.* 77: 76–85

Ogrinc, G., Mutha, S., and Irby, D.M. (2002) Evidence for longitudinal ambulatory care rotations: a review of the literature. *Acad Med.* 77: 688–693

Ogur, B., Hirsh, D., Krupat, E., and Bor, D. (2007) The Harvard Medical School-Cambridge integrated clerkship: an innovative model of clinical education. *Acad Med.* 82: 397–404

Okuda, Y., Bryson, E.O., DeMaria, S. Jr., et al. (2009) The utility of simulation in medical education: what is the evidence? *Mount Sinai J Med.* 76: 330–343.

Organization for Economic Co-operation and Development (2011) *Health at a glance 2011. OECD indicators (2011)* [Online] http://www.oecd.org/dataoecd/24/8/49084488.pdf Accessed 28 March 2012

Pangaro, L. (2006) A shared professional framework for anatomy and clinical clerkships. *Clin Anat* 19: 419–428

Papa, F.J. and Harasym, P.H. (1999) Medical curriculum reform in North America, 1765 to the present: a cognitive science perspective. *Acad Med.* 74: 154–164

Papadakis, M.A., Teherani, A., Banach, M.A., et al. (2004) Disciplinary action by medical boards and prior behavior in medical schools. *N Engl J Med.* 353: 2673–2682

Park, J.H., Son, J.Y., Kim, S., and May, W. (2011) Effect of feedback from standardized patients on medical students' performance and perceptions of the neurological examination. *Med Teach.* 33: 1005–1010

Paolo, A.M. and Bonaminio, G.A. (2003) Measuring outcomes of undergraduate medical education: residency directors' ratings of first-year residents. *Acad Med.* 78: 90–95

Parmelee, D.X. (2010) Team-based learning: moving forward in curriculum innovation: a commentary. *Med Teach.* 32: 105–107

Parmelee, D.X. and Michaelsen, L.K. (2010) Twelve trips for doing team-based learning (TBL). *Med Teach.* 32: 118–122

Pelling, S., Kalen, A., Hammar, M., and Wahlström, O. (2011) Preparation for becoming members of health care teams: findings from a 5-year evaluation of a student interprofessional training ward. *J Interprof Care.* 25: 328–332

Peters, A.S., Feins, A., Rubin, R., Seward, S., Schnaidt, K., and Fletcher, R.H. (2001) The longitudinal primary care clerkship at Harvard Medical School. *Acad Med.* 76: 484–488.

Pham, H.H., Simonson, L., Elnicki, M., Fried, L.P., Goroll, A.H., and Bass, E.B. (2004) Training U.S. medical students to care for the chronically ill. *Acad Med.* 79: 32–41

Preamble to the Constitution of the World Health Organization as adopted by the International Health Conference, New York, 19–22 June, 1946; signed on 22 July 1946 by the representatives of 61 States (Official Records of the World Health Organization, no. 2, p. 100) and entered into force on 7 April 1948. [Online] http://www.who.int/about/definition/en/print.html Accessed 2 May 2012

Pruitt, S.D. and Epping-Jordan, J.E. (2005) Preparing the 21st century global healthcare workforce. *BMJ.* 330: 637–639

Putnam, C.E. (2006) Reform and innovation: A repeating pattern during a half century of medical education in the USA. *Med Educ.* 40: 227–234.

Quattrochi, J., Pasquale, S., Cerva, B., and Lester, J. (2002). Learning Neuroscience: An Interactive Case-Based Online Network (ICON). *J Sci Educ Technol.* 11: 15–38

Rabinowitz, H.K., Diamond. J.J., Markham, F.W., and Wortman, J.R. (2008) Medical school programs to increase the rural physician supply: a systematic review and projected impact of widespread replication. *Acad Med.* 83: 235–243

Rand Europe, Ernst & Young, LLP. (2012) *National Evaluation of the Department of Health's Integrated Care Pilots. Final Report: Full Version.* Prepared for the Department of Health. March 2012. [Online] http://www.rand.org/content/dam/rand/pubs/technical_reports/2012/RAND_TR1164.pdf Accessed 30 March 2012

Reeves, S., Zwarenstein, M., Goldman, J., et al. (2010) The effectiveness of interprofessional education: key findings from a new systematic review. *J Interprof Care.* 24: 230–241

Regehr, G. and Norman, G.R. (1996) Issues in cognitive psychology: implications for professional education. *Acad Med.* 71: 988–1001

Rider, E.A., Nawotniak, R.H., and Smith, G. (2007) *A Practical Guide to Teaching and Assessing the ACGME Core Competencies.* Marblehead (MA): HCPro, Inc.

Rourke, J.T.B. (2002) Building the new Northern Ontario rural medical school. *Aust J Rural Health.* 10: 112–116

Ruiz, J.G., Mintzer, M.J., and Leipzig, R.M. (2006) The impact of e-learning in medical education. *Acad Med.* 81: 207–212

Schmidt, H.G. (1993) Foundations of problem-based learning: some explanatory notes. *Med Educ.* 27: 422–432

Schmidt, H.G. (1989) The rationale behind problem-based learning. In H. G. Schmidt, M. Lipkin Jr., M.W. de Vries, and J.M. Greep (eds.). *New Directions for Medical Education* (pp. 105–111). New York: Springer-Verlag

Schuwirth, L.W.T., Southgate, L., Page, G.G., et al. (2002) When enough is enough: a conceptual basis for fair and defensible practice performance assessment. *Med Educ.* 36: 925–930

Simpson, D., Fincher, R.M., Hafler, J.P., et al. (2007) Advancing educators and education: defining the components and evidence of educational scholarship. *Med Educ.* 41: 1002–1009

Siu, A.L., Mayer-Oakes, S.A., and Brook, R.H. (1985) Innovations in medical curricula: templates for change? *Health Affairs.* 4(2): 60–71

Srinivasan, M., Li, S.T.T., Meyers. F.J., et al. (2011) 'Teaching as a competency': competencies for medical educators. *Acad Med.* 86: 1211–1220

Steinert, Y., Mann, K., Centeno, A., et al. (2006) A systematic review of faculty development initiatives to improve teaching effectiveness in medical education: BEME guide no. 8. *Med Teach.* 28: 497–526

Stern, D.T. and Papadakis, M. (2006) The developing physician—becoming a professional. *N Engl J Med.* 355: 1794–1799

Strasser, R.P., Lanphear, J.H., McCready, W.G., Topps, M.H., Hunt, D.D., and Matte, MC. (2009) Canada's new medical school: the Northern Ontario School of Medicine: social accountability through distributed community engaged learning. *Acad Med.* 84: 1459–1464

Stratton, T.D., Rudy, D.W., Sauer, M.J., Perman, J.A., and Jennings, C.D. (2007) Lessons from industry: one school's transformation toward 'lean' curricular governance. *Acad Med.* 82: 331–340

Swing, S.R. (2007) The ACGME outcome project: retrospective and prospective. *Med Teach.* 29: 648–654

Talbot, C.H. (1970) Medical Education in the Middle Ages. In C.D. O'Malley (ed.) *The History of Medical Education* (pp. 73–87). UCLA Forum in Medical Sciences, Number 12. Berkeley: University of California Press

Tamblyn, R. (1999) Outcomes in medical education: what is the standard and outcome of care delivered by our graduates? *Adv Health Sci Educ.* 4: 9–25

ten Cate, O., Snell, L., Mann, K., and Vermunt, J. (2004) Orienting teaching toward the learning process. *Acad Med.* 79: 219–228

The Association of Faculties of Medicine of Canada (2010) *The Future of Medical Education in Canada (FMEC): a Collective Vision for MD Education.* Ottawa: The Association of Medical Faculties of Canada

Thistlethwaite, J. (2012) Interprofessional education: a review of context, learning and the research agenda. *Med Educ.* 46: 58–70

Vernon, D.T.A. and Blake, R.L. (1993) Does problem-based learning work? A meta-analysis of evaluative research. *Acad Med.* 68: 550–563

Wass, V., van der Vleuten, C., Shatzer, J., and Jones, R. (2001). Assessment of clinical competence. *Lancet.* 357: 945–949

Whelan, G.P., Boulet, J.R., McKinley, D.W., et al. (2005) Scoring standardized patient examinations: lessons learned from the development and administration of the ECFMG Clinical Skills Assessment (CSA). *Med Teach.* 27: 200–206

Wile, M.Z. and Smith, C.K. (2000) Case Western Reserve University School of Medicine. In: *Medical Education: Ten Stories of Curriculum Change*. New York: Milbank Memorial Fund. [Online] http://www.milbank.org/reports/americanmedicalcolleges/0010medicalcolleges.html#casewestern Accessed 28 March 2012

Wilkinson, T.J. and Frampton, C.M. (2004) Comprehensive undergraduate medical assessments improve prediction of clinical performance. *Med Educ.* 38: 1111–1116

Worley, P. and Murray, R. (2011) Social accountability in medical education—an Australian rural and remote perspective. *Med Teach.* 33: 654–658

CHAPTER 29

Postgraduate medical education

Jamiu O. Busari and Ashley Duits

If we have learnt anything from the past decade of reform it is that the postgraduate training of doctors can't simply be fitted in round service: it takes planning and hard work.

Graeme Catto

Reproduced from *British Medical Journal*, Catto G, 'Specialist registrar training: Some good news at last', 320, p. 817, Copyright 2000, with permission from BMJ Publishing Group Ltd.

Introduction

Postgraduate medical education (PME) is the phase of medical training where doctors, after having obtained a formal medical qualification, can develop additional competencies in a defined area of their choice. PME has developed from a setting similar to an apprenticeship, where junior doctors work in a (clinical) learning environment with more experienced colleagues (or teachers), who are also being responsible for their instruction and supervision. The training in this context is conducted according to the existing and relevant regulations specified by the local universities, specialist boards and/or national medical societies or institutes for postgraduate medical training.

Over the last few decades, PME has witnessed increasing convergence in training methods with emphasis on both practical training and theory. Modern principles of medical education have exerted increasing influence in several countries as witnessed by the wave of curricular reform in Europe, North America, and Australia (WFME 2003; CPMEC 2006; GMC 2009; Royal College of Physicians and Surgeons of Canada 2005; SDMCG 2000; Reenen van et al. 2009).

Sophisticated educational programmes have emerged as a result, the components of which are planned clinical or practical rotations, expert supervision, theoretical teaching, research experience, systematic assessments, and evaluation. The convergence of the principles for postgraduate training worldwide has also been promoted by the increased interactions between universities and other educational institutions, regulatory bodies, medical societies, and medical associations. These, in turn, have been influenced by the increased mobility of physicians and the fast growing internationalization of the medical workforce.

Historical perspective of PME

The origins of Western medical education can be traced from the Greek and Roman times to the influence of Christian, Muslim, and Jewish authorities in the early Middle Ages. In the 16th and 17th centuries, the education and practice of medicine was defined by renowned physicians such as: William Harvey, the English physician who described the systemic circulation; Vesalius, the Flemish surgeon and anatomist who noted that the heart had four chambers, the liver two lobes, and that the blood vessels originated in the heart, not the liver; and van Leeuwenhoek, the Dutch microbiologist, who was the first to observe and describe single-celled organisms, which he originally referred to as animalcules and that are now referred to as micro-organisms.

It was not until the beginning of the last century that major changes in medical education occurred following the discoveries of 19th century researchers like Koch, Virchow, and Pasteur. Of significant influence in the development of medical education in the early 1900s, however, was the work of William Osler and Abraham Flexner, both of whom are considered pioneers in the development of medical education, as it exists today.

Pioneers in the development of PME

Sir William Osler, (12 July 1849–29 December 1919) was a physician and one of the founding professors at Johns Hopkins Hospital. Osler was the first Professor of Medicine and founder of the Medical Service at Johns Hopkins Hospital. He created the first residency programme for specialty training of physicians, and was the first to bring medical students out of the lecture halls for bedside clinical training (Epstein and Hundert 2002).

Abraham Flexner, born in Louisville, Kentucky (13 November 1866–21 September 1959), was an American educator. The Flexner Report, published in 1910, reformed medical education in the United States (Flexner 1910). The report examined the state of American medical education and led to far-reaching reforms in the way doctors were trained as well as to the closure of most rural medical schools and all but two of America's African American medical colleges. Ironically, one of the schools, Louisville National Medical College was located in his own hometown of Louisville (Johnston 1984).

Flexner later conducted a related study of medical education in Europe. According to Bonner (2002, pp. 182–186), Flexner's work came to be 'nearly as well known in Europe as in America'. With funding from the Rockefeller foundation, he worked toward restructuring the nation's medical schools. Bonner went on stating that 'Flexner exerted a decisive influence on the course of medical training and left an enduring mark on some of the nation's most renowned schools of medicine'. Remarkably, Flexner worried that 'the imposition of rigid standards by accrediting groups was making the medical curriculum a monstrosity' and that medical students were moving through it with 'little time to stop, read, work or think'. (Bonner 2002)

Consequences of the Flexner Report

The Flexner Report is now remembered for its effect in creating a single model of medical education, characterized by a philosophy that has largely survived to the present day. 'An education in medicine', wrote Flexner, 'involves both learning and learning how; the student cannot effectively know, unless he knows how'. (Bonner 2002) Although the report is over 100 years old, many of its recommendations are still relevant—particularly those concerning the physician as a 'social instrument…whose function is fast becoming social and preventive, rather than individual and curative'. To a remarkable extent, the present day aspects of the medical profession in North America shown in fig. 29.1 are consequences of the Flexner Report.

Definition of PME

As indicated earlier in this chapter, PME is a phase of medical training that is limited to a specified period of time, and which cannot be completely separated from continuing medical education (CME) or continuous professional development (CPD) (see fig. 29.2). The shaping, reshaping and development of a professional in response to the changing societal and individual needs within the context of the evolution of medical science and healthcare delivery, is a lifelong process. This process starts when the physician, as a student, is admitted to medical school and persists for as long as he or she is engaged in professional medical activities.

While it is difficult to provide a concise definition of PME, a description that satisfactorily depicts the concept is that it is the phase after basic undergraduate medical training where physicians enrol in additional supervised medical education, in preparation for independent professional practice. It comprises of preregistration, vocational, or professional training, as well as specialist, subspecialist and other formalized training programmes for defined expert tasks. Upon completion of the formal postgraduate training, a degree, diploma or certificate is usually granted. In general, PME often requires additional theoretical education in addition to the practical clinical aspects of the learning process, which can be organized in various ways. This can either be closely connected

- ◆ At least 6, and preferably 8 years of post-secondary and university-based formal instruction for physicians
- ◆ Medical training that adheres closely to the scientific method and is thoroughly grounded in human physiology and biochemistry. In addition, medical research that adheres fully to the protocols of scientific research (Beck 2004)
- ◆ A significant increase in quality of the professional competency of physicians (Barzansky 1992)
- ◆ Establishment of medical schools only after permission of the state government, and the size of existing medical schools being subject to state regulation
- ◆ Each state branch of the American Medical Association oversees all conventional medical schools located within the state
- ◆ Medical practice in the USA and Canada is a highly paid and well-respected profession

Figure 29.1 Present day aspects of the medical profession in North America.

with a local clinical training programme or organized through regional, national, or international theoretical courses. In most cases, universities, specialist boards, medical societies, and colleges or institutes for PME manage these programmes.

CPD meanwhile refers to the process of continuously developing the multifaceted competencies inherent in, and required for medical practice following at least a formal undergraduate medical training. It is drawn from the various domains of knowledge and skills (e.g. medical, managerial, social, or personal) so that a high quality of professional performance can be guaranteed. Although it is often used to designate the period commencing the completion of postgraduate training, CPD is a much more, far-reaching activity that is carried out during the entire professional life of the physician after graduation and is characterized by self-directed learning that rarely involves supervised training typical of undergraduate medical training.

Early years of postgraduate training versus higher specialist training

PME is currently undergoing major changes—the old model of learning through an apprenticeship relationship is being challenged. The number of hours that residents are expected to spend training per week as well as the length of their training programmes are under close scrutiny. A seamless (medical) educational curriculum is needed that will take students through their basic undergraduate medical training into the early general postgraduate training and then on to the higher specialist or fellowship training. This process should aim at producing fully trained doctors who can improve the

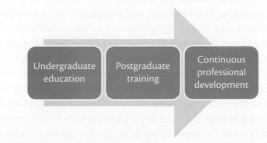

Figure 29.2 The medical education continuum.

healthcare of the population that they serve and develop new skills through a process that is demonstrable to the public.

There is a wealth of educational theory in the medical literature about how best to deliver medical training and how to assess training outcomes in PME. The principles of good medical education and training, however, encompass many different elements and clear learning outcomes should be outlined so that there is no doubt as to what competencies are expected of those entering the training programmes. The assessment systems are expected to closely match the curriculum and should be fair, reliable and valid. The curricula should reflect the skills, knowledge, care, and behaviour expected of physicians and the clinical teachers must possess the appropriate teaching skills and attitudes. In addition, postgraduate medical education and training should reflect the diversity of the society in which the doctor is practising. This includes patient-focused care, learner-centred education, and equal accessibility to education and training for everyone in society.

While the objective of PME is broad and generic in nature, the principal aim of higher specialist training is to provide the physician, who has completed basic training, with an educational programme that will prepare him or her for independent practice, either as a consultant or as a senior member of an academic department.

While the needs of the trainee physician will differ depending on the type of consultant post to which they aspire, they all need the opportunity to engage in diverse and challenging clinical practice. This will enable them to develop their clinical skills to the point where proficient independent practice is achieved and academic pursuits, including participation in original research, sustained. All higher specialist trainees need experience in management, teaching and multidisciplinary teamwork. Training must occur in well-organized local schemes, which offer a variety of training placements under the supervision of skilled and competent trainers.

The exposure to wide clinical experience, to academic and research work and participation in teaching, management and audit should enable trainees to undertake professional practice informed by a scientific, objective spirit, which will enable them to evaluate developments in their specialty throughout their professional lives. They should develop the habit of self-directed learning that will motivate ready participation in continuing professional development.

There are, however, a few challenges facing higher specialist training. A recent exploratory study on curriculum and assessment in higher specialist training (Bullock et al. 2004) showed that there is an apparent lack of connection between curriculum documentation, teaching and learning methods, and assessment. Also, the authors discovered that while there is a general recognition that training focuses on producing good surgeons or clinicians, the wider skills and processes required by a consultant, such as team working, teaching, management, and communication with patients and other staff, are under-recognized in existing curricula. This is despite the growing recognition of the importance of such areas within medicine (General Medical Council 1998; Department of Health 2001). A third issue that emerged was the importance of assessment—the quality, reliability and validity of postgraduate medical examinations were questioned. The authors argued that if higher specialist training aims to prepare doctors for the consultant role, there is a need to work towards an agreement on a wider range of key skills, which should then be reflected in the curriculum.

Changes and trends in PME

For the past 100 years, PME has been based on the concept of residency as articulated by the exemplary work of physicians and educators like Osler, Flexner, Welch, and Halsted. Prior to this period however, there was no known formalized structure of medical education. Therefore, whether or not a student gained the medical experience that was required was dependent mostly on the whim of the professor or 'master physician'. This was because medical training at the time was an apprenticeship in which the professor expected and often demanded virtual indentured servitude. Unfortunately, the available educational experiences offered by others during this vocational period were too brief to be of value.

In the late 19th century, William Halsted, an American surgeon and one of the celebrated big four at Johns Hopkins Hospital propagated a 'residency' model for training physicians to correct the inadequacies of unstructured training. The residency experience was considered an important advance in medical training and the fundamental requirements of a Halsted residency were a fixed period of time for training, structured educational content, actual experience with patients, increasing responsibility for patient care during training, and a period of supervised practice after formal training. Halsted also introduced a selection process for choosing residents based on merit, and a curriculum of specified length and content that focused on learning from graduated responsibility for patient care.

One can gain a better understanding of how the changes and trends in postgraduate medical education have evolved over the years; however, by using the analogy of discourses (Hodges 2006). Discourses, as depicted by Hodges, are thought models that people use as ways of seeing the world. They act like lenses or filters that help us to order our world by giving meaning to our work in such a way that we can communicate it to others and act in certain ways. According to Hodges, the competent doctor in the 1700s was a member of a guild carrying a blade for bloodletting and emetics for purging, and whose objective was to balance the humours of the body. In the 1800s the competent doctor was the gentleman with a walking stick, diagnosing patients by looking at their tongue, and smelling their urine. At the time, it was unusual to find women practising the craft. By 1950 a competent doctor, still most likely to be a man, wore a white coat, discussed a woman's health with her husband, and withheld the true diagnosis from a dying patient to prevent unnecessary worry. In the 21st century, professional competency no longer accommodates bloodletting, smelling urine, and withholding diagnoses as good clinical practice.

Hodges argues that what has changed in the practice and training of physicians over the years, is not the competency of physicians, but the discourses constructing what is understood as competent medical practice. This remark triggers a rethinking and re-examination of what we consider to be 'competent medical practice' and how medical education has evolved. Particularly, when one takes the discourse of competence being a measure of a physician's ability to memorize factual knowledge and apply this in the treatment of illness and disease that was characteristic of the period before the 1960s, to the period thereafter when competence was perceived as the ability to demonstrate proficiency in clinical performance. The 1980s witnessed a series of shifts that included a drive for models of accountability, and an explosion in the growth of dedicated institutions and medical educators in the field of measurement and evaluation, resulting in the discourse that focused on the psychometric reliability of tests as a measure of physician competence. However since the 1990s the discourse of competence has moved to the physician's ability to reflect effectively using portfolios and reflective exercises such as diaries, reflective essays, and learning contracts (Callaghan et al. 2007).

A lot of the proposals that Osler and Flexner propagated in the last century have significantly influenced the way postgraduate medical education has been defined, especially in the US, Canada, and the UK. The key elements of these proposals include the recommendations for a strong training in biomedical sciences for all medical students made up of a preclinical and clinical phase of the curriculum, medical education taking place in multifaculty universities and clinical experience and teaching being attained through formal clinical clerkships and rotations for students.

These proposals have also initiated several changes in the framework of medical curricula, with widespread curricular reform, and robust models for competency based medical training in several countries (GMC 2009; Cooke et al. 2010). While a significant amount of these changes have been fully integrated in many postgraduate medical training programmes in the last 30 years, several concerns related to the reform in PME have also arisen (GMC 2009; Bleakely et al. 2011).

Some of these concerns are related to the management of the ever-increasing body of scientific and medical knowledge, both in the volume of material on individual subjects and the number of subjects considered relevant (*knowledge management*), the tendency for individual subjects to be seen as silos of knowledge rather than as being intimately linked (*holistic versus atomistic knowledge*), and observations that newly qualified doctors are well grounded in knowledge, but much less well equipped in practical, clinical skills, and essential interpersonal skills (*cognitive versus clinical skills*). Other concerns include the changing expectations of patients, policy makers and employers (*social accountability*), changes in the pattern of delivery of healthcare (*value based healthcare*) (Porter 2010), the development of formal postgraduate education and training in all disciplines (*professional medical education*), and the importance of interprofessional and team-based care delivery (*team-based learning and practice*). In response to these concerns a number of initiatives have taken place—these include:

* The development of outcomes-based frameworks and standards for undergraduate and/or postgraduate programmes such as *Tomorrow's Doctors*, CanMEDS, World Federation of Medical Education, the Scottish Doctor, the Dutch Kaderbesluit, the Swiss competency framework. All of these define the essential outcomes required of graduates (Sottas 2011; WFME 2003; Frank 2005; GMC 2009; SDMCG 2000; Reenen van et al. 2009). These frameworks require achievement of particular competencies rather than reliance on local decisions or on time served.

* Integrated curricula, which are often organ- or systems-based. Integration can be horizontal (across disciplines that are traditionally taught in the same phase of the preclinical/clinical divide) or vertical (across different curricular years, including across the preclinical/clinical divide), or both. Vertically integrated curricula are characterized by early clinical experience and by 'science' content being delivered all the way across the course.

* Recognition that not all students learn in the same way and that differing curricular models are necessary.

* Recognition that the trainees' understanding and ability to apply knowledge are essential.

* Increasing delivery of education in community settings rather than entirely in hospitals.

* Development of assessment methods, which are robust and more appropriate. This includes deriving pass marks by standard setting procedures and blueprinting assessments against curricular outcomes.

* Increased recognition of curricular components relating to ethical and professional behaviour

* Professionalization of teaching and training.

Competency-based training

Although most of these concepts have formed the basis of postgraduate medical education worldwide, assessment of a physician's competency to practise never became universal. A major disadvantage of the residency system was that, in the past, the time required for training in each specialty was arbitrarily chosen, based on the opinions of expert physicians. Little attention was paid to the actual time required to learn a particular procedure or fully understand how to treat a particular condition; consequently, there were no measures of the time needed to acquire the desired competencies. In an attempt to compensate for these shortcomings, fellowships were created and like the regular postgraduate training programmes consisted of arbitrary durations of training, leaving the ultimate decision of competency attainment and professionalism to the judgement of the programme director.

Currently, the situation in PME has changed and many medical institutions have adopted competency-based medical education as an educational process that results in a proven competency in the acquisition and application of specific skills, knowledge, and attitudes. These attributes are required for effective performance in the practice of medicine. It is important to note that the acquisition of these skills and knowledge is not dependent on the length of training or clinical experiences of the trainee. Rather, it requires a definition of what is required by the trainee to practise competently, as well as verification that the trainee can assume complete care of a particular patient. Since the attainment of competency is an individual process and not one that is based on the assumption that all trainees progress at the same speed, it means that some trainees may achieve the desired competencies sooner than would be expected for the required period of training.

Distinguishing competence from competency

In the last decade 'competency' has become a familiar and accepted concept in PME, and therefore it is worthwhile examining its definition and how it is applied in medical education. It is also important to note that there is a difference between 'competence' and 'competency', which could spark off debates, both about how competent an individual is and what their level of competency is in a specific area.

Competence is a generic term referring to a person's overall ability in performing a task. It is what a person needs to know and do in performing a particular job, role or function (Clinton et al. 2005). According to Epstein and Hundert, competence in medicine is 'the habitual and judicious use of communication, knowledge, technical skills, clinical reasoning, emotions, values, and reflection in daily practice for the benefit of the individuals and communities being served'. (Epstein and Hundert 2002) Competence is not considered to be an achievement but rather a habit of lifelong learning (Leach 2002b). It is seen as contextual, reflecting the relationship between a person's abilities and the tasks he or she is required to perform in a particular situation (Leach 2002a; Klass 2000). Common contextual factors include the practice setting, the nature of the patient's presenting symptoms, the patient's educational level, and other demographic characteristics of the patient and of the physician. Many aspects of competence, such as history taking and clinical reasoning, are also content-specific and not necessarily generalizable to all situations. Therefore a trainee's clinical reasoning may appear to be competent in areas in which their base of knowledge is well organized and accessible (Bordage and Zacks 1984) but may appear to be much less competent in unfamiliar territory (Busari and Arnold 2009; Bordage and Zacks 2002). Competence is also developmental. Habits of mind and behaviour and practical wisdom are gained through deliberate practice (Ericsson 2004) and reflection on experience (Epstein 1999, 2003).

Competency, on the other hand, refers to specific capabilities, such as leadership, that an individual demonstrates while performing a task and it involves the collective application of an individual's knowledge, skills and attitudes. Competency is not intended to reduce the value of professional qualifications to a lowest common denominator, but is a way of standardizing how knowledge, skills, and abilities are combined in describing what aspects of performance are (considered) important in particular areas. Despite the differences however, both competence and competency are important when assessing an individual's 'work attributes' as a whole (Worth-Butler et al. 1994).

Developing and implementing PME

There are several reports in the literature that demonstrate a mismatch between the professional competencies of medical doctors and the healthcare priorities that communities define for themselves. Rigid and outdated medical educational programmes have been partly responsible for this, which have led to major changes in the under and postgraduate medical curricula over time. Of particular note is the transition of change through science-based curricula (at the start of the 20th century) to problem-based curricula (at the end of the 20th century), and finally ending as outcome or competency based curricula due to the shift in both medically and non-medically related expectations (Frenk et al. 2010)—see fig. 29.3.

All the changes being highlighted in PME today are expected, on the one hand, to align the tasks of the trained or modern physician with modern clinical practice and the changing health requirements of the community, and on the other, to align with the social and cultural expectations of society at large. It is also the expectation that the modern physician should possess specific competencies that are required to effectively address current healthcare challenges—some of which include the ageing and changing patient population, chronic and emerging infectious diseases, patient empowerment and behaviour, and cultural diversity (Trappenburg 2006). These specific challenges demand a clear definition of the level of professionalism a physician should demonstrate and have led to attempts by several groups to explicitly formulate the principles of professionalism.

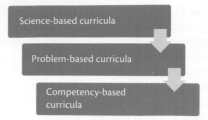

Figure 29.3 Evolving curricula.

The European Federation of Internal Medicine, the American College of Physicians-American Society of Internal Medicine (ACP-ASIM) Foundation, and the American Board of Internal Medicine (ABIM) Foundation have made an effort in this direction by initiating the Medical Professionalism Project that has proposed several fundamental principles (primacy of patients' welfare, patient autonomy, and social justice) and a set of principal professional responsibilities centred on patients' interests (professional competence, honesty, confidentiality, appropriate relationships, quality of care, access to care, fair resource management, scientific pursuit, trust, and confidentiality). Furthermore, commitment to quality improvement, health equity, and cost-effectiveness has also been firmly advocated. It is clear that as a professional the modern medical doctor should constantly address both individual patient and societal needs (Medical Professionalism Project 2002).

There are a few key issues that need to be addressed Some of these issues include the development of reliable assessment tools and the training of faculty to effectively apply them in practice (Nasca and Heard 2010; Ginsburg et al. 2010). While direct observation and formative feedback are essential educational skills that instructors should possess, learners on the other hand. Learners need to master skills such as self-directed assessment and also be the driving force behind their individual learning programmes. Hence, the curriculum, the assessment process and the evaluation system as a whole must be aligned with a certain measure of certainty, to ensure that the acquired knowledge is applied effectively in patient care.

Curriculum

Introducing competency-based medical education in postgraduate medical education requires significant changes at all stages of training. The ultimate goal should be a clear demonstration that the learner is fit to advance in training or to be fully entrusted to practice as an autonomous medical professional (Iobst et al. 2010). As the definition of successful curriculum completion has changed from time spent on rotations to the acquisition of predefined abilities, competency-based medical education primarily focuses on educational outcomes with more liberty being given to the teaching programme and the student's learning approach. In this context, the student is primarily responsible for driving the educational process.

Curriculum development should actively involve faculty because of the strict and specific requirements of the assessment procedures. Furthermore, considering the workplace requirements, the practical implementation of the curriculum in daily clinical practice should be guaranteed. Clearly, medical educational institutions should assure that instructional activities form an integral part of the daily routine of the clinical staff. In addition to the professional and practice requirements, it is important to ensure that the curriculum is aligned with or is within the framework of the legal system of a country.

Finally, there are several educational formats that have been used in designing competency-based curricula (Ringsted et al. 2003; Leung 2002; Scheele et al. 2008). In one case for example, the content of the curriculum was divided into logical units or 'themes'. These themes were defined by tasks or activities that the trainees needed to fulfil (and be assessed on) with the help of specific assessment methods based on CanMEDS roles (Scheele et al. 2008). As a result a more effective planning of corresponding rotations could be established.

Teaching skills

It was almost 50 years ago that Bloom suggested that learning the content of any concept could occur at many levels of expertise—from simple recitation of information that we do not really understand to knowing information so well that we can list it, discuss it, analyse it, use it in a variety of situations and extrapolate it's use to other similar problems (Bloom 1974). Hence, in the clinical learning environment, if we expect our learners to master the clinical material they are being taught and also use the information appropriately in the clinical setting, we need to give them the opportunities to practise and not just expect them to know facts about a topic.

The goal of teaching is to facilitate learning and to ensure that the trainees achieve the desired goal of the educational process. However, when the emphasis of teaching is on the content of the subject and the person teaching it, then the teaching is classified as *teacher-centred* and *content-oriented*. The teacher is the key person in this session and is concerned, primarily, with the transmission of information. When the focus of teaching is not about transmitting information or imparting knowledge, but about facilitating learning, then the teaching is considered to be *student-centred* and *learning-oriented*. The adult learning model actively illustrates the latter approach where the responsibility for learning is placed in the hands of the learners, who are exposed to situations or stimuli that rouse prior knowledge and experiences (David and Patel 1995). This teaching process involves stimulating the learners to learn, through being dealt with respectfully and being acknowledged as adults. The passive role of the teachers in this process also motivates and induces readiness to learn.

The instructional methods that are chosen to achieve learning often depend on who is being taught, for example whether it is the novice learner, such as a third-year medical student or a group of learners with multiple levels of training experience—from preclinical students, to senior residents, and fellows during a grand round. The methods used to create meaningful learning experiences for multilevel learners may differ from those used for a uniform group. For example, the learners in a uniform group are more likely to have similar backgrounds and experiences, as opposed to the mixed group whose participants may range from students with no prior experience to fellows with vast experience—creating a bigger challenge for the instructor.

In addition to possessing the necessary teaching skills, clinical educators should also understand that different instructional methods work better in particular circumstances. Furthermore, with the increasing need for trainees to be taught at sites remote from the main campus, it is important to be aware of educational strategies used for distance learning.

Currently, in PME, many faculty members are not well trained in teaching or assessment skills. There is a need therefore for recurring training programmes where educators can develop their teaching competencies. The ability to perform reliable, reproducible and valid assessments should be ensured by regular and specific staff training as well as by setting up clearly defined performance criteria. These criteria should also take into consideration local situations that include the culture and social context. Several reports have shown the effectiveness of such an approach, with some even recommending making participation in courses on clinical training mandatory for senior doctors (Mortensen et al. 2010). Special attention should be given to circumstances within the curriculum where coaching occurs by colleague trainees (albeit seniors) who are not considered completely competent in supervision.

Finally, when deciding on which instructional method to use in any educational process, it is helpful to define what the specific learning outcomes of the curriculum would be. These specific learning outcomes otherwise called 'intended learning outcomes' form the building blocks of any curriculum, and the choice of the method to be used depends on what we want to teach the learner (content), whom we are teaching (learner), the level of competence prior to the educational encounter (prior or antecedent knowledge), and the level of competence expected to be achieved after the educational encounter (intended learning outcome) (fig. 29.4).

Assessment

Effective assessment is a central requirement in PME. It has several facets that focus on the needs of students, teachers, institutions, patients, and society. Not only is assessment necessary for the trainees who require feedback, it also serves as a performance indicator for teachers and institutions and facilitates the process of complying with the regulations of official accrediting institutions and bodies (Norcini et al. 2011).

Assessment (according to Miller's pyramid) should be of a direct nature in order to ensure a clear demonstration of the acquired level of professional development. The process of assessment itself should involve clearly predefined levels of competence that facilitate the advancement of the trainee through the sequential phases of the training programme. The training programmes, as a result, require some degree of flexibility, as not all learners advance at the same rate (ten Cate and Scheele 2007). The challenge in setting up

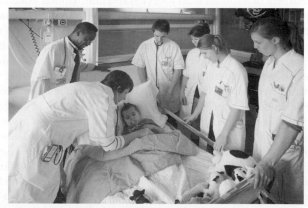

Figure 29.4 Postgraduate medical education in action.

such programmes is in how to develop a multidimensional curriculum that satisfies all the requirements and definitions and that clearly captures and facilitates the interaction between the teacher and learner.

Part of the assessment procedure should include self-assessments by the trainee. This has been described as 'the process of interpreting data about one's own performance and comparing them to an explicit or implicit standard' (Epstein and Hundert 2002) and should also be clearly formulated in relation to the competency requirements. As self-assessment by trainees can be inaccurate it should be complemented by performance criteria and/or multisource feedback (Regehr and Eva 2006; Davis et al. 2006). It should also be supported with feedback from external sources, including that of faculty (Wall et al. 2012). A safe learning environment is a prerequisite for fostering trainee self-activity (Bellande et al. 2010).

Over time a vast collection of assessment tools (related to varying medical competency areas), educational approaches, and technological innovations have had an impact on postgraduate assessment. However, it has become evident that specific criteria should also be defined to guarantee effective educational approaches, assessment methods, and assessment tool selection. In order to effectively introduce assessment into PME, issues like feasibility (e.g. finding time in busy clinical schedules to perform a sufficient number of assessments and feedback sessions) and the fidelity of assessment scores should be carefully evaluated. Special attention should be given to the 'newer' competencies, which reflect the changes in societal expectations of the medical doctor's role and focus on patient centeredness and professional attitude, responsibilities and ethics. Recently, consensus criteria for a framework of good assessment have been developed and address the issues of validity or coherence, reproducibility or consistency, equivalence, feasibility, educational effect, catalytic effect and acceptability for both individual and system assessment (Norcini et al. 2011). It should be mentioned though, that further research is still needed to define effective assessment criteria for the professional competencies.

Special attention should be given to the tools used for assessment purposes. In designing the tools one should strive to have learners demonstrate the level of competence as concretely as possible. Although considerable effort has been put into the design and development of existing tools so as to prevent assessor subjectivity in trainee assessment (examples of such tools include in-training evaluation reports (ITERs), clinical exams, objective structured assessment of technical skills (OSATS) and mini-clinical evaluation exercise (CEX)), they all still require significant assessor judgement (Chaudhry et al. 2008). Although there is ongoing debate on the required psychometric characteristics of the available tools, it is clear that faculty should receive appropriate training in the effective use and interpretation of these tools (Ginsburg et al. 2010).

A relatively new and important tool in competency assessment is the portfolio (Friedman Ben David et al. 2001). Portfolios, in which learning evidence is collected, have been introduced to promote trainee responsibility and stimulate self-assessment. Evidence of learning would mainly consist of the results from trainee assessment programmes and details on acquired knowledge and skills. Trainee and responsible staff can then review and comment on the portfolio. At the end of the review a personal development plan for the ensuing training period can be formulated.

The daily constraints on educational activities resulting from the clinical responsibilities of individual supervisors on the wards should also be addressed, and effective programmes dealing with these constraints supported. Some groups have proposed that general competencies be further defined with specific activity observations (like entrustable professional activities (EPAs)) bridging the observed tension between theory and practice and making the general competencies in the daily working environment more concrete for assessment by the supervisors (ten Cate and Scheele 2007). In essence, specific educational goals within a discipline or part of a defined rotation need to be identified and a minimum set of specific observations or EPAs selected to assess the trainees' competencies in specific areas—graded by importance, characteristics and risks of the tasks for daily practice (Scheele et al., 2008). Furthermore, attention should be given to the assessment of 'newer' roles such as manager, health advocate and collaborator.

In general, the assessment procedure should lead to both global and specific outcomes. Global outcomes relate to the progress of the trainee regarding the curriculum-defined competencies; the specific outcomes concentrate on the medical specialty requirements in patient care. Therefore a comprehensive system for collating evidence of the trainee's personal development (e.g. using a portfolio) would facilitate the assessment process by faculty and also help in the joint development of a tailor-made personal development plan.

Lastly, the final assessment of trainees should address their readiness to bear full professional responsibility in patient care and should preferably take place by direct observation during the delivery of care.

Feedback

In competency-based residency training the learning path is nonhierarchical and should take place in a safe environment where supervisors and trainees can easily interact. The trainee is actively involved in the development of their individual training plans, which should include frequent and accurate tutor feedback sessions and the supervisors should be available to facilitate this process where and when necessary. Competency-based PME requires feedback to be formative (in contrast to the more summative approach of traditional postgraduate medical education). Furthermore it is well accepted that frequent and direct observation of the trainee by the tutor ensures accuracy of feedback. Technical developments have added some flexibility to this requirement and make time-delayed direct observation possible (Klein et al. 2012).

Accreditation

Accreditation is a critical element for ensuring quality and accountability in PME. Interestingly, however, until recently there have been few published studies of its effectiveness (Norcini and van Zanten 2010). A good process requires that the quality of PME programmes be evaluated regularly, using reliable external accreditation criteria. This process of continuous evaluation and improvement also demands that relevant authorities ensure that the competencies that trainees are expected to achieve are relevant to the individual and collective healthcare requirements of patients and the community (WFME 2003). Furthermore, evaluating social accountability and increasing public participation in the accreditation process should help to align professional outcomes with societal needs. According to the World Health Organization, social accountability of medical training refers to 'the obligation of the programme to direct its educative, research and service activities towards addressing priority health concerns of the community, region and/or nation for which they have a mandate to serve' (Fleet et al. 2008). Of note and probably unknown to many, the Flexner report in 1910, already emphasized such a contract between the physician and his community and the importance of this commitment to society.

Accreditation processes should ideally take local issues into account and not focus only on administrative compliance. They should strive to foster continuous quality improvement—rigid, episodic, and prescriptive standards can paradoxically impede innovative, effective, and efficient programme development (Norcini and Banda 2011).

Challenges

When implementing modern curricula the training of faculty is a major endeavour. It is of the utmost importance that the proposed curriculum and stated values are in accordance with the working and learning environment (also described as 'the hidden curriculum') in order to achieve the proposed goals (Hafferty 1998, Lempp and Seale 2004). In a recent seminal study that involved different stakeholders in medical education, four main areas were identified as defining the process of implementation of new, competency based, PME programmes (Wallenburg et al. 2010). These perspectives were described as accountability, educational, work–life balance, and trust-based. The accountability perspective focuses on the transparency and accountability of modern programmes and relies on formal regulation of training and monitoring. The educational perspective stresses the formalization of the educational process and more than the other perspectives, stresses residents' responsibilities for their own learning. Interestingly the work–life balance perspective gave primary attention to the life–work balance of the professional. As expected the nowadays prominent part-time work issue was given great importance within this perspective. Finally, the trust-based perspective relates to the classic view of medical training based on role models and trust.

A clear understanding of the existing perspectives of the available faculty and other stakeholders would greatly facilitate the design of an effective faculty-training programme. One should also realize that the type of training hospital (academic or regional) also influences faculty and the educational environment—with varying prioritization of medical training and daily patient care (Wallenburg et al. 2010). All in all, deep insight is necessary for effective change management strategies in order to effectively implement competency-based training programmes.

It is still not clear, from a departmental and individual physician's point of view, how (and if) PME can influence the educational culture sufficiently to effectively ensure daily practice-related teaching and learning. As shown by a recent report on the Danish reform of PME, only a limited effect could be observed over a three and a half year period in the daily clinical training practice and educational culture (Mortensen et al. 2010). In particular, small effects were observed on structural educational issues such as course attendances and preparation of individual learning plans. Further studies are therefore needed to design effective ways of improving the educational environment for postgraduate medical education.

Assessment tools like the Postgraduate Educational Environment Measure (PHEEM) and the Dutch Residency Educational Climate Test (D-RECT) could be used for validating the educational climate and/or environment (Wall et al. 2009; Boor et al. 2011). Accreditation bodies should also emphasize the importance of educational courses and clinical training and value them equally with other academic courses or programmes as this would influence the educational environment positively.

Quality assurance remains of the utmost importance in postgraduate medical education and the use of recognized international quality assurance systems is strongly advocated to achieve this— e.g. WFME standards (WFME, 2003). This would facilitate regular and standard national and international evaluations, comparisons, and benchmarking (Soemantri et al. 2010).

One of the real challenges facing competency-based PME is the consolidation of the shift from the traditional, time specific, modular rotations to a more flexible, competency-driven training with the opportunity for early or delayed completion of the trainee's programme, which in turn is dependent on individual progress in the various competency domains. Regarding professionalism and the medical educational continuum, PME should prepare the trainee for lifelong learning through CPD programmes. Exploiting the possibilities of novel learning techniques provided by technological advances such as virtual simulators and e-learning can provide additional flexibility and offer new educational opportunities for both faculty and trainees.

Finally, ongoing evaluation and research in medical education will continue to provide essential information on proposed PME programmes and the adequacy and applicability of programme-defined competencies. The Best Evidence Medical Education (BEME) initiative (Issenberg et al. 2005) is a valuable development in this area. Of interest also is the effectiveness of the different tools used to measure trainee competency—this is currently being addressed in the United States by the Milestones Project (Nasca and Heard 2010).

Conclusions

- The modern day physician should be able to competently address patient and public health requirements as well as manage care in line with the changing expectations of the society at large.

- Effective postgraduate medical education requires the use of competency-based training methods and reliable and valid assessment strategies.

- Safe learning environments are a prerequisite for modern postgraduate medical training.

- Faculty and clinical staff should be well trained and have their proficiency in teaching and designing educational outcomes evaluated regularly.

- Clinical teachers should be actively involved in curriculum development in order to safeguard practical implementation in the clinical workplace.

References

Barzansky, B. (1992) *Abraham Flexner: Lessons from the past with applications for the future*. New York, Westport, CT: Greenwood Press

Beck, A.H. (2004) STUDENTJAMA. The Flexner report and the standardization of American medical education. *JAMA*. 291: 2139–2140

Bellande, B.J., Winicur, Z.M.,, and Cox, K.M. (2010) Commentary: Urgently needed: a safe place for self-assessment on the path to maintaining competence and improving performance. *Acad Med.* 85: 16–18

Bleakely, A., Bligh, J., and Browne, J. (2011) *Medical Education for the Future: Identity, power and location.* Dordrecht: Springer

Bloom, B.S.E. (1974) *Taxonomy of educational objectives : The classification of educational goals handbook 1: Cognitive domain* New York: Longman

Bonner, T. (2002) *Iconoclast: Abraham Flexner and a Life in Learning.* Baltimore, MD: Johns Hopkins University Press

Boor, K., van der Vleuten, C., Teunissen, P., Scherpbier, A., and Scheele, F. (2011) Development and analysis of D-RECT, an instrument measuring residents' learning climate. *Med Teach.* 33: 820–827

Bordage, G. and Zacks, R. 1984. The structure of medical knowledge in the memories of medical students and general practitioners: categories and prototypes. *Med Educ.* 18: 406–416

Bordage, G. and Zacks, R. (2002) *Clinical Reasoning.* Dordrecht, the Netherlands: Kluwer Academic

Bullock, A.D., Burke, S.E., and Wall, D. (2004) Higher Specialist Training: a study of curriculum and assessment within four specialties. *Med Teach.* 26(2): 174–177

Busari, J.O., and Arnold, A. (2009) Educating doctors in the clinical workplace: unraveling the process of teaching and learning in the medical resident as teacher. *J Postgrad Med.* 55: 278–283

Callaghan, K., Hunt, G., and Windsor, J. (2007) Issues in implementing a real competency-based training and assessment system. *N Z Med J.* 120: U2510

Chaudhry, S.I., Holmboe, E., and Beasley, B.W. (2008) The state of evaluation in internal medicine residency. *J Gen Intern Med.* 23: 1010–1015

Clinton, M., Murrells, T., and Robinson, S. (2005) Assessing competency in nursing: a comparison of nurses prepared through degree and diploma programmes. *J Clin Nurs.* 14: 82–94

Cooke, M., Irby, D.M., and O'Brien, B.C. (2010) *Educating Physicians : a call for reform of medical school and residency.* San Francisco, CA: Jossey-Bass; Chichester: John Wiley & Sons Ltd[distributor]

CPMEC (2006) *Australian Curriculum Framework for Junior Doctors* [Online]. http://curriculum.cpmec.org.au/index.cfm Accessed 5 March 2013

David, T.J. and Patel, L. (1995) Adult learning theory, problem based learning, and paediatrics. *Arch Dis Child.* 73: 357–363

Davis, D.A., Mazmanian, P.E., Fordis, M., Van Harrison, R., Thorpe, K.E., and Perrier, L. (2006) Accuracy of physician self-assessment compared with observed measures of competence: a systematic review. *JAMA.* 296: 1094–1102

Department of Health (2001) *Working together – learning together. A framework for lifelong learning for the NHS.* London: DOH

Epstein, R. (2003) Mindful practice in action (I): Technical competence, evidence-based medicine, and relationship-centered care. *Families. Systems.. and Health.* 21: 1–9

Epstein, R.M. (1999) Mindful practice. *JAMA.* 282: 833–839

Epstein, R.M. and Hundert, E.M. (2002) Defining and assessing professional competence. *JAMA.* 287: 226–235

Ericsson, K. (2004) Deliberate practice and the acquisition and maintenance of expert performance in medicine and related domains. *Acad Med.* 79: S70–S81

Fleet, L.J., Kirby, F., Cutler, S., Dunikowski, L., Nasmith, L., and Shaughnessy, R. (2008) Continuing professional development and social accountability: a review of the literature. *J Interprof Care.* 22(Suppl 1): 15–29

Flexner, A. (1910) Medical Education in the United States and Canada: A report to the Carnegie Foundation for The Advancement of Teaching. *Carnegie Foundation Bulletin.* New York: Carnegie Foundation

Frank, J.R. (ed.) (2005) The CanMEDS 2005 physician competency framework. Better standards. Better physicians. Better care. Ottawa: The Royal College of Physicians and Surgeons of Canada [Online] http://www.royalcollege.ca/portal/page/portal/rc/common/documents/canmeds/resources/publications/framework_full_e.pdf Accessed 6 March 2013

Frenk, J., Chen, L., Bhutta, Z.A., et al. (2010) Health professionals for a new century: transforming education to strengthen health systems in an interdependent world. *Lancet.* 376: 1923–1958

Friedman Ben David, M., Davis, M.H., Harden, R.M., Howie, P.W., Ker, J., and Pippard, M.J. (2001) AMEE Medical Education Guide No. 24: Portfolios as a method of student assessment. *Med Teach.* 23: 535–551

Ginsburg, S., McIlroy, J., Oulanova, O., Eva, K., and Regehr, G. (2010) Toward authentic clinical evaluation: pitfalls in the pursuit of competency. *Acad Med.* 85: 780–786

GMC (1998) *Maintaining Good Medical Practice.* London: General Medical Council

GMC (2009) *Tomorrow's Doctors: Outcomes and standards for undergraduate medical education.* London: General Medical Council

Golub RM. (2010) Are you sure this is right? Insights into the ways trainees act, feel, and reason. *JAMA.* 304(11): 1236–1238

Hafferty, F.W. (1998) Beyond curriculum reform: confronting medicine's hidden curriculum. *Acad Med.* 73: 403–407

Hodges, B. (2006) Medical education and the maintenance of incompetence. *Med Teach.* 28: 690–696

Iobst, W.F., Sherbino, J., Cate, O.T., et al. (2010) Competency-based medical education in postgraduate medical education. *Med Teach.* 32: 651–656

Issenberg, S.B., McGaghie, W.C., Petrusa, E.R., Lee Gordon, D., and Scalese, R.J. (2005) Features and uses of high-fidelity medical simulations that lead to effective learning: a BEME systematic review. *Med Teach.* 27: 10–28

Johnston, G.A., Jr (1984) The Flexner Report and black medical schools. *J Natl Med Assoc.* 76: 223–225

Klass, D. (2000) Reevaluation of clinical competency. *Am J Phys Med Rehabil.* 79: 481–486

Klein, D., Staples, J., Pittman, C., and Stepanko, C. (2012) Using electronic clinical practice audits as needs assessment to produce effective continuing medical education programming. *Med Teach.* 34: 151–154

Leach, D.C. (2002a) Building and assessing competence: the potential for evidence-based graduate medical education. *Qual Manag Health Care.* 11: 39–44

Leach, D.C. (2002b) Competence is a habit. *JAMA.* 287: 243–244

Lempp, H., and Seale, C. 2004. The hidden curriculum in undergraduate medical education: qualitative study of medical students' perceptions of teaching. *BMJ.* 329: 770–773

Leung, W.C. (2002) Competency based medical training: review. *BMJ.* 325: 693–696

Medical Professionalism Project (2002) Medical professionalism in the new millennium: a physicians' charter. *Lancet.* 359: 520–529

Mortensen, L., Malling, B., Ringsted, C., and Rubak, S. (2010) What is the impact of a national postgraduate medical specialist education reform on the daily clinical training 3.5 years after implementation? A questionnaire survey. *BMC Med Educ.* 10: 46

Nasca, T.J., and Heard, J.K. (2010) Commentary: trust, accountability, and other common denominators in modernizing medical training. *Acad Med.* 85: 932–934

Norcini, J., Anderson, B., Bollela, V., et al. (2011) Criteria for good assessment: consensus statement and recommendations from the Ottawa 2010 Conference. *Med Teach.* 33: 206–214

Norcini, J.J., and Banda, S.S. 2011. Increasing the quality and capacity of education: the challenge for the 21st century. *Med Educ.* 45: 81–86

Norcini, J., and Van Zanten, M. (2010) An overview of accreditation. certification. and licensure processes. In P. Peterson and E. Barry McGaw (eds) *International Encyclopedia of Education.* 3rd edn. Oxford: Elsevier

Porter, M.E. (2010) What is value in health care? *N Engl J Med.* 363: 2477–2481

.Reenen Van, R., Rooyen Den, C., and Schelfhout-Van Deventer, V. (2009) *Modernisering medische vervolgopleidingen: nieuw kaderbesluit CCMS* [Online]. Koninklijke Nederlandsche Maatschappij tot bevordering der Geneeskunst. http://knmg.artsennet.nl/artikel/Modernisering-medische-vervolgopleidingen-nieuw-kaderbesluit-CCMS.htm Accessed 5 March 2013

Regehr, G., and Eva, K. (2006) Self-assessment, self-direction, and the self-regulating professional. *Clin Orthop Relat Res.* 449: 34–38

Ringsted, C., Ostergaard, D., and Scherpbier, A. (2003) Embracing the new paradigm of assessment in residency training: an assessment programme for first-year residency training in anaesthesiology. *Med Teach.* 25: 54–62

Scheele, F., Teunissen, P., Van Luijk, S., et al. (2008) Introducing competency-based postgraduate medical education in the Netherlands. *Med Teach.* 30: 248–253

SDMCG (2000) Learning Outcomes for the Medical Undergraduate in Scotland: A foundation for competent and reflective practitioners. In: The Scottish Deans' Medical Curriculum Group (ed.) [Online] http://www.scottishdoctor.org/node.asp?id=phase1 Accessed 6 March 2013

Soemantri, D., Herrera, C., and Riquelme, A. (2010) Measuring the educational environment in health professions studies: a systematic review. *Med Teach.* 32: 947–952

Sottas, B. (2011) Learning outcomes for health professions: the concept of the Swiss competencies framework. *GMS Z Med Ausbild.* 28: Doc11

ten Cate, O. and Scheele, F. (2007) Competency-based postgraduate training: can we bridge the gap between theory and clinical practice? *Acad Med.* 82: 542–547

Trappenburg, M. (2006) Societal neurosis in health care. In J.W.K.T Duyvendak and M. Kremer (eds) *Policy. People and the New Professional: De-Professionalisation and Re- Professionalisation in Care and Welfare.* Amsterdam, the Netherlands: Amsterdam University Press

Wall, D., Clapham, M., Riquelme, A., et al. (2009) Is PHEEM a multi-dimensional instrument? An international perspective. *Med Teach.* 31: e521–e527

Wall, D., Singh, D., Whitehouse, A., Hassell, A., and Howes, J. (2012) Self-assessment by trainees using self-TAB as part of the team assessment of behaviour multisource feedback tool. *Med Teach.* 34: 165–167

Wallenburg, I., Van Exel, J., Stolk, E., Scheele, F., De Bont, A., and Meurs, P. (2010) Between trust and accountability: different perspectives on the modernization of postgraduate medical training in the Netherlands. *Acad Med.* 85: 1082–1090

WFME (2003) Postgraduate medical education. *World Federation for Medical Education. Global standards for Quality Improvement.* Copenhagen: World Federation of Medical Education

Worth-Butler, M.M., Murphy, R.J.L., and Fraser, D.M. (1994) Towards an integrated model of competence in midwifery. *Midwifery.* 10: 225–231

CHAPTER 30

Continuing professional development

Karen V. Mann and Joan M. Sargeant

The education of the doctor which goes on after he has his degree is,after all, the most important part of his education.

Reproduced from Boston Medical and Surgical Journal, 131:140, 1894

Introduction

The term continuous professional development (CPD) came to the fore in the United Kingdom in 1993 (Karle et al. 2011). CPD refers to an array of educational activities that health professionals undertake to maintain, develop, and enhance the knowledge, skills, professional performance, and relationships they use to provide care for patients and the public (Davis et al. 2003; 2009; Institute of Medicine 2010). CPD evolved from the more narrowly focused and traditional concept of didactic continuing medical education (CME); it addresses not only the clinical domain, but also additional professional practice competencies (e.g. communication, collaboration, and professional) and it emphasizes self-directed lifelong learning and learning from practice) (Stanton 1997). The overarching goal remains to enhance patient care and improve health outcomes. In this chapter, we will use the term CPD (which usually incorporates CME activities). However, where the traditional term CME is more appropriate, we will also include that.

Although traditionally less visible than undergraduate and postgraduate education, CPD has emerged as the longest, and arguably most important part of the educational continuum. Societal expectations, commitment to patient safety, and the rapid pace and breadth of growth of knowledge have made the need to maintain and enhance competence clear and non-negotiable. Today's CPD is characterized by a broad array of learning opportunities, a combination of self- and other directed learning, and varied educational formats, both synchronous and asynchronous. CPD is now understood as development extending beyond medical knowledge into all aspects of the professional role. Adult development continues throughout the life span and occurs not just in conferences and classrooms, but in workplaces, and in the course of practice. Rather than learning *to* practise, we increasingly understand that learning *in* practice is fundamental (Sfard 1999). Moreover, CPD is shifting from a focus solely on learning to focus on practice change and improvement, and integration with initiatives in quality improvement and knowledge translation. Lastly, a rich research enterprise has developed to answer important questions about how to enhance learning that will support physicians across their professional lifetimes and how to determine the impact of this learning.

Overview

Our purpose in this chapter is to lay out the theoretical foundations of CPD, to describe traditional and emerging modes of CPD, the evidence-base for its value, and recent influences upon the field. In doing so, we hope to convey the significant shifts occurring in the field, transforming both content and educational approaches. We will begin with an overview of the development of our understanding of CPD, followed by briefly presenting theories and frameworks which have informed that understanding. In keeping with the shift from interest in how physicians learn to how that learning is transferred to practice, we will present selected approaches to understanding how this translation can be facilitated. We will describe the relationships that are developing between knowledge translation, quality improvement (QI) and CPD. We will present information about the evidence for CPD and the various teaching and learning approaches which are available to practitioners. We will also explore external influences and the regulation of CPD as it is developing internationally, and the skills required of physicians in the maintenance of competence.

Theoretical foundations

The goal of effective learning in CPD is that physicians are able to incorporate new learning appropriately into practice and, through that change, contribute to improved health outcomes. The challenge for CPD educators then, is to understand how physicians learn and to develop educational interventions and programmes that will support effective learning.

Ways of understanding learning in medicine have been strongly rooted in the positivist tradition of the profession. They also reflect the profession's values of autonomy and individuality in their emphasis on the individual learner. It is unsurprising then, that for several decades after formal CME began, it relied heavily on transmission of new knowledge, to be added to each individual's existing knowledge, therefore bringing them 'up to date'. This model assumed that having knowledge was necessary, but was also sufficient to enable physicians to change their behaviour in ways that would improve their practice and the outcomes for their patients.

A sentinel event in understanding how physicians learn occurred in response to the question posed to North American continuing education leaders of the early 1980s. It was a simple question: 'Does CME work?' but it reflected an awareness that some physicians were not keeping up and that their practice was inadequate.

The result of this challenge was the study of 'change and learning in the lives of physicians' (Fox et al. 1989), which involved interviews with 356 physicians, in which they reflected on a recent learning experience, and on how they had learned. Almost 800 individual incidents of learning were gathered, which were synthesized into a model of learning and change. This model stimulated a major shift in understanding physicians' learning, and how CME could support and enhance the effectiveness of their learning, and their ability to make changes in their practice.

Several 'change study' findings contribute to our understanding of physician learning today. The study identified different forces for change—professional, personal, and social. Professional forces were the most likely to lead to change, and included a desire for enhanced competence, or changes in the clinical environment. Personal forces, such as the desire for wellbeing were also important, as were social factors, such as relationships with colleagues. Changes varied in magnitude and difficulty, ranging from small changes, often in response to regulation, to more major, even transformative changes. The model also described the ways in which physicians identified the need for learning and the gap between their current and desired performance. Lastly, three stages in making change emerged: preparing for the change, making the change, and sustaining the change (fig. 30.1). The study and the model it generated provided a way of understanding learning that extended beyond acquiring knowledge and highlighted the complexity of incorporating new learning effectively.

Several other approaches to learning have guided the development of CPD interventions. These are summarized in the following sections.

Adult learning theory and principles

Adult learning theory, or andragogy (Knowles 1980), is underpinned by three main assumptions:

1. Adult learners bring considerable experience to their learning

2. They are more commonly motivated by internal desires and goals than by external goals and rewards, and

3. They are motivated to learn about practical matters that relate to their roles and goals in everyday life.

Although adult learning theory has been criticized (Norman 1999), it brings together several pedagogical approaches which are viewed as important in CPD (Mann et al. 2011). These include: self-direction and lifelong learning; reflection and reflective practice;

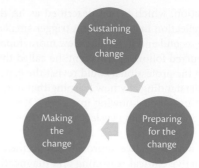

Figure 30.1 Stages in making change.

experiential learning; and enquiry-based learning. Adult learning principles can provide an important context for the development of educational interventions (Hean et al. 2009).

Self-directed and lifelong learning

The importance of physicians being self-directed, ongoing learners has increased, particularly in the context of incremental rates of growth of knowledge and information, and inevitable changes and improvements in practice. Although they do not completely overlap, embedded in these two approaches to learning is the shared goal that professionals will be able to determine their own learning needs, gather resources to meet them, undertake the new learning, and evaluate their own effectiveness as learners. A parallel goal underlying this approach is that learners will be self-directed, in that they will be motivated to determine needs, and continue their development, through their professional life.

Learners in CPD may be self-directed in the educational courses and resources they choose, and in their individual learning in the course of their work. Self-direction and self-regulation are fundamental components of societal expectations of professionals. Almost universally, medical education earlier in the continuum of education has statements of the importance of self-direction and self-regulation and the goal of producing graduating physicians who are self-directed and capable of self-regulation (Candy 1991).

Reflective practice and learning from experience

The importance of learning from experience has long been acknowledged and that assumption underlies a pervasive means of learning in medical education at all levels, dating back to Flexner's recommendations (Flexner 1910). Kolb (1984) identified learning from experience as a cycle, involving concrete experience, and its transformation by the learner through reflection, abstract conceptualization, and opportunities for applying learning in practice.

Our current ideas of learning from experience are informed significantly by the work of Schön (1987). Based on studies of professionals and how they learned in the course of their work, he developed the idea of the reflective practitioner, who learned through engagement in two types of reflection. Schön's model included a cycle, beginning with knowledge that individuals acquire through formal and informal learning, called 'knowing-in-action'. This knowledge is available to the practitioner as they encounter the usual challenges of practice. However, sometimes a surprise occurs, prompting two kinds of reflective thinking. The first is 'reflection in action', which Schön described as 'in the moment' thinking. This reflection in action might trigger small adjustments at the time. The second and in Schön's view more important reflective activity occurred following the event; he called this 'reflection on action', when the professional could revisit the experience, with the goals of understanding any new learning that might result and incorporating it into their knowing in action. Other models proposed similar iterative learning cycles, notably those of Boud et al. (1985).

For some, a more reflective approach has seemed contrary to the logico-deductive clinical reasoning and diagnostic models in medicine, and has not fitted comfortably into more scientific ways of knowing. However, interest in reflection and reflective practice has been renewed as its role in learning has been examined (Mann et al. 2009), and evidence of its contributions to competent practice accumulates. Reflective approaches have been shown to reduce diagnostic error in complex cases (Mamede and Schmidt 2008), to be integral to clinical reasoning and expertise development, to allow for integration of new knowledge, and to promote understanding of one's practice in a broader context. Lastly, reflection has emerged as a critical component of self-regulation, particularly facilitating the acceptance and use of feedback (Sargeant et al. 2008, 2009). Evidence of its greater acceptance is seen across the medical education continuum, in goal statements, in the introduction and use of portfolios for learning and assessment. In CPD, most notable is the requirement for a demonstration of reflective activity to achieve accreditation of an activity, for both provider and attendee (Royal College of Physician and Surgeons of Canada 2012; College of Family Physicians of Canada 2012).

Learning in practice and work-based learning

Recently, attention has focused increasingly on the learning that occurs through participating in the activities of professional practice. Work-based learning and work-based assessment are being explored at all levels (Norcini and Burch 2007). Their importance at the CPD level is tied both to an emerging understanding of the learning that occurs in the course of work, and the increasing professional oversight and regulation that accompanies the emphasis on maintenance of competence.

The works of Eraut (2000, 2007) and Billett (2001, 2004) have informed our understanding of how learning occurs at work. Both propose that learning occurs from and in interaction with others, and is tied closely to the specific culture and context which exists in the workplace.

Self-regulation, self-awareness, and self-assessment

Self-regulation is fundamental to both societal and professional expectations of physicians. Self-regulation is of interest at the level of the profession; however, in terms of its relevance to learning, most work has been conducted at the individual level. Initiatives in continuous improvement, maintenance of competence, lifelong learning, and work-based learning share reliance on professionals' self-assessment capability. The literature has demonstrated consistently that individuals are poor at assessing their own performance accurately (Eva and Regehr 2005).Considerable work has been undertaken to understand the complex ways in which people make self-assessments, and to enhance the effectiveness of that activity (Sargeant et al. 2010). Despite its inaccuracy, individuals' self-assessment of their performance exerts a powerful influence on the learning they undertake, the feedback they seek, and their acceptance and use of that feedback. For CPD providers, the importance of enhancing self-assessment is central to the goal of ongoing development of maintenance of competence.

Learning in communities of practice: a sociocultural view

Learning in medical education, and particularly in CPD, has concentrated on the individual learner. When doctors did almost all of their learning individually, this was appropriate; however, large numbers of physicians now choose to learn in groups, as a means of maintaining currency and improving practice. This method of learning evolved from the model of problem-based learning (Premi et al. 1994) and was based on similar educational principles of motivation to learn, of sharing experience and knowledge in the group, and of building understanding and knowledge collaboratively. More recently, sociocultural theories have provided important insights into medical education. These theories approach learning as resulting from participation in a community of practice: learners begin at the periphery of a community of practice and gradually becoming more central members of the community as they gain knowledge and assume responsibility (Lave and Wenger 1991; Wenger 1998). In this view of learning, knowledge is developed collaboratively and shared and distributed across the community. Physicians who are learning in communities of practice are able to share, appraise, and build knowledge together.

Complexity theory

Theories to support learning in CPD have also recognized the environment in which learning occurs. Complexity and systems theories arise from social psychology (Ross et al. 1991); they view the individual, social system and environment as interacting dynamically. In contrast, today's healthcare systems are based solidly upon a traditional scientific foundation. Physicians and health professionals traditionally 'deliver' care to patients who in turn respond to the care (Sweeney 2002). Such a perspective has also shaped medical education: educators 'deliver' programmes to learners with the intent that the learners respond by using their new learning to improve. Linear models overlook the interaction of individual elements and the importance of values and personal and social influences.

Healthcare and education no longer fit such a linear model and complexity theory provides a useful lens for understanding them. The main tenets include:

1. Complex systems consist of multiple components and are understood by observing the interaction of the components.

2. Interaction among components can produce unpredictable behavior.

3. Complex systems interact with and are influenced by the environment.

4. Interactions between components of the system are non-linear.

Grasping such concepts helps us to understand the dynamic nature of medical education and the healthcare system in which it occurs, and the influence of the external system and environment upon learning and change.

Theories informing practice change

Changing behaviour is a complex undertaking. It requires attention to the cognitive, affective, or emotional aspects and to the practical aspects of learning and change. We now turn to approaches which have developed to enhance the likelihood of change.

Davies, Walker, and Grimshaw (2010) conducted a systematic review of the use of theory in the design of guideline dissemination strategies and interpretations of the results of rigorous evaluations. The authors found that theory use was poorly justified in the design of interventions and urged that theory be more explicitly used to understand barriers to change, design effective interventions, and explore mediating and moderating variables and influences.

Three such approaches are presented:

* The PRECEDE model (Green and Kreuter 1991)
* The Stages of Change Theory (Prochaska and DiClemente 1983)
* The Theory of Planned Behaviour (Ajzen 1991).

The PRECEDE Model: Predisposing, Reinforcing and Enabling Causes in Educational Diagnosis and Evaluation

This model (Green and Kreuter 1991) was developed originally in the field of health education, to provide a means of systematically planning, implementing and understanding factors that influence the effect of health education programmes, particularly upon behavioural change.

Three groups of factors influencing change are described. Predisposing factors provide the foundation and motivation for change; they include knowledge, attitudes, and beliefs. Enabling factors promote conditions for making change, for example, relevant skills, access, and availability of resources and support. Reinforcing factors provide a continuing incentive to sustain a change; for example, reminders, refresher sessions, and positive responses from others, especially peers. The PRECEDE model has been found to be effective in guiding and assessing the effects of CME interventions and of health-behaviour related interventions in a variety of fields.

Stages of Change Theory

Stages of Change Theory views behaviour change as a dynamic process, rather than a single event. The Transtheoretical model proposed by Prochaska and DiClemente (1983), and often referred to as the 'readiness to change' model, is a well-known example. Originally developed in relation to addictive behaviour, this model identifies five stages as a person successfully changes behaviour. These are precontemplation, contemplation, preparation, action, and maintenance. The 'readiness to change' model is the foundation for motivational interviewing, which health professionals may employ to help patients change unhealthy lifestyles. Arguably, practice behaviours are also deeply embedded and resistant to change, and so the model has been applied to physicians as well.

A key aspect of the model is that individuals at different stages of change may require different approaches. In the precontemplation and contemplation stages just providing information may be useful; however, in the preparation and action stages, skills training and advice or support to deal with barriers may be required. Once a new behaviour is in place, the maintenance stage can be helped by environments that provide support and reinforce behaviour.

Theory of planned behaviour

The theory of planned behaviour (Ajzen 1991; Ramsay et al. 2010) has been widely used to predict individual behaviours. It has been one of the most used theories to understand the determinants of professional behaviour. In this theory an individual's intention to perform a behaviour is the proximal predictor of behaviour. Three factors influence intention: attitude (a person's overall evaluation of the behaviour), subjective norm (a person's own estimate of the social pressure to perform or not perform the target behaviour), and perceived behavioural control (the extent to which a person feels able to enact the behaviour). There are two aspects to perceived control: the first is how much control over the behaviour a person has; the second is how confident they feel about being able to perform the behaviour. Perceived behavioural control also has a direct effect on behaviour. Grimshaw and colleagues (2011) have used this model extensively to explore specific practice behaviours.

Domains influencing behaviour change

From multiple theories and frameworks of both individual and organizational behaviour change, British psychologists have used a rigorous process to identify and clarify 12 domains influencing behaviour and behavioural change, and the constructs within each domain (Michie et al. 2005). The domains include: knowledge; skills; social or professional role and identity; beliefs about capabilities; beliefs about consequences; motivation and goals; memory, attention, and decision processes; environmental context and resources; social influences; emotion; behavioural regulation; and nature of the behaviours. It is notable that only two of these domains, knowledge and skills, are those addressed by traditional continuing education programmes. Recognizing that the other ten domains that influence change are outside the realm of traditional education helps to explain why education alone so often does not result in performance change and improvement.

Implications for CPD professionals

Despite Lewin's oft quoted maxim that 'there is nothing so practical as a good theory' (Lewin 1951), it is generally difficult to transform theory directly into practice. In education the task is further complicated by the many conceptions of learning that exist, and the endless variety of changes they hope to predict and explain. There are, however, important principles that can be taken from them to guide our practice. These are summarized in table 30.1).

CPD design, implementation, and evaluation

From a consideration of how and why physicians learn and change, we now turn to design and implementation of CPD.

Traditionally, CPD has been designed and implemented using curriculum design models derived from general education theory and practice. Kern et al.'s (1998) model has six steps: identify a problem; conduct a needs assessment; set goals and objectives based on identified needs; select educational strategies to meet the goals; implement and evaluate; and give feedback to inform the programme. We will describe each step briefly (Davis et al. 2003).

Identifying a problem refers to the clinical issue or health problem to be addressed; for example, obesity in children. A needs assessment is conducted to determine the specific features of the problem for the target audience (e.g. family physicians, specialists, healthcare teams) in a particular setting. Needs assessments can be considered as subjective (e.g. a survey seeking the views and impressions of members of the target audience regarding their learning needs) or objective (i.e. as determined by practice audit, population health, or performance data). From needs assessment results, specific goals and objectives for the educational activity are defined, and appropriate learning strategies selected to enable the objectives to be met. For example, brief didactic sessions can provide knowledge updates, while case-based discussions or other problem-solving activities can foster comprehension and application of knowledge. If new skills are to be acquired (whether clinical or communication skills) learning strategies would include opportunities for skills practice with feedback.

While the model described fits formal CPD programme planning for groups, CPD also takes place at the individual level as an individually initiated and designed activity. Moore (2008) summarized theories and evidence on how individuals learn and constructed a process of five steps: recognize an opportunity for learning, search for resources, engage in learning, try out what was learned, and incorporate what was learned into practice. With increasing focus now being placed upon physician self-directed learning and upon learning from one's practice; such a model is helpful in describing this process.

Table 30.2 provides a way of thinking about CME activities based upon the size of the target population and gives examples of some strategies. Before describing each of these types of programme, we will briefly review the evidence for effective CPD.

Table 30.1 Implications of theories, perspective and frameworks of learning and change for CPD

Theories, perspectives and frameworks	Implications for CPD
Perspectives with a focus on learning	
Curriculum development (Kern et al. 1998)	Designing, implementing and evaluating learning activities proceeds in a systematic process beginning with needs identification
Adult learning theory (Knowles 1980)	Experience, personal goals, and practical needs motivate individual learning
Self-direction and lifelong learning (Candy 1991)	Learners can identify their own learning needs and undertake and evaluate their learning
Perspectives with a focus on behaviour change	
Knowledge translation (Graham and Logan 2006; Graham et al. 2006)	Translating learning into practice and enabling behaviour change is a complex activity requiring understanding of personal and system influences. Education is only one of many activities to promote change
PRECEDE model of change (Green and Kreuter 1991)	Three groups of factors influence individual behaviour change: predisposing, enabling, reinforcing
Stages of change or 'readiness' to change (Prochaska and DiClemente 1983)	Individuals appear to proceed through five stages when making a change: pre-contemplation, contemplation, preparation, action, maintenance
Theory of planned behaviour, (Aizen 1991)	An individual's intention to change is the most likely predictor of change, and is influenced by three individual factors: attitude, subjective norm, perceived control
Psychological domains influencing behaviour change (Michie et al. 2005)	Of 12 identified individual and institutional domains influencing change, only two are directly impacted by education; i.e. knowledge and skills. This further highlights the complexity of influences upon change
Perspectives informing both learning and behaviour change	
Change and learning in lives of physicians (Fox et al. 1989)	Multiple factors influence physician learning and their ability to change their practice. Change is a process rather than an event
Reflective practice and learning from experience (Kolb 1984; Schön 1987)	Learning occurs powerfully through experience. Reflection is integral to learning from practice and making change to one's practice based on that learning
Self-regulation and self-assessment, (Eva and Regehr 2005; Sargeant et al. 2010)	While self-regulation is fundamental to professional practice, individuals are generally poor at self-assessing their own performance. External feedback and reflection upon it can enable informed self-assessment
Learning in practice and workplace learning (Eraut 2007; Billet 2004)	Learning occurs through the process of engaging in work; i.e., in the activities of professional practice. A challenge is to make this learning explicit and enable it
Communities of practice (Wenger 1998)	Learning is a social activity and individuals can learn through their participation in a community of practice
Complexity (Sweeney and Griffiths 2002)	Both environmental and personal factors influence learning and one's ability and willingness to change

Table 30.2 Strategies for CME based on number of learners

Population size	Types of CPD programmes
Large groups	Lectures, conferences, webinars
Small groups	Workshops, small group learning, journal clubs
Individual learning	Academic detailing, audit and feedback, reading the literature, literature reviews

Effectiveness of CPD activities

Evaluating the impact of CPD activities upon physicians' practice and patient outcomes is central to determining their effectiveness. To answer this question, over 15 years ago, Davis and colleagues (Oxman et al. 1995; Davis et al. 1995) began a series of systematic reviews to determine the impact of traditional educational activities. They found that didactic sessions like lectures, the mainstay of traditional CME, were the least effective in promoting change in practice. More effective were small group sessions, which enable interaction, and educational interventions combined with other activities like sending reminders.

Other researchers (Mazmanian et al. 2009; Davis et al. 2009; Grol et al. 2003) have explored more broadly the influence of CPD in improving patient outcomes. A recent Cochrane review demonstrated that educational meeting or workshop formats improve physician performance and patient outcomes by only small observed effects (Forsetlund et al. 2009). Some CPD knowledge providers offer a variety of other evidence-based learning formats including practice audits, academic detailing, and reminders, but these too have generally small or small to moderate observed effects (Davis et al. 2009; O'Brien et al. 2007).

CPD activities

With this evidence in mind, we will now briefly review the learning activities identified in Table 30.2. Large group activities include the traditional didactic or lecture presentations of CPD meetings, conferences, and clinical rounds held by hospital departments. Video-conferencing, computers, and the internet enable new forms of large group activity. Webinars are live interactive sessions presented using various software programs that enable participants to hear and see the presentation and to interact with the speaker and other participants by text and/or voice. They enable participants in diverse locations, locally and internationally, to participate in an activity. Large group sessions are best used for sharing information; for example, raising awareness about new evidence and emerging trends. Their effectiveness in helping physicians consider how they might apply the new information presented in their practice can be enhanced by interactivity (e.g. by providing cases for discussion, posing questions for participants to discuss in groups of two or three, or by stimulating individual reflection on practice through directed questions).

Examples of common small group activities include workshops, journal clubs, and other formal small group learning sessions. Workshops support activity and learning through interacting with other participants and with the material presented. Because of the high degree of interaction, workshops are considered more effective for changing attitudes and perceptions and for enabling physicians to see how they might change their practice. Workshops are also effective for learning and practising skills such as communication, interpersonal, critical thinking, and patient management skills.

Journal clubs are educational groups that meet to discuss and critique a particular research article. One person generally takes responsibility for presenting a review and leading the discussion.

The Practice Based Small Group Learning Program is a Canadian programme offering accredited CME through the Foundation for Medical Practice (Practice Based Small Group Information 2012). Through trained facilitators and evidence-based materials, small groups engage in discussion of cases to learn about the management of various clinical problems. Discussions also stimulate reflection on one's practice and address strategies for applying new knowledge and changing practice (Armson et al. 2007).

Individual activities include journal reading, academic detailing, and practice audit and feedback, among others. In academic detailing a trained healthcare professional visits physicians in their practice settings to provide education on a specific topic. The academic detailers are usually pharmacists but can be nurses or physicians— see fig. 30.2. Sessions are usually one-on-one but may take place in small groups, formats that allow tailoring the session to the needs of the learners and that encourage discussion of educational messages. The information provided is rigorously evidence-based and balanced. Systematic reviews have found that academic detailing leads to about a 6% absolute increase in practice change (O'Brien et al. 2007). Physicians who use academic detailing report that its evidence-based approach has led them to more critically evaluate information from other CME programmes, pharmaceutical representatives, and journal articles, but not advice from specialists (Allen et al. 2007).

In a practice audit, individual physicians conduct an audit of records of their patients with a particular health problem (e.g. diabetes) to determine if they are meeting clinical practice guidelines or standards; they then receive feedback on how their care compares to recommended care on the various measures. While not a traditional CME event, learning takes place through seeing the comparison between one's own practice with the standards; and when a gap exists, it can be a stimulus to change one's practice (O'Brien et al. 2007).

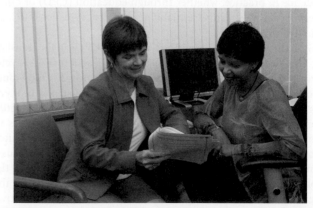

Figure 30.2 Education session with an academic detailer in the physician's office.

Evaluation of educational outcomes

Whether group or individual learning, evaluation of CPD activities is linked to the learning goal or objectives; i.e., how can achievement of the objectives be measured? A traditional framework for evaluation of educational outcomes identifies them at four levels: reaction of participants, learning (knowledge and skills), behaviour change, and impact on the organization—which for CPD includes impact on patient outcomes (Kirkpatrick 2007).

Moore (2003, 2008) expanded upon the four-level Kirkpatrick framework to create a six-level model for assessing educational outcomes of CPD activities. He added a new Level 1, participation, and most significantly, expanded upon the learning level by including Miller's pyramid (Miller 1990) of progressive levels of competence. These levels differentiate the ways of knowing: i.e. 'knows', 'knows how', 'shows how', and 'does', discriminations which are helpful in thinking about the outcomes of acquiring knowledge.

Knowledge translation and evaluation of outcomes

Evaluating the impact of CPD upon physicians' behaviour or performance in practice, and upon organizational and patient outcomes, also links CPD to the developing field of knowledge translation (KT) or implementation science. KT refers broadly to the ways that knowledge is applied in practice, and specifically to application of evidence in clinical practice to improve patient outcomes, provide more effective health services, and strengthen healthcare systems (Graham et al. 2004). KT activities have focused upon enabling individual physicians and health professionals to change their practice and improve patient outcomes by applying best evidence (Eccles et al. 2005).

While the ultimate goals of both KT and CPD are to improve patient care and outcomes, the paths towards these goals differ. For CPD, the path as described earlier has been traditionally through education and learning. For KT, the path is through interventions in addition to education which can more directly promote behaviour change. It is timely, though, to consider the fields of CPD and KT and how they can each inform the other, especially in light of the shared goal of improving patient care and health outcomes. It is now estimated that 30% to 40% of patients do not receive care informed by best evidence and that 20% to over 50% receive care that is inappropriate (Grol 2001; Grol et al. 2003; McGlynn et al. 2003). Strategies to enhance application of evidence in practice, whether through education (CPD) or other interventions (KT), are essential if new clinical evidence is to lead to improvement.

Graham et al. (2006) identified a seven-step cycle for translating knowledge into action, the knowledge-to-action (KTA) cycle, derived from a review of planned action theories for individual behaviour and identification of common elements across the theories described previously. The steps in the KTA cycle are: identify a problem, adapt knowledge to local context, assess barriers to knowledge use; select, tailor, implement interventions; monitor knowledge use; evaluate outcomes; and sustain knowledge use. Common elements to CPD are problem identification, focusing the problem, planning for appropriate intervention, implementing the intervention, and evaluating the outcomes. The focus of KT activities is behaviour change and the specific identification and mitigation of barriers, only one of which may be lack of knowledge.

To further emphasize the complexity of change, Harrison (2004) proposed a systems-based framework for enhancing CPD and translation of new evidence into physician practice, driven by concerns for patient safety and rising costs. Systems theory, similar to complexity theory, focuses on how a system and its components receive information from the environment, process it, and produce outputs into the environment. Relationships are important (i.e. relationships among individuals and between individuals and the organization). Harrison proposes the interaction of six types of systems in translating new information into physician practice, emphasizing just how difficult a task it is to change practice.

Meta-analyses are helpful in determining and comparing outcomes of interventions, whether focused on education or other methods of inducing change; however, they do not really help us understand why something does or does not work, and they do not consider the influence of the context. Approaches enabling understanding of 'why' specific interventions work as well as 'if' they work can be helpful. Qualitative studies conducted either alone or as components of mixed-method studies can begin to explore the factors, both individual and contextual, that influence an intervention and its outcomes. For example, Kennedy et al. (2004) describe a study following a CPD intervention to explore translation of the new knowledge into practice. They tested knowledge through multiple-choice questions and behaviour through standardized patient encounters, followed by exploration of knowledge–behaviour discrepancies through interviews. Two factors explained the gap in applying knowledge to practice—level of certainty and sense of urgency—suggesting that focusing on these in CPD interventions may enhance application of new knowledge in practice. Notably, perceptions of certainty and urgency are not traditionally included in CPD content.

Realist evaluation (Pawson and Tilley 1997) is a comprehensive approach to studying complex social interventions (e.g. education or behaviour change) in complex social environments (e.g. busy healthcare settings). Realist evaluation asks the questions 'why does a programme work?', 'for whom?', and 'under what circumstance?' In addition to outcomes, it attends particularly to the explanatory components of whether an intervention works or not, components generally overlooked in comparative outcome studies. It recognizes that it is the interaction between the intervention and the context which leads to the outcome, not just the intervention itself. We believe this is a helpful perspective for CPD and KT (Sales 2009). Realist evaluation is also theory-based—i.e. it strives to make explicit the relationships between the intervention, context, and outcomes. Its goals are also consistent with recent calls for CPD research to be more theoretically and scientifically based, and to include the study of context and of influencing conditions (Institute of Medicine 2010).

External influences on CPD

Multiple external factors influence the provision of and physician participation in CPD (fig. 30.3). These are both formal organizational requirements for CPD, and more informal systems changes (e.g. influence of quality improvement and patient safety movements). Central among the formal influences are national CPD programme accreditation requirements, professional requirements for maintenance of certification, and more recently, regulatory requirements for revalidation. We will begin by discussing each of these, followed by a discussion of emerging influences, including

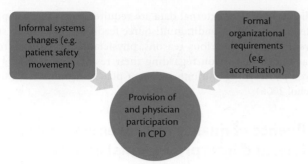

Figure 30.3 External factors that influence the provision of and physician participation in CPD.

quality improvement, patient safety and interprofessional education, and relationships across the educational continuum.

National accreditation of CPD/CME activities

The USA and Canada have national accreditation requirements for CPD, which influence the structure and content of formal CPD programmes offered by Faculties of Medicine, professional associations, and other organizations. In the US, the organization is the Accreditation Council for CME (ACCME) (2012b). Both countries have traditionally required that CPD programmes be designed using needs assessments of the target population, and a planning committee including representatives of the target population; that sessions are interactive; that content is not biased by private industry influence; and that programmes be evaluated. A significant more recent addition to these requirements in both Canada and the USA is evaluation demonstrating that the programme is actually influencing physicians' behaviour. This has happened in response to public and political demands that formal CPD needs to have greater impact, needs to produce behaviour change, and ultimately be seen to be improving patient care and outcomes (Institute of Medicine 2010).

The impact of these requirements is that CPD programmes are transitioning from solely 'learning' activities where the goal is to share new knowledge, to 'behaviour change activities' and knowledge translation interventions, where the goal is to change physicians' practice. Hence, CPD activities and evaluations are including a focus upon changing practice. Strategies to enhance consideration of behaviour change range from self-reports, such as 'Intention to change' questionnaires following an education intervention (Wakefield et al. 2003) to chart audit to determine if care and outcomes changed as a result of the intervention (O'Brien et al. 2007).

Maintenance of certification

Across professional and regulatory associations in many countries, guidance is provided and requirements identified for physicians regarding the amount and type of CPD, professional and practice assessment, and other activities in which they must engage.

In Canada, the two national certifying colleges, the College of Family Physicians of Canada (CFPC) and the Royal College of Physicians and Surgeons of Canada (RCPSC), have recognized the need for lifelong learning as a fundamental component of maintaining competence and hence certification. Their maintenance

of certification programmes require their members to participate in and document their continuing professional development activities (College of Family Physicians of Canada 2012; Royal College of Physicians and Surgeons of Canada 2012). These programmes are available to non-member physicians. They provide a Canadian standards-based framework for ongoing professional development.

The RCPSC Maintenance of Certification (MOC) Program for specialist physicians (Royal College of Physicians and Surgeons of Canada 2012) is an evidence-informed educational initiative designed to support, enhance, and promote the continuing professional development activities of MOC Program participants, based on the principles of lifelong learning. Programme participants are responsible for designing and implementing a personal CPD plan that is relevant to their professional roles and responsibilities. The MOC Program provides strategies and tools to document the learning activities and outcomes that enhance practice and help to develop a learning plan for the future. A central purpose of the MOC Program is to enable specialists to build evidence-informed practices that enhance the quality of specialty care. As well, the MOC Program enables the identification, documentation, and validation of learning outcomes and practice enhancements for purposes such as relicensure or privilege to practise.

Within the RCPSC MOC, there are three sections of learning activities: (1) Group learning—accredited group learning activities, e.g. rounds, journal clubs, conferences; (2) Self-learning—planned learning in response to a need (e.g. fellowships, personal learning projects); scanning for new evidence (e.g. reading, internet search); and systems learning through contributions to standards or patient safety (e.g. practice guideline development, quality committee), and (3) Assessment—formal knowledge assessment or performance assessment (chart audit, multisource feedback, or simulation).

Through these three general categories of activities, the MOC Program promotes a learning culture that includes reflection, inquiry, peer review and assessment of knowledge, competence and performance across the entire spectrum of roles. The revisions align with an emphasis upon physicians' reflecting upon and learning in response to their practice and performance. While group learning as in large conferences or meetings is still acknowledged and forms a section of learning activities, it is no longer the predominant mode.

Similarly, the CFPC maintenance of certification programme, MAINPRO (The College of Family Physicians of Canada 2012), has transitioned from providing CME credit solely for group activities to providing it also for individual reflective practice and improvement activities, in which physicians document a practice question, conduct a scholarly perusal of the literature to address the question, and describe how the findings will influence their practice.

In the USA, the American Board of Internal Medicine (ABIM) requires an alternate mode of performance assessment, participation in a Performance Improvement Module (PIM) (American Board of Internal Medicine 2012; Duffy 2008). PIMs involve a formatted audit of one's practice, completion of patient and office systems questionnaires, a review of a report compiling practice findings, physician reflection upon the report, development of a plan for practice change, and monitoring of progress. Again, the emphasis is upon learning from, and improving, one's practice.

In the UK, the focus is upon developing a personal learning plan from standardized data collected about one's performance. The General Medical Council (GMC) defines good medical practice (General Medical Council 2012a) and provides guidelines and principles for identifying learning needs based on a portfolio approach to data collection, and for developing, implementing, evaluating, and documenting learning plans and activities. Physicians collect performance data through, for example, multisource feedback, patient questionnaires, critical incidents, and practice reviews. They then meet with a peer coach or mentor to discuss their findings, identify care gaps and develop a personal learning plan (General Medical Council 2012b).

A theme in all these efforts is the move to individual physician practice-based learning, through identifying learning needs via their patient practice and professional interactions, and planning, undertaking, and evaluating actions designed to meet those needs. While lectures are still timely and appropriate for transmission of information, and for use as one of many learning approaches, the notion of practice-based individualized self-directed learning is becoming predominant.

Emphasis on performance assessment

Congruent with ideas of learning from practice, individual performance assessment is now also considered as a data source for learning and improvement. Regulatory authorities, responsible by legislation for assuring their public of physicians' competence, are now formally linking participation in their performance assessment programmes to physicians' development and practice improvement. For example, in Canada, the multisource feedback programme, Physician Achievement Review implemented in Alberta and Nova Scotia and being considered by other provinces, provides a confidential report to each physician of their individual scores compared to the provincial means. Physicians are expected to use the results of these obligatory assessments to plan and implement their continued development and improvement.

In the UK, as already noted, the GMC requires use of a portfolio of activities for data collection about one's performance and subsequent development of a Personal Learning Plan. The ABIM similarly requires its members to develop an improvement plan using the results of their practice assessment. Increasingly the emphasis is upon using data from one's own practice to inform continued learning and development.

Informed self-assessment

The concept of purposefully collecting data about one's practice to inform self-assessment of clinical performance is important. Studies show that people are generally poor self-assessors of their performance (Kruger et al. 1999) and that physicians are no exception (Davis et al. 2006). This means that physicians' assessments of their practice and learning needs in the absence of objective practice data can often be flawed, and hence may not be a reliable source for identifying gaps in practice. In response the notion of 'informed self-assessment' has been identified. It describes a process by which practitioners and learners purposefully collect, analyse, and interpret data to use to inform their self-assessment and self-directed learning (Sargeant et al. 2010; Lockyer 2011).

Reliable sources of external data are required, such as those provided through chart audit, multisource feedback, and patient surveys. Further, for various reasons, physicians may benefit from a facilitated discussion regarding their results and coaching to develop a learning and improvement plan (Sargeant et al. 2011; Nichol 2006).

Influence of quality improvement, patient safety, and interprofessional education

Quality improvement initiatives

QI incorporates organizational and cross-disciplinary level approaches to improving systems and processes within healthcare institutions (Deming 1986). Similar to CME, the goal is improving healthcare and patient outcomes, generally through addressing systems and patient care delivery problems which arise. Many opportunities exist for synergy between CPD and QI initiatives; for example, to identify where an educational approach may provide the solution to a healthcare problem (Kitto et al. 2011, 2013; Shojania et al. 2012). The USA is leading in formally linking CPD to QI initiatives through the national accreditation criteria (Accreditation Council for Continuing Medical Education 2012a; Association of American Medical Colleges 2012). The Association of American Medical Colleges' (AAMC) goal is to provide guidance for CPD professionals as they move CME from a primarily conference-based model to one which employs best educational methods, QI, and performance improvement (PI) principles to close the clinical care gap.

Patient safety

Similar to QI initiatives, patient safety initiatives seek to improve patient care and outcomes by reducing the potential for error. The patient safety literature tells us that most medical errors are avoidable and many can be prevented by enhancing collaboration among health professionals (Institute of Medicine 2000). This literature also demonstrates that traditional models of healthcare in which departments and professions operate in silos can contribute to increased patient risk and reduced quality of care. Hence, it emphasizes the imperative for interprofessional education and collaboration.

Interprofessional education and collaborative practice

The impetus to provide more collaborative care and team-based practice has continued to gain momentum. Indeed, in the past few years, several influential reports have argued that interprofessional education (IPE) and collaborative practice are key to addressing patient safety issues, communicable and chronic diseases, emergency and disaster care, mental health needs, and the need for more trained healthcare providers globally (WHO 2010; Frenk et al. 2010). In 2011, the Interprofessional Education Collaborative identified four overarching competencies for collaborative practice. These included: values and ethics; roles and responsibilities; interprofessional communication, and interprofessional teamwork and team-based care (Interprofessional Education Collaborative 2011a). The same group advanced a set of enabling recommendations to enhance the development of IPE competencies (Interprofessional Education Collaborative 2011b).

Interprofessional education initiatives in continuing education have proven to be complex. There have been challenges in developing programmes that are relevant to all health professionals, and reports suggest that physicians have been less likely to attend events that are designed to be truly interprofessional (Mann et al. 2009). Interestingly, the evidence of beneficial effects on care has been most often demonstrated at the post-licensure level; however, the evidence as assessed through a recent Cochrane review is modest (Reeves et al. 2010).

The Interprofessional Education Collaborative (2011b) identified reinforcing factors, including emphasis on the quality of care, focus on the patient, the promise of healthcare reform, an ageing society, and rapidly evolving scientific knowledge. However, transfer of learning to the workplace and motivation to participate are hampered by the absence of role models, existing reimbursement systems, logistical barriers, resistance to change, and differing professional cultures (Schmitt et al. 2011). For CPD, there is also the challenge of developing appropriate assessments, accreditation processes, and standards.

Above all, in the view of Schmitt et al. (2011), IPE for practicing professionals should present more refined and sophisticated models rather than a repetition of what has been learned before or remediation for those not previously exposed.

Relationships across the continuum of education

Finally, we strongly support the growing connection of CPD with other levels of medical education. (Association of American Medical Colleges 2012) Many of the challenges are common to all levels. These include: selecting appropriate and best evidence-based educational strategies; providing opportunities for feedback that can be used to enhance learning and performance; developing and utilizing effective assessment strategies; supporting critical thinking, self-appraisal and identification and addressing of learning needs; and recognizing the need for development in roles beyond the 'clinical expert' role. Every level faces the challenges of social accountability and supporting the growth of professional competence and professional identity. Considering the educational trajectory as a whole offers important opportunities for increased understanding of how each level of education can complement the others. In particular CPD, encompassing an understanding of competence and effective learning in practice, can inform learners' preparation at the undergraduate and postgraduate levels.

Conclusions

◆ Changing physician behaviour is a complex undertaking. It requires attention to the cognitive aspects, the affective or emotional aspects, and the practical aspects of learning and change. It is a process, rather than a single event.

◆ Knowing what to do is not enough. Changing practice behaviour involves identifying learning needs, and developing appropriate strategies to assist learners in meeting them.

◆ In addition to knowledge, physician learners require a variety of meta-cognitive skills. These skills include the capacity to be reflective, to self-assess their practice and performance, and to direct their own learning.

◆ A variety of educational strategies are available to support learners. To be most effective, they must be carefully selected and appropriately implemented.

◆ Significant shifts are occurring in this field, transforming both content and educational approaches, focusing on practice change and improving health outcomes.

References

Accreditation Council for CME (ACCME) (2012a) *Why should providers engage within a system or framework for quality improvement?* [Online] http://www.accme.org/education-and-support/video/faq/why%C2%A0should-providers-engage-within-system-or-framework-quality Accessed 12 April 2012

Accreditation Council for CME (ACCME) (2012b) *Accreditation criteria.* [Online] http://www.accme.org/requirements/accreditation-requirements-cme-providers/accreditation-criteria Accessed 12 April 2012

Accreditation Council for CME (ACCME) (2012c) *Recommendations by focus area.* [Online] https://www.aamc.org/initiatives/cme/lifelong/ Accessed 12 April 2012

Allen, M., Ferrier, S., O'Connor, N., and Fleming, I. (2007) Family physicians perceptions of academic detailing: a quantitative and qualitative study. *BMC Med. Educ.* 7 (36): 1–9

Ajzen, I. (1991) The theory of planned behaviour. *Organizational Behaviour and Human Decision Processes.* 50: 179–211

American Board of Internal Medicine. (2012) *American Board of Internal Medicine.* [Online] http://www.abim.org/pim/ [Accessed 12 April 2012].

Armson, H., Kinzie, S., Hawes, D., et al. (2007) Translating learning into practice: lessons from the practice-based small group learning program. *Canadian Family Physician*, 53 (9), 1477–1485.

Association for American Medical Colleges. (2012) *Continuing Education and Performance Improvement (CE/PI)* [Online] https://www.aamc.org/initiatives/cme Accessed 12 April 2012

Billett, S. (2001) Learning through work: workplace affordances and individual engagement. *J Workplace Learn.* 13: 209–214

Billett, S. (2004) Workplace participatory practices: conceptualizing workplaces as learning environments. *J Workplace Learn.* 16: 312–324

Boud, D., Keogh, R., and Walker, D. (1985) *Reflection: Turning Experience into Learning.* London: Kogan Page

Candy, P.C. (1991) *Self-Direction for Lifelong Learning: a Comprehensive Guide to Theory and Practice.* San Francisco CA: Jossey-Bass

College of Family Physicians of Canada (2012) *Continuing Professional Development (CPD)* [Online] http://www.cfpc.ca/CPD/ Accessed 12 April 2012

Davies, P., Walker, A.E., and Grimshaw, J.M. (2010) A systematic review of the use of theory in the design of guideline dissemination and implementation strategies and interpretation of the results of rigorous evaluations. *Implement Sci.* 5: 14

Davis, D., Barnes, D.E., and Fox, R. (2003) *The Continuing Professional Development of Physicians: From Research to Practice.* Chicago IL: AMA Press

Davis, D., Bordage, G., Moores, LK., et al. (2009) The science of continuing medical education: terms, tools, and gaps: effectiveness of continuing medical education: American College of Chest Physicians Evidence-Based Educational Guidelines. *Chest.* 135(Supplement 3): 8S–16S

Davis, D. and Galbraith, R. (2009) American College of Chest Physicians Health and Science, Policy Committee. Continuing medical education effect on practice performance: effectiveness of continuing medical education: American College of Chest Physicians Evidence-Based Educational Guidelines. *Chest.* 135(Supplement 3): 42S–48S

Davis, D.A., Mazmanian, P.E., Fordis, M., et al. (2006) Accuracy of physician self-assessment compared with observed measures of competence: a systematic review. *JAMA.* 296: 1094–1102

Davis, D.A., Thomson, M.A., Oxman, A.D., and Haynes, R.B. (1995) Changing physician performance. a systematic review of the effect of continuing medical education strategies. *JAMA*. 274: 700–705

Deming, W.E. (1986) *Out of Crisis*. Cambridge, MA: Massachusetts Institute of Technology

Duffy, F.D., Lynn, L.A., Didura, H., et al. (2008) Self-assessment of practice performance: development of the ABIM practice improvement module. *J Continuing Educ Health Prof*. 28(1): 38–46

Eccles, M., Grimshaw, J., Walker, A., Johnston, M., and Pitts, N. (2005) Changing the behavior of healthcare professionals: the use of theory in promoting the uptake of research findings. *J Clin Epidemiol*. 58(2): 107–112

Eraut, M. (2000) Non-formal learning and tacit knowledge in professional work. *Br J Educ Psychol*. 70: 113–136

Eraut, M. (2007) Learning from other people in the workplace. *Oxford Rev Educ*. 33: 403–422

Eva, K. and Regehr, G. (2005) Self-assessment in the health professions: a reformulation and research agenda. *Acad Med*. 80(10): S46–S54

Flexner, A. (1910) *Medical Education in the United States and Canada*. Washington DC: Science and Health Publications

Forsetlund, L., Bjorndal, A., Rashidian, A., et al. (2009) Continuing education meetings and workshops: effects on professional practice and health care outcomes. *Cochrane Database Systematic Reviews England*. 2, 2, CD003030

Fox, R., Mazmanian, P., and Putnam, R.W. (1989) *Change and Learning in the Lives of Physicians*. New York: Praeger

Frenk J, Chen, L., Bhutta, Z.A., et al. (2010) Health professionals for a new century: transforming education to strengthen health systems in an interdependent world. *Lancet*. 376: 1923–1958

General Medical Council (2012a) *Good Medical Practice*. [Online] http://www.gmc-uk.org/guidance/good_medical_practice.asp Accessed 12 April 2012

General Medical Council (2012b) Draft CPD guidance for consultation. [Online] http://www.gmc-uk.org/Draft_CPD_guidance_for_consultation_Oct_11.pdf_44814603.pdf Accessed 12 April 2012

Graham, I.D. and Logan, J. (2004) Innovations in knowledge transfer and continuity of care. *CJNR*. 36(2): 89–103

Graham, I.D., Logan, J., Harrison, M.B., et al. (2006) Lost in knowledge translation: time for a map? *J Cont Educ Health Prof*. 26(1): 13–24

Green, L.W. and Kreuter, M.W. (1991) *Health Promotion Planning: An Educational and Environmental Approach*. Toronto: Mayfield Publishing Group

Grimshaw, J.M., Eccles, M.P., Steen, N., et al. (2011) Applying psychological theories to evidence-based clinical practice: identifying factors predictive of lumbar spine x-ray for low back pain in UK primary care practice. *Implement Sci*. 6: 55

Grol, R. (2001) Successes and failures in the implementation of evidence-based guidelines for clinical practice. *Med Care*. 39: 1146–1154

Grol, R. and Grimshaw, J. (2003) From best evidence to best practice: effective implementation of change in patients' care. *Lancet*. 362: 1225–1230

Harrison, R.V. (2004) Systems-based framework for continuing medical education and improvements in translating new knowledge into physicians' practices. *J Cont Educ Health Prof*. 24: S50–S62

Hean, S., Craddock, D., and O'Hallaran, C. (2009) Learning theory and interprofessional education. *Learn Health Social Care*. 8: 250–262

Institute of Medicine (2000) *To Err is Human: Building a Safer Health System*. Washington, DC: National Academic Press

Institute of Medicine (2010) *Redesigning Continuing Education in the Health Professions*. Washington DC: National Academies Press

Interprofessional Education Collaborative (2011a) *Core Competencies for Interprofessional Collaborative Practice*. Report of an Expert Panel. May 2011. Washington DC

Interprofessional Education Collaborative (2011b) *Team Based Competencies. Building a Shared Foundation for Education and Clinical Practice*. Proceedings of a Conference. 16-17 Feb 2011. Washington DC

Karle, H., Paulos, G., and Wentz, D., (2011) Continuing professional development: concepts, origins and rationale. In: D. Wentz (ed.) *Continuing Medical Education: Looking Back, Planning Ahead* (pp. 281–290). Lebanon NH: Dartmouth College Press

Kennedy, T., Regehr, G., Rosenfield, J., Roberts, SW., and Lingard, L. (2004) Exploring the gap between knowledge and behavior: a qualitative study of clinical action following an educational intervention. *Acad Med*. 79: 386–393

Kern, D.E., Thomas, P.A., Howard, D.M., and Bass, E.B. (1998) *Curriculum Development for Medical Education: A Six-Step Approach*. Baltimore, MD: Johns Hopkins University Press

Kitto, S.C., Sargeant, J., Reeves, S., and Silver, I. (2011) Towards a sociology of knowledge translation: the importance of being dis-interested in knowledge translation. *Adv Health Sci Educ*. 17: 289–299

Kitto, S., Bell, M., Peller, J., et al. (2013) Positioning continuing education: boundaries and intersections between the domains continuing education, knowledge translation, patient safety and quality improvement. *Adv Health Sci Educ*. 18; 144–156

Kirkpatrick, J.D. (2007) *Implementing the Four Levels: A Practical Guide for Effective Evaluation of Training Programs*. San Francisco CA: Berrett-Koehler

Knowles, M. (1980) *The Modern Practice of Education: From Pedagogy to Andragogy*. 2nd edn. New York, NY: Cambridge Books

Kolb, D. (1984) *Experiential Learning: Experience as the Source of Learning and Development*. Englewood Cliffs, NJ: Prentice Hall

Kruger, J. and Dunning, D. (1999) Unskilled and unaware of it: how difficulties in recognizing one's own incompetence lead to inflated self-assessments. *J Personality Soc Psychol*. 77: 1121–1134

Lave, J. and Wenger E. (1991) *Situated Learning. Legitimate Peripheral Participation*. Cambridge, UK: Cambridge University Press

Lewin, K. (1951) *Field Theory in Social Science: Selected Theoretical Papers*. New York NY: Harper and Row

Lockyer, J, Armson, H., Chesluk, B., et al. (2011) Feedback data sources that inform physician self assessment. *Med Teach*. 33(2): e113–e120

Mamede, S., Schmidt, H., and Penaforte, J.C. (2008) Effects of reflective practice on the accuracy of medical diagnoses. *Med Educ*. 42: 468–475

Mann, K., Dornan, T., and Teunissen, P. (2011) Perspectives on learning. In T. Dornan, K. Mann, A. Scherphier, and J. Spencer (eds) (2011) *Medical Education: Theory and Practice* (pp. 17–38). Edinburgh UK: Elsevier

Mann, K., Gordon, J.J., and MacLeod, A.M. (2009) Reflection and reflective practice in health professions education: a systematic review of the literature in the health professions. *Adv Health Sci Educ Theory Pract*. 14: 595–621

Mann, K., Sargeant, J., and Hill, T. (2009) Knowledge translation in interprofessional education: what difference does IPE make to practice? *Learn Health Soc Care*. 8: 154–164

Mazmanian, P.E., Davis, D.A., and Galbraith, R. (2009) American College of Chest Physicians Health and Science Policy Committee. Continuing medical education effect on clinical outcomes: effectiveness of continuing medical education: American College of Chest Physicians Evidence-Based Educational Guidelines. *Chest*. 35: 49S–55S

McGlynn, E.A., Asch, S.M., Adams, J., et al. (2003) The quality of health care delivered to adults in the United States. *N Engl J Med*. 348: 2635–2645

Michie, S., Johnston, M., Abraham, C., et al. (2005) Making psychological theory useful for implementing evidence based practice: a consensus approach. *Qual Safety Healthcare*. 14: 26–33

Miller, G.E. (1990) The assessment of clinical skills/competence/performance. *Acad Med*. 65: S63–S67

Moore, D.E. (2003) *A Framework for Outcomes Evaluation in the Continuing Professional Development of Physicians*. United States: American Medical Association

Moore, D.E. (2008) *How Physicians Learn and How to Design Learning Experiences for Them: an approach based on an interpretive review of evidence*. Proceedings of a Conference: Continuing Education in the Health Professions. New York NY: Josiah Macy, Jr. Foundation, pp. 30–63

Nelson, M.S. (1995) The physician as learner: linking research to practice. *JAMA*. 274(9): 775

Nichol, M.B. (2006) The role of outcomes research in defining and measuring value in benefit decisions. *J Managed Care Pharm.* 12(6): 19–23

Norcini, J. and Burch, V. (2007) Workplace-based assessment as an educational tool: AMEE Guide No. 31. *Med Teach.* 29: 855–871

Norman, G. (1999) The adult learner: a mythical species. *Acad Med.* 74: 886–889

O'Brien, M.A., Rogers, S., Jamtvedt, G., et al. (2007) Educational outreach visits: effects on professional practice and health care outcomes. *Cochrane Database Systematic Reviews.* 4, CD000409

Oxman, A.D., Thomson, M.A., Davis, D.A., and Haynes, R.B. (1995) No magic bullets: a systematic review of 102 trials of interventions to improve professional practice. *Can Med Ass J.* 153: 1423–1431

Pawson, R. and Tilley, N. (1997) *Realistic Evaluation.* Thousand Oaks CA: Sage Publications Inc

Practice Based Small Group Information (2012) *The Foundation for Medical Practice Web Site.* [Online] http://www.fmpe.org/en/programs/pbsg.html Accessed 12 April 2012

Premi, J., Shannon, S., Hartwick, K., Lamb, S., Wakefield J., and Williams J. (1994) Practice-based small-group CME. *Acad Med.* 69: 800–882

Prochaska, J.O. and DiClemente C.C. (1983) Stages and processes of self-change of smoking: toward an integrative model of change. *J Consult Clin Psychol.* 51: 390–395

Ramsay, C.R., Thomas, R.E., Croal, B.L., et al. (2010) Using the theory of planned behaviour as a process evaluation tool in randomized trials of knowledge translation strategies: a case study from UK primary care. *Implement Sci.* 29: 71

Reeves, S. Zarenstein, M., Goldman, J., et al. (2010) The effectiveness of interprofessional education: key findings from a recent systematic review. *J Interprof Care.* 24: 230–241

Ross, L. and Nisbett, R.E. (1991) *The Person and the Situation: Perspectives of Social Psychology.* Philadelphia: Temple University Press: McGraw-Hill

Royal College of Physicians and Surgeons of Canada (2012) *A Continuing Commitment to Lifelong Learning: A Concise Guide to Maintenance of Certification.* [Online] http://royalcollege.ca/moc Accessed 6 March 2013

Sales, A. (2009) *Quality Improvement.* Oxford UK: Blackwell Publishing Ltd

Sargeant, J., Mann, K., Sinclair D, van der Vleuten C., and Metsemakers, J. (2008) Understanding the influence of emotions and reflection on multi-source feedback and use. *Adv Health Sci Educ Theory Pract.* 13: 275–288

Sargeant, J., Armson, H., Chesluk, B., et al. (2010) The processes and dimensions of informed self-assessment: a conceptual model. *Acad Med.* 85: 1212–1220

Sargeant, J., McNaughton, E., Mercer, S., Murphy, D., Sullivan, P., and Bruce, D.A. (2011) Providing feedback: exploring a model (emotion, content, outcomes) for facilitating multisource feedback. *Med Teach.* 33: 744–749

Schmitt, M., Baldwin, D.C., and Reeves, S. (2011) Continuing interprofessional education. Collaborative learning for collaborative practice. In D. Wentz (ed.) *Continuing Medical Education: Looking Back, Planning Ahead* (pp. 300–316). Lebanon NH: Dartmouth College Press

Schön, D. (1987) *Educating the Reflective Practitioner.* San Francisco CA: Jossey-Bass

Sfard, A. (1999) On two metaphors for learning and the dangers of choosing just one. *Educ Res.* 27: 2–13

Shojania, K.G. (2012) Continuing medical education and quality improvement: a match made in heaven? *Ann Intern Med.* 156: 305–308

Stanton, F., and Grant, J. (1997) *The Effectiveness of Continuing Professional Development.* London England: Joint Centre for Medical Education and Open University

Sweeney, K., and Griffiths, F. (eds) (2002) *Complexity and Healthcare: An Introduction.* Abingdon, UK: Radcliffe Medical Press Ltd

Wakefield, J., Herbert, C.P., Maclure, M., et al. (2003) Commitment to change statements can predict actual change in practice. *J Cont Educ Health Prof.* 23: 81–93

Wenger, E. (1998) *Communities of Practice.* Cambridge UK: Cambridge University Press

World Health Organization (2010) *Health Professions Networks, Nursing and Midwifery Human Resources for Health. Framework for Action on Interpersonal Education and Collaborative Practice* (WHO/HRH/HPN/10.3). Geneva, Switzerland: World Health Organization

CHAPTER 31

Remediation

David Mendel, Alex Jamieson, and Julia Whiteman

Dysfunctional doctors should be helped back to practise wherever appropriate.

Donald Irvine

Reproduced from *British Medical Journal*, Donald Irvine,
'The performance of doctors. II: Maintaining good practice,
protecting patients from poor performance', 314, p. 1613,
Copyright 1997, with permission from BMJ Publishing Group Ltd

Background

In the context of medical practice, remediation has been defined as 'the process of addressing performance concerns (knowledge, skills, and behaviours) that have been recognized, through assessment, investigation, review, or appraisal, so that the practitioner has the opportunity to return to safe practice' (Academy of Medical Royal Colleges 2009, p. 2). Typically, the remediation of medical practitioners can be viewed as a process with three components—identification of performance deficiencies, provision of educational interventions and reassessment of performance (Hauer et al. 2009).

Before considering how medical practitioners can be remediated, we will first explore how underperformance is defined and identified and then consider the range of possible underlying causes.

Defining and identifying underperformance

The importance of protecting patients from underperforming doctors has become increasingly recognized in the past decade and forms a component of clinical governance, the process by which health services assure their standards of care. Underperformance may be recognized at any career stage, from undergraduate medical training through to retirement.

Doctors in training grades are subject to supervision and one might therefore assume that underperformance would be managed. However, uncertainty on thresholds for concern, fear of challenge, lack of documentation and an absence of remediation may all be barriers to responding to performance concerns in this group (Dudek et al. 2005). Paice (2006) has described early signs of trainees in difficulty including ward rage and 'the disappearing act'; these should trigger an increased level of supervision and attention to underlying causes.

Following the completion of specialist training, the idea that a doctor's performance should be subject to periodic scrutiny, in a manner analogous to airline pilots, is a relatively recent development, although it is expected, and even assumed to be occurring, by the public (St George et al. 2004).

The prevalence of underperforming doctors is uncertain and dependant on where the defining cut-off point is placed and what methodology is applied for assessment (Williams 2006, p. 174). Existing assessment programmes typically operate at three levels (Finucane et al. 2003):

- Level 1—Screening whole populations of doctors, using tools such as appraisal, peer review visits or re-licensing examinations.

- Level 2—Targeting 'at risk' groups, e.g. older doctors, isolated practitioners.

- Level 3—Assessing individuals whose performance has given rise to concern, e.g. through complaints or other governance processes.

The General Medical Council (GMC), in the UK, judges performance against its published guidance on 'Good Medical Practice' (GMC 2008), setting out the standards expected of all practising doctors, and has developed, level three, 'fitness to practise' assessments that are viewed as robust and defensible to challenge (Southgate et al. 2001). Complaints to regulators, however, generally identify a small minority of practising doctors (GMC 2011; NCAS 2009).

Level one assessments, such as peer reviews of practising doctors in Canada (Goulet et al. 2002; Hall et al. 1999; McAuley et al. 1990; Norton and Faulkner 1999), may begin to reveal the prevalence of underperformance. Williams (2006) estimates a prevalence of between 6 and 12% based on medical errors, medicolegal actions, quality control and medical record studies. This high prevalence of underperformance has not been found in UK studies to date (Bahrami and Evans 2001; Joesbury et al. 2001; Taylor 1998), but the UK is planning to commence level one screening for all doctors from the end of 2012 in the form of revalidation. This will utilize evidence from a 5-year cycle of annual appraisals, conducted by trained peers, triangulated with performance information from other clinical governance processes. It is uncertain how this process will compare with other level one screening programmes such as peer review visits in Canada or relicensing examinations in the USA.

Finucane et al. (2003) surveyed assessment programmes in Canada, Australia, New Zealand, and the UK during 2001. All assessments were carried out by statutory regulators, some deliberately at arm's length from licensing authorities. Level one assessment constitutes screening, but level three is high stakes and requires rigorous assessment. Assessment tools varied widely and involved a trade-off between reliability and validity on the one hand and cost and acceptability on the other. Case discussion, doctor interviews, medical records review, use of standardized/simulated patients, and direct observation were the most popular methods.

Assessments by regulators usually describe performance but do not explain why underperformance has arisen (Cox et al. 2006). The National Clinical Assessment Service (NCAS), in the UK, provides an assessment service which aims to seek holistic explanations for doctors' performance concerns and includes a focus on context (National Patient Safety Agency 2006). Analysis of NCAS (2009) cases over eight years cite clinical difficulties, misconduct and health, with most involving more than one area, implying that remediation interventions need to address more than simply knowledge and skills. However, while making full and holistic level three assessments prior to remediation is theoretically attractive, the accompanying expense and delay reduces their acceptability and feasibility.

The methods by which we identify underperformance may have important consequences. Intrusive assessment programmes risk damaging professional morale, and targeting at risk groups may be discriminatory (St George et al. 2004). Practitioners may come to attention because standards and expectations have evolved, or accountability has been enhanced, rather than because of any change in their performance. Most remediation programmes focus on the small minority of doctors identified from complaints to regulators, whose difficulties are likely to be at the severe end of the spectrum. It is uncertain whether resources match potential need, as opposed to identified need, or if the most appropriate doctors are being referred (Humphrey and Locke 2007).

Determinants of doctors' performance

Having considered how underperformance may be identified, we will now review some of the determinants of doctors' performance, beginning with some theoretical considerations.

Miller (1990), writing with reference to the assessment of clinical skills, proposed a triangle in which knowledge ('knows') and competence ('knows how') form a wide base to underpin performance ('shows how') and action ('does'). Rethans et al. (2002) suggest that 'shows how' should be referred to as 'competency', rather than as 'performance', because, while Miller's triangle assumes that competence predicts performance, in reality the relationship is far more complicated and is influenced by both systemic and individual factors. Klass (2007) also describes a 'situational' rather than 'attributional' model of competence and performance: this recognizes that doctors' performance is subject to complex influences and fluctuations.

The determinants of doctors' performance can be classified as: individual (internal) factors and work-associated (external) factors (Cox et al. 2006, p. 159). We will examine the role of each of these elements (table 31.1).

Individual factors

Health

The impact of health on doctors' performance has received relatively little attention (Harrison and Sterland 2006) but it is estimated that

Table 31.1 The determinants of doctors' performance

Individual (internal) factors	Work-associated (external) factors
Health	Climate
Personality and attitudes	Culture
Undergraduate education received	Team working and leadership
Impact of CPD	Workload, sleep, and shift work

up to 15% of doctors' fitness to practise will be impaired through health at some stage in their careers. Eight percent of concerns referred to the GMC in 2010 concerned health, including mental and behavioural illness, physical illness and adapting practice when ill (GMC 2011). Of 1472 cases investigated by NCAS between December 2007 and March 2009, 24% of concerns related to health problems, amongst which mental health issues and alcohol misuse were prominent (National Patient Safety Agency 2009).

Surveys from around the world have suggested that doctors may be reluctant to consult their colleagues about their health (Harrison and Sterland 2006). Mental health, stress and emotional problems are present in a significant minority and self-prescribing is also prevalent (Bruguera et al. 2001; Davidson and Schattner 2003).

Both the GMC (2011) and NCAS (2009) receive more concerns about older doctors, a finding replicated in North America (Kohatsu et al. 2004). Given that cognition is known to decline with age, the role of cognitive deficits in underperforming doctors is an important consideration. Gibson et al. (2006) point out that assessment of cognition is complex and multifaceted. There is no existing quick questionnaire able to assess higher functions for doctors in this context and specialist occupational health assessment, backed up by neuropsychiatry and neuropsychology, is necessary.

Cognitive impairment was found in a significant minority of 45 physicians with performance difficulties referred to the regulator in Ontario, Canada and was sufficient to explain their failure to improve with remediation (Turnbull et al. 2006). The authors noted that referencing to neuropsychological scores for an age-matched population underestimates the impairment. If referencing was made to age independent measures, it strongly predicted both performance on competency tests and success in remediation. Arguably, neuropsychological testing prior to remediation could save expending valuable resources on remediation for doctors who might be better served by a career change or retirement.

Doctors are known to suffer from higher rates of occupational stress, depression and substance misuse when compared with the general population or other professions, while levels of psychosis and personality disorders are similar (Firth-Cozens 2006a). Stress above threshold levels consistently affects around 28% of doctors, compared with 18% in the general population (Firth-Cozens 2003), and it impacts on patient care (Firth-Cozens 2001; Taylor et al. 2007).

Misuse of drugs and alcohol are important health factors, known to be prevalent in a significant minority that may also affect doctors' performance (Brooks et al. 2011). Stress, easy access to drugs, personality traits prevalent in doctors, and the increasing prevalence of substances misuse within society in general, are all potential underlying causes (Ghodse and Galea 2006). The NHS Practitioner Health Programme (2010), which provides a comprehensive specialist service to doctors in London, saw 184 patients in its first year of operation, of which 62% had mental health problems, 36% addiction problems, and 2% physical problems alone.

Personality and attitudes

Descriptions of disruptive doctors and how to manage their behaviour originate from North America (Swiggart et al. 2009). In the USA disruptive behaviour, which can be seen as a dysfunctional response to stress, is a leading cause of referral to regulators (Adshead et al. 2011).

The Five Factor Model of Personality, known as the 'Big Five' is widely researched and regarded as a good predictor of job performance (Barrick et al. 2001).The trait of conscientiousness—being hard working, organized, and self-disciplined—is the most consistently valid predictor of performance and its measurement has been advocated as a tool to measure professionalism in medical students (McLachlan et al. 2009). Emotional stability, being resilient and relaxed under pressure, is also a predictor of work performance. Extroversion may be related to performance in client-facing occupations, which would include many areas of medicine (Firth-Cozens and King 2006). Personality characteristics may show a U-shaped curve, in that in either extreme they may be counterproductive (Firth-Cozens and King 2006). Disruptive behaviours may arise from overplayed strengths.

Doctors referred for remediation frequently express feelings that they have been treated unjustly and may exhibit emotional responses, related to loss of professional status, seen in bereavement (Whiteman and Trompetas 2005). Chronic embitterment syndrome describes a condition in which a single act of perceived injustice leads to chronic symptoms of anger, ruminations, and helplessness (Sensky 2009).This condition may be seen as post-traumatic and precipitated by a specific life event, in this case feelings of entitlement thwarted by a perceived gross injustice (Linden et al. 2008).

Medical education and continous professional development

Undergraduate education

Communication skills teaching are now a core part of the curriculum in most medical schools (*Tomorrow's Doctors* (GMC 2003)). It is recognized that teaching communication skills to medical students improves skills in relationship building, organization, time management, patient assessment, negotiation, and shared decision-making. (Paice 2006;Yedidia et al. 2003). In addition medical undergraduates in the UK now have opportunities for small group learning and self-directed learning and for the linking of learning to practice wherever possible, with experience of patient contact in all years of the curriculum (GMC 2003 paras 100–105). All of this should prepare undergraduates for later stages in professional life where effective team working, and the ability to learn from practice, and to reflect critically on one's own practice, are key to maintaining levels of performance (Steward 2009, p. 234).

This is in contrast to the experience of previous generations of doctors whose undergraduate teaching was fact-based and didactically delivered, with no teaching of communication skills, and a prevailing ethos within medical culture tending to impose on students 'unrealistic expectations [of themselves], denial, indirect communication patterns, rigidity, and isolation' (McKegney 1989). This early formative professional experience when added to other

factors such as situations of isolated clinical practice can leave practitioners unprepared to meet the challenges of maintaining standards of clinical practice in an ever-changing world of increasing patient demand and accountability

Continuous professional development (CPD)

With the completion of postgraduate specialty training, doctors assume a greater level of autonomy and in parallel take individual responsibility for their ongoing learning.

In the UK a culture of learning has developed in the last 10–15 years which has had an enabling influence on practitioners in this respect. The publication in 1998 of the 'Chief Medical Officer's Review of Continuing Professional Development in General Practice' (Calman 1998) was an endorsement by policy makers of the concept of lifelong learning, of the value of learning in interprofessional teams, of the use of personal development plans to give direction to learning, of the value of linking learning to practice, of learning being evidence-based, and of the importance of educational leadership at all levels (fig. 31.1). The NHS Appraisal system introduced in the UK in 2002 (Department of Health 2002) has facilitated the development of a growing awareness and understanding among doctors of the nature and value of continuing professional development in its many forms (Schostak et al. 2010).Thus the policy context has become more favourable over the last 15 years for the fostering and promotion of continuing professional development in medicine.

External factors

Climate and culture

Within organizations, the term climate is used to describe the experience of the work environment and the term culture to describe the values which produce manifestations that include hierarchy, informal practices, rituals and common narratives, including jargon (West and Spendlove 2006). While in may seem obvious that organizational culture will affect the performance of individuals, there is a lack of high-quality studies that demonstrate direct effects (West and Spendlove 2006).

There is, however, evidence that suggests national culture may be important.

In the UK, doctors referred to the GMC with an international primary medical qualification, both in the European Union (EU) and outside were more likely to receive high impact decisions (suspension or erasure) than doctors whose primary medical qualification

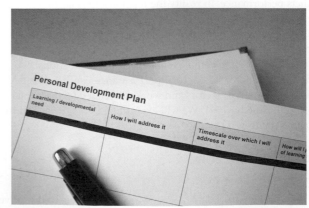

Figure 31.1 Formulating a personal development plan.

was in the UK (Humphrey et al. 2011). In 2010 non-UK qualified doctors were no more likely than their UK qualified colleagues to be the subject of a complaint to the GMC and, although ethnicity data held by the GMC is incomplete, there is no evidence that ethnicity is related to the likelihood of a doctor facing a complaint (GMC 2011). Referrals to NCAS in the UK are also higher for non-white doctors who qualified outside the UK, but there was no suggestion that non-white doctors who qualified in the UK were being referred disproportionately (workforce comparators being available in the hospital and community sectors, but not for general practice where data on ethnicity was not available) (National Patient Safety Agency 2009).

While the data must be interpreted cautiously, it can be argued that culture may be playing an important role in the difficulties experienced by medical graduates working internationally. Practices in healthcare in different countries vary widely, and medical theory and practice is closely interwoven with cultural traditions (Hofstede et al. 2010). Dimensions of culture, deeply embedded value systems that are learned in childhood, whilst differing in individuals, show clear trends across different countries (Hofstede et al. 2010). These dimensions, based on large surveys of value preferences, can help us to understand the difficulties experienced by doctors working outside their own culture (Freeman and Jalil 2011).

For example, 'power distance' describes the extent to which people are expected to behave and be treated equally in a society. Doctors coming from 'high power distance' societies have a relationship with teachers based on assumed authority and may be unfamiliar with the expectation of 'low power distance' societies where learners are self-directed and willing to challenge their teacher's assertions. Similar considerations apply to relationships with patients and the extent to which power and decision-making in consultations is shared. A number of cultural dimensions may be implicated in other difficulties relating to respecting boundaries, probity and standards of governance.

Language competence may also be an issue for international medical graduates (GMC 2011).

Team working and leadership

Teams are groups of people who share responsibility for specific tasks and their effectiveness is commonly understood in terms of an input–process–output model. There is evidence to support a number of input factors when creating teams, and process factors to maximize the effective output of individual members. These include time to reflect on functioning, creativity through tolerating constructive conflict and uncertainty, mutual support, and effective leadership (West and Borrill 2006).

Leadership can usefully be defined as creating 'the conditions for people to thrive, individually and collectively, and achieve significant goals' (Pendleton and Furnham 2012, p. 2). In the context of remediation, we are concerned with the impact of leadership on team members and, while good leadership may benefit patient care (Firth-Cozens 2006b), negative leadership traits, possibly resulting from overplayed strengths, can cause disruption. Maladaptive patterns, resulting from leadership pressures, have been likened to the exaggerated responses seen in personality disorders (Pendleton and Furnham 2012, p. 146).

Another personality related issue, 'hubris syndrome', has been suggested to arise from overplayed confidence amongst individuals in positions of power, leading to recklessness, inattention to detail and restlessness (Owen 2006). While Owen's (2006) focus is on politicians, the same dysfunctional behaviours may be observed in disruptive medical leaders.

Workload, sleep, and shift work

Workload, sleep deprivation, and shift working, frequently in combination, can all adversely affect doctors' performance with potentially severe consequences (Smith 2006). For example, studies have shown that junior doctors working in intensive care make fewer serious medical errors when extended shifts of over 24 hours are reduced (Landrigan et al. 2004); the speed and accuracy of laparoscopic surgeons' performance is impaired after a night on call (Grantcharov et al. 2001); and surgeons operating after less than 6 hours sleep availability have higher complication rates (Rothschild et al. 2009).

However, reducing working times and shift lengths may inadvertently create new problems, for instance implementing the European Working Time Directive, has created difficulties with rotas and training time availability, particularly in some acute specialities (Temple 2010)

Medical care needs to be provided on a 24-hour basis and the effects on performance of long hours and sleep deprivation can potentially be ameliorated through either systemic intervention, such as changing work patterns, or individually with advice on measures such as sleep hygiene.

However, despite extensive research, there remains uncertainty on precisely how long a person can safely work, the impact of different shift systems, and which individual interventions are effective in reducing the adverse effects of shift and night work (Smith 2006)

What constitutes effective remediation?

Having explored the factors that are thought to influence doctors' performance, we will now focus on remediation processes and what we know about their effectiveness. We will first consider the pedagogic theory behind remediation, and then review the evidence to support common interventions.

Pedagogic theory

Conceptually there are three broad overlapping learning theories. Behaviourist (associative) perspectives emphasize learning as a process, constructivist (cognitive) perspectives emphasize learning as developing understanding, and the situative perspective emphasises learning as a social practice (Mayes and De Freitas 2007). We will consider the particular issues that influence the pedagogy of remediation, tracing the journey through assessment, motivation to change, learning, and reassessment.

Prior to remediation an assessment is undertaken, either globally or limited to specific areas of concern, and learning needs are described, but not necessarily accepted by the doctor concerned, with variable consideration given to the underlying causes of underperformance. Learner motivation is determined by a combination of expectancy and value, with extrinsic factors, including social motivation, and intrinsic factors, based on interest in the subject (Biggs 2003). In remediation powerful extrinsic motivation may arise from the threat to a doctor's career by the regulator, with its accompanying loss of status and power. Extrinsic motivation of this kind may be helpful, but does not necessarily imply a deep interest in real change.

'Phenomenography' seeks to understand the learner's perspective (Biggs 2003) and draws from the work of Marton and Saljo (1976) who observed 'deep' and 'surface' approaches to learning. Deep learning, which reflects a real interest in the subject, contrasts with superficial learning that implies learning by rote. This describes the approach to a particular task, and is not an attribute of the learners themselves. Harnessing deep and genuine interest in learning and developing new skills appears important to successful remediation. Frequently, this requires enabling doctors to move on from feelings of bitterness and passivity and to take real ownership of their learning (Whiteman and Jamieson 2007). Motivational interviewing approaches, which engage the collaboration of the leaner, are more likely to be helpful than confrontation (Cohen and Rhydderch 2007). Formulation of a personal development plan creates a personal curriculum and facilitates the doctor taking ownership of learning (Whiteman and Jamieson 2007). Powerful motivation to remain in medical practice may not be helpful in cases where a career change, or retirement, is the most realistic option.

Learners tend to work towards the requirements of assessment, and a well designed curriculum utilizes this observation. The assessment should be clearly linked to the aims and objectives of the programme and require deep learning for success—a concept described as 'constructive alignment' (Biggs 2003). For doctors' remediation this implies realistic reassessment of both competence and performance, and typically this includes simulated consultations, triangulated by written tests of applied knowledge, and direct observation of practice in workplace based assessments.

Experiential learning, a cornerstone of most remediation programmes, is conceived as a cycle, with the learner constructing knowledge through experience, reflection, building on existing theory, and then reapplying the learning in new situations (Kolb 1984). Within this constructivist conception, behaviourist techniques, such as the use of feedback and reinforcement are widely used. Effective feedback needs to describe specific behaviours and not the person. Tools which meet this criterion include 'agenda led outcomes based analysis' which invites the learner to ask for help, agree objectives, review performance descriptively, and act out alternatives. This reduces the risk of negative feedback when working in groups and is also effective in one-to-one situations (Silverman et al 2004).

Analysing learning styles is popular in general practice education and may provide useful insights into how we learn, described as 'metacognition'. They are based on preferences for activities within the learning cycle and may have links with personality, for instance extroverts preferring active and pragmatic activities and introverts are more drawn towards reflection and theorizing (Kolb 1984). Numerous tools are available, with variable reliability and validity, but their usefulness has been contested (Coffield et al. 2004). Providing evidence of effectiveness is methodologically challenging. Since personality is cited as a factor in underperformance, working with personality assessments may also be helpful (Cohen and Rhydderch 2007).

One-to-one learner–trainer relationships are typical in remediation, often supplemented by small group work, and cost, together with locating suitable placements, may be an issue. Lectures convey information to large numbers of learners cheaply, but risk being teacher-centred and didactic (Biggs 2003) and it is doubtful whether they are effective on their own in developing complex skills. E-learning is an alternative, which, in practice, also risks becoming a means of transmitting information rather than a means of education (Biggs 2003, p. 213), but it can potentially be 'blended' effectively with other modalities such as small-group work (Littlejohn and Pegler 2007). Where courses are used in remediation, deep learning may be encouraged through clear objectives and reflection on how the learning will be used in practice.

Constructivists see learning as a complex outcome determined by both the learner's perceptions and input, and the teacher's approach, and varying according to the learning material (Biggs 2003; Ramsden 2003). This conception recognizes that multiple influences are involved, and is not prescriptive in advocating any one approach but places the focus on what the learner is achieving. Freire's (1996, p. 60) aphorism that 'liberating education describes acts of cognition, not transferrals of information' complements this thinking,

The pedagogy of remediation outlined so far has been based on constructivism and behaviourism but situative approaches, emphasizing learning as a social practice, are also important. Learners are seen as 'legitimate peripheral participants' in a 'community of practice' in which they progress from practising a limited range of skills to becoming responsible for more complex and complete practice tasks (Lave and Wenger 1991). In remediation, previously independent practitioners can be seen as having been relegated from full to peripheral participants and their progress in retraining determines their future reintegration as full members of the medical community. This process of socialization involves modelling attitudes, values, and behaviours, and for doctors with performance difficulties, who have frequently worked in poorly performing and dysfunctional teams, working within a new community of practice may be helpful. At the end of remediation it is important, and sometimes challenging, to provide maintenance for the individual in a new team in which the improved practice can continue.

Evidence

Having reviewed the pedagogic theories that underpin remediation we will now consider what interventions have been shown to be effective, an area that is less well researched than assessment (Cohen and Rhydderch 2007).

We have made reference to Kirkpatrick's (1998) four levels, which provide a useful framework to measure educational outcomes, based on:

- Level one—learners' reaction to teaching
- Level two—learners' changes in knowledge, skills and attitudes
- Level three—behavioural changes in practice
- Level four—results for the organization and clients.

A variety of terms to describe the processes used in remediation, including 'mentoring', 'educational supervision', 'clinical supervision', and 'coaching' are used interchangeably and inconsistently by organizations involved and in the literature; it is helpful to have clear definitions of what is intended (Clark et al. 2006) (fig. 31.2). Remedial interventions typically comprise three different patterns, depending on the practitioner's needs and the potential risks to patient safety. Professional support such as mentorship and supervision, whilst the doctor is continuing to practise, may be suitable for practitioners with relatively minor performance issues, who are working in a suitably safe environment. Full retraining, typically in a training practice, may be indicated for practitioners with more significant performance difficulties or who are practising in potentially unsafe contexts. Finally, support outside service provision may be needed for practitioners who have been suspended by regulators (Whiteman and Jamieson 2007, p. 667).

We will review the common interventions applied in remediation, focusing in each case on the supporting evidence of benefit and then consider examples of remediation programmes from around the world. We assume that, before starting remediation, any health issues affecting performance will have been addressed, ongoing health support provided if needed, and appropriate reasonable adjustments made in the workplace in consultation with occupational health.

Mentoring and coaching

Mentoring may be defined as 'regular guidance and support offered by a more experienced colleague' (Clark et al. 2006) and this may include help with career plans and relationships as well as clinical issues. Mentoring relationships are regarded as confidential, and mentors are not expected to write reports about clients (GMC 2010). Mentors are often, but not necessarily, working in the same organization or field as the mentee (Oxley and Standing Committee on Postgraduate Medical and Dental Education 1998), and the relationship is typically voluntary. Confusingly, the term is widely used in the literature to describe a variety of supervisory relationships (Oxley et al. 2003).

Coaching may be defined simply as 'unlocking a person's potential to maximise their own performance' (Clark et al. 2006). The emphasis in coaching is on the formative aspects of enhancing

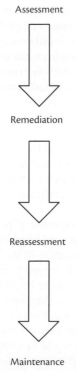

Assessment

Remediation

Reassessment

Maintenance

Figure 31.2 The remediation process.

performance and typically, as with mentoring, relationships tend to be voluntary and confidential.

A review of the benefits of mentoring for doctors (Oxley et al. 2003) noted that the bulk of the literature on this subject comes from the USA and centres on academic faculty development. In the UK, mentoring is described with enthusiasm by authors, and there is widespread agreement that it is beneficial. Mentoring within remediation is not specifically cited and research on mentoring in underperformance appears to be lacking (Purkiss et al. 2008).

A Dutch study (Overeem et al. 2010) of peer mentoring in doctor performance assessments, utilizing 360-degree feedback reports from peers, found that, whilst mentors used strategies to encourage reflection and enable mentees to integrate their peers' views into their self-assessments, they reported difficulty in disregarding their own views of their colleagues.

Empirically, it makes sense to recommend mentoring for some doctors with performance difficulties, particularly when issues with relationships, team working, and career choices are prominent, but it is not possible to cite evidence demonstrating benefits from this intervention. Mentoring is commonly prescribed as part of remediation by regulators (GMC 2010) and it is unclear whether the mentoring relationship is affected by being prescribed rather than being voluntary.

Clinical and educational supervision

Difficulties surround the definition of supervision, and the distinction between 'clinical supervision' and 'educational supervision'. A broad definition of clinical supervision is 'an exchange between practising professionals to enable the development of professional skills' (Clark et al. 2006). This purposefully encompasses a wide variety of formal and informal contexts and leaves open the issues of monitoring and accountability. Proctor's (1994) view of supervision as normative, when it focuses on rules and standards, formative, when it focuses on development, and restorative, when it seeks to sustain colleagues in their roles is useful and allows for a balance of each element depending on the context. The essential aims of supervision can also be seen as ensuring patient safety and promoting professional development and this comprises three functions—education, support, and administration (Kilminster and Jolly 2000, p. 829).

Educational supervision can be defined as 'organised clinical supervision taking place in the context of a recognised training' (Clark et al. 2006). As well as supportive and developmental roles, it implies a normative function of assessing progress against required standards and providing reports. It has also been described as a process similar to a series of regular appraisals (Lloyd and Becker 2007, p. 375).

The published evidence base for the benefits of supervision is typically highly context specific, for example there is evidence of its benefits in surgery (Fallon et al.1993), emergency department medicine (Sox et al. 1998), and outpatients (Gennis and Gennis 1993). There is some limited evidence for the benefits of educational supervision, which is a newer concept, and implies a broader less hands-on approach, in trainee contexts (Kilminster and Jolly 2000) but not specifically in relation to remediation.

Remediation programmes

A recent survey of remediation programmes in Australia, Canada, New Zealand, the UK, and the USA provides an overview of current practice in the major Anglophone nations (Humphrey and Locke 2007). The 15 programmes surveyed differed widely in:

+ age, with most having been established in the last decade
+ size, with nine assessing less than 20 doctors per year
+ funding and
+ the impetus behind their establishment.

In most cases the aims centred on improving deficits in doctors' performance but the programmes varied in relation to the emphasis placed on overall performance, as opposed to specific areas of deficit, and only a minority of programmes made reference to enhancement, defined as 'increasing, heightening, intensifying or adding value to knowledge' (Humphrey and Locke 2007).

Programmes varied in the extent to which they assessed underlying influences on performance, such as health, personality and cognition. With the exception of the Individual Support Unit in Wales (Cohen et al. 2005), their remediation processes were framed purely educationally. NCAS was exceptional in focusing beyond the individual to make recommendations about team working (Berrow et al. 2007). Direct involvement in the remediation process varied and, whilst exit assessments were frequently systematic and intense, information on outcomes was not sought. None of the programmes carried out any long-term systematic follow up, making it impossible to assess how effective they were in maintaining improved performance or addressing the original concerns in the future.

The evidence base relating to the effectiveness of CPD interventions in general suggests that they work best when they involve active learning, with the opportunity to deliberately practise new skills and receive individualized feedback (Mansouri and Lockyer 2007). Relatively few studies have focused on outcomes in remediation specifically.

Hauer et al.'s (2009) thematic review of remediation across the continuum of medical careers found seven studies on medical students, and two on training grade doctors, all of which used examinations of knowledge and skills to assess and reassess the participants. The outcomes were therefore at Kirkpatrick level two and did not assess changes in behaviour. Four studies of remediation in practising doctors, all from Canada, were reported. None measured outcomes at Kirkpatrick's level four, improvement in outcomes for patients, but three demonstrated positive changes in behaviour. None of the studies included a control group of poor performers who did not receive remediation and methodological weaknesses arose from potential observer bias.

A small study from Ontario found negative findings (Hanna et al. 2000) in five moderate to severely underperforming doctors given a 3-year individualized remediation programme, including state of the art educational interventions with proven benefits in other contexts. One doctor improved, whilst three actually deteriorated, and the authors speculate that, given the subjects were older, cognitive decline may have been a factor. This finding is consistent with the suggestion that cognitive assessment may be advisable prior to embarking on extensive remediation programmes for older doctors (Turnbull et al. 2000; Turnbull et al. 2006).

Reassessment of performance

Because regulators and other bodies involved in remediation have developed assessments that are robust and defensible against legal challenge, paradoxically it may be easier to measure outcomes for doctors receiving remediation than their colleagues experiencing generic CPD. However, passing an assessment, which could be considered as demonstrating learning and behaviour changes at a specific end point, does not necessarily ensure continuing changes in practice or improved health outcomes for patients. Hauer et al. (2009) lament the lack of research available on the outcomes of remediation, both in the short and long term.

Putting the evidence into practice

We will now summarize the themes from the literature to provide practical suggestions for remediation of underperformance in practice. It is axiomatic that the first our first priority should always be the safety of patients.

Concerns about performance can arise in any stage of the medical life cycle, from undergraduate studies through to retirement. Tackling concerns early makes sense empirically and may be facilitated by formal policies for addressing underperformance in trainees (Anderson et al. 2011; Lusznat et al. 2010). Once doctors complete specialist training, governance becomes more problematic: the prevalence of underperformance, how it can be most effectively identified, and where remedial resources are best concentrated, remains uncertain. This is likely to be an issue of growing importance as the ongoing development of clinical governances systems, including revalidation of doctors, increases medical professional accountability.

We have argued that the determinants of underperformance are complex and include personal and systemic factors as well as knowledge and skills. This presents particular challenges and, given the complexity of many cases, educational work with underperforming doctors is challenging and requires high levels of skill and patience. Many doctors referred for remediation express anger, and a belief that they have not received justice from assessing authorities. Some individuals, who have tried to function in unacceptable workplace environments, will have a degree of justification. Supervision to support case workers through these complexities may be helpful (Whiteman and Jamieson 2007) and the London Deanery Professional Support Unit provides supervision utilizing a model based on narrative and systemic techniques (Launer and Halpern 2006).

Educational interventions in remediation are less well researched than assessment, and literature reviews emphasize that, whilst there is much good practice in different areas, approaches frequently lack uniformity.

From a pedagogical perspective if practitioners are underperforming and in need of remedial interventions a key factor in their ability to change their situation is the ability to take control of their own learning. First, they need to have a clear understanding of their situation before they can begin to change it. Second, they need to be able to appreciate the importance of their own active involvement in their learning. Freire (1996, p. 33) is clear on the significance of active personal involvement through 'praxis: reflection and action upon the world in order to transform it'. Freire's (1996, p. 90) notion of conscientization (from the Portuguese *conscientização*), an awakening of critical awareness as a precursor to change, is analogous to the idea of andragogy promoted by Knowles (1973, p. 45). Knowles' first assumption of andragogy is that of 'self-concept: as a person matures his self concept moves from one of being a dependent personality toward one of being a self-directed human being'.

In addition to such self-direction the autonomous practitioner/learner needs to understand the value of experience as a resource for learning, not only as an individual but as a member of a team. For older practitioners with personal experience of a traditional didactically based undergraduate medical education, especially if they have worked in a degree of isolation of whatever kind in later professional life, and have had no exposure to more recent ideas about learning, this can be a difficult step to take. They need to be able to trust their own experience, and the experience of others, in contexts such as practice-based interprofessional clinical case discussion, as a legitimate source of professional learning for all participants. The concept of individual experiential learning is thoroughly examined by Kolb (1984). The value and nature of team-based learning is well expressed by Lave and Wenger (1991, p. 15):

> learning is a process that takes place in a participation framework, not in an individual mind. This means among other things, that it is mediated by the differences of perspective among the co-participants. It is the community, or at least those participating in the learning context, who 'learn' under this definition. Learning is, as it were, distributed among co participants, not a one-person act.

As a recent study has shown, if a practitioner is underperforming clinically they are also likely to possess identifiable characteristics of both isolation, including little discernible involvement in educational activities, and lack of insight (Holden et al. 2012). The challenges for remediation programmes with such practitioners are significant.

Remediation is a litigious area and requires boundaries, lines of accountability and decision making that is defensible to challenge. Delivery of remediation by a body that is independent of the assessing authority may be helpful in achieving this (Cohen and Rhydderch 2007) and clear, evidence-based documentation is essential throughout the process.

Conclusions

♦ Concerns about a doctor's performance can arise at any stage in the medical lifecycle, from undergraduate and postgraduate training through to retirement.

♦ The prevalence of underperformance, how it can be most effectively identified, and where remedial resources are best concentrated, remains uncertain.

♦ The determinants of underperformance are complex and frequently include personal and systemic factors as well as knowledge and skills.

♦ Educational interventions in remediation are less well researched than assessment, and approaches frequently lack uniformity.

♦ Educational work with doctors whose performance has given cause for concern is challenging and requires high levels of skill and patience.

♦ A broad range of pedagogic concepts can be applied to remediation, with the doctor's development of insight and readiness to change being critical.

References

Academy of Medical Royal Colleges, The Academy Remediation Working Group, London (2009) *Remediation and Revalidation* [Online] http://www.aomrc.org.uk/publications/statements/doc_download/63-remediation-and-revalidation.html Accessed 15 March 2012

Adshead, G., Old, P., and Wadman, K. (2011) Personality and behaviour. In: *NCAS Annual Conference 2011: Disruptive behaviour—Tackling concerns about practitioner behaviour.* [Online] www.ncas.nhs.uk/EasySiteWeb/GatewayLink.aspx?alId=128942 Accessed 22 March 2013

Anderson, F., Cachia, P.G., Monie, R., and Connacher, A.A. (2011) Supporting trainees in difficulty, a new approach for Scotland, *Scottish Med J.* 56(2) 72

Bahrami, J. and Evans, A. (2001) Underperforming doctors in general practice: a survey of referrals to UK Deaneries. *Br J Gen Pract.* 51(472): 892

Barrick, M.R., Mount, M.K., and Judge, T.A. (2001) Personality and performance at the beginning of the new millennium: What do we know and where do we go next? *Int J Selection Assess.* 9(1–2): 9–30

Berrow, D., Humphrey, C., Field, R., et al. (2007) Clarifying concerns about doctors' clinical performance: what is the contribution of assessment by the National Clinical Assessment Service? *J Health Org Manag.* 21(2–3): 333–343

Biggs, J. (2003) *Teaching for Quality Learning at University.* 2nd edn. London: Open University Press

Brooks, S.K., Chalder, T., and Gerada, C. (2011) Doctors vulnerable to psychological distress and addictions: Treatment from the Practitioner Health Programme. *J Ment Health.* 20(2) 157–164

Bruguera, M., Guri, J., Arteman, A., Grau Valldosera, J., and Carbonell, J. (2001) Care of doctors to their health care: Results of a postal survey, *Medicina Interna.* 117(13): 492–494

Calman, K. (1998) A Review of Continuing Professional Development in General Practice, a report by the Chief Medical Officer , Department of Health [Online] http://www.publications.doh.gov.uk/pub/docs/doh/cmodev.pdf Accessed 23 February 2012

Clark, P., Jamieson, A., Launer, J., Trompetas, A., Whiteman, J., and Williamson, D. (2006) Intending to be a supervisor, mentor or coach? Which, what for and why? *Educ Prim Care.* 17: 109–116

Coffield, F., Moseley, D., Hall, E., and Ecclestone, K. 2004, Should we be using Learning Styles? What research has to say to practice. [Online] http://www.voced.edu.au/content/ngv12401 Accessed 15 March 2012

Cohen, D. and Rhydderch, M. (2007) Assessment when performance gives rise to concern. Abingdon: Radcliffe Publishing, p. 150

Cohen, D., Rollnick, S., Smail, S., Kinnersley, P., Houston, H., and Edwards, K. 2005, Communication, stress and distress: evolution of an individual support programme for medical students and doctors. *Med Educ.* 39(5): 476–481

Cox, J., King, J., Hutchinson, A., and McAvoy, P. (2006) *Understanding Doctors' Performance.* Abingdon: Radcliffe Publishing

Davidson, S.K. and Schattner, P. L. 2003, Doctors' health-seeking behaviour: a questionnaire survey. *Med J Aust.* 179(6): 302–305

Department of Health (2002) Appraisal for General Practitioners: Guidance. [Online] http://www.dh.gov.uk/en/Publicationsandstatistics/Publications/PublicationsPolicyAndGuidance/DH_4006979 Accessed 9 December 2007

Dudek, N.L., Marks, M.B., and Regehr, G. (2005) Failure to fail: the perspectives of clinical supervisors. *Acad Med.* 80(10): S84

Fallon, W.F., Wears, R.L., and Tepas III, J.J. (1993) Resident supervision in the operating room: does this impact on outcome? *J Trauma.* 35(4): 556

Finucane, P.M., Bourgeois-Law, G.L.A., Ineson, S.L., and Kaigas, T.M. (2003) A Comparison of Performance Assessment Programs for Medical

Practitioners in Canada, Australia, New Zealand, and the United Kingdom. *Acad Med.* 78(8): 837–843

Firth-Cozens, J. (2001) Interventions to improve physicians' well-being and patient care. *Soc Sci Med.* 52(2): 215–222

Firth-Cozens, J. (2003) Doctors, their wellbeing, and their stress. *BMJ.* 326(7391): 670–671

Firth-Cozens, J. (2006a) A perspective on stress and depression. In: J. Cox, J. King, P. Hutchinson, et al. (eds) *Understanding Doctor's Performance* (pp. 22–37). Abingdon: Radcliffe

Firth-Cozens, J. (2006b) Leadership and the quality of healthcare. In: J. Cox, J. King, P. Hutchinson, et al. (eds) *Understanding Doctors' Performance* (pp. 123–133). Oxford: Radcliffe

Firth-Cozens, J. and King, J. (2006) Are psychological factors linked to performance? In: J. Cox, J. King, P. Hutchinson, et al. (eds) *Understanding Doctors' Performance* (pp. 67–77). Abingdon: Radcliffe

Freeman, R. and Jalil, M. (2011) 5th Meeting of UK Performance Group hosted by Wessex Deanery, 19 May 2011, Unpublished

Freire, P. (1996) *Pedagogy of the Oppressed.* London: Penguin Books

Gennis, V.M. and Gennis, M.A. (1993) Supervision in the outpatient clinic. *J Gen Intern Med.* 8(7): 378–380

Ghodse, H. and Galea, S. (2006) Misuse of drugs and alcohol. In: J. Cox et al. (eds) *Understanding Doctor's Performance* (pp. 38–45). Abingdon: Radcliffe

Gibson, K., Kartsounis, L., and |Kopelman, M. 2006, Cognitive impairment and performance. In: J. Cox, J. King, P. Hutchinson, et al. (eds) *Understanding Doctors' Performance* (pp. 48–60). Abingdon: Radcliffe Publishing

GMC (2003) *Tomorrow's Doctors.* [Online] http://www.gmc-uk.org/education/undergraduate/tomorrows_doctors_2009.asp Accessed 15 March 2012

GMC (2008) GMC: Guidance on Good Practice. [Online] http://www.gmc-uk.org/guidance/index.asp Accessed 5 March 2013

GMC (2010) Glossary of Terms used in Fitness to Practise Actions. [Online] http://www.gmc-uk.org/Glossary_of_Terms_used_in_Fitness_to_Practise_Actions.dot.pdf_25416199.pdf Accessed 5 March 2013

GMC (2011) The State of Medical Education and Practice 2011. [Online] http://www.gmc-uk.org/publications/10471.asp Accessed 15 March 2012

Goulet, F., Jacques, A., Gagnon, et al. (2002) Performance assessment. Family physicians in Montreal meet the mark! *Can Fam Phys.* 48(8): 1337

Grantcharov, T.P., Bardram, L., Peter, F.J., and Rosenberg, J. 2001, Laparoscopic performance after one night on call in a surgical department: prospective study. *BMJ.* 323(7323): 1222–1223

Hall, W., Violato, C., Lewkonia, R., et al. (1999) Assessment of physician performance in Alberta: the Physician Achievement Review. *CanMed Ass J.* 161(1): 52

Hanna, E., Premi, J., and Turnbull, J. (2000) Results of remedial continuing medical education in dyscompetent physicians. *Acad Med.* 75(2): 174–176

Harrison, J. and Sterland, J. (2006) The impact of health on performance. In: J. Cox, J. King, P. Hutchinson, et al. (eds) *Understanding Doctors' Performance* (pp. 4–21). Abingdon: Radcliffe

Hauer, K. E., Ciccone, A., Henzel, T. R., et al. 2009, Remediation of the deficiencies of physicians across the continuum from medical school to practice: a thematic review of the literature. *Acad Med.* 84(12): 1822

Hofstede, G.H., Hofstede, G.J., and Minkov, M. (2010) *Cultures and Organizations: Software for the Mind.* New York: McGraw-Hill Professional

Holden, J., Cox, S., and Hargreaves, S. (2012) Avoiding isolation and gaining insight, [Online] http://careers.bmj.com/careers/advice/view-article.html?id=20006663 BMJ Careers Accessed 23 February 2012

Humphrey, C., Hickman, S., and Gulliford, M.C. (2011) Place of medical qualification and outcomes of UK General Medical Council fitness to practise process: cohort study. *BMJ.* 342: 1817

Humphrey, C. and Locke, R. (2007) *Provision of Assessment and Remediation for Physicians About Whom Concerns Have Been Expressed: An international survey.* London: National Clinical Assessment Service

Irvine, D. (1997) The performance of doctors. II: Maintaining good practice, protecting patients from poor performance. *BMJ.* 314: 1613

Joesbury, H., Mathers, N., and Lane, P. (2001) Supporting GPs whose performance gives cause for concern: the North Trent experience. *Fam Pract.* 18(2): 123

Kilminster, S.M. and Jolly, B.C. 2000, Effective supervision in clinical practice settings: a literature review. *Med Educ.* 34(10): 827–840

Kirkpatrick, D.L. (1998) *Evaluating Training Programs: The Four Levels.* San Francisco: Berrett-Koehler

Klass, D. (2007) A performance-based conception of competence is changing the regulation of physicians' professional behavior. *Acad Med.* 82(6): 529–535

Knowles, M. (1973) *The Adult Learner: A Neglected Species.* Houston, TX: Gulf Publishing

Kohatsu, N.D., Gould, D., Ross, L.K., and Fox, P.J. (2004) Characteristics associated with physician discipline: a case-control study. *Arch Intern Med.* 164(6): 653

Kolb, D.A. (1984) *Experiential Learning: Experience as the Source of Learning and Development.* New Jersey: Prentice-Hall

Landrigan, C.P., Rothschild, J.M., Cronin, J.W., et al. (2004) Effect of reducing interns' work hours on serious medical errors in intensive care units. *N Engl J Med.* 351(18): 1838–1848

Launer, J. and Halpern, H. (2006) Reflective practice and clinical supervision: an approach to promoting clinical supervision among general practitioners. *Work Based Learn Prim Care.* 4(1): 69–72

Lave, J. and Wenger, E. (1991) Practice, person, social world. In: J. Lave, and E. Wenger *Situated Learning—Legitimate Peripheral Participation* (pp. 45–54). Cambridge: Cambridge University Press

Linden, M., Baumann, K., Rotter, M., and Schippan, B. (2008) Diagnostic criteria and the standardized diagnostic interview for posttraumatic embitterment disorder (PTED). *Int J Psychiatry Clin Pract.* 12(2): 93–96

Littlejohn, A. and Pegler, C. (2007) *Preparing for Blended e-Learning.* London: Routledge

Lloyd, B.W. and Becker, D. (2007) Paediatric specialist registrars' views of educational supervision and how it can be improved: a questionnaire study. *JRSM.* 100(8): 375

Lusznat, R., King, J., and du Boulay, C. (2010) The Wessex Deanery Strategy for Professional Support. [Online] http://www.wessexdeanery.nhs.uk/docs/Professional%20Support%20Strategy%202011.doc Accessed 5 March 2013

Mansouri, M. and Lockyer, J. (2007) A meta-analysis of continuing medical education effectiveness. *J Continuing Educ Health Prof.* 27(1): 6–15

Marton, F. and Saljo, R. (1976) On qualitative differences in learning: I and ll. *Br J Educ Psychol.* 46(1 & 2) 4–11, 128–148

Mayes T and De Freitas S (2007) Learning and e-learning: The role of theory. In: H. Beetham and R. Sharpe (eds) *Rethinking Pedagogy for a Digital Age: designing and delivering e-learning* (pp. 13–25). London: Routledge

McAuley, R.G., Paul, W.M., Morrison, G.H., Beckett, R.F., and Goldsmith, C.H. (1990) Five-year results of the peer assessment program of the College of Physicians and Surgeons of Ontario. *CMAJ.* 143(11): 1193

McKegney, C.P. 1989, Medical education: a neglectful and abusive family system. *Fam Med.* 21(6): 452

McLachlan, J.C., Finn, G., and Macnaughton, J. (2009) The conscientiousness index: a novel tool to explore students' professionalism. *Acad Med.* 84(5): 559

Miller, G.E. (1990) The assessment of clinical skills/competence/performance. *Acad Med.* 65(9): s63–s67

National Patient Safety Agency (2006) *National Clinical Assessment Service. Establishing the effectiveness and value of NCAS services.* [Online] http://www.ncas.npsa.nhs.uk/EasySiteWeb/GatewayLink.aspx?alId=9410. Accessed 15 March 2012

National Patient Safety Agency (2009) *NCAS Casework The first eight years.* [Online] http://www.ncas.npsa.nhs.uk/news/first-eight-years/ Accessed 15 March 2012

Norton, P.G. and Faulkner, D. (1999) A longitudinal study of performance of physicians' office practices: data from the Peer Assessment Program in Ontario, Canada. *The Joint Commission Journal on Quality Improvement.* 25(5): 252

Overeem, K., Driessen, E.W., Arah, O.A., Lombarts, K.M., Wollersheim, H.C., and Grol, R.P.T.M. (2010) Peer mentoring in doctor performance assessment: strategies, obstacles and benefits. *Med Educ.* 44(2): 140–147

Owen, L.D. (2006) Hubris and nemesis in heads of government. *J Roy Soc Med.* 99(11): 548

Oxley, J., Fleming, B., Golding, L., Pask, H., and Steven, A. (2003) Mentoring for doctors: enhancing the benefit, Improving Working Lives for Doctors, Doctors Forum. London: Department of Health

Oxley, J. and Standing Committee on Postgraduate Medical and Dental Education (1998) *Supporting Doctors and Dentists at Work: an enquiry into mentoring.* London: SCOPME.

Paice, E. (2006) The role of education and training. In: J. Cox et al. (eds) *Understanding Doctors' Performance* (pp. 78–90). Abingdon: Radcliffe

Pendleton, D. and Furnham, A. (2012) *Leadership All you Need to Know,* Basingstoke: Palgrave McMillan

Practitioner Health Programme (2010) *NHS Health Practitioner Programme. Report on the first year of operation.* London: NHS Specialised Commissioning Group

Proctor, B. (1994) Supervision—competence, confidence, accountability. *Br J Guidance Counselling.* 22(3): 309–318

Purkiss, V., Poll, D., Hill, K., Young, D., and Tinker, R. (2008) The development of a team to provide mentorship for underperformance. *Educ Prim Care.* 19(2): 197–201

Ramsden, P. (2003) *Learning to Teach in Higher Education.* 2nd edn. London: Routledge

Rethans, J.J., Norcini, J.J., Baron-Maldonado, M., et al. (2002) The relationship between competence and performance: implications for assessing practice performance. *Med Educ.* 36(10): 901–909

Rothschild, J.M., Keohane, C.A., Rogers, S., et al. (2009) Risks of complications by attending physicians after performing night time procedures. *JAMA.* 302: 14, 1565.

Schostak, J., Davis, M., Hanson, J., et al. (2010) *The Effectiveness of Continuing Professional Development.* London: College of Emergency Medicine

Sensky, T. (2009) Chronic embitterment and organisational justice. *Psychother Psychosom.* 79(2): 65–72

Silverman, J., Kurtz, S., and Draper, J. (2004) *Skills for Communicating with Patients.* 2nd edn. Abingdon: Radcliffe

Smith, L. (2006) Workload, sleep and shift work. In: J. Cox, J. King, P. Hutchinson, et al.(eds) *Understanding Doctor's Performance* (pp. 134–158). Abingdon: Radcliffe

Southgate, L., Cox. J., David, T., et al. (2001) The assessment of poorly performing doctors: the development of the assessment programmes for the General Medical Council's Performance Procedures. *Med Educ.* 35(Suppl 1): 2–8

Sox, C.M., Burstin, H.R., Orav, E.J., Conn, A., et al. (1998) The effect of supervision of residents on quality of care in five university-affiliated emergency departments. *Acad Med.* 73(7): 776

St George, I., McAvoy, P., and Kaigas, T.B. (2004) Assessing the competence of practicing physicians in New Zealand, Canada, and the United Kingdom: progress and problems. *Fam Med.* 36(3): 172–177

Steward, A. (2009) *Continuing your Professional Development in Lifelong Learning.* London and New York: Continuum

Swiggart, W.H., Dewey, C.M., Hickson, G.B., Finlayson, A.J., and Spickard Jr, W.A. 2009, A plan for identification, treatment, and remediation of disruptive behaviors in physicians. *Frontiers Health Serv Manag.* 25(4): 3

Taylor, C., Graham, J., Potts, H., Candy, J., Richards, M., and Ramirez, A. (2007) Impact of hospital consultants' poor mental health on patient care. *Br J Psychiatry.* 190(3): 268

Taylor, G. (1998) Underperforming doctors: a postal survey of the Northern Deanery. *BMJ.* 316(7146): 1705

Temple, J. (2010) Time for training: a review of the impact of the European Working Time Directive on the quality of training. London: Medical Education England

Turnbull, J., Carbotte, R., Hanna, E., et al. (2000) Cognitive difficulty in physicians. *Acad Med.* 75(2): 177–181

Turnbull, J., Cunnington, J., Unsal, A., Norman, G., and Ferguson, B. (2006) Competence and cognitive difficulty in physicians: a follow-up study. *Acad Med.* 81(10): 915–918

West, M. and Borrill, C. (2006) The influence of team working. In: J. Cox, J. King, P. Hutchinson, et al. (eds) *Understanding Doctors' Performance* (pp. 106–122). Abingdon: Radcliffe

West, M. and Spendlove, M. (2006) The impact of culture and climate in healthcare organisations. In: J. Cox, J. King, P. Hutchinson, et al. (eds) *Understanding Doctors' Performance* (pp. 91–105). Abingdon: Radcliffe

Whiteman, J. and Jamieson, A. (2007) Remediation with trust, assurance and safety. *Educ Prim Care.* 18(6): 665–673

Whiteman, J. and Trompetas, A. (2005) Deanery performance work in primary care, In: I. Hastie and N. Jackson (eds) *Postgraduate Medical Education and Training: A guide for primary and secondary care* (pp. 177–184), Abingdon: Radcliffe Publishing

Williams, B.W. (2006) The prevalence and special educational requirements of dyscompetent physicians. *J Cont Educ Health Prof.* 26(3): 173–191

Yedidia, M.J., Gillespie, C.C., Kachur, E., et al. (2003) Effect of communications training on medical student performance. *JAMA.* 290(9): 1157–1165

CHAPTER 32

Transitions in medical education

Michiel Westerman and Pim W. Teunissen

Anyone who knows anything about being a medical student and a preregistration house officer recognises that you learn more in a fortnight as a house officer when the chips are down than in six months as a student.

NRC Roberton

Reproduced from *British Medical Journal*, NRC Roberton, 'LMSSA: a back door entry into medicine?', 294, p. 1096, Copyright 1987, with permission from BMJ Publishing Group Ltd.

Introduction

Transitions are a double-edged sword. Medical students or doctors transitioning from one phase of medical education to the next or from one post to another have to cope with changes that range from hardly noticeable to mind-boggling. For instance, transitions may involve getting to know new colleagues, finding your way around in a new physical setting, figuring out differences in etiquette, traditions, and routines, learning new skills and knowledge to suit the needs of a different population of patients, and managing the impressions others form of you. In short, transitions represent both threats and opportunities. According to Wilkie and Raffaelli, each transition involves a 'fundamental re-examination of who and what we are, even if this processing is occurring at a largely unconscious level' (Wilkie and Raffaelli 2005, pp. 107–114). In this process of adjustment lies an opportunity to learn, but it may also lead to stress and even high levels of burn-out (Bogg et al. 2001; Teunissen and Westerman 2011a).

In this chapter a transition is defined as a period of change in which medical students or medical doctors experience some form of discontinuity in their professional life space, forcing them to respond by developing new behaviours or changing their professional life space in order to cope with the new situation. Apart from the impact transitions may have on individuals within the alleged medical education continuum, transitions have been a driving force behind many curriculum redesigns and even educational paradigm shifts. Moreover, the way in which medical students and doctors perceive transitions can be seen as a window into the merits and failings of the medical educational system. As an object of study, transitions are of practical as well as scientific importance (Teunissen and Westerman 2011b). Transitions will never be eliminated, so understanding the processes of smooth and disruptive transitions offers valuable lessons that are helpful in preparing future doctors for their responsibilities and guiding their continuing workplace education. From a scientific point of view, transitions are a research subject on the crossroads of many disciplines. Fields such as sociology, anthropology, and organizational and social psychology have long histories of studying how people adapt to new environments and cope with transitions. Transitions within in medical education offer a highly relevant context where theoretical concepts from other fields can be tested and refined.

This chapter explores the nature of three major transitions within the medical education continuum (Molenaar et al. 2009): the transition from preclinical education to clinical education, the shift from being a medical student to becoming a junior doctor, and, finally, the transition from registrar to medical specialist or general practitioner. We will not cover the transition from high school to medical school or smaller transitions throughout, for instance, specialty training where trainees move from one rotation to the next (Bernabeo et al. 2011).

After reviewing the origins of the three major transitions within the medical education continuum, we elaborate on the current state of the science for each of the transitions. Building on this overview of the literature, we characterize the way in which medical education researchers have problematized transitions. We contrast this with the problematization of transitions in the fields of sociology, organizational studies, and pedagogy. This juxtaposition of approaches to the study of transitions results in a number of practical and research implications for understanding transitions in the medical education domain.

Transitions within medical education and their origin, evolution, and characteristics

History of transitions within medical education

In the beginning of the 20th century, medical education found itself on the threshold of major reform. In 1908 the Council on Medical Education (instituted in 1904 by the American Medical Association) invited the Carnegie Foundation for the

Advancement of Teaching to survey the quality of medical schools and their programmes in both the United States and Canada. At that time over 150, mainly commercial, medical schools existed and the quality of medical education varied enormously throughout the country. Large numbers of inadequately trained physicians settled into medical practice, leading to great variations in practice and in some instances poor health care quality (Beck 2004). At the beginning of the 20th century the scientific method of systemized empirical medicine was finding its way into medicine and the American Medical Association was struggling with the dilemma of how best to implement this approach into medical training. The educationalist Abraham Flexner was invited to investigate all medical schools in North America and Canada in order to evaluate the system and formulate recommendations for reform. Looking back, Flexner's report had a major impact on the design of medical curricula throughout the world and laid the foundation for many of the transitions within the medical educational continuum that medical students and doctors are dealing with today (Flexner 1910).

In his revolutionary report Flexner recommended that after a number of years of preclinical training in fields such as anatomy, physiology, and pathology a clinical phase of medical training within teaching hospitals should follow. In the preclinical years students had to be trained in formal analytic reasoning which was, and still is, typical within the natural sciences (Cooke et al. 2006). Flexner argued that after the mastery of analytical reasoning, students had to enter the clinical setting: 'the facts are locked up in the patient. To the patient therefore, the medical student must go' (Flexner 1910). Within this clinical phase students could learn from real patients, and develop their clinical and diagnostic skills, under the supervision of experienced physicians. Thus, the transition from preclinical to the clinical stage of medical education became a fact. Postgraduate medical training as we know it nowadays did not exist at the time of Flexner. At that time only a small number of physicians specialized into a specific discipline after graduation from medical school. However, Flexner already foresaw the value of advanced training and specialization. And the rapid development and expansion of scientific biomedical knowledge gave rise to the institutionalization of postgraduate medical curricula. This resulted into additional transitions, one when leaving medical school and starting as a junior doctor in postgraduate training and another one after completion of specialty training and commencing work as a medical specialist or general practitioner.

In the following paragraphs we will present the main issues that are described within the medical educational literature within each of these transitions and how they have developed over time.

Characteristics and their development within the three major transitions

The transition from preclinical to clinical medical training

Throughout the 20th century medical curricula worldwide were largely based on Flexner's report and consisted of three to four years of preclinical education followed by a period of clinical training in teaching hospitals. Most medical schools had lecture-based curricula in which the essentials of anatomy, physiology, and pathology were taught to the student in order to prepare them for their clinical training. However, in the late 1960s the student centred pedagogy of problem-based learning (PBL) was developed in Canada

and would be adopted in the following decades as the new pedagogical perspective in (medical) education worldwide (Neville and Norman 2007; Norman and Schmidt 1992; Walton and Matthews 1989). Furthermore, in the 1990s undergraduate curricula entered another reform process by the shift from a process model of education towards an outcome based model or competency based education (Harden 2002, 2007; Newble et al. 2005).

The problems of transfer and role uncertainty

Throughout the years students have experienced the transition from preclinical to clinical training as a dynamic period. Although students report that learning from real patients is motivating and exciting, they also describe this transition as intense and stressful (Prince et al. 2005; Walker et al. 1981). The intensity and stressfulness of this transition could be explained by a number of reasons. First, students struggle with the fact that they are uncertain about their role and responsibilities in the clinical setting, and therefore struggle to adapt to that role and its accompanying responsibilities. This starts with basic struggles, such as not knowing how to address other healthcare providers because students do not know whether the other is a nurse, specialist registrar, or a hospital consultant (O'Brien et al. 2007). Also, students experience a sudden increase in working hours upon entrance of the clinical training phase and therefore have limited hours available for studying (while they still need to pass their examinations) (Radcliffe and Lester 2003). This is one of the signs of the clash between the learning orientation of university-based medical education and the performance orientation of workplace-based medical training (Teunissen and Westerman 2011b).

Another issue within the transition from non-clinical training to the clinical phase of medical school is that students struggle with the transfer of knowledge into practice. Students find it difficult to mobilize and use their previously gathered knowledge and skills for clinical reasoning purposes (Brown 2010; Prince et al. 2000). The problems of transfer and role uncertainty have been topics of interest in transition research mainly within the comparison of students from a PBL curriculum versus more traditional, lecture-based, curricula and their levels of preparation for clinical practice. The results derived from these studies are ambivalent. Medical students educated within a PBL curriculum seem to be more confident and less intimidated by the novelties of the clinical workplace than their colleagues trained in a lecture-based curriculum and therefore struggle less with role uncertainties (Hayes et al. 2004; O'Neill et al. 2003). On the other hand, one of the aims of PBL is the integration of both basic and applied sciences in order to stimulate the clinical functioning of their students. Research does not indicate that PBL curricula succeed in this integration (Prince et al. 2000). Research shows that levels of preclinical knowledge and skills are not associated with performance on transition to the clinical training phase (van Hell et al. 2008). This implies that the problem of transferring knowledge and skills into the clinical setting cannot just be explained by feelings of unpreparedness due to a lack of knowledge and skills. In contrast, it seems that more individual characteristics are important in how the transition progresses. An explanation for the problem of transfer could be that students need to amend their way of learning. Where there was a structured programme in the university years, allowing the students to internalize their medical knowledge and skills in an ordered way, students are now dependent on the hectic clinical context in which they are responsible for their own learning and development (Teunissen and Westerman

2011a). In order to do so, students need to develop a more self-directed and experiential way of learning in which they take control over their own development. A study from White shows that PBL does seem to help medical students develop self-regulating learning capacities and that students with these capacities are more comfortable with the creation of their own learning (White 2007).

The role of the individual

As mentioned earlier, it appears that within the transition to the clinical phase of training a lot depends on how the individual student handles the uncertainties concerning expectancies, role, and social integration. Several studies investigated which individual characteristics would facilitate a smooth transition. For instance, mature students are found to show higher levels of confidence and are less likely to feel intimidated and overwhelmed by these uncertainties, due to psychological hardiness derived from previous life experiences (Shacklady et al. 2009). Another example is that female students perceive the transition as more challenging, because they feel that they need to show more competence in patient care in comparison to male students in order to overcome a male-dominated culture in the hospital (Babaria et al. 2009).

In order to better prepare medical student for the clinical phase of their training, some medical schools offer transition courses in which basic clinical skills, knowledge, and tasks are covered and students are trained in the application of different coping strategies (Jacobs et al. 2005; Matheson et al. 2010; O'Brien and Poncelet 2010; Poncelet and O'Brien 2008). However, there is a paucity of evidence on the effectiveness of such transitional programmes, although students do report high levels of satisfaction with them.

The transition from medical student to junior doctor or into postgraduate training

Along with the student-centred pedagogy of PBL in the 1990s came the introduction of early clinical experience. Early clinical experience is defined as human contact with real patients in a social or clinical context within an early stage in the medical career (Littlewood et al. 2005). The implementation of vertically integrated medical curricula aims to alleviate, amongst others, the transition from medical student to junior doctor or from medical student directly into postgraduate training (Wijnen-Meijer et al. 2010). Early clinical experience has proven to be influential in career choice after medical schools and in obtaining a post within postgraduate training (Dornan et al. 2006; Yardley et al. 2010). Furthermore, there are indications that early clinical experience increases the self awareness and confidence of medical students and therefore facilitates the transition into the clinical setting (Dornan and Bundy 2004). However, despite early clinical experience and vertically integrated curricula, the transition from medical school into postgraduate training remains an issue within the medical trajectory. We will next describe the most prominent issues within this transition.

Preparedness and role identification

Various studies have identified different challenges when starting as a newly qualified doctor. First, a lack of preparedness is reported within different domains, for instance inadequate basic medical skills, such as prescribing, initiating treatment, or practical skills like using insulin in patients with diabetes (Conn et al.2003; Matheson and Matheson 2009; Nikendei et al. 2008; Wall et al. 2006). Other researchers also identified a lack of preparedness in

time management and communication skills (including breaking bad news to patients) (Bogg et al. 2001; Hannon 2000).

Besides these feelings of unpreparedness within clinical or non-clinical domains that contribute to the intensity of the transition, junior doctors struggle with the identification of their new roles and responsibilities (Brennan et al. 2010; Tallentire et al. 2011). This is similar to the uncertainty about roles and position described earlier within the transition from preclinical to clinical training. However, the focus of this struggle has shifted from uncertainty about the role of other team members towards a struggle with their own position and responsibility for patient care. Junior doctors often perceive a gap between the amount of responsibility imposed upon them and the amount they feel they are ready for (Tallentire et al. 2011). Next to uncertainty in performing (practical) medical tasks (Brown et al. 2007), the changed relationship with patients also adds to junior doctors' struggle to cope in their new role (Prince et al. 2004). These struggles exemplify a role shift for the junior doctor. Their role has shifted from that of a learner, who is mainly focused on their own professional development and who may use patient encounters merely to learn from, to that of a caregiver who has clinical responsibility for the patient (Teunissen and Westerman 2011b). Junior doctors often perceive that they provide suboptimal patient care and also realize that they do not make optimal use of their work experience as a learning opportunity, leading to feelings of guilt and uncertainty (Hannon 2000). This struggle with the identification of the new professional role was described in the famous sociological work from 1961 'Boys in White' (Becker et al. 1961), which describes how students struggle with the identification of their professional role and struggle to perform their patient care tasks; and at the same time expect themselves to learn.

A stressful stage

Combined, these stressors of unpreparedness and the struggle with role identification lead to an intense transition as is illustrated by research findings in the United Kingdom showing that 25% of junior doctors were experiencing burnout (Bogg et al. 2001). This percentage is similar to that in a study performed 15 years earlier which found that 28% of junior doctors showed evidence of depression (Firth-Cozens 1987). In dealing with the different stressors and uncertainties, junior doctors indicate that the amount of support received during the start as a junior doctor is pivotal (Calman and Donaldson 1991; Lempp et al. 2004). In order to gain further insight into the influential factors within the transition to junior doctor several studies investigated the influence of certain personality traits and how these facilitate or impede the transition. For instance, high scores on the personality traits conscientiousness and extraversion are associated with higher levels of feeling prepared for practice amongst junior doctors and high scores on neuroticism are negatively associated with perceived preparedness (Cave et al. 2009). Furthermore, students who lack flexibility or have a shy or unmotivated appearance are at risk for a slower development into their professional role, since they can be reluctant to ask questions in order to learn, or can withdraw from clinical team activities aimed at patient care (Wilkinson and Harris 2002). In response to the difficulties of starting junior doctors, most researchers state that this transition should be smoothed out by interventions such as curriculum changes or transitional courses. However, the fact that research on transitions in the 1960s and recent research findings described in this paragraph show great resemblance, suggests that the stressors within this transition cannot merely be averted by curriculum changes or interventions, but that another approach to these problems is needed. For that reason, some recent papers explicitly postulate that this phase should not be merely viewed as a stressful period full of potential threats. These authors see transitions as inevitable and stress that they could be used as a unique learning opportunity that provide the individual with a chance for rapid personal development (Kilminster et al. 2010, 2011; Teunissen and Westerman 2011a).

The transition from specialty trainee to hospital consultant

The transition from specialty trainee to independent practice as a hospital consultant is the last major transition that can be discerned within the medical education trajectory. As mentioned, postgraduate training at the time of Flexner was not formally institutionalized and was only applicable to a small number of graduated medical students. Throughout the rest of the 20th century postgraduate curricula developed worldwide to the point at which almost everywhere medical school was followed by a number of years of specialization into a specific discipline within medicine, ranging from family medicine to neurosurgery. Initially, learning within these years of specialization was largely based on the master–apprentice model (Ludmerer and Johns 2005; Sylvia et al 2008). However, since the mid 1990s there has been a worldwide shift toward competency-based curricula in postgraduate medical education (Bannon 2006; Ludmerer and Johns 2005; Scheele et al. 2008). The majority of research on the transition to hospital consultant addressed study populations that had not been trained within competency-based curricula. Therefore, we cannot describe how this shift to competency-based postgraduate curricula might influence the transition from specialty training to hospital consultant. Furthermore, in comparison to the previously described transitions, the literature on the transition to hospital consultant is sparse.

Two sides of the coin

The transition from specialty training to independent practice as a new hospital consultant signifies the end of a long educational trajectory, but at the same time marks the onset of a new stage within the medical career. New consultants perceive this transition as twofold. On one hand they experience emotions of success and achievement, but high levels of uncertainty and distress are reported at the same time (Westerman et al. 2010). The challenges new consultants are faced with are final responsibility for patient care, responsibility in management tasks, and being an educational supervisor. A number of studies report that new consultants perceive they are adequately prepared by their specialty training for clinical tasks, such as medical knowledge and skills, but when it comes to the non-clinical tasks such as handling financial issues, leadership, management, and education their level of preparation is lacking (Beckett et al. 2006; Brown et al. 2009; Higgins et al. 2005; McKinstry et al. 2005; Morrow et al. 2009; Westerman et al. 2013). The confrontation with the tasks and responsibilities that they are unacquainted with is often situated within a new context of an unknown hospital with new colleagues and a new organizational structure and culture, which adds to the intensity of this period (Westerman et al. 2010).

As a result of the novelties within this transition to hospital consultant and the shift toward final responsibility, the transition is described as a period in which a process of 'fundamental re-examination of who and what you are' takes place in order to adapt oneself to the new situation (Brown et al. 2009; Wilkie and Raffaelli2005, pp. 107–114). This re-examination signifies the process of professional identity development that is initiated in this transition and which progresses throughout the first few years as a new hospital consultant.

Several studies describe different interventions aimed at alleviating the intense transition, either by providing support through mentoring for new consultants (Roberts et al. 2002) or providing specific training aimed at developing non-clinical skills (MacDonald and Cole 2004). Again, statements have been made that a better alignment between specialty training and starting as a hospital consultant could result in a less intense transition (Brown et al. 2009). The effectiveness of these interventions remains to be investigated.

Different perspectives on transitions

In this section we will present four different perspectives on transitions from four research fields: medicine, social psychology, organizational studies, and pedagogy. By presenting the way in which transitions are conceptualized and studied within these different perspectives we create a frame of reference for discussing how transitions within the medical educational continuum can be viewed and approached. Simultaneously, we can use insights from research fields outside medicine to inform future research or measures aimed at facilitating or enabling healthcare professionals to benefit from transitions (fig. 32.1).

The four different perspectives are derived from various literature fields, all with different research traditions and approaches to transitions. In order to facilitate the comparison and categorization of insights from these different perspectives, we use Foucault's concept of problematization (Alvesson and Sandberg 2011). Foucault described problematization as thinking differently and viewing a given fact or situation as a problem. By critically reflecting on a situation and presenting it to oneself as a problem, new ways of conceptualizing that situation will emerge and therefore new answers to the problem might arise (Healy 2005). By characterizing the problematization features in each of the four domains, we pave the way for formulating a different approach to transitions in the medical domain and a concomitant future research agenda. Each of the

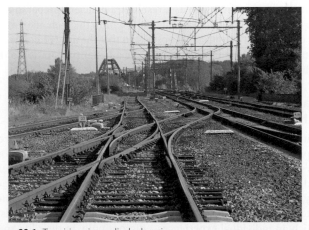

Figure 32.1 Transitions in medical education.
Reproduced with permission from Tom Visée.

following paragraphs will describe how transitions within each of the four fields are conceptualized, after which we will characterize the way in which transitions are 'problematized'.

As the first of four perspectives, we will present how the three major transitions within the medical education literature, as described earlier, are being researched. Second, we will describe two perspectives on transitions stemming from social psychological and sociological research. The first originates from an individual psychological approach to transitions, looking at how people perceive and cope with changes in their life span. The latter of the two perspectives will conceptualize transitions from a contextual and organizational point of view and will look at how newcomers transition into a new work setting. As a fourth perspective we will present different concepts derived from sociocultural pedagogy and examine their take on how people learn from and develop within new situations.

Transitions as interruptions of the medical education continuum

Throughout the years a steady but relatively small number of papers have been published addressing the different transitions within the medical education continuum. In the majority of these papers transitions are described from an individual perspective, the person who is transitioning. The general conclusion is that transitions are stressful and problematic stages within the medical trajectory (Teunissen and Westerman 2011a). Transitions are often viewed as undesired interruptions of a continuum, and proposed interventions aim at curriculum alterations in order to better align training with the next stage in the professional's medical trajectory. Furthermore, it appears that the rationale for investigating transitions is to evaluate the preceding training in terms of efficiency and degree of preparation. For instance, several studies have investigated if students trained in a student-centred curriculum have better communication or clinical skills than students from a traditional curriculum (O'Neill et al. 2003; Willis et al. 2003). Few studies address possibilities of aiding the individual within the transition. Although recently, some authors have argued that transitions should be viewed as learning opportunities instead of a threat for the person in transition (Kilminster et al. 2011; Teunissen and Westerman 2011b).

This predominant view on transitions as threats, or problematic situations, often results in interventions aimed at eliminating the transition. More specifically, the problems that arise within the transition are mainly seen as a result of a deficient preparation of the transitioning individual. Therefore, within the domain of medical education, it is repeatedly postulated that the answer lies in curriculum alterations in order to achieve a better preparation of the individual for the next phase of their career.

Transitions as key characteristics of human development

Within social psychology and sociological research, different approaches to human development are maintained. The second perspective that we will present stems from these research fields and is often described as transition psychology or life course sociology, in which human development is inextricably bound to different transitions (George 1993). Transitions are defined as periods in which an individual experiences a discontinuity in their life-space that requires new behavioural responses in order to effectively cope

with that new situation (Adams et al. 1976; Blair 2000; Higgins 1995). Therefore, transitions can be ignited by different life-events such as; school entrance, marriage, divorce, parenthood, retirement, or entering a new work position.

Several conceptual frameworks or transition models exist that provide insight into the different phases present within transitions and the psychological processes therein. Adams et al. described a seven-phase transition model with concomitant effects on self-esteem of the person in transition (Adams et al. 1976). Another, more practical model, is that of Nicholson who describes transitions as a cyclical process in which four phases can be identified i.e. preparation, encounter, adjustment, and stabilization (Nicholson 1990, pp. 83–108). For example, a medical student is prepared by his preclinical training (phase 1) for entering the clinical setting, and upon entrance he encounters (phase 2) a multitude of novel tasks, and expectations. In order to overcome and master these novel tasks, the student needs to adjust and change (phase 3), after which a new stable phase will begin (phase 4).

Since transition psychology and life course sociology approach transitions as psychological developmental processes, numerous studies have been conducted into individual psychological characteristics that can facilitate or impede these developments. For instance, several studies have shown that personality traits like extroversion (Kling et al. 2003; Schlossberg 1981) or optimism (Brissette et al. 2002) are associated with a smoother transition and lower stress levels. Furthermore, Vardi shows that self-esteem and an internal locus of control (i.e. the personal beliefs as to what extent one can control or influence events that affect them), are associated with a smoother transition (Vardi 2000).

When we apply Foucault's concept of problematization, we can postulate that transition psychology and life course sociology conceptualize transitions as initiators of human development, which provide the individual with the possibilities of adaptation and personal growth. This perspective on human development, in which transitions take centre stage contrasts with the medical education domain in which transitions are often viewed as threats that should be prevented, as described in the preceding paragraphs. Therefore, the psychological perspective on transitions could provide us with insight and tools to better support and direct the individual throughout the transition. The commonality between medical education research and this individual developmental approach to transitions lies in their neglect of the relationship between individuals in transition and the context in which the transition is situated. When personality traits are viewed as strong predictors for the progression through transitions, this could results in a more or less static approach to transitions when these traits are seen as stable through time. This contradicts with a more sociocultural perspective on transitions, in which the individual and the new context are interrelated and continuously changing.

Transitions within an organizational context

The third perspective on transitions comes from organizational psychology, more specifically organizational socialization research. This area of research originates from the work of Maanen van and Schein (1979) and has gradually developed into an established area of interest within human resource management. Organizational socialization is concerned with both the content and process of learning through which newcomers develop into a new role or position within an organization (Chao et al. 1994).

Multiple studies have been performed to gain a better insight into how newcomers tend to socialize and integrate within a new setting, in order to inform measures aimed at increasing employee engagement, productivity, and satisfaction with the organization (Saks and Gruman 2011). Morrison recognized that newcomers within an organization are actively in search for information in order to develop themselves within four specific domains; task mastery, role clarification, acculturation, and social integration (Kammeyer-Mueller and Wanberg 2003; Morrison 1993, pp. 173–183). These domains show great similarity to the largest hurdles present within transitions in medical education. Especially, the domains of role clarification and acculturation are identified as prominent in different medical transition studies (Brown et al. 2009; Tallentire et al. 2011; Westerman et al. 2010). The similarity between these concepts of how newcomers develop into a new setting and characteristics within transitions in medical education, underpins the usefulness of these insights in interventions aimed at facilitation of medical students or doctors in transition.

Another key characteristic of how transitions are depicted within organizational socialization research is that transitions are considered social processes in which the interaction and forming of relationships with new colleagues are essential for reducing role uncertainty of the newcomer and therefore facilitate integration and socialization (Fang et al. 2011; Feldman 1976; Morrison 2002; Yellin 1999). This focus on socialization and transitions as social processes was already acknowledged by Becker in his famous work 'Boys in White: Student Culture in Medical School' in the 1960s in which he describes how medical students struggle to adapt to and integrate with clinical supervisors, nurses and fellow students upon entering the clinical setting (Becker et al. 1961).

When we apply the problematization approach to the organizational socialization perspective on transitions, we can draw the following conclusions. Transitions are social processes in which the newcomer is in search of information regarding their new tasks, role, and the existing culture. The rationale for most organizational socialization research is to enhance and improve both productivity and engagement of newcomers within the organization. Although this approach results in valuable insights and strategies for supporting individuals in transition, the focus on role clarification and social interaction does not address the problem of transfer, as present within the medical education domain. For example the medical student struggles to transfer previously acquired knowledge into practice for clinical reasoning purposes.

Transitions in the light of constructivist pedagogy

The fourth outlook on transitions that we review is a pedagogical one. Of course, pedagogy, the science of teaching and learning, covers a range of perspectives. We focus on the link between Piagetian and Vygotskian constructivist theory.

The basic need for equilibrium is an important feature in the work of Jean Piaget. Although Piaget (1896–1980) was a biologist by study, he mainly researched cognitive development processes and the nature of intelligence. In his work he looked at how children solve problems and challenging tasks by carefully observing their approaches. Piaget described how children and adults' interactions with their environment leads to experiences that either fit their reference mental model or not. In case of an experience that fits expectations, it will be easily assimilated. However, when people, students or doctors in our case, find themselves in a transition

phase, they may experience new and unexpected things, leading to disequilibrium. People react differently to disequilibrium, for example with confusion or anger, but eventually will find a new equilibrium by learning, changing behaviour or changing the setting (Piaget 1950). The scope of change is probably the result of the novelty of the experience and the degree of effort an individual chooses to put into the new situation (Newell and Simon 1972).

Another constructivist theorist is Vygotsky. Often being named as the father of sociocultural learning theory, he conceptualized learning and teaching as a social and cultural phenomenon rather than as a process in the heads of individuals (Kozulin et al. 2003). Vygotsky described the concept of the 'zone of proximal development' (ZPD), which denotes 'the distance between the actual developmental level as determined by independent problem solving and the level of potential development as determined through problem solving under adult guidance or in collaboration with more capable peers' (Vygotsky 1978, pp. 79–91).

Chaiklin has identified several aspects of the zone of proximal development concept that show how well it aligns with transitions in medical education (Chaiklin 2003). By describing these characteristics in relation to transitions, it becomes clear how the concept of ZPD offers yet another take on transitions in medical education. Chaiklin differentiates between an objective ZPD and a subjective ZPD. In our case, the objective ZPD would refer to the (psychological) functions that need to be formed during a given period in order enter the next period. For instance, when starting as a specialist registrar, one has to develop the ability to diagnose and treat patients and be prepared to carry responsibility for decisions that affect patients. Moreover, the age of specialist registrars may coincide with starting a family, or buying a house for the first time. These aspects of the transition are not dependent on any individual doctor and therefore constitute the objective ZPD. The subjective ZPD refers to the extent to which a person's capabilities are realizing the requirements of the next phase. It helps to identify the development an individual person needs to make. Vygotsky's ZPD explains why people may respond differently to the same transitions. From a problematization viewpoint, the ZPD focuses on the potential of individuals in a given transition with its inherent requirements, rather than on already existing capabilities. Using ZPD, one looks at what will be possible as a result of the transition, not backwards looking for explanations as to why a transition exists. It is also a concept that combines a focus on individual capabilities with the possibilities and restrictions afforded by the context in which a transition takes place.

Interventions and future research

The following three major transitions within the medical education continuum are described in this chapter: the transition from preclinical to clinical medical training, from medical student to specialty trainee, and from specialty trainee to independent practice as hospital consultant. These transitions have been shown to be highly demanding stages within the medical career and are characterized by numerous challenging novelties ranging from unknown tasks and new roles with accompanying responsibilities, to new contexts and unfamiliar colleagues. The intensity of these transitions is illustrated by the high stress levels and burnout that have been repeatedly reported (Bogg et al. 2001; Firth-Cozens 1987).

Research into these transitions can function as a lens for the merits and failings of our educational system, since they provide information on the alignment between the content of training programs and the actual work within the next stage of the medical career. In the medical education domain transitions are mainly conceptualized as problems or possible threats that should be amended, most often by means of curriculum alterations. Without doubt, it is pivotal that medical education prepares future physicians optimally within the medical and generic competencies needed for their further careers. However, these proposed measures tend to overlook the fact that transitions are situated within a context and culture with its accompanying social features and uncertainties, which do not necessarily change by means of curricular changes. Approaching transitions as individual problems that can be solved through better preparation by training fails to take into account the psychological and social forces in play within these transitions. In this chapter, we have reviewed approaches to transitions from other disciplines that could inform both future research and development of interventions. Several of these perspectives stemming from the psychology and sociology literature, are presented in this chapter and illustrate how transitions are viewed as opportunities for personal development and acknowledge the complex interplay between the transitioning individual with his coping strategies, the preparation received through prior training, the context, and the sociocultural character of transitions.

Interventions

Since transitions are characterized by an intricate interplay between the preparation received through training, psychological characteristics that influence individual perceptions and coping strategies, and contextual factors such as support received from colleagues, friends, and the organization, multiple interventions can be deployed aimed at the facilitation of medical professionals in transition.

Evidently, medical training programmes, both undergraduate and postgraduate, should strive towards an optimal alignment between the content of the programme and the competencies needed within the next phase of the medical trajectory. Training programmes need to focus on both conceptual and practical medical competencies as well as generic competencies, such as communication, collaboration, management, and professional skills. When one views transitions as recurrent, inevitable and possibly worthwhile phases within the careers of all medical doctors, then some preparation for dealing with transitions is indispensable. Although many curricula try to stimulate self-directed learning, the necessary skills are rarely explicitly trained. A more explicit focus on self-directed learning and coping skills for an imminent transition might benefit many medical students and doctors.

Psychological factors such as personality traits and coping strategies that have proven to be influential facilitators or inhibitors within transitions are not likely to be altered by means of curriculum alterations or transitional courses. Therefore, another category of interventions could aim to increase support and guidance for medical students, trainees, and consultants in transition. This could be achieved by measures ranging from mentoring programs to peer support groups and organizational orientation programmes offered upon entrance. For example, Roberts et al. describe the beneficial effect of mentoring for newly appointed consultants in psychiatry in helping them to adapt to their new post (Roberts et al. 2002). Another example stems from the organizational psychology research literature in which organizational socialization programmes are shown to be effective in getting new employees engaged within the organization and in improving newcomer well-being (Saks and Gruman 2011).

These proposed interventions all aim to alleviate the transition by either establishing better preparation of skills and competencies needed to meet the requirements of the new post, or by increasing the amount of support during the transition. However, a third category of interventions could be postulated, although we acknowledge it might be more difficult to bring about. These interventions should aim to empower and equip students and trainees in such a way that they will be better able to adapt and handle themselves within a new context, role or setting and use transitions as opportunities for rapid personal development, which resonates with Chaiklin's description of Vygotsky's zone of proximal development (Chaiklin 2003).

Future research

Multiple possibilities can be identified for future research into transitions within the medical trajectory; we will briefly discuss several options. However, before describing these concrete areas of future research we want to plead for future research, which first of all aims to clarify rather than describe certain phenomena present within transitions. Clarification research anchored within a conceptual framework—i.e. research aimed at identifying how and why things work in relation to existing theories (Bordage 2009; Cook et al. 2008) is needed since plenty remains poorly understood within transitions and the development of measures aimed at facilitation of transitions is therefore hampered. We have presented different theoretical perspectives that can be used as conceptual frameworks for the future study of transitions in the medical domain, ranging from psychological concepts covering human development to notions from the organizational literature addressing the entrance of newcomers to a novel setting.

As described throughout this chapter, transitions are characterized by an intricate interplay between preparation received through prior training, psychological characteristics that influence individual perception and coping strategies, and contextual factors. As a result of this interplay tangible areas for future research can be identified and result in a better understanding of transitions. First of all, future research could address how trainees or consultants cope with the disruptive elements and changes they are faced with and which coping strategies or psychological traits can be identified as facilitators or inhibitors of transitions. Second, in addressing the contextual factors in force within transitions, future research could pay attention to the role of social support and focus on how hospitals can best facilitate the entrance of newcomers within their organization. Third, transitions and research thereof can function as a lens through which we can look at the effectiveness of medical training programmes and so function as an evaluation tool for curricula. Therefore, transition research enables the investigation of the influence of received prior training on the progression of transitions. For instance, future research could address the importance of generic competencies within transitions. Or, it could be investigated whether competency based education does indeed better prepare future doctors for the real world and altering societal demands in comparison to more traditional process-based curricula (i.e. lecture-based and focused on knowledge acquisition). In addition, resulting from a better understanding of transitions within the medical trajectory, evidence-based interventions could be implemented and so form an additional future domain of research. For instance, the beneficial effect of mentoring programmes or peer support groups on individuals in transition should be studied. Finally, future research could address the recently described approach to transitions as learning opportunities (Kilminster et al. 2011) and further investigate how transitions can be transformed from threats towards a learning opportunities, and how students or new consultants can best be guided trough this phase while learning from it.

The investigation of transitions demands an approach consisting of multiple methodologies and methods. Most studies performed on transitions, both qualitative and quantitative, have been based on a cross-sectional design. However, a cross-sectional approach does not allow the actual investigation of a process—which constitutes the essence of transitions (Thomson and Holland 2003). Longitudinally designed studies should be performed to investigate the progression of individuals throughout transitions. Within this follow-up both qualitative and quantitative data can be gathered—depending on the research questions. Finally, the follow up of cohorts of students or trainees could result in a better understanding of these transitions within the medical career since it allows for a generalization from individual experiences and perceptions towards concepts or insights that apply to larger groups.

Conclusions

+ In transitioning from one phase of medical education to the next, individuals have to cope with changes ranging from novel clinical and non-clinical tasks, to a novel role with its accompanying responsibility and new colleagues.

+ Transitions are characterized by an intricate interplay between educational, psychological and contextual factors.

+ Transitions can function as a lens for the merits and failings of the current medical educational system.

+ Contemporary perspectives on transitions within medical education approach transitions as threats that should be prevented instead of opportunities for personal and professional development.

+ Adjacent research stemming from psychology provides valuable insights into how individuals in transitions can be supported.

References

Adams, J., Hayes, J., and Hopson, B. (1976) *Transition, understanding and managing personal change*. Martin Robertson and Company, London.

Alvesson, M., and Sandberg, J. (2011) Generating research questions through problematization. *Acad Manag Rev*. 36: 247–271

Babaria, P., Abedin, S., and Nunez-Smith, M. (2009) The effect of gender on the clinical clerkship experiences of female medical students: results from a qualitative study. *Acad Med*. 84: 859–866

Bannon, M. (2006) What's happening in postgraduate medical education? *Arch Dis Childh*. 91: 68–70

Beck, A.H. (2004) The Flexner Report and the Standardization of American Medical Education. *JAMA*. 291: 2139–2140

Becker, H.S., Blanche, G., Hughes, E.C., and Strauss, A.L. (1961) *Boys in White: Student Culture in Medical School*. Chicago: University of Chicago Press

Beckett M., Hulbert D., and Brown R. (2006) The new consultant survey 2005. *Emerg Med J*. 23: 461–463

Bernabeo, E.C., Holtman, M.C., Ginsburg, S., Rosenbaum, J.R., and Holmboe, E.S. (2011) Lost in transition: the experience and impact of frequent changes in the inpatient learning environment. *Acad Med*. 86: 591–598

Blair, S.E.E. (2000) The centrality of occupation during life transitions. *Br J Occup Ther*. 63: 19–25

Bogg, J., Gibbs, T., and Bundred, P. (2001) Training, job demands and mental health of pre-registration house officers. *Med Educ*. 35: 590–595

Bordage, G. (2009) Conceptual frameworks to illuminate and magnify. *Med Educ*. 43: 312–319

Brennan, N., Corrigan, O., Allard, J. et al. (2010) The transition from medical student to junior doctor: today's experiences of Tomorrow's Doctors. *Med Educ*. 44: 449–458

Brissette, I., Scheier, M.F., and Carver, C.S. (2002) The role of optimism in social network development, coping, and psychological adjustment during a life transition. *J Personality Soc Psychol*. 82: 102–111

Brown, J. (2010) Transferring clinical communication skills from the classroom to the clinical environment: perceptions of a group of medical students in the United Kingdom. *Acad Med*. 85: 1052–1059

Brown, J., Chapman, T., and Graham, D. (2007) Becoming a new doctor: a learning or survival exercise? *Med Educ*. 41: 653–660

Brown, J., Ryland, I., Shaw, N., and Graham, D. (2009) Working as a newly appointed consultant: a study into the transition from specialist registrar. *Br J Hosp Med (Lond)*. 70: 410–414

Calman, K.C. and Donaldson, M. (1991) The pre-registration house officer year: a critical incident study. *Med Educ*. 25: 51–59

Cave, J., Woolf, K., Jones, A., and Dacre, J. (2009) Easing the transition from student to doctor: how can medical schools help prepare their graduates for starting work? *Med Teach*. 31: 403–408

Chaiklin, S. (2003) The zone of proximal development in Vygotsky's analysis of learning and instruction. In A. Kozulin, B. Gindis, V.S. Ageyev, et al. (eds) *Vygotsky's Educational Theory in Cultural Context* (pp. 39–64). Cambridge: Cambridge University Press

Chao, G.T., O'Leary-Kelly, A.M., Wolf, S., Klein, H.J., and Gardner, P.D. (1994) Organizational Socialization: Its content and consequences. *J Appl Psychol*. 79: 730–743

Conn, J.J., Dodds, A.E., and Colman, P.G. (2003) The transition from knowing to doing: teaching junior doctors how to use insulin in the management of diabetes mellitus. *Med Educ*. 37: 689–694

Cook, D.A., Bordage, G., and Schmidt, H.G. (2008) Description, justification and clarification: a framework for classifying the purposes of research in medical education. *Med Educ*. 42: 128–133

Cooke, M., Irby, D.M., Sullivan, W., and Ludmerer, K.M. (2006) American Medical Education 100 Years after the Flexner Report. *N Engl J Med*. 355: 1339–1344

Dornan, T. and Bundy, C. (2004) What can experience add to early medical education? Consensus survey. *BMJ*. 329: 834

Dornan, T., Littlewood, S., Margolis, S.A., Scherpbier, A., Spencer, J., and Ypinazar, V. (2006) How can experience in clinical and community settings contribute to early medical education? A BEME systematic review. *Med Teach*. 28: 3–18

Fang, R., Duffy, M.K., and Shaw, J.D. (2011) The organizational socialization process: review and development of a social capital model. *J Manag*. 37: 127–152

Feldman, D.C. (1976) A contingency theory of socialization. *Adm Sci Q*. 21: 433–452

Firth-Cozens, J. (1987) Emotional distress in junior house officers. *BMJ*. 295: 533–536

Flexner, A. (1910) *Medical Education in the United States and Canada: A report to the Carnegie Foundation for the Advancement of Teaching [Carnegie Foundation Bulletin No.4]*. New York: Carnegie Foundation for the Advancement of Teaching

George, L.K. (1993) sociological perspectives on life transitions. *Annu Rev Sociol.* 19: 353–373

Hannon, F.B. (2000) A national medical education needs' assessment of interns and the development of an intern education and training programme. *Med Educ.* 34: 275–284

Harden, R.M. (2002) Developments in outcome-based education. *Med Teach.* 24: 117–120

Harden, R.M. (2007) Outcome-based education: the future is today. *Med Teach,* 29, 625–629.

Hayes, K., Feather, A., Hall, A. et al. (2004) Anxiety in medical students: is preparation for full-time clinical attachments more dependent upon differences in maturity or on educational programmes for undergraduate and graduate entry students? *Med Educ.* 38: 1154–1163

Healy, P. (2005) Foucault: Problematization, Critique and Dialogue. In P. Healey (ed.) *Rationality, hermeneutics, and dialogue: toward a viable postfoundationalist account of rationality* (pp. 64–87). Aldershot: Ashgate Publishing Ltd

Higgins, E.T. (1995) The four a's of life transition effects: attention, accessibility, adaptation, and adjustment. *Social Cognition.* 13: 215–242

Higgins, R., Gallen, D., and Whiteman, S. (2005) Meeting the non-clinical education and training needs of new consultants. *Postgrad Med J.* 81: 519–523

Jacobs, J.C., Bolhuis, S., Bulte, J.A., Laan, R., and Holdrinet, R.S. (2005) Starting learning in medical practice: an evaluation of a new Introductory Clerkship. *Med Teach.* 27: 408–414

Kammeyer-Mueller, J.D. and Wanberg, C.R. (2003) Unwrapping the organizational entry process: Disentangling multiple antecedents and their pathways to adjustment. *J Appl Psychol.* 88: 779–794

Kilminster, S., Zukas, M., Quinton, N., and Roberts, T. (2010) Learning practice? Exploring the links between transitions and medical performance. *J Health Organ Manag.* 24: 556–570

Kilminster, S., Zukas, M., Quinton, N., and Roberts, T. (2011) Preparedness is not enough: understanding transitions as critically intensive learning periods. *Med Educ.* 45: 1006–1015

Kling, K. C., Ryff, C. D., Love, G., and Essex, M. (2003) Exploring the influence of personality on depressive symptoms and self-esteem across a significant life transition. *J Pers Soc Psychol.* 85: 922–932

Kozulin, A., Gindis, B., Ageyev, V.S., and Miller, S.M. (2003) Socio-cultural theory and education: Students, teachers and knowledge. In A. Kozulin, B. Gindis, V.S. Ageyev et al. (eds) *Vygotsky's Educational Theory in Cultural Context* (pp. 1–12). Cambridge: Cambridge University Press

Lempp, H., Cochrane, M., Seabrook, M., and Rees, J. (2004) Impact of educational preparation on medical students in transition from final year to PRHO year: a qualitative evaluation of final-year training following the introduction of a new year 5 curriculum in a London medical school., *Med Teach.* 26: 276–278

Levinson, D.J., Darrow, C., Klein, E., Levinson, M., and McKee, B. (1978) *The Seasons of a Man's Life*. New York: Ballantine Books

Littlewood, S., Ypinazar, V., Margolis, S. A., Scherpbier, A., Spencer, J., and Dornan, T. (2005) Early practical experience and the social responsiveness of clinical education: systematic review. *BMJ.* 331: 387–391

Ludmerer, K.M. and Johns, M.M.E. (2005) Reforming graduate medical education. *JAMA.* 294: 1083–1087

Maanen van, J. and Schein, E.H (1979) toward a theory of organizational socialization. *Res Organ Behav.* 1: 209–264

MacDonald, J. and Cole, J. (2004) Trainee to trained: helping senior psychiatric trainees make the transition to consultant. *Med Educ.* 38: 340–348

Matheson, C. and Matheson, D. (2009) How well prepared are medical students for their first year as doctors? The views of consultants and specialist registrars in two teaching hospitals. *Postgrad Med J.* 85: 582–589

Matheson, C., Matheson, D., Saunders, J., and Howarth, C. (2010) The views of doctors in their first year of medical practice on the lasting impact of a preparation for house officer course they undertook as final year medical students., *BMC Med Educ.* 10: 48

McKinstry, B., Macnicol, M., Elliot, K., and Macpherson, S. (2005) The transition from learner to provider/teacher: the learning needs of new orthopaedic consultants. *BMC Med Educ.* 5: 17

Molenaar, W. M., Zanting, A., van Beukelen, P. et al. (2009) A framework of teaching competencies across the medical education continuum. *Med Teach.* 31: 390–396

Morrison, E.W. (1993) Longitudinal study of the effects of information seeking on newcomer socialization. *J Appl Psychol,* 78: 173–183

Morrison, E. W. (2002) Newcomers' relationships: the role of social network ties during socialization. *Acad Manage J,* 45, 1149–1160.

Morrow, G., Illing, J., Burford, B., and Kergon, C. (2009) Are specialist registrars fully prepared for the role of consultant? *Clin Teach.* 6: 87–90

Neville, A.J.M. and Norman, G.R.P. (2007) PBL in the undergraduate MD program at McMaster University: three iterations in three decades. *Acad Med.* 82: 370–374

Newble, D., Stark, P., Bax, N., and Lawson, M. (2005) Developing an outcome-focused core curriculum. *Med Educ.* 39: 680–687

Newell, A. and Simon, H.A. (1972) *Human problem solving*. Englewood Cliffs, NJ: Prentice Hall

Nicholson, N. (1990) The transition cycle: causes, outcomes, processes and forms. In Fisher, S., and Cooper, C.L. (eds) *On the Move: the Psychology of Change and Transition* (pp. 83–108). New York: John Wiley & Sons Inc.

Nikendei, C., Kraus, B., Schrauth, M., Briem, S., and Junger, J. (2008) Ward rounds: how prepared are future doctors? *Med Teach.* 30: 88–91

Norman, G.R. and Schmidt, H.G. (1992) The psychological basis of problem-based learning: a review of the evidence. *Acad Med.* 67: 557–565

O'Brien, B., Cooke, M., and Irby, D.M. (2007) Perceptions and attributions of third-year student struggles in clerkships: do students and clerkship directors agree? *Acad Med.* 82: 970–978

O'Brien, B.C. and Poncelet, A.N. (2010) Transition to clerkship courses: preparing students to enter the workplace. *Acad Med.* 85: 1862–1869

O'Neill, P.A., Jones, A., Willis, S.C., and McArdle, P.J. (2003) Does a new undergraduate curriculum based on Tomorrow's Doctors prepare house officers better for their first post? A qualitative study of the views of pre-registration house officers using critical incidents. *Med Educ.* 37: 1100–1108

Piaget, J. (1950) *The Psychology of Intelligence*. London: Routledge

Poncelet, A. and O'Brien, B. (2008) Preparing medical students for clerkships: a descriptive analysis of transition courses. *Acad Med.* 83: 444–451

Prince, K.J., Boshuizen, H.P., van der Vleuten, C.P.M., and Scherpbier, A.J. (2005) Students' opinions about their preparation for clinical practice., *Med Educ.* 39: 704–712

Prince, K.J., Van de Wiel, M., Scherpbier, A.J., van der Vleuten, C.P.M., and Boshuizen, H.P. (2000) A qualitative analysis of the transition from theory to practice in undergraduate training in a PBL-medical School. *Adv Health Sci Educ Theory Pract.* 5: 105–116

Prince, K.J., Van de Wiel, M., van der Vleuten, C.P.M., Boshuizen, H.P., and Scherpbier, A.J. (2004) Junior doctors' opinions about the transition from medical school to clinical practice: a change of environment. *Educ Health.* 7: 323–331

Radcliffe, C. and Lester, H. (2003) Perceived stress during undergraduate medical training: a qualitative study. *Med Educ.* 37: 32–38

Roberts, G., Moore, B., and Coles, C. (2002) Mentoring for newly appointed consultant psychiatrists. *Psychiatr Bull.* 26: 106–109

Saks, A.M. and Gruman, J.A. (2011) Getting newcomers engaged: the role of socialization tactics. *J Manag Psychol.* 26: 383–402

Scheele, F., Teunissen, P., Van, Luijk, S. et al. (2008) Introducing competency-based postgraduate medical education in the Netherlands. *Med Teach.* 30: 248–253

Schlossberg, N.K. (1981) A model for analyzing human adaptation to transition. *Couns Psychol.* 9: 2–18

Shacklady, J., Holmes, E., Mason, G., Davies, I., and Dornan, T. (2009) Maturity and medical students' ease of transition into the clinical environment. *Med Teach.* 31: 621–626

Sylvia, R.C., Richard, L.C., and Yvonne, S. (2008) Role modelling—making the most of a powerful teaching strategy. *BMJ.* 336: 718–721

Tallentire, V.R., Smith, S.E., Skinner, J., and Cameron, H.S. (2011) Understanding the behaviour of newly qualified doctors in acute care contexts. *Med Educ,* 45, 995–1005.

Teunissen, P.W. and Westerman, M. (2011a) Opportunity or threat; ambiguity in the consequences of transitions in medical education. *Med Educ.* 45: 51–59

Teunissen, P.W. and Westerman, M. (2011b) Junior doctors caught in the clash: the transition from learning to working explored. *Med Educ.* 45: 968–970

Thomson, R. and Holland, J. (2003) Hindsight, foresight and insight: The challenges of longitudinal qualitative research. *Int J Soc Res Methodol.* 6: 233–244

van Hell, E.A., Kuks, J.B., Schonrock-Adema, J., van Lohuizen, M.T., and Cohen-Schotanus, J. (2008) Transition to clinical training: influence of pre-clinical knowledge and skills, and consequences for clinical performance. *Med Educ.* 42: 830–837

Vardi, Y. (2000) Psychological empowerment as a criterion for adjustment to a new job. *Psychol Rep.* 87: 1083–1093

Vygotsky, L.S. (1978) Interaction between learning and development. M. Lopez- Morillas, (Trans) In M. Cole, V. John-Steiner, S. Scribner, et al. (eds) *Mind in Society: The Development of Higher Psychological Processes* (pp. 79–91). Cambridge, MA: Harvard University Press

Walker, L.G., Haldane, J.D., and Alexander, D.A. (1981) A medical curriculum: evaluation by final-year students. *Med Educ.* 15: 377–382

Wall, D., Bolshaw, A., and Carolan, J. (2006) From undergraduate medical education to pre-registration house officer year: how prepared are students? *Med Teach.* 28: 435–439

Walton, H.J. and Matthews, M.B. (1989) Essentials of problem-based learning. *Med Educ.* 23: 542–558

Westerman, M., Teunissen, P.W., Fokkema, J.P.I., et al. (2013) The transition to hospital consultant and the influence of preparedness, social support, and perception; a structural equation modeling approach. *Med Teach.* Mar 25. [Epub ahead of print]

Westerman, M., Teunissen, P.W., van der Vleuten, C.P.M., et al. (2010) Understanding the transition from resident to attending physician: a transdisciplinary, qualitative study. *Acad Med.* 85: 1914–1919

White, C.B. (2007) Smoothing out transitions: how pedagogy influences medical students' achievement of self-regulated learning goals. *Adv Health Sci Educ Theory Pract.* 12: 279–297

Wijnen-Meijer, M., ten Cate, O.T., van der Schaaf, M. and Borleffs, J.C. (2010) Vertical integration in medical school: effect on the transition to postgraduate training. *Med Educ.* 44: 272–279

Wilkie, G., and Raffaelli, D. (2005) In the deep and: making the transition from SpR to consultant. *Adv Psychiatr Treat.* 11: 107–114

Wilkinson, T.J. and Harris, P. (2002) The transition out of medical school—a qualitative study of descriptions of borderline trainee interns. *Med Educ.* 36: 466–471

Willis, S.C., Jones, A., and O'Neill, P.A. (2003) Can undergraduate education have an effect on the ways in which pre-registration house officers conceptualise communication? *Med Educ.* 37: 603–608

Yardley, S., Littlewood, S., Margolis, S.A., et al. (2010) What has changed in the evidence for early experience? Update of a BEME systematic review. *Med Teach.* 32: 740–746

Yellin, L.L. (1999) Role acquisition as a social process. *Sociol Inquiry.* 69: 236–256

PART 7

Selection

CHAPTER 33

Selection into medical education, training and practice

Fiona Patterson

Must it always be only in rueful valedictory repentance that the gatekeepers of medical education come to see what they have been doing?

Henry Dicks

Introduction

As selection is the first assessment for entry into medical education, there has been growing interest in how best to design and validate selection methods and systems. A large number of research papers have been published exploring selection methods as predictors of performance at medical school, and there is an emerging literature exploring selection practices for postgraduate training. This chapter outlines the key concepts associated with selection and the relative accuracy of different selection methods for medical education. Following this review, some considerations for a future research agenda are offered.

Assessments used in a selection context are different from those of professional licensure examinations. In licensure examinations, the aim is to assess end-of-training capability, where judgements are made by trained examiners about an individual's capacity to perform a job with competence. In theory, all candidates can pass the assessment. By contrast, in selection settings, if the number of candidates outweighs the number of available posts, then the assessment is geared towards ranking individuals. Potentially, if the competition is high, competent candidates may not be awarded a post.

In assessment for selection the intention is to *predict* who will be a competent doctor; in other words, to identify those individuals who will successfully complete training *before* training commences. Furthermore, undergraduate and postgraduate selection may have different goals; undergraduate courses selecting primarily on academic ability and postgraduate selection focusing more on job-fit. It cannot be assumed that those with high academic ability alone can be turned into good doctors via medical training—other skills and qualities need to be present from the start. Certain abilities and attributes may become more important late in the education and training pathway, such as leadership and decision-making.

Recently there has been much debate about the admissions processes of medical schools (Prideaux et al. 2011). Faced with limited student places and large numbers of applicants, most schools have traditionally relied on academic criteria in admission procedures. Almost universally, high academic achievement is a minimum entry requirement. This assumes that the skills required to be a good doctor are trainable given a good level of academic ability. However, researchers recognize that future clinicians should not be selected solely on academic performance criteria (Greengross 1997; Hughes 2002; Reede 1999). This follows the so-called (and somewhat artificial) divide in criteria between *cognitive* (e.g. clinical knowledge) and *non-cognitive* attributes (e.g. empathy, communication, integrity) (Prideaux et al. 2011). Conceptually, a key issue is whether schools should aim to select individuals who will make successful students or those who will make competent clinicians (McManus 2003). Clearly, success as a student and competence as a doctor are not mutually exclusive, and the former is not necessarily a precursor of the latter.

Of the limited research evidence available at postgraduate level, selection criteria vary within and between specialties, and also within and between countries. An important consideration in designing selection systems is the reactions of key stakeholders to the methods used (e.g. reactions towards the use of interviews versus IQ tests). This relates to the *political* validity of selection systems, where the levels of stakeholder acceptance of the methods used are an important aspect of decision-making; stakeholders include not only the applicants and recruiters, but also wider stakeholders such as government, regulatory bodies and the general public (Patterson et al. 2012a).

Key concepts in selection

The selection process

Figure 33.1 outlines the main elements involved in designing and implementing a selection system. The process starts by conducting a thorough analysis of the relevant knowledge, skills, abilities and attributes associated with performance in the target role. This information is used to construct a person specification (and job description where appropriate). This is used to decide which selection instruments are best used to elicit applicant behaviour related to the selection criteria. In deciding to apply for a post (or a place at medical school), applicants will engage in *self-selection* where they can make an informed judgement about whether the particular role suits their skills and abilities.

This in-depth job analysis is the cornerstone of producing an effective selection process, as the aim is to accurately identify appropriate selection criteria. In job analysis studies, researchers use various methods, such as direct observation and interviews with job incumbents (Patterson et al. 2000). Having defined these criteria at an entry level appropriate for the career stage (e.g. entry to specialty training), this information is used to guide choice of selection methods. Outputs from this analysis should detail the responsibilities in the target job and provide information about the particular competencies and characteristics required of the jobholder.

The importance of conducting a thorough job analysis cannot be understated; job analysis has been described by some as the basis for virtually all human resource activities necessary for the successful functioning of organizations (Mirabile 1990; Morgeson and Campion 1997; Oswald 2003; Siddique 2004). In a postgraduate medical selection context, job analysis studies conducted in the UK have identified a wide range of attributes beyond clinical knowledge and academic achievement that need to be considered to ensure that doctors train and work within a specialty for which they have a particular aptitude (Patterson et al. 2008). These findings support the notion that identification of both the generic core

skills (competencies) common to all specialties and the specialty-specific competencies that differentiate specialties will inform the development of robust postgraduate selection criteria and provide the basis of a reliable, valid and legally defensible selection system (Patterson et al. 2008). Once selection decisions are made, and the appointed applicants enter training, information on the performance of trainees related to the original selection criteria should be used to examine the predictive validity of the selection instruments (i.e. the extent to which selection scores are correlated with subsequent in-training assessments and work performance).

Figure 33.1 emphasizes that best practice selection is a two-way selection process. In order to attract the best trainees, both medical schools and hospitals have become increasingly aware that evaluating candidates' reactions to the selection process is essential, particularly in relation to perceptions of fairness. Since large resources are often spent on selection, its utility should be evaluated. In addition, information collected at selection can be used to design tailored development plans for trainees.

The core elements of best practice in selection are clear, yet research shows that there are two elements in the process that are often not conducted effectively. First, many organizations fail to conduct a thorough job analysis to identify precisely the key knowledge, skills and behaviours associated with competent performance in the target role. Second, validation studies are rarely conducted in organizations, as they are time consuming and difficult to administer. These studies often require tracking the performance of trainees over several years—from selection to medical school through to senior posts. In medical education and training, far more validation research has taken place in undergraduate selection. Here, research has explored the predictive validity of various cognitive

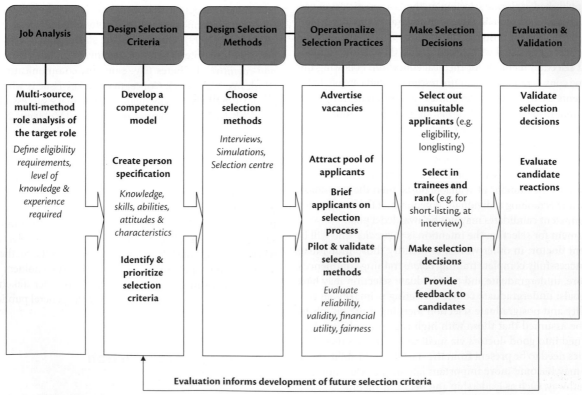

Figure 33.1 The selection process.

factors (e.g. prior academic performance on knowledge tests) with respect to exam performance (Ferguson et al. 2002). The criteria used to judge performance at medical school are potentially more readily observed as there are standardized assessments involved.

Research demonstrates that best practice in selection is an iterative process. Results from evaluation studies should be used to review the original selection criteria and choice of selection methods. Furthermore, feedback can be used to make continual improvements to selection systems, so as to enhance accuracy and fairness.

Conducting validation studies in selection and the criterion problem

Executing validation studies is complex in practical terms, since researchers rarely use one single predictor to make selection decisions. Applicants are judged on multiple selection criteria (depending on their stage in the education pathway). Given the multifaceted nature of the role of a doctor, recruiters are likely to design multiple selection tools to assess selection criteria. Therefore, recruiters must decide whether a job applicant must score highly on all selection criteria (non-compensatory) or whether high scores on some criteria can make up for low scores on another (compensatory). In practice, recruiters might assign different weightings to various selection criteria, depending on the nature of the job role. For example, if clinical knowledge is the most important criterion and an applicant does not achieve a certain score they may not be considered further.

In theory, the way to assess criterion-related validity (i.e. the extent to which scores on a selection measure predict some future outcome) is to use a predictive (or follow-up) study design. This design involves collecting predictor information for candidates (from selection tools, e.g. interview ratings, test scores) and then following-up to gather data on their performance (e.g. during their first year of employment or exams at medical school). Predictive validity is then assessed by examining the correlation between scores at selection and subsequent criterion data (e.g. through relevant work-based assessments). Cohen (1988) defined validity coefficients below $r = 0.1$ as being weak, below $r = 0.3$ as being moderate, and above $r = 0.5$ as being strong. Research shows it is unusual in field studies to obtain validity coefficients in excess of $r = 0.5$ (Salgado et al. 2001). Nevertheless, research consistently shows that validity coefficients of considerably less than $r = 1.0$ can provide a basis for improved selection practices (Anastasia and Urbina 1997). This means that relatively low correlations between selection and criterion data may still provide useful information to drive improvements in selection procedures.

Conducting validation studies in practice presents a variety of problems. One major problem is in accessing the appropriate outcome data to validate the selection process. Often, the criteria used to measure performance in the job role do not match the criteria used for selection. Conversely, sometimes the criterion and predictor are similar (e.g. using knowledge-based tests to predict exam performance in medical school), which may lead to problems of common method variance and content overlap. Ideally, predictor scores should not be used to make selection decisions until after a predictive validation study has been conducted. Practically, this is difficult to achieve and so piloting is essential to conduct an appropriate validation. Box 33.1 presents three sources of error that are important to consider when conducting validation studies

---

Box 33.1 Sources of error in validation studies

Sampling error

If relatively small samples are used in validation studies, the results obtained may be unduly influenced by the effects of small numbers of people within the sample whose results may be unusual.

As sample size increases, more reliable results are obtained.

Poor measurement precision

The measurement of attributes at both the predictor (i.e. selection method) and criterion (i.e. job performance) stages of the validation process is subject to unsystematic error. This error (unreliability) in the scores obtained will reduce the ceiling for the observed correlation between predictor and criterion: the error is unsystematic and random, thus this element of the predictor or criterion score will not correlate systematically with anything. This means that as reliability decreases, the maximum possible correlation between predictor and criterion will decrease.

Restricted range of scores

The sample of people used in a validation study may not provide the full range of theoretically possible scores on the predictor or criterion measures or both. A restricted range of scores has a straightforward statistical effect on limiting the size of the linear correlation between two variables. So, like unreliability, range restriction in a sample serves to reduce the magnitude of the observed correlation coefficient.

---

in selection—including sampling, measurement precision, and restriction of range issues.

Validity of selection procedures

Any single validation study is unlikely to provide a definitive answer regarding the validity of a selection method. This is because a particular study can only be conducted on a sample of relevant people and has to be conducted at a particular time, using specific measures. There are therefore likely to be specific factors, such as sampling, measures, and timing of the study, that will influence the results in some way. To estimate the validity of a particular selection procedure, more than one study, design is needed, so that error is minimized. Most selection systems combine several predictors, such as applicants' scores on interviews, as well as academic achievements.

In validation studies, a key consideration is the value of adding another predictor in increasing the predictive power of the selection process. This is known as *incremental validity*. For example, recruiters may want to know how validity is improved as a result of using a personality test (rather than relying solely on interview scores). Information on the incremental validity of a specific selection tool is valuable as it allows organizations to conduct a cost–benefit analysis of including additional tools.

Candidate reactions and organizational justice theory

Of crucial importance are *candidates' reactions* to different recruitment methods (Hausknecht et al. 2004). Considerable research has attempted to determine applicants' view on selection methods. Research tends to explain the different factors that affect applicant reactions using theories of *organizational justice*. *Distributive justice* focuses on perceived fairness regarding equity (i.e. where the selection outcome is consistent with the applicant's expectation) and equality (i.e. the extent to which applicants have the same opportunities in the selection process). *Procedural justice* refers to the formal characteristics of the selection process, such as information and feedback offered, job-relatedness of the selection procedures, and the level of ability of the staff involved in the selection process (i.e. recruiter effectiveness) (Anderson et al. 2001).

Four main factors seem to account for positive applicant reactions. These relate to the extent to which selection methods:

+ are based on a thorough job analysis and appear job-relevant

+ are not personally intrusive

+ do not contravene procedural or distributive justice expectations

+ allow applicants to meet in person with the recruiters

The research literature also shows that applicants prefer multiple opportunities to demonstrate their skills (as in selection centres) and prefer selection systems that are administered consistently for all applicants. In particular, when competition ratios are high, applicant reactions and candidate expectations of fair play are crucial.

Within a medical selection context, researchers have used organizational justice theory to examine candidate reactions to a UK postgraduate selection process over three years (Patterson et al. 2011b). The researchers found that candidates perceived high-fidelity selection methods (e.g. selection centres and work simulations) as being more job-relevant and fairer than low-fidelity methods (e.g. machine marked clinical problem-solving tests and situational judgement tests). However, this presents organizations with a justice dilemma, as while high-fidelity methods encourage positive candidate reactions, they are also considerably more expensive than low-fidelity measures, especially for high volume selection. Therefore, both the cost and the justice perspectives should be taken into account when designing selection systems (Patterson et al. 2011b). In practice, most selection systems use a combination of different tools to balance both the validity and utility of the process.

Fairness

Fair selection and recruitment are based on three principles: (1) having objective and valid criteria (developed through an appropriate job analysis); (2) accurate and standardized assessment by trained personnel; and (3) monitored outcomes (see fig. 33.2). Research has explored the extent to which selection procedures are fair to subgroups of the population (such as minority ethnic groups and women). First, it should be made clear that a test is not unfair or biased simply because members of different subgroups obtain different scores on the tests. Men and women have different mean scores for height; this does not mean that rulers are unfair measuring instruments. However, since it is important for selection criteria to be job-related, it would be unfair to use height as a selection criterion for a job if the job could be done by people of any height. Normally the extent to which a selection method is related to job performance can be estimated by validation research and it is clear, therefore, that fairness and validity are closely related.

Research has found that international differences in attainment are a consistent feature of medical education (Woolf et al.

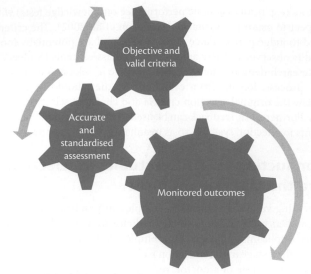

Figure 33.2 Fair selection and recruitment.

2011)—particularly in postgraduate exams, where international medical graduates tend to score lower than domestic medical graduates (Eva et al. 2010). However, researchers have not been able to provide a satisfactory explanation of the *causal factors* underlying this phenomenon.

Selection methods

Over several decades, many different selection methods have been reviewed by researchers in several different occupational groups (Campion et al. 1997; Lievens and Thornton 2005; Salgado and Anderson 2002). There has been a great emphasis on identifying which methods are the most reliable and valid. However, current thinking in medical selection advocates a shift away from focusing on method validity and more towards the development of *multimethod selection systems* and *programmatic approaches* (van der Vleuten and Schuwirth 2005). The following section reviews the most prominent methods used in medical selection and the concept of selection systems design.

Interviews and multiple mini-interviews

Interviews are ubiquitous in the selection processes of a variety of professions (Campion et al. 1997). Interviews are used at different stages of the selection process, either as the sole method of selection, or in conjunction with other methods. Interviews can vary in terms of:

+ purpose

+ duration

+ mode of administration (e.g. telephone, face-to-face, video, webcam)

+ number of interviewers (i.e. one-to-one or panel)

+ degree of structure (i.e. unstructured, semi-structured, or structured)

Research consistently shows that criterion-related validity is highest for interviews that are structured, ask relevant and standardized questions based on thorough role analysis, and use a panel of interviewers who are trained in best practice interview techniques and the use of validated scoring criteria (Campion et al. 1988; Goho and Blackman 2006; McDaniel et al. 1994).

Meta-analytic studies have found that structured interviews are valid predictors of job performance (McDaniel et al. 1994; Wiesner and Cronshaw 1988). Research evidence also suggests that structured interviews have incremental validity over cognitive ability tests (Cortina et al. 2000; Schmidt and Hunter 1998) and result in relatively small differences between ethnic groups (Bobko et al. 1999). Adding structure to an interview may also increase the chances of an organization successfully defending a lawsuit (Posthuma et al. 2002).

On the other hand, u interviews are prone to potential biases and errors, including:

* stereotyping

* first impressions (e.g. making a judgement solely on first impressions, rather than allowing the candidate a chance to demonstrate their skills—'I know if they are the right person immediately')

* halo and horns effects (e.g. selectors being unduly influenced by one positive or negative characteristic of the applicant)

* leniency

All of these aspects are likely to distort interviewers' ratings of candidates (Edwards et al. 1990).

Unfortunately, unstructured interviews are still widely used for selection in a variety of occupations, despite their low reliability, low predictive validity, and thus poor legal defensibility (Klehe 2004; Terpstra et al. 1999; Williamson et al. 1997). Despite the evidence supporting interviews as good predictors of general job performance, there is limited research on the reliability and validity of interviews for medical school admissions. Meta-analyses show that, over a 14-year period, inte-rater interviewer reliability of structured medical school selection interviews (i.e. the extent to which interviewers giving similar scores to similar interview performances) ranged from 0.27 to 0.38 (Kreiter et al. 2004). Furthermore, a high degree of variability has been identified between interview formats and the characteristics they purport to measure, meaning different types of interviews may assess different interviewee characteristics (Albanese et al. 2003). In addition, postgraduate interviews have been shown to be susceptible to interviewer bias, whereby candidates are awarded preferential ratings if their personality inventory scores are similar to those of the interviewers (Quintero et al. 2009). However, a 5-year longitudinal study into the development and implementation of the Canadian Dental Association structured interview (Meredith et al. 1982) showed that an average inter-rater reliability of 0.81 can be achieved by:

* carrying out a thorough job analysis to identify key competencies

* using a critical incident technique to develop relevant structured interview questions

* training the interviewers appropriately

This finding shows how the reliability and validity of an interview is dependent on the approach to conducting a thorough job analysis and developing interview questions in partnership with key stakeholders, based on identified competencies.

The multiple mini-interview (MMI) is a relatively new approach to constructing interviews for medical school admissions. MMIs build on the format of the objective structured clinical examination (OSCE). MMIs comprise a series of short testing stations, each of which employs a single standardized short interview scenario and a single rater (interviewer). The primary purpose of the MMI is to overcome problems with the test–retest reliability of traditional interview techniques (Eva and Reiter 2004).

The MMI has been investigated psychometrically at a number of centres internationally and has been shown to have good reliability and validity (Eva et al. 2004a, b, 2009; Roberts et al. 2008). Moreover, candidate and interviewer reactions have been positive (Kumar et al. 2009; Razack et al. 2009). MMIs have been successfully implemented in several schools worldwide (Harris and Owen 2007; Lemay et al. 2007; Roberts et al. 2008). and have been shown to be reliable and valid in selecting suitable candidates for postgraduate positions (Hofmeister et al. 2009). Investigation is ongoing into the financial utility of the MMI for selecting students into medical and dental programmes (van der Vleuten 1996). However, initial findings suggest that MMIs are cost-effective, but require more physical space than traditional interviews (Rosenfeld et al. 2008). There is emerging consensus on the credibility, feasibility and acceptability of MMIs as an undergraduate and postgraduate medical selection tool (Dore et al. 2010; Dowell et al. 2012; Prideaux et al. 2011). Although, it has been argued that for the MMI method to be valid, the design of MMI stations should be closely mapped to outputs from a thorough job analysis study (Patterson and Ferguson, 2012).

References

Large-scale empirical studies consistently show that references tend to be unreliable and ineffective at predicting job performance (McCarthy and Goffin 2001; Ferguson et al. 2003; Muchinsky 1979). Despite these findings, references are widely used in selection in a variety of occupations, including medicine, and it is likely that they will continue to be used as an additional guide in the selection process (Muchinsky 1979; IRS Employment Review 2002). In practice, employers tend to value references, even though references tend to be poor at differentiating between candidates. In a medical selection context, there is limited evidence that references (or personal statements) are reliable, and there is no evidence that references measure anything different from interviews (Prideaux et al. 2011). Anecdotally, low scores on reference reports can be informative. Practically, recruiters tend to favour references as an employment record rather than for use in ranking candidates.

In the UK, references for undergraduate applicants are used. However, the reliability is often questionable given recent changes in data legislation, which remove the confidentiality that existed previously (Hughes 2002). In studying predictive validity, Ferguson and colleagues (2003) showed that references obtained though the Universities and Colleges Admissions Service (UCAS) did not predict pre-clinical or clinical performance. However, medical schools differ in terms of the weight placed on references obtained through the UCAS application (Parry et al. 2006).

CVs and application forms

The curriculum vitae (CV) is often the first form of contact between an applicant and an organization, and can be influential on the outcomes of the subsequent selection process. CVs usually comprise 'hard' verifiable items, such as education and work experience, and 'soft' items, such as candidates' interests. However, despite their wide use, the non-standardized nature of CVs leaves their predictive validity questionable at best (Highhouse 2008).

Application forms are often used as an alternative to CVs because they are a more structured method for short-listing candidates. The information obtained through application forms is collected in a systematic way, making it easier for employers to objectively assess a candidate's suitability for a given post, and to compare applicants. Application forms may include questions on biographical information, educational background, previous work experience, and competencies identified through a job analysis. Application forms are a crucial part of the selection process and the quality of information obtained varies according to the design of the form. Research shows that structured application forms can provide valid information about a candidate, and demonstrate incremental validity as a predictor of future performance beyond the contribution of clinical problem solving tests, as long as they are based on appropriate selection criteria obtained through a job analysis (Patterson et al. 2009a). However, the validity of application forms is threatened by the developing industry of online resources and organizations that provide model answers to questions (Plint and Patterson 2010).

Academic records

Academic criteria are a major component of selection into medical school in several countries. Traditionally, selection for admission to medical school is based on predicted or actual school-end examination results, such as A-levels in the UK. One problem associated with using A-level grades for selection is in discriminating amongst students who obtain similarly high A-level results (McManus et al. 2005). Another concern is that entry into medical school is socially exclusive, partly because A-level results might reflect type of schooling and social class (Nicholson 2005). In the USA and Canada, students apply to medical school at postgraduate level (graduate entry). However, academic grades such as grade point average (GPA) remain the main criterion for selection, although they are usually considered in combination with other predictors, such as the Medical College Admission Test (MCAT).

Some authors have shown that academic criteria, such as A-level grades, correlate with dropout rates, career progression, and success at postgraduate membership and fellowship exams (Arulampalam et al. 2007; Ferguson et al. 2002; Lumb and Vail 2004; McManus 1997; McManus and Richards 1986; McManus et al. 2005). These findings are in contrast with earlier studies, which questioned the long-term predictive validity of academic ratings (Reede 1999). Research suggests pre-admission academic grades, such as A-levels or GPAs, are related to academic performance at medical school (Kreiter and Kreiter 2007). However, the relationship of pre-admission academic grades to long-term outcome measures of doctors' performance is less clear (Ferguson et al. 2002; McManus 1997).

General mental ability and aptitude tests

Tests of *general mental ability* (GMA) and tests of specific cognitive abilities (e.g. numerical, verbal and spatial reasoning) are increasingly popular in selection procedures (Hodgkinson and Payne 1998; Ryan et al. 1999; Salgado et al. 2001). GMA and cognitive ability tests are robust predictors of job performance and training success across a wide range of occupations (Bertua et al. 2005;

Salgado et al. 2003). However, there are concerns regarding fairness, since GMA tests can result in marked racial differences in test performance (Murphy 2002; Outtz 2002).

Aptitude tests are standardized tests designed to measure the ability of a person to develop skills or acquire knowledge. They are used to predict future performance in a given activity (Cronbach 1984). Like tests of GMA, aptitude tests measure an individual's overall performance across a broad range of mental abilities. Aptitude tests often include items measuring more specialized abilities, such as verbal and numerical skills. These can predict academic, training, or job performance. Aptitude tests, which include specific ability tests and a knowledge component, are increasingly popular in medicine. In the UK, concerns over the discriminatory power of A-levels led to the introduction of additional selection methods, such as specific medical knowledge tests (Parry et al. 2006) and intellectual aptitude tests (e.g. the Oxford Medicine Admission test). The use of aptitude tests for medical school selection is also increasing across several countries (McManus et al. 2005). The outlook is somewhat different at postgraduate level though, where aptitude tests are rarely used. This is not surprising given that most applicants, particularly in the USA, have already passed an aptitude test for entry into medical school, so there is a danger of obtaining redundant information. At this stage, arguably, a high level of cognitive ability is a necessary but not a sufficient condition to predict who will be a competent physician.

In a selection context—especially with respect to widening access—it is important to distinguish between GMA, in terms of:

- *crystallized* intelligence (i.e. knowledge-based intelligence acquired via schooling)

- *fluid* intelligence (i.e. biologically-based cognitive skills, such as processing speed or inductive reasoning) (Ackerman 2003; Ackerman and Heggestad 1997; Blair 2006)

It has been argued that tests of fluid intelligence should be used for medical school admissions to widen access, so as to identify raw talent independent of education (Tiffin et al. 2012). However, other researchers argue that knowledge-based measures may be better predictors of subsequent exam performance (McManus 2005).

Personality inventories

The last 20 years have seen a substantial increase in the use of personality and related tests in personnel selection, for a broad spectrum of jobs (Barrick et al. 2001; Ones et al. 2007). Over several decades of research, personality researchers have agreed a general taxonomy of personality traits, the Big Five model, which is based on five factors or traits:

- extroversion (i.e. outgoing, sociable, impulsive)

- emotional stability (i.e. calm, relaxed)

- agreeableness (i.e. trusting, cooperative, helpful)

- conscientiousness (i.e. hardworking, dutiful, organized)

- openness to experience (i.e. artistic, cultured, creative)

Some research has shown that important relationships exist between measures of personality and job or academic performance (Barrick et al. 2001). In particular, conscientiousness has been shown to be a positive predictor of pre-clinical medical school exam results (Ferguson et al. 2003; Ferguson et al. 2000; Lievens et al. 2002), which shows incremental validity over knowledge-based assessments (Ferguson et al. 2000; Ferguson et al. 2003). Still, the use of personality tests to assess characteristics of job applicants remains controversial. Critics argue that the predictive validity of personality traits for job performance is often low (Tett et al. 1999) and that, personality tests used by organizations are often poorly chosen (Murphy and Dzieweczynski 2005). Furthermore, there exist concerns that 'faking', or responding in a socially desirable way, can compromise the validity of personality tests (Birkeland et al.200; Rosse et al. 1998), although there is evidence which suggests that this is not always the case (Hough et al. 1990).

In medicine, concerns over the strong reliance on academic predictors have led to the search for alternative selection methods. Specifically, there is a growing interest in the role of personality tests in selection at undergraduate level. The Personal Qualities Assessment (PQA) has been piloted for use in medical school selection in Australia and Scotland (Nicholson 2005), and has been shown to be effective at differentiating candidates (Lumsden et al. 2005; Powis 2009; Powis et al. 2005). However, further research into the predictive and construct validity of the PQA is required (Prideaux et al. 2011). Practically, in high stakes selection, best practice is to use personality assessment to drive more focused questioning at interviews, rather than as a screening tool in isolation.

Situational judgement tests

Selection practices within medicine have tended to focus on assessing academic ability alone, and yet research clearly shows that a range of non-academic attributes (such as integrity, empathy, and resilience) are important for effective performance as a clinician (Lumsden et al. 2005; Prideaux et al. 2011). Even so, it is difficult to measure non-academic attributes on the scale required to assess the large numbers of applicants into medical positions. For example, the reliability of interviews and selection centres in assessing non-academic attributes is variable (Albanese et al. 2003; Patterson and Ferguson 2012). Moreover, there is little research evidence to indicate the predictive validity of personality questionnaires in selection (Prideaux et al. 2011).

In response to the need to assess non-academic attributes, recruiters have turned to situational judgement tests (SJTs). These have proved to be a popular selection tool among many occupational groups (Lievens et al. 2008), due to the growing research evidence showing SJTs to be a valid and reliable method for assessing a range of non-academic attributes (Christian et al. 2010; Lievens and Sackett 2007; Patterson et al. 2012).

SJTs are usually machine-markable tests designed to assess individuals' judgement regarding situations encountered in the workplace. Candidates are presented with a set of hypothetical work-based scenarios and asked to make judgements about possible responses. SJT scenarios are typically derived from job analysis studies (Patterson et al. 2009a), to ensure that test content reflects the most important situations that a candidate may face in the job. The scenarios used in SJTs are concerned with testing awareness about what is effective behaviour in a given situation. A variety of response formats can be used in SJTs and these are typically classified into one of two formats: (1) knowledge-based (i.e. *what should you do/what is the best option*) and (2) behavioural tendency (i.e. *what would you most likely do*). Response alternatives can be presented in either a written (low-fidelity) or a video-based (medium-fidelity) format (Christian et al. 2010; Lievens et al. 2008). Unlike interviews and personality tests, SJTs offer a standardized way of objectively assessing non-academic attributes. This makes it possible to make comparisons between candidates, whilst at the same time facilitating positive candidate reactions due to the job-relatedness of the situations (Lievens and Sackett 2007).

There is emerging evidence to suggest that SJTs are a useful method to evaluate a range of professional attributes that have been shown to be important predictors of job performance in medicine (Koczwara et al. 2012; Lievens and Patterson 2011; Patterson et al. 2009b). For example, an SJT measuring empathy, integrity and resilience is used to select doctors applying for training in general practice in the UK (Plint and Patterson 2010), and an SJT is used to measure applicants' interpersonal awareness in medical school admissions in Belgium (Lievens et al. 2005a). Not only do SJTs offer an objective way of reliably assessing non-academic attributes, they are also low cost compared to alternative methods, such as patient simulations in selection centres.

Selection centres

A selection centre (SC) is a selection *method*, not a place. SCs (often called assessment centres) involve a combination of selection techniques, such as written exercises, interviews, and work simulations, to assess candidates across a number of key skills, attitudes, and behaviours. Candidates are usually assessed in groups or individually by multiple assessors. The SC is different from an OSCE. In an OSCE, each station assesses a candidate in one key skill, and is usually observed by one assessor. By contrast, the SC allows the candidate multiple situations (interview, work simulation, or written exercise) to demonstrate a key skill, and to be observed by a number of trained assessors. Thus, a fairer and more reliable assessment can be made (due to multiple observations of key behaviours by multiple observers). With careful design, the increased reliability should equate to greater validity (Jefferis 2007) and more positive candidate reactions.

SCs were first used during World War II to select military personnel. However, it was not until the 1950s that the idea developed as a selection method, when the American company AT&T applied SCs to identify people with managerial potential. Since then, SCs have been widely used in recruitment. SCs are especially popular for graduate recruitment, with IRS Employment Review estimating that over half of recruiters, and over 95% of large organizations employing more than 10 000 individuals, use selection centres for graduate recruitment (IRS Employment Review 2004). It is only recently that SCs have been used in medicine (Patterson et al. 2001). In the UK, Patterson and colleagues have pioneered the use of SCs to select GPs and the results have shown good predictive validity in this context (Patterson et al. 2005). This work has been extended to select doctors for postgraduate training in other specialties, such as obstetrics and gynaecology, and paediatrics (Randall et al. 2006a, b). Patterson and colleagues have also piloted the use of SCs in the UK for graduate entry to medical school (Kidd et al. 2006).

Research shows that a carefully designed and run SC can be effective at predicting job performance across a wide range of occupations (Damitz et al. 2003; Lievens et al. 2005b; Schmidt and Hunter 1998; Schmitt et al. 1984). As described earlier, gains are made in reliability and validity because SCs make use of a combination of different exercises (using a multi-trait, multi-method approach) and use standardized scoring systems to measure the selection criteria. Scoring should be directly linked to the selection criteria (not the exercise scores) and the information gathered should be interpreted in context by trained assessors. Well-executed SCs have incremental validity over cognitive ability tests (Dayan et al. 2002; Krause et al. 2006; Lievens et al. 2003) and they tend to be viewed positively by candidates (Macan et al. 1994; Rynes and Connerley 1993). Thus, careful design and implementation of an SC is crucial for the assessment to live up to its reputation and to be cost-effective (Algera and Grueter 1989; Woodruffe 2000).

Table 33.1 summarizes the research evidence on the utility of different selection tools. The evidence on each of the techniques listed also includes an estimate of extent of usage across all occupational groups, and likely applicant reactions to each. Note that there are international differences in the extent of use of the methods, which is also influenced by differences in employment law.

Design of selection systems

Selection systems design concentrates on an overall programme of assessment, comprising a combination of methods (each with their distinctive psychometric properties) to make decisions about candidate selection. The focus of selection systems design is not on how much validity a single assessment method adds; rather it is concerned with *for what purpose a selection method is most valid*.

The aim of selection systems design is to develop a bespoke selection process that uses methods that assess the relevant competencies identified through a multi-source, multi-method job analysis. For example, research into the use of selection systems design for postgraduate training has shown that integration of domain specific knowledge tests, low-fidelity SJTs, and high-fidelity selection centres work in combination to provide higher incremental validity, beyond that of any of these measures if used in isolation (Lievens and Patterson 2011). In addition, for the selection system to be credible, all job-relevant stakeholders should be involved in every step of the design process, from the job analysis to the design of the selection methods, through to the design of the outcome measures. This stakeholder involvement adds contextual relevance to the selection system and encourages organizational ownership of the selection programme. Box 33.2 outlines some of the difficulties associated with establishing the credibility and stakeholder ownership of a new selection system, by describing the shift away from localized selection towards nationally coordinated standardized tailored assessments. There are various factors that contribute to the success of selection systems design. Notably, it is not just the

selection methods that have to be corporately owned and validated; the system supporting the process is also critical for success (Plint and Patterson 2010).

Key issues in selection systems design are utility and cost efficiency, especially in systems with large numbers of applicants, as this could seriously limit the opportunities to use certain selection methods (Prideaux et al. 2011). Investment in the development of bespoke selection measures may be expensive at the outset, but in the medium to long-term, this investment can translate into significant gains in utility. For example, switching from a hand-scored application form method to a machine-markable test developed in partnership with key stakeholders can significantly reduce costs (Lievens and Patterson 2011; Irish et al. 2011; Patterson et al. 2009a, b).

There is a specific consideration that is also particularly relevant to national medical school selection: *political validity*. Political validity relates to the influence that stakeholder groups outside of an organization have on the design and development of its selection systems (Patterson and Zibarras 2011; Patterson et al. 2012b). For example, in most countries there are various perspectives that must be taken into account when developing medical selection systems. These include: professional trade unions, regulators, professional bodies, employer associations, the general public, politicians, and the government. This means that the design, development, and implementation of any new selection system requires acceptance from a variety of important stakeholders, who often have different views on how selection practices should be administered.

At present, there are some selection practices that display little or no predictive validity (e.g. a lottery system for entry into medical school, or referees' reports for advanced level selection). However, these practices are viewed as politically valid because various groups of important stakeholders consider them credible. For example, the introduction of a lottery system for medical selection addresses a political agenda of widening access into medical school by removing from the process, variables such as socioeconomic status, access to education, and family income. Similarly, using unstructured referees' reports for selection into advanced levels of postgraduate training addresses the employers' political agenda of obtaining senior medics' personal appraisals of candidates' characters, which is often perceived as being more credible than performance on high-fidelity selection tools. Although a selection method may be viewed as politically valid, this is no guarantee of predictive validity (which

Table 33.1 The relative accuracy of different selection techniques.

Selection method	Evidence for criterion-related validity	Applicant reactions	Extent of use
Structured interviews	High	Moderate to positive	High
Cognitive ability	High	Negative to moderate	Moderate
Personality tests	Moderate	Negative to moderate	Moderate
Work sample tests	High	Positive	Low
Selection centres	High	Positive	Moderate
Handwriting	Low	Negative to moderate	Low
References	Low	Positive	High

Box 33.2 From the 'good old days' of medical selection to specialty-tailored assessments

Selection practices for postgraduate training in the UK would typically involve short-listing a large number of unstructured CVs, followed by a series of unstructured panel interviews using a variety of non-standardized, person specifications for each of the medical specialties (Plint and Patterson 2010; Field 2000). This lack of standardization and the emphasis on medical school performance ratings led to legal challenges (Highhouse 2008). From a selection perspective, research has found that medical school performance alone could not be used effectively to predict success in postgraduate specialty training (Ferguson et al. 2002; McManus et al. 2003), because other qualities were required (Eva and Reiter 2005).

In 2006, a national approach to selection was adopted that developed standardized person specifications for each of the postgraduate specialties, and in 2007 a move was recommended towards specialty-tailored assessments at SCs (Tooke 2007). SCs use multi-trait, multi-method approaches (Lievens et al. 2003) that assess candidates on various criteria, and are considered to have high reliability and predictive validity (Schmidt and Hunter 1998; Robertson and Smith 2001). Based on this recommendation, fair and transparent national selection programmes for entry into UK medical specialty training have been carefully developed using international best practice methods and the involvement of key stakeholders. By using SCs and machine-marked tests, the new national selection programmes have shown good predictive validity (Patterson et al. 2009b; Gale et al. 2010), favourable candidate reactions (Gilliland 1993), and substantial savings in recruitment costs (Crawford 2005). Despite these positive outcomes, some UK doctors still refer to the time before the national coordination of the recruitment process as 'the good old days'. This shows how important it is to encourage stakeholder buy-in, and highlights the importance of involving all stakeholder groups at all stages when developing a new selection system.

can be empirically demonstrated). This means that while the stakeholders might be satisfied with the selection method, there is still a risk of the wrong people being selected.

The way to address this is through effective selection systems design, such as that illustrated by the programme exploring widening entry into medicine. For example, medical schools in the UK that use the UK Clinical Aptitude Test (UKCAT) as part of their admissions process are attempting to reduce the relative disadvantage faced by certain socioeconomic groups (Tiffin et al. 2012). Despite efforts to improve social mobility through access to higher education in the UK, access to medicine is still largely restricted to those from advantaged backgrounds (only 5% of entrants have parents from a non-professional background). There has been a push to widen participation in medicine, which led to the development of the UKCAT in 2006. The UKCAT assesses skills such as verbal reasoning and decision analysis and is designed to ensure that candidates have the most appropriate mental abilities for a career in medicine (fig. 33.3). In the USA, some schools have developed community outreach programmes that comprise special preparation and enrichment programmes; these act within comprehensive strategies of recruitment and retention (Acosts and Olsen 2006). By incorporating these additional training and assessment programmes into selection systems design, more members of underrepresented socioeconomic communities are now being admitted into medical school (Thomson et al. 2003).

Future research

Selection in medicine is a relatively new research topic, and there are still many unchartered territories. The discipline of medicine is changing dramatically and the skills relevant to many specialties are changing rapidly. For example, in surgery, the use of laparoscopes and other technologies has transformed many surgical procedures. With rapid developments in technology, it is likely that the pace of change will increase. As a result, since the career path for a physician is long and complex, it is difficult to define appropriate selection criteria for student selection that are also relevant to physicians of the future. Research must involve more job analysis studies to define the knowledge, skills, abilities and attitudes relevant for

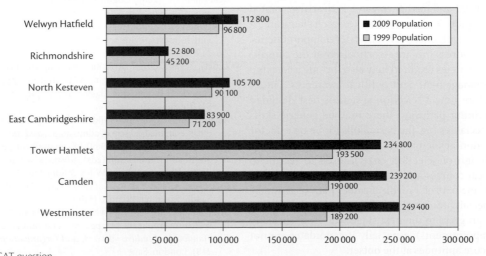

Figure 33.3 Sample UKCAT question.
Reproduced from Brian Holmes, Marianna Parker, and Katie Hunt, Score Higher on the UKCAT, 2012, p. 83, with permission from Oxford University Press.

physicians in general, and to explore differences between special-ties. In many countries, the enhanced focus on patient satisfaction has highlighted the requirement for empathy and communication skills, where doctors work in partnership with patients. In this way, given that medicine involves a specialized career path, the demands on individuals entering a career in medicine are high.

Designing an accurate selection system is a complex process. It should be acknowledged that medical education and training is a continual process, and that the predictive validity of selection tests may not be stable at all points in the career pathway. A fac-tor may be identified as an important predictor for undergraduate training but may not be predictive for aspects of specialty training. For example, conscientiousness is a positive predictor for under-graduate pre-clinical training but a negative predictor for under-graduate clinical performance (Ferguson et al. 2003). Similarly, other evidence shows that openness to experience is important to GP training performance, but is not important for undergraduate training performance. The real challenge is to integrate this knowl-edge and to develop selection systems that are internally reliable from undergraduate selection through to selection for specialty training.

Future research must account for contemporary theoretical mod-els of adult intellectual development and skills acquisition, which attempt to integrate cognitive and non-cognitive factors. One such model is PPIK theory (Ackerman 1996), which asserts that adult intellectual ability is a function of four factors:

* process (e.g. basic mental capacities, such a processing speed)
* personality (e.g. extroversion or conscientiousness)
* interests (e.g. preferences for science or art)
* knowledge (e.g. factual knowledge, as contained in A-levels)

Specifically, PPIK theory proposes a developmental trajectory to understand adult intellectual functioning, where personality, intellect and interests operate concurrently. For example, a per-son's interests may influence the types of knowledge they seek out. This approach may help us to understand what motivates people to study medicine, and their choice and aptitude for later specialty training.

The selection gateways to progress in medical training should be preceded by accurate careers information. The process of self-selec-tion is crucially important and further research is clearly warranted in this area. When exploring the selection research literature, it is notable that little research exists for senior-level appointments. Future research must address this area, particularly at the consult-ant level, where competencies required may also include leadership of teams, resource management, and political awareness. Future research should explore how a selection system is best designed across the whole training pathway. There may be generic skills required across all specialties (i.e. the basic skills for being a doctor including cognitive, non-academic and behavioural skills). These should guide the design of selection criteria used to recruit to undergraduate medical courses at the outset of training. It should not be assumed that one part of a medical career path (e.g. under-graduate to initial specialty training) will fully prepare an applicant with all the skills to progress to the next stage (e.g. from specialty training to senior appointments), especially if candidates are not selected to have the core aptitudes at the outset.

Conclusions

♦ Best practice in the design of selection systems involves two fun-damental elements: (a) conducting a thorough job analysis, and (b) conducting validation research to assess the predictive valid-ity of the selection instruments. The design of selection systems should also be a two-way, iterative process, whereby candidates' evaluations of the selection process are used to make improve-ments to the system. Research shows that candidates tend to prefer high-fidelity selection methods, such as simulation exer-cises in selection centres. This can present a 'justice dilemma' for employers who also need to balance the costs of implementing high-fidelity selection methods with the costs of implementing low-fidelity methods with sufficient validity, such as machine-marked aptitude tests.

♦ An in-depth job analysis, which identifies appropriate selection criteria for a particular role, is fundamental to producing an effec-tive selection system. This analysis should detail responsibilities in the target job and provide information about the particular competencies and characteristics required of the jobholder. The identification of selection criteria should also be used to guide the choice of selection methods.

♦ Once selection decisions are made, and appointed applicants have started working in the role, information should be col-lected on employees' job performance. This information should be related back to the original selection criteria, so as to examine the predictive validity of the selection instruments.

♦ A relatively large amount of research exists on the predictive validity of various cognitive factors in relation to exam per-formance at medical school. Relatively less research has been conducted looking into the predictive validity of factors predict-ing performance of doctors at subsequent stages of the medical career pathway. Further research is required to explore the extent to which selection methods can predict a range of work perform-ance and training outcomes in the long-term.

References

Ackerman, P.L. (1996) A theory of adult intellectual development: Process, personality, interests, and knowledge. *Intelligence.* 22(2): 227–257

Ackerman, P.L. (2003) Cognitive ability and non-ability trait determinants of expertise. *Educ Res.* 32(8): 15–20

Ackerman, P.L. and Heggestad, E.D. (1997) Intelligence, personality, and interests: evidence for overlapping traits. *Psychol Bull.* 121(2): 219–245

Acosts, D. and Olsen, P. (2006) Meeting the needs of regional minority groups: the University of Washington's programs to increase the American Indian and Alaskan native physician workforce. *Acad Med.* 81(10): 863–870

Albanese, M.A., Snow, M.H., and Skochelak, S.E. et al. (2003) Assessing personal qualities in medical school admissions. *Acad Med,* 78(3), 313–321.

Algera, J. and Grueter, M. (1989) Job analysis for personnel selection. In: M. Smith and I. Robertson (eds) *Advances in Selection and Assessment* (pp. 7–30). Chichester: John Wiley & Sons Ltd

Anastasia, A. and Urbina, S. (1997) *Psychological Testing.* 7th edn. Upper Saddle River, NJ: Prentice Hall

Anderson, N., Born, M., and Cunningham-Snell, N. (2001) Recruitment and selection: Applicant perspectives and outcomes. In N. Anderson (ed.) *Handbook of Industrial Work and Organizational Psychology* (pp. 200–218). London: Sage

Arulampalam, W., Naylor, R.A., and Smith, J.P. (2007) A hazard model of the probability of medical school drop-out in the UK. *Roy Stat Soc*. 167: 157–178

Barrick, M.R., Mount, M.K., and Judge, T.A. (2001) Personality and performance at the beginning of the new millennium: What do we know and where do we go next? *Int J Selection Assess*. 9: 9–30

Bertua, C., Anderson, N., and Salgado, J. F. (2005) The predictive validity of cognitive ability tests: A UK meta-analysis. *J Occ Org Psychol*. 78(3): 387–409

Birkeland, S.A., Manson, T.M., Kisamore, J.L., et al. (2006) A meta-analytic investigation of job applicant faking on personality measures. *Int J Selection Assess*. 14: 317–335

Blair, C. (2006) How similar are fluid cognition and general intelligence? A developmental neuroscience perspective on fluid cognition as an aspect of human cognitive ability. *Behav Brain Sci*. 29: 109–160

Bobko, P., Roth, P.L., and Potosky, D. (1999) Derivation and implications of a meta-analytic matrix incorporating cognitive ability, alternative predictors, and job performance. *Personnel Psychol*. 52(3): 561–589

Campion, M.A., Palmer, D.K., and Campion, J.E. (1997) A review of structure in the selection interview. *Personnel Psychol*. 50: 655–702

Campion, M.A., Pursell, E.D., and Brown, B.K. (1988) Structured interviewing: raising the psychometric properties of the employement interview. *Personnel Psychol*. 41(1): 25–42

Christian, M., Edwards, B., and Bradley, J. (2010) Situational judgement tests: constructs assessed and a meta-analysis of their criterion-related validities. *Personnel Psychol*. 63: 83–117

Cohen, J. (1988) Statistical power analysis for the social sciences. 2nd edn. London: Earlbaum.

Cortina, J.M., Goldsten, N.B., Payne, S.C. et al. (2000) The incremental validaty of interview scores over and above cognitive ability and conscientiousness scores. *Personnel Psychol*. 53(2): 325–351

Crawford, M.E. (2005) Reassuring evidence on competency based selection. *BMJ*. 330(7493): 714

Cronbach, L.J. (1984) *Essentials of Psychological Testing*. 4th edn. New York: Harper and Row

Damitz, M., Manzey, D., Kleinmann, M. et al. (2003) Assessment center for pilot selection: Construct and criterion validity and the impact of assessor type. *Appl Psychol*. 52(2): 193–212

Dayan, K., Kasten, R., and Fox, S. (2002) Entry-level police candidate assessment center: An efficient tool or a hammer to kill a fly? *Personnel Psychol*. 55: 827–849

Dicks, H.V. (1965) Medical education and medical practice. *BMJ*. 2: 818

Dore, K.L., Kreuger, S., Ladhani, M., et al. (2010) The reliability and acceptability of the Multiple Mini-Interview as a selection instrument for postgraduate admissions. *Acad Med*. 85(10): 60–63

Dowell, J., Lynch, B., Till, H., et al. (2012) The multiple mini-interview in the U.K. context: 3 years of experience at Dundee. *Med Teach*. 34(4): 297–304

Edwards, J.C., Johnson, E.K., and Molidor, J.B. (1990) The interview in the admission process. *Acad Med*, 65(3): 167–177

Eva, K. and Reiter, H. (2004) Where judgement fails: pitfalls in the selection process for medical personnel. *Adv Health Sci Educ*. 9(2): 161–174

Eva, K.W. and Reiter, H.I. (2005) Reflecting the relative values of community, faculty and students in the admissions tools of medical school. *Teach Learn Med*. 17: 4–8

Eva, K., Reiter, H., Rosenfeld, J., et al. (2004a) The relationship between interviewers' characteristics and ratings assigned during a multiple mini-interview. *Acad Med*. 79(6): 602–609

Eva, K., Rosenfeld, J. and Reiter, H. et al. (2004b) An admissions OSCE: the multiple mini-interview. *Med Educ*. 38(3), 314–326.

Eva, K., Reiter, H., Trinh, K. et al. (2009) Predictive validity of the multiple mini-interview for selecting medical trainees. *Med Educ*. 43(8): 767–775

Eva, K., Wood, T., Riddle, J. et al. (2010) How clinical features are presented matters to weaker diagnosticians. *Med Educ*. 44(8): 775–785

Ferguson, E., Sanders, A., O'Hehir, F., et al. (2000) Predictive validity of personal statements and the role of the five factor model of personality in relation to medical training. *J Occ Organis Psychol*. 73: 321–344

Ferguson, E., James, D., and Madeley, L. (2002) Factors associated with success in medical school: systematic review of the literature. *BMJ*. 324(7343): 952–957

Ferguson, E., James, D., O'Hehir, F., et al. (2003) Pilot study of the roles of personality, references, and personal statements in relation to performance over the five years of a medical degree. *BMJ*. 326(7386): 429–432

Field, S. (2000) Vocational training; the dawn of a new era? *Educ Gen Pract*.11: 38

Gale, T.C.E., Roberts, M.J., Sice, P.J., et al. (2010) Predictive validity of a selection centre testing non-technical skills for recruitment to training in anaesthesia. *Br J Anaesth*. 105(5): 603–609

Gilliland, S.W. (1993) The perceived fairness of selection systems: An organizational justice perspective. *Acad Manag Rev*. 18(4): 694

Goho, J. and Blackman, A. (2006) The effectiveness of academic admission interviews: an exploratory meta-analysis. *Med Teach*. 28(4): 335–340

Greengross, S. (1997) What patients want from their doctors. In: I. Allen, P. Brown, and P. Hughes (eds) *Choosing Tomorrow's Doctors* (pp. 9–12). London: Policy Studies Institute

Harris, S. and Owen, C. (2007) Discerning quality: using the multiple mini-interview in student selection for the Australian National University Medical School. *Med Educ*. 41(3): 234–241

Hausknecht, J.P., Day, D.V., and Thomas, S.C. (2004) Applicant reactions to selection procedures: An updated model and meta-analysis. *Personnel Psychol*. 57(3): 639–683

Highhouse, S. (2008) Stubborn reliance on intuition and subjectivity in employee selection. *Industrial Organiz Psychol*. 1(3): 333–342

Hodgkinson, G.P. and Payne, R.L. (1998) Graduate selection in three European countries. *J Occ Organiz Psychol*. 71(4): 359–365

Hofmeister, M., Lockyer, J., and Crutcher, R. (2009) The multiple mini-interview for selection of international medical graduates into family medicine residency education. *Med Educ*. 43(6): 573–579

Hough, L.M., Eaton, N.K., Dunnette, M.D., Kamp, J.D., and McCloy, R.A. (1990)Criterion related validities of personality constructs and effect of response distortion on those validities. *J Appl Psychol*. 75: 581–595

Hughes, P. (2002) Can we improve on how we select medical students? *J Roy Soc Med*. 95(1): 18–22

Irish, B., Carr, A.S., Sowden, D., et al. (2011) Recruitment into specialty training in the UK [Online] (updated 12 Jan 2011) http://careers.bmj.com/careers/advice/view-article.html?id=20001789 Accessed 28 June 2012

IRS Employment Review (2002) Of good character: supplying references and providing access. *IRS Employment Review*. 754: 6–34

IRS Employment Review (2004) Graduate Recruitment 2004/05: upturn and optimism. *IRS Employment Review*. 811: 8–40.

Jefferis, T. (2007) Selection for specialist training: what can we learn from other countries? *BMJ*. 334: 1302–1304

Kidd, J., Fuller, J., Patterson, F., et al. (2006) Selection Centres: Initial description of a collaborative pilot project. Proceedings for the Association for Medical Education in Europe (AMEE) Conference, September, Genoa, Italy

Klehe, U.C. (2004) Choosing how to choose: Institutional pressures affecting the adoption of personnel selection procedures. *Int J Selection Assess*. 12(4): 327–342

Koczwara, A., Patterson, F., Zibarras, L., et al. (2012) Evaluating cognitive ability, knowledge tests and situational judgement tests for postgraduate selection. *Med Educ*. 46(4): 399–408

Krause, D.E., Kersting, M., Heggestad, E., et al. (2006) Incremental validity of assessment center ratings over cognitive ability tests: A study at the executive management level. *Int J Selection Assess*. 14: 360–371

Kreiter, C. and Kreiter, Y. (2007) A validity generalization perspective on the ability of undergraduate GPA and the medical college admission test to predict important outcomes. *Teach Learn Med*. 19(2): 95–100

Kreiter, C., Yin, P., Solow, C., et al. (2004) Investigating the reliability of the medical school admissions interview. *Adv Health Sci Educ*. 9(2): 147–159

Kumar, K., Roberts, C., Rothnie, I., et al. (2009) Experiences of the multiple mini-interview: a qualitative analysis. *Med Educ.* 43(4): 360–367

Lemay, J.-F., Lockyer, J., Collin, V., et al. (2007) Assessment of non-cognitive traits through the admissions multiple mini-interview. *Med Educ.* 41(6): 573–579

Lievens, F. and Patterson, F. (2011) The validity and incremental validity of knowledge tests, low-fidelity simulations, and high-fidelity simulations for predicting job performance in advanced-level high-stakes selection. *J Appl Psychol.* 96(5): 927–940

Lievens, F. and Sackett, P. (2007) Situational judgment tests in high-stakes settings: issues and strategies with generating alternate forms. *J Appl Psychol.* 92(4): 1043–1055

Lievens, F. and Thornton, G.C. (2005) Assessment centres: recent developments in practice and research. In: A. Evers, O. Smit-Voskuijl, and N. Anderson (eds) *Handbook of Personnel Selection* (pp. 243–264). Oxford: Blackwell

Lievens, F., Buyse, T., and Sackett, P. R. (2005a) The operational validity of a video-based situational judgment test for medical college admissions: Illustrating the importance of matching predictor and criterion construct domains. *J Appl Psychol.* 90(3): 442–452

Lievens, F., Van Keer, E., and De Witte, M. (2005b) Assessment centers in Belgium: The results of a study on their validity and fairness. *Psychologie du Travail et des Organisations.* 11: 25–33

Lievens, F., Peeters, H., and Schollaert, E. (2008) Situational judgment tests: a review of recent research. *Personnel Rev.* 37(4): 426–441

Lievens, F., Coetsier, P., De Fruyt, F., et al. (2002) Medical students' personality characteristics and academic performance: A five-factor model perspective. *Med Educ.* 36: 1050–1056

Lievens, F., Harris, M., Van, K., et al. (2003) Predicting cross-cultural training performance: the validity of personality, cognitive ability, and dimensions measured by an assessment center and a behavior description interview. *J Appl Psychol.* 88(3): 476–489

Lumb, A. and Vail, A. (2004) Comparison of academic, application form and social factors in predicting early performance on the medical course. *Med Educ.* 38(9): 1002–1005

Lumsden, M., Bore, M., Millar, K., et al. (2005) Assessment of personal qualities in relation to admission to medical school. *Med Educ.* 39: 258–265

Macan, T.H., Avedon, M.J., Paese, M., et al. (1994) The effects of applicants' reactions to cognitive ability tests and an assessment center. *Personnel Psychol.* 47: 715–738

McCarthy, J.M. and Goffin, R.D. (2001) Improving the validity of letters of recommendation: An investigation of three standardized reference forms. *Military Psychol.* 13(4): 199–222

McDaniel, M.A., Whetzel, D.L., Schmidt, F.L., et al. (1994) The validity of employment interviews: A comprehensive review and meta-analysis. *J Appl Psychol.* 79(4): 599–616

McManus, I.C. (1997) From selection to qualification: how and why medical students change. In: I. Allen, P. Brown, and P. Hughes (eds) *Choosing Tomorrow's Doctors* (pp. 60–79). London: Policy Studies Institute

McManus, I.C. (2003) Commentary: How to derive causes from correlations in educational studies. *BMJ.* 326(7386): 429–432

McManus, I.C. and Richards, P. (1986) Prospective survey of performance of medical students during preclinical years. *BMJ.* 293(6539): 124–127

McManus, I.C., Smithers, E., Partridge, P., et al. (2003) A levels and intelligence as predictors of medical careers in UK doctors: 20 year prospective study. *BMJ.* 327(7407): 139–142

McManus, I.C., Powis, D., Wakeford, R., et al. (2005) Intellectual aptitude tests and A-levels for selecting UK school leaver entrants for medical school. *BMJ.* 331(7516): 555–559

Meredith, K.E., Dunlap, M.R., and Baker, H.H. (1982) Subjective and objective admissions factors as predictors of clinical clerkship performance. *Med Educ.* 57(10, Pt 1): 743–751

Mirabile, R.J. (1990) The power of job analysis. *Training.* 27(4): 70–72,74

Morgeson, F.P. and Campion, M.A. (1997) Social and cognitive sources of potential inaccuracy in job analysis. *J Appl Psychol.* 82(5): 627–655

Muchinsky, P.M. (1979) The use of reference reports in personnel selection: a review and evaluation. *J Occ Psychol.* 52(4): 287–297

Murphy, K.R. (2002) Can conflicting perspectives on the role of g in personnel selection be resolved? *Human Performance.* 15(1–2): 173–186

Murphy, K.R. and Dzieweczynski, J.L. (2005) Why don't measures of broad dimensions of personality perform better as predictors of job performance? *Human Performance.* 18: 343–357

Nicholson, S. (2005) The benefits of aptitude testing for selecting medical students. *BMJ.* 331(7516): 559–560

Ones, D.S., Dilchert, S., Viswesvaran, C., et al. (2007) In support of personality assessment in organizational settings. *Personnel Psychol.* 60(4): 995–1027

Oswald, F.L. (2003) Job analysis: Methods research and applications for human resource management in the new millennium. *Personnel Psychol.* 56(3): 800–803

Outtz J (2002) The role of cognitive ability tests in employment selection. *Human Performance.* 15: 161–171

Parry, J., Mathers, J., Stevens, A., et al. (2006) Admissions processes for five year medical courses at English schools: review. *BMJ.* 332(7548): 1005–1009

Patterson, F. and Ferguson, E. (2012) Testing non-cognitive attributes in selection centres: how to avoid being reliably wrong. *Med Educ.* 46(3): 240–242

Patterson, F. and Zibarras, L. (2011) Exploring the construct of perceived job discrimination and a model of applicant propensity for case initiation in selection. *Int J Selection Assess.* 19(3): 251–257

Patterson, F., Ferguson, E., Lane, P., et al. (2000) A competency model for general practice: implications for selection, training, and development. *Br J Gen Pract.* 50(452): 188–193

Patterson, F., Ferguson, E., Lane, P., et al (2001) A new competency based selection system for general practitioners. *BMJ.* 323: 2–3

Patterson, F., Ferguson, E., Lane, P., et al. (2005) A new selection system to recruit general practice registrars: preliminary findings from a validation study. *BMJ.* 330(7493): 711–714

Patterson, F., Ferguson, E., and Thomas, S. (2008) Using job analysis to identify core and specific competencies: implications for selection and recruitment. *Med Educ.* 42(12): 1195–1204

Patterson, F., Baron, H., Carr, V., et al. (2009a) Evaluation of three short-listing methodologies for selection into postgraduate training in general practice. *Med Educ.* 43: 50–57

Patterson, F., Carr, V., Zibarras, L., et al. (2009b) New machine- marked tests for selection into core medical training: evidence from two validation studies. *Clin Med.* 9: 417–420

Patterson, F., Denney, M.-L., Wakeford, R., et al. (2011a) Fair and equal assessment in postgraduate training? A future research agenda. *Br J Gen Pract.* 61(593): 712–713

Patterson, F., Zibarras, L., Carr, V., et al. (2011b) Evaluating candidate reactions to selection practices using organisational justice theory. *Med Educ.* 45(3): 289–297

Patterson, F., Lievens, F., Kerrin, M., Zibarras, L., and Carette, B. (2012a) Designing selection systems for medicine: Implications for the political validity of high stakes selection methods. *Int J Selection Assess.* 20(4): 486–496

Patterson, F., Ashworth, V., Zibarras, L., et al. (2012b) Evaluating the effectiveness of situational judgement tests to assess non-academic attributes in selection. *Med Educ.* 46(9): 850–868

Plint, S. and Patterson, F. (2010) Identifying critical success factors for designing selection processes into postgraduate specialty training: the case of UK general practice. *Postgrad Med J.* 86(1016): 323–327

Posthuma, R.A., Morgeson, F.P., and Campion, M.A. (2002) Beyond employment interview validity: a comprehensive narrative review of recent research and trends over time. *Personnel Psychol.* 55(1): 1–81

Powis, D. (2009) Personality testing in the context of selecting health professionals. *Med Teach.* 31(12): 1045–1046

Powis, D., Bore, M., Munro, D., et al. (2005) Development of the personal qualities assessment as a tool for selecting medical students. *J Adult Cont Educ.* 11(1): 3–14

Prideaux, D., Roberts, C., Eva, K., et al. (2011) Assessment for selection for the health care professions and specialty training: Consensus statement and recommendations from the Ottawa 2010 Conference. *Med Teach.* 33(3): 215–223

Quintero, A., Segal, L., King, T., et al. (2009) The personal interview: assessing the potential for personality similarity to bias the selection of orthopaedic residents. *Acad Med,* 84(10): 1364–1372

Randall, R., Davies, H., Patterson, F., et al. (2006a) Selecting doctors for postgraduate training in paediatrics using a competency based assessment centre. *Arch Dis Childh.* 91(5): 444–448

Randall, R., Stewart, P., Farrell, K., et al. (2006b) Using an assessment centre to select doctors for postgraduate training in obstetrics and gynaecology. *Obstet Gynaecol.* 8(4): 257–262

Razack, S., Faremo, S., Drolet, F., et al. (2009) Multiple mini-interviews versus traditional interviews: stakeholder acceptability comparison. *Med Educ.* 43(10): 993–1000

Reede, J.Y. (1999) Predictors of success in medicine. *Clin Orthopaed Rel Res.* 362: 72–77

Robertson, I.T. and Smith, M. (2001) Personnel selection. *J Occ Organiz Psychol.* 74(4): 441–472

Roberts, C., Walton, M., Rothnie, I., et al.(2008) Factors affecting the utility of the multiple mini-interview in selecting candidates for graduate-entry medical school. *Med Educ.* 42: 396–404

Rosenfeld, J., Reiter, H., Trinh, K., et al. (2008) A cost efficiency comparison between the multiple mini-interview and traditional admissions interviews. *Adv Health Sci Educ.* 13(1): 43–58

Rosse, J.G., Stecher, M.D., Miller, J.L., et al. (1998)The impact of response distortion on pre-employment personality testing and hiring decisions. *J Appl Psychol.* 83: 634–644

Ryan, A.M., McFarland, L., and Baron, H. (1999) An international look at selection practices: nation and culture as explanation for variability in practice. *Personnel Psychol.* 52(2): 359–392

Rynes, S.L. and Connerley, M.L. (1993) Applicant reactions to alternative selection procedures. *J Business Psychol.* 7(3): 261–277

Salgado, J.F. and Anderson, N. (2002)Cognitive and GMA testing in the European Community: Issues and evidence. *Human Performance.* 15: 75–96

Salgado, J., Anderson, N., Moscoso, S., et al. (2003) A meta-analytic study of general mental ability validity for different occupations in the European community. *J Appl Psychol.* 88(6): 1068–1081

Salgado, J.F., Viswesvaran, C., and Ones, D. (2001) Predictors used for personnel selection: an overview of constructs, methods, and techniques. In: N. Anderson, D. S. Ones, H. K. Sinangil, et al. (eds) *Handbook of Industrial. Work and Organizational Psychology.* Volume 1 (pp. 99–165). London: Sage

Schmidt, F.L. and Hunter, J.E. (1998) The validity and utility of selection methods in personnel psychology: Practical and theoretical implications of 85 years of research findings. *Psychol Bull.* 124(2): 262–274

Schmitt, N., Gooding, R.Z., Noe, R.A., et al. (1984) Meta-analyses of validity studies published between 1964 and 1982 and the investigation of study characteristics. *Personnel Psychol.* 37: 407–422

Siddique, C. (2004) Job analysis: a strategic human resource management practice. *Int J Human Resource Manag.* 15(1): 219–244

Terpstra, D.A., Mohamed, A.A., and Kethley, R.B. (1999) An analysis of Federal court cases involving nine selection devices. *Int J Selection Assess.* 7(1): 26–34

Tett, R.P., Jackson, D.N., Rothstein, M., et al. (1999) Meta-analysis of bi-directional relations in personality-job performance research. *Human Performance.* 12: 1–29

Thomson, W., Ferry, P., King, J., et al. (2003) Increasing access to medical education for students from medically underserved communities: one program's success. *Acad Med.* 78(5): 454–459

Tiffin, P.A., Dowell, J.S., and McLachlan, J.C. (2012) Widening access to UK medical education for under-represented socioeconomic groups: modelling the impact of the UKCAT in the 2009 cohort. *BMJ.* 344: e1805

Tooke, J. (2007) Aspiring to Excellence: Findings and recommendations of the independent inquiry into modernising medical careers. *MMC Inquiry* [Online] (Updated 28 Feb 2008) http://www.mmcinquiry.org.uk/ Accessed 28 June 2012

van der Vleuten, C.P.M. (1996) The assessment of professional competence: developments, research and practical implications. *Adv Health Sci Educ.* 1: 41–67

van der Vleuten, C. and Schuwirth, L. (2005) Assessing professional competence: from methods to programmes. *Med Educ.* 39: 309–317

Wiesner, W.H. and Cronshaw, S.F. (1988) A meta-analytic investigation of the impact of interview format and degree of structure on the validity of the employment interview. *J Occ Psychol.* 61(4): 275–290

Williamson, L.G., Campion, J.E., Malos, S.B., et al. (1997) Employment interview on trial: Linking interview structure with litigation outcomes. *J Appl Psychol.* 82(6): 900–912

Woodruffe, C. (2000) *Development and Assessment Centres: Identifying and Developing Competence.* 3rd edn. London: Institute of Personnel and Development

Woolf, K., Potts, H.W., and McManus, I.C. (2011) Ethnicity and academic performance in UK trained doctors and medical students: Systematic review and meta-analysis. *BMJ.* 342: 901

CHAPTER 34

Study dropout in medical education

Gilbert Reibnegger and Simone Manhal

The reward for work well done is the opportunity to do more.

Jonas Salk (1956)

Introduction

Medical education is an important issue of considerable public interest (Finucane and McCrorie 2010; Walsh 2011); it is essential in order to train new medical doctors, thereby securing sustained and continuing healthcare. Medical education is more expensive than most other study programmes. To be successful in medical education, students are required to possess strong personal characteristics and abilities, both of cognitive and non-cognitive nature. Dropout in medical education is therefore an important topic for society, for medical schools, for the medical profession, and for the individual students and their families.

In publicly funded medical education, dropout means economic loss to society: directly because of lost investment, and indirectly because of the risk that the required flow of new doctors entering the healthcare system might be reduced. For medical schools students dropping out of study without achieving graduation results in direct economic loss and, even more dangerously, bear the risk of a reduction of public funding and, thus, poorer quality of teaching in the future. A high rate of dropout in a medical school could be seen as an indicator of general deficiencies and weaknesses of the educational system at the institution. Student attrition wastes the resources of the school and adversely affects the morale of the remaining students and staff (Simpson and Budd, 1996). For the individual students and their families, economic losses will result from dropout, but also more serious consequences are likely to occur such as reduced opportunities for future careers because of absent formal qualifications. In addition, severe psychological problems might arise from the emotional trauma and the frustrating experience of having failed.

As a consequence, all relevant stakeholders, society, the medical profession, medical schools as well as medical teachers and students, have strong reasons to keep dropout in medical education as low as possible (fig. 34.1).

It is, therefore, somewhat surprising that the scientific literature dealing with the issue of dropout in medical education is relatively scarce: the first systematic review of scientific work on dropout in medicine has just been published (O'Neill et al. 2011a). This chapter summarizes some recent pieces of scientific work on the problem of dropout. The chapter does not claim to provide an exhaustive picture of the existing relevant literature; rather, we shall try to figure out the most promising predictors for study dropout. Generally, in many scientific investigations dropout was not the primary variable of interest for the authors; rather, most frequently investigators primarily intended to identify predictors and determinants for study success as measured, for example, by better study achievements, better marks, or more rapid completion of study. The question of outright withdrawal from study without ever achieving graduation, therefore, was frequently treated as a side issue.

In addition to giving an account of the relevant literature, we shall have an eye on the statistical methods employed in most available papers on study success or dropout, and we shall provide an argument to make more use of so-called waiting time analysis techniques (in clinical medicine known as 'survival analysis'), as these statistical tools seem to be particularly appropriate to analyse the 'waiting times' involved in studying time-dependent phenomena such as study success or dropout.

Rough estimation of the size of the problem

Evaluation of the dropout rate in medical education is complicated by the long time interval between admission of a student and their graduation. Nevertheless, in many countries attrition rates in medical schools are quite low, and hence, the selection process for admission might represent a major hurdle to becoming a doctor (Carlson 1991; Spooner 1990). As we shall demonstrate later, Austria's medical education system constituted one rare exception to this rule because the open admission policy, which had been held in this country until 2005, was 'paid for' by extraordinarily high dropout rates exceeding 50% of the admitted students.

In the UK, earlier estimates for medical student wastage range between 0.5 and 13% (Green et al. 1993). Comparable data from the USA indicate the risk to lie between 2 and 16% (Daugherty et al. 1990; Fogelman and Van der Zwagg 1981; Gupta 1991; Herman and Veloski 1981; Hojat et al. 1996; McCaghie 1990; Stetto et al. 2004; Strayhorn 1999), and in Australia and New Zealand data

Dropout can result in						
Emotional trauma	Reduced career opportunities	Poor morale in schools	Interruptions to healthcare workforce planning	Loss of funding for school	Economic loss to society	Economic loss to student and family

Figure 34.1 Why dropout is important.

range between 8 and 14.8% (Collins and White 1993; Lipton et al. 1988; Neame et al. 1992; Powis et al. 1988; Ward et al. 2004). For the Netherlands, figures are reported ranging from 12.3 to 20.1% (Cohen-Schotanus et al. 2006; Urlings-Strop et al. 2009), and a 16.7% dropout rate was reported in one study from South Africa (Iputo and Kwizera 2005).

Potential predictor variables for study dropout in medical education

Dropout, in medical as well as in other fields of education, is generally supposed to be a complex phenomenon, and many factors may contribute to the failure to complete a course. Screening the literature for variables that may function as predictors of dropout, therefore, yields a multitude of potential factors, partly associated with personal and/or sociodemographic attributes of the individual student, partly determined by medical school, by educational characteristics, and other causes.

For decades, the path-analysis model (Tinto 1975, 1987, 1992) has been the most dominant theory on dropout in university studies. According to this theory, the student's academic preparedness and their perceived academic and social integration within a study programme are the strongest determinants of retention or dropout. As additional factors, the student's personal characteristics, such as entry qualifications, psychological attributes and others, as well as more external factors like family background are acknowledged in Tinto's theory. However, educational variables are not adequately included in the theory.

An interesting overview of some of the reasons that may lead to dropout in medical education was provided by Simpson and Budd (1996, pp. 172–178): they surveyed the situation in one medical school by retrospectively assessing the records of all students who dropped out prematurely between 1983 and 1992.

During the studied time period, 238 students failed to complete their medical education. These were 14% of the total intake of 1714 students during that period. Among the students leaving there were 146 (61%) males, and 92 (39%) females, but among the admitted students there were 891 (52%) males and 823 (48%) females; thus the probability for dropout was significantly higher in males ($P = 0.0018$). One hundred and twelve of the 238 (47%) students left the study programme voluntarily, and 126 (53%) were asked to withdraw for academic reasons. Academic difficulties were therefore the most common reasons for dropout. Seventy-one (30%) students who dropped out reported personal problems; 21 (9%) had a mixture of personal and academic problems; 20 (8%) left because of illness; and 13 students had documented psychiatric or psychological problems.

It is interesting to see that the most important reason for dropout was a change of the student's opinion about a medical career, or that they or their teachers felt that they were not suited to medicine.

Accordingly, two students left because they were unable to cope with the dissection of cadavers. A few students reported that they had never wanted to study medicine but had been persuaded to do so by their families.

The study by Simpson and Budd (1996, pp.172–178) is also of interest because they tried to follow the further path of the students after dropout from the programme: 168 (71%) transferred to another degree programme; 140 of them chose a science-based degree; 21 transferred to an arts degree; 6 to another medical school (2 transferred to dentistry); and 1 went to veterinary college. The outcome of the remaining 70 students was unknown.

Previous academic performance was also found to be a good, albeit not perfect predictor of academic success by another systematic review of existing literature (Ferguson et al. 2002), but this report also points out the paucity of data other than previous academic performance that might be predictive for success in medical education.

Arulampalam et al. (2004a, pp. 492–503) conducted a study of factors influencing the probability of medical students in the UK dropping out during their first year of study; they analysed 51 810 students. They focused on dropout during the first year of study on the basis of a prior analysis of the cohorts entering medical schools in 1985 and 1986 (Arulampalam et al. 2004b); about half of all dropouts occurred in the first year of study, and the effects of the factors influencing first year dropout differed from those in later dropout. Following Tinto's path analysis model (Tinto 1975, 1987, 1992) the authors included control variables indicating the prior academic preparedness of the students, their social background and personal attributes. Prior qualifications and the type of school attended were also included.

The overall first year dropout rate was determined to be 3.8%. Male sex was identified as a risk factor for dropout; other factors being constant, the probability for dropout was 0.3% higher for men. In contrast, age at study entry over 21 years was associated with a 1.2% reduction in dropout risk in comparison to ages up to 19 years.

The family background of medical students was not a significant predictor for dropout in the study by Arulampalam et al. (2004a, pp. 492–503) with one exception: having a parent employed as a medical doctor was associated with a 0.75% reduction of dropout risk. This could reflect greater commitment to the study and/or better preparedness and prior information of such students.

Similarly, having an academic degree prior to entering medical school was a strong predictor of reduced dropout risk. In this group dropout probability was reduced by about 2%. While raw data suggested significant effects of social background on the dropout risk, multivariate analyses showed that in fact prior qualifications at school were independent predictors of dropout and, via their statistical associations with social background, were indeed responsible for the observed effects. Interestingly, particularly high scores in biology, chemistry, and physics were found to be predictors of a lower dropout probability in first year medical education: achieving one grade higher in one of these subjects reduced the dropout risk by 0.38%. Interestingly, high attainments in other subjects such as English were not correlated with the risk of dropout. Notably, students who scored well in subjects other than biology, chemistry, and physics were more likely to drop out of medical education and were more likely to transfer degree course. Furthermore, the analyses revealed that there was no significant effect of the type of school on dropout probability, nor was there any statistically significant interaction between the effects of high school achievements and school type.

The same authors later published another study (Arulampalam et al. 2007) where they extended the scope of their investigation by including on the one hand three cohorts beginning medical study in the years 1990 to 1992 and on the other hand the three cohorts starting from 1998 to 2000. Again, the first year dropout was the variable of interest. A major goal of this successor study was a comparison of the results of the analyses over a decade of time.

The authors first noted a marked increase in the numbers of students admitted to medical education: while in the period from 1990 to 1992 on average 4125 students were admitted per year, this figure rose to 4876 in the later 3-year period. Importantly, the dropout rate also increased from 3.5% in the early cohorts to 4.9% in the later cohorts. Accordingly, there were some profound differences between the results found in the early as compared to the later cohorts; for example, while in the 1990–1992 cohorts males were at lower risk of dropout (3.33% versus 4.05% in females), in the later cohorts there was little difference between the sexes with males now showing 0.09% higher dropout risk than females.

Age effects were insignificant for the early cohorts but were significant for the late cohorts. Among the cohorts having started from 1998 to 2000, the authors on the basis of a multivariate model defined a 'default student' as a white female aged 18 or 19 years, not disabled and from a social background in which neither parent is a doctor. For this 'default' group, a dropout probability of 3.1% was found.

While no significant overseas student effects in dropout rate were found in the early cohorts, in the late cohorts overseas female students were less likely to drop out by 1.9% than an average female student.

In agreement with Tinto's theory (Tinto 1975, 1987, 1992) of the role of social integration, in both groups of cohorts students living on campus were found to be less prone to study dropout by about 1.7%. Recorded disability was not found to be a significant predictor for dropout. Ethnic background was not available for the early cohorts, but was recorded only for the later cohorts. Indian females were found to have a dropout risk about 1.9% smaller than that of Caucasian females; for Indian versus Caucasian males, no differences were detected. Other minority ethnic groups were less likely to drop out by 0.8% points. In females, the 'protective' effect of having a parent working as medical doctor was confirmed (about 1% smaller dropout probability); in men, no effect was seen.

As in their first investigation, the authors again found a remarkably strong effect of having an academic degree before entering medical education; dropout risk in such students was 2.4% smaller than in school leavers.

Similarly, the importance of prior qualifications, particularly in biology was confirmed. Each extra A-level grade in biology reduced the dropout risk by about 0.86%; the comparable figures for chemistry and physics were about 0.5% points each. Also, having studied mathematics lowered the dropout probability by about 0.5%, regardless of grade.

Interestingly, further in-depth analyses of the data revealed that not all the observed student characteristics were able to explain the increase of the dropout rate over the time period studied; rather, most of this increase could be associated with medical school effects. As explanations, the authors mention less effective admission policies, changing curricula, greater costs of attending medical school, and a growing mismatch between student and school characteristics. Of course, unobserved student characteristics could also have been responsible for the noted increase in dropout. In conclusion, the authors cited living on campus, having a parent who was a doctor, and better prior qualifications, as the main predictors of a high probability of retention in medical education.

Yates and James (2007, pp. 65–73) tried to determine risk factors for poor performance on the undergraduate course. They included in their investigation all 594 medical students entering their programme over 3 consecutive years. Admission criteria were unchanged during this period, and all students should have left the course before data collection. Nineteen students left or had their course terminated in the first 2 years, and nine students failed to complete their clinical course. Another 34 students spent more than the usual 5 years before graduating as a doctor. Unfortunately, the study focused mainly on poor versus good study performance, and did not make separate analyses for dropout. Poorer school performance was found to be a predictor for poor performance in the preclinical course, whereas non-Caucasian ethnicity was associated with more problems in the clinical course (but was a risk factor throughout). Males and students with a late offer of a place were also at higher risk for poor performance.

Admission and student selection

The majority of studies on dropout in medical education published in the past decade laid their focus on the association between personal attributes of the students at study entry and study success, or study dropout. Consequently, selection of students for admission to medical education is the main theme of these investigations.

Not surprisingly, selection of medical students prior to admission has been deemed a major determinant for study success or failure in undergraduate medical education and, consequently, for subsequent professional behaviour (Lancet [Editorial] 1984, Lazarus and Van Niekerk 1986). It is commonly agreed that the educational process in medicine, requiring the construction of appropriate knowledge, skills and attitudes for healthcare delivery, has to rest on solid foundations such as the cognitive abilities and personal attributes of the applicants admitted to study. Certainly, the selection of medical schools entrants is of pivotal importance (Sade et al. 1985). The recent literature review by O'Neill et al. (2011a, pp. 440–454), for example, analyses 13 key investigations on dropout of medical students in detail, and only one of these 13 papers was found not to consider prior qualifications, admission test scores or interview scores as potential predictors of dropout.

As a consequence, selection of students before admission to medical education is of importance also for study dropout. When screening the literature available, one can discern three different scientific questions:

- What is the impact of selection of students versus open admission?

* How does active selection compare with mere restriction of available study places by non-discriminating methods such as a lottery?

* How do different methods of selection compare with each other?

We shall consider these questions separately (fig. 34.2).

What is the impact of selection of students versus open admission?

Today, in virtually all countries, admission to medical education is restricted. However, for many decades Austria's university admission system was an exception. Every Austrian citizen who successfully passed secondary school was generally entitled to be admitted to whatever university course they wanted, including medicine. As in many other studies, open admission in medicine led to quite unsatisfactory consequences; since the capacities and resources of universities and faculties were limited and by no means adapted to the steadily increasing number of students, study conditions were poor. Among other limitations and weaknesses, students as well as faculty were frustrated, mass lectures were predominant, small-group and bedside teaching were exceptions rather than the rule. Consequently, Austrian medical students exceeded the scheduled study time of 6 years by 50% or more, and approximately half of the students failed and dropped out from medical education.

As recently described by Reibnegger et al. (2010, 2011), students from other countries were admitted to Austrian universities only after they proved they had also been admitted to the same course of study in their country of origin. Since citizens from other member states of the European Union were included in these regulations, European law was violated and in 2005, the European Court ruled that Austria's policy of foreign student admission to its universities had to be changed. After the court's decision, it was feared that Austrian medical universities would be overwhelmed by German students; in Germany with its about 10-fold population size, admission to medical education is restricted by a selection system based on secondary school marks, and in both countries the native tongue is German. In order to avoid this, Austrian law was changed; for a

> What is the impact of selection of students versus open admission?
>
> How does active selection compare with mere restriction of available study places by non-discriminating methods such as a lottery?
>
> How do different methods of selection compare with each other?

Figure 34.2 Factors that may influence study dropout.

few studies, including medicine and dentistry, admission tests and restriction of study places became legally possible.

This fundamental change in admission policy for medical education in a whole country made a 'real life experiment' possible, namely, the scientific study of the effects of installing selection of medical students by admission tests on a number of interesting phenomena, such as study progress and dropout, in comparison with open admission. The first detailed analyses were reported from the Medical University of Graz (Reibnegger et al. 2010, 2011) (fig. 34.3). At that medical school, an admission test was developed for the selection of applicants. The test was based on the performances of the applicants on a composite multiple choice test: the main part asks for secondary school-level knowledge of biology, chemistry, mathematics and physics. Furthermore, the test comprises an assessment of comprehension of scientific texts, and since 2010, a situational judgment test where the applicants are presented a vignette describing a critical incident in a medical context and then have to choose the optimum of several alternatives of possible action.

The effects of this new admission test on study progress (Reibnegger et al. 2010) as well as on dropout (Reibnegger et al. 2011) were indeed dramatic. Whereas, for example, the fraction of students who were able to successfully complete the first part of the study programme (scheduled as the first two study semesters) among unselected and openly admitted students from the cohorts starting in academic years 2002–2003 to 2004–2005 was only about 20 to 25%, this fraction on average rose to more than 80% among the later student cohorts having started in 2005–2006 to 2007–2008 and having been actively selected. By survival analysis techniques of data on 2532 students, the effect of the selection procedure versus open admission proved to be highly significant: the semi-empiric Cox proportional hazards technique (Cox 1972)

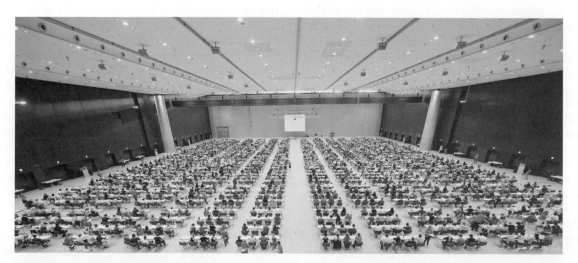

Figure 34.3 More than 1700 applicants sitting the 2011 admission test at the Medical University of Graz in the City Hall of Graz, Austria.

yielded a hazard ratio of 4.47 (SE, 0.28, $P \ll 0.0001$), meaning that the 'hazard' of a selected student to complete the first part of study is four to five times higher than that of an openly admitted student throughout the observation time. The 'hazard' or 'hazard rate' is defined as the instantaneous conditional rate per unit time for the interesting event (here: successful completion of the first part of study) to occur at time t, given that a person has 'survived' (i.e. not experienced the terminating event) up to time t.

As expected, dropout rates were markedly influenced by the change in admission policy: data were obtained from the study history of all 2860 students admitted to the human medicine diploma programme from academic years 2002–2003 to 2008–2009, observed until end of February, 2010 (Reibnegger et al. 2011). Of these, 1971 were openly admitted, and 889 were admitted after admission testing. Within the observation period, 764 of 1971 openly admitted students (38.8%) dropped out in contrast to only 41 of 889 selected students (4.6%). This difference between both groups is highly significant. Of course, one has to bear in mind the longer observation period for openly admitted students; nevertheless, survival analysis techniques, which account explicitly for the time variable, confirm the overwhelmingly significant effect of the installation of a selection procedure. For example, a Cox regression analysis of the data yields a hazard ratio of 0.145 (SE 0.0234); meaning, that the dropout risk in the selected student group is only about 14.5% of that in the openly admitted students, with a 95% confidence interval ranging from 10.6 to 19.9%.

The same analysis, when including sex and age as possible predictors of dropout, confirms the statistically independent and strong effect of the absence of a selection process as the most dominant predictor for study dropout. The respective hazard ratios and their 95% confidence intervals were 0.139 (0.1 to 0.2) for selection or, equivalently, $0.139^{-1} = 7.2$ (5.2 to 9.8) for the lack of selection, 1.9 (1.7 to 2.2) for ages older than the 75th age percentile of 20.89 years, and 1.7 (1.4 to 1.9) for female sex. Obviously, age and sex are significant modulators of the dropout risk, but their effects are relatively small in comparison to absence versus presence of student selection.

Moreover, in a Cox regression analysis using open versus selected admission as stratum variable, the effects of sex and age remain significant only in the openly admitted students; in selected students both variables are no longer significant. The same result is obtained using a flexible parametric Royston–Parmar survival analysis (Royston and Parmar 2002).

Interestingly, these effects of sex and age found by Reibnegger et al. (2011, pp. 1040–1048) in the Austrian context of open admission were just the opposite of the effects of these variables in the study by Arulampalam et al. (2004a, pp. 492–503) on medical students in the UK; in the Austrian open admission situation before 2005, being female and being older indicated significantly higher dropout risk, while in the British environment these variables were predictive of lower risk. This discrepancy underscores the profoundly different historical environment of both studies; the situation in a university system after decades of open admission is, not surprisingly, completely different from the circumstances in systems having long-standing experience, with prior definition of the number of available study places and with diverse selection methods for choosing their students.

One can safely conclude that absence versus presence of a selection process before admission to medical education is one of the most important, if not the largest, single factor in determining the risk of dropout. However, the investigations by Reibnegger et al. (2010, 2011) do not answer important questions regarding the optimum selection method. Are the observed effects just caused by the restriction of the number of available study places and, hence, an improved study situation due to a much better fit of the number of admitted students with the available resources and capacities? (Note that at the Medical University of Graz in the years before 2005 the number of new students openly admitted each year was on average 700, while since the installation of the selection process only 336 students are admitted for the programme each year.) Or is there also a significant and independent contribution of the chosen selection method?

The next section deals with the question as to whether selection by chance has the same potential to reduce study dropout as an active selection process based on cognitive or non-cognitive abilities of the applicants.

Active selection versus admission by lottery

There are some who believe that selection processes resemble a lottery, and that random selection of students for admission may ultimately produce similar study achievements as those chosen by the existing selection procedures. Norman (2004, pp. 79–82) in particular questions the use of autobiographic letters, interviews and other admission methods, which have been consistently shown to be of limited value.

In the Netherlands since the 1970s, students were selected on the basis of a state-run lottery where the probability for admission of a student was determined by chance but also modulated by school marks; the higher your marks, the more tickets you got. Since 1999, the best students have unrestricted access to medical schools, and medical schools are allowed to select up to 50% of their students on the basis of other criteria. Urlings-Strop et al. (2009, pp. 175–183) used this unique national situation for an interesting controlled experiment at Erasmus MC Medical School; they performed a prospective study comparing 389 students who had been admitted by selection and 938 students who had been admitted by weighted lottery. The students comprised the cohorts starting in four subsequent academic years from 2001 to 2004. The selection was a two step process, combining non-cognitive and cognitive abilities of the students. The main study outcome measures were dropout rates, study rate as determined by credits per year, and mean grade per first examination per year. In the paper, the authors describe the first results of the study; they analysed the data collated after 4 years of employing the lottery-selection strategy for admission. From the 1327 students admitted, 164 failed, yielding an overall dropout rate of 12.3%. The authors concluded that the relative risk for dropping out of medical school in the preclinical phase was 2.6 times higher for lottery-admitted students than for selected students (95% confidence interval of the relative risk ranging from 1.6 to 4.2).

In a later paper (Urlings-Strop et al. 2011) the investigation was expanded to include the clinical phase of medical school. By this second analysis, in comparison to selected students a twice as high dropout rate for the lottery-admitted students could be confirmed. In addition, achievements were higher in selected students; they achieved a very high grade about 1.5 times more frequently than students admitted after lottery.

According to the results by Urlings-Strop et al. (2009, 2011) we have good evidence that selection just by chance is clearly less effective at reducing the probability of dropout than active selection based on personal characteristics. Furthermore, academic achievements are better in actively selected students than in lottery-admitted students.

Effects of different selection methods on study dropout in medical education

The qualifications of a student at entry to the programme are generally regarded to constitute an important predictor for study success or dropout. The problem one faces when screening the published literature is the broad heterogeneity of the selection processes and criteria used in different settings: some put more weight on cognitive attributes, while others focus predominantly on personality tests, aptitude tests and others (Benbassat and Baumal 2007).

How should the qualifications of a student before admission be measured? Should we rely on school grades, or should we actively test before admission? In the latter case, how should we construct the tests? Should we concentrate on cognitive abilities, on explicit knowledge, or should we rely on aptitude testing, on interviews, or on other measures of psychosocial characteristics of the applicants?

Selection based on cognitive characteristics typically is measured by grade point average or performance on standardized knowledge tests, such as the Medical College Admission Test (MCAT) in North America, which was introduced in 1928 and has undergone successive revisions to improve its contents and predictive validity (Association of American Medical Colleges 2012; Callahan et al. 2010; McCaghie 2002), or the Graduate Australian Medical School Admission Test (GAMSAT) in Australia and the UK (Australian Council for Educational Research 2012). Non-cognitive qualities typically comprise all other qualities that might be required from applicants. The list of such qualities seems to be never-ending; more than 80 such qualities were identified by a literature review (Albanese et al. 2003). Despite different opinions concerning the relative weight that should be given to cognitive versus non-cognitive characteristics in selecting medical students, most authors agree that a broad scope of assessment including academic achievement and personal characteristics is desirable (Institute for International Medical Education 2002). Eva et al. (2009, pp. 767–775) recently gave strong arguments that cognitive and non-cognitive tests, although sometimes appearing to be independent of each other, eventually do not really yield mutually exclusive characteristics in an individual—in the sense that cognitive tests always produce asocial 'bookworms' or non-cognitive tests select social 'butterflies' who are not capable of rational thinking. Rather, with more and deeper delving into medical education, it becomes more difficult to claim independence between cognitive and non-cognitive domains.

With regard to study dropout, most investigations available agree in stating that poorer qualifications at study entry are predictive of higher risk for dropout (Arulampalam et al. 2004a, b, 2007; Gough and Hall, 1975; Powis et al., 1992; Strayhorn 1999; Urlings-Strop et al. 2009; Ward et al. 2004;). As reviewed by O'Neill et al. (2011a), odds ratios for dropout in 9 of 13 quality-assessed papers in which lower entry qualifications were found, ranged from 1.65 to 4.00. Rarely, no or insignificant associations were observed between entry qualifications and dropout risk (Cohen-Schotanus et al. 2006; Iputo 2005).

Recently, O'Neill et al. (2011b, pp. 1111–1120) compared testing at admission versus selection by highest grades in six subsequent cohorts of 1544 medical students admitted to the University of Southern Denmark during the years 2002 to 2007. Half of the students were admitted on the basis of their prior achievement of the highest grades, the other half sat a composite admission test consisting of a knowledge test on a broad spectrum of domains, and they had to attend a semi-structured interview. Dropout was defined as the termination of studies at the school within 2 years of starting for any reason. Univariate and multivariate logistic regression analyses revealed that none of the various sociodemographic variables were independent dropout predictors. Students who were admitted based on admission test (rather than based on high grades), students who attended a grammar school and students who assigned first priority for medicine upon application had a decreased probability for dropout.

In conclusion, it seems safe to state that better entry qualifications—cognitive and/or non-cognitive—are an effective means to prevent premature withdrawal from medical education; the paper by O'Neill et al. (2011b, pp. 1111–1120) even suggests that testing before admission seems to be superior to relying purely on previous school achievements.

Miscellaneous considerations

As has become evident, over the decades various authors have tried to identify quite diverse predictor variables for dropout in medical education. In the preceding sections, we have discussed some of these potential factors with a predominant focus laid on selection of students and their qualifications at entry. In this section, we shall summarize results obtained on variables other than those associated with selection and admission tests.

Sociodemographic variables

According to the literature review by O'Neill et al. (2011a, pp. 440–454), among 10 of 13 quality assessed papers on dropout in medical education that considered gender as a potential predictor, there were only three reporting an association between gender and dropout risk (Arulampalam et al. 2004a,b, 2007; Stetto et al. 2004). However, results were contradictory. In openly admitted Austrian students (Reibnegger et al., 2011) women were found to carry a higher risk of dropout but in Austrian students admitted after selection by a knowledge test, the effect vanished. Similarly, age effects were unclear. Several studies investigated ethnicity, but again, no conclusive evidence for or against a significant effect of ethnicity could be identified. Social class has never been found to be a clear-cut indicator of dropout with the exception that having a parent who works as medical doctor, seems to be associated with smaller risk of dropout, at least in women (Arulampalam et al. 2004a, b, 2007).

Few studies dealt with psychological or perceptional scale variables as potential predictors for study dropout; there is some indication that students who are more resilient, more self-reliant and more 'thick skinned' and 'uninhibited' are more likely to successfully complete medical education (Ward et al. 2004). A systematic literature review on several indicators of psychological distress among US and Canadian medical students was presented (Dyrbye et al. 2006) but unfortunately gives no evidence regarding potential effects of psychological issues on dropout.

Academic struggling also seems to indicate higher risk for premature termination of medical education (Hojat et al. 1996; Stetto et al. 2004). A remarkably strong association was found between dropout and failure of a student to master the curriculum within the expected time period. Moreover, failing at least one basic science course in the beginning of the study or achieving only low grades in the first year of study also were significant predictors of higher dropout probability.

There are some studies indicating that active learning curricula or problem-based curricula might be associated with better study results, both in terms of shorter time to graduation and of reduced dropout rates (Iputo and Kwizera 2005; Schmidt et al. 2009).

Failure time analysis techniques in investigations on study dropout and related problems in medical education research

Investigations on students' success or failure to complete a study programme inevitably involve observations over prolonged time intervals. 'Waiting times' from start of study to graduation or premature withdrawal from study therefore constitute an important variable in such research attempts. When one screens the available literature on dropout and related topics in medical education it becomes evident that various types of regression analyses (mostly univariate and multivariate variants of linear or logistic regression techniques) are used for statistical analysis. However, a certain group of statistical techniques, which are deliberately designed to handle time-dependent data, are only rarely applied. In this section, we shall therefore provide a brief summary of these methods, which in clinical medicine are well-known under the heading 'survival analysis', and we shall provide arguments why these methods appear particularly promising for the type of problems we meet in medical education research.

Survival analysis—or, more generally, analysis of failure times—represents a field of statistics extensively used by clinical researchers. Survival analysis tells researchers not just about average survival times of groups of patients, but—probably even more importantly—also enables qualitative identification and quantitative description of single or multiple predictive factors influencing and modulating survival times.

In medical education research, however, this type of statistical analysis is only rarely used. This is a pity since in educational research we are frequently confronted with time-dependent data. Quite often a basic observation on students is the time elapsing from one well-defined event, such as, for example, the start of a study programme or a course, to another well-defined event, for example, graduation, attaining a well-defined competency, passing a well defined examination, or—negatively—dropping out from study. Such times are called waiting times.

What makes waiting times special? Why are 'normal' statistics frequently insufficient to handle such data? First, waiting time distributions are always positively valued (there is no 'negative waiting time'), and frequently they are strongly skewed and non-Gaussian. For example, while the bulk of students of a certain cohort will graduate more or less at the time prescribed by the curriculum, there may be some students requiring extraordinarily long times to succeed: the distribution of completion times of study programmes is frequently positively skewed. Second, in waiting time problems the phenomenon of statistical censoring is common. Reasons may be that we wish to analyse our data without waiting until even the last student reaches the terminating event. Some students may have dropped out from study without ever reaching graduation. How should we proceed with such observations? Should we delete such students from our analysis? This could pose major statistical problems, however. Moreover, individuals not reaching the terminating event nevertheless contribute valuable information. Let us suppose, the waiting time is the time from study start to graduation. A student dropping out after 3 years would present a censored observation of 3 years because we know that the waiting time for him or her is 3 years plus an undetermined further amount of time.

Waiting time analysis consists of a set of non-parametric, semi-parametric, and parametric statistical methods designed to handle these two typical difficulties. Most frequently, we do not know the theoretical distribution of waiting times underlying the data available. The most direct approach to analyse waiting times, the so called 'product limit method' which in honor of its inventors is also termed the Kaplan–Meier method, does not make any assumptions about underlying distributions but solves the problem in a nonparametric way (Kaplan and Meier 1958). The method provides estimates for the cumulative probabilities of the event occurring—or not occurring—only at the discrete time points when an event actually occurs. Since we do not postulate a specific distribution of the waiting times, we have no knowledge about the behaviour of these probabilities between the experimentally observed time points. For graphical visualization of the results of a Kaplan–Meier procedure it is therefore common to use step functions. Also the semiparametric Cox regression technique does not make explicit assumptions regarding the distribution underlying the waiting times (Cox 1972). However, by applying the so-called proportional hazards assumption, the technique enables the estimation the predictive strength(s) of one or more explanatory variables of different scale qualities (interval, ordinal, and nominal) on the hazard function, which underlies the cumulative probabilities of occurrence or non-occurrence of the event in a most elegant way. Thus, univariate and multivariate analyses of the single or combined predictive effects of potentially important predictor variables are easily made. Even the inclusion of time-dependent predictor variables is possible. The terminus 'semiparametric' is owed to the fact that no parametric assumptions are made regarding the baseline cumulative probabilities but the effects of the potential predictor variables are modelled in a parametric form, whereby the parameters are estimated by fitting the model to the observed data. In fact, in most applications in medicine, a combination the Kaplan–Meier (for estimating the cumulative probabilities, i.e. the 'survival' or 'failure' curves) and the Cox method (for judging the predictive strengths of predictors, alone or in combination) has become state of the art.

Parametric models for waiting time analysis make explicit assumptions regarding the distribution function underlying the observed waiting times. Thus, we assume that waiting times follow a distribution whose probability density function can be written down explicitly as a function of certain parameters which can be determined by fitting the model to the observed data. In contrast to survivor curves obtained by the Kaplan–Meier technique or Cox models, parametric models, once fitted, allow easy construction of smooth curves of for example the probability density functions of the event occurring or not occurring, or the hazard functions.

In past decades, at least in medical context, classical parametric models were rarely used compared with their nonparametric and semiparametric counterparts. One of the major reasons for this was the lack of flexibility of these models, which in many instances prevented a satisfactory fit to real life datasets. Quite recently, however, a number of statistical tools has been developed overcoming the limitations of classical parametric models (Royston and Parmar 2002). Fortunately, these technically more advanced models are easily accessible in one of the major commercial statistical software packages (Royston and Lambert 2011).

These recent developments are of considerable interest since suitable parametric models, if at hand, possess several advantages over the (semi)parametric approaches: they allow the estimation of the baseline cumulative probability functions and their variances occur in a smooth, continuous manner (the functions are not just step functions being defined only at discrete time points but they vary smoothly over time). Consequently, 'smooth' estimation and visualization of many other important features like hazard and probability functions, hazard and probability difference functions, hazard ratios and more from such models have become feasible.

We have successfully employed survival analysis methods in recent studies on study success as well as study dropout in medical education (Reibnegger et al. 2010, 2011), and from our experiences, we recommend making stronger use of these statistical techniques in the realm of medical educational research. Waiting time analysis enables important insights into time-dependent phenomena, and it has the capacity to identify potential predictive variables as well as their relative strengths in a statistically correct manner also in interim analysis scenarios or in situations with censored data. The construction of meaningful prognostic models is possible: these are typically multiple regression models enabling the prediction of future outcomes given the values of several covariates measured at or before the time origin (which, in our case, could be the start of a study program or a specified course).

There are many excellent sources available on waiting time analysis. One example is a text by Kleinbaum and Klein (2005). Both the theory and practical applications of using a commercial statistical package are presented in a more recent book (Cleves et al. 2008).

Conclusions

- O'Neill et al. (2011b, p. 1116) conclude from their recent investigation on study dropout in medical education that—according to existing literature—'lower entry qualifications...seemed to be the only consistent predictors of dropout'.

- Taking the Austrian experience (Reibnegger et al. 2011) into account we may add that by far the strongest factor associated with high risk of dropout is whether there is a selection process at all. Open admission, no doubt, is the worst choice, resulting in absurdly high dropout rates exceeding 50% and more.

- The question of how to select still remains open; recently, for example, interesting work has been published indicating that combining, for example school achievements with structured interviews can provide additional predictive power (Lambe and Bristow 2011).

- Selection of students has been, and remains, a hot topic, and political as well as medical school authorities should be aware of their responsibility both towards the applicants and towards society in general (Norman 2004).

References

Albanese, M.A., Snow, M.H., Skochelak, S.E., Huggett, K.N., and Farrell, P.M. (2003) Assessing personal qualities in medical school admissions. *Acad Med.* 78: 313–321

Arulampalam, W., Naylor, R.A., and Smith, J.P. (2004a) Factors affecting the probability of first year medical student dropout in the UK: a logistic analysis for the intake cohorts of 1980-92. *Med Educ.* 38, 492–503.

Arulampalam, W., Naylor, R.A., and Smith, J.P. (2004b) A hazard model of the probability of medical school dropout in the United Kingdom. *J Roy Stat Soc.* 167: 157–178

Arulampalam, W., Naylor, R.A., and Smith, J.P. (2007) Dropping out of medical school in the UK: explaining the changes over ten years. *Med Educ.* 41: 385–394

Association of American Medical Colleges (2012) Medical College Admission Test. [Online] https://www.aamc.org/students/applying/mcat Accessed 22 March 2012

Australian Council for Educational Research. Graduate Australian Medical School Admissions Test. [Online] http://www.gamsat-ie.org/ Accessed 22 March 2012

Benbassat, J., and Baumal, R. (2007) Uncertainties in the selection of applicants for medical school. *Adv Health Sci Educ.* 12: 509–521

Callahan, C.A., Hojat, M., Veloski, J., Erdman, J.B., and Gonella, J.S. (2010) The predictive validity of three versions of the MCAT in relation to performance in medical school, residency, and licensing examinations: a longitudinal study of 36 classes of Jefferson Medical College. *Acad Med.* 85: 980–987

Carlson, C.A. (1991) International medical education. Common elements in diverging systems. *JAMA.* 266: 921–923

Cleves, M., Gutierrez, R., Gould, W., and Marchenko, Y. (2008) *An Introduction to Survival Analysis Using Stata.* 2nd edn. College Station (Texas): Stata Press

Cohen-Schotanus, J., Muijtjens, A.M.M., Reinders, J.J., Agsteribbe, J., van Rossum, H.J.M., and van der Vleuten, C.P.M. (2006) The predictive validity of grade point average scores in a partial lottery medical school admission system. *Med Educ.* 40: 1012–1019

Collins, J.P., and White, G.R. (1993) Selection of Auckland medical students over 25 years: time for change. *Med Educ.* 27: 321–327

Cox, D.R. (1972) Regression models and life tables (with discussion). *J Roy Stat Soc.* 34: 187–220

Daugherty, S.R., Eckenfels, E.J, and Schmidt, J.L. (1990) Longitudinal analysis of admission decisions. *Acad Med.* 65: S1–S2

Denenberg, D. and Roscoe, L. (2001) *50 American Heroes Every Kid Should Meet!* Millbrook Press, Minneapolis, p. 99

Dyrbye, L.N., Thomas, M.R., and Shanafelt, T.D. (2006) Systematic review of depression, anxiety, and other indicators of psychological distress among U.S. and Canadian medical students. *Acad Med.* 81: 354–373

Eva, K.W., Reiter, H.I., Trink, K., Wasi, P., Rosenfeld, J., and Norman, G.R. (2009) Predictive validity of the multiple mini-interview for selecting medical trainees. *Med Educ.* 43: 767–775

Ferguson, E., James, D., and Madeley, L. (2002) Factors associated with success in medical school: systematic review of the literature. *BMJ.* 432: 952–957

Finucane, P., and McCrorie, P. (2010) Cost-effective undergraduate medical education. In: K. Walsh (ed.) *Cost effectiveness in Medical Education* (pp. 5–13). Abingdon: Radcliffe

Fogelman, B.Y.S., and Van der Zwagg, R. (1981) Demographic, situational and scholastic factors in medical school attrition. *South Med J.* 74: 602–606

Gough, H.G., and Hall, W.B. (1975) An attempt to predict graduation from medical school. *J Med Educ.* 50: 940–950

Green, A., Peters, T.J., and Webster, D.J. (1993) Preclinical progress in relation to personality and academic profiles. *Med Educ.* 27: 137–142

Gupta, G.C. (1991) Student attrition. A challenge for allied health education programmes. *JAMA.* 266: 963–967

Herman, M.W., and Veloski, J.J. (1981) Premedical training, personal characteristics and performance in medical school. *Med Educ.* 15: 363–367

Hojat, M., Gonnella, J.S., Erdmann, J.B., and Veloski, J.J. (1996) The fate of medical students with different levels of knowledge: are the basic medical sciences relevant to physician competence? *Adv Health Sci Educ.* 1: 179–196

Institute for International Medical Education (2002) Global minimum essential requirements in medical education. Report of the Core Committee. *Med Teach.* 24: 130–135

Iputo, J.E., and Kwizera, E. (2005) Problem-based learning improves the academic performance of medical students in South Africa. *Med Educ.* 39: 388–393

Kaplan, E.L., and Meier, P. (1958) Nonparametric estimation from incomplete observations. *J Am Stat Ass.* 53: 457–481

Kleinbaum. D.G, and Klein, M. (2005) *Survival Analysis. A Self-Learning Text.* (2nd ed.) New York (New York): Springer Science + Business Media, LLC.

Lambe, P., and Bristow, D. (2011) Predicting medical student performance from attributes at entry: a latent class analysis. *Med Educ.* 45: 308–316

Lancet (Editorial) (1984) Medical student selection in the UK. *Lancet.* 24: 1190–1191

Lazarus, J. and van Niekerk, J.P. (1986) Selecting Medical Students: a rational approach. *Med Teach.* 8: 343–357

Lipton, A., Huxham, G., and Hamilton, D. (1988) School results as predictors of medical school achievements. *Med Educ.* 22: 381–388

McCaghie, W.C. (1990) Perspectives in medical school admission. *Acad Med.* 65: 136–139

McCaghie, W. (2002) Assessing readiness for medical education: evolution of the Medical College Admission Test. *JAMA.* 288: 1085–1090

Neame, R.L., Powis, D.A., and Bristow, T. (1992) Should medical students be selected only from recent school-leavers who have studied science? *Med Educ.* 26: 433–440

Norman, G. (2004) Editorial—The morality of medical school admission. *Adv Health Sci Educ.* 9: 79–82

O'Neill, L., Hartvigsen, J., Wallstedt, B., Korsholm, L., and Eika, B. (2011b) Medical school dropout—testing at admission versus selection by highest grades as predictors. *Med Educ.* 45: 1111–1120

O'Neill, L.D., Wallstedt, B., Eika, B., and Hartvigsen, J. (2011a) Factors associated with dropout in medical education: a literature review. *Med Educ.* 45: 440–454

Powis, D.A., Neame, R.L.B., Bristow, T., and Murphy, L.B. (1988) The objective structured interview for medical student selection. *BMJ.* 96: 765–768

Powis, D.A., Waring, T.C., Bristow, T., and O'Connell, D.L. (1992) The structured interview as a tool for predicting premature withdrawal from medical school. *Aust N Z J Med.* 22: 692–698

Reibnegger, G., Caluba, H.-C., Ithaler, D., Manhal, S., Neges, H.M., and Smolle, J. (2010) Progress of medical students after open admission or admission based on knowledge tests. *Med Educ.* 44: 205–214

Reibnegger, G., Caluba, H.-C., Ithaler, D., Manhal, S., Neges, H.M., and Smolle, J. (2011) Dropout rates in medical students at one school before and after the installation of admission tests in Austria. *Acad Med.* 86: 1040–1048

Royston, P, and Lambert, P.C. (2011) *Flexible Parametric Survival Analysis Using Stata: Beyond the Cox Model.* College Station (Texas): Stata Press

Royston, P., and Parmar, M.K.B. (2002) Flexible parametric proportional-hazards and proportional-odds models for censored survival data, with application to prognostic modelling and estimation of treatment effects. *Stat Med.* 21: 2175–2197

Sade, R.M., Stroud, M.R., Levine, J.H., and Fleming, G.A. (1985) Criteria for selection of future physicians. *Ann Surg.* 201: 225–230

Schmidt, H.G., Cohen-Schotanus, J., and Arends, L.R. (2009) Impact of problem-based, active learning on graduation rates for 10 generations of Dutch medical students. *Med Educ.* 43: 211–218

Simpson, K.H. and Budd, K. (1996) Medical student attrition: a 10-year survey in one medical school. *Med Educ.* 30: 172–178

Spooner, C.E. (1990) Help for the gatekeepers: comment and summation on the admission process. *Acad Med.* 65: 183–188

Stetto, J.E., Gackstetter, G.D., Cruess, D.F., and Hooper, T.I. (2004) Variables associated with attrition from Uniformed Services University of the Health Sciences Medical School. *Military Med.* 169: 102–107

Strayhorn, G. (1999) Participation in a pre-medical summer programme for under-represented minority students as a predictor of academic performance in the first three years of medical school: two studies. *Acad Med.* 74: 435–447

Tinto, V. (1975) Dropout from higher education: a theoretical synthesis from recent research. *Rev Educ Res.* 45: 89–125

Tinto, V. (1987) *Leaving College: Rethinking the Causes and Cures of Student Attrition.* Chicago: University of Chicago Press

Tinto, V. (1992) Student attrition and retention. In: B.R. Clarke, and G. Neave (eds) *Encyclopedia of Higher Education* (pp. 1697–1709). 3rd edn. Oxford: Pergamon Press

Urlings-Strop, L.C., Stijnen T., Themmen, A.P.N., and Splinter, T.A.W. (2009) Selection of medical students: a controlled experiment. *Med Educ.* 43: 175–183

Urlings-Strop, L.C., Themmen, A.P.N., Stijnen T., and Splinter, T.A.W. (2011) Selected medical students achieve better than lottery-admitted students during clerkship. *Med Educ.* 45: 1032–1040

Walsh, K. (2011) Test results can predict more than just test results. *Med Educ.* 45: 538

Ward, A.M., Kamien, M., and Lopez, D.G. (2004) Medical career choice and practice location: early factors predicting course completion, career choice and practice location. *Med Educ.* 38: 239–248

Yates, J., and James, D. (2007) Risk factors for poor performance on the undergraduate medical course: cohort study at Nottingham University. *Med Educ.* 41: 65–73

PART 8

Assessment

CHAPTER 35

Principles of assessment

Lambert W. T. Schuwirth and Julie Ash

We need to assess in a real context, with all the intricacies of that.

Cees van der Vleuten

Reproduced from Medical Education, Lisa Pritchard, 'Accidental Hero', 39, pp. 761-762, Copyright 2005, with permissions from Association for the Study of Medical Education and Wiley

Introduction

You are a clinician in an academic hospital. A student is doing his clinical rotations under your supervision. He has examined a patient, Mr Johnson. The student tells you that he has taken Mr Johnson's blood pressure and that it was 160/100 mmHg. The student also tells you that he has informed Mr Johnson that his blood pressure was far too high and should immediately be treated, because he would certainly develop serious cardiovascular disease in the future if not treated.

You wonder whether the student's reasoning is completely correct.
Well, in fact, it is not. The student has made serious mistakes. First, there is agreement that a single blood pressure measurement is insufficient to draw conclusions from (Llabre et al. 1988). Second, you do not know whether the blood pressure was taken correctly. Did the student use the right cuff and the right technique? Third, it is a big leap of faith to give a prediction to someone that they are sure to develop cardiovascular disease. And finally, the message has probably upset the patient so much that the next blood pressure measurement will probably be higher. The student has made errors in sampling (only one take), probably in measurement techniques, in predictive validity and in so-called consequential validity. And we have not even addressed the subject of the validity of using a cuff, stethoscope, and sphygmomanometer for the measurement of someone's blood pressure.

Here is another case.
You are a clinician in an academic hospital. A student is doing his clerkships under your supervision. He sits an examination in your discipline. The student has to obtain a minimum score of 60% in order to pass the examination. He scores 59%. The reason why you examine the student is to determine whether he will be a good doctor later. You tell the student that he failed the test and that he has to study much harder because otherwise he will not become a good doctor.

We wonder whether your reasoning is completely correct.
Well, in fact, it is not. In this case you would make the same errors as the student in the first example, but just in a different context. One test is never enough and there may be many sampling errors involved. The test may be imperfectly constructed and thus pick up aspects that have nothing to do with medical competence (some test items may benefit the student who has good exam technique for example). The conclusion as to whether someone will become a good doctor based on the result of one test is ill-grounded to say the least. Finally, every test has an influence on students' learning behaviour even before it is actually run.

This chapter will deal with some basic principles about testing and assessment which will help in making well-informed decisions when designing, implementing or changing a part of an assessment programme, or the programme as a whole.

Purposes of assessment

Assessment never takes place in a vacuum; it is always done with specific purposes in mind. This may seem obvious, but it does require anyone who is involved in designing or adapting assessment programmes to be well aware of the purposes of their programme. Only then can a credible evaluation of the quality of the assessment programme—to the extent to which it is effective and efficient in optimally attaining its goals—be done (fig. 35.1).

Of course, the most obvious and most frequently mentioned purpose of assessment is to determine whether students have learned enough during the course to allow them to progress to the next study phase or to graduate. Despite the many developments in formative assessment and assessment for learning there is still reason enough to keep this purpose in mind. Society expects and often funds us as educators to 'produce' competent professionals and is therefore entitled to expect us to be accountable for the quality of our graduates. Also, the individual students want information as to how they are doing and how likely they are to end up as sufficiently competent professionals—regardless of their often voiced

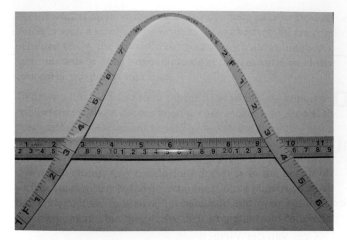

Figure 35.1 Assessment.

Pre-assessment effects relate to the influence on learning exerted by students' expectations about the upcoming assessment. This may be based on knowledge of old tests, cues from lectures or information from the student grapevine.

True assessment effects relate to the learning that occurs at the time students sit examinations. During examinations students are required to remember subject matter they have learnt. This is an active process which leads to a better storage of the topic in the student's memory and allows for better retrieval afterwards (Larsen et al. 2008).

Post-assessment effects concern the learning that takes place because of the assessment results and the feedback provided about strengths and weaknesses of the candidate.

Figure 35.2 Learning effects of assessment.

antipathy to tests. The central question, however, is not whether this is a relevant goal but how best this goal can be achieved. When an assessment programme relies merely on a series of selective tests, the results of which are added up to determine the level of quality of the graduates, even in the more senior years, the efficiency of the process may be questioned. For example, it is plausible to assume that those students who would not be capable of becoming a competent professional would have been sifted out in the more junior years. Continuing to aim the entire assessment programme in the more senior years at detecting the—possibly rare—'bad apples' is spending considerable resources for little return. In medicine this is often described as a number-needed-to-treat problem.

But of course, most agree that the mere fact of having an assessment programme is what seems to make students study in the first place, and we think this is a fair assumption. It is further a generally held opinion that the driving force of assessment on students' learning is even stronger than the that of the official curriculum (Cilliers et al. 2012; Frederiksen 1984; Newble and Jaeger 1983). Typically, we as teachers chide our students for this strategic economical attitude to study and think it not becoming of the true scholar or the professional we want to educate (Boud 1990).

But frankly, this attitude is not helpful, and we would encourage all medical educators to consider this matter further. First, we may ask ourselves whether such strategic students are really behaving unprofessionally. Many students do realize that learning for the examinations does differ from learning to become a good doctor (Cilliers et al. 2010), but they also know that if they do not study specifically to the examinations they will never become a doctor. Most of us recognize the same tension that sometimes arises between conducting a scientific study for the purpose of publication and doing a study that we are scientifically interested in. A second consideration, raised some time ago (Boud 1990), is whether our assessment really promotes the development of academic values and habits typical of the lifelong independent learners we want our students to be. It is clear that, if the assessment programme only serves to determine at the end of a module whether a student has learned enough, it does not help inform the students about what they need to do to become the best doctor they can be (but only about whether they have achieved a bare minimum). Providing such limited information at those crucial moments in the course is not optimally conducive to using assessment to steer students' learning in any direction.

So it is fair to say that if the purpose of the assessment is to steer students' learning in a desired direction, assessment needs to be ongoing and programmatic (Dannefer and Henson 2007; Fishlede et al. 2007; Schuwirth and van der Vleuten 2011; van der Vleuten and Schuwirth 2005). Such assessment needs to be informative, not only as to where the students are at this moment in their professional development, but also as to what they need to do to improve optimally. Three aspects of the learning effects of assessment can be distinguished: pre-assessment effects, true assessment effects, and post assessment effects (Gielen et al. 2003)—see fig. 35.2.

Still, it is safe to state that the empirical literature on how assessment exactly drives student learning is scarce. Newble and Jaeger (1983) provide one of the few more systematic reports on how a change in assessment in their institute has led to a change in student learning behaviour; but with their design, they were unable to unpick exactly which factors exerted this influence. The same applies to the studies reported in the often-cited overview paper by Frederiksen (1984). Recently, studies by Cilliers et al. (Cilliers et al. 2010, 2012a, b) have provided us with a model of the relationships between the assessment factors that influence student learning, the mechanisms by which this influence is exerted and the possible consequences. These studies demonstrate that the relationship between assessment and learning is much more complicated than one would intuitively believe—however further studies have demonstrated the model to be robust across contexts (Cilliers et al. in press a, b).

There are some generic lessons to be drawn from the research.

First, when looking at the factors associated with the assessment itself it is important to consider not only the content of the assessment and its format (Hakstian 1971; Stalenhoef-Halling et al. 1990), but also the scheduling and the role each assessment piece plays in the regulatory structure (Cohen-Schotanus 1999). Compensatory rules, for example, will lead some students who performed well initially to slacken off in later assessments, whereas conjunctive rules (requiring a pass at every examination to progress) can lead to a more minimal effort approach to each examination (a bare pass is enough).

A second factor of concern is the personal interpretations and experiences of students undergoing assessments. Although there is ample evidence in the literature that there are no real differences in what multiple-choice and open-ended questions test (Norman et al. 1987; Norman 1989; Schuwirth et al. 1996; Ward 1982), the perception of students is that they are different types of tests and students report that they prepare differently for them (Hakstian 1971; Stalenhoef-Halling et al. 1990).

A final factor to consider is what the steering effect of assessment could be. Cilliers et al. (2010, 2012) distinguish influences on the nature of cognitive processing activities (i.e. what students do to learn the material) and metacognitive regulation activities (such as allocation, distribution and quantity of their learning efforts).

So, in all it is not enough to just change the assessment process if one wants to influence student learning—you must also address the perceptions of students and their ability to control the learning process.

Of course, it would be inefficient if we were to collect all this valuable assessment information without using it to its full advantage. Evaluating the combined information resulting from our assessments can also tell us something about the quality of our education. If, for example, the majority of the students fail an examination a further enquiry into the quality of the education or the assessment is in order. Another indicator of problems with educational quality may be a pattern breach, such as a year group progressing well through the course and then suddenly struggling to pass a certain topic. Again, this may be sufficient reason to have a closer look at that particular topic. We want to stress here that these results can only serve as a flag and always need further information gathering before any decision on the educational quality of the topic can be made. Especially with small student numbers there may be variations in group performance without actually meaning that there is an educational problem.

Another—quite popular—way of describing the purposes of assessment is the distinction between formative and summative functions. In this, the formative function refers to all the information the assessment process provides to students to improve their learning and to teachers to improve their teaching. The summative function signifies the decision-making function of assessment. Formerly, there was shared opinion that one should not mix formative and summative functions within one assessment method, mainly because the summative function would overshadow the formative function. In other words, students who have passed the test would not consider the feedback anymore because it has become irrelevant to them.

But this poses a problem if we want to approach assessment from the viewpoint of 'assessment *for* learning' (Schuwirth and van der Vleuten 2011; Shepard 2009; van der Vleuten and Schuwirth 2005). In this, assessment is seen as an integral part of the learning process and is used to optimize the learning of each individual student. It may be clear that in order for any assessment to be able to exert such an influence it has to carry stakes—so it has to count for something and be taken seriously—*and* it has to be maximally informative. This cannot be achieved without a programme of assessment, in which most, if not all, assessments combine both formative and summative functions (Schuwirth and Van der Vleuten 2012a; van der Vleuten and Schuwirth 2005; Van der Vleuten et al. 2012). This broader programmatic approach is needed because purely summative assessment (which in its extreme meaning would imply only telling the student whether they have passed or not) simply has too little information to be a useful addition to an assessment programme. Purely formative assessment on the other hand (with no stakes at all) may eventually not be taken seriously by teachers and students, because

it does not count and it involves a lot of work. In order to combine formative and summative functions of assessment some rules are useful. First, a distinction must be made between assessment moments and decision moments. The assessment moments can be informative and add information to a dossier or portfolio until the moment a decision needs to be made about the student's progress (Dijkstra et al. 2010, 2012; van der Vleuten and Schuwirth 2005). Because all assessment in a programme contributes to a high-stakes decision each assessment therefore, carries some stakes in itself. Second, when the function of the test is—at least partly—to influence and improve student learning, then both the assessment scores and the demonstration of the effective learning need to be elements of the summative function. In other words summative information should include evidence of learning and improvement. If, for example, a mini-CEX (Norcini et al. 1995, 2003) is used to provide feedback, not only should the scores on each particular mini-CEX carry weight and be used for progress decisions, but also it has to be assessed whether students really have used the feedback to formulate learning goals and whether they have actually achieved their learning goals. If a student fails to do so this should have consequences. So, all this must be the objective of the summative function (and, of course, in the end the decision as whether this has led to sufficient improvement to meet agreed standards).

Finally, the learning and assessment environment should be safe; in that it accepts that students make mistakes and that these are useful for them to learn from. This is easier said than done because many students are high achievers who in the past have been extensively rewarded for a good performance orientation. An assessment *for* learning programme, however, would require them to adopt much more a learning-orientated approach in which mistakes help identify learning needs—this is not an easy conversion.

Methods of assessment

One way of the defining quality of an assessment programme is to evaluate the extent to which it is fit for its purpose (Brown 2004; Dijkstra et al. 2010); in other words how well the different assessment instruments are used and combined to fulfil the purposes of the assessment programme.

Often, assessment programmes are described in terms of the assessment formats, such as multiple-choice tests, orals, computer-based tests or essays. This is surprising because there is good evidence that it is not the format of the assessment that decides what it actually tests, or what its validity is, but the content (Norman et al. 1985; Norman 1989; Schuwirth et al. 1996; Schuwirth and van der Vleuten 2011; Ward 1982). A question such as: 'what is the lower normal value in mmol/l for the haemoglobin level for a normal health young male adult?' is an open-ended question, but is hardly considered tapping into what is commonly seen as higher-order cognitive skills. On the other hand one might consider the question shown in box 35.1.

This is a multiple choice question but one can hardly argue that it is a mere fact. In the first example a simple (but possibly relevant) fact was asked and in the second a deliberation or analogy. We want to stress that this is not an issue of what is more relevant—facts or deliberations—but it is clear that there is good supportive evidence that case-based items elicit different thinking operations than isolated items (Schuwirth et al. 2001) regardless of the response format (Schuwirth and van der Vleuten 2009).

> **Box 35.1** Multiple choice question
>
> A researcher conducted a predictive validity study. For this she compared the results on a first year test in an undergraduate medical curriculum with the combined actual clerkship ratings from 10 different rotations four years later. She studied the results of 300 students and found that 20 of them obtained an overall unsatisfactory rating during their clerkships. Of these 20 students, 16 (80%) also had an unsatisfactory result during the first sitting of the test in year 1. If we were to compare this figure of 80% with an epidemiological parameter and use the first year test as the diagnostic test, than this figure best represents:
>
> **A** sensitivity
>
> **B** specificity
>
> **C** positive predictive value
>
> **D** negative predictive value
>
> **E** relative risk
>
> **F** attributive risk
>
> Answer: A sensitivity

The most important lesson from this is that when designing assessment it is essential first to focus on what the items ask (the stimulus) and then on how the answer is captured (the response format) (Schuwirth and van der Vleuten 2009). Of course, the response format must fit the stimulus. A case describing a patient with complaints of fatigue, polyuria, and polydipsia (with the intent to assess whether students would spontaneously think of the diagnosis diabetes mellitus) combined with a multiple-choice question—'which of the following diagnoses should you spontaneously consider?'—is an obvious example of what we mean by a misalignment between stimulus and response format.

So, if the response format has to follow the stimulus, problems arise when item writers are forced to follow the opposite route; for example if they are required to produce multiple-choice items only. Writing good multiple-choice items to test higher-order cognitive skills is not easy (Case and Swanson 1996) and requires using a problem or case and a question asking for a decision (Schuwirth et al. 1999, 2001). This may tempt authors to flee into asking basic facts (Downing and Haladyna 1997; Elstein 1993; Ferland et al. 1987; Harden et al. 1976; Joorabchi and Chawhan 1975; Kolstad and Kostad 1985). We believe this to be one of the main reasons why there is the widespread misconception that closed question formats (of which the multiple choice question is but one example) are unfit for the assessment of higher-order cognitive skills or clinical reasoning. Another reason is the so-called cueing effect. This cueing effect—first described in the mid-1950s (Hurlburt 1954)—suggests that, in contrast to open-ended questions, a multiple-choice question can be answered correctly simply by recognizing the correct option rather than from having to produce it spontaneously. The vast number of studies in this field (Anbar 1991; Blackwell et al. 1991; Bridgeman 1992; Case and Swanson 1993; Forsdyke 1978; Hettiaratchi 1978; Hull et al. 1995; Hurlburt 1954; Joorabchi and Chawhan 1975; Kolstad and Kostad 1985; Maguire et al. 1997; McCarthy 1966; McCloskey and Holland 1976; Newble et al.

1979, 1995; Norman et al. 1985, 1987, 1996; Peitzman et al. 1990; Rothman and Kerenyi 1980; Ruch and Stoddard 1925; Schuwirth et al. 1996; Veloski et al. 1993; Ward 1982) are best summarized by the conclusion that, generally, scores on open-ended tests are lower than on multiple-choice tests with similar content but that the (disattenuated) correlations between scores are perfect (1.00). In other words, open-ended questions may be a bit more difficult but they do not provide unique information about the candidate over what would have been elicited with multiple-choice questions. Here it is important to bear in mind again that these were comparisons in which the content was similar and the factor studied was just the format. The results do not negate our earlier suggestion to determine the content first and then find the most suitable format.

Another main category of assessment methods are the observation-based methods, such as the oral examination, objective structured clinical exams (OSCEs), mini clinical evaluation exercise (mini-CEX), and other workplace-based assessment methods. Here, a crucial point is the way the assessors convert their observation of students' performance into judgements or scores. There are several important principles to heed here.

A first is that subjectivity is not equal to unreliability. It has long been thought that the unreliability of the unstandardized orals or bedside examinations until the 1960s was due to the subjectivity of the assessor. This has given rise to the worldwide popularity of the OSCE (Harden and Gleeson 1979). Research into OSCEs, however, then showed that the unreliability of unstructured examinations was not so much due to the examiner's subjective judgements but to case-specificity (Swanson 1987; Swanson and Norcini 1989; van der Vleuten and Swanson 1990). Case or domain specificity means that the performance of a candidate on one particular case or OSCE station is a poor predictor of performance on any other given case (Eva et al. 1998; Eva 2003; Swanson et al. 1987; Swanson and Norcini 1989). This is a difficult issue. First, because it is counterintuitive. We like to think about clinical problem-solving in terms of generic ability, preferably as one that can be taught. So, the finding that the ability is not generic but dependent on the specific knowledge about the problem at hand is not what we expected (Chase and Simon 1973; Chi et al. 1982; Polsen and Jeffries 1982). It has taken quite a long time for this notion to become common knowledge, simply because counterintuitive research findings take longer to permeate to educational practice than intuitive ones. Second, it means that we cannot rely on short tests. High-stakes tests based on one case or only a few items are notoriously unreliable due to domain specificity (Clauser et al. 2008; van der Vleuten et al. 1991).

Further light was shed on the influence of subjectivity on reliability by comparative research between checklists and rating scales (Hodges et al. 1999). In the original design of OSCEs a checklist approach was suggested to make the assessment objective. This, however, led to great concern amongst teachers because they often felt that although they ticked all the boxes on the checklist their personal judgement was that the student did not really perform well. Research comparing checklist to rating scales showed that global rating scales overall produced even slightly higher reliabilities (Hodges et al. 1999). This is a finding that has made its way to educational practice quite easily, because it aligned with the teachers' gut feeling.

So in all, it can be concluded that observation-based assessment can be reliable and valid if there is some structure (but not too much), a good sampling across different cases or assignments and if trained examiners are used with sufficient content knowledge to judge a candidate's performance.

These principles have given rise to the development of workplace-based assessment methods such as the mini-CEX (Norcini et al. 1995; Norcini et al. 2003) or direct observation of procedural skills (DOPS). They are all based on the notion that an expert examiner who observes the clinical performance of a candidate in the authentic setting can make a judgement about performance. Again, the central issue is to obtain sufficient individual observations to enable a reliable decision with respect to the level of competence and/or performance of a candidate. Typically, 7–11 observations are needed for this (Williams et al. 2003).

A final point we want to discuss here is the examiner and their role. In the previous paragraphs we have often referred to the expert examiner. It is becoming increasingly clear that this expertise does not only refer to content expertise—which of course is needed—but also to expertise in their role as an examiner. Research is demonstrating increasingly that examiner expertise resembles diagnostic expertise to a remarkable extent (Berendonk et al. 2012; Govaerts et al. 2011; Govaerts et al. 2012). Therefore, good observation-based assessment—especially for high-stakes assessment—requires extensive training of the examiners.

Psychometrics

Psychometrics have long been at the heart of assessment and it is fair to say that they have dominated the way our assessments were designed and conducted. In the past few years, however, there has been an ever louder call for a broader view on the quality of assessment rather than only a psychometrical one (Dochy and McDowell 1997; Hodges 2006; Schuwirth and van der Vleuten 2006, 2012b). This is not to say that psychometrics as a view on the quality of assessment should be done away with, quite the contrary, they remain a powerful set of tools in the armamentarium of assessment. Therefore, in this section we want to discuss the principles of validity and reliability or generalizability before moving to additional approaches.

Validity

Validity is often described as the extent to which a test or assessment actually measures or assesses what it is purported to measure, and better, the meaningfulness of the interpretation of test results (Downing and Haladyna 2004). This may sound easier than it is, because, other than for example body height, many of the things we want to measure in assessment cannot be observed directly. Instead, these have to be inferred from behaviour of the candidate (Cronbach and Meehl 1955). Although this is probably perfectly clear in aspects such as professionalism, which have to be inferred from professional behaviour, it is also true of knowledge. We are interested in the knowledge that students have but can only test the knowledge they can demonstrate on the test.

The most intuitive approach to validity is the so-called criterion validity; the question whether the score on a test predicts future performance well enough (C. F, Kane 2001). This is often the underlying thought when medical educators are asked to what extent these new educational methods and assessments really produce better doctors. For assessment in medical education it may not appear strange to ask this question, after all it is so analogous

to the predictive values of diagnostic tests. Yet, there is a difference. In epidemiology there is often a gold standard, i.e. an outcome that can clearly be measured or observed. In educational assessment this is much more difficult for several reasons. The first is what we have already described; the characteristic we want to assess cannot be observed directly and has to be inferred from what we *can* observe. The implication of this is that we need a way to validate a gold standard as well, and if we would have only criterion validation for this then we would have to find another gold standard and validate this one as well, needing yet another gold standard. This would entail an infinite loop of validation studies. A second reason is that medical competence is a quite nebulous and multifaceted concept, entailing elements of knowledge, skills, problem-solving ability, attitudes, professionalism, realism, meta-cognitive regulation skills and many more. So it is probably impossible to define a single measurable parameter that could be used as an outcome measure to compare test results with.

This has led to a second development in our thinking about validity in the education context, namely that validity is determined by the combined judgements of experts. So when we take professionalism as an example, an assessment method for professional behaviour contains those items and judgements on which experts agree constitute professional behaviour. The major criticism to this approach was that expert judgement may be flawed by all kinds of biases (Plous 1993), especially when the judges were asked to validate their own assessments. Still, this approach has never been completely abandoned (Ebel 1983), and it still supports our efforts in blueprinting, item construction and quality control. In other words, it helps us to build validity into a test.

Cronbach and Meehl (1955) then advocated the construct validity approach. In this line of thinking the characteristics we want to assess are seen as constructs, invisible human characteristics which we assume exist but which we cannot observe directly and to which we ascribe certain features. The most well-known psychological construct is intelligence. It cannot be observed directly yet we assume it to be present—and measurable—in all humans. We also assume some features of intelligence, such as intelligent people learn faster, have better memory skills and are better able to deal with abstract concepts. A typical clinical construct is blood pressure. Blood pressure cannot be observed directly, and you may seriously question as to whether there is really a physical phenomenon that is 120 over 80 mmHg, but we measure blood pressure and take actions on it (Llabre et al. 1988). From this it may become clear that, first, any assessment can only be valid *for* a certain goal and not be valid per se, just like a thermometer is only a valid instrument for measuring temperature and not sodium levels. Second, and more important, is to realize that before one can start validating an instrument a good theoretical framework needs to be formed about the construct.

So, if we want to validate a new instrument assumed to measure for example clinical problem-solving we will first have to define what clinical problem-solving is and what its features are. In this case we will have to use the cognitive literature on problem solving, understanding

- ◆ the role of knowledge (Boshuizen and Schmidt 1992; Chi et al. 1982; Ericsson and Charness 1994; Eva 2004)

- ◆ the use of scripts (Boreham 1994; Marewski et al. 2009; Schmidt and Boshuizen 1993b)

- ◆ the influence of increasing efficiency and

◆ the intermediate effect (the finding that intermediates frequently outperform experts on long simulation-based assessments) (Schmidt et al. 1988; Schmidt and Boshuizen 1993a).

The second step would then be to collect evidence supporting our contention that our new assessment method really assesses the construct we want to assess. In line with Popper's criterion of falsifiability we need to design critical experiments with a maximal probability of refuting our claim of validity. Only if these falsification attempts fail can we claim that further evidence for our validity arguments. It may be clear from this that a validity procedure is never really finished and validity is never 100% guaranteed much like a scientific theory is never 100% proven.

Finally, we want to highlight the currently most dominant theory on validity; the one formulated by Kane (Kane 2001, 2006). In his view demonstrating validity must be seen as a chain of arguments linking raw observations to a construct. Four types of inferences are important in his view. The first inference is from observation to score (e.g. does the score or judgement an examiner gives really reflect their true judgement or is it, for example, influenced by trying to avoid the extra workload that often accompanies failing a student). The second inference concerns the representativeness of the observed score of the so-called universe score—i.e. the score a student would obtain had they been given all possible relevant items on the topic. The third inference is from universe score to target domain. In our example this could be clinical decision making—i.e. the observation that a student makes the right selection in a series of cases leading us to infer that the student is a good decision maker. Finally, an inference must be made that a student who makes the right decisions in many cases does this based on good clinical reasoning (and for example not on good guessing) (Schuwirth and van der Vleuten 2012a).

Reliability

The main reason why we have highlighted Kane's theory in the previous section (and not another theory such as Messick's (Messick 1994)) is because Kane's theory demonstrates so nicely the relationship between reliability (as a measure for the second inference from observed scores to universe scores) and validity. It shows that an assessment method cannot be valid if it is not reliable (if one of the essential steps in the series of arguments is missing the whole argument fails) but also why an assessment method can be reliable despite being invalid (if one of the other arguments fail). Therefore, we think it is warranted to spend a separate section on reliability.

In the dominant theories about assessment the concept of 'reproducibility' of scores is used as a measure for reliability. So, it is based on the question whether the score on a second similar test would be comparable to that on the present test. In test theory, the notion of a parallel test is used. This is a hypothetical test on the same topic and with equally difficult yet different questions. If the student hypothetically would sit the original test and then sit the parallel test and both tests were perfectly reliable the scores would be similar on both tests.

So what does similar mean? Well, there are three levels of conclusions related to reproducibility that one may want to draw. The first and least stringent is that the same students who pass and fail the first test would pass and fail on the parallel test. The second would be that the rank ordering from best-performing to most poorly performing student on both tests would be the same. The third—and most stringent—requirement would be that the students would obtain the same scores on the original and the parallel test, so if a student scored 63% on the original they would also score 63% on the parallel test.

Unfortunately, this parallel test is a hypothetical one, which creates a problem when we want to use it in the non-hypothetical real world. Therefore, to approach this test–retest correlation, a split-half method can be used. In this, the test is randomly subdivided into two halves and the scores of all students on these halves are compared to each other by calculating a split-half correlation. To be precise, this correlation must be corrected for test length because each of the halves contains, of course, only half the number of items from the original test. A further caveat is that each subdivision, even if it is random, is only one of all possible subdivisions and could therefore lead to a spuriously high or low correlation. An alternative would be to make as many split halves as there are possible (and take the mean of all correlations) or to split the test in as many parts as possible and use the mean of all intercorrelations (Haertel 2006). The latter is the basis for the famous Cronbach's alpha; probably the most often used—and unfortunately also misused (Cronbach and Shavelson 2004)—measure for reliability.

Thus far this may sound a credible approach—it is certainly a coherent train of thoughts. Yet there are limitations which may not be visible on first sight and therefore we want to highlight some of them. First, split-half correlations and Cronbach's alpha are based on the notion of test–retest correlation, and therefore they do not take into account possible differences in difficulty between the original test and the parallel test. So, when one wants to make an inference about a test—such as whether students would obtain the same score on a parallel test—a correlational approach is not sufficient and will lead to an overestimation of the actual reliability (and may lead to gross mistakes in determining the grades of students). This means that for criterion-referenced scoring (which is probably most often used in educational tests), a correlation-based method will overestimate the true reproducibility (Colliver et al. 1989). A second important factor to take into account is that measures such as Alpha are in fact based on the internal consistency of the test or the intercorrelations between items and on test–retest correlations. So they can only be suitable measures for reliability under the assumption that the whole universe, from which the test is a sample, is internally consistent. To explain this further we need to explain that every test is only a sample of items from an almost infinite universe of relevant items, and thus if we want the test to be internally consistent in order to be reliable, we also state that we expect the universe to be internally consistent. If the items of a test must agree with each other on the level of knowledge of a candidate and they are expected to lead to one single result or number describing this knowledge, then we assume that we would also be able to describe that candidate's knowledge in one result or number—had they answered all the questions from the universe. So test-retest and internal consistency approaches to reliability are only trustworthy if we assume the universe from which they are a sample is internally consistent. This may seem an abstract notion but perhaps a clinical analogy may help to clarify this (Schuwirth and van der Vleuten 2012a). Suppose we use a homogenized blood sample in a test tube to test the reliability of a newly developed haemoglobin tester. Suppose we take three subsamples from the test tube and do three independent haemoglobin measurements with the new instrument. Since the sample is homogenized we assume repeated measurements will yield the same results, but if the results varied we would rightfully conclude that the instrument is unreliable. However, if we were to take three subsamples from an erythrocyte sedimentation rate (ESR) column—one from the plasma portion, one from the white cell portion, and one from the red cell portion—and we get the same results for all three haemoglobin measurements we would also doubt the reliability of the instrument because we expect different results. So our expectation of the nature of the universe (homogenized like the test tube or variable like the ESR column) determines whether we can credibly use internal consistency as a measure of reliability. That this is more than just a philosophical play of mind is becoming increasingly clear in competency-based educational settings, where much debate is going on about the nature of competencies and their homogeneity (Albanese et al. 2008; Govaerts 2008).

A more flexible approach to reliability is generalizability theory (Brennan 1983). This theory is based on the idea that in a test there is variation—or better still variance—in students' scores, which is partly based on variance in the ability of students and partly on variance in other aspects of the test. Examples of such variance components would be

◆ systematic variance in item difficulty (the question 'which lung has three lobes?' is easier for all students than 'name the amino acid sequence of insulin') or

◆ systematic variance in examiner leniency (hawks versus doves).

From the scores of all candidates on all items statistical estimates can be made about the contribution of all components of variance towards the total variance. Of course the different components vary with the type of test. In a standard multiple-choice test for example the components are shown in fig. 35.3.

In our example the error cannot be disentangled from the person × item interaction; there is no way, for example, of telling from the data whether student A really thought item 2 was harder than average or whether they were just distracted.

It will be clear that for a generalizability analysis to be performed well the researcher has to have clear idea as to what the specific components are that need to be included. In an OSCE with two examiners per station, there are students (P), cases (I), judges (J), and all their two-way interaction effects (PI, PJ, IJ), and a three-way interaction effect (PIJ) which is, again, intertwined with general error. The researcher also has to make decisions as to whether the factors are crossed or nested and whether they are random (i.e. drawn from a theoretically infinite universe) or fixed (from a limited universe). These are not decisions that can be made arbitrarily but need careful considerations because they determine the types of generalizations a researcher can make. We can give an example to illustrate this. If a researcher wants to determine whether the students' scores would be the same if they were given the whole universe of testable items (admissible observations in generalizability terminology, or population at risk in epidemiological terms) the systematic item difficulty would have to be included in the analysis. If, on the other hand, the researcher only wants to infer whether the rank ordering of students' performance on the test is sufficiently equal to the rank ordering on their performance on a universe test, the item variance component can be left out (the interaction of course cannot be left out, because it is non-systematic). So depending on the type of generalizations some factors need to be included and others have to be left out. This is in contrast to the so-called classical test theory, the theory in which, amongst others, split-halves and Cronbach's alpha are used. In this theory the reliability inference (test–retest correlation) is more or less built into the procedure.

These two theoretical approaches—classical test theory and generalizability theory—are two of the dominant psychometric ways of estimating whether the test as a sample of items or assignments is sufficiently reliable—i.e. whether the test scores are sufficiently representative of the universe scores. More generically, they tell us whether the breadth and the size of the sample are large enough to allow us to draw conclusions about students that would be reproducible; i.e., the same if we had presented the students with the

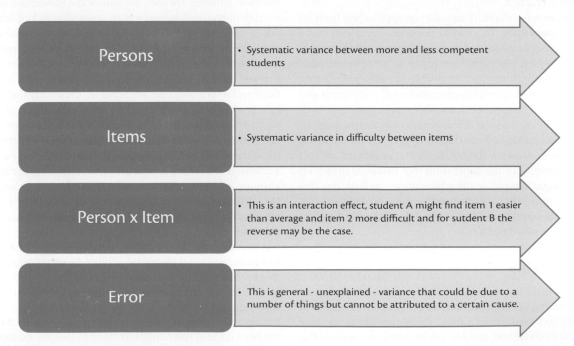

Figure 35.3 Components that can make up variance.

whole universe of possible items. In most papers and professional discussions the word reliability is used in assessment to indicate reliability in the psychometric sense. Moreover, it is often seen as synonymous with the second validity inference; i.e. the inference from observed scores to universe scores (Kane 2006). Unfortunately, it often seems to be forgotten that other, non-psychometric, arguments can also be made to support such inferences. In the next paragraph we will describe such other approaches.

As we have already described, the most often employed reliability arguments are based on the assumption of homogeneity of the universe. This begs the question: 'what if we have reason to assume that the universe is not homogeneous?' or 'what if we cannot or do not want to express the assessment results numerically, such as with portfolios?' In such cases it is better to rely on measures that carefully determine whether more information is needed to represent the universe or whether saturation of information is reached. This is equivalent to the diagnostic principle not to over-diagnose or over-test. In our medical training we were taught never to order extra diagnostic tests if the diagnosis and/or the management of the patient had already been sufficiently established, or when it was unlikely that the outcome of the additional diagnostic procedure would change our decisions. This idea, to determine whether a new observation is really going to contribute unique information, is another way of looking at 'reliability' (we have used the quotation marks here to indicate that we do not mean reliability in the strict psychometric sense). In portfolio assessment for example, this means that the judges do not all have to concur with each other. In fact, 'reliability' is reached when it is sufficiently plausible that adding another examiner's judgement will not provide us with unique information about the quality of a student's portfolio (Driessen et al. 2005). So in this approach judges may differ and each highlight a different aspect of the quality of the portfolio, but if it is unlikely that an extra judge will provide us with a unique additional view it is no longer useful to collect judgements and one is safe to argue that sufficient universe representation is reached.

Finally, increasingly reliability can also be approached from an organizational framework. This can be done for example by using organizational procedures and safety nets to ensure that the assessment leads to the best representation of the universe score. Such procedures encompass second opinions, appeals procedures, supervision of assessors, careful documentation of judgements and transparency. These, due process measures in conjunction with good assessor training and the development of sufficient assessor expertise, all ensure that any conclusion a teacher or a certifying committee want to draw on the results of an assessment are sufficiently representative of the conclusion that would be drawn on the basis of a larger sample or the whole universe. Basically, this means that the conclusions are trustworthy, more credible or, actually, more reliable—in the traditional meaning of the word: 'information that can be relied upon'.

Standard setting

We have tried to make the case that reliability cannot be determined well without making assumptions as to what the assessment tries to capture; it requires assumptions about the nature of the universe from which the assessment is a sample of items or assignments. We have further tried to explain that psychometric analyses can be used as one of the methods to support arguments underpinning a validity inference but that there are many more.

The same is true for standard setting. Although we often wish that there were a truth in standard setting much like it is a truth that the Earth revolves around the Sun, we have to acknowledge that standards are constructed by people (Norcini and Shea 1997). What is considered a good doctor today was probably not a good doctor 50 years ago; what is considered a good working knowledge of anatomy now is probably different from what we considered a good working knowledge of anatomy 30 years ago. It is therefore fair to say that the whole process of standard setting is mainly a process of capturing well enough what our current expectations of students and graduated doctors are. This makes it immediately clear that there is no one single best method for standard setting. We would even go further and argue that it is unlikely that there will ever be a single standard setting method that is the best for all methods of assessment. Instead, we want to argue that for each assessment method and perhaps for each context a specific standard setting method needs to be chosen (and perhaps adapted). Of each of the over 30 existing methods (Berk 1986; Cusimano 1996; Livingston and Zieky 1982) the strengths and weaknesses have to be considered. Plausible arguments have to be made—which can be supported by statistics—as to why a certain method for standard setting is most appropriate for the assessment at hand.

Thus far you may have noticed that we have not even used the terms absolute or relative methods of standard setting at all. There is good reason for this, because when it comes to principles there is not a big difference between them. Both approaches start with assumptions about the 'borderline students'. In more absolute methods such as Angoff (Angoff 1971), Nedelsky (Nedelsky 1954), Ebel (Ebel 1972), Borderline, Borderline regression (Kaufman et al. 2000; Kramer et al. 2003), and contrasting groups the judges have to form an opinion as to what can be expected from a borderline student, whereas in more relative methods such as Hofstee (Hofstee 1983), and other methods that 'grade on the curve' the scores of students are used to capture the borderline student. The overlap in concepts between both types of standard setting methods is also reflected in common practices in assessment. If, for example, we were to find that 100% of the students repeatedly fail a test we would seriously reconsider the standard that was set for that test. And even if the teachers claim that the test is not too difficult and it tests only relevant material, eventually they will have to give in or be forced to lower their standards, which, of course, is a norm-referenced action. On the other hand, if a norm-referenced test repeatedly would yield a 100% pass, eventually the content of the test will be carefully scrutinized to see if it is too easy (which is a criterion-referenced approach). Therefore, if no method is 100% absolute or 100% relative it is better to look at other aspects of the various methods to underpin the defensibility of the method we want to use in a given situation. We will only describe these generally.

A first basis for arguments for the defensibility of a standard set to a particular test is its reproducibility. But note, where in reliability of assessment the main inference is whether the *same* students would achieve a comparable result on *another* test, in standard setting the question is whether *another* group of judges would reach a comparable standard on *the same* set of items. Interesting work has been done in this field. Norcini and Shea, for example, demonstrated that an Angoff standard-setting procedure is reproducible

(Norcini and Shea 1992). An Angoff procedure requires a panel of judges to review all the items for a test and try to estimate for each item the probability that a hypothetical borderline student (a student who is barely competent enough to pass) would answer the question correctly (Angoff 1971). Norcini and coworkers showed that not only would the same panel of judges come to a similar standard on the same test if they performed the Angoff procedure roughly one year later, but also that different panels of similar experts would come to the same decision on the same test (Angoff 1971). In another study they demonstrated that varying the subspecializations of Angoff judges (who were judging a test covering a broad content area) did not significantly influence the estimate of the performance of borderline students (Norcini et al. 1988).

So, one would be led to conclude that Angoff is stable and therefore the best method, but this is not necessarily so. Verhoeven et al. for example, demonstrated that the cut-off score derived by Angoff panels differed substantially between recently graduated doctors and experienced faculty members (Verhoeven et al. 2002). Their study demonstrated that not just any panel would do, the credibility of an Angoff rating depends on the credibility of the judges performing the procedure. It is therefore fair to say that if the judges cannot establish their credibility as experts for setting the standards (for example because they have not had sufficient contact with students to be able to picture the borderline students or because they lack the content knowledge to understand the items) the standard will not be credible.

A second factor is the decision whether the standard is needed before the test or whether it can be set afterwards. Although there may be logistical reasons to set the standard before the test administration, often acceptability issues play a major role. The decision to choose a method that will produce a standard before the administration of the test precludes the use of any method that is derived from the results (for example any grading on the curve method) or that needs direct observation of student performance (such as the borderline regression method in OSCEs (Kaufman et al. 2000)). Therefore, we urge care before ruling out potentially powerful methods; the desire to please students, teachers or other stakeholders (over selecting the most meaningful method) is not necessarily the best argument in education. A more important argument is the validity of the information being used in setting the standard. Methods that rely on judges' imagination of the borderline student and how they would perform on an item are less defensible than methods that are based on actual observation of performance. It is for this reason that some researchers argue for the use of actual performance data in a second Angoff round as an extra reality check for the judges (Norcini 2003) or why a borderline regression method is more defensible for an OSCE than an Angoff method (Kaufman et al. 2000; Kramer et al. 2003).

In standard setting not only is the credibility of the judges important but also the credibility of the information on which the standards are based. For methods that are based on the actual performance of students it is necessary that there be enough students on whose data to base the norm. Although there is no clear cutoff number above which norm-referenced methods are sufficiently credible it is clear that 10 is too few and 10,000 is probably abundant. A good way of checking this in a certain context is to compare the fluctuations in proportions of passing and failing students in subsequent tests within the same cohort of students to those proportions between cohorts of student on the same or equated tests.

Verhoeven and his colleagues, for example, demonstrated that correlation in item scores between student cohorts of different universities were considerably higher than such correlations within student cohorts on comparable subsequent tests. (Verhoeven et al. 1998) This means that in his study—using progress testing—two cohorts of 250 medical students were far more comparable to each other than two consecutive progress tests were (van der Vleuten et al. 1996).

Of course contributing to the credibility of the underlying information is the sheer amount of it. Any opportunity to give useful information to inform judges or standard setters either before the test administration or afterwards should be taken (Norcini and Shea 1997; Norcini 2003). The general rule governing the whole domain of assessment—the higher the stakes of the decisions, the richer the information these decisions require—applies to standard setting as well (Dijkstra et al. 2012). Of course, one needs to ensure that the extra information is handled correctly. It is, for example, a good idea to feed back actual test results to an Angoff panel and offer the judges the chance to change their ratings, but one has to take care not to lure them into providing a judgement that just concurs with the actual performance data. In short, adding extra sources of information can decrease random error in the process of arriving at a standard but one must take care not to introduce systematic bias. Increased error will show up in reliability analyses, increased bias will not. So, we cannot stress enough that a good process is needed to ensure the quality of the standard-setting process.

A final point is the issue of due diligence. Norcini and Shea (1997) introduce this aspect quite explicitly. Standards must be credible to the stakeholders. A process that is laborious and involves the efforts of many experts has more stakeholder credibility than a standard which is automatically produced by a particular statistical procedure. In a similar vein a standard setting procedure must be easy enough to explain to all stakeholders. Sometimes complicated methods are suggested which are plausible and rational but which are difficult to explain.

Conclusions

- Assessment is always a matter of gathering information to support human judgement about the progress or competency of candidates. One cannot design or conduct assessment in a vacuum; one cannot claim to assess reflection or clinical reasoning without giving some thought as to what reflection or clinical reasoning are.

- If assessment is a process of forming a value judgement about candidates, this process should be seen as producing a series of arguments supporting how we use what can be observed about candidates (i.e. their behaviour) to infer what we think are their competencies. So not only do we infer professional values from observing professional behaviour, but also we infer knowledge from observing the scores on a multiple-choice test.

- The notion of the collection of different types of information and combining them in different ways underlies the currently popular notion of programmatic assessment (van der Vleuten and Schuwirth 2005; Van der Vleuten et al. 2012).

- No single instrument can paint the whole picture of a candidate's competence so an array of methods is needed in a programme.

◆ No individual method is perfect—so methods have to be combined in such a way that the weaknesses of one method are compensated for by the strengths of another. Such a combination of methods will be broad enough to capture even such an elusive concept as medical competence.

◆ To draw a final analogy to healthcare; to capture the concept of competence without deconstructing competence into 'atoms', the programme of assessment should be broad and flexible—just as the array of diagnostic methods in healthcare are able to capture the concept of health without having to break the idea of health down into atoms. Any conclusions drawn as to the health of a patient are similarly based on a combination of numerical, qualitative, deductive, inductive, probabilistic and even authority-based arguments, but they derive their strengths from coherence, transparency and credibility. Single methods and single theoretical approaches can be used to support this process but never to dominate it.

References

Albanese, M.A., Mejicano, G., Mullan, P.,et al. (2008) Defining characteristics of educational competencies. *Med Educ.* 42 (3): 248–255

Anbar, M. (1991) Comparing assessments of students' knowledge by computerized open-ended and multiple-choice tests. *Acad Med.* 66(7): 420–422

Angoff, W.H. (1971) Scales, norms and equivalent scales. In: R.L. Thorndike (ed.) *Educational Measurement* (pp. 508–600). Washington DC: American Council on Education

Berendonk, C., Stalmeijer, R.E., and Schuwirth, L.W.T. (2012) Expertise in performance assessment: assessors' perspectives. *Med Educ.* Advanced EPub, doi: DOI 10.1007/s10459-012-9392-x

Berk, R.A. (1986) A consumer's guide to setting performance standards on criterion-referenced tests. *Rev Educ Res.* 56(1): 137–172

Blackwell, T., Ainsworth, M., Dorsey, N., et al. (1991) A comparison of short-answer and extended-matching questions scores in an OSCE, *Acad Med.* 66(9): s40–s42

Boreham, N.C. (1994) The dangerous practice of thinking, *Med Educ.* 28: 172–179

Boshuizen, H. and Schmidt, H.G. (1992) On the role of biomedical knowledge in clinical reasoning by experts; intermediates and novices. *Cogn Sci.* 16: 153–184

Boud, D. (1990) Assessment and the promotion of academic values. *Studies Higher Educ.* 15(1): 101–111

Brennan, R.L. (1983) *Elements of Generalizability Theory.* Iowa City IA: ACT Publications

Bridgeman, B. (1992) A comparison of quantitative questions in open-ended and multiple-choice formats. *J Educ Measurement.* 29(3): 253–271

Brown, S. (2004) Assessment for learning. *Learn Teach Higher Educ.* 1; 81–89

Case, S.M. and Swanson, D.B. (1993) Extended-matching items: a practical alternative to free response questions. *Teach Learn Med.* 5(2): 107–115

Case, S.M. and Swanson, D.B. (1996) Constructing written test questions for the basic and clinical sciences. (http://www.nbme.org/publications/item-writing-manual-download.html) Accessed 6 March 2013

Chase, W.G. and Simon, H.A. (1973) Perception in chess. *Cogn Psychol.* 4(1): 55–81

Chi, M.T.H., Glaser, R., and Rees, E. (1982) Expertise in problem solving. In: R.J. Sternberg (ed.) *Advances in the Psychology of Human Intelligence* (pp. 7–76). Hillsdale NJ: Lawrence Erlbaum Associates.

Cilliers, F.J., Schuwirth, L.W., Adendorff, H.J., Herman, N., and van der Vleuten, C.P. (2010) The mechanisms of impact of summative assessment on medical students' learning. *Adv Health Sci Educ.* 15: 695–715

Cilliers, F.J., Schuwirth, L.W.T., and van der Vleuten, C.P.M. (2012a) A model of the pre-assessment learning effects of assessment is operational in an undergraduate clinical context. *BMC Med Educ.* 12(9): DOI: 10.1186/1472-6920-12-9

Cilliers, F.J., Schuwirth, L.W.T., Herman, N., Adendorff, H.J., and van der Vleuten C.P.M. (2012b) A model of the pre-assessment learning effects of summative assessment in medical education. *Adv Health Sci Educ.* 17: 39–53

Cilliers, F.J., Schuwirth, L.W.T., and van der Vleuten, C.P.M. (in press a) Evidence for the validity of a model of the pre-assessment learning effects of consequential assessment. *Med Educ.* in press

Cilliers, F.J., et al. (in press b) Generalizability findings for a model of the pre-assessment learning effects of assessment in new contexts. *Med Teach.* in press

Clauser, B.E., Margolis, M.J., and Swanson, D.B. (2008) Issues of validity and reliability for asessments in medical education. In: Holmboe ES and Hawkins RE (eds) *Evaluation of Clinical Competence* (pp. 10–23). Philadelphia, PA: Mosby Elsevier

Cohen-Schotanus, J. (1999) Student assessment and examination rules. *Med Teach.* 21(3): 318–321

Colliver, J., Verhulst, S., Williams, R., et al. (1989) Reliability of performance on standardized patient cases: a comparison of consistency measures based on generalizability theory. *Teach Learn Med.* 1(1): 31–37

Cronbach, L.J. and Meehl, P.E. (1955) Construct validity in psychological tests, *Psychol Bull.* 52(4): 281–302

Cronbach, L. and Shavelson, R.J. (2004) My current thoughts on coefficient alpha and successor procedures. *Educ Psychol Measurement.* 64(3): 391–418

Cusimano, M.D. (1996) Standard setting in medical education. *Acad Med.* 71(10 Suppl): S112–S120

Dannefer, E.F. and Henson, L.C. (2007) The portfolio approach to competency-based assessment at the Cleveland Clinic Lerner College of Medicine. *Acad Med.* 82(5): 493–502

Dijkstra, J., van der Vleuten, C.P.M., and Schuwirth, L.W.T. (2010) A new framework for designing programmes of assessment. *Adv Health Sci Educ.* 15: 379–393

Dijkstra, J., Galbraith, R., Hodges, B., et al. (2012) Expert validation of fit-for-purpose guidelines for designing programmes of assessment. *BMC Med Educ.* 12(20): DOI 10.1186/1472-6920-12-20

Dochy, F.R.J.C. and McDowell, L. (1997) Introduction: assessment as a tool for learning. *Studies Educ Eval.* 23(4): 279–298

Downing, S.M. and Haladyna, T.M. (1997) Test item development: validity evidence from quality assurance procedures. *Appl Measurement Educ.* 10(1): 61–82

Downing, S.M. and Haladyna, T.M. (2004) Validity threats: overcoming interference with proposed interpretations of assessment data. *Med Educ.* 38(3): 327–333

Driessen E., Van der Vleuten, C.P.M., Schuwirth, L.W.T., et al. (2005) The use of qualitative research criteria for portfolio assessment as an alternative to reliability evaluation: a case study, *Med Educ.* 39(2): 214–220

Ebel, R.L. (1972) *Essentials of Educational Measurement.* Englewood Cliffs, NJ: Prentice-Hall

Ebel, R.L. (1983) The practical validation of tests of ability. *Educ Measurement: Issues Pract.* 2(2): 7–10

Elstein, A.E. (1993) Beyond multiple choice questions and essays: The need for a new way to assess clinical competence. *Acad Med.* 68(4): 244–248

Ericsson, K.A. and Charness, N. (1994) Expert performance. *Am Psychol.* 49(8): 725–747

Eva, K.W. (2003) On the generality of specificity. *Med Educ.* 37: 587–588

Eva, K.W. (2004) What every teacher needs to know about clinical reasoning. *Med Educ.* 39: 98–106

Eva, K.W., Neville, A.J., and G.R., Norman (1998) Exploring the etiology of content specificity: Factors influenceing analogic transfer and problem solving., *Acad Med.* 73(10): s1–s5

Ferland, J.J., Dorval, J., and Levasseur, L. (1987) Measuring higher cognitive levels by multiple choice questions: a myth?, *Med Educ.* 21(2): 109–113

Fishlede, A.J., Henson, L.C., and Hull, A.L. (2007) Cleveland Clinic Lerner College of Medicine: An innovative approach to medical education and the training of physician investigators. *Acad Med.* 82(4): 390–396

Forsdyke, D.R. (1978) A comparison of short and multiple choice questions in the evaluation of students of biochemistry. *Med Educ.* 12(5): 351–356

Frederiksen, N. (1984) The real test bias: Influences of testing on teaching and learning. *Am Psychol.* 39(3): 193–202

Gielen, S., Dochy, F., and Dierick, S. (2003) Evaluating the consequential validity of new modes of assessment: The influences of assessment on learning, including pre-, post- and true assessment effects. In: Segers M, Dochy F, and Cascallar E (eds) *Optimising New Modes of Assessment: In Search of Qualities and Standards* (pp. 37–54). Dordrecht: Kluwer Academic Publishers

Govaerts, M.J.B. (2008) Educational competencies or education for professional competence? *Med Educ.* 42(3): 234–236

Govaerts, M.J.B., Schuwirth, L.W.T., Van der Vleuten, C.P.M., et al. (2011) Workplace-based assessment: effects of rater expertise. *Adv Health Sci Educ.* 16(2): 151–165

Govaerts, M.J.B., Van de Wiel, M.W.J., Schuwirth, L.W.T., Van der Vleuten, C.P.M., and Muijtjens, A.M.M. (2012) Raters' performance theories and constructs in workplace-based assessment. *Adv Health Sci Educ.* Epub, doi: DOI 10.1007/s10459-012-9376-x

Haertel, E.H. (2006) Reliability. In: Brennan RL (ed.) *Educational Measurement* (pp. 65–110) Westport: ACE/Praeger

Hakstian, R.A. (1971) The effects of type of examination anticipated on test preparation and performance. *J Educ Res.* 64(7): 319–324

Harden, R.M. and Gleeson, F.A. (1979) Assessment of clinical competence using an objective structured clinical examination (OSCE). *Med Educ.* 13(1): 41–54

Harden, R.M., Brown, R.A., Biran, L.A., et al. (1976) Multiple choice questions: to guess or not to guess, *Med Educ.* 10: 27–32

Hettiaratchi, E. (1978) A comparison of student performance in two parallel physiology tests in multiple choice and short answer forms, *Med Educ.* 12: 290–296

Hodges, B., Regehr, G,, McNaughton, N., Tiberius, R., and Hanson, M.(1999) OSCE checklists do not capture increasing levels of expertise, *Acad Med.* 74(10): 1129–1134

Hodges, B. (2006) Medical education and the maintenance of incompetence, *Med Teach.* 28(8): 690–696

Hofstee, W.K.B. (1983) The case for compromise in educational selection and grading. In: S.B. Anderson and J.S. Helmick (eds) *On Educational Testing* (pp. 109–127). San-Francisco: Jossey-Bass

Hull, A.L., Hodder, S., Berger, B., et al. (1995) Validity of three clinical performance assessments of internal medicine clerks. *Acad Med.* 70(6): 517–522

Hurlburt, D. (1954) The relative value of recall and recognition techniques for measuring precise knowledge of word meaning, nouns, verbs, adjectives. *J Educ Res.* 47(8): 561–576

Joorabchi, B. and Chawhan, A.R. (1975) Multiple choice questions. The debate goes on. *Br J Med Educ.* 9(4): 275–280

Kane, M.T. (2001) Current concerns in validity theory. *J Educ Measurement.* 38(4): 319–342

Kane, M.T. (2006) Validation. In: Brennan RL (ed.) *Educational Measurement* (pp. 17–64). Westport: ACE/Praeger

Kaufman, D.M., Mann, K.M., Muijtjens, A.M.M., et al. (2000) A comparison of standard-setting procedures for an OSCE in undergraduate Medical Education. *Acad Med.* 75: 267–271

Kolstad, R.K. and Kostad, R.A. (1985) Multiple-choice test items are unsuitable for measuring the learning of complex instructional objectives. *Scientia Paedagogica Experimentalis.* 22(1): 68–76

Kramer, A., Muijtjens, A., Jansen, K., et al. (2003) Comparison of a rational and an empirical standard setting procedure for an OSCE. *Med Educ.* 37: 132–139

Larsen, D.P., Butler, A.C., and Roediger, H.L. (2008) Test-enhanced learning in medical education. *Med Educ.* 42: 959–966

Livingston, S.A. and Zieky, M.J. (1982) *Passing Scores: A manual for setting standards of performance on educational and occupational tests.* Princeton NJ: Educational Testing Service

Llabre, M.M., Ironson, G.H., Spitzer, S.B. et al. (1988) How Many Blood Pressure Measurements Are Enough? An application of generalizability theory to the study of blood pressure reliability. *Psychophysiology.* 25(1): 97–106

Maguire, T.O., Skakun, E.N. , and Triska, O.H. (1997) Student thought processes evoked by multiple choice and constructed response items. In: Scherpbier, A., Van der Vleuten, C., Rethans, J.. and Van der Steeg, L. (eds) Advances in Medical Education: Proceedings of the seventh Ottawa Conference on Medical Education (pp. 618–621). Dordrecht, The Netherlands: Kluwer Academic Publishers

Marewski, J.N., Gaissmaier, W., and Gigerenzer, G. (2009) Good judgements do not require complex cognition. *Cognitive Processing.* 11(2): 103–121

McCarthy, W.H. (1966) An assessment of the influence of cueing items in objective examinations. *J Med Educ.* 41: 263–266

McCloskey, D.I. and Holland, R.A. (1976) A comparison of student performances in answering essay-type and multiple-choice questions. *Med Educ.* 10(5): 382–385

Messick, S. (1994) The interplay of evidence and consequences in the validation of performance assessments. *Educ Res.* 23(2): 13–23

Nedelsky, L. (1954) Absolute grading standards for objective tests. *Educ Psychol Measurement.* 14(1): 3–19

Newble, D.I., Baxter, A., and Elsmlie, R.G. (1979) A comparison of multiple-choice tests and free-response tests in examinations of clinical competence. *Med Educ.* 13: 263–268

Newble, D.I. and Jaeger, K. (1983) The effect of assessments and examinations on the learning of medical students. *Med Educ.* 17: 165–171

Newble, D.I., van der Vleuten, C.P.M., and Norman, G.R. (1995) Assessing clinical problem solving. In: J. Higgs and M. Jones (eds) *Clinical Reasoning in the Health Professions* (pp. 168–178). Oxford: Butterworth-Heinemann Ltd

Norcini, J.J. (2003) Setting standards on educational tests. *Med Educ.* 37: 464–469

Norcini, J.J. and Shea, J.A. (1992) The reproducibility of standards over groups and occasions. *Appl Measurement Educ.* 5: 63–72

Norcini, J.J. and Shea, J.A. (1997) The credibility and comparability of standards. *Appl Measurement i Educ.* 10(1): 39–59

Norcini, J.J., Shea, J.A., and Kanya, T.D. (1988) The effect of various factors on standard setting, *J Educ Measurement.* 25(1): 57–65

Norcini, J., Blank, L.L., Arnold, G.K., et al. (1995) The Mini-CEX (Clinical Evaluation Exercise);a preliminary investigation. *Ann Intern Med.* 123(10): 795–799

Norcini, J.J, Blank, L.L., Duffy, F.D., et al. (2003) The mini-CEX: A method for assessing clinical skills. *Ann Intern Med.* 138(6): 476–481

Norman, G.R. (1989) Reliability and construct validity of some cognitive measures of clinical reasoning. *Teach Learn Med.* 1(4): 194–199

Norman, G., Swanson, D., and Case, S. (1996) Conceptual and methodology issues in studies comparing assessment formats, issues in comparing item formats. *Teach Learn Med.* 8(4): 208–216

Norman, G., Tugwell, P., Feightner, J., et al. (1985) Knowledge and clinical problem-solving. *Med Educ.* 19: 344–356

Norman, G.R., Smith, E.K.M., Powles, A.C., et al. (1987) Factors underlying performance on written tests of knowledge, *Med Educ.* 21: 297–304

Peitzman, S.J., Nieman, L.Z., and Gracely, E.J. (1990) Comparison of 'fact-recall' with 'higher-order' questions in multiple-choice examinations as predictors of clinical performance of medical students. *Acad Med.* 65(9 Suppl): S59–S60

Plous, S. (1993) *The Psychology of Judgment and Decision Making.* New York: McGraw-Hill

Polsen, P. and Jeffries, R. (1982) Expertise in problem solving. In: R.J. Sternberg (ed.) *Advances in the Psychology of Human Intelligence* (pp. 367–411). Hillsdale NJ: Lawrence Erlbaum Associates

Pritchard, L. (2005) Accidental hero. *Med Educ.* 39(8): 761–762

Rothman, A.I. and Kerenyi, N. (1980) The assessment of an examination in pathology consisting of multiple-choice, practical and short essay questions. *Med Educ.* 14(5): 341–344

Ruch, G. and Stoddard, G. (1925) Comparative reliabilities of five types of objective examinations. *J Educ Psychol.* 16: 89–103

Schmidt, H.G. and Boshuizen, H.P. (1993a) On the origin of intermediate effects in clinical case recall. *Memory Cogn.* 21(3): 338–351

Schmidt, H.G. and Boshuizen, H.P. (1993b) On acquiring expertise in medicine. Special Issue: European educational psychology. *Educ Psychol Rev.* 5(3): 205–221

Schmidt, H.G., Boshuizen, H.P.A., and Hobus, P.P.M. (1988) Transitory stages in the development of medical expertise: The 'intermediate effect' in clinical case representation studies. *Proceedings of the 10th Annual Conference of the Cognitive Science Society.* Montreal, Canada: Lawrence Erlbaum Associates, pp. 139–145

Schuwirth, L.W.T. and van der Vleuten, C.P.M. (2006) A plea for new psychometrical models in educational assessment. *Med Educ.* 40(4): 296–300

Schuwirth, L.W.T. and van der Vleuten, C.P.M. (2009) Written assessment. In: J.A. Dent and R.M. Harden (eds) *A Practical Guide for Medical Teachers.* 4th edn. Edinburgh: Churchill Livingstone

Schuwirth, L.W.T. and van der Vleuten, C.P.M. (2011) Programmatic assessment: from assessment of learning to assessment for learning. *Med Teach.* 33(6): 478–485

Schuwirth, L.W.T. and van der Vleuten, C.P.M. (2012a) Assessing competence: extending the approaches to reliability. In: Hodges, B.D. and Lingard, L. (eds) *The Question of Competence* (pp. 113–130). Ithaca NY: Cornell University Press

Schuwirth, L.W.T. and van der Vleuten, C.P.M. (2012b) Programmatic assessment and Kane's validity perspective. *Med Educ.* 46(1): 38–48

Schuwirth, L.W.T., van der Vleuten, C.P.M., and Donkers, H.H.L.M. (1996) A closer look at cueing effects in multiple-choice questions. *Med Educ.* 30: 44–49

Schuwirth, L.W.T., Blackmore, D.B., Mom, E.M.A., et al. (1999) How to write short cases for assessing problem-solving skills. *Med Teach.* 21(2): 144–150

Schuwirth, L.W.T., Verheggen, M.M., Van der Vleuten, C.P.M., et al. (2001) Do short cases elicit different thinking processes than factual knowledge questions do? *Med Educ.* 35(4): 348–356

Shepard, L. (2009) The role of assessment in a learning culture. *EducRes.* 29(7): 4–14

Stalenhoef-Halling, B.F., Van der Vleuten, C.P.M., Jaspers, T.A.M., et al. (1990) A new approach to assessing clinical problem-solving skills by written examination: Conceptual basis and initial pilot test results. In: W. Bender, R.J. Hiemstra, A. Scherpbier, et al. (eds.) *Teaching and Assessing Clinical Competence, Proceedings of the fourth Ottawa Conference* (pp. 552–557). Groningen, The Netherlands: Boekwerk Publications

Swanson, D.B. (1987) A measurement framework for performance-based tests. In: I. Hart and R. Harden (eds) *Further Developments in Assessing Clinical Competence* (pp. 13–45). Montreal: Can-Heal publications

Swanson, D.B. and Norcini, J.J. (1989) Factors influencing reproducibility of tests using standardized patients. *Teach Learn Med.* 1(3): 158–166

Swanson, D.B., Norcini, J.J., and Grosso, L.J. (1987) Assessment of clinical competence: written and computer-based simulations. *Assess Eval Higher Educ.* 12(3): 220–246

Van der Vleuten, C.P.M. and Swanson, D. (1990) Assessment of clinical skills with standardized patients: State of the art. *Teach Learn Med.* 2(2): 58–76

Van der Vleuten, C.P.M. and Schuwirth, L.W.T. (2005) Assessing professional competence: from methods to programmes. *Med Educ.* 39(3): 309–317

Van der Vleuten, C.P.M., Norman, G.R., and De Graaf, E (1991) Pitfalls in the pursuit of objectivity: issues of reliability. *Med Educ.* 25: 110–118

Van der Vleuten, C.P.M., Verwijnen, G.M., and Wijnen, W.H.F.W. (1996) Fifteen years of experience with progress testing in a problem-based learning curriculum. *Med Teach.* 18 (2): 103–110

Van der Vleuten, C.P.M., Schuwirth, L.W.T., Driessen, E.W., et al. (2012) A model for programmatic assessment fit for purpose. *Med Teach.* 34: 205–214

Veloski, J., Rabinowitz, H., and Robeson, M. (1993) A solution to the cueing effects in multiple choice questions: the Un-Q-format. *Med Educ.* 27: 371–375

Verhoeven, B.H., Verwijnen, G., Scherpbier, A., et al. (1998) An analysis of progress test results of PBL and non-PBL students. *Med Teach.* 20(4): 310–316

Verhoeven, B.H., Verwijnen, G., Muijtjens, A., et al. (2002) Panel expertise for an Angoff standard setting procedure in progress testing: item writers compared to recently graduated students. *Med Educ.* 36: 860–867

Ward, W.C. (1982) A comparison of free-response and multiple-choice forms of verbal aptitude tests. *Appl Psychol Measurement.* 6(1): 1–11

Williams, M., Klamen, D, and McGaghie, W. (2003) Cognitive, social and environmental sources of bias in clinical performance ratings. *Teach Learn Med.* 15(4): 270–292

CHAPTER 36

Setting standards

Danette W. McKinley and John J. Norcini

A good decision is based on knowledge and not on numbers.
Plato, Early Dialogues.

Introduction

Tests serve a variety of different purposes. In some instances, they are used by an instructor to determine what students have learned. In other cases, they are used to provide feedback or to determine which candidates are admitted to a programme or awarded a license or other qualification. These uses also include the evaluation of faculty by students. While the goals of an assessment may vary, in educational programmes there are often decisions associated with the use of these instruments—decisions regarding the competency or proficiency of individuals.

Deciding on a standard, the score that separates success from failure on these assessments, is a matter of translating a description of the characteristics denoting the desired level performance into a number that applies to a particular test. The purpose of this chapter is to provide a detailed description of the types of approaches that can be used to make decisions about the relationship between test performance and a construct, for example 'competence'. The chapter will begin by clarifying the distinction between scores and standards. This is followed by an overview of assessment methods currently used in medical education and a presentation of common assessment goals. This information will provide a context for the more detailed presentation of standard setting methods that follows.

Scores versus standards

There is a difference between scores and standards that is useful to establish before describing the various methods of setting standards. These terms are often used loosely and are defined in a variety of ways. For purposes of this chapter, a *score* describes the performance of an examinee along an underlying trait or continuum. In contrast, a *standard* refers to how good the performance needs to be for a particular purpose (Kane 1998b; Norcini 1994; Norcini and Guille 2002). Standards reflect an idea or conceptualization of a construct. For example, in an exit examination from medical school, the standard reflects the desirable characteristics of those considered 'competent' and able to progress to the next level of training.

The distinction between scores and standards is fundamental to an understanding of the process for deriving the passing score. In a sense, the pass–fail point is the operationalization of the standard.

The nature of the standard will vary depending on the purpose of the assessment.

Assessment purposes and stakes

When the purpose of the assessment is to gather information about individuals (e.g. a classroom test) and/or to provide feedback to examinees regarding their progress towards instructional goals, the stakes are generally considered to be low, meaning that errors of measurement are unlikely to have significant adverse consequences for the individual being tested. Even when assessment results are aggregated to determine whether instructional goals are met (for example, within or across departments), the stakes may be low. In contrast, when assessment results are used to make decisions of importance (e.g. graduation, promotion, retention), the stakes are higher, and errors of measurement are less tolerable (American Educational Research Association 1999). In these high stakes decision-making settings, greater rigour must be employed to ensure that the inferences are justified and the conclusions drawn are unbiased.

Although there are circumstances where passing scores must be established (e.g. licensure examinations), standard setting has been criticized for a variety of reasons. One criticism is that the task presented to judges seems impossible, that is, conceptualizing the standard and then predicting examinee performance may be beyond panellists' capability (Shepard 1980). Another criticism has been that panellists in cut score studies may be providing their opinions about how much examinees need to know in order to meet the conceptual standard defined, rather than basing their judgements on evidence (Zieky 2001). However, for some assessments, the purpose is not only to determine a level of knowledge or ability, but to provide information regarding those who meet criteria that define proficiency. When assessment results will be interpreted regarding the placement of examinees in an ordered fashion, it is necessary to set standards (Hambleton 2001). Both the purpose and the stakes associated with the assessment are essential to decisions about standard-setting. The purpose drives the need for standards in the first place and, along with the stakes, determines how credible and rigorous the process needs to be. As described in the next section, assessment purposes and stakes may also influence the choice of standard type.

Types of standards

There are two types of standards: relative (sometimes called norm-referenced) and absolute (sometimes called criterion-referenced) (Livingston and Zieky 1982). Relative standards are established based on a comparison of those who take the assessment with each other. For example, when the cut score is set based on the number or percentage of examinees that will pass, the standard is relative. This type of standard setting is typically used in selection for employment or admission to educational programmes where a limited number of positions are available.

Relative standards are rarely used in high stakes examinations (e.g. graduation, certification, or licensure) because the ability of the groups of test takers could vary over time and the content of the assessment may also vary over time. To avoid the disadvantages associated with this method, absolute standard setting approaches are more commonly used in competence testing.

Absolute standards are set by determining the amount of test material that must be answered correctly (or performed correctly) in order to pass. For example, if the examinee must answer 75% of the items on a multiple-choice test correctly in order to pass the standard is absolute. When absolute standards are used it is possible for all examinees to pass or for all examinees to fail.

Framework for guiding the standard setting process

The purposes of the assessments that require decisions are quite varied and include selection, student testing, licensure, initial certification or registration, and continuing assessment of competence. In creating a process for setting standards, it is important to give consideration to

1. Who sets the standards
2. The methods they use and
3. The evidence that is collected to support the argument that the cut scores established are credible (Norcini and Shea 1997).

This section will provide an overview of the concerns that govern the selection and implementation of establishing cut off scores.

Who sets the standards?

The characteristics of those chosen to set standards are likely to have the most effect on the credibility and defensibility of the resulting standards (Norcini and Shea 1997). For tests where there is much at stake for the examinees, it is important to have several different standard-setters involved in the process. They must be familiar with the goals or purpose of the assessment and should be knowledgeable in the field (Jaeger 1991). Depending on the aim of the assessment, they would ideally represent a mix of the roles relevant to the discipline (e.g. teachers, clinicians, academics, generalists, specialists). In addition, they would be balanced in terms of personal characteristics such as age, race, and gender. Finally, it is essential to avoid including any standard setters who might have a conflict of interest (e.g. representatives of pharmaceutical companies that have products appearing in the assessment).

What standard setting method is used?

The characteristics of the process of selecting the pass–fail point of an assessment contributes to the evidence of the credibility of the standard and its associated cut score (Norcini and Guille 2002; Norcini and McKinley 2009). The method selected should be easy to explain to those participating in the process and should be supported by research. The process should be designed to meet assessment goals. Those participating should be engaged in thoughtful effort (due diligence). Methods that are based on global judgements and done quickly are not as defensible, but the process should not take many days either. The process should show that considerable effort was made in conceptualization of the standard and determination of the score associated with that standard. What follows is a detailed explanation of these desirable characteristics of the standard setting process.

Based on information

Methods for setting standards can be based entirely on results (e.g. outcomes), entirely on judgements of experts, or on a combination of the two. Because there are not many circumstances when a 'gold standard' is available in medical education, it is rare for assessments of students or professionals to base cut scores solely on empirical results. There are, however, a few exceptions. In the case of admissions testing, outcome data (e.g. successful completion of a course), may be available. Typically, in this situation, relative standards are being used.

Many methods allow a cut score to be based solely on the judgement of experts, without reference to performance data or consequences (e.g. the difficulty of the questions or the pass rate). Some participants in the standard setting process may become uncomfortable when data are presented, thinking that it introduces 'bias' by skewing their judgements in an undesirable way. It should be emphasized that methods for establishing cut scores are not intended to determine 'truth', but to create a plausible decision point based on expert judgement. Decisions that are based on all available information are likely to be more credible. Therefore, processes that permit expert judgement in light of performance data are preferable.

Aligned with assessment goals

The method must produce standards that are consistent with the purpose of the assessment. Methods that produce relative standards are to be used when the purpose is to select a specific number of examinees. Methods that produce absolute standards are to be used when the purpose is to judge competence.

Demonstrates 'due diligence'

Methods that require those participating in the standard setting process to expend thoughtful effort will demonstrate due diligence, and this lends credibility to the final result. A process that is too short is unlikely to be convincing to the stakeholders, and one that is too long will be inefficient and expensive.

Based on research

When the method used to set standards is supported by prior research literature, the results produced will be more credible. Ideally, the research should show that cut scores obtained are reasonable compared to those produced by other methods, are the same when replicated over different groups of judges, are free of potentially biasing effects, and are sensitive to differences in test difficulty and content.

Easily described and executed

The process is enhanced if the method is easy to explain and implement. If the judges' task is too challenging, the likelihood of variability in the results increases. Use of a process that is easily explained and logistically straightforward decreases the amount of training time needed for the judges, allowing more time for fulfilling the 'due diligence' goal described earlier. It is also likely to increase judges' agreement and consistency, ensuring fairness in decisions.

What evidence supports the standard?

In setting standards, the nature and definition of, for example, the 'competent' physician or the 'unsatisfactory' medical student varies with time, place, and many other factors. Therefore, standards on educational tests reflect judgements that are made in the context of a particular assessment, its purpose, and the concerns of society and the profession. Because standards are based on judgements and there is no 'gold standard' to use in determining satisfactory performance or competence, it is not possible to determine whether the 'right' cut point has been set. Instead, collecting evidence which establishes the credibility and defensibility of the cut score is paramount.

The *Standards for Education and Psychological Testing* (American Educational Research Association 1999) provides detailed information on specific criteria to judge the quality of the evidence related to the *consequences of testing* (e.g. are there any benefits associated with the assessment programme such as improvement in patient outcomes). These consequences are typically a direct result of the cut scores established for the assessment programme components. Gathering evidence to support the validity of decisions based on assessment scores is an essential component of judging the quality of an assessment programme.

This view of validity has been shown to rest on a series of assertions and assumptions that support the interpretation of the assessment scores (Kane 2006). The four components of Kane's inferential chain of evidence of validity are labelled *scoring*, *generalization*, *extrapolation*, and *interpretation/decision*. The *interpretation/decision* component of the argument requires evidence to be procured to establish that the theoretical framework required for score interpretation can be supported. Additionally, where decision rules are employed (e.g. pass/fail), evidence to support the procedure, and the efficacy of the ensuing placement or categorization of those being assessed, should be gathered.

The collection of data to provide evidence supporting the interpretations made from scores is an essential part of an assessment programme. Based on interviews with assessment experts, a framework for designing an assessment programme was developed by Dijkstra et al. (2010), and included a component that was labelled 'taking action'. Through the use of multiple assessment instruments, a large amount of data from different sources is made available. When high-stakes decisions are to be made, the use of data from multiple assessments is advisable (American Educational Research Association 1999). Action is taken when interpretation of the data

is made, assigning value to the information collected. The resulting decisions based on the data may vary from pass–fail decisions to provision of feedback and remediation.

Methods for setting standards

There are generally two categories of methods for setting absolute standards: test-centred and examinee-centred (Livingston and Zieky 1982; Jaeger 1989; Hambleton et al. 2000). Test-centred approaches to standard setting require the judges to make decisions based on examination content, while examinee-centred approaches focus judgements on examinee performance. During the 1980s, methods were proposed that combined absolute and relative methods, and these are called compromise methods. This section describes several test-centred, examinee-centred, and compromise methods, along with the strengths and weaknesses of each. Table 36.1 provides an abbreviated description of these approaches to standard setting.

Selection of an approach to set the cut score will be dependent on a number of factors, including the availability of experts capable of providing judgements, test materials, test results, and the time needed to conduct the meeting and to compile the results of the standard setting process. Although there has been extensive research comparing methods, none of the results support the use of one method over another. While it is not possible to identify the 'best' method, there are considerations that should be taken into account when evaluating the process of establishing a cut score. In addition to the factors identified earlier in this chapter (fit for purpose; based on informed judgement; demonstrates due diligence; supported by research; easily understood and implemented) that support the credibility of the standard setting process (Norcini and Shea 1997; Norcini and Guille 2002; Norcini and McKinley 2009), there are a number of other guidelines to be used in appraising the standard setting process and its results. Hambleton (2001) provides a comprehensive list of factors to consider in the overall evaluation of the standard setting process.

Test-centred approaches

Test-centred methods are those in which the actual examination material is used to establish the cut score. These methods have been studied extensively with multiple-choice examinations, and there has been some research conducted with constructed-response and other forms of performance-based assessment. The three approaches that have been most extensively studied in the field of medical education are the Nedelsky (1954), Angoff (1971), and Ebel (1972) methods. It is interesting to note that these investigators were not necessarily studying the establishment of passing scores. In most cases, the methods they used to determine a passing score were secondary to the focus of their efforts, and in fact, the description of the Angoff method was essentially a footnote. Still, these methods provided the basis for further research in setting cut scores.

Nedelsky's method

This method can only be used with multiple-choice items since it is based on assumptions about guessing, and it requires judges to consider incorrect responses (Nedelsky 1954). The task involves review

Table 36.1 Description of standard setting methods

Type	Method	Description
Test-centred	Nedelsky (1954)	Judges asked to identify options that the borderline examinee can eliminate as incorrect.
	Angoff (1971)	Judges asked the percentage of borderline examinees who will select the correct option. Alternately, judges are asked whether the borderline examinee will respond correctly (Y/N).
	Ebel (1972)	Judges' task is to provide ratings of importance as well as difficulty. Within category, judges estimate the percentage of borderline examinees who would respond correctly.
Examinee-centred	Contrasting groups	Using a different measure, examinees are divided into two or more categories and scores on the assessment of interest are compared to determine the degree of overlap. The median score (50% point) within a category (e.g. competent) identifies the cut score. Alternately, panellists can review examinee performance without knowledge of scores, determining whether the performance can be considered passing or failing. The cut score is the intersection of the two score distributions.
	Borderline groups	Experts observe examinees (or review representations of their performance) and determine if this represents failing, clear pass, or borderline performance. The cut score is the median score of the group whose performance is considered 'borderline'.
	Generalized examinee centred (Cohen et al. 1999)	Panellists review samples of examinee performance and provide ratings for two or more points on a rating scale. The ratings are used to generate a regression model where judges' ratings are used predict the cut score.
	Analytic judgement (Plake and Hambleton 2001)	Panellists classify performance for two or more categories. The average score for all performances within a category is the cut score. This approach is typically used to set test level standards.
Compromise methods	Hofstee (1983)	Panellists are asked to identify 1. Lowest acceptable fail rate 2. Highest acceptable fail rate 3. Lowest acceptable cut score 4. Highest acceptable cut score The judgements are averaged across all panellists and graphically compared to the score distribution, and the intersection of the four data points with the score distribution defines the cut score

of test content in order to identify those incorrect options that the borderline test taker would be able to eliminate as incorrect. The approach assumes that the borderline test taker responds by first eliminating those options that are incorrect, reducing the number that need to be considered in selecting a final answer. That is, the approach assumes that the borderline examinee is able to eliminate some of the options, and then guesses at random (Livingston and Zieky 1982).

To compute the passing score, there are two steps. First, for each item, eliminate the incorrect options. Then, the borderline test taker's expected score is calculated as 1 divided by the number of remaining options. For example, if there is a five-choice item, and two options are eliminated, the item score is 1/3, or 0.33. In the second step in the process, these expected scores are summed across all items to generate the cut score for the entire test. The two steps will provide the cut score for one judge. To combine the scores, the test-level scores of individual judges can be averaged. Alternately, the median value of all judges can be calculated; this value will be less affected by extremes (low or high) among the judges.

Maguire et al. (1992) provided an example the application of the Nedelsky method to the Medical Council of Canada's Qualifying Examination, a multiple-choice test. Their rationale was that the task of eliminating options was consistent with clinical reasoning—even the barely passing student would be able to eliminate

dangerous or unwarranted options in multiple-choice items. They proposed using a correction to the item-level estimates, where the correct response is given a weight of 2, and a plausible distractor (one that might be chosen by the borderline student) is given a weight of 1. The item score is 1 divided by the sum of the option weights. They found that for the 57 items that were used in two different examination administrations, the agreement in the cut score was reasonable. They concluded that the use of the Nedelsky procedure with a correction was credible given the stability of the results, and the appropriateness of the approach for the assessment task.

Angoff's method

Angoff (1971) described an approach for setting the passing score in the following manner: the cut-score panellists would read the item and determine whether the minimally competent candidate would choose the correct response. First, it is necessary to define the 'minimally competent candidate'. Then, all test materials are reviewed item-by-item, and judgements are made regarding whether the minimally competent candidate would correctly respond to the item. The count of the items that judges predicted the minimally competent candidate would answer correctly would be the cut score. In a footnote, he acknowledged that it might be difficult for the judges to simply answer whether the minimally competent candidate would choose the correct response. To avoid this potential problem, he suggested that they could think of a number of minimally competent candidates and determine the proportion of those examinees who would answer the item correctly. In this way, they would provide estimates of the probability of the minimally competent candidates choosing the correct response, and the mean of these estimates, across judges and items, would be the cut score.

Over time, this approach has been modified to include participant training using a sample of the test items. Judges are given feedback based on two sets of data: the estimates of their peers and aggregated examinee performance. Typically, discussion ensues, and participants are permitted to change their estimates. Once training is completed, judges are usually asked to complete ratings for each task and examinee independently, and then their ratings are shared and discussed. Following this discussion, judges are free to change their ratings. In standard setting studies using data from performance-based assessments (Norcini et al. 1993), the judges are asked to determine the probability that a minimally competent test taker will adequately manage the task. Averaging across judges to obtain a passing score for each case derives the passing score, and the average across cases is the projected test-level cut score.

Yudkowsky et al. (2008) compared the original Angoff method with a modified version where judges were able to provide a 'maybe' response to the question of whether the borderline examinee would or would not perform the task adequately. The authors wanted to determine the effect of permitting judges to note that the borderline examinee may have a 50–50 chance of performing the task correctly. They found that, for the standardized patient exam used as the focus of the research, about 10% of the checklist items were rated 'maybe', suggesting that judges used the option in a limited fashion and that the 'cognitive complexity' of the standard setting task was reduced (Yudkowsky et al. 2008, p. S15). The authors concluded that the method was a useful alternative to the traditional Angoff, where judges are asked to estimate the percentage of borderline examinees that will correctly perform a task or correctly respond to an item.

In contrast, Jalili et al. (2011) found that the three-level Angoff produced cut scores that were unacceptably high, and the consistency of the judgements was substantially lower when compared to the traditional Angoff (Yes/No) approach. That is, for the objective structured clinical examination (OSCE) that was studied by these authors, the results of the three-level Angoff were more variable. They concluded that although the approach could be considered 'faculty-friendly' (Jalili et al. 2011, p. 1207), the cut scores generated would result in unacceptably high fail rates. This suggests that additional research is warranted to determine the settings in which the use of the original and modified Angoff approaches are appropriate.

Ebel's method

Ebel (1972) proposed that the determination of the passing score should take account of both the relevance of the item content as well as their difficulty. In this method, judges identify the characteristics of the minimally competent examinees and review test content. They then evaluate each item and classify it according to whether the content relevance was essential, important, minimal, or questionable, and whether the item was easy, of medium difficulty,

or hard. When all items are classified, the judges estimate the proportion of the hypothetical minimally competent candidates who would choose the correct responses within each category (i.e., for the easy essential items, the easy important items, and so on).

All three of the test-centred methods presented here have certain elements in common:

- those familiar with the characteristics of a hypothetical borderline examinee are asked to judge test items or content
- the characteristics of a borderline examinee define the standard
- judges are trained in the method selected
- judgements are made individually, and may be discussed to promote consensus and
- judgements are combined to select a cut score.

There is debate about whether it is advisable to provide judges with performance data; some critics assert that introduction of performance data prevents the method from being 'absolute'. However, research has shown that, in the absence of performance data, judges establish cut scores that are unrealistically high (Downing et al. 2006; Clauser et al. 2009). Consequently, for examinations that have already been administered, it is advisable to provide the judges with data that indicates the difficulty of the items. One strategy is to provide the proportion of correct responses (p-value) for all test takers, and the p-value for those in the lowest quintile of total test scores to give some indication of how discriminating the items are. Alternately, it is feasible to have the judges rate the items without knowing the correct answer on the first round but giving them the answers and data during a second round. In this way, it would be similar to having them take the exam themselves, which may affect their perceptions about item difficulty and relevance.

The time involved in conducting a standard setting study with multiple-choice examinations using these methods is considerable. Training, practice, the provision of empirical information, and obtaining revised judgements from subject matter experts can be expensive and logistically complex. The Nedelsky approach could not be used with an assessment that did not present the judges with incorrect options and can only be used with multiple-choice examinations. The Ebel method could involve more than one meeting, since both relevance and difficulty ratings are needed. The Angoff method has been used with standardized patient and OSCE examinations, usually at the case level, and typically with those instruments that assess history-taking and physical examination skills. Downing et al. (2003) provided a comparison of four methods and found that the four approaches they considered produced different cut scores. They concluded that the original method proposed by Angoff (1971) that they called the 'Direct Borderline' method was acceptable, and importantly, easy for medical educators to implement.

One feature that the three test centred approaches have in common is the requirement that judges estimate the percentage of examinees that will select the correct response. The application of test-centred methods to determine cut scores for assessments of performance (e.g. observations, standardized patient examinations) can be taxing. Application of these methods to performance-based assessment can take considerably longer, making it more difficult to recruit and retain expert judges for the process. Open-ended item formats are not as amenable to this judgement task since the 'correct' response can be obtained in a number of different ways. Further, the judges' task of selecting the correct response and eliminating distractors bears little resemblance to the task of determining the percentage of examinees that would display competent performance. In a study that required panellists to provide expected scores on three dimensions used to score each task (Hambleton and Plake 1995), the authors indicated that panellists applying Angoff's method to a performance-based assessment wanted to develop a policy for which a specified number of tasks needed to be passed in order to pass the examination overall. The panellists also thought that the method forced the separation of the assessment into isolated parts. They preferred to see performance across examinees by task in order to see patterns of performance across the dimensions measured. This suggests that panellists prefer review of performance at the task level, rather than at the scoring criteria within task level.

Another challenging aspect of performance-based assessment is that relatively few tasks can be presented, because testing time is limited. Examinee performance can vary greatly from task to task. Because fewer tasks can be presented to examinees in a reasonable time, task specificity is often a concern in performance-based assessment (Haertel and Linn 1996). Task specificity can reduce the consistency in examinee scores and can reduce the generalizability of results (Traub 1994). The matter of task specificity requires that quite a number of tasks be reviewed in order for the passing score to generalize to the construct of interest. When planning the standard setting process, it is important to ensure that the performances selected for review are representative of the full range of scores, and the tasks are representative of those defining the content area being measured.

Despite these issues (task specificity and the nature of the judgement task), the Angoff method is frequently modified for use with performance-based assessments (Dauphinee and Blackmore 1994; Morrison et al. 1996; Norcini et al. 1993). For some performance-based measures (e.g. communication skills), other methods may be more appropriate. Application of these methods to performance-based assessment can take considerably longer, making it more difficult to recruit and retain expert judges for the process. In the next section of the chapter, we provide an overview of alternate methods where judgements are made about test takers, rather than test content.

Examinee-centred approaches

There are methods that have been used with both multiple choice questions and performance-based assessments that focus on the review of examinee performance. As with test-centred approaches, these methods also require the specification of knowledge and skills that typify competent (and incompetent) performance. Examinee-centred approaches include the contrasting groups method (Livingston and Zieky 1982), the borderline group method (Livingston and Zieky 1982), the generalized examinee-centred method (Cohen et al. 1999), the examinee paper selection method, the holistic or booklet method, the analytic judgment method, the dominant profile method, the judgemental policy capturing method, and the direct judgement method (Hambleton et al. 2000). The focus of this chapter is on examinee-centred methods more commonly used in medical education; a more thorough overview appears in Hambleton et al. (2000). In the next section, a description of the contrasting groups, borderline groups, generalized

examinee-centred methods, and analytic judgment methods will be presented.

Contrasting groups method

The contrasting groups method requires panellists to review examinee work and classify the entire performance of an examinee as acceptable or unacceptable (Livingston and Zieky 1982). Traditionally, information external to the test is used to classify the examinees in these categories (Hambleton et al. 2000). Scores from the test on which performance standards are being established are then used to generate distributions (one for each category), and the distributions are compared to determine their degree of overlap. This is done by tabulating the percentage of test takers in each category and at each score level who are considered 'competent'. The passing score is the point at which about 50% of the test takers are considered competent. This method can be challenging to use when there is no external measure that predefines the groups.

One variation of this method is to have the panellists judge the performance of examinees on the test of interest without knowledge of their test scores (Clauser and Clyman 1994). Panellists are asked to review samples of examinee performance and determine whether the sample is indicative of passing or failing performance. The cut score is then identified as the intersection of the two score distributions based on whether the performance was judged as passing or failing. Another variation is to regress the number of judges rating the performance as competent to the test scores, and set the passing score at the point at which 50% of the panellists rated the performance as competent (Burrows et al. 1999).

In an innovative approach, Shea et al. (2009) applied the method to teacher evaluations. In this study, the panellists were familiar with teaching responsibilities and qualities needed for promotion and appointment. Students provided web-based feedback and reports were available for faculty members by department, faculty rank, and setting (i.e. classroom or clinical). The judges' task was to sort dossiers of teacher performance into four groups: 'superior', 'excellent', 'satisfactory', and 'unsatisfactory'. Cut scores for each category were established by calculating the means of all judges, and identifying the mean between the average scores of two adjacent groups. For example, if the average score for 'superior' dossiers was 85% and the average score for 'excellent' dossiers was 80%, the cut score for the 'superior' category would be 82.5%. The authors found that the results were reproducible, the standards were consistent with expectations, and that the information produced was useful for identifying faculty eligible for promotion, as well as those in need of remediation.

Borderline group method

The borderline group method requires the identification of the characteristics (e.g. knowledge, skills, and abilities) of the 'borderline' examinee just as in the test-centred approaches. The 'borderline' examinee is one whose knowledge and skills are not quite adequate, but are not inadequate (Livingston and Zieky 1982). Actual examinee performances are categorized by panellists as clear fail, borderline, or clear pass. The passing score is then set at the median (i.e. 50th percentile) score of the borderline group (e.g. Rothman and Cohen 1996). Research supports the credibility and applicability of this method, particularly to performance-based tests of clinical skills (e.g. Rothman et al. 1996), but it requires that experts rate performance as the test is administered, or that video recording of the test occurs. A large number of examinees should be included in the administration to reduce the statistical error associated with the cut score. That is, for smaller samples, the variation in judgement of what constitutes failing performance is likely to be larger, increasing the error associated with the cut score. When smaller groups of examinees are tested, other approaches may be more useful, and result in the generation of more credible cut scores.

Generalized examinee-centred method

In this method, proposed by Cohen et al. (1999), samples of examinee responses are evaluated by panellists using a rating scale. Ratings can have as few as two categories (e.g. adequate vs. inadequate) or several categories (e.g. minimal, partially proficient, proficient, advanced). The rating scale is associated with the categories needed for the particular assessment. The judgements and test scores are used to 'develop a functional relation (linear or nonlinear) between the rating scale and the test score scale' (Cohen et al. 1999, p. 347). The authors argue that this approach 'seeks to make examinee-centred standard setting more efficient by using all the ratings to set each cut score' (Cohen et al. 1999, p. 347). When compared to the contrasting groups and borderline group methods, the sample rated represents the full range of scores from the test of interest. Another advantage to this approach is that it is not dependent on another criterion measure to identify the groups. The authors also assert that this method does not require the large samples needed by the contrasting groups and borderline methods. Since all rated performances are included in the estimation of the cut score, smaller samples can be drawn for rating, providing that they are representative of the range of test scores.

A similar approach that has the advantage of using all examinee scores is the borderline regression method. In this method, checklist scores are regressed on the global ratings made by examiners in the administration of the test (Wood et al. 2006). This approach has the advantage of using ratings for all examinees. The midpoint of the rating scale is used to predict the cut score for each station and then averaged to derive the test standard. A similar approach that has been studied involved having judges rate each performance as 'adequate' or 'inadequate'. A regression analysis is used to identify the station score at which 50% of the judges rated the performance as adequate and 50% rated the performance as inadequate (McKinley et al. 2005). These approaches will require the use of statistical software to derive the passing score based on the panellists' (or examiners') judgements. Another potential issue with this approach is that it is based on the relationship between panellists' judgements and test scores. To the extent that a linear (or nonlinear) relationship exists, passing scores can be derived. If the variance in panellists' judgement cannot be attributed to the assessment task, the error associated with the resulting cut score will be high, and would suggest deficiencies in the process (e.g. definition of the standard or task content).

Analytic judgement method

Plake and Hambleton (2001) described the use of an approach that establishes the cut score based on panellists' classifications of samples of examinees' performance. Examinees' performance samples representing the entire range of scores are provided for each task in the assessment. Panellists are not aware of examinee scores. In their study, seven classifications were made:

> Labels on the classification scale identify locations on the performance scale, such as below basic, basic, proficient, and advanced; and then each of these categories can be further divided into low, middle, and high, for example

> Plake and Hambleton 2001, p. 290.

This method is especially useful when the assessment consists of more than one component (e.g. history-taking, physical examination, and communication skills). Each component of the assessment is independently rated. Following initial ratings, panellists discuss their ratings, and wide discrepancies amongst panellists are identified. The purpose of the discussion is to allow panellists to provide their rationale, since there may be elements of an examinee's response that were overlooked by the other panellists. The cutoff score for a performance category is the average score of the performances within that classification:

> For example, for setting a proficient standard, all of the papers classified high basic and low proficient are used in calculating the average score. This average score is used as the performance standard

> (Plake and Hambleton 2001, p.290.

The authors note that results of field trials employing this method are promising. The panellists (and policymakers) were satisfied with the approach because it relied on the judgements of experts (in this case, classroom teachers and school administrators) reviewing actual student performance. They noted that disadvantages of the approach included the large number of performance samples needed for the process as well as the logistics involved in selecting and managing all of the samples required.

A similar approach was used by Ross et al. (1996) in research on standard setting with a standardized patient examination. Once the judges in the study provided ratings for each case, they were asked to make test-level decisions for each examinee based on the performance samples they had reviewed. The consistency of the ratings based on the results of generalizability analyses and level of agreement based on calculation of kappa coefficients suggested that the judges were capable of performing the task consistently. In addition, the authors were able to determine that judges used a compensatory model in setting test level standards. That is, poor performance on one task could be offset by better performance on another task. This finding can be of considerable importance when scores on tasks are averaged to produce a total test score.

The examinee-centred methods presented here have the advantage of asking panellists to rate actual examinee performance. Rather than imagining the hypothetical examinee who embodies the description of the standard, panellists make judgements about actual performances. This holistic approach to setting cut scores for performance-based assessments closely parallels the scoring task. However, it can be logistically challenging to ensure that there is adequate sampling of tasks and examinee performances.

Whether the cut score is established using a test-centred or an examinee-centred method, additional information is sometimes used to support the judgements made and to determine the final cut score(s). Compromise methods were developed to explicitly combine the use of test results (failure rate) and test content. These methods can be used to set passing scores or to adjust them once the panellists have provided their judgements (Cizek 1996). The next section of the chapter presents two compromise methods for establishing passing scores.

Compromise methods

Although results from the standard setting panellists are the most important elements in determining the cut score, additional information is often used to determine the final cut score that will be applied to examinations (Geisinger 1991; Geisinger and McCormick 2010). One type of information that is considered is the pass–fail rate for the cut score. The compromise approaches proposed by Hofstee (1983), Beuk (1984), and De Gruijter (1985) explicitly ask the panellists to consider both the cut score and the passing (or failing) rate. Each approach assumes that the judges have an opinion about what constitutes an 'acceptable' cut score and passing rate.

Hofstee suggested that the chosen cut score was only one out of a universe of possible cut scores. In addition, it is feasible to plot all possible failure rates. To ensure that panellists have considered these data, the standard that is being set (e.g. minimal competence or proficiency) is discussed, the details of the examination process are reviewed, and the panellists are asked to answer four questions:

1. What is the *lowest* acceptable percentage of students who fail the examination? (Minimum fail rate; f_{min}).

2. What is the *highest* acceptable percentage of students who fail the examination? (Maximum fail rate; f_{max}).

3. What is the *lowest* acceptable percent correct score that would be considered passing? (Minimum cut score; k_{min}).

4. What is the *highest* acceptable percent correct score that would be considered passing? (Maximum cut score; k_{max}).

The four data points are calculated by averaging across all judges. The percentage of examinees that would pass for every possible value of the cut score on the test is graphed and the four data points are plotted, based on the four judgements of the standard setting panel. Figure 36.1 provides an example of application of the Hofstee method. In this example, 140 students took a 50-item end of year test. The curve in the chart shows the projected failure rate based on percent correct scores on the test. Instructors were asked the four questions listed earlier:

1. What is the *lowest* acceptable percentage of students who fail the examination? Average: 20%

2. What is the *highest* acceptable percentage of students who fail the examination? Average: 30%

3. What is the *lowest* acceptable percent correct score that would be considered passing? Average: 60%

4. What is the *highest* acceptable percent correct score that would be considered passing? Average: 75%

Using the information from the judges, two points are plotted: the intersection of the lowest acceptable fail rate and the highest acceptable percentage correct score; and the intersection of the highest acceptable fail rate and the lowest acceptable percentage correct score (see fig. 36.1). These two points create a line that intersects the curve that is defined by percentage correct score and projected failure rate. The passing score is found by following the dotted line from the intersection to the x-axis (percentage correct scores). The fail rate is found by following the dotted line from the intersection to the y-axis (percentage fail).

In a modification of Hoffstee's method, Beuk (1984) suggested that the panellists report to what extent each of their judgements should be considered in deriving the final cut score (fig. 36.2). That is, panellists are asked the degree to which their decisions are examinee-oriented or test-oriented. The means and standard deviations of both the cut scores and acceptable pass rates are computed. The mean passing rate and mean cut score are plotted. The point on the chart where these two points intersect is identified. The compromise consists of using the ratio of the standard deviation

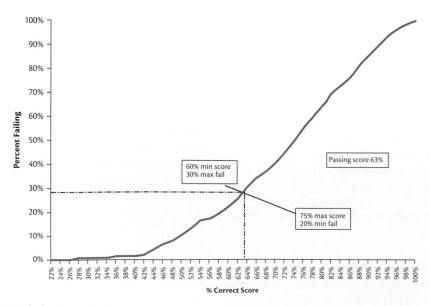

Figure 36.1 Example of Hofstee standard setting method

of pass rate to the standard deviation of cut score. The point where the distribution of scores intersects the line generated based on the slope constitutes the cut score. De Gruijter (1985) further suggested that an additional question be posed to panellists, that of the level of uncertainty regarding these two judgements. Beuk's and De Gruijter's methods have not been reported in the literature for medical education, but the Hofstee method has been used by a number of researchers.

Schindler et al. (2007) reported on the 'successful' use of the Hofstee approach to set cut scores for a surgery clerkship. Because the goal was to set a cut score for the clerkship as a whole instead of individual assessments (multiple-choice examinations, OSCE, clerkship grades, ratings of professionalism) the standard setting panel determined that the use of the Hofstee was appropriate. The use of multiple, related assessments led the group to conclude that compensatory standards would be set, although a breech in professionalism could result in failing. Panellists reviewed score distributions for all students as well as those who had failed in previous years, along with scoring rubrics and examination materials, before they responded to the four questions in the Hofstee method. The authors found that there was a high level of agreement amongst the judges, and that the pass rate derived was reasonable when applied to previous clerkship data.

Implementing and evaluating the methods

There are several considerations in selecting judges for participation in the standard setting process. The first is to ensure adequate representation of stakeholder groups to the extent possible. In medical education, when evaluation of clinical knowledge is the focus, panels typically consist of both practicing physicians and physician educators. This approach ensures that the judges can be considered experts in the content area involved and are familiar with the demands that are typical of those being assessed (Jaeger 1991).

Second, the number of judges empanelled also supports conclusions regarding the representativeness of panel members. If the number of judges is large enough, they can be split into groups, permitting an analysis of the generalizability of results and review

of examination materials or examinee performances (Hambleton 2001). Whenever possible, dividing the panellists into subgroups allows the comparison of the cut scores derived, and a check for consistency in the judgements across groups. Determining the error associated with the judgements is an essential part of the process (American Educational Research Association 1999; Geisinger and McCormick 2010). Collection of information about the qualifications and characteristics of the panellists is necessary to provide evidence of their expertise and to show that key stakeholders had a role in the process.

Training the judges in the method to be used is crucial (Kane 1998a; Hambleton 2001; Raymond and Reid 2001). Training typically consists of discussions of the performance standard and purpose of the assessment, and an orientation to the method selected. Often, the panellists take the test, or some portion of it, themselves. The quality of the training has been shown to relate to the stability of the cut score (Norcini and Shea 1992). The standard setting study should be evaluated by panellists over the course of the process. That is, the judges should provide feedback to facilitators regarding their understanding of the performance standard identified and their confidence in the result of the process. To help anticipate any problems in training or in time and resource allocation (e.g. space for materials, development of a data collection tool), a pilot study of the process should be conducted. Having a field trial will ensure that problems can be anticipated, and that a realistic estimate of the time needed can be obtained.

A detailed description of the process provides evidence of the appropriateness of the performance standard and the method used to derive the cut score. Information on participant training and a clear description of performance categories (standards) should be included in the description. When feasible, data provided to the participants as part of deriving the cut score should include information on the consequences or impact on test takers.

Finally, evidence of the effect of the performance standard should be collected. Such evidence includes information on the procedure, consistency of the judgements, feedback provided by the panellists, and comparison to other measures of similar knowledge and skills. An approach that has been used to validate the cut

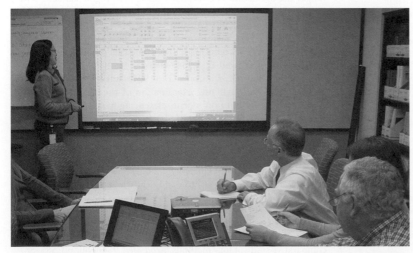

Figure 36.2 Setting the standard

scores generated by standard setting studies has been applied by a number of researchers (Sireci 1995; Sireci et al. 1997; Violato et al. 2003). Violato et al. (2003) compared the results of cluster analysis to established cut scores for a multiple-choice test that was derived using the Nedelsky method, and a performance-based assessment, where the Ebel approach was used to set the cut score. They found that the results of the cluster analysis provided support for the methods that had been used on a certification examination in optometry, and that the results of the statistical analysis were more consistent with the results based on the Ebel method. Because cluster analysis can be used to statistically identify two or more groups based on test results, their research is an example of the collection of empirical evidence of the validity of the resulting cut scores. Table 36.2 provides a brief summary of guidelines for evaluating the standard setting process.

Establishing performance standards has a long history in education and licensure. The comparison of methods, the effect of various factors on the resulting cut scores, and innovative uses of standard setting approaches have all been presented in the literature. The choice of method should be related to the purpose and content of the assessment. No research has identified one method as superior in all cases (Livingston and Zieky 1982; Downing et al. 2006). Guidelines have been provided to assist in the selection of a method and the evaluation of the process. It is important to keep in mind that standard setting consists of judgements made in a particular context, and that there is no 'right' answer to be obtained. Rather, careful consideration of the factors involved in establishing cut scores is paramount in the process. This could include deliberation on whether standards should be compensatory, the effect of use of the examination and cut scores over time (test and cut score equating), how changes in the profession affect the interpretation of the results, and what can be done with those who do not pass the assessment.

Conclusions

♦ Standard setting is the process of translating a description of the characteristics denoting the desired level performance into a number that applies to a particular test.

♦ Selection of a standard setting method is dependent on the goals and stakes associated with the assessment.

♦ Because the cut score is based on judgement, it can be categorized as arbitrary; however, judgements need not be capricious.

♦ A successful standard setting process is based on information, aligned with assessment goals, demonstrates due diligence, is based on research, is easily described and executed.

♦ There are a variety of methods that meet these criteria, and these generally fall into two categories: test-centred and examinee-centred.

References

American Educational Research Association (1999) *Standards for Educational and Psychological Testing*. Washington DC: American Educational Research Association

Angoff, W.H. (1971) Scales, norms, and equivalent scores. In: R.L. Thorndike (ed.) *Educational Measurement* (pp. 508–600). Washington, DC: American Council on Education

Beuk, C.H. (1984) A Method for Reaching a Compromise Between Absolute and Relative Standards in Examinations. *J Educ Measurement*. 21(2): 147–152

Burrows, P.J., Bingham, L., and Brailovsky, C.A. (1999) A modified contrasting groups method used for setting the passmark in a small scale standardised patient examination. *Adv Health Sci Educ: Theory Pract*. 4(2): 145–154

Cizek, G.J. (1996) Setting passing scores. *Educ Measurement: Issues Pract*. 15(2): 20–31

Clauser, B.E. and Clyman, S.G. (1994) A contrasting-groups approach to standard setting for performance assessments of clinical skills. *Acad Med*. 69(10 Suppl): S42–S44

Clauser, B.E., Mee, J., Baldwin, S.G., Margolis, M.J., and Dillon, G.F. (2009) Judges' use of examinee performance data in an Angoff standard-setting exercise for a medical licensing examination: an experimental study. *J Educ Measurement*. 46(4): 390–407

Cohen, A.S., Kane, Michael T., and Crooks, T.J. (1999) A generalized examinee-centred method for setting standards on achievement tests. *Appl Measurement Educ*. 12(4): 343–366

Dauphinee, W.D. and Blackmore, D.E. (1994) Setting minimal passing standards for the qualifying examination of the Medical Council of Canada: the transition from norm-referencing to criterion-referencing. In A.I. Rothman and R. Cohen (eds) *Proceedings of the Sixth Ottawa Conference on Medical Education* (pp. 245–247). Toronto: University of Toronto Bookstore

De Gruijter, D.N.M. (1985) Compromise Models for Establishing Examination Standards. *J Educ Measurement*. 22(4): 263–269

Dijkstra, J., Van der Vleuten, C.P.M., and Schuwirth, L.W.T. (2010) A new framework for designing programmes of assessment. *Adv Health Sci Educ*, 15(3): 379–393

Downing, S.M., Lieska, N.G., and Raible, M.D. (2003) Establishing passing standards for classroom achievement tests in medical education: a comparative study of four methods. *Acad Med*. 78(10 Suppl): S85–S87

Table 36.2 Guidelines for evaluating the standard setting process

Based on information	Assessment purpose and type(s) of instruments used are essential elements of information provided to panellists.
	Provide data to the participants regarding the consequences of the process and cut score derived.
Aligned with assessment goals	Consistency in the definition of the performance standard and the goals of the assessment programme is necessary. The selection of a method to determine the cut score should be directly related to assessment goals: selection of a predefined number of examinees requires use of relative standards; operationalizing a conceptual standard (e.g. 'excellence') dictates use of absolute standards.
Demonstrates due diligence	Training of participants is essential. Sufficient time is needed to practise the method, including reaching consensus on the definition of the standard. Careful deliberation by panellists ensures that, although arbitrary, judgements are not capricious.
Based on research	Methods that have been reported in the literature should be used, and if revised, pilot testing of the modified method should be conducted.
Easily described and executed	Judges should thoroughly understand the task. Feedback should be solicited to evaluate their understanding and confidence in the process. A detailed description of the procedures should be provided, along with results of the process.

Downing, S.M., Tekian, A., and Yudkowsky, R. (2006) Procedures for establishing defensible absolute passing scores on performance examinations in health professions education. *Teach Learn Med.* 18(1): 50–57

Ebel, R. (1972) *Essentials of Educational Measurement.* 2nd edn. Englewood Cliffs NJ: Prentice-Hall

Geisinger, K.F. (1991) Using standard-setting data to establish cutoff scores. *Educ Measurement Issues Pract.* 10(2): 17–22

Geisinger, K.F. and McCormick, C.M. (2010) Adopting cut scores: post-standard-setting panel considerations for decision makers. *Educ Measurement Issues Pract.* 29(1): 38–44

Haertel, E. and Linn, R. (1996) Comparability. In G. W. Phillips (ed.) *Technical Issues in Large-Scale Performance Assessment* (pp. 59–78). Washington, DC: National Center for Education Statistics, US Department of Education

Hambleton, R.K. (2001) Setting performance standards on educational assessments and criteria for evaluating the process. In G. Cizek (ed.) *Setting Performance Standards: Concepts, Methods, and Perspectives* (pp. 89–116). Mahwah NJ: Lawrence Erlbaum Associates

Hambleton, R.K., Jaeger, R.M., Plake, B.S., and Mills, C. (2000) Setting performance standards on complex educational assessments. *Appl Psychol Measurement.* 24(4): 355–366

Hambleton, R.K. and Plake, B.S. (1995) Using an extended Angoff procedure to set standards on complex performance assessments. *Appl Measurement Educ.* 8(1): 41–55

Hofstee, W.K.B. (1983) The case for compromise in educational selection and grading. In S.B. Anderson and J.S. Helmick (eds.), *On Educational Testing* (pp. 109–127). San Francisco: Jossey-Bass

Jaeger, R.M. (1989) Certification of student competence. In R.L. Linn (ed.) *Educational Measurement* (pp. 485–514). New York: American Council on Education and Macmillan

Jaeger, R.M. (1991) Selection of judges for standard-setting. *Educ Measurement Issues Pract.* 10(2): 3–14

Jalili, M., Hejri, S.M., and Norcini, J.J. (2011) Comparison of two methods of standard setting: the performance of the three-level Angoff method. *Med Educ.* 45(12): 1199–1208

Kane, M.T. (1998a) Choosing between examinee-centered and test-centered standard-setting methods. *Educ Assess.* 5(3): 129–145

Kane, M.T. (1998b) Criterion bias in examinee-centered standard setting: some thought experiments. *Educ Measurement Issues Pract.* 17(1): 23–30

Kane, M.T. (2006) Validation. In R.L. Brennan (ed.) *Educational Measurement* (pp. 17–64). Westport CT: American Council on Education and Praeger

Livingston, S.A. and Zieky, M.J. (1982) *Passing Scores: A manual for setting standards of perfromance on education and occupational tests.* Princeton, NJ: Educational Testing Service

Maguire, T., Skakun, E., and Harley, C. (1992) Setting standards for multiple-choice items in clinical reasoning. *Eval Health Prof.* 15(4): 434–452

McKinley, D.W., Boulet, J.R., and Hambleton, R.K. (2005) A work-centred approach for setting passing scores on performance-based assessments. *Eval Health Prof.* 28(3): 349–369

Morrison, H. McNally, H., Wylie, C., McFaul, P., and Thompson, W. (1996) The passing score in the objective structured clinical examination. *Med Educ.* 30(5): 345–348

Nedelsky, L. (1954) Absolute grading standards for objective tests. *Educ Psychol Measurement.* 14(1): 3–19

Norcini, J.J. (1994) Research on standards for professional licensure and certification examinations. *Eval Health Prof.* 17(2): 160–177

Norcini, J.J. and Guille, R. (2002) Combining tests and setting standards. In G.R. Norman, C.P.M. Van der Vleuten, and D.T. Newble (eds) *International Handbook of Research in Medical Education* (part

two, (pp. 811–834). Kluwer International Handbooks of Education. Dordrecht, the Netherlands: Kluwer Academic Publishers

Norcini, J.J. and McKinley, D.W. (2009) Standard setting. In J.A. Dent and R.M. Harden (eds) *A Practical Guide for Medical Teachers* (pp. 311–317). Edinburgh; New York: Elsevier Churchill Livingstone

Norcini, J.J. and Shea, J.A. (1992) The reproducibility of standards over groups and occasions. *Appl Measurement Educ.* 5(1): 63–72

Norcini, J.J. and Shea, J.A. (1997) The credibility and comparability of standards. *Appl Measurement Educ.* 10(1): 39–59

Norcini, J.J. Stillman, P.L., Sutnick, A.I., et al. (1993) Scoring and standard setting with standardized patients. *Eval Health Prof.* 16(3): 322–332

Plake, B.S. and Hambleton, R.K. (2001) The analytic judgement method for setting standards on complex performance assessments. In G. Cizek (ed.) *Setting Performance Standards: Concepts, Methods, and Perspectives* (pp. 283 312). Mahwah N.J.: Lawrence Erlbaum Associates

Raymond, M.R. and Reid, J. (2001) Who made thee a judge? Selecting and training participants for standard setting. In G. J. Cizek (ed.) *Setting Performance Standards: Concepts, Methods, and Perspectives* (pp. 119–158). Mahwah NJ: Lawrence Erlbaum Associates

Ross, L.P. Clauser, B.E., Margolis, M.J., Orr, N.A., and Klass, D.J. (1996) An expert-judgment approach to setting standards for a standardized-patient examination. *Acad Med.* 71(10 Suppl): S4–S6

Rothman, A.I., Blackmore, D., Cohen, R., and Reznick, R. (1996) The consistency and uncertainty in examiners' definitions of pass/fail performance on OSCE stations. *Eval Health Prof.* 19(1): 118–124

Rothman, A.I. and Cohen R. (1996) A comparison of empirically- and rationally-defined standards for clinical skills checklists. *Acad Med.* 71(10 Suppl): S1–S3

Schindler, N., Corcoran, J., and DaRosa, D. (2007) Description and impact of using a standard-setting method for determining pass/fail scores in a surgery clerkship. *Am J Surg.* 193(2): 252–257

Shea, J.A. Bellini, L.M., McOwen, K., and Norcini, J.J. (2009) Setting standards for teaching evaluation data: an application of the contrasting groups method. *Teach Learn Med.* 21(2): 82–86

Shepard, L. (1980) Standard setting issues and methods. *Appl Psychol Measurement.* 4(4): 447–467

Sireci, S.G. (1995) *Using Cluster Analysis to Solve the Problem of Standard Setting.* New York: US Department of Education, Educational Resources Information Center (ERIC): ERIC Documents (ED395991)

Sireci, S.G., Robin, F., and Patelis, T. (1997) *Using Cluster Analysis to Facilitate the Standard Setting Process.* Chicago IL: Educational Resources Information Center (ERIC) (ED414292)

Traub, R.E. (1994) Facing the challenge of multidimensionality in performance assessment. In A.I. Rothman and R. Cohen (eds) *Proceedings of the Sixth Annual Ottawa Conference on Medical Education* (pp. 9–11). Toronto: University of Toronto Bookstore

Violato, C., Marini, A., and Lee, C. (2003) A validity study of expert judgment procedures for setting cutoff scores on high-stakes credentialing examinations using cluster analysis. *Eval Health Prof.* 26(1): 59–72

Wood, T.J., Humphrey-Murto, S.M., and Norman, G.R. (2006) Standard setting in a small scale OSCE: a comparison of the modified borderline-group method and the borderline regression method. *Adv Health Sci Educ.* 11(2): 115–122

Yudkowsky, R., Downing, S.M., and Popescu, M. (2008) Setting standards for performance tests: a pilot study of a three-level Angoff method. *Acad Med.* 83(10 Suppl): S13–S16

Zieky, M.J. (2001) So much has changed: how the setting of cutscores has evolved since the 1980s. In: G. Cizek (ed.) *Setting Performance Standards: Concepts, Methods, and Perspectives* (pp. 19–52). Mahwah NJ: Lawrence Erlbaum Associates

CHAPTER 37

Choosing instruments for assessment

Sean McAleer and Madawa Chandratilake

No single examination format will guarantee acceptability, feasibility, validity, and reliability, but care in identifying the strengths and weaknesses of each approach and clear objectives for the assessment should help staff select a useful range of tests.

Stella Lowry

Introduction

The professional abilities desired of a doctor are multiple and diverse. As there is no single magical assessment instrument to assess them all, several assessment instruments—i.e. an assessment toolkit, are used to assess students or trainees in every medical education programme. The fundamental step in selecting instruments is defining the purpose of assessment. No assessment instrument is 100% appropriate or inappropriate for a given purpose. Rather, certain instruments are stronger contenders than others in comprehensive attainment of the purpose concerned. Several educational, formal, and moral obligations should be considered in setting up the purposes of assessment.

Although the ultimate goal of every assessment is the provision of feedback for further learning, traditionally, the assessments are dichotomously defined as to: provide feedback (formative), and make pass/fail decisions (summative) (Epstein 2007). Traditionally, there has been more emphasis on the latter—i.e. assessment *of* learning (Lynch et al. 2004). However, there is a growing emphasis towards assessment *for* learning—i.e. where the main purpose of an assessment is to provide feedback for future learning and development (Lynch et al. 2004). Criterion-based summative assessments are essential to ensure the social accountability of the medical profession. Similarly, students should be given meaningful feedback on their abilities and actions. Although the primary goal of each assessment instrument may be either formative or summative the overall toolkit of assessment instruments should consider both aspects.

Until recently, the assessments in medical education have focused primarily on medical knowledge, practical skills, and clinical skills. Professionalism has been an opportunistic and implicit component of such assessments, which has had minimal impact on pass/fail decisions (Arnold 2002; Ginsburg et al. 2000). With enhanced emphasis on the social accountability of medicine, patients must be convinced that doctors are both safe and professional (Boelen and Woollard 2009). Therefore, fitness to practise medicine is defined as clinical competence, lack of impairments, and professionalism (Parker 2006). The toolkit should, therefore, contain instruments to cover all these outcomes.

It is widely acknowledge that 'assessment drives learning', especially at undergraduate and postgraduate levels (Epstein 2007). Therefore, the instrument chosen should emphasize the educationally desirable direction that teachers expect their students to follow. For example, if more time is allocated for learning clinical skills in wards, and students are assessed on knowledge using a multiple choice question (MCQ) examination, then they will be more likely to use the library than practice their clinical skills. Conversely, they will learn clinical skills by spending more time on the wards, if they are assessed using an objective structured clinical examination (OSCE). Therefore, the assessments should reflect the educationally desirable direction expressed in the curriculum outcomes.

Once the purpose(s) of the assessment is determined, the array of instruments available should be evaluated to select the most appropriate.

Selecting the instruments

What, why, how, where, who, and *when* are important questions to address when choosing your assessment instruments. The first three are key questions and should be answered sequentially. *What* determines the outcomes and competencies; the *why* should set the purpose (e.g. formative, summative or both); the *how* depends on both *what* and *why*, and helps determine the assessment methods (written, practical or both). These three important questions influence the latter three: *where* (the assessment setting), *who* (the assessors, e.g. teachers, peers, or patients), and *when* (the timing, e.g. during or at the end of the course).

The framework for assessing clinical ability introduced by Miller (1990) is widely used as a means to discuss different assessment instruments meaningfully. In his framework the *know* and *knows how* levels represent the knowledge domain. At the *knows* level, the assessments focus on lower-order thinking (i.e. the ability to memorize and comprehend), while at the *knows how* level the focus is on higher-order thinking (i.e. thinking skills such as problem-solving). Usually, these levels of ability are assessed away from patients in an examination hall or computer suite environment. At the *shows how* level, competence—i.e. the demonstration of the capacity to do—is assessed. The assessment usually takes place in simulated environments (e.g. clinical skills centres) using simulated materials (e.g. manikins and simulated patients). At the *does* level the performance of the candidate is assessed in authentic settings like the workplace—with the involvement of actual patients. This outline of how to use different assessment instruments assumes that they are used as they should be. The quality of the assessment items will determine the ultimate level assessed by each instrument (e.g. a poorly developed OSCE station may merely assess knowledge rather than competence).

Assessment of cognitive ability

Cognitive ability is assessed using written and oral instruments. In written assessment instruments, the candidates are expected to either construct their responses: e.g. essays, modified essays, short answer questions, or select a response from a given list of options (e.g. multiple choice questions).

Constructed response questions

The essay

'Like the novel, the essay is a literary device for saying almost everything about almost anything' (Huxley 1959, preface). In terms of its use as an assessment tool this quote is damning indeed. The essay is a form of written assessment that is longevity personified. It has been used to assess knowledge, but has been shown to have a number of disadvantages that in most contexts largely outweigh the pluses. It is now rarely used in medical schools for, while it is easy to set, it is time consuming to mark. It is also difficult to be consistent in scoring. For example it is not uncommon for two markers to give vastly different scores to the same essay. Unless you can demonstrate adequate reliability it is best to avoid using essays (Schuwirth and van der Vleuten 2003). Many essay-type exams use double markers. One way of testing for reliability is to see how well the scores given by each marker agree. There is also the problem relating to adequate sampling. If you have a broad range of learning outcomes then you will need to set several essay titles to ensure representative sampling.

When, if ever, should we consider using the essay as a method of assessment? There are a variety of situations that favour the essay. For instance, if only a few students are being assessed then the time factor becomes less of a problem; or if the learning outcomes focus on written expression and organizational skills then the essay may be considered (Ebel 1972). They can also be useful for exploring attitudes to certain topics such as euthanasia. However, the bottom line is to check whether you can measure your learning outcomes better through more objective written tests, if not then the essay may be an option.

If you do decide on using the essay then consider the following:

- Make sure that the question clearly defines what is required of the student.
- Do not allow for a choice of essay—i.e. make it clear that all essay questions must be answered.
- To help increase inter-rater reliability develop a scoring grid based on the ideal answer.
- Have a clear policy on how to deal with irrelevant material and make this known to the students. This will prevent them writing everything they know about the topic.
- Do not use the essay to assess factual recall—this can be achieved best through other tests.

The modified essay

The modified essay question (MEQ) became quite popular in the 1980s in both undergraduate and postgraduate medical education (Feletti and Smith 1986; Rabinowitz 1987). It has its basis in situations that occur in clinical practice and it aims to test problem solving and clinical decision making. The usual type of MEQ involves about 8 to 10 short essay questions—responses may vary from 50 to 200 words per question. A case scenario is presented followed by a related question. The paper is basically a number of open-ended questions following a developing clinical situation. To construct such an exam one would look (as always) at the learning outcomes and develop linked scenarios related to these outcomes. The full set of questions should then be reviewed by your colleagues and a comprehensive answer to each agreed upon. This procedure will allow for clear marking schedules ensuring better reliability than the longer essay question. An example of the layout for a MEQ based around general practice is shown in box 37.1.

Obviously the scenarios would be more detailed and the questions more specific but you can see how one could cover quite a few issues using 10 or 12 questions. MEQs can also be used as an aid to learning (e.g. as an additional resource for a lecture or a catalyst for small group discussion).

Criticism has been levelled at their inability to target the assessment of higher cognitive skills (Palmer and Devitt 2006) and there is some evidence to suggest that carefully constructed MCQs are better able to assess higher cognitive levels than MEQs (Khan and Aljarallah 2011).

Box 37.1 Sample MEQ

Question 1: Jenny Smith is a 30-year-old woman married to John for 3 years. They have been trying unsuccessfully to start a family. Jenny comes to see you and asks . . .

How would you deal with Jenny's request and what would your concerns be?

Question 2: Her husband John comes to see you the following day and talks about their relationship. He asks you for advice on . . .

How would you deal with this situation?

Short answer questions (SAQ)

In answering the essay question students are allowed freedom to write whatever they wish but with SAQ the task facing the student is more structured and the responses are limited. SAQ require students to provide a concise answer to a given question, usually a few words or at most a sentence or two. The more information required in an answer, the more difficulties there will be in ensuring a high level of reliability. SAQ are usually easy to construct, have a low probability of guessing, can cover a wide range of outcomes quite efficiently and are used mainly as a way of measuring factual recall or comprehensioin of information. There are however limitations. Complex issues can be diffcult to address. It can be challenging to construct the question so that there is only one correct answer—anticipating all possible correct answers is not as easy as it seems.

There are a variety of formats available. Some use a case vignette, followed by specific questions related to the scenario described: e.g. what disease does this patient have? what other treatments should be considered? Others will merely ask a direct question: e.g. what are the three main causes of death in Scotland? They can be used in quizzes, in self assessments and in progess testing (Rademakers et al. 2005). When constructing SAQ keep the item brief and unambiguous and use direct questions if possible. It is also recommended that you use a precise structured marking scheme. With numerical answers always ensure that you specify the unit of value required. Indicate to the candidate the length of response that is required: e.g. 'your answer should be no more than 20 words', and also the number of marks on offer.

SAQs can be computer marked but it is a mechanical process and the assessment engines used will look for model answers in the responses. If the answers are complex in their content and there is more than one way in which the response can be written then they will be unsuitable for such marking. However , if the answers are precise and brief then computerised marking is feasible (Leacock and Chodorov 2003; Siddiqi et al. 2010).

Selected response questions

True/false format

True/false questions were once a widely practised selected response format primarily because of their ability to cover a large content area and their relative ease of construction (Chandratilake et al. 2011). They exist in several forms; the most common form is a stem with a cluster of items (usually four to five), each of which is to be indicated as either true or false by the candidates. However, this format has been losing its popularity since the late 1980s, as educational researchers highlighted several of its limitations. It was demonstrated to be inappropriate to make pass / fail decisions in many assessment settings (Downing 1992). The key weaknesses highlighted were as follows:

◆ There is a high chance of guessing the correct answer (Downing 1992). As the answer should either be 'true' or 'false', a candidate, who is completely ignorant of the topic, has 0.5 probability of getting the item correct. Therefore, a candidate can score 50% of the marks for an entire exam purely by guessing. The greater the opportunity for guessing the lesser the reliability (Nnodim 1992). Although assessors attempted to discourage guessing by awarding negative marks for incorrect answers, reliability did not improve. In fact, awarding negative marks is educationally unsound; punishment does not discourage behaviour to the same extent that

rewards encourage behaviour; the marks obtained will not reflect the actual performance of candidates; and awarding negative marks tends to benefit risk takers (Chandratilake et al. 2011).

◆ Usually, the intention of an assessor is to award marks for knowing the correct answer. However, in the context of true/false items, candidates can still score marks by recognizing that an item is incorrect, but still not know what the correct answer is (Downing 1992; Frisbie 1973; Schuwirth and van der Vleuten 2003).

◆ They are weak in discriminating between high and low performers (Downing 1992). In medical education, knowledge tests are used not only to make pass/fail decisions but also to rank candidates who pass the exam and to award those who perform with distinction. Therefore, the discrimination ability of a test, i.e. the ability of the test to distinguish between high and low performers, is important. Several studies (Ebel 1980; Oosterhof and Glasnapp 1974) have demonstrated that the true/false assessment format has less discrimination power compared to other selected response formats. The discrimination power of true/false MCQs may be reduced further if negative marks are awarded.

◆ Focusing on areas that are absolutely true or false may lead to the assessment of trivial knowledge (Case and Swanson 2002; Downing 1992). In using the true/false format, the statements should be either absolutely true or absolutely false. However, for many clinical problems, there are no such clear-cut distinctions. The true false/format is not appropriate for the assessment of 'grey areas'. Therefore, the true/false format tends to encourage the assessment of trivial facts rather than assessing the ability to solve clinical problems (Downing 1992; Downing et al. 1995; Scouller and Prosser 1994). Although, memorization of facts is essential, the ultimate goal of medical education is solving clinical problems (Spencer and Jordan 1999). Furthermore, in attempting to construct true or false statements, especially the ones which are focused on problem solving, the assessors tend to make more technical flaws than in other MCQ formats (Albanese 1993; Schuwirth and van der Vleuten 2003). These cues can provide an edge for test-wise candidates (Scouller and Prosser 1994).

◆ They may not encourage learning around the general topic area (Schuwirth and van der Vleuten 2004). Candidates, who are assessed by the true/false format, attempt to memorize specific material, but do not read around the subject matter even when they are provided with feedback on the answers (Rees 1986). Therefore, this format provides minimum support for deep learning.

Multiple choice questions (MCQs)

The MCQ is probably the best known of the objective tests and consists of a stem and/or lead and a number of options, usually five (Case and Swanson 1998). There are two basic types—the correct answer type and the single best answer type. Examples of both types are shown in Box 37.2.

You can see from the example in Box 37.2 that the single best answer type can present problems as it can be challenging to develop an option that is clearly the best. Always ensure that you have strong evidence to support your choice of correct answer. This question allows you address higher cognitive levels and not just recall of facts.

The advantages of MCQs are well documented (Collins 2006; McCoubrie 2004; Palmer and Devitt 2006). If they are carefully constructed they can measure a range of learning outcomes and

---

Box 37.2 Sample MCQs

Correct answer type

Who wrote 'The Greatest Benefit to Mankind?'

A. Cole Porter

B. Roy Porter

C. Hall Porter

D. Suzi-May Porter

E. Oh Mr. Porter

Answer B. Roy Porter

The single best answer type

A 2-year-old girl who has had a febrile illness and a proven urinary tract infection on two prior occasions has been diagnosed once again with pyelonephritis. Which is the single most appropriate investigation to perform?

A. Antegrade pyelogram

B. CT scan

C. DMSA scan

D. X-ray KUB

E. IVU

Answer C. DMSA scan

---

ensure that there is good sampling. They are easy to mark and many MCQ exams are now delivered on-line (Nicol 2007), which allows a large numbers of students to be tested cost effectively (Bull and McKenna 2004). They can be set to assess different cognitive levels, they can be designed with a diagnostic end in mind, and also used to encourage deep learning (Draper 2009; Johannesen and Habib 2010; Schultheis 1998). Another advantage is the fact that performance statistics are readily available through software packages.

However, there is a tendency to use 'recall' type questions, which merely encourage rote learning. Setting questions to assess the higher levels of Bloom's taxonomy (Bloom 1956) takes time and effort. Creativity cannot be easily tested as fixed choices do not allow for freedom of expression. There is also the difficulty of constructing four plausible distractors. Having an MCQ with two or three options that are obviously incorrect increases the probability of guessing correctly. When constructing MCQs there are some key do's and don'ts. The stem should be meaningful and describe a problem in a succinct and clear fashion. It is imperative that a question should contain only one best or correct answer. Avoid negative stems where possible and ensure that all the options are grammatically linked to the stem. Try to avoid terms such as 'all of the above' or 'none of the above'. With the former all one needs to do is identify two options that are correct and this will indicate that 'all of the above' is the correct answer. Using the latter term as the correct answer only tests the candidate's ability to rule out wrong answers. Also, avoid imprecise terms such as sometimes, frequently or often as they are open to different interpretations. Creating effective distractors can be a challenging task. Just (2009) makes the point that how well one constructs distractors will impact on the difficulty level of the question. Four plausible distractors will decrease the chances of guessing

the correct answer. Distractors based on common student errors or misconceptions can prove ideal. Another tip is to ensure that all of the options are roughly similar in length.

Extended matching question format

Extended matching questions (EMQs) are referred to as a modified type of MCQ that have more than five options (Case and Swanson 1993). The standard EMQ format consists of four components: a theme, a list of options, multiple stems, and a lead-in. The *theme* is the general topic covered by the EMQ, and the list of *options* usually comprise eight to 12 homogeneous response choices (e.g. lists of diagnoses, investigations, or test results). The *stems* are clinical vignettes. Usually three stems are included in a standard EMQ. The *lead-in* is the question and the student must select one of the options which best suits. In a well-constructed EMQ the list of items are plausible and short, the lead-in is presented as a question, and the stems are relatively long. In writing EMQs, many item writers find it easy to begin with selecting a theme and proceed sequentially with writing the lead-in, developing the option list, formulating the stems, and reviewing the items with peer feedback (Case and Swanson 1993). For a standard EMQ a testing time of 1 minute per stem is advised. However, the length and the complexity of the problem presented in a stem may warrant longer or

---

Box 37.3 Sample EMQ

Theme: Urinary tract infection

A. Antegrade pyelogram

B. CT scan

C. DMSA scan

D. DTPA

E. Helical CT

F. Hippuran renogram

G. Isotope GFR

H. IVU

I. KUB

J. MAG 3 scan

K. MCUG

L. MRI

M. MRU

N. Retrograde pyelogram

O. Retrograde urethrogram

For each of the following scenarios which is the single most appropriate investigation to perform?

1. A 2-year-old girl who has had a febrile illness and a proven urinary tract infection on two prior occasions has been diagnosed once again with pyelonephritis. (C)

2. A 7-year-old with a straddle injury presents with retention of urine, gross scrotal swelling, and perineal bruising. (O)

3. A 7-year-old with known moderate hypertension presents with continuous wetting from birth. (M)

shorter time allocations (Case and Swanson 1993). Box 37.3 shows an example of an EMQ.

EMQs are recommended for assessment in the basic sciences and clinical medicine (Case and Swanson 1998). Although this format has been used to assess factual knowledge (Lukic et al. 2001) it may be best used for the assessment of problem-solving ability (Case and Swanson 1998; Coderre et al. 2004). EMQs have been used successfully for both formative (Lukic et al. 2001) and summative (Beullens et al. 2002) purposes. EMQs have been shown to be effective in assessing clinical reasoning (Beullens et al. 2005), specifically the hypothetico-deductive type (Heemskerk et al. 2008), and clinical decision making (Case and Swanson 1993).

The EMQ format has several practical and educational advantages. Its structured nature may make writing questions relatively easy (Case and Swanson 1993). A selected number of options together with a stem can be conveniently converted to a single best or single correct answer type MCQ if necessary. The themes can be used to organize the assessment content meaningfully and representatively (e.g. patient presentations), thus enhancing the validity of the assessment. The case vignettes can assess higher-order thinking (e.g. problem-solving) more than factual recall (Coderre et al. 2004). With a higher number of options and reduced chance of guessing, EMQs are powerful at discriminating between high and low performers (Beullens et al. 2002; Case and Swanson 1993). Therefore, high reliabilities can be achieved with fewer items and/or shorter testing times, provided that the quality of question remains high. The marks obtained by students for EMQs correlate highly with marks for skills assessments such as OSCEs (Wass et al. 2001b). However, item writers may need to be trained on how best to write EMQs in order to improve the quality. Using EMIs for the assessment of factual knowledge may not be cost effective as other question formats may be just as effective and not so time consuming to produce.

Orals and viva voce

In the standard oral or viva examinations, two or more examiners pose questions about a wide area of a given medical discipline within a limited time (Jayawickramarajah 1985). The exam format is similar to an interview and there is no involvement of patients (Davis and Karunathilake 2005). Based on the responses, the examiners score the examinee either independently or by achieving consensus (see fig. 37.1). Oral examinations are probably the only

component of an exam in which the questions and responses are not recorded (Jayawickramarajah 1985).

They have been used in both undergraduate and postgraduate medical education to make high stake decisions (e.g. deciding pass/fail or awarding merits) for decades. Some (Sandars 1998; Wass et al. 2003) argue that they assess in-depth knowledge of the subject, clinical or practical problem-solving, communication skills, and professional attitudes better than other assessment methods. In the assessment of knowledge, they may be effective at assessing the 'construction' of a response by the examinee rather than the selection of a response from a given set of options—as in MCQs (Chirculescu et al. 2007). However, their use as a summative assessment method has been severely criticized for a number of reasons. The evidence suggests that oral and viva examinations mostly assess factual recall and not higher-order thinking such as problem-solving or clinical reasoning (Jayawickramarajah 1985). The format is inherently subjective—the questions may be based on the whims of an examiner on the day (Cobourne 2010). The haphazard nature of the questions posed by the examiners to different examinees within the allocated time slot raises issues relating to validity and reliability. The questions may not adequately deal with the subject matter; since candidates are not asked identical questions, comparison or generalizability of the competence of examinees becomes challenging (Cobourne 2010). In a viva exam, the examiners may be influenced by other factors, rather than the actual performance of the examinee, such as command of language, level of anxiety, personal appearance, or personality, which may have no bearing on clinical competence (Davis and Karunathilake 2005). A structured approach to the viva, however, may improve its reliability (Tutton and Glasgow 1989). If each candidate is asked the same questions by the same examiners who are trained and use clearly defined criteria a more standardized exam will result. An alternative to having two pairs of examiners throw random questions at candidates for 30 minutes would be 10 examiners each spending 6 minutes with a candidate with their own set questions.

The seating arrangement used in many standard oral examinations can be quite confrontational (Jayawickramarajah 1985). In such instances candidates may feel they are in the witness box being grilled by a particularly aggressive barrister. The whole examination set up may make examinees more stressed than other methods of assessment (Jayawickramarajah 1985). However, viva examinations at undergraduate level have not necessarily been perceived as an unfair method of assessment especially by students who have faced such examinations for the purpose of obtaining a merit or a distinction (Duffield and Spencer 2002).

Although oral examinations may not be appropriate for high stakes assessments in undergraduate and postgraduate medical education, they may still be useful for formative purposes primarily because of the close one-to-one contact they provide for the feedback provider and recipient (Cobourne 2010).

Assessment of clinical ability

Both competence (e.g. the OSCE) and performance (e.g. workplace-based assessments) assessments primarily use structured clinical observations in simulated or workplace environments. The clinical observations are structured by introducing checklists or rating scales. Both contain a series of items. Checklists require the assessors to indicate a yes/no answer (e.g. done/not done, observed/not observed) and are better at assessing the stepwise completion of a

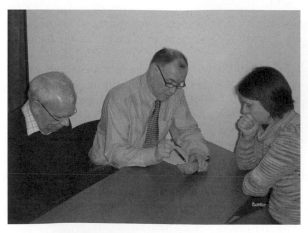

Figure 37.1 Oral examinations: inter-rater reliability can be a major problem.

task. Therefore, they are more suitable for the early stages of training (e.g. for the assessment of basic clinical tasks in early undergraduate years) (Chipman and Schmitz 2009). Rating scales, on the other hand, require the assessors to consider the quality of each step of a given task. Therefore, they are more appropriate than checklists in assessing clinical skills during the later years of undergraduate education, and right throughout postgraduate training and continuing medical education (Hodges et al. 1999; Regehr et al. 1998). Most importantly, rating scales are useful in assessing attitudes and professionalism.

Rating scales

Although the discussion here is focused mainly on rating scales, most of the principles are also applicable to the use of checklists.

In the context of assessments, rating scales contain a set of characteristics, qualities, competences, or outcomes to be judged and they put in place a systematic procedure for reporting observers' judgements. For assessors, they provide a common frame of reference for measuring all students or trainees on the same set of characteristics or outcomes. There are several advantages of using rating scale based assessments: they are flexible and can be used in multiple settings and at different times; the cost of developing rating scales is relatively low; they have the potential to be used as a basis for providing feedback; and they can be used in workplace environments unobtrusively. However, there are several disadvantages. They need to be completed by more than one assessor for the judgements to be credible and reliable (e.g. multisource feedback). The predictive validity of rating scales remains inconclusive. For example, there is no firm evidence to suggest that a rating scale that purports to measure empathy and warmth will have a strong positive correlation with a future measure of this trait (Hemmerdinger et al. 2007).

Several human errors may threaten the discriminatory power of judgements made using rating scales—see fig. 37.2 (McLaughlin et al. 2009). Therefore, steps should be taken to minimize these errors in developing and utilizing rating scales.

Error of leniency

Some assessors may be stricter or more lenient than others which results in unfairness. This error can be minimized by using multiple assessors and the provision of feedback to assessors about their ratings.

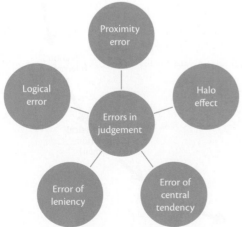

Figure 37.2 Errors that threaten the discriminatory power of judgments.

Error of central tendency

Certain assessors make their judgements around the mid points of the rating scale and avoid using the extremes. Increasing the number of categories in the rating scale to more than five (DeVellis 2003), anchoring categories with appropriate descriptors (Archer et al. 2008), and providing training to assessors in advance, will help reduce this error.

Halo effect

At times, the performance of candidates under assessment may be marred by candidates' previous performance or behaviour during training (McLaughlin et al. 2009). This happens particularly when candidates are known to the assessors as students or trainees, but can be minimized by assessor training.

Proximity error

When related but distinct items are next to each other in the rating scale the assessors' judgement of one may influence the other. For example, when reflective ability is placed just after professionalism, the assessor may judge the professionalism of a candidate based on their reflective ability and may give the same or similar ratings to both items, without explicitly thinking about professionalism. Placing closely related items well apart will be an effective countermeasure.

Logical error

At times, although the related items (e.g. empathy and the ability to communicate) are placed apart assessors may be influenced by their rating of one in rating the other (e.g. someone with great empathy is a great communicator, or vice versa). Making the assessors clear about the construct represented by each item will help minimize this error.

In addition, assessors may assess students or trainees without actually observing the specified task, behaviour or attitude. In workplace environments, this may happen due to several reasons: the assessors not having adequate time or interaction with candidates to make an informed judgement, having too many items in the rating scale that cannot be observed within a structured assessment setting, or poor integration of assessments into the formal training.

A range of assessment instruments have been developed to assess clinical ability—these use checklists and/or rating scales. *Competence* is largely assessed using OSCEs. *Performance* may be effectively assessed with newer workplace based assessment instruments (which are dealt with in the workplace based assessment chapter)

Objective structured clinical examinations (OSCEs)

In searching for a fair and practical way to assess skills Harden and colleagues (1975) developed an innovative instrument for assessing clinical skills in undergraduate medical students at Dundee. Harden and Gleeson (1979) later described this approach where students move around a structured set of tasks, many involving simulated patients and are observed by examiners using checklists. A wide range of competencies can be measured: e.g. history taking, physical examination, communications skills, counselling skills, data interpretation, and practical procedures. The term 'station' is used to describe the setting for the specific task undertaken and most OSCEs incorporate around 15 to 20 stations and each station lasts about 5–10 minutes on average. All students go through the same stations and it is important that each task can be carried out in the given time. It is also essential to pilot all the stations before using them in an exam setting so that examiners are familiar with the marking schedules and the logistics are checked. There are some stations that will not require the presence of an examiner (e.g. data or X-ray interpretation), and it is important that the student has clear instructions about how to proceed. Thorough training of simulated patients is essential if there is to be a consistency in their performance. You may be able to use real patients or actors but the message is the same—they must have a standardized approach to each student.

The checklist is a list of actions that need to be carried out to complete the task. It should not be too lengthy as too many items make will make it difficult to use and impact on inter-rater reliability. If necessary the checklist can be weighted so that certain key items contribute more to the overall mark. Keep the checklist as simple as possible by only including those really important actions and keep the range of possible response to a minimum—e.g. carried out successfully, not carried out. If you wish to assess attitudes or professional values then you might wish to include a global rating scale. Here the assessor uses a rating to indicate the level of empathy or rapport a student may have with a patient. The scale could range from 1 to 5 or 1 to 10, but it is important to clearly describe the type of rating used (Hodges and McIlroy 2003). Regehr et al. (1998) compared the psychometric properties of global ratings and checklists. They concluded that 'global rating scales scored by experts showed higher inter-station reliability, better construct validity, and better concurrent validity than did checklists . In those situations where you have access to expert, well trained examiners you might well consider their use. Figure 37.3 shows the format of an 18 station OSCE with 5-minute stations. This will allow for 16 students to be assessed objectively within an 90 minutes period.

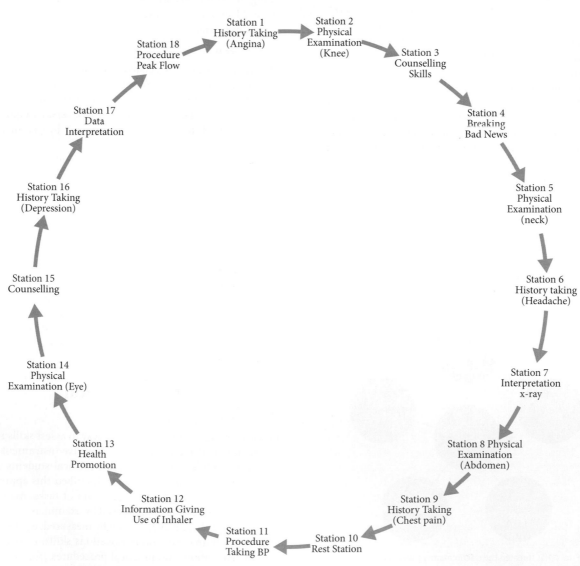

Figure 37.3 The layout of an eighteen station OSCE.

OSCEs are now used worldwide to assess both postgraduate and undergraduate students across a wide range of specialties from psychiatry (Park et al. 2004) to anaesthesiology (Hanna et al. 2005), and indeed they are used in a wide variety of professions such as dentistry (Mossey et al. 2001), veterinary medicine (Bark and Cohen 2002; Bark and Shahar 2006), and nursing (McWilliam and Botwinski 2010). The OSCE has its challenges; the recruitment of administrative, technical, and clinical staff; finding an environment that will allow for a large number of different tasks to be carried out in relative privacy; ensuring the smooth flow of students from station to station; and developing clear guidance for all concerned. The planning needs to be done well in advance and backup resources should always be in place as it is surprising how often equipment can fail to work when it is needed. You should calculate the costs in advance—if you have not got the resources or the manpower then running an OSCE is simply not feasible (Poenaru et al. 1997; Reznick et al. 1993).

Long cases

In the conventional long case, candidates are required to interview a real patient and perform a physical examination—usually for a period of 30 to 60 minutes (Ponnamperuma et al. 2009). During this encounter, which is not under the observation of examiners, candidates are expected to gather and interpret relevant information to arrive at a diagnosis. Subsequently, they present their findings to a panel of examiners and face an unstructured interview about the patient. The examiners provide a global rating based on the presentation of findings by the candidate and their performance in the follow-up interview. This method of assessment has been used mainly in final year undergraduate assessments, and in postgraduate assessments (Wass et al. 2001a).

The main strength of this assessment method is its enhanced authenticity in terms of context, as it is almost similar to a real doctor–patient consultation, and in terms of entirety, as it helps assess the ability of the candidate to approach and deal with a patent as a whole (Wass and van der Vleuten 2004). It tends to assess the skills of eliciting and interpreting relevant information, clinical reasoning, and problem-solving (Epstein 2007; Hardy et al. 1998), which cannot be assessed by oral or written knowledge tests, or short skills assessments (Hardy et al. 1998). These strengths support its educational impact and validity to some extent.

However, long cases have been criticized for their poor psychometric rigor, which has led to questions about their use especially in high-stakes summative assessments. Usually, in long case assessments, the clinical competence of the candidate is determined by their performance in a single patient encounter, which represents only a single core clinical problem. Such performance neither confirms nor predicts the candidate's ability to manage patients presenting with different clinical problems or presentations; the ability to solve clinical problems has been demonstrated to be content specific (Eva 2011). Therefore, several patients with different clinical problems are required to adequately sample a given clinical discipline, and each patient should be seen by every candidate. In practice, it is impossible to provide the same patient to all candidates in every exam setting. In many situations, two candidates in the same cohort see two different patients—i.e. they take two different examinations, which make comparisons between the two candidates impossible. The long cases have been demonstrated to have poor reliability. The main issue, however, is with inter-case reliability rather than inter-rater reliability (Wass and van der Vleuten 2004). To simply increase the number of patients and to make the same set of patients available to all candidates in a long case examination may be unfeasible in terms of time, resources and ethical grounds (it would be unethical for several candidates to examine the same patient). On the other hand, the assessment of candidates based solely on follow-up interviews after unobserved encounters with patients may only assess the knowledge of candidates and not their clinical competence (van der Vleuten 2000).

To overcome some of these weaknesses, the long cases have been modified and made more structured. When examiners observed the encounter between the candidate and patient, the marks given for observations correlated highly with the final global score, but correlated poorly with the marks given for presentations (Wass and Jolly 2001). The agreement between assessors on the marks given for the observation component was higher than their agreement on marks given for the presentation (Wass and Jolly 2001). Even with the structured format of long cases, at least 160 minutes of testing time per candidate may be necessary to achieve a reliability acceptable for high-stakes examinations—e.g. a generalizability coefficient of 0.8 (Wass et al. 2001a).

Although the psychometric issues challenge the use of this format for summative examinations, the high authenticity, holistic approach to patient management and interactive component with real patients make it highly recommended for providing feedback to trainees and students (Ponnamperuma et al. 2009).

Short cases

Short cases are usually used together with long cases in an examination. They are a series of system- or region-based examinations with the objectives of assessing the candidate's ability to elicit physical signs, use correct procedures for physical examination, interpret physical signs, and build rapport with patients (Hardy et al. 1998). Candidates usually examine three to five patients within 10 to 15 minutes (Hardy et al. 1998; Wass et al. 2001c). The examiners rate candidates globally based on their presentations at each case, but they may or may not have observed the performance of candidates. Short cases have been demonstrated to elicit different thinking processes when compared to questions assessing factual knowledge (Schuwirth et al. 2001). Scoring may be more reliable if the short cases are more structured, for example if the assessor observes candidates during their performance (Wass et al. 2001c). Again, if the number of short cases completed by a given candidate does not cover all organ systems, the issue with generalizability of performance may arise—threatening the validity of the format.

Epilogue

We have developed a basic table (table 37.1) which will allow you to quickly see the pros and cons associated with each instrument and its domain of reference. It is not always straightforward and the table is just a guide to the choices available.

Table 37.1 The pros and cons of assessment instruments

Assessment instrument	Domain	Pros	Cons
Essay	Higher levels of knowledge Can also assess thinking skills	Easy to construct	Time-consuming to mark Writing skills can influence the grades Problems with reliability Subjective Poor content validity
MEQ	Factual knowledge and comprehension Problem-solving skills	Useful as a formative tool	Construction can be time consuming Careful training for markers recommended
SAQ	Factual knowledge and comprehension Problem-solving skills	Avoids cueing and guessing	Clear marking criteria required
True/false	Factual knowledge and comprehension	Easy to mark Can be used to cover broad content areas	Susceptible to guessing Limited in its feedback Encourages rote learning
MCQ	Factual knowledge, comprehension, and application	Good content validty High reliability Easy to mark	Writing higher order questions may be challenging May promote rote learning
EMQ	Factual knowledge, comprehension and application Problem-solving skills	Good content validity High reliability Easy to mark	Writing higher-order questions may be challenging
Orals	Knowledge Can also assess clinical reasoning/professionalism	Can be used to discriminate borderline/distinction candidates	Time consuming Can be unreliable Subjective Examiner training needed
OSCE	Clinical skills Communication	Objective Good validity and reliability	Less authentic Expensive in terms of resources
Short cases	Clinical skills Diagnositic skills	Authentic Useful as a formative tool	Problems with validity and reliability
Long cases	Clinical skills Diagnostic skills Clinical reasoning	Authentic Holistic approach to patient management Useful as a formative tool	Problems with validity and reliability

Conclusions

- Identify the learning outcomes you wish to assess.

- Establish the purpose of the assessment; summative or formative or both. Attempt to provide constructive feedback in every assessment.

- It is not always possible to separate knowledge, skills, and attitudes; you may need to use more than one assessment instrument.

- Positive educational impact and feasibility are just as important as validity and reliability.

- The better the assessment the deeper the learning.

References

Albanese, M.A. (1993) Type K and other complex multiple-choice items: An analysis of research and item properties. *Educ Measurement Issues Pract.* 12: 28–33

Archer, J., Norcini, J., Southgate, L., Heard, S., and Davies, H. (2008) mini-PAT (Peer Assessment Tool): a valid component of a national assessment programme in the UK? *Adv Health Sci Educ Theory Pract.* 13(2): 181–192

Arnold, L. (2002) Assessing professional behavior: yesterday, today, and tomorrow. *Acad Med.* 77(6): 502–515

Bark, H., and Cohen, R. (2002) Use of an objective, structured clinical examination as a component of the final-year examination in small animal internal medicine and surgery. *J Am Vet Med Ass.* 221(9): 1262–1265

Bark, H. and Shahar, R. (2006) The use of the Objective Structured Clinical Examination (OSCE) in small-animal internal medicine and surgery. *J Vet Med Educ.* 33(4): 588–592

Beullens, J., Struyf, E., and Van Damme, B. (2005) Do extended matching multiple-choice questions measure clinical reasoning? *Med Educ,* 39(4): 410–417

Beullens, J., Van Damme, B., Jaspaert, H., and Janssen, P. J. (2002) Are extended-matching multiple-choice items appropriate for a final test in medical education? *Med Teach.* 24(4): 390–395

Bloom, B.S. (1956) *Taxonomy of educational objectives: the classification of educational goals; Handbook I.Cognitive domain.* New York: McKay

Boelen, C. and Woollard, B. (2009) Social accountability and accreditation: a new frontier for educational institutions. *Med Educ.* 43(9): 887–894

Bull, J. and McKenna, C. (2004) *Blueprint for Computer-assisted Assessment.* London: Routledge Falmer

Case, S. and Swanson, D. (1993) Extended Matching Items: a practical alternative to free-response questions. *Teach Learn Med.* 5(2): 107–115

Case, S. and Swanson, D. (1998) *Constructing Written Test Questions for the Basic and Clinical Sciences.* Philadelphia: National Board of Medical Examiners

Case, S.M. and Swanson, D.B. (2002) *Constructing Written Test Questions for the Basic and Clinical Sciences.* Philadelphia: National Board of Medical Examiners

Chandratilake, M., Davis, M., and Ponnamperuma, G. (2011) Assessment of medical knowledge: The pros and cons of using true/false multiple choice questions. *Natl Med J Ind.* 24(4): 225–228

Chipman, J.G. and Schmitz, C. C. (2009) Using objective structured assessment of technical skills to evaluate a basic skills simulation curriculum for first-year surgical residents. *J Am Coll Surg.* 209(3): 364–370

Chirculescu, A.R.M., Chirculescu, M., and Morris, J. F. (2007) Anatomical teaching for medical students from the perspective of European Union enlargement. *J Anat.* 210(5): 638–638

Cobourne, M.T. (2010) What's wrong with the traditional viva as a method of assessment in orthodontic education? *J Orthodont.* 37(2): 128–133

Coderre, S.P., Harasym, P., Mandin, H., and Fick, G. (2004) The impact of two multiple-choice question formats on the problem-solving strategies used by novices and experts. *BMC Med. Educ.* 4: 23

Collins, J. (2006) Writing multiple-choice questions for continuing medical education activities and self-assessment modules. *Radiographics.* 26: 543–551

Davis, M.H., and Karunathilake, I. (2005) The place of the oral examination in today's assessment systems. *Med Teach.* 27(4): 294–297

DeVellis, R.F. (2003) *Scale Development: Theory and Application.* London: Sage Publications

Downing, S.M. (1992) True-false, alternate-choice, and multiple-choice items. *Educ Measurement Issues Pract.* 11: 27–30

Downing, S.M., Baranowski, R.A., Grosso, L.J., and Norcini, J.J. (1995) Item type and cognitive ability measured: The validity evidence for multiple true-false items in medical specialty certification. *Appl Measurement Educ.* 8: 187–197

Draper, S.W. (2009) Catalytic assessment: understanding how MCQs and EVS can foster deep learning. *Br J Educ Tachnol.* 40(2): 306–315

Duffield, K.E. and Spencer, J.A. (2002) A survey of medical students' views about the purposes and fairness of assessment. *Med Educ.* 36(9): 879–886

Ebel, R.L. (1972) *Essentials of Educational Measurement.* New Jersey: Prentice Hall

Ebel, R.L. (1980) Are true-false items useful? In R. L. Ebel (ed.) *Practical Problems in Educational Measurement* (pp. 145–156). Lexington, MA: D.C. Heath

Epstein, R.M. (2007) Medical education—Assessment in medical education. *N Engl J Med.* 356(4): 387–396

Eva, K.W. (2011) On the relationship between problem-solving skills and professional practice elaborating professionalism (pp. 17–34). In C. Kanes (ed.) Dordrecht: Springer Netherlands

Feletti, G.I. and Smith, E.K.M. (1986) Modified essay questions—are they worth the effort. *Med Educ.* 20(2): 126–132

Frisbie, D.A. (1973) Multiple choice versus true-false: A comparison of reliabilities and concurrent validities. *J Educ Measurement.* 10: 297–304

Ginsburg, S., Regehr, G., Hatala, R., et al. (2000) Context, conflict, and resolution: a new conceptual framework for evaluating professionalism. *Acad Med.* 75(10 Suppl): S6–S11.

Hanna, M.N., Donnelly, M.B., Montgomery, C.L., and Sloan, P.A. (2005) Perioperative pain management education: A short structured regional anesthesia course compared with traditional teaching among medical students. *Regional Anesth Pain Med.* 30(6): 523–528

Harden, R.M. and Gleeson, F.A. (1979) Assessment of clinical competence using an objective structured clinical examination (OSCE). *Med Educ.* 13(1): 41–54

Harden, R.M., Stevenson, M., Downie, W.W., and Wilson, G.M. (1975) Assessment of clinical competence using objective structured examination. *BMJ.* 1(5955): 447–451

Hardy, K.J., Demos, L.L., and McNeil, J.J. (1998) Undergraduate surgical examinations: an appraisal of the clinical orals. *Med Educ.* 32(6): 582–589

Heemskerk, L., Norman, G., Chou, S., Mintz, M., Mandin, H., and McLaughlin, K. (2008) The effect of question format and task difficulty on reasoning strategies and diagnostic performance in Internal Medicine residents. *Adv Health Sci Educ.* 13(4): 453–462

Hemmerdinger, J. M., Stoddart, S. D., and Lilford, R. J. (2007) A systematic review of tests of empathy in medicine. *BMC Med Educ.* 7: 24

Hodges, B., and McIlroy, J.H. (2003) Analytic global OSCE ratings are sensitive to level of training. *Med Educ.* 37(11): 1012–1016

Hodges, B., Regehr, G., McNaughton, N., Tiberius, R., and Hanson, M. (1999) OSCE checklists do not capture increasing levels of expertise. *Acad Med.* 74(10): 1129–1134

Huxley, A. (1959) *Collected Essays.* New York: Harper and Row.

Jayawickramarajah, P.T. (1985) Oral examinations in medical education. *Med Educ.* 19(4): 290–293

Johannesen, M., and Habib, L. (2010) The role of professional identity in patterns of use of multiple-choice assessment tools, *Technology, Pedagogy and Education,* 19(1): 93–109

Just, S. (2009) Writing distractors for multiple choice questions. http://www.pedagogue.com/articles/writing_distractors_SBJ.htm Accessed 9 April 2013

Khan, M.Z., and Aljarallah, B.M. (2011) Evaluation of modified essay questions (MEQ) and multiple choice questions (MCQ) as a tool for assessing the cognitive skills of undergraduate medical students. *Int J Health Sci Qassim University.* 5(1): 45–50

Leacock, C., and Chodorov, M. (2003) C-rater: automated scoring of short answer questions. *Computers and Humanities.* 37(4): 389–406

Lowry, S. (1993) Medical education: assessment of students. *BMJ.* 306: 54

Lukic, I.K., Gluncic, V., Katavic, V., Petanjek, Z., Jalsovec, D., and Marusic, A. (2001) Weekly quizzes in extended-matching format as a means of monitoring students' progress in gross anatomy. *Ann Anat.* 183(6): 575–579

Lynch, D.C., Surdyk, P.M., and Eiser, A.R. (2004) Assessing professionalism: a review of the literature. *Med Teach.* 26(4): 366–373

McCoubrie, P. (2004) Improving the fairness of multiple-choice questions: a literature review. *Med Teach.* 26(8): 709–712

McLaughlin, K., Vitale, G., Coderre, S., Violato, C., and Wright, B. (2009) Clerkship evaluation—what are we measuring? *Med Teach.* 31(2): 36–39

McWilliam, P. and Botwinski, C. (2010) Developing a Successful Nursing Objective Structured Clinical Examination. *J Nursing Educ.* 49(1): 36–41

Miller, G.E. (1990) The assessment of clinical skills, competence and performance *Acad Med.* 65(9): s63–s67

Mossey, P.A., Newton, J.P., and Stirrups, D.R. (2001) Scope of the OSCE in the assessment of clinical skills in dentistry. *Br Dent J.* 190(6): 323–326

Nicol, D. (2007) E-assessment by design: using multiple-choice tests to good effect. *J Further Higher Educ.* 31(1): 53–64

Nnodim, J.O. (1992) Multiple-choice testing in anatomy. *Med Educ.* 26: 301–309

Oosterhof, A.C., and Glasnapp, D.R. (1974) Comparative reliabilities and difficulties of the multiple-choice and true-false formats. *J Exp Educ.* 42: 62–64

Palmer, E., and Devitt, P. (2006) Constructing multiple choice questions as a method for learning. *Anns Acad Med Singapore.* 35(9): 604–608

Park, R.S., Chibnall, J.T., Blaskiewicz, R.J., Furman, G.E., Powell, J.K., and Mohr, C.J. (2004) Construct validity of an objective structured clinical examination (OSCE) in psychiatry: Associations with the clinical skills examination and other indicators. *Acad Psychiatry.* 28(2): 122–128

Parker, M. (2006) Assessing professionalism: theory and practice. *Med Teach.* 28(5): 399–403

Poenaru, D., Morales, D., Richards, A., and O'Connor, H. M. (1997) Running an objective structured clinical examination on a shoestring budget. *Am J Surg.* 173(6): 538–541

Ponnamperuma, G.G., Karunathilake, I.M., McAleer, S., and Davis, M.H. (2009) The long case and its modifications: a literature review. *Med Educ.* 43(10): 936–941

Rabinowitz, H.K. (1987) The modified essay question—an evaluation of its use in a family medicine clerkship. *Med Educ.* 21(2): 114–118

Rademakers, J, Ten Cate, T.J., and Bär, P.R. (2005) Progress testing with short answer questions. *Med Teach.* 27(7): 578–582

Rees, P.J. (1986) Do Medical-Students Learn from Multiple-Choice Examinations. *Med Educ.* 20(2): 123–125

Regehr, G., MacRae, H., Reznick, R. K., and Szalay, D. (1998) Comparing the psychometric properties of checklists and global rating scales for assessing performance on an OSCE-format examination. *Acad Med.* 73(9): 993–997

Reznick, R.K., Smee, S., Baumber, J.S., Cohen, R., Rothman, A., Blackmore, D., and Berard, M. (1993) Guidelines for estimating the real cost of an objective structured clinical examination. *Acad Med.* 68(7): 513–517

Sandars, J. (1998) *MRCGP: approaching the new modular examination approach to the oral examination component.* Knutsford UK: Pastest.

Schultheis, N.M. (1998) Writing cognitive educational objectives and multiple-choice test questions. *Am J Health-System Pharm.* 55(22): 2397–2401

Schuwirth, L.W.T., and van der Vleuten, C.P.M. (2003) ABC of learning and teaching in medicine—Written assessment. *BMJ.* 326(7390): 643–645

Schuwirth, L.W.T., and van der Vleuten, C.P.M. (2004) Different written assessment methods: what can be said about their strengths and weaknesses? *Med Educ.* 38(9): 974–979

Schuwirth, L.W.T., Verheggen, M.M., van der Vleuten, C.P.M., Boshuizen, H.P.A., and Dinant, G.J. (2001) Do short cases elicit different thinking processes than factual knowledge questions do? *Med Educ.* 35(4): 348–356

Scouller, K. and Prosser, M. (1994) Students' experiences in studying for multiple choice question examinations. *Studies Higher Educ.* 19: 267–279

Siddiqi, R., Harrison, C.J., and Siddiqi, R. (2010) Improving teaching and learning through automated short-answer marking. *IEEE Trans Learn Technol.* 3(3): 237–249

Spencer, J.A. and Jordan, R.K. (1999) Learner centred approaches in medical education. *BMJ.* 318(7193): 1280–1283

Tutton, P J.M. and Glasgow, E.F. (1989) Reliability and predicitve capacity of examinations in anatomy and improvement in the reliability of viva voce (oral) examinations by the use of structured rating system. *Clin Anat.* 2(1): 29–34

van der Vleuten, C. (2000) Validity of final examinations in undergraduate medical training. *BMJ.* 321(7270): 1217–1219

Wass, V. and Jolly, B. (2001) Does observation add to the validity of the long case? *Med Educ.* 35(8): 729–734

Wass, V. and van der Vleuten, C. (2004) The long case. *Med Educ.* 38(11): 1176–1180

Wass, V., Jones, R., and van der Vleuten, C. (2001a) Standardized or real patients to test clinical competence? The long case revisited. *Med Educ.* 35(4): 321–325

Wass, V., McGibbon, D., and van der Vleuten, C. (2001b) Composite undergraduate clinical examinations: how should the components be combined to maximize reliability. *Med Educ.* 35(4): 326–330

Wass, V., van der Vleuten, C., Shatzer, J., and Jones, R. (2001c) Assessment of clinical competence. *Lancet.* 357(9260): 945–949

Wass, V., Wakeford, R., Neighbour, R., and van der Vleuten, C. (2003) Achieving acceptable reliability in oral examinations: an analysis of the Royal College of General Practitioners membership examination's oral component. *Med Educ.* 37(2): 126–131

CHAPTER 38

Test-enhanced learning

Douglas P. Larsen and Andrew C. Butler

The active recall of a fact from within is, as a rule, better
than its impressions without.
                    Edward Thorndike (Thorndike, 1906, p. 123)

Introduction

A chief resident faced a difficult educational task. The residents in
the programme did not feel that they adequately understood, recognized, or knew how to treat rare metabolic diseases. The chief resident collaborated with a faculty member who had special expertise
in this area to create two 1-hour didactic conferences that reviewed
the diseases. The faculty member provided an extensive overview
and many case examples. After the conferences, the residents felt
that they had learned the material, and they were grateful that their
educational need had been met. No further formal exposure to the
material occurred.

This example illustrates a fundamental misconception about
learning that is ubiquitous in medical education—the assumption
that performance during learning (or immediately afterwards) will
be maintained. Both objective assessments (e.g. tests) and subjective judgements (e.g. feelings of mastery) during learning are often
poor predictors of long-term retention because they reflect the
accessibility of knowledge at a given moment rather than how well
that knowledge has been stored in memory (Bjork and Bjork 1992).
This misconception undermines the critical educational objective
of helping clinicians to acquire and retain the large body of medical
knowledge that they will need to apply in the future.

With this misconception in mind, educators must consider how
likely it is that the residents in the real-life scenario above remembered the material that was taught in the conferences. Based on
what we know from cognitive science, the answer is probably little or nothing at all, which is troubling because much of medical
education occurs through similar methods and settings. For example, residents at most teaching hospitals in the United States spend
at least 8 hours a week in formal didactic conferences. In fact, in
the United States, the Accreditation Council on Graduate Medical
Education (ACGME) mandates these conferences (ACGME 2011,
p. 7). Yet studies have shown no difference in knowledge between
clinicians who attended such conferences and peers who did not
(Cacamese et al. 2004; FitzGerald and Wenger 2003; Picciano et al.
2003; Winter et al. 2007). The same problem exists at all levels of
medical education. Students spend countless hours in classrooms
prior to their clinical years and then spend several hours a week
in didactic sessions during their clinical rotations. Practising

physicians are required by regulatory agencies to spend a certain number of hours each year at continuing medical education
conferences.

The challenge for medical education is to develop and implement
learning methods that produce long-term retention of knowledge
that can be flexibly recalled and applied in the future. This chapter
reviews one such method, called *test-enhanced learning* (Roediger
and Karpicke 2006a, Larsen et al. 2008, Roediger and Butler 2011)
Test-enhanced learning is based on the finding that retrieving
information from memory produces superior long-term retention, commonly referred to as the *testing effect*. Although practising
retrieval of information is often implemented as a test, it can take
many forms and is not limited to traditional paper or electronic
tests. A large body of research in cognitive science and related fields
has shown the testing effect to be a robust and replicable finding.
In fact, the evidence is so strong that the Institute of Education
Sciences from the Department of Education in the US has recommended using retrieval practice to promote retention at all levels of
education (Pashler et al. 2007).

The goals of this chapter are to introduce the idea of test-
enhanced learning, review the main findings in the literature, and
provide some guidance as to how test-enhanced learning might be
implemented in medical education.

Overview of test-enhanced learning

In education, tests are typically synonymous with assessment—
most educators and students consider testing a tool for assessing
student learning and providing feedback to guide future activities
(Black and William 1998). As conceptualized within test-enhanced
learning, testing has a different purpose: to directly increase retention and understanding by the act of taking the test. The memory
retrieval that occurs while taking a test is often thought to be a
neutral event—similar to measuring someone's weight. Much
like stepping on scale does not change a person's weight, memory
retrieval during a test is assumed to sample one's knowledge but
leave it unchanged. Research in cognitive science indicates that
this assumption is false; rather, the act of retrieving information
from memory actually changes memory (Bjork 1975), leading to
superior retention over time and better understanding (Roediger

and Butler 2011; Roediger and Karpicke 2006a). Although it is difficult to divorce testing from assessment, the mnemonic benefits of retrieval practice suggest that testing is a powerful learning tool.

A brief history of testing effect research

The idea that practising memory retrieval promotes long-term retention dates back many centuries. Consider the following statement: 'Exercise in repeatedly recalling a thing strengthens the memory'. Although this quotation sounds as though it could be part of this chapter, it is actually from Aristotle's classic treatise on memory—*De Memoria et Reminiscentia* (Hammond 1902, p. 202). The first empirical demonstration of the mnemonic benefits of testing in a controlled experiment occurred just over a hundred years ago (Abbott 1909). Over the next 30 years, educational psychologists became interested in applying this phenomenon to the classroom (Gates 1917; Jones 1923–1924; Spitzer 1939). However, interest dwindled in the second half of the 20th century and testing effect research became sporadic despite the publication of many important studies (Carrier and Pashler 1992; Glover 1989; Tulving 1967; Wheeler and Roediger 1992). More recently, there has been a resurgence of interest in the phenomenon (Roediger and Butler 2011; Roediger and Karpicke 2006a).

Robustness and replicability

The findings in recent studies have firmly established that the phenomenon is robust and replicable. One powerful example comes from a recent study by Karpicke and Roediger (2008, pp. 966–968) in which they examined various methods for learning foreign vocabulary with flash cards. They gave undergraduate students Swahili–English word pairs (e.g. *mashua–boat*) to learn through repeatedly studying and testing the pairs until each pair had been successfully recalled once. After a pair had been recalled, it was assigned to one of four types of additional practice: (1) repeated studying and testing, (2) repeated studying only, (3) repeated testing only, and (4) no further activity. One week later, the students were given a final cued recall test in which they had to recall the English translations when prompted with the Swahili words. The results were striking; repeated testing only produced a much higher level of correct recall relative to repeated studying only and no further activity. Interestingly, additional study had little or no effect on retention—repeated studying and testing did not improve correct recall relative to repeated testing only, and the repeated study only was marginally better than no further activity.

The rapid accumulation of studies has allowed researchers to quantify the effect of retrieval practice (Bangert-Drowns, Kulik and Kulik 1991; Phelps 2012; Rawson and Dunlosky 2011). Phelps (2012, pp. 21–43) recently conducted a meta-analysis that included several hundred studies conducted over the past 100 years. He found that the mean effect size related to testing was either moderate ($d = 0.55$) or large ($d = 0.88$), depending on how the effect size was calculated. When testing was more frequent and post-test feedback was provided, the effect of testing on achievement was even larger.

Most studies on the testing effect have sought to examine the benefits of retrieval practice by comparing it to a restudy control condition (Butler and Roediger 2007; Carrier and Pashler 1992; Glover 1989). Restudy is an ideal comparison activity because it usually involves reprocessing all of the to-be-learned material (whereas testing involves reprocessing only what can be recalled) and it is

common in education (Karpicke et al. 2009). However, one possible criticism is that restudy could be considered a more passive task than testing. With this criticism in mind, several recent studies have compared retrieval practice to other more active learning strategies, such as note-taking, concept-mapping, self-explanation, and various mnemonic techniques (Fritz et al. 2007a; Karpicke and Blunt 2011; Larsen et al. 2013; McDaniel et al. 2009). All of these studies have found benefits of testing relative to these other learning strategies.

A host of studies have also demonstrated the durability of testing effects. Although many studies have used relatively short retention intervals ranging from minutes to a few days, other studies have examined retention over much longer intervals. These studies have found reliable benefits of testing after periods ranging from several weeks (Butler and Roediger 2007; Kromann et al. 2009; Rawson and Dunlosky 2011) to more than 6 months (Carpenter et al. 2009; Larsen et al. 2009; 2012, 2013; McDaniel et al. 2011). In fact, one small study demonstrated that the benefits of retrieval can last up to 5 years (Bahrick et al. 1993).

Generalizability

The generalizability of test-enhanced learning is also well established with respect to several important variables: learners, materials, and performance measures. Concerning learners, the testing effect has been obtained in many different demographics that have a wide variety of characteristics and abilities. The mnemonic benefits of retrieval practice have been demonstrated across the age spectrum from young children (Fritz et al. 2007b) to older adults (Tse et al. 2010). The testing effect has also been observed with medical students (Kromann et al. 2009; Larsen et al. 2012; Rees 1986) and medical residents (Larsen et al., 2009). In terms of differences in student knowledge and ability, testing seems to benefit learners regardless of their level of prior knowledge (Carroll et al. 2007) or their memory ability and intelligence (Brewer and Unsworth 2012); however, there is some indication that the magnitude of the testing effect may be reduced in individuals with greater prior knowledge, memory ability, and/or intelligence.

The testing effect also generalizes across many types of materials. Traditional laboratory studies of retrieval practice have often used simple materials, such as word pairs (Karpicke and Roediger 2008) or general knowledge facts (Butler et al. 2008). However, the benefits of testing have been shown to extend to a variety of more complex materials. For example, studies have found testing effects using texts (Kang et al. 2007), lectures (Butler and Roediger 2007), multimedia presentations (Johnson and Mayer 2009), and maps (Carpenter and Pashler, 2007). The benefits of testing also seem to extend to inductive function learning (Kang et al. 2011), identifying bird species (Jacoby et al. 2010), and various skills like resuscitation (Kromann et al. 2009). In addition, it is important to note that the phenomenon seems to transcend knowledge domains, having been observed with materials from a variety of disciplines such as history (Carpenter et al. 2009), science (McDaniel et al. 2007), and medicine (Larsen et al. 2009).

Finally, one other variable that is critical to generalizability is the outcome measure used to assess the benefits of retrieval practice. Most testing effect studies have used a final assessment that is an exact repetition of the same test that was given during learning. In recent years, researchers have begun to explore whether the effects of testing extend beyond the retention of information to the understanding and use of that information. Transfer of knowledge involves applying previously learned information to a new context

(Barnett and Ceci 2002), an important outcome for educational purposes. Many testing effect studies have shown that practising retrieval improves transfer of knowledge (Butler 2010; Johnson and Mayer 2009; Karpicke and Blunt 2011; Larsen et al. 2012; McDaniel et al. 2009). Overall, these studies suggest that testing can improve both the retention and understanding of material, enabling the application of knowledge to a variety of contexts.

Theoretical mechanisms

When discussing theoretical explanations for the mnemonic benefits of retrieval practice, it is important to distinguish between the direct and indirect effects of testing. Direct effects of testing refer to the improved retention and understanding that result from the act of successfully retrieving information from memory (i.e. the focus of this chapter). In contrast, the indirect effects of testing refer to a host of other ways in which testing can influence learning. For example, testing can help students to assess what they know and do not know, providing valuable feedback that they can use to guide future study. In addition, frequent testing can motivate students to study and attend class (Fitch et al. 1951; Mawhinney et al. 1971), helping them to avoid putting off studying until the last minute (Michael 1991).

One of the first formal hypotheses put forth to explain the testing effect focused on differences in the amount of exposure to the material. In many early testing effect studies, the experimental group would study material and then take a test, while the control group would simply study the material, and then both groups would take a final test to measure retention. Based on this comparison, some researchers pointed out that the testing group received two exposures to the material (they were re-exposed to the material that they retrieved on the test), and this difference may be driving the effect (Thompson et al. 1978; Slamecka and Katsaiti 1988). However, many subsequent studies have disproven this idea by showing that testing still produces a benefit when the control group has the opportunity to re-study the material and total exposure to the material is matched (Carrier and Pashler 1992; Glover 1989; Karpicke and Roediger 2008).

Other theories that have attempted to explain the testing effect have focused on how the act of retrieval affects memory, and these theories can be categorized into two groups. One group of theories revolves around the idea that the mnemonic benefits of testing result from the reprocessing of the material that occurs during retrieval (Carpenter 2009; Pyc and Rawson 2009). When a memory is retrieved, the memory trace is elaborated and new retrieval routes are created, making it more likely it will be successfully retrieved again in the future. The amount of effort that is involved in retrieving information is considered to be an index of the amount of reprocessing that occurs; this notion of retrieval effort helps to explain why production tests (e.g. short answer tests), which require more effort, tend to produce better retention than recognition tests (e.g. multiple choice questions), which require less effort (Butler and Roediger 2007; Kang et al. 2007).

A second group of theories centres on the relationship between initial learning and the final test, invoking a principle called transfer-appropriate processing (Morris et al. 1977; Roediger et al. 2002). Transfer-appropriate processing posits that memory performance is enhanced when the cognitive processes that are engaged during learning match the processes that are required during retrieval. With respect to the testing effect, this principle applies because the cognitive processes engaged while taking an initial test provide a better match for the final retention test relative to the processes engaged while restudying the material (the traditional control condition). When considering how integral memory retrieval is to the application of knowledge outside the classroom, the principle of transfer-appropriate processing suggests that students should be engaging in activities during learning that provide retrieval practice.

Overall, there is ample evidence to support both groups of theories, and it is important to note that they are not mutually exclusive. Further development of theory is ongoing and many researchers are now concentrating on gaining a better understanding of the underlying mechanisms that produce the mnemonic benefits of retrieval practice. In the future, we expect that these psychological theories will be enriched by new evidence and ideas from cognitive neuroscience that specify possible brain mechanisms (Roediger and Butler 2011).

Finally, it is important to briefly touch on a few of the theories that have been put forth to explain some of the indirect effects of testing. A full review of these theories is beyond the scope of this chapter. However, one important category of theories about the indirect effects of testing focuses on metacognition. Agrawal et al. (2012, pp. 326–335) have argued that the act of taking a test and reviewing feedback stimulates self-monitoring to identify areas of unexpected results. This rehearsal influences subsequent studying behaviour, thereby facilitating further learning and long-term retention (Kulhavy and Stock 1989). Similarly, Pyc and Rawson (2010, p. 335; 2012, pp. 737–746) have suggested that testing enables learners to discover whether the strategy that they used to encode the to-be-remembered information was effective—an idea that they refer to as the mediator effectiveness hypothesis. When learners take a test and fail to retrieve a piece of information, they can subsequently use a different strategy to encode the information. Finally, Butler et al. (2008, pp. 918–928) have shown that receiving feedback after a test can help to improve metacognition by making learners better able to distinguish between test responses that are correct and incorrect. They argue that feedback is important for low-confidence correct responses because it helps the learner to correct a metacognitive error (i.e. thinking that a response is incorrect when it is actually correct).

Implementing test-enhanced learning in medical education

The following section discusses some of the factors that influence the efficacy of retrieval practice, while also offering practical recommendations for using test-enhanced learning in the classroom and clinic (fig. 38.1).

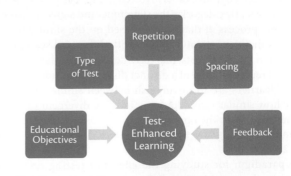

Figure 38.1 Factors that influence test-enhanced learning.

Aligning retrieval practice with educational objectives

When considering the implementation of test-enhanced learning, it is important to recognize that the principle of retrieval practice can be broadly applied to a variety of activities beyond simple written tests. For example, retrieval practice occurs when students answer questions orally, attempt to diagnose a patient, or perform a surgical technique. The key aspect of the activity is that the information, procedure, or skill is retrieved from memory. Although educators have a wide range of possible activities from which to choose, the form of retrieval practice must be tailored to the educational objectives in order for learning to be optimized. As with all good educational planning, educators must ask themselves: 'What do I want my students *to know*? What do I want them *to be able to do*?' These questions help to identify the type of learning that is needed in a given situation. Learning may focus on declarative facts, concepts (grouping and categorization of facts), principles (rules that determine how facts are applied), problem-solving (principles that lead to the solution of novel situations), or psychomotor tasks (Smith and Ragan 2005, pp. 78–82). Once the type of learning is identified, the educator must match the form of retrieval practice to the desired type of learning.

Learning facts is often derided as a 'lower' form of learning. This position neglects the reality that much of the practice of medicine is based on the knowledge of facts. For example, physicians must learn the characteristics of diseases, drug dosing and side effects, and what constitutes 'normal' and 'abnormal' on a clinical test. Much of the research on test-enhanced learning has focused on learning and retaining factual knowledge. For instance, Larsen et al. (2009, pp. 1174–1181) investigated the effects of three short-answer written tests at 2-week intervals after a didactic conference covering the diagnosis and treatment of two different neurological conditions. They found that repeated testing led to better retention of these facts after 6 months when compared to repeated studying. Similarly, Turner et al. (2011, pp. 731–737) demonstrated that after a life support course, four unannounced oral tests given over the telephone significantly improved the retention of factual knowledge at 2 months compared to a control group that only received a single oral test. The oral tests were given without feedback so that the groups only differed in their amounts of retrieval practice. In practical terms, educators must have clear idea of which facts are foundational and applicable to a clinical learning objective and then make sure that learners have opportunities to retrieve these facts from memory.

Concept learning is another critical aspect of medical education. One of the main cognitive tasks involved in making a medical diagnosis is to correctly categorize the symptoms and signs of a patient's illness. This process of diagnosis is based on the similarities and differences that the patient possesses with different disease categories based on 'illness scripts' that have developed as the practitioner's mental representation of a distinct disease (Schmidt and Rikers 2007). If learners are to distinguish between similar diseases or identify how similar symptoms may indicate divergent diagnoses, then they must have the opportunity to practise sorting these concepts and identifying how to apply them to a given case (Smith and Ragan 2005, p. 178).

One paradigm for studying the effects of testing on concept learning in the cognitive psychology literature uses bird species identification (Jacoby et al. 2010). In studies in this field, testing was shown to improve the recognition of both studied and novel exemplars of bird species, and the classification of these exemplars as well. Testing is thought to improve learning in these cases by enabling students to practise the identification of key details that distinguished birds from each other or characteristics that allowed them to be grouped together. These findings are important because they demonstrate that testing can improve the ability of subjects to identify the relationships between key elements of knowledge—a key characteristic of 'deeper' levels of learning (Marton and Saljo 1976).

Jacoby et al. (2010, pp. 1441–1451) also demonstrated the effects of testing on subjects' awareness of their levels of knowledge (i.e. metacognition). They found an increase in the ability of subjects to determine how well they had learned the material and to predict which categorization tasks would be more difficult than others (known as classification judgement learning). These findings closely complement the work described earlier by Agrawal et al. (2012, pp. 326–335), regarding the effects of testing on enhancing self-monitoring and also the mediator shift-hypothesis developed by Pyc and Rawson (2010, pp. 335; 2012, pp. 737–746). Improved ability to predict classification difficulty has particularly important implications for both education and clinical practice. If learners are able to predict which concepts are difficult to classify, they can direct further study towards those topics. In clinical medicine, practitioners would be more aware of when a particular diagnosis can be difficult, and therefore would take more care in order to avoid errors.

In terms of practical application in medical education, concepts could be tested through clinical case scenarios. Learners must be exposed to a sufficient number of cases to be able to learn to make the distinctions between similarities and differences. Learners should see examples that fit in the category and counter-examples that do not fit (Smith and Ragan 2005, pp. 176–178). Too often in case-based learning only a single case is presented, which is unlikely to allow learners to develop a clear set of rules to be applied to future cases. Learners need repeated retrieval attempts to form and verify mental rules regarding the relationships between the pieces of information that they have learned.

Testing that allows learners to practise application can facilitate the application of knowledge. Although much less research has been directed at how testing can be used to achieve these educational objectives, some studies have begun to investigate whether retrieval practice can facilitate transfer of learning (Butler 2010; Johnson and Mayer 2009; Karpicke and Blunt 2011; Larsen et al. 2012; McDaniel et al. 2009). For example, Butler (2010, pp. 1118–1133) demonstrated that repeated retrieval practice on facts and concepts improved the ability to apply knowledge to novel situations. After studying scientific texts, learners were asked questions that required them to retrieve facts and concepts from the texts. Performance on a final application test 1 week later demonstrated improved transfer of learning for facts and concepts that were tested compared to facts and concepts that were repeatedly studied. Importantly, an additional experiment showed that learners who engaged in repeated testing were better able to apply concepts that they had learned to novel situations in an unrelated knowledge domain.

In addition to the purely cognitive domains of learning, testing has been shown to produce increased retention in the area of psychomotor skills. One of the first studies to examine test-enhanced learning in the medical education literature investigated the effects of testing on cardiopulmonary resuscitation. Kromann et al. (2009, pp. 21–27) found that a single test at the end of a cardiac resuscitation course improved retention by almost 10% at 2 weeks compared to students who had received the traditional training. Follow-up at 6 months continued to show an effect on retention with a clinically relevant effect size ($d = 0.40$) (Kromann et al. 2010). Another example with real-life application is the work done by Wayne et al. (2006a, pp. 251–256). The researchers demonstrated that simulation-based repeated retrieval practice by internal medicine residents led to mastery of advanced cardiac life support protocols. This mastery level was maintained without significant decrement for at least 14 months (Wayne et al. 2006b). Importantly, real-life performance in cardiac resuscitation was superior for residents trained with simulation-based deliberate practice compared to non-simulation trained residents (Wayne et al. 2008).

As some of our examples demonstrate, retrieval practice in medical education can have a direct impact on the care that patients receive. Educators should plan for and carry out retrieval practice based on specific educational objectives. Figure 38.2 shows some examples.

Type of test

Educators who implement test-enhanced learning must use the test format that will have the greatest impact. Tests can be separated into two categories: production tests and recognition tests (fig. 38.3). Production tests, such as short answer and essay tests, involve generating a response from memory. In contrast, recognition tests, such as multiple-choice and true–false tests, involve selecting a response from information that is provided. Both types of test have been shown to improve retention (McDaniel et al. 2011). However, production tests generally produce better long-term retention than recognition tests (Glover 1989; Kang et al. 2007). Butler and Roediger (2007, pp. 604–618) gave students either a short-answer test or a multiple-choice test after watching a videotaped lecture. When retention was measured on a final test 1 month later, the initial short-answer test produced better performance than the initial multiple-choice test.

The superior retention that results from production tests can be explained by the idea of retrieval effort. That is, production tests tend to require considerable mental effort to generate the information, whereas recognition tests involve simply selecting the correct information. One form of production test that requires substantial effort is the free recall test. Free recall tests require learners to generate information with relatively few or no cues. For example, a free

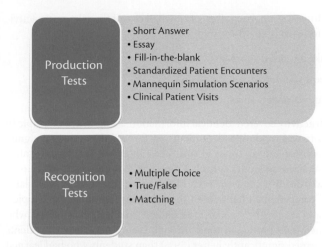

Figure 38.3 Examples of production and recognition tests.

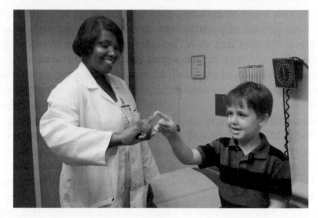

Figure 38.4 Patient encounters (both real and simulated) should be considered retrieval practice opportunities that should be incorporated into test-enhanced learning.

recall test might be given to students asking them to name all of the nerves in the human body. One reason that free recall tests are particularly effective is that learners have to retrieve the organization of the information as well as the individual items. As a result, free recall tests can induce learners to create better organizational structures of knowledge (Zaromb and Roediger, 2010).

Although studies in the cognitive psychology laboratory often use relatively simple free recall tests (e.g. essays), free recall can be implemented in many more complex ways that directly correspond to processing that educators target in medical education. One such example is the use of mechanical simulation in psychomotor skills learning (Kromann et al. 2009; 2010; Wayne et al. 2006b; 2008). During manikin simulation, learners must retrieve and apply their knowledge with few or no explicit cues. Of course, the various symptoms and signs manifested by the manikin clearly provide some implicit cues, but retrieval is largely self-directed because the learner must remember both the information (e.g. the specific steps to take during a medical intervention) and the organization of that information (e.g. the correct ordering of the steps).

Another way of implementing free recall in medical education is through standardized patient encounters (fig. 38.4). In a study by Larsen et al. (2012), students learned the necessary information to diagnose and treat patients with three neurological conditions in a

Knowledge of declarative facts

Concepts used to categorize groups of facts

Transfer of learning to new contexts

Principles used in problem-solving

Interactions with patients in live encounters

Procedural skills learned on simulation models with anticipation of real-life application

Figure 38.2 Examples of educational objectives that retrieval practice can help to achieve.

teaching session. Next, they performed one of three learning activities for each of the three topics:

◆ take a written short-answer test

◆ see a standardized patient, or

◆ study a review sheet.

Each activity covered identical information. Assignment of a topic to activity was randomized. Students performed the activity assigned to each topic four times at one-week intervals. Six months after initial learning students took a final test that consisted of seeing a standardized patient for each of the three topics. One week later they completed a final written short-answer test on all three topics. On average for the standardized patient final test, the students who learned their particular topic through seeing standardized patients performed significantly better (59%) than students who had learned the same topic through written testing (49%) or studying a review sheet (43%). Interestingly, on the final written test, students who learned the topic through standardized patients and through written tests performed equivalently (both 61% retention on average) and better than students who learned the topic through studying a review sheet (48%). One possible explanation for the difference in the pattern of results across the two types of test is that the written test provided more cues for the students relative to the standardized patient test. That is, learning by seeing a standardized patient was essentially like taking a free recall test—students had to retrieve both the information itself and the organization for the information. In contrast, learning by taking a written test led students to be more dependent on the cues provided by the test. Thus, when students had not had practice retrieving the organization of the material, they had more difficulty in the final standardized patient test relative to the final written test in which cues were provided. This finding highlights the need to make sure that the type of retrieval that is practised during learning is a good match for the way in which the information will need to be retrieved and used in the future.

Patient encounters (simulated or real) should be planned for as retrieval practice opportunities. In some cases, the structured practice and feedback afforded by simulated patients may produce superior results, even compared to actual patient encounters. For example, Safdieh et al. (2011, p. 5634) examined performance of second year students on a neurological exam by comparing a group that received their school's standard curriculum of small groups and lectures and a group that received the standard curriculum plus a single standardized patient session dedicated to practising the neurological exam. The final outcome measure was based on an OSCE in which students performed a neurological exam with a standardized patient. Students who practised the exam with a standardized patient demonstrated superior performance compared to students who had received the standard curriculum—a durable effect that persisted over 2 years. Interestingly, the intervention group even outperformed students in the control group who had completed their neurology clerkship, during which they would have had repeated opportunities to practice their neurological exam on actual patients.

The differential effectiveness of instructor-generated practice relative to student-generated practice is also suggested by findings of Larsen et al. (2012). In this study, 71% of students reported studying the review sheets by self-quizzing. However, despite these efforts, the study group performed worse than both the written testing and standardized patient groups. While the differences

between instructor-generated and student-generated testing needs to be more thoroughly explored in future studies, there are several reasons to suspect that student-generated testing may not be as beneficial as instructor-generated testing. First, student-generated testing often occurs immediately after the student is exposed to the material. For example, students might read a passage, cover it up, and then try to recall what was just read. Or they might listen to a lecture on the physical exam and then practise it right away in a small group. Recall is relatively easy when attempted immediately after study—the resulting high level of performance can inflate students' judgements of learning and generate an illusion of competence (Bjork 1994). However, the level of performance immediately after learning is a poor indicator of future retention.

Another potential problem is that when the principle of retrieval effort is considered, immediate retrieval from working or short-term memory is much easier than retrieval from long-term memory (Bjork 1994). Thus, the more difficult recall engendered by an instructor-generated test would be expected to produce greater retention. Another point that may influence the efficacy of student-generated versus instructor-generated testing is the fact that learners will often stop quizzing themselves once they have successfully recalled an item (Kornell and Bjork 2008). Karpicke and Roediger (2007, pp. 151–162) demonstrated that repeated retrieval after a successful initial recall event produces much better retention. Repeated instructor-generated tests may force a learner to continue to practise retrieval after they would have stopped on their own.

Overall, a review of the findings regarding the type of test indicates that once educators have identified their educational objectives, they must think broadly about the types of retrieval practice that will best help them achieve these objectives. Tests should be designed to require the generation of information rather than the recognition of information. In addition, tests should be designed to approximate the settings in which the learning will be applied in the future. Mechanical simulation and simulated patient encounters appear to provide increased retention that surpasses written testing when considering eventual clinical application. However, it is important to note that it may be the type of test (free recall versus cued recall) that is driving the superiority of simulation testing. Although self-testing is better for students than simply studying material by re-reading, instructors must recognize that incorporating retrieval practice opportunities as part of the formal curriculum may produce better results than solely relying on self-testing.

Repetition

Educators must also think about the frequency with which tests are given to students. Although a single test is better than no test, repeated testing will produce greater long-term retention. Several of the examples discussed above show how single tests (especially in the psychomotor domain) have lasting effects. Kromann et al. (2010, pp. 395–401) demonstrated that a single test with cardiac resuscitation led to improved performance with a clinically relevant effect size even after 6 months. The study by Safdieh et al. (2011, p. 5634) showed that a single test with standardized patients produced superior neurological exam performance approximately two years later. Clearly, a single test is effective.

Nevertheless, a multitude of studies have found that even higher levels of retention are possible with repeated retrieval practice. For example, retention on final recall generally improves as the number of successful retrievals of the information increases (Karpicke and Roediger, 2007; Wheeler and Roediger 1992). Item analyses in the study by Larsen et al. (2012) have also found that a higher number of successful retrieval events was associated with a greater likelihood of retention 6 months after initial learning. When considered with regard to the principle of repetition, the study by Karpicke and Roediger (2008, pp. 966–968) described in the first part of the chapter is particularly instructive. Note that in this experiment students learned all word pairs sufficiently well to be recalled at least once— essentially a single test. As the results clearly show, additional study after successful retrieval produced no benefit, yet repeated testing after the first successful retrieval generated superior retention.

Repeated retrieval practice is embedded within the concept of deliberate practice—the idea that deliberate effort to improve performance in a specific domain is critical to becoming an expert in that domain. Deliberate practice has emerged from the simulation literature as a key component of successful simulation (Issenberg et al. 2005). Indeed, the word *practice* implies repeated effort. Deliberate practice includes well-defined learning objectives, which leads to repeated practice with clear outcome measures (McGaghie et al. 2011), and it forms an iterative process of feedback and monitoring that leads to further practice until mastery is reached. In the Best Evidence Medical Education (BEME) review of simulation-based education (Issenberg et al. 2005), deliberate practice was found to be a key element that leads to improvement in patient care. In a meta-analysis of simulation-based medical education compared with traditional curricula, McGaghie et al. (2011, pp. 706–711) demonstrated a combined effect size with a correlation coefficient of 0.71 in favour of improved skill learning through deliberate practice using simulation compared to traditional curricula. Despite the clear benefits of deliberate practice, it is not universally applied. A survey of all anesthesia residents in Canada found that while 94% of residencies used high-fidelity manikin simulation in training, 81% of residents reported not utilizing repeated practice of the simulation scenarios (Price et al. 2010).

Unfortunately, repetition (let alone repeated retrieval practice) is rarely planned into medical education curricula. The importance of repetition becomes apparent when one considers the trajectory of forgetting that naturally occurs once information is learned. Ebbinghaus, the 19th century psychologist, was the first to describe the forgetting curve in which large amounts of forgetting occur quickly, followed by a more slow and steady decline in retention (Ebbinghaus 1967/1885). Ebbinghaus' finding has been confirmed by countless studies over the years, and it is illustrated by the study by Larsen et al. (2009, pp. 959–966), who investigated the effects of repeated tests at 2 week intervals on long-term retention of information that resident physicians learned in a didactic conference. In this study, retention dropped an average of 24% after two weeks between initial learning and a follow-up test with feedback. A third test 2 weeks later showed no further decline—rather, there was a slight increase in performance. Six months after initial learning, performance on the final test declined only slightly compared to the third test. Thus, these results indicate that residents did initially forget some of the information, but testing helped to mitigate forgetting.

Overall, the findings reviewed in this section indicate that repeated testing helps to promote even better long-term retention than a single test. Repeated retrieval practice coupled with feedback maintains initial learning while also fostering further learning, thus resulting in even higher levels of performance (Karpicke and Roediger 2007; Larsen et al 2012, 2013). Repetition also allows the learner to take full advantage of feedback, and to practise to correct errors.

Spacing

The principle of repetition is linked with the concept of spacing or distributing practice over time. An extensive body of literature has demonstrated that spaced practice improves retention of information and motor skills compared to massed practice (Cepeda et al. 2006; Dempster 1989). Spacing is beneficial when implemented within a single learning session (Pyc and Rawson 2009), across multiple sessions compared to a single session (Rohrer and Taylor 2006), and using longer intervals relative to shorter intervals between sessions (Carpenter et al. 2009). Unfortunately, there is no easy recommendation regarding the optimal interval between practice attempts because it seems to depend on the interval over which the information must be retained. Recent meta-analyses indicate that a spacing interval that is 10–20% of the retention interval maximizes retention (Cepeda et al., 2006; 2008).

An important study by Cepeda et al. (2008, pp. 1095–1102) demonstrates the importance of adequate spacing during learning. Subjects were trained to recall 32 disparate trivia facts. Next, they were randomized to receive a second learning session at intervals of from 0 to 105 days. In the second learning session, they were asked to retrieve the facts two times, each with feedback. Subjects were randomized to a final recall test at intervals of 7, 35, 70, and 350 days after the second learning session. The results showed an interaction between the practice interval (i.e. the delay between initial and second learning sessions) and the retention interval (i.e. the delay between the last practice session and final recall). The effect of spacing formed an asymmetric U function. For all intervals, final test performance (i.e. retention) initially improved as the practice interval increased. However, this benefit began to slowly decrease after a point, which was different for each retention interval. Thus, the point of maximal retention that occurred right before the effect began to decline marks the point of optimal spacing (the top of the upside-down U).

Cepeda et al. (2008, pp. 1095–1102) found that a ratio of 10–20% between the practice interval and the retention interval maximized retention. For retention of 7, 35, 70, and 350 days, the optimal spacing was found to be 1, 11, 21, and 21 days, respectively. Although it is unclear if these exact numbers would be equally applicable to all types of education, the principles demonstrated in the study have important practical applications. If educators want learners to retain information for long periods of time (months to years), then they must space practice over weeks and months.

The effects of spacing have been demonstrated in medical education literature also. Using online multiple choice questions covering core topics in urology delivered by email to urology residents, Kerfoot (2009, pp. 2671–2673) demonstrated that spaced learning improved retention over a two-year period compared to massed learning. In another study, Schmidmaier et al. (2011, pp. 1101–1110) investigated a test-enhanced learning paradigm with students using four back-to-back cycles of short answer testing using electronic flashcards covering topics in clinical nephrology. Students who used the repeated testing performed significantly better on a cued-recall test 1 week after initial learning, compared to students who had simply restudied the material. However, there was no difference between the groups at 6 months. These findings stand in contrast to other medical education studies that have found significant differences between testing and control groups at intervals of 2 to 6 months (Larsen et al. 2009; 2012; 2013; Turner et al. 2011). The major difference between these studies, which showed a long-term improvement of retention, and the study Schmidmaier et al. (2011, pp. 1101–1110) conducted was the interval over which tests were spaced during learning. The studies that showed effects over long retrieval intervals used intervals of 1–2 weeks, whereas Schmidmaier et al. (2011, pp. 1101–1110) used much shorter intervals. The differential outcomes of these studies illustrates the findings of Cepeda et al. (2008, pp. 1095–1102)—longer spacing intervals during learning are critical to promoting retention over longer retention intervals.

The study by Larsen et al. (2009, pp. 1174–1181) used 2-week testing intervals and saw a dramatic drop in retention within the first 2 weeks. Subsequent studies by the same group (Larsen et al. 2012, 2013) used 1-week testing intervals and increased the number of testing events from three to four. The more recent studies did not show the dramatic drop in performance during initial learning that was found with the two-week interval. By the end of the initial learning phase in these two newer studies, performance was greater than or equal to performance immediately after learning. The end result was better long-term retention on the final test (albeit comparing across studies with several other differences).

Although these studies did not directly compare different testing intervals, they still illustrate an important practical point. Optimal spacing is a delicate balance—the next test should be delayed long enough to make it effortful and promote retention, but not so long that the information will be forgotten. Different types of memories (i.e. procedural skills versus factual knowledge) may be forgotten at different rates, and therefore the optimal practice interval is likely to differ depending on what students need to learn.

Feedback

For repetition and spacing to have maximal impact on learning from tests, feedback must be provided. Feedback is critical because it helps the learner to close the gap between actual and desired learning (Bangert-Drowns et al. 1991; Hattie and Timperley 2007). Providing feedback after a test enables students to correct memory errors (Butler and Roediger 2008) and maintain correct responses (Butler et al. 2008). Although testing improves retention even without feedback (Glover, 1989; Roediger and Karpicke 2006b; Karpicke and Roediger 2008), feedback can enhance the benefits of testing, especially when learners fail to retrieve the correct response (Kang et al. 2007).

Before discussing the benefits of feedback, it is important to stress that testing increases retention even without feedback. Many studies have found that testing without feedback enhances retention in laboratory settings (Butler and Roediger 2008; Karpicke and Roediger 2010; Roediger and Karpicke 2006b) as well as in real-life medical education settings (Turner et al. 2011). The fact that testing without feedback improves retention is evidence that retrieval has a direct effect on memory, thereby improving retention even in the absence of further studying or exposure to information.

Nevertheless, providing feedback after a test can further improve retention relative to testing without feedback (Butler et al. 2007; Butler and Roediger 2008). For example, Karpicke and Roediger (2010, pp. 116–124) showed when repeated testing was coupled with feedback, the level of retention rose by 25% or more compared to testing without feedback. This finding is an example of

an indirect effect of testing—improved learning through the studying of feedback materials. Agrawal et al. (2012, pp. 326–335) have demonstrated that testing provides important opportunities for monitoring learning because students realize the limits of their knowledge when they confront test questions. Feedback allows learners to then build on those realizations and focus their learning on correcting errors. The act of attempting retrieval before re-studying information may be important to effective learning from feedback. Kornell et al. (2009, pp. 989–998) showed that if learners attempted and failed to answer a difficult question before studying the answer to the question, they remembered more than if they studied the question and answer together. Students are conscious of the learning process from tests. In the study by Larsen et al. (2012), when students were asked how testing affected their learning, they reported that testing allowed them to verify their levels of knowledge, correct mistakes, and work on improved performance.

The timing of feedback may also be an important factor in determining retention. Although many educators and researchers assume that feedback must be given immediately in order to be effective (Mory 2004), recent studies have shown that delaying feedback may be more beneficial (Butler et al. 2007; Butler and Roediger 2008; Metcalfe et al. 2009). However, one critical assumption in recommending delayed feedback is that all of the feedback is fully processed. Often, students are not motivated to go over feedback when it is given after a delay; if full processing of the feedback cannot be guaranteed, then it may be better to give immediate feedback.

The forms of feedback can be as varied as the forms of testing. In addition to the traditional forms of formal testing with formal answers (whether electronic or paper), educators must think about simulation and clinical practice as well. Feedback and debriefing have long been considered important elements of learning from simulation (Rudolph et al. 2008). In a clinical setting, testing may take the form of oral questions given by a supervising clinician or may take the form of a patient encounter. In all of these setting educators should consider what types of feedback are provided. For patient encounters in particular, educators must consider whether clinical supervision is provided in a way that provides meaningful feedback—either from direct observation of clinical activities by the supervising physician or from thorough discussion and follow-up. Feedback amplifies the direct effects of testing and makes tests even more powerful learning interventions.

Conclusions

- Test-enhanced learning represents a powerful learning tool that could be utilized to improve medical education.

- Retrieval practice can take many forms, ranging from written tests to actual patient encounters.

- The form of testing used should be closely aligned with educational objectives.

- Production tests (e.g. short-answer, free recall or simulation) tend to promote better long-term retention than recognition tests (e.g. multiple choice tests).

- Use repeated retrieval practice spaced out over time whenever possible, with intervals that are close enough to prevent forgetting but long enough to require some effort to recall.

- Provide feedback after each test to facilitate learning and improve metacognition.

References

Abbott, E.E. (1909) On the analysis of the factors of recall in the learning process. *Psychol Monogr.* 11: 159–177

Accreditation Council for Graduate Medical Education (2011) *Common Program Requirements.* Chicago, IL: [Online]http://www.acgme.org/acWebsite/dutyHours/dh_dutyhoursCommonPR07012007.pdf Accessed 19 April 2012

Agrawal, S., Norman, G.R., and Eva, K.W. (2012) Influences on medical students' self-regulated learning after test completion. *Med Educ.* 46: 326–335

Bahrick, H.P., Bahrick, L.E., Bahrick, A.S., and Bahrick, P.E. (1993) Maintenance of foreign language vocabulary and the spacing effect. *Psychol Sci.* 4: 316–321

Bangert-Drowns, R.L., Kulik, J.A., and Kulik, C.C. (1991) Effects of frequent classroom testing. *J Educ Res.* 85: 89–99

Bangert-Drowns, R.L., Kulik, C.C., Kulik, J.A., and Morgan, M. (1991) The instructional effect of feedback in test-like events. *Rev Educ Res.* 61: 213–238

Barnett, S.M., and Ceci, S.J. (2002) When and where do we apply what we learn? A taxonomy for far transfer. *Psychol Bull.* 128: 612–637

Bjork, R.A. (1975) Retrieval as a memory modifier. In: R. Solso (ed.) *Information Processing and Cognition: The Loyola Symposium* (pp. 123–144). Hillsdale, NJ: Lawrence Erlbaum Associates

Bjork, R.A. (1994) Memory and metamemory considerations in the training of human beings. In: J. Metcalfe & A. Shimamura (eds) *Metacognition: Knowing about Knowing* (pp. 185–205). Cambridge, MA: MIT

Bjork, R.A., and Bjork, E.L. (1992) A new theory of disuse and an old theory of stimulus fluctuation. In: A. Healy, S. Kosslyn, and R. Shiffrin (eds) *From Learning Processes to Cognitive Processes: Essays in Honor of William K. Estes* (Vol. 2, pp. 35–67). Hillsdale, NJ: Erlbaum

Black, P., and William, D. (1998) Assessment and classroom learning. *Assessment in Education: Principles, Policy, and Practice.* 5: 7–74

Brewer, G.A., and Unsworth, N. (2012) Individual differences in the effects of retrieval from long-term memory. *J Memory Language.* 66: 407–415

Butler, A.C. (2010) Repeated testing produces superior transfer of learning relative to repeated studying. *J Exp Psychol: Learn Memory Cogn.* 36: 1118–1133

Butler, A.C., and Roediger, H.L., III (2007) Testing improves long-term retention in a simulated classroom setting. *Eur J Cogn Psychol.* 19: 514–527

Butler, A.C., and Roediger, H.L., III (2008) Feedback enhances the positive effects and reduces the negative effects of multiple-choice testing. *Memory Cogn.* 36: 604–616

Butler, A.C., Karpicke, J.D., and Roediger, H.L., III (2007) The effect of type and timing of feedback on learning from multiple-choice tests. *J Exp Psychol Appl.* 13: 273–281

Butler, A.C., Karpicke, J.D., and Roediger, H.L., III (2008) Correcting a metacognitive error: Feedback enhances retention of low confidence correct responses. *J Exp Psychol Learn Memory Cogn.* 34: 918–928

Cacamese, S.M., Eubank, K.J., Hebert, R.S., and Wright, S.M. (2004) Conference attendance and performance on the in-training examination in internal medicine. *Med Teach.* 26: 640–644

Carpenter, S.K. (2009) Cue strength as a moderator of the testing effect: The benefits of elaborative retrieval. *J Exp Psychol: Learn Memory Cogn.* 35: 1563–1569

Carpenter, S.K. and Pashler, H. (2007) Testing beyond words: Using tests to enhance visuospatial map learning. *Psychonomic Bull Rev.* 14: 474–478

Carpenter, S.K., Pashler, H., and Cepeda, N.J. (2009) Using tests to enhance 8th grade students' retention of U. S. history facts. *Appl Cogn Psychol.* 23: 760–771

Carrier, M., and Pashler, H. (1992) The influence of retrieval on retention. *Memory Cogn.* 20: 632–642

Carroll, M., Campbell-Ratcliffe, J., Murnane, H., and Perfect, T. (2007) Retrieval-induced forgetting in educational contexts: Monitoring, expertise, text integration, and test format. *Eur J Cogn Psychol.* 19: 580–606

Cepeda, N.J., Pashler, H., Vul, E., Wixted, J.T., and Rohrer, D. (2006) Distributed practice in verbal recall tasks: A review and quantitative synthesis. *Psychol Bull.* 132: 354–380

Cepeda, N.J., Vul, E., Rohrer, D., Wixted, J.T., and Pashler, H. (2008) Spacing effect in learning: A temporal ridgeline of optimal retention. *Psychol Sci.* 19: 1095–1102

Dempster, F.N. (1989) Spacing effects and their implications for theory and practice. *Educ Psychol Rev.* 1: 309–330

Ebbinghaus, H. (1967) *Memory: A Contribution to Experimental Psychology* (H. A. Ruger and C. E. Bussenius, Trans.) New York: Dover (Original work published 1885)

Fitch, M.L., Drucker, A.J., and Norton, J.A. (1951) Frequent testing as a motivating factor in large lecture courses. *J Educ Psychol.* 42: 1–20

FitzGerald, J.D., and Wenger, N.S. (2003) Didactic teaching conferences for IM residents: who attends, and is attendance related to medical certifying examination scores? *Acad Med.* 78: 84–89

Fritz, C.O., Morris, P.E., Acton, M., Voelkel, A.R., and Etkind, R. (2007a) Comparing and combining retrieval practice and the keyword mnemonic for foreign vocabulary learning. *Appl Cogn Psychol.* 21: 499–526

Fritz, C.O., Morris, P.E., Nolan, D., and Singleton, J. (2007b) Expanding retrieval practice: An effective aid to preschool children's learning. *Q J Exp Psychol*, 60, 991–1004.

Gates, A.I. (1917) Recitation as a factor in memorizing. *Arch Psychol.* 6(40): 1–104

Glover, J.A. (1989) The 'testing' phenomenon: Not gone but nearly forgotten. *J Educ Psychol.* 81: 392–399

Hammond, W.A. (1902) *Aristotle's Psychology: A Treatise on the Principle of Life: (De Anima and Parva Naturalia)* Macmillan: New York

Hattie, J. and Timperley, H. (2007) The power of feedback. *Rev of Educ Res.* 77: 81–112

Issenberg, S.B., McGaghie, W.C., Petrusa, E.R., Lee, G.D., and Scalese, R.J. (2005) Features and uses of high-fidelity medical simulations that lead to effective learning: A BEME systematic review. *Med Teach.* 27: 10–28

Jacoby, L.L., Wahlheim, C.N., and Coane, J.H. (2010) Test-enhanced learning of natural concepts: effects on recognition memory, classification, and metacognition. *J Exp Psychol Learn Memory Cogn.* 36: 1441–1451

Johnson, C.I. and Mayer, R.E. (2009) A testing effect with multimedia learning. *J Educ Psychol.* 101: 621–629

Jones, H.E. (1923–1924) The effects of examination n the performance of learning. *Arch Psychol.* 10: 1–70

Kang, S.H.K., McDaniel, M.A. and Pashler, H. (2011) Effects of testing on learning of functions. *Psychonomic Bull Rev.* 18: 998–1005

Kang, S.H.K., McDermott, K.B. and Roediger, H.L., III (2007) Test format and corrective feedback modulate the effect of testing on memory retention. *Eur J Cogn Psychol.* 19: 528–558

Karpicke, J.D., and Blunt, J.R. (2011) Retrieval practice produces more learning than elaborative studying with concept mapping. *Science.* 331: 772–775

Karpicke, J.D. and Roediger, H.L., III (2007) Repeated retrieval during learning is the key to long-term retention. *J Memory Language.* 57: 151–162

Karpicke, J. D. and Roediger, H. L., III (2008) The critical importance of retrieval for learning. *Science.* 15: 966–968

Karpicke, J. D. and Roediger, H. L. III (2010) Is expanding retrieval a superior method for learning text materials? *Memory Cogn.* 38: 116–124

Karpicke, J.D., Butler, A.C., and Roediger, H.L., III (2009) Metacognitive strategies in student learning: Do students practice retrieval when they study on their own? *Memory.* 17: 471–479

Kerfoot, B.P. (2009) Learning benefits of on-line spaced education persist for 2 years. *J Urol.* 181: 2671–2673

Kornell, N. and Bjork, R. A. (2008) Optimising self-regulated study: The benefits—and costs—of dropping flashcards. *Memory.* 16: 125–136

Kornell, N., Hays, M.J., Bjork, R.A. (2009) Unsuccessful retrieval attempts enhance subsequent learning. *J Exp Psychol Learn Memory Cogn.* 35: 989–998

Kromann, C.B., Jensen, M.L., and Ringsted, C. (2009) The effects of testing on skills learning. *Med Educ.* 43: 21–27

Kromann, C.B., Jensen, M.L., and Ringsted, C. (2010) The testing effect on skills might last 6 months. *Adv Health Sci Educ.* 15: 395–401

Kulhavy, R.W., and Stock, W.A. (1989) Feedback in written instruction: The place of response certitude. *Educ Psychol Rev.* 1: 279–308

Larsen, D.P., Butler, A.C., Lawson, A.L., and Roediger, H.L., III (2012) The importance of seeing the patient: Test-enhanced learning with standardized patients and written tests improves clinical application of knowledge. *Adv Health Sci Educ.* doi: 10.1007/s10459-012-9379-7 (published online ahead of print)

Larsen, D.P., Butler, A.C., and Roediger, H.L., III (2008) Test-enhanced learning in medical education. *Med Educ.* 42: 959–966

Larsen, D.P., Butler, A.C., and Roediger, H.L., III (2009) Repeated testing improves long-term retention relative to repeated study: A randomized, controlled trial. *Med Educ.* 43: 1174–1181

Larsen, D.P., Butler, A.C., and Roediger, H.L., III (2013) Comparative effects of test-enhanced learning and self-explanation on long-term retention. *Med Educ.* 47: 674–682

Marton, F. and Saljo, R. (1976) On qualitative differences in learning: I—outcome and process. *Br J Educ Psychol.* 46: 4–11

Mawhinney, V.T., Bostow, D.E., Laws, D.R., Blumenfeld, G.J., and Hopkins, B.L. (1971) A comparison of students studying-behavior produced by daily, weekly, and three-week testing schedules. *J Appl Behav Analysis.* 4: 257–264

McDaniel, M.A., Agarwal, P.K., Huelser, B.J., McDermott, K.B., and Roediger, H.L., III (2011) Test-enhanced learning in a middle school science classroom: The effects of quiz frequency and placement. *J Educ Psychol.* 103: 399–414

McDaniel, M.A., Anderson, J.L., Derbish, M.H., and Morrisette, N. (2007) Testing the testing effect in the classroom. *Eur J Cogn Psychol.* 19: 494–513

McDaniel, M.A., Howard, D.C., and Einstein, G.O. (2009) The read-recite-review study strategy: Effective and portable. *Psychol Sci.* 20: 516–522

McGaghie, W.C., Issenberg, S.B., Cohen, E.R., Barsuk, J.H., and Wayne, D.B. (2011) Does simulation-based medical education with deliberate practice yield better results than traditional clinical education? A meta-analytic comparative review of the evidence. *Acad Med.* 86: 706–711

Metcalfe, J., Kornell, N., and Finn, B. (2009) Delayed versus immediate feedback in children's and adults' vocabulary learning. *Memory Cogn.* 37: 1077–1087

Michael, J. (1991) A behavioral perspective on college teaching. *The Behavior Analyst.* 14: 229–239

Morris, C.D., Bransford, J.D., and Franks, J.J. (1977) Levels of processing versus transfer-appropriate processing. *J Verbal Learn Verbal Behav.* 16: 519–533

Mory, E.H. (2004) Feedback research review. In: D. Jonassen (ed.) *Handbook of Research on Educational Communications and Technology* (pp. 745–783). Mahwah, NJ: Erlbaum

Pashler, H., Bain, P., Bottge, B., et al. (2007) *Organizing instruction and study to improve student learning: A practice guide* (NCER 2007–2004) Washington, DC: National Center for Education Research, Institute of Education Sciences, US Department of Education

Picciano, A., Winter, R., Ballan, D., Bimberg, B., Jacks, M., and Laing, E. (2003) Resident acquisition of knowledge during a noontime conference series. *Fam Med.* 35: 418–422

Phelps, R.P. (2012) The effect of testing on student achievement, 1910–2010. *Int J Testing.* 12: 21–43

Price, J.W., Price, J.R., Pratt, D.D., Collins, J.B., and McDonald, J. (2010) High-fidelity simulation in anesthesiology training: a survey of Canadian anesthesiology residents' simulator experience. *Can J Anesthesiol.* 57: 134–142

Pyc, M.A., and Rawson, K.A. (2009) Testing the retrieval effort hypothesis: Does greater difficulty correctly recalling information lead to higher levels of memory? *J Memory Language.* 60: 437–447

Pyc, M.A., and Rawson, K.A. (2010) Why testing improves memory: Mediator effectiveness hypothesis. *Science.* 330: 335

Pyc, M.A., and Rawson, K.A. (2012) Why is test–restudy practice beneficial for memory? an evaluation of the mediator shift hypothesis. *J Exp Psychol Learn Memory Cogn.* 38 737–746

Rawson, K.A., and Dunlosky, J. (2011) Optimizing schedules of retrieval practice for durable and efficient learning: How much is enough? *J Exp Psychol Gen.* 140: 283–302

Rees, P.J. (1986) Do medical students learn from multiple choice examinations? *Med Educ.* 20: 123–125

Roediger, H.L., III and Butler, A.C. (2011) The critical role of retrieval practice in long-term retention. *Trends Cogn Sci.* 15: 20–27

Roediger, H.L., III and Karpicke, J.D. (2006a) The power of testing memory: Basic research and implications for educational practice. *Perspectives Psychol Sci.* 1: 181–210

Roediger, H.L., III and Karpicke, J.D. (2006b) Test-enhanced learning: Taking memory tests improves long-term retention. *Psychol Sci.* 17: 249–255

Roediger, H.L., III, Gallo, D.A., and Geraci, L. (2002) Processing approaches to cognition: The impetus from the levels of processing framework. *Memory.* 10: 319–332

Rohrer, D. and Taylor, K. (2006) The effects of overlearning and distributed practice on the retention of mathematics knowledge. *Appl Cogn Psychol,* 20: 1209–1224

Rudolph, J.W., Simon, R., Raemer, D.B., and Eppich, W.J. (2008) Debriefing as formative assessment: Closing performance gaps in medical education. *Acad Emerg Med.* 15: 1–7

Safdieh, J.E., Lin, A L., Aizer, J., et al. (2011) Standardized patient outcomes trial (SPOT) in neurology. *Med Educ Online.* 16: 5634

Schmidmaier, R., Ebersbach, R., Schiller, M., Hege, I., Holzer, M., and Fischer, M. R. (2011) Using electronic flashcards to promote learning in medical students: Retesting versus restudying. *Med Educ.* 45: 1101–1110

Schmidt, H.G., and Rikers, R.M.J.P. (2007) How expertise develops in medicine: knowledge encapsulation and illness script formation. *Med Educ.* 41: 1133–1139

Slamecka, N.J., and Katsaiti, L.T. (1988) Normal forgetting of verbal lists as a function of prior testing. *J Exp Psychol Learn Memory Cogn.* 14: 716–727

Smith, P.L., and Ragan, T.J. (2005) *Instructional Design.* Hoboken, NJ: John Wiley and Sons, Inc.

Spitzer, H.F. (1939) Studies in retention. *J Educ Psychol.* 30: 641–656

Thompson, C.P., Wenger, S.K., and Bartling, C.A. (1978) How recall facilitates subsequent recall: A reappraisal. *J Exp Psychol Human Learn Memory.* 4: 210–221

Thorndike, E.L. (1906) The principles of teaching based on psychology. New York: A. G. Seiler

Tse, C.-S., Balota, D.A., and Roediger, H.L. III. (2010) The benefits and costs of repeated testing on the learning of face-name pairs in healthy older adults. *Psychology and Aging.* 25: 833–845

Tulving, E. (1967) The effects of presentation and recall of material in free-recall learning. *J Verbal Learn Verbal Behav.* 6: 175–184

Turner, N.M., Scheffer, R., Custers, E., and Cate, O.T. (2011) Use of unannounced spaced telephone testing to improve retention of knowledge after life-support courses. *Med Teach.* 33: 731–737

Wayne, D.B., Butter, J., Sidall, V.J., et al. (2006a) Mastery learning of advanced cardiac life support skills by internal medicine residents using simulation technology and deliberate practice. *J Gen Intern Med.* 21: 251–256

Wayne, D.B., Siddall, V.J., Butter, J., Fudala, M.J., Wade, L.D., and Feinglass, J., (2006b) A longitudinal study of internal medicine residents' retention of advanced cardiac life support skills. *Acad Med.* 81: S9–S12

Wayne, D.B., Didwania, A., Feinglass, J., Fudala, M.J., Barsuk, J.H., and McGaghie, W.C. (2008) Simulation-based education improves quality of care during cardiac arrest team responses at an academic teaching hospital: A case-control study. *Chest.* 133: 56–61

Wheeler, M.A., and Roediger, H.L., III. (1992) Disparate effects of repeated testing: Reconciling Ballard's (1913) and Bartlett's (1932) results. *Psychol Sci.* 3: 240–245

Winter, R.O., Picciano, A., Bimberg, B., et al. (2007) Resident knowledge acquisition during a block conference series. *Fam Med.* 39: 498–503

Zaromb, F.M. and Roediger, H.L. (2010) The testing effect in free recall is associated with enhanced organization processes. *Memory Cogn.* 38: 995–1008.

CHAPTER 39

Assessing learners' needs

Casey B. White, Lou Ann Cooper, Mary Edwards, and Jennifer Lyon

Learning needs assessment can be undertaken for many reasons, so its purpose should be defined and should determine the method used and the use made of findings.

Janet Grant

Introduction

The assessment of learners' needs is a challenging but critical component of educational programmes. This chapter is intended to be a resource for educators who want to know how best to assess and meet the needs of their learners. Because needs assessment is dynamic and continuous throughout the educational process, we discuss needs assessment in contexts that comprise the primary elements of education and curriculum design, including: learning objectives; teaching and learning methods and approaches; mentoring; assessment of learning; and program evaluation. Learners' needs must be assessed at each of these points for education to have maximum impact (fig. 39.1).

Certain fundamentals should be integrated across the educational continuum; these are addressed at the start of this chapter so as not to emphasize them repetitively in each of the subsequent sections.

Self-regulated (or self-directed) learning

A major function of education should be the development of lifelong learning skills, and self-regulation is a fundamental component of effective lifelong learning (Zimmerman 2002). Thus, in medical education and practice, nurturing self-regulated learning is vital to meeting students' needs, particularly as they advance into clinical clerkships and residency. Self-regulated learning is a cycle with three phases: planning (choose strategies based on goals), practising (implement strategies), and evaluating (determine effectiveness of each strategy in achieving goals). Results of the evaluation are then used for adjustments in the next cycle (Zimmerman 2002; Chalkin 2003). In studies that link goal-setting to self-regulating strategies and self-regulating strategies to achievement, researchers have also reported that self-regulated learning has three distinct elements (Pintrich 1995, 1999):

- controlling available resources
- controlling or modifying self-efficacy or anxiety related to learning and

- controlling cognitive learning strategies such as deep level processing (King 1996).

Zimmerman (2000) reported that self-regulated learning involves self-awareness and self-motivation, the use of specific processes such as setting goals and monitoring progress, and self-motivation qualities such as self-efficacy and intrinsic interest (Zimmerman 2000). Self-regulatory processes can be integrated, practised, tested, and modified by learners under the guidance of teachers, mentors, and others. Evolving research on self-regulation in learning has revealed a social element that includes connections with and feedback from others in the classroom or learning environment (Patrick and Middleton 2002; Chalkin 2003), and that self-regulated learning occurs when students are encouraged to reflectively and strategically engage in learning activities in environments that foster self-regulation (Butler 2002). Unfortunately, despite the evidence, implementing the practice of self-regulated learning remains a challenge for educators (Zimmerman et al. 1996).

Medical educators can help their students become autonomous learners by intentionally integrating opportunities for them to construct their own knowledge (Baxter Magolda 1999) through active and experiential learning activities (Kolb 1984; Lave and Wenger 1991) and to practice goal-setting and self-regulation strategies that can enhance effective learning (Pintrich 1999; Zimmerman 2000). Key to self-regulated learning is the ability to diagnose one's own learning needs, and to address those needs appropriately. Medical educators must be prepared to do their part to help learners become more self-regulating. This includes understanding underlying theory and relevant evidence, making choices about teaching, learning, and assessment that foster acquisition of self-regulating behaviours and providing feedback to learners.

Reflection

Literature on the reflective practitioner dates back to the early 20th century (Dewey 1933). However, in spite of its long history,

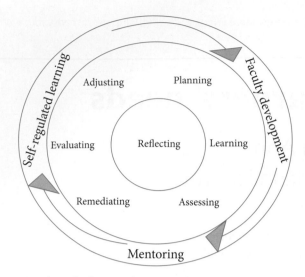

Figure 39.1 The cycle of assessing learning needs.

efforts to help learners acquire skills for reflection have not been fully embraced (Nothnagle et al. 2011). This is due in part to poor training and lack of skills among faculty who are charged with helping students learn how to reflect (McGrath and Higgins 2006).

Many approaches to encourage reflection have been tried (fig. 39.2). However, even when time is set aside to foster reflection, students will not achieve fully developed reflective practice skills without effective facilitation, clear objectives, and appropriate learning environments (Boud 2001).

One problem with achieving learning outcomes related to reflection is the lack of real healthcare contexts in preclinical medical education—this shortcoming makes discussions and writing assignments appear superficial (Law 2011). However, trying to develop reflective practice skills among clinical students is difficult as students are then under pressure to learn clinical skills (Nothnagle et al. 2011).

Electronic portfolios have shown some promise. A recent review of the literature reported that portfolios can help meet learning outcomes across diverse domains that include improved integration of theory with practice, improvement in organizational skills, and better self-awareness and reflection (Buckley et al. 2010).

Mentoring

Formative assessment of learning needs can be conducted effectively within the context of one-to-one interactions between an individual student and instructor, particularly when the interaction is part of a continuing relationship. Such mentoring relationships

Reflective writing assignments (Wald et al. 2012)

Discussing clinical problems

Deliberate practice (Duvivier et al. 2011)

Reflective practice groups (Platzer et al. 1997a, b)

Illness narratives (Charon and DasGupta 2011) and

Electronic portfolios (Challis 2005)

Figure 39.2 Approaches to encourage reflection.

are considered a vital component of student development and students have consistently expressed their desire for mentors (Hauer et al. 2005). The structure of the mentoring relationship can vary, depending on personal and professional needs, available time, and interest of both students and faculty. Four models described in the literature include: apprenticeship (teaching by a more experienced professional), cloning (role-modelling; grooming a successor), nurturing (creating a safe environment), and friendship (peer mentoring) (Ratnapalan 2010).

Regardless of whether the mentoring relationship is developed through formal or informal agreement, there are a number of requirements for success. Qualities of an effective mentor include: good interpersonal skills; knowledge and experience in relevant specialities; the ability to challenge as well as support; an open mind; and willingness to spend time to build and nurture the relationship (Taherian and Shekarchian 2008). A good mentee must respect the mentor's time and effort by being responsible, punctual, and following through on tasks and advice. The mentee must be willing to communicate openly; accept critique in a positive spirit; accept challenges; respect boundaries; and participate fully in establishing goals and making decisions (Rose et al. 2005).

Faculty development

Many educational programmes fail because faculty directly involved in educating students are not sufficiently prepared to do so—they lack training in educational theory and cannot apply that theory in learning contexts (ten Cate et al. 2011; Wilkerson and Irby 1998). Deans often make assumptions that faculty with an interest in teaching naturally possess skills such as writing learning objectives, facilitating learning through discussion, monitoring individual and team progress, providing effective feedback (Kogan et al. 2012), and assessing progress and achievement against objectives (Murdoch-Eaton and Whittle 2012). In addition, faculty often have limited understanding of how to address problems created when students experience academic difficulties, particularly in learning more advanced cognitive skills such as clinical reasoning (Audetat et al. 2012; ten Cate et al. 2011).

Just as the quality of teaching skills matters, so does the quality of programmes designed to help faculty become better teachers (Pernar et al. 2012; Stenfors-Hayes et al. 2011). In addition to informational websites and publications with teaching tips (McKeatchie and Svinicki 2005), there are workshops conducted by those involved in medical education at their home institutions (UVA 2012) and at regional and national meetings (AAMC/MERC 2012), and there are a growing number of institutions that offer graduate degree programmes in health sciences education (UIowa 2005; UIC 2011). In 1996 there were seven of these masters programmes worldwide—as of 2013 there are 76. Along with the growth in the number of programmes, there is a growing expectation that future leaders in medical education will need more formal credentials (Tekian and Harris 2012).

As medical education evolves based on accreditation requirements and changes in healthcare delivery, faculty instructors must be prepared to implement educational approaches that provide opportunities for learners to develop self-regulating habits, so that they are prepared to assess and address their own learning needs. Approaches will put increasing emphasis on learners' participation in and responsibility for their own learning.

Planning

Planning comprises considering what is to be learned, how it will be learned, and how learning will be assessed. Needs assessment helps educators identify what is to be learned—well-written learning objectives guide faculty and students toward achievement of those objectives.

Needs assessment

An assessment of learning needs should be conducted to gather information about learners, including their level of prerequisite knowledge or gaps in learning, and to devise an appropriate intervention (Kaufman et al. 1993; Morrison et al. 2006). Needs assessments also provide data about the effectiveness of previous instruction and can provide the basis for the development of learning objectives. Learning objectives, in turn, guide the choice of learning activities, assessment methods and outcomes for programme evaluation. Needs assessments can be formal or informal—most include elements of both (Grant 2002; Walsh 2006).

Informal and formal approaches to needs assessment and data collection provide flexibility for assessing learners' needs in medical education (Grant 2002). In addition to the types of needs assessments described below, medical educators are making use of other approaches to determine needs including reflection on action (or in action), self-assessment (in diaries, logs, and periodic reviews), peer review, observation, and practice review (Grant 2002). A common practice in conducting a needs assessment is to assess the health needs of the community in order to align educational objectives with the health of the population (Kanashiro et al. 2007).

Framing a formal needs assessment as a research project can help medical educators with limited experience navigate the process. The four major phases of needs assessment are planning, data collection, data analysis and reporting—see fig. 39.3 (Bradshaw 1972; Grant 2002; Morrison et al. 2006). Performing formal needs assessment will guide the planning process and ensure that learners' needs are reflected throughout the instructional process.

The first stage is planning. Decisions made during this phase include selecting participants and deciding on data collection and analysis methods.

The second stage is data collection. This will involve using a variety of methods to collect quantitative and qualitative data. Data collected may be criterion-referenced (comparing the learners' data with expected standards) or comparative (comparing the learners' data with that of their peers).

The third stage is data analysis; this is determined by the types of data collected. For quantitative data this means selecting the correct statistical tests. For qualitative data this means reviewing comments for themes.

The fourth and final stage is reporting. Results should be reported in the format best suited for the data and the audience.

Learning outcomes

Information from needs assessments informs subsequent decisions relevant to curricular planning and the development of instructional content. Perhaps the most critical step in developing learner-centred instruction is developing learning outcomes. Learning outcomes serve multiple functions. First, they guide educators in designing learning that is appropriate and effective for the audience. Second, they guide decisions about assessing student learning because the assessments should measure whether or not outcomes have been achieved. Lastly, they serve as a guide to help students manage their own learning by clearly stating the expected outcomes.

Taxonomies can provide useful guidance. Educators have classified learning into three domains: knowledge, skills, and attitudes (Bloom 1956; Harrow 1972; Krathwohl et al. 1964; Simpson 1972). When assessing learners' needs and designing or modifying instruction it is important to consider all three domains.

Individualized learning plans

In learner-centred education, personal learning plans can equip learners with autonomy over what and how they are learning. They provide learners with self-generated information on learning needs. From a theoretical standpoint, personal learning plans are aligned with principles of adult learning theory and should assist students in achieving deeper learning (Marton and Säljö, 1984a, b).

There are various formats for personal learning plans, but a common feature is the learner's creation of personal learning outcomes as a part of guiding and assessing their own learning (Challis 2000; Walsh 2006). Personal learning outcomes are developed by students and intended to state what they wish to achieve from instruction. Learning plans also include the strategies they will use to achieve learning outcomes, plans to assess progress, and timelines. Vital to the success of learning plans is clear guidance and feedback as the plan is developed, and feedback on progress toward achievement of outcomes (Challis 2000).

Learning

Learning theory and methods

There is a broad range of theories about how learning occurs and how best to provide instruction that supports learning. For many years, the more traditional format was a *behaviourist* approach, which looks for observable behaviour change as evidence of learning (Skinner 1938; Watson 1914). Behaviourist instruction is generally didactic, with the instructor as the expert imparting knowledge to the learner. In contrast to behaviourism, the *constructivist* approach is based on the belief that learning is the result of an interaction

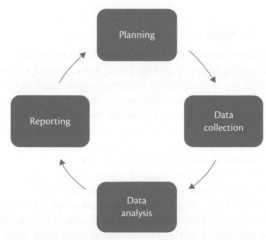

Figure 39.3 Phases of needs assessment.

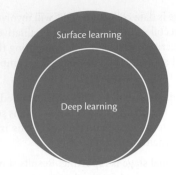

Figure 39.4 Surface and deep learning.

between experiences and ideas (Piaget 1950, 1967; Shepard et al. 2005; Swanwick 2010). Instruction based on constructivist principles promotes the learners' construction of new knowledge based on their previous experiences, and views the learner as an active participant in the learning process with the instructor as facilitator. Social learning theory emphasizes the social context of learning (Lave and Wenger 1991; Swanwick 2010; Vygotsky 1978), through which the student is exposed to the authentic setting, where they observe experienced clinicians and become acclimatized to the environment.

Recent curriculum redesign in medical schools has focused on adopting more active approaches to learning (Abbott et al. 2010; Barondess 1985; Barzansky et al. 2000; Borkan et al. 2009; Cunningham et al. 2006; Des Marchais 1993; Fields et al. 1998; Jones et al. 2001; Miflin 1999). Particular elements in active learning such as giving responsibility to learners helps prepare students for the clinical clerkships in which they are expected to be responsible for their learning. As residents they will also be expected to self-assess their knowledge and skills and develop plans for addressing deficits.

Learning can be surface or deep (fig. 39.4). Surface learning involves rote memorization of discrete data without conceptual integration, while deep learning incorporates new information into existing knowledge and makes conceptual connections (Heijne-Penninga et al. 2008; Papinczak et al. 2008; Svirko and Mellanby 2008). Medical students have expressed a preference for active learning approaches (Śniadecki et al. 2011; Usmani et al. 2011; Van Hell et al. 2009), and research shows improved performance and deeper learning when information is more closely integrated into the context of medical practice (Dornan et al. 2007; Findlater et al. 2012). For example, one study found that 72% of students preferred learning radiology through active techniques (Zou et al. 2011).

In spite of known benefits and student preference for learning in a clinical context, active learning can be a challenging adjustment for students. It also requires additional effort and planning on the part of educators, who must be deliberate in assuring that methods will help students to achieve outcomes (Abraham et al. 2011; Smith and Mathias 2007). Developing active, critical, self-regulating learning habits requires a great deal of effort, motivation, and flexibility from both students and instructors (Karakitsiou et al. 2012). Medical educators need to assess student readiness; need to understand how to encourage active learning and critical thinking skills; and carefully watch—and be ready to support—individuals who struggle with the transition to active learning.

Learning styles

One way to assess learning needs is to identify students' learning styles. Multiple tools, such as the VARK inventory (visual, audio, read/write, kinetic) (Fleming 2001), Kolb's Learning Styles Inventory (Kolb 1984), and the Myers Brigg Type Indicator (Myers and Myers 1980), can be used to identify individual preferences. However, although most educators agree that 'individuals differ in regard to what mode of instruction or study is most effective for them' (Pashler et al. 2010), there is significant controversy about whether tailoring instructional methods to match students' preferences actually improves learning (Pashler et al. 2010). There is also increasing evidence that many learners cannot be categorized within one particular style. Not only are individuals often multimodal (i.e. comfortable learning through more than one style), their preferences may also vary over time, circumstance and context (Gurpinar et al. 2011). For example, in a study of first-year medical students using the VARK inventory, researchers found that while the students do have preferences for particular ways of learning, the majority preferred multiple modes (Lujan and DiCarlo 2006). Overall, there is agreement that students do have learning preferences and can also benefit from being exposed to a variety of learning formats. Providing resources in a variety of modes gives learners choice and a sense of control over their learning, which is vital to development of self-regulated learning habits.

Learning resources

Use of electronic devices for the delivery of learning resources has become commonplace in medical education, and provides enormous flexibility to meet students' needs and to review how effectively needs have been met (Glicksman et al. 2009; Kröncke, 2010; McNulty et al. 2009; Poulton et al. 2009). As technology continues to develop, point-of-care mobile resources that provide just in time access to important information are becoming increasingly deployed in medical education (Boruff and Bilodeau 2012; Brunet et al. 2011; Chatterley and Chojecki 2010, Davies et al. 2012; Flannigan and McAloon, 2011).

Understanding learning preferences and making adjustments to accommodate multiple styles is an important and continuously evolving element of assessing learners' needs. Faculty should also be involved in selecting learning resources. They should evaluate whether students have the skills necessary to find, assess, and use available resources to ensure that they have the opportunity to succeed.

Study strategies

Just as students vary in their preferences for learning, they also vary in their approaches to studying. Here, self-regulated learning and motivation are important, as study strategies tend to be unique and can be dynamic depending on the material to be learned, the timing, the environment, the available resources, and the peer-interactions (Ward et al. 2011; Yeung and Dixon-Woods 2010). For example, a student might adopt one approach for memorizing facts and another for developing a hands-on skill.

Specific strategies can include visualization, mnemonics and other memory devices, conceptual building (layering concepts upon each other), diagramming (mental or physical drawing), hands-on rehearsal (developing physical as well as mental memory), or speaking/listening/discussion (Lonka et al. 1994; White and Gruppen 2007). The selection of learning strategies is closely linked with learning style, as a student with a visual learning preference will be more likely to select more visually oriented study techniques. However, the same student, needing to learn a skill or acquire knowledge that requires a different technique will, in many cases, adapt a learning strategy to meet that need (Pandey and Zimitat 2007; Ward et al. 2011). Additional learning strategy choices focus on the learning environment and timing. Factors affecting a student's choice of setting may include the level of noise, solitary versus group study, location (indoor or outdoor), privacy (home, library cubicle, public café), time of day (or night), length of period devoted to learning, and how often the student studies (White et al. 2007).

Difficulties can evolve in any setting where students have not fully developed or applied their metacognitive skills, resulting in selection of inappropriate or less effective learning strategies (Reid et al. 2005). Students might not effectively connect study strategy with learning style, environment, timing, available resources, or other personal or professional factors, particularly if motivation is limited. Instructors can help by acting as role models and providing additional monitoring of student learning activity, effective formative feedback, and motivational support (Kenny et al. 2003; Maudsley, 2001; McKimm and Swanwick 2009, White et al. 2007).

Learning environment

The importance and influence of the physical and intellectual learning environments in medical education are well documented (Boor et al. 2008; Genn, 2001a, b; Roff 2005; Veerapen and McAleer 2010). The physical learning environment (including the campus, classrooms, libraries, study rooms, clinical spaces, and laboratories) is usually influenced by the curriculum, learning needs, and content. Spaces such as lecture halls are necessary for larger group activities, whereas quiet spaces might be more appropriate for individual acquisition of data. Small group discussion tends to be more effective in smaller spaces, although there are small group pedagogies (e.g. think-pair-share) that can work in large group spaces. For experiential or situated learning, context is essential—and it may be simulated or authentic. There are also emotional, intellectual and personal elements to learning environments that provide a culture of encouragement for learners while fostering a spirit of inquiry, discovery, and collaboration within the educational culture (Genn, 2001a, b).

The clinical context is the most authentic and the most challenging environment. The transition from more traditional preclinical education to clinical training can be stressful for students (Godefrooij et al. 2010; Prince et al. 2005). Although patient care in the real world is vital to clinical training, when the two are in conflict, patient care trumps education. Thus, it is critical that students in the clinical environment possess the skills to manage their own learning, including the ability to self-assess their strengths and weaknesses (White et al. 2007).

When assessing learners' needs it is important to have an understanding of various elements including

- the ways in which learning occurs
- how learning styles can impact instructional approaches
- learning resources
- study strategies and
- the learning environment.

The ways in which these elements interact to influence learning impacts the assessment of learners' needs.

Assessing

It is often said that assessment drives the curriculum—largely because it plays an integral role in communicating important curricular outcomes. To be effective, assessment should provide learners with meaningful feedback on their strengths and weaknesses that they can then use in directing their own learning; it should also provide critical information to instructors, who can then identify specific learning needs. An assessment programme should be subjected to critical review to include evidence of validity, reliability, educational impact, cost, and acceptability (Schuwirth and van der Vleuten 2010; Van der Vleuten et al. 1996).

Formative and summative assessment

If students are to play a role in assessing and addressing their own learning needs (and they should be expected to do this), they will need feedback against which to gauge their own assessment. Although it can take many forms, feedback is generally defined as formative or summative. Formative feedback supports and enhances learning; it is designed to reinforce good performance and to improve poor performance (Cantillon and Sargeant 2008). Summative feedback is documentation of achievement based on overall behaviour, given at the end of an educational experience (Bienstock et al. 2007).

Formative assessment

In medical education learners have consistently complained that they do not receive sufficient feedback (De et al. 2004). There is evidence that learners do not recognize feedback when they are getting it, and part of the reason for that might be that educators are not providing feedback that is effective (Bing-You and Trowbridge 2009). In particular, we all have a psychological need to protect our egos so we try to see ourselves in the best light possible; this is one reason that self-assessment is so difficult for many (Baumeister 1998; Kruger and Dunning 1999). Negative feedback that feels like a personal attack can trigger emotions such as anger, guilt and self-doubt. These emotions can in turn block feedback from reaching the learner at a cognitive level, where it can be internalized, reflected upon and used to improve performance (Bing-You and Trowbridge 2009).

There is ample evidence to guide instructors in providing formative feedback that achieves the goal of helping learners understand their own strengths and weaknesses so they can improve their performance. Fairly simple guidelines advise that feedback should be a two-way conversation between learner and teacher; should be well timed; should be based on first-hand data about specific behaviours; should be phrased in descriptive and non-evaluative language; and should address decisions and actions rather than intentions and interpretations (Ende 1983).

Summative assessment

In the educational literature, there has been much less attention paid to summative feedback. Because summative feedback involves passing judgement about achievement compared with standards, it is often viewed negatively (Taras 2005). These judgements carry high stakes, and can lead students to focus on learning for external rewards, rather than motivating them to learn for learning's sake

(Joughin 2010). This extrinsic motivation has also been linked to surface learning, while deep learning is generally what medical educators hope to achieve with their students (Entwistle 1997).

Another concern about summative assessment is whether the grade that is assigned is a fair representation of student achievement (Yorke 2010). The more complex the learning to be judged, the more difficult it is to establish standards that accurately measure learning. To make matters more complicated, theorists argue that learners might not have direct, conscious access to all they know because knowledge is tacit and distributed and may not be easily captured for formal assessment (Knight 2002). Yet another concern about summative assessment is that it can become completely separated from formative assessment (Taras 2005), in fact so much so that some researchers have claimed that summative and formative have split into 'two mutually exclusive entities' based on their separate functions (Bloom 1971).

These issues are all relevant to medical education, particularly in the assessment of clinical skills and knowledge. Medical schools struggle to ensure that scoring in the clinical setting is coherent and standardized (Adler et al. 2011; Huntley et al. 2012; Karabilgin et al. 2012). To ensure valid and reliable assessment, many schools have adopted objective structured clinical examinations (OSCEs), in which performance is scored by trained faculty or standardized patients. However, checklists frequently used to measure OSCE performance can have too much granularity, which can threaten validity, especially in the measurement of more complex, higher order domains (Gupta et al. 2011; Ponton-Carss et al. 2011; Weissman 2011).

Careful steps need to be taken to ensure reliability and validity of scoring instruments for summative assessments. To avoid making judgements based on measurements that are inadequate or not standardized, researchers recommend using multiple methods to assess clinical performance, making sure there are adequate observations on which to base the summative assessment, and faculty development to improve standardization (Gupta et al. 2011; Lee and Wimmers 2011).

Written examinations (MCQs)

Written examinations that employ 'single-best option' multiple choice questions (MCQs) select items from a range of all possible questions. The items selected must be representative of the content domain (Downing 2002) and without technical flaws (Downing 2005). When the number of items is too small or the content sampled is too narrow, reliability can be affected. The reliability of MCQ tests is sensitive to test length, how well the items discriminate, time factors, and the homogeneity of the test-takers (Downing 2004).

Examinations using MCQs are cost efficient and make efficient use of time to assess knowledge and its application. Locally developed MCQ examinations can be tailored to specific learning objectives, and results can be used to evaluate the relative strengths and weaknesses of individual learners for both formative and summative feedback.

Classroom assessment

Classroom assessment techniques (CATs) are designed to help instructors and their students monitor learning against course objectives. CATs are a method of formative assessment focused on learning rather than teaching (Angelo and Cross 1993). The process is focused on answering three fundamental questions:

- What are essential knowledge, skills and attitudes am I trying to teach (learning objectives)?
- How well are my students learning?
- How effectively am I teaching?

Specific techniques include 'the one-minute paper' (what is the most important thing you learned during this class?) and 'the muddiest point' (what was confusing to you today?) (Angelo and Cross 1993; Holladay, 2002). Important elements of CAT methodology include reporting back to students what was learned from their feedback, and a willingness to modify teaching/learning approaches based on the feedback.

A significant advantage of CATs is that instructors are not surprised after an assessment to discover that students have not necessarily learned what has been taught. Information from standard test performance is difficult to use to improve learning because often the information is acquired too late to be useful (Leahy et al. 2005). CATs allow instructors time to identify learning gaps and to address them prior to a graded assessment.

Workplace assessment

Workplace-based assessment is critical in medical education because it involves assessing critical knowledge, skills, and behaviours in authentic settings (Holmboe and Hawkins 2008). Typically, methods used for workplace-based assessment fall into one of three categories: observation, discussion of clinical cases, or feedback from peers, coworkers and patients (also known as 360 degree assessment) (fig. 39.5).

There are significant reliability (and thus validity) problems associated with rater-based observation and assessment, and in particular with rater-based assessment of clinical performance (Van Der Vleuten 2000). The bias inherent in human judgement is revealed in significant variations amongst raters in behaviours they notice, their ability to identify true competence and even their agreement on what behaviours and what level of performance provide evidence that competencies have been achieved (Sadler 2009; Williams et al. 2003; McGill et al. 2011). This variability in ratings influences the reliability of oral and written feedback that learners receive from clinical instructors (Kogan et al. 2012). However, an important element of workplace-based assessment is the opportunity it provides for observation followed by formative assessment and feedback,

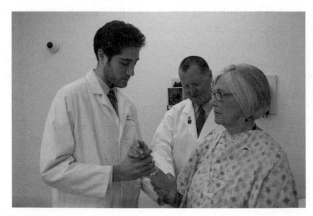

Figure 39.5 Assessing learning needs in the clinical environment.

which have significant potential for identifying learners' needs and developing a plan for addressing those needs.

There is currently no consensus in the literature linking observation with improvements in performance. Studies examining multisource workplace feedback provide the strongest evidence linking workplace-based assessment with improved performance (Fidler et al. 1999; Smither et al. 2005). However, some studies have found that recipients of multisource feedback were unlikely to make practice changes, even if scores indicated changes were needed (Lockyer et al. 2003).

Additional studies examining the reliability and validity of workplace assessment are needed. In the meantime, low inter-rater reliability among those assessing clinical skills based on observation, and limited exploration and use of multisource feedback approaches, has led to more widespread use of OSCEs.

Objective structured clinical examinations (OSCEs)

OSCEs are used in medical education to assess the knowledge, skills, and attitudes of students in the contexts of history taking, physical examination, and professional behaviours. They date back to the late 1970s, when they were described as 'a timed examination in which students interact with a series of simulated patients in stations that may involve history-taking, physical examination, counselling or patient management' (Harden and Gleeson 1979).

OSCEs typically have a series of stations, each of which presents a clinical challenge. Research recommends the use of a larger number of stations and multiple scorers to improve reliability. Standardized patients are commonly used in OSCE stations; sometimes these individuals are trained actors (Norman et al. 1982), but often they are not (Rubin and Philp, 1998). There are advantages in the use of standardized patients versus real patients—training reduces variability in challenges presented to students (Norman et al. 1985), they can simulate scenarios that would be distressing to real patients, and they are available and adaptable. There are also several disadvantages—they tend to become 'textbook patients' who do not portray the idiosyncrasies of real patients (Wallace et al. 2002), and the costs can be high (Hodges et al. 1997).

OSCEs can be used to provide formative or summative feedback to learners so that gaps in knowledge, skills and behaviours can be addressed; however, they can also provide feedback to instructors about potential weaknesses in a curriculum (Casey et al. 2009). Because of the evidence that well-designed OSCEs are feasible, reliable, and valid (Hodges et al. 1998), medical schools around the world have adopted them, as has the National Board of Medical Examiners (USMLE 2012). Researchers caution, however, that OSCEs are most reliable when they incorporate a relatively large number of stations and more than one scorer is used to judge performance.

Self-assessment

The use and benefits of self-assessment as a tool to enhance learning are well documented in the academic literature (Claxton 1995; Darrow et al. 2002; Schunk 1990). Self-assessment is a skill that can lead to improvements in metacognitive development and academic achievement; it can also have positive effects on teacher-learner relationships that in turn enhance learning.

Self-assessment can also empower students to become more responsible for their own learning (Banta et al. 1996). It can encourage them to identify and address their own learning needs. When combined with self-reflection, self-assessment can help students

better understand themselves as learners, which can in turn increase motivation and knowledge (Wlodkowski and Ginsberg 1995). Assessing one's own progress, even against standards set by experts, begins a shift of responsibility for learning from teacher to student that also shifts the power differential in the learning process (Baxter Magolda 1999; Kegan 1994).

Educators caution that self-assessment must be integrated thoughtfully and meaningfully into curricula in order to reap benefits; it must be 'part of more pervasive cultural shifts in the classroom' (Shepard 2000). In fact, self-assessment is often described in the context of approaches to teaching that are more active than the traditional classroom setting, in which teachers lecture and students take notes. Also, self-assessment is often combined with a student-centred approach to learning that engages students in developing individual portfolios for learning and/or taking some responsibility for peer assessment. There is evidence of a variety of positive self-assessment outcomes: these include improved cognitive performance; non-cognitive changes (Gordon 1992); more independent approaches to learning; increased self-assessment accuracy; and better critical thinking (King and Kitchener 1994 and Baxter Magolda 1999).

This research and its outcomes were not applied to medical education for many years. However, a growing focus on lifelong learning has led to medical education's accrediting agencies now mandating changes in educational practices across the continuum of medical education. Medical schools are expected to provide their students with opportunities for active learning that integrate self-assessment into the formative assessment process, and residents are expected to integrate formative feedback with self-generated feedback into their daily practice (ACGME 2011). It is now common for students to participate in approaches such as collaborative learning, peer teaching, team-based learning and simulation—all of which increase their responsibility for their own learning, and integrate ongoing self-assessment of progress toward goals.

The struggling learner

Learning outcomes guide assessment and should specifically describe performance that indicates satisfactory mastery of content (Morrison et al. 2006). When assessments indicate that students have not mastered content as expected, their self-efficacy and motivation to learn can be affected (Pintrich 2003). As importantly, they can be at risk for subsequent deficiencies, as new content builds upon previous content.

Once struggling learners have been identified it is necessary to determine the root cause of the deficiencies in order to begin a remediation process. Problem learners can be classified into four categories: affective, cognitive, structural, and interpersonal (Chesser-Smyth 2005; Cleland et al. 2010; Quirk 1994; Tooth et al. 1989; White et al. 2009). Affective problems are a result of the learner dealing with external personal issues that affect their memory, motivation, and attention. Cognitive problems include issues with written communication, spatial perception, oral communication, integrating information, and knowledge acquisition. Cognitive learning problems are the most straightforward to remediate because they have clear-cut causes. Structured learning problems relate to the learner's time management and study skills. Interpersonal learning problems involve difficulties interacting with others (Quirk 1994; White et al. 2009).

In order for remediation to succeed, learners must play a critical role in helping themselves improve performance. Reflection on reasons for performance that does not meet expected standards and attribution of causes underlying poor performance are critical. Learners who remediate most successfully attribute their performance to their own insufficient effort and believe that they can control and so improve their performance (Weiner 1980, 1992). Students should be encouraged to reflect upon their performance and discuss why it did not meet expectations (Saxena et al. 2009; Sayer et al. 2002; Winston et al. 2010).

Remediation strategies should be based upon the nature of the problem—examples include additional academic tutoring, one-on-one mentoring, establishing personal goals and learning plans, review of study strategies, and online tutorials. While remediation typically occurs after a performance deficit is noted on a summative assessment, remediation after formative assessment is most effective (Cleland et al. 2010). Effective self-assessment provides learners with important information about their own progress; if they are able to self-identify gaps in their learning, they are in essence identifying learning needs, and can then request additional support and remediation (White et al. 2009).

Evaluating

Programme evaluation is an essential component of the educational process that 'closes the loop', thus ensuring that the curriculum is evolving to meet the needs of both learners and institution. Rather than a focus on the learning needs of specific individuals, in order to identify curricular areas where teaching and learning can be improved, the goals of evaluation are more commonly linked to aggregated outcomes (Morrison 2003). Evaluation methods can be applied to a single educational module or classroom activity, individual courses or clerkships, or the entire programme of medical education (Frye and Hemmer 2012).

Kirkpatrick (2006) describes an evaluation framework that has gained traction in medical education. As modified by Freeth et al. (2002), Kirkpatrick's levels of evaluation consist of: (1) reaction (learner satisfaction), (2) learning outcomes (changes in attitudes, knowledge or skills acquired), (3) behaviour (performance improvement; behaviour applied in subsequent work roles), and (4) results (patient/health outcomes). The model promotes the value of measuring outcomes at multiple levels and makes an important distinction between learning and the application of knowledge and skills; it also recognizes the need to align evaluation results with institutional goals. The model has been criticized because it does not explicitly address the context and processes of learning and it assumes that evidence collected at higher levels is superior to that at lower levels (Holton 1996; Yardley and Dornan 2012).

There are alternatives to Kirkpatrick's levels of evaluation that include an examination of the educational process and context variables. The 3-P model of learning and teaching is learner-centred (Biggs 1993) and includes

- presage factors (sociopolitical context for education, individual characteristics of the teachers and learners)
- process factors (strategies/approaches to learning) and
- product factors (learning outcomes).

Student context refers to students' motivation, values and expectations, learning styles, and prior knowledge and skills. Teacher context includes the classroom or institutional teaching environment, the structure and content of the curriculum, the teaching methods, and the evaluations. Process is the approach to learning that results from interaction between the student and teacher contexts. Learning outcomes are the result of interactions between presage and process factors.

Other models that are frequently used in the evaluation of medical education programmes include the logic model (Logic Model Development Guide 2003) and the CIPP (context, inputs, processes, and products) model (Stufflebeam 2000). A logic model is based on systems theory and can be useful in both the planning and evaluation of an educational programme or its individual components. In the course of alternating the focus among context, inputs, and process, the CIPP model provides formative evaluation focused on programme improvement.

Evaluation methods should incorporate quantitative and qualitative data to examine both educational processes and outcomes. For effective decision-making, the evaluation plan should also include both formative and summative methods. Formative evaluation focuses on monitoring programme activities and short-term outcomes and provides information for the purpose of improvement of the educational programme (e.g., mid-course corrections). Programme evaluation tends to focus on learning outcomes; however, understanding how students learn can contribute much to improving what they learn (Wilkes and Bligh, 1999). In summative evaluation, the focus is on demonstrating effectiveness by examining intermediate and long-term learning outcomes and process objectives, and on determining value by appraising key quality indicators (Cook 2010).

Conclusions

- Assessing learners' needs is a dynamic cyclical process that occurs throughout all phases of education: planning, learning, assessing and evaluating.

- Ongoing and comprehensive faculty development is critical to effective teaching and learning.

- Learners must develop skills and habits to effectively monitor their progress, assess their performance against goals, and adjust strategies as needed to achieve goals.

- External feedback provides learners with key information on their progress—mentoring relationships can help in this regard.

References

AAMC/MERC (2012) *Medical Education Research Certificate (MERC) Program* [Online]. Washington, DC. https://www.aamc.org/members/gea/merc/ Accessed 7 January 2012

Abbott, A., Sullivan, M., Nyquist, J., Mylona, E., and Taylor, C. (2010) A 'medical student practice profile' as the foundation for a case-based curriculum revision. *Teach Learn Medic.* 22: 307–311

Abraham, R.R., Fisher, M., Kamath, A., Izzati, T.A., Nabila, S., and Atikah, N.N. (2011) Exploring first-year undergraduate medical students' self-directed learning readiness to physiology. *Adv Physiol Educ.* 35: 393–395

ACGME (2011) *The Accreditation Council for Graduate Medical Education Approved Standards* [Online]. ACGME. http://www.acgme-2010standards.org/index.html Accessed 24 May 2012

Adler, M.D., Vozenilek, J.A., Trainor, J.L., et al. (2011) Comparison of checklist and anchored global rating instruments for performance rating of simulated pediatric emergencies. *Simulation in Healthcare.* 6: 18

Angelo, T.A., and Cross, K.P. (1993) *Classroom Assessment Techniques*. San Francisco: Jossey-Bass Publishers

Audetat, M.C., Dory, V., Nendaz, M., et al. (2012) What is so difficult about managing clinical reasoning difficulties? *Med Educ*. 46: 216–227

Banta, T.W., Lund, J.P., Black, K.E., and Oblander, F.W. (1996) *Assessment in Practice: Putting principles to work on college campuses*. San Francisco: Jossey-Bass

Barondess, J.A. (1985) The GPEP Report: I. Preparation for Medical School. *Ann Intern Med*. 103: 138–139

Barzansky, B., Jonas, H.S., and Etzel, S.I. (2000) Educational programmes in US medical schools, 1999–2000. *JAMA*. 284: 1114–1120

Baumeister, R.F. (1998) *The Self*. New York: McGraw-Hill

Baxter Magolda, M.B. (1999) *Creating Contexts for Learning and Self-authorship: Constructive-Developmental Pedagogy*. Nashville, TN: Vanderbilt University Press

Bienstock, J.L., Katz, N.T., Cox, S.M., Hueppchen, N., Erickson, S., and Puscheck, E.E. (2007) To the point: medical education reviews—providing feedback. *Am J Obstet Gynecol*. 196: 508–513

Biggs, J.B. (1993) From theory to practice: a cognitive systems approach. *Higher Educ Res. Devel*. 12: 73–85

Bing-You, R.G., and Trowbridge, R.L. (2009) Why medical educators may be failing at feedback. *JAMA*. 302: 1330–1331

Bloom, B.S. (1956) *Taxonomy of Educational Objectives; the classification of educational goals*. New York: Longmans, Green

Bloom, B.S. (1971) *Handbook on Formative and Summative Evaluation of Student Learning*. New York: McGraw-Hill

Boor, K., Scheele, F., van der Vleuten, C.P.M., Teunissen, P.W., Den Breejen, E.M.E., and Scherpbier, A.J.J.A. (2008) How undergraduate clinical learning climates differ: a multi-method case study. *Med Educ*. 42: 1029–1036

Borkan, J., Feldmann, E., Dollase, R., and Gruppuso, P. (2009) Redesigning the clinical curriculum at the Warren Alpert Medical School of Brown University. *Med Health. Rhode Island*. 92: 300

Boruff, J.T. and Bilodeau, E. (2012) Creating a mobile subject guide to improve access to point-of-care resources for medical students: a case study. *J Med Lib Ass JMLA*. 100: 55

Boud, D. (2001) Using journal writing to enhance reflective practice. *New Directions for Adult and Continuing Education*. 2001: 9–18

Bradshaw, J. (1972) The concept of social need. *New Society*. 30: 640–643

Brunet, P., Cuggia, M., and Le Beux, P. (2011) Recording and podcasting of lectures for students of medical school. *Studies in Health Technology and Informatics*. 169: 248

Buckley, S., Coleman, J., and Khan, K. (2010) Best evidence on the educational effects of undergraduate portfolios. *Clin Teach*. 7: 187–191

Butler, D.L. (2002) Qualitative approaches to investigating self-regulated learning: contributions and challenges. *Educ Psychol*. 37: 59–63

Cantillon, P. and Sargeant, J. (2008) Teaching rounds: giving feedback in clinical settings. *BMJ*. 337: 1292–1294

Casey, P.M., Goepfert, A.R., Espey, E.L., et al. (2009) To the point: reviews in medical education—the Objective Structured Clinical Examination. *Am J Obstet Gynecol*. 200: 25–34

Chalkin, S. (ed.) (2003) *The Zone of Proximal Development in Vygotsky's Analysis of Learning Instruction*. Cambridge: Cambridge University Press

Challis, M. (2000) AMEE Medical Education Guide No. 19: Personal learning plans. *Med Teach*. 22: 225–236

Challis, D. (2005) Towards the mature ePortfolio: Some implications for higher education. *Can J Learn Technol* [Online], 31(3) Web.18. http://www.cjlt.ca/index.php/cjlt/article/view/93/87 Accessed 18 Apr 2012

Charon, R. and DasGupta, S. (2011) Narrative medicine, or a sense of story. *Lit Med*. 29: vii–xiii

Chatterley, T. and Chojecki, D. 2010. Personal digital assistant usage among undergraduate medical students: exploring trends, barriers, and the advent of smartphones. *J Med Lib Ass JMLA*. 98: 157

Chesser-Smyth, P.A. (2005) The lived experiences of general student nurses on their first clinical placement: A phenomenological study. *Nurse Educ Pract*. 5: 320–327

Claxton, G. (1995) What kind of learning does self-assessment drive? Developing a 'nose' for quality: comments on Klenowski (1995). *Assess Educ*. 2: 339–343

Cleland, J., Mackenzie, R., Ross, S., Sinclair, H., and Lee, A. (2010) A remedial intervention linked to a formative assessment is effective in terms of improving student performance in subsequent degree examinations. *Med Teach*. 32: 185–190

Cook, D.A. (2010) Twelve tips for evaluating educational programs. *Med Teach*. 32: 296–301

Cunningham, C.E., Deal, K., Neville, A., Rimas, H., and Lohfeld, L. (2006) Modeling the problem-based learning preferences of McMaster University undergraduate medical students using a discrete choice conjoint experiment. *Adv Health Sci Educ*. 11: 245–266

Darrow, A.A., Johnson, C.M., Miller, A.M., and Williamson, P. (2002) Can students accurately assess themselves? Predictive validity of student self-reports. *Update: Applications of Research in Music Education*. 20: 8–11

Davies, B.S., Rafique, J., Vincent, T.R., et al. (2012) Mobile Medical Education (MoMEd)—how mobile information resources contribute to learning for undergraduate clinical students: a mixed methods study. *BMC Med Educ*. 12: 1

De, S.K., Henke, P.K., Ailawadi, G., Dimick, J.B., and Colletti, L.M. (2004) Attending, house officer, and medical student perceptions about teaching in the third-year medical school general surgery clerkship. *J Am Coll Surg*. 199: 932–942

Des Marchais, J. (1993) A student-centred, problem-based curriculum: 5 years' experience. *Can Med Ass J*. 148: 1567

Dewey, J. (1933) *How We Think, a Restatement of the Relation of Reflective Thinking to the Educative Process*. Boston: D.C. Heath

Dornan, T., Boshuizen, H., King, N., and Scherpbier, A. (2007) Experience-based learning: a model linking the processes and outcomes of medical students' workplace learning. *Med Educ*. 41: 84–91

Downing, S. (2005) The effects of violating standard item writing principles on tests and students: the consequences of using flawed test items on achievement examinations in medical education. *Adv Health Sci Educ*. 10: 133–143

Downing, S.M. (2002) Threats to the validity of locally developed multiple-choice tests in medical education: construct-irrelevant variance and construct underrepresentation. *Adv Health Sci Educ*. 7: 235–241

Downing, S.M. (2004) Reliability: on the reproducibility of assessment data. *Med Educ*. 38: 1006–1012

Duvivier, R.J., van Dalen, J., Muijtjens, A.M., Moulaert, V.R., van der Vleuten, C.P., and Scherpbier, A.J. (2011) The role of deliberate practice in the acquisition of clinical skills. *BMC Med Educ*. 11: 101

Ende, J. (1983) Feedback in clinical medical education. *JAMA*. 250: 777–781

Entwistle, N. (1997) Reconstituting approaches to learning: A response to Webb. *Higher Educ*. 33: 213–218

Fidler, M., Lockyer, J.M., Toews, J., and Violato, C. (1999) Changing physicians practices: The effect of individual feedback. *Acad Med*. 74: 702–714

Fields, S.A., Toffler, W.L., Elliott, D., and Chappelle, K. (1998) Principles of clinical medicine: Oregon Health Sciences University School of Medicine. *Acad Med*. 73: 25

Findlater, G.S., Kristmundsdottir, F., Parson, S.H., and Gillingwater, T.H. (2012) Development of a supported self-directed learning approach for anatomy education. *Anat Sci Educ*. 5: 114–121

Flannigan, C., and McAloon, J. (2011) Students prescribing emergency drug infusions utilising smartphones outperform consultants using BNFCs. *Resuscitation*. 82: 1424–1427

Fleming, N.D. (2001) *Teaching And Learning Styles: VARK Strategies*. Christchurch, New Zealand: Neil Fleming

Freeth, D., Hammick, M., Koppel, I., Reeves, S., and Barr, H. (2002) *A Critical Review of Evaluations of Interprofessional Education.*. London: UK Centre for the Advancement of Interprofessional Education

Frye, A.W. and Hemmer, P.A. (2012) Program evaluation models and related theories: AMEE Guide No. 67. *Med Teach*. 34: e288–e299

Genn, J. (2001a) AMEE Medical Education Guide No. 23 (Part 1): Curriculum, environment, climate, quality and change in medical education—a unifying perspective. *Med Teach.* 23: 337–344

Genn, J. (2001b) AMEE Medical Education Guide No. 23 (Part 2): Curriculum, environment, climate, quality and change in medical education—a unifying perspective. *Med Teach.* 23: 445–454

Glicksman, J.T., Brandt, M.G., Moukarbel, R.V., Rotenberg, B., and Fung, K. (2009) Computer - assisted teaching of epistaxis management. *The Laryngoscope.* 119: 466–472

Godefrooij, M., Diemers, A., and Scherpbier, A. (2010) Students' perceptions about the transition to the clinical phase of a medical curriculum with preclinical patient contacts; a focus group study. *BMC Med Educ.* 10: 28

Gordon, M.J. (1992) Self-assessment programmes and their implications for health professions training. *Acad Med.* 67: 672–679

Grant, J. (2002) Learning needs assessment: assessing the need. *BMJ.* 324: 156–159

Gupta, S., Bassett, P., Man, R., Suzuki, N., Vance, M.E., and Thomas-Gibson, S. (2011) Validation of a novel method for assessing competency in polypectomy. *Gastrointestinal Endoscopy.* 75: 568–585

Gurpinar, E., Bati, H., and Tetik, C. (2011) Learning styles of medical students change in relation to time. *Adv Physiol Educ.* 35: 307–311

Harden, R.M., and Gleeson, F.A. (1979) Assessment of clinical competence using an objective structured clinical examination (OSCE). *Med Educ.* 13: 41–54

Harrow, A.J. (1972) *A Taxonomy of the Psychomotor Domain: a guide for developing behavioral objectives.* New York: D. McKay Co

Hauer, K.E., Teherani, A., Dechet, A., and Aagaard, E.M. (2005) Medical students' perceptions of mentoring: a focus-group analysis. *Med Teach.* 27: 732–734

Heijne-Penninga, M., Kuks, J.B., Hofman, W.H., and Cohen-Schotanus, J. (2008) Influence of open- and closed-book tests on medical students' learning approaches. *Med Educ.* 42: 967–974

Hodges, B., Regehr, G., Hanson, M., and McNaughton, N. (1997) An objective structured clinical examination for evaluating psychiatric clinical clerks. *Acad Med.* 72: 715–721

Hodges, B., Regehr, G., Hanson, M., and McNaughton, N. (1998) Validation of an objective structured clinical examination in psychiatry. *Acad Med.* 73: 910–912

Holladay, C.J. (2002) Classroom assessment techniques by Thomas Angelo and K. Patricia Cross. San Francisco: Jossey Bass Publishers, 1993. *Adv Physiol Educ.* 26: 57–57

Holmboe, E.S., and Hawkins, R. (2008) *Direct Observation by Faculty. Practical Guide to the Evaluation of Clinical Competence.* Philadelphia. PA: Mosby-Elsevier, pp. 110–129

Holton, E.F. (1996) The flawed four-level evaluation model. *Hum Resource Devel Q.* 7: 5–21

Huntley, C.D., Salmon, P., Fisher, P.L., Fletcher, I., and Young, B. (2012) LUCAS: a theoretically informed instrument to assess clinical communication in objective structured clinical examinations. *Med Educ.* 46: 267–276

Jones, R., Higgs, R., De Angelis, C., and Prideaux, D. (2001) Changing face of medical curricula. *Lancet.* 357: 699–703

Joughin, G. (2010) The hidden curriculum revisited: a critical review of research into the influence of summative assessment on learning. *Assess Eval Higher Educ.* 35: 335–345

Kanashiro, J., Hollaar, G., Wright, B., Nammavongmixay, K., and Roff, S. (2007) Setting priorities for teaching and learning: an innovative needs assessment for a new family medicine program in Lao PDR. *Acad Med.* 82: 231

Karabilgin, O.S., Vatansever, K., Caliskan, S.A., and Durak, H. İ. (2012) Assessing medical student competency in communication in the pre-clinical phase: Objective structured video exam and SP exam. *Patient Education and Counseling.* 87(3): 293–299

Karakitsiou, D.E., Markou, A., Kyriakou, P., et al. (2012) The good student is more than a listener—The 12+1 roles of the medical student. *Med Teach.* 34: e1–e8

Kaufman, R.A., Rojas, A.M., and Mayer, H. (1993) *Needs Assessment: A User's Guide.* Englewood Cliffs, NJ: Educational Technology Publications

Kegan, R. (1994) *In Over Our Heads: The Mental Complexity Of Modern Life.* Cambridge, MA: Harvard University Press

Kenny, N.P., Mann, K.V., and MacLeod, H. (2003) Role modeling in physicians' professional formation: reconsidering an essential but untapped educational strategy. *Acad Med.* 78: 1203

King, L.A. (1996) Who is regulating what and why? Motivational context of self-regulation. *Psychol Inquiry.* 7: 57–60

King, P.M., and Kitchener, K.S. (1994) *Developing Reflective Judgment: understanding and promoting intellectual growth and critical thinking in adolescents and adults.* San Francisco: Jossey-Bass Publishers

Kirkpatrick, D.J. (2006) *Evaluating Training Programs: The Four Levels.* San Francisco: Berren-Koehler

Knight, P.T. (2002) Summative assessment in higher education: practices in disarray. *Studies Higher Educ.* 27: 275–286

Kogan, J.R., Conforti, L.N., Bernabeo, E.C., Durning, S.J., Hauer, K.E., and Holmboe, E.S. (2012) Faculty staff perceptions of feedback to residents after direct observation of clinical skills. *Med Educ.* 46: 201–215

Kolb, D.A. (1984) *Experiential Learning: experience as the source of learning and development.* Englewood Cliffs, NJ: Prentice-Hall

Krathwohl, D.R., Bloom, B.S., and Masia, B.B. (1964) *Taxonomy of Educational Objectives, Handbook II: Affective Domain.* New York: David McKay Company

Kröncke, K.D. (2010) Computer-based learning versus practical course in pre-clinical education: Acceptance and knowledge retention. *Med Teach.* 32: 408–413

Kruger, J., and Dunning, D. (1999) Unskilled and unaware of it: how difficulties in recognizing one's own incompetence lead to inflated self-assessments. *J Personality Soc Psychol.* 77: 1121

Lave, J. and Wenger, E. (1991) *Situated Learning: Legitimate Peripheral Participation.* CambridgeUK; New York: Cambridge University Press

Law, S. (2011) Using narratives to trigger reflection. *Clin Teach.* 8: 147–150

Leahy, S., Lyon, C., Thompson, M., and Williams, D. (2005) Classroom assessment: minute by minute, day by day. *Educ Leadership.* 63: 19–24

Lee, M., and Wimmers, P.F. (2011) Clinical competence understood through the construct validity of three clerkship assessments. *Med Educ.* 45: 849–857

Lockyer, J., Violato, C., and Fidler, H. (2003) Likelihood of change: A study assessing surgeon use of multisource feedback data. *Teach Learn Med.* 15: 168–174

Lonka, K., Lindblom-YlÄnne, S., and Maury, S. (1994) The effect of study strategies on learning from text. *Learn Instruct.* 4: 253–271

Lujan, H.L., and DiCarlo, S.E. (2006) First-year medical students prefer multiple learning styles. *Adv Physiol Educ.* 30: 13–16

Marton, F., and Säljö, R. (1984a) Approaches to learning. In F. Marton, D. Hounsell, and N. Entwistle (eds) *The Experience of Learning: Implications for teaching and studying in higher education.* 3rd (Internet) edition (pp. 39–58). Edinburgh: University of Edinburgh, Centre for Teaching, Learning and Assessment

Marton, F., and Säljö, R. (1984b) Cognitive focus during learning. In F. Marton, D. Hounsell, and N. Entwistle (eds) *The Experience of Learning: Implications for teaching and studying in higher education.* 3rd (Internet) edition (pp. 56–80). Edinburgh: University of Edinburgh, Centre for Teaching, Learning and Assessment

Maudsley, R.F. (2001) Role models and the learning environment: essential elements in effective medical education. *Acad Med.* 76: 432

McGill, D.A., van der Vleuten, C.P., and Clarke, M.J. (2011) Supervisor assessment of clinical and professional competence of medical trainees: a reliability study using workplace data and a focused analytical literature review. *Adv Health Sci Educ Theory Pract.* 16: 405–425

McGrath, D., and Higgins, A. (2006) Implementing and evaluating reflective practice group sessions. *Nurse Educ Pract.* 6: 175–181

McKeatchie, W., and Svinicki, M. (2005) *Teaching Tips: Strategies, research, and theory for college teachers.* Boston: Houghton Mifflin

McKimm, J., and Swanwick, T. (2009) Assessing learning needs. *Br J Hosp Med*. 70: 349

McNulty, J.A., Sonntag, B., and Sinacore, J.M. (2009) Evaluation of computer-aided instruction in a gross anatomy course: A six-year study. *Anat Sci Educ*. 2: 2–8

Miflin, B.-M., Campbell, C.-B., and Price, D.-A. (1999) A lesson from the introduction of a problem-based, graduate entry course: the effects of difference views of self-direction. Medical Education 33: 801–807

Morrison, G.R., Ross, S.M., and Kemp, J.E. (2006) *Designing Effective Instruction*. Hoboken, NJ: John Wiley & Sons Inc.

Morrison, J. (2003) ABC of learning and teaching in medicine: evaluation. *BMJ*. 326: 385–387

Murdoch-Eaton, D., and Whittle, S. (2012) Generic skills in medical education: developing the tools for successful lifelong learning. *Med Educ*. 46: 120–128

Myers, I.B., and Myers, P.B. (1980) *Gifts Differing: Understanding Personality Type*. Mountain View, CA: Davies-Black Publishing

Norman, G.R., Neufeld, V R., Walsh, A., Woodward, C.A., and McConvey, G.A. (1985) Measuring physicians performances by using simulated patients. *J Med Educ*. 60: 925–934

Norman, G.R., Tugwell, P., and Feightner, J.W. (1982) A comparison of resident performance on real and simulated patients. *J Med Educ*. 57: 708–715

Nothnagle, M., Anandarajah, G., Goldman, R.E., and Reis, S. (2011) Struggling to be self-directed: residents' paradoxical beliefs about learning. *Acad Med*. 86: 1539–1544

Pandey, P. and Zimitat, C. (2007) Medical students' learning of anatomy: memorisation, understanding and visualisation. *Med Educ*. 41: 7–14

Papinczak, T., Young, L., Groves, M., and Haynes, M. (2008) Effects of a metacognitive intervention on students' approaches to learning and self-efficacy in a first year medical course. *Adv Health Sci Educ Theory Pract*. 13: 213–232

Pashler, H., McDaniel, M., Rohrer, D., and Bjork, R. (2010) Learning styles: Concepts and evidence. *Psychol SciPublic Interest*. 28: 105

Patrick, H., and Middleton, M. J. 2002. Turning the kaleidoscope: what we see when self-regulated learning is viewed with a qualitative lens. *Educ Psychol*. 37: 27–39

Pernar, L.I., Beleniski, F., Rosen, H., Lipsitz, S., Hafler, J., and Breen, E. (2012) Spaced education faculty development may not improve faculty teaching performance ratings in a surgery department. *J Surg Educ*. 69: 52–57

Piaget, J. (1950) *The Psychology of Intelligence*. London: Routledge, and Paul

Piaget, J. (1967) *Six Psychological Studies*. New York: Random House

Pintrich, P.R. (1995) Understanding self-regulated learning. *New Directions Teach Learn*. 1995: 3–12

Pintrich, P.R. (1999) The role of motivation in promoting and sustaining self-regulated learning. *Int J Educ Res*. 31: 459–470

Pintrich, P.R. (2003) A motivational science perspective on the role of student motivation in learning and teaching contexts. *J Educ Psychol*. 95: 667

Platzer, H., Blake, D., and Snelling, J. (1997a) A review of research into the use of groups and discussion to promote reflective practice in nursing. *Res Post-Compulsory Educ*. 2: 193–204

Platzer, H., Snelling, J., and Blake, D. (1997b) Promoting reflective practitioners in nursing: a review of theoretical models and research into the use of diaries and journals to facilitate reflection. *Teach Higher Educ*. 2: 103–121

Ponton-Carss, A., Hutchison, C., and Violato, C. (2011) Assessment of communication, professionalism, and surgical skills in an objective structured performance-related examination (OSPRE): a psychometric study. *Amn J Surg*. 202(4): 433–440

Poulton, T., Conradi, E., Kavia, S., Round, J., and Hilton, S. (2009) The replacement of 'paper' cases by interactive online virtual patients in problem-based learning. *Med Teach*. 31: 752–758

Prince, K.J.A H., Boshuizen, H., Van Der Vleuten, C.P.M., and Scherpbier, A.J.J.A. (2005) Students' opinions about their preparation for clinical practice. *Med Educ*. 39: 704–712

Quirk, R (1994), Educational issues in the design of courses based on competency standards: A discussion paper. St Leonards, New South Wales, Australia: NSW TAFE Commission Ratnapalan, S. (2010) Mentoring in medicine. *Can Fam Physician*. 56: 198

Reid, W., Duvall, E., and Evans, P. (2005) Can we influence medical students' approaches to learning? *Med Teach*. 27: 401–407

Roff, S. (2005) Education environment: a bibliography. *Med Teach*. 27: 353–357

Rose, G.L., Rukstalis, M.R., and Schuckit, M.A. (2005) Informal mentoring between faculty and medical students. *Acad Med*. 80: 344–348

Rubin, N.J., and Philp, E.B. (1998) Health care perceptions of the standardized patient. *Med Educ*. 32: 538–542

Sadler, D.R. (2009) Indeterminacy in the use of preset criteria for assessment and grading. *Assess Eval Higher Edu*. 34: 159–179

Saxena, V., O'Sullivan, P.S., Teherani, A., Irby, D.M., and Hauer, K.E. (2009) Remediation techniques for student performance problems after a comprehensive clinical skills assessment. *Acad Med*. 84: 669

Sayer, M., Chaput De Saintonge, M., Evans, D., and Wood, D. (2002) Support for students with academic difficulties. *Med Educ*. 36: 643–650

Schunk, D.H. (1990) Goal setting and self-efficacy during self-regulated learning. *Educ Psychol*. 25: 71–86

Schuwirth, L.W.T., and van der Vleuten, C.P.M. (2010) How to design a useful test: the principles of assessment. In T. Swanwick (ed.) *Understanding Medical Education: Evidence, Theory and Practice*. Oxford: Wiley-Blackwell

Shepard, L.A. (2000) The role of assessment in a learning culture. *Educ Res*. 29: 4–14

Shepard, L.A., Flexer, R.J., Hiebert, E.H., Marion, S.F., Mayfield, V., and Weston, T.J. 2005. Effects of introducing classroom peflormance assessments on student learning. *Educ Measurement Issues Pract*. 15: 7–18

Simpson, E. (1972) *The Psychomotor Domain*. Washington DC: Gryphon House

Skinner, B.F. (1938) *The Behavior of Organisms: An Experimental Analysis*. Cambridge, MA: B.F. Skinner Foundation

Smith, C.F. and Mathias, H. (2007) An investigation into medical students' approaches to anatomy learning in a systems-based prosection course. *Clin Anat*. 20: 843–848

Smither, J.W., London, M., and Reilly, R.R. (2005) Does performance improve following multisource feedback? A theoretical model, meta-analysis and review of empirical findings. *Pers Psychol*. 58: 33–66

Śniadecki, M., Kiszkielis, M., and Wydra, D. 2011. Surgery course evaluation. expectations of medical students in surgery rotation? From bench to bedside. *Polish J Surg*. 83: 554–561

Stenfors-Hayes, T., Hult, H., and Dahlgren, L.O. (2011) What does it mean to be a good teacher and clinical supervisor in medical education? *Adv Health Sci Educ Theory Pract*. 16: 197–210

Stufflebeam, D.L. (2000) The CIPP model for program evaluation. In: Stufflebeam, D. L., Madaus, G. F. and Kellaghan, T. (eds) *Evaluation Models: Viewpoints on Educational and Human Services Evaluation*. 2nd edn (pp. 325–365). Norwell, MA: Kluwer Academic Publishers

Svirko, E. and Mellanby, J. (2008) Attitudes to e-learning, learning style and achievement in learning neuroanatomy by medical students. *Med Teach*. 30(9-10): e219–e227

Swanwick, T. (Ed.) (2010) *Understanding Medical Education: Evidence, Theory and Practice*. Hoboken, NJ: Wiley-Blackwell.

Taherian, K. and Shekarchian, M. (2008) Mentoring for doctors. Do its benefits outweigh its disadvantages? *Med Teach*. 30: e95–e99

Taras, M. (2005) Assessment–summative and formative–some theoretical reflections. *Br J Educ Studies*. 53: 466–478

Tekian, A., and Harris, I. (2012) Preparing health professions education leaders worldwide: A description of masters-level programs. *Med Teach*. 34: 52–58

ten Cate, T.J., Kusurkar, R.A., and Williams, G.C. (2011) How self-determination theory can assist our understanding of the teaching and learning processes in medical education. AMEE Guide No. 59. *Med Teach*. 33: 961–973

Tooth, D., Tonge, K., and McManus, I. (1989) Anxiety and study methods in preclinical students: causal relation to examination performance. *Med Educ*. 23: 416–421

UIC (2011) *College of Medicine at Chicago: Master of Health Professions Education* [Online]. http://chicago.medicine.uic.edu/departments___programmes/departments/meded/educational_programmes/mhpe/ Accessed 22 January 2012

UIowa (2005) *University of Iowa Master in Medical Education (MME)* [Online]. http://www.uiowa.edu/admissions/graduate/programmes/programme-details/med-educ.html Accessed 25 May 2012

Usmani, A., Omaeer, Q., and Sultan, S.T. (2011) Mentoring undergraduate medical students: Experience from Bahria University Karachi. *J Pakistan Med Ass*. 61: 790

USMLE (2012) *United States Medical Licensing Examination* [Online]. Federation of State Medical Boards (FSMB) and National Board of Medical Examiners. http://www.usmle.org/ Accessed 24 May 2012UVA (2012) 'NXGen' Faculty Development: Teach the Teachers [Online]. http://www.medicine.virginia.edu/education/medical-students/UMEd/faculty-development-nxgen-teach-the-teachers Accessed 8 January 2012

Van Der Vleuten, C. (2000) Validity of final examinations in undergraduate medical training. *BMJ*. 321: 1217–1219

Van der Vleuten, C., Verwijnen, G., and Wijnen, W. (1996) Fifteen years of experience with progress testing in a problem-based learning curriculum. *Med Teach*. 18: 103–110

Van Hell, E.A., Kuks, J.B.M., Raat, A., Van Lohuizen, M.T., and Cohen-Schotanus, J. (2009) Instructiveness of feedback during clerkships: Influence of supervisor, observation and student initiative. *Med Teach*. 31: 45–50

Veerapen, K., and McAleer, S. (2010) Students' perception of the learning environment in a distributed medical programmeme. *Med Educ Online*. 15: 51–68

Vygotsky, L. (1978) *Interaction between Learning and Development. Mind and Society*. Cambridge, MA: Harvard University Press

Wald, H.S., Borkan, J.M., Taylor, J.S., Anthony, D., and Reis, S.P. (2012) Fostering and evaluating reflective capacity in medical education: developing the REFLECT rubric for assessing reflective writing. *Acad Med*. 87: 41–50

Wallace, J., Rao, R., and Haslam, R. (2002) Simulated patients and objective structured clinical examinations: review of their use in medical education. *Adv Psychiatr Treat*. 8: 342–348

Walsh, K. (2006) How to assess your learning needs. *JRSM*. 99: 29–31

Ward, A., Litman, D., and Eskenazi, M. (2011) Predicting change in student motivation by measuring cohesion between tutor and student. *Proceedings of the 6th Workshop on the Innovative Use of NLP for Building Educational Applications* (pp. 136–141). Available from: ACM Portal ACM Digital Library

Watson, J.B. (1914) *Behavior: An Introduction to Comparative Psychology*. New York: H. Holt and Company.

Weiner, B. (1992) *Human Motivation: Metaphors, Theories. and Research*. New York: Sage Publications, Inc.

Weiner, E.S. (1980) 'The Diagnostic Evaluation of Writing Skills' (DEWS): Application of DEWS criteria to writing samples. *Learning Disability Quarterly*. 3: 54–59

Weissman, S.H. (2011) The difficulty of assessing students' competence in patient care. *Acad Med*. 86: 1485

White, C.B. and Gruppen, L.D. (2007). *Self-regulated Learning in Medical Education*. Edinburgh, UK: ASME—Association for the Study of Medical Education

White, C.B., Ross, P.T., and Gruppen, L.D. 2009. Remediating students' failed OSCE performances at one school: The effects of self-assessment, reflection, and feedback. *Acad Med*. 84: 651

Wilkerson, L., and Irby, D.M. (1998) Strategies for improving teaching practices: a comprehensive approach to faculty development. *Acad Med*. 73: 387–396

Wilkes, M., and Bligh, J. (1999) Evaluating educational interventions. *BMJ*. 318: 1269–1272

Williams, R.-G., Klamen, D.-A., and McGaghie, W.-C. (2003) Cognitive, social and environmental sources of bias in clinical performance ratings. *Teaching and Learning in Medicine*. 15: 270–292

Winston, K.A., Van Der Vleuten, C.P.M., and Scherpbier, A.J.J.A. (2010) At-risk medical students: implications of students' voice for the theory and practice of remediation. *Med Educ*. 44: 1038–1047

W. K. Kellogg Foundation (1998) *Logic Model Development Guide* [Online]. W. K. Kellogg Foundation http://www.wkkf.org/knowledge-center/resources/2006/02/wk-kellogg-foundation-logic-model-development-guide.aspx Accessed 4 April 2013

Wlodkowski, R.J., and Ginsberg, M.B. (1995) *Diversity. and Motivation: Culturally Responsive Teaching*. San Francisco: Jossey-Bass

Yardley, S., and Dornan, T. 2012. Kirkpatrick's levels and education 'evidence'. *Med Educ*. 46: 97–106

Yeung, K., and Dixon-Woods, M. (2010) Design-based regulation and patient safety: A regulatory studies perspective. *Soc SciMed*. 71: 502–509

Yorke, M. (2010) How finely grained does summative assessment need to be? *Studies Higher Educ*. 35: 677–689

Zimmerman, B.J. (2000) Attainment of self-regulation: A social cognitive perspective. In Boekaerts, M., Pintrich, P., and Zeidner, M. (eds) *Handbook of Self-regulation* (pp. 13–35). San Diego, CA: Academic Press,.

Zimmerman, B.J. (2002) Becoming a Self-regulated learner: an overview. *Theory into Practice*. 41: 64–72

Zimmerman, B.J., Bonner, S., and Kovach, R. (1996) *Developing Self-regulated Learners [electronic resource]: beyond achievement to self-efficacy*. Washington, DC: American Psychological Association

Zou, L., King, A., Soman, S., et al. (2011) Medical students' preferences in radiology education: a comparison between the Socratic and didactic methods utilizing powerpoint features in radiology education. *Acad Radiol*. 18: 253–256

CHAPTER 40

Self-regulated learning in medical education

Timothy J. Cleary, Steven J. Durning,
Larry D. Gruppen, Paul A. Hemmer,
and Anthony R. Artino, Jr.

> From the start, the aim of revalidation has been to enable
> doctors to show that they are up to date and fit to practise,
> and to encourage improvement through meaningful
> reflection based on evidence drawn from practice.
>
> Graeme Catto
>
> Reproduced from *British Medical Journal*, Catto G, 'GMC
> and the future of revalidation: Building on the GMC's achievements', 330, p. 1205,
> Copyright 2005, with permission from BMJ Publishing Group Ltd.

Introduction

Most trainees succeed in completing medical school and residency training and develop into successful physicians, at least by our current performance standards. Although this speaks highly of our curricula, assessment, teaching, and learning practices, medical educators and researchers recognize many unresolved challenges that still need to be addressed. For example, a noteworthy percentage of medical trainees and physicians underperform in clinical situations (Frellsen et al. 2008; Greenburg et al. 2007). Underperformance could manifest itself early—for example by failing exams—or during the latter stages of training and practice—for example by making incorrect diagnostic or treatment decisions (Institute of Medicine 2000). These latter behaviours are particularly problematic because of their adverse effect on patient care.

Attention should not be solely placed on underperforming professionals, as even competent physicians can improve their competence through lifelong learning. Several medical education researchers have argued that medical educators must instil a belief among trainees that professional responsibility entails continually striving to improve their skills throughout their careers (Brydges and Butler 2012). In medical education, these lifelong learning skills, such as seeking out professional development opportunities and independently reflecting on, practising, and refining one's medical abilities, are similar to what others have called self-directed practice (Li et al. 2010; Slotnick 2001; White and Gruppen 2007). Unfortunately, physicians often demonstrate poor awareness of their strengths and weaknesses; they can exhibit weak motivation and may lack the necessary strategic skills to proactively and strategically enhance their abilities (Eva and Regehr 2005). Thus, developing effective ways to engage all students and physicians in these reflective and regulatory skills should be an important goal in medical education (Brydges and Butler 2012).

In addition, others have argued that medical educators need to re-examine the types of assessments that are used to evaluate the competence of trainees—such as multiple choice questions (MCQs), objective structured clinical exams (OSCEs), and essays (Durning et al. 2011a). These assessments are effective for assessing some aspects of knowledge, skills and attitudes but may be less useful in generating feedback to inform the nature of remedial activities. Thus, while common assessment approaches may identify 'at-risk' trainees, the results do not necessarily inform a tailored remediation plan, nor does performance on such exams account for the variance in trainee outcomes, such as in academic achievement, clinical competence, and patient care (Durning et al. 2011a). Another concern is that most medical education research tends to either be largely atheoretical or reliant on theories that focus primarily on the individual learner as the reason for 'failure', often to the exclusion of environmental or social factors (Durning and Artino 2011).

Although these issues related to individual and contextual factors are distinct and represent a major challenge for medical educators, from our perspective, many of them can be understood and addressed through a lens of self-regulation theory and research.

From a social-cognitive perspective, self-regulated learning (SRL) is a multidimensional process incorporating a set of inter-related and contextualized thoughts, actions, and feelings that a person strategically uses to reach personal goals (Bandura 1986; Zimmerman 2000). Individuals integrate their thoughts, actions, and feelings so that they effectively manage and take control over their own learning and performance. Social-cognitive models of SRL as well as other SRL frameworks have been used by researchers and practitioners to guide assessment and intervention activities across a wide array of domains (Boekaerts et al. 2000; Zimmerman and Schunk 2011).

At the outset, it is important for medical educators to consider two important points about SRL:

♦ SRL is a process that can be applied to virtually any domain or activity involving performance and mastery and

♦ SRL skills can be explicitly taught through instruction, guided practice, and remedial tutoring (Butler 1998; Graham and Harris 2009).

Given these basic premises, theoretical models of SRL should appeal to medical educators because they can provide a conceptual framework from which to understand and address the many thorny issues in medical education we have described.

The purpose of this chapter is to provide an overview of SRL theory and research and to describe its relevance to medical education. We will review some of the core similarities among different theoretical perspectives on SRL, but devote most attention to a social-cognitive perspective that emphasizes SRL as a contextualized, situation-specific, 'cyclical' process. We underscore the conceptual and empirical advantages of this cyclical account of SRL and provide specific examples to illustrate each component of the regulatory process. To conclude, we provide specific guiding principles for medical education research and practice and discuss some broad implications of SRL theory for the field in general.

Theories of self-regulation

Theories of SRL are concerned with explaining how individuals become masters of their cognition (thinking and beliefs), affect (emotion), behaviour, and environment as they learn or perform (Carver 2004; Puustinen and Pulkkinen 2001; Vohs and Baumeister 2004; Zimmerman 2000). Although it is beyond the scope of this chapter to review all of the theoretical models of SRL, it is important to note that there are wide variations among theories regarding the nature of human motivation, the role of environment and how self-regulatory skills develop (Zimmerman and Schunk 2001). As an example, *information processing theory* (Winne 2001) places primary importance on how individuals think about, interpret, and understand information as well as the cognitive tactics they use to optimize learning. In this model, motivation and the role of environment have traditionally not been strongly emphasized; indeed, in medical education these domains have often been minimized. In contrast, *operant or behavioral* theories tend to place primary importance on environmental factors, such as reinforcement and modeling, to explain behaviour (Mace et al. 2001), yet de-emphasize the role of cognition and beliefs because they cannot be directly measured.

There is also disagreement about several core aspects of SRL, such as whether it is primarily a conscious process or if automaticity plays a critical role (Vohs and Baumeister 2004). Interestingly,

this latter point parallels the recent debate in the clinical reasoning literature, where most investigators now see clinical reasoning as having both automatic (non-analytic reasoning) and effortful, conscious processes (analytic reasoning) (Norman 2005).

Despite the many differences that exist across models of self-regulation, we are primarily concerned with areas of commonality and points of symmetry (fig. 40.1). Many theorists conceptualize SRL in terms of a *cyclical feedback loop* (Carver 2004; Winne 2001; Zimmerman and Schunk 2001). Although the precise nature and specific processes of the loop can vary across theoretical perspectives, the core function of the loop is to allow individuals to gather information that is used to evaluate performance. From a cyclical perspective, the quality of learning or performance is maximized when individuals learn to use different regulatory processes, such as goal-setting, self-monitoring, and self-evaluation in an integrated way, throughout the process of performing an activity. Thus, if students need to master venepuncture, a cyclical account of self-regulation predicts that mastery will most likely occur when they prepare prior to practising venepuncture, engage in monitoring activities during the venepuncture activity, and reflect on the outcome of the procedure (Cleary and Sandars 2011).

A second core feature of many current theories of SRL is the explicit link between individuals' *motivation* and the quality of their regulatory engagement during learning (e.g. effort, choice, and persistence). Contemporary theories do not simply address *how* individuals learn and perform; they also explain *why* those individuals choose to do so (Bandura 1997; Pintrich 2000; Zimmerman 2000). Although many factors have been linked to motivated behaviours, much emphasis is placed on the role of environment as well as individuals' self-motivation beliefs including:

♦ confidence about performing specific tasks (self-efficacy)

♦ interest or level of enjoyment (task interest)

♦ perceptions of ability as fixed or changeable over time (conceptions of ability)

♦ reasons for their struggles or successes (causal attributions for why they obtained a particular outcome) and

♦ reasons why they perform activities—e.g. for learning or mastery (learning has its own rewards) or for external reasons (getting good grades from supervisors).

The medical education literature has recognized the importance of some of these motivational processes. Recent studies have suggested that students who adopt a performance goal orientation (primary focus on performance and outcomes) as well as those

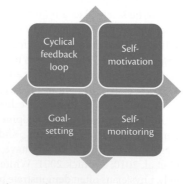

Figure 40.1 Core features of SRL models.

who exhibit low levels of self-efficacy will tend to exhibit weaker achievement and performance than those who possess a mastery orientation (primary focus on enjoyment of learning as a process) and possess high levels of confidence (Artino et al. 2012). In addition, preliminary work suggests that students' self-efficacy beliefs relate to their performance in medical school (Artino et al. 2010, 2011). When one also considers the higher than typical rates of burnout and depression among students, residents and practising physicians relative to the general public (Dyrbye et al. 2010; Goebert et al. 2009), there is compelling evidence that researchers need to further explore how these motivational beliefs and other factors impact the extent to which students engage in and regulate their learning.

Third, most SRL models depict self-regulation as a *goal-directed activity*. That is, self-regulated individuals do not haphazardly use strategies or randomly attempt to learn, but rather strategically and purposefully engage in particular behaviours to attain well-defined and personally meaningful outcomes. When individuals set goals, such as performing a procedure in a flawless manner, they benefit from both a motivational and self-regulatory perspective. That is, personal goals energize behaviour because they represent what one ultimately hopes to attain. However, they also represent the standard against which individuals determine whether they have attained success or demonstrated progress, thereby facilitating the process of self-evaluation (Zimmerman 2008a).

Perhaps the most essential aspect of SRL models, however, is the emphasis placed on *self-monitoring* (Epstein et al. 2008; Winne 2001; Zimmerman and Schunk 2001). While self-regulated individuals are motivated to set goals and to engage in specific learning activities, they also strive to keep track of their behaviours and progress. Self-monitoring acts as a core feedback mechanism in SRL models because it is through this process that individuals increase their self-awareness and gather the requisite information to effectively evaluate how they performed on a particular task. For example, students who graph the number of errors they make when performing a procedure are much more likely to display greater awareness of their skills than those who do not engage in this type of monitoring (Epstein et al. 2008). Having access to self-monitored performance data is crucial to being able to accurately self-evaluate and to subsequently adapt strategy use during future performance attempts.

A social-cognitive account of SRL

Although there are many viable models of SRL that underscore the features outlined earlier, we focus on a social-cognitive model because, from our perspective, this framework possesses a number of desirable characteristics that appear to be directly linked with emergent trends and key goals of medical education. First, social-cognitive models emphasize SRL as a contextualized skill that can be taught and improved (Bandura, 1986). Given the complexity of the contexts in which medical education and clinical care takes place (Bleakley et al. 2012), it is interesting to note the growing evidence that SRL varies across contexts and that individuals will often interpret and respond to similar situations in distinct ways (Bong 2005; Cleary and Chen 2009; Hadwin et al. 2001; Winne and Jamieson-Noel 2002). Thus, to understand SRL in medical education, one needs to situate this process in the context of well-defined activities. To emphasize this point, recent work in medical education has shown that physicians tend to differentially respond to patients with the same chief complaint and the same underlying diagnosis, in part because of the influence of contextual features (Durning et al. 2010b, 2012; Eva 2003; Eva et al. 1998).

Depicting behaviour as a social event differs in many respects from an information-processing perspective, which is, arguably, the pervading view in medical education (Bleakley et al. 2012; Durning and Artino 2011). In contrast to placing primary emphasis on the knowledge or metacognitive skills of the actor (e.g. student), social-cognitive theorists emphasize how these person-related variables interact in reciprocal ways with their behaviours and the environment in which they learn or perform. More specifically, human functioning is conceptualized in terms of reciprocal interactions between *personal* (e.g. beliefs, expectations, attitudes, and prior knowledge), *behavioural* (e.g. individual actions, choices, and verbal statements) and *environmental* factors (e.g. resources, consequences of actions, other people, and physical settings) (Bandura 1986).

Another desirable feature of a social-cognitive model is its emphasis on the importance of vicarious learning (learning by watching others perform tasks) and the corresponding instructional techniques of modelling and demonstration. In addition to research in educational psychology showing the importance of modelling as an instructional tool (Schunk et al. 2008; Schunk and Swartz, 1993), the recent discovery of the mirror neuron system (activation of the same areas of the brain when watching someone perform the task on their own) also supports this component of the theory (Glenberg 2011).

Finally, as previously mentioned, social-cognitive models of SRL have been studied and applied across a variety of contexts. Although many self-regulation intervention programmes borrow from different theoretical paradigms, social-cognitive assumptions pervade many of these programmes (Bembenutty et al. 2013). From our perspective, medical educators can benefit from conceptualizing many of the professional activities in our field from the general lens of social-cognitive theory as well as various models emanating from this perspective, including dynamic, cyclical accounts of SRL.

Zimmerman's three-phase cyclical feedback loop

Social-cognitive researchers have defined SRL as self-generated thoughts, feelings, and actions that are planned and cyclically adapted to attain personal goals (Zimmerman 2000). Dissecting this definition reveals several core elements. For example, SRL is a goal-directed process involving the integration of multiple subprocesses, such as self-monitoring and self-evaluation. The definition also suggests that even though the source of SRL can have social origins (e.g. influence of supervisors), at a more fundamental level, self-regulatory actions are generated and directed by the self. Of greatest importance to this chapter, however, is the phrase *planned and cyclical adapted*. This phrase suggests a temporal process whereby individuals think and plan prior to learning and then subsequently adjust or modify their learning or performance to reach personal goals. This notion is similar to deliberate practice, particularly the phase when the trainee no longer needs their coach to successfully practise and perform the task (Ericsson 2006). What truly makes an individual regulatory in nature is their skill in *proactively* and *strategically modifying* what and how they approach particular tasks.

From Zimmerman's 2000 perspective, self-regulation is best conceptualized as a cyclical process involving forethought (before the task), performance (during the task) and self-reflection (after the task). Forethought phase processes, which include individuals' goals and strategic plans, occur *prior to* engaging in learning. For example, a resident who proactively reviews his clinic schedule and each patient's medical problems in order to develop appropriate goals is exhibiting adaptive forethought. Forethought processes not only set the stage for learning or performance, they often become the benchmarks or standards against which individuals judge success and failure.

From this cyclical model perspective, however, learners will not automatically put their strategic plans into action (i.e. performance). They need to possess the necessary motivation to do so. That is, individuals who possess high levels of confidence in their abilities to perform specific tasks (self-efficacy), positive perceptions of enjoyment or interest in the activities (task interest), and strong beliefs that engaging in those activities will lead to desired outcomes (outcome expectations) are likely to implement their strategic plan and to engage in other types of regulatory processes during learning. For example, a clinician who has been part of a successful quality improvement (QI) project in her hospital and who perceives that she now possesses the necessary skills to meet the needs of patients (self-efficacy) and sees the benefits of these types of initiatives for both her own productivity and patient care (outcome expectations), is more likely to devote her efforts in other QI initiatives.

During attempts to learn or demonstrate skill (performance or *during* phase of the cycle) highly self-regulated individuals will not only implement their forethought (*before*) plans and strategies but will often use various self-control tactics to manage their attention, behaviours, and learning. For example, a medical student who is struggling to find the necessary time to study for a physiology course or who becomes increasingly bored or frustrated during studying, may use a calendar to manage time, or take a series of study breaks or use self-reinforcement (e.g. 'if I study for two hours, I can eat my favorite dessert') to maintain attention during learning. Self-regulated individuals are also keen on self-monitoring their behaviours, thoughts, and potential barriers to learning. Self-monitoring is the information hub of the feedback loop, as it serves as the basis for individuals to make appropriate judgements and reactions following performance.

In the final phase of this feedback loop (*after* phase), learners evaluate whether or not their goals were reached (self-evaluation), identify the reasons for this level of performance (attributions), and draw conclusions about how to adapt prior to future learning or performing clinical tasks (adaptive inferences). Self-reflection is particularly important because it is during this phase when learning can become short-circuited or can continue to progress amidst challenges. From a conceptual point of view, a single iteration of the feedback loop is completed when a person's reflective judgements impact how they will approach subsequent learning.

As an illustration of how these three cyclical phases might occur, consider Dr Smith, who has been a primary care internist for 13 years and is part of a thriving practice in a lower-middle class suburb. He sees a reasonable range of problems in his practice and has a good referral network for complicated cases. In the following scenario, Dr Smith is considered to be a sophisticated self-regulated learner.

Forethought—identifying a problem and devising a strategic plan

Recently, the local healthcare system had distributed a new protocol for asthma treatment. Over the years Dr Smith had noticed asthma guidelines in medical journals and had scanned them briefly. However, he recently overheard several colleagues talking about similar guidelines that had been implemented by their own systems. Reflecting on his own practice he recognized that it deviated from these proposed guidelines (task analysis). Although at first glance Dr Smith reasoned that the variation did not appear to be important to patient outcomes, upon more careful analysis of his professional goals and the adequacy of his established protocols, he recognized that his asthma protocols were not meeting standards. In addition, given his realization that his practice would be undergoing substantial scrutiny over the next few years (task value), he recognized the need to adapt and modify his practice based on the recommended changes. In order to accomplish this, Dr Smith established as his primary goal, to establish an effective, clear asthma plan based on best practice guidelines and to do so within 2 months. To accomplish this goal, he decided to enlist a variety of tactics (planning), such as devoted reading time regarding the asthma guidelines, consultation with his respiratory consultant and informal discussions with colleagues.

Forethought commentary

The changing landscape of asthma treatment helped Dr Smith realize the need to develop more clear goals and strategies for his practice—essential forethought phase processes. However, what aided Dr Smith was his high level of insight regarding his own practice as well as the quality of his motivation beliefs. Because he perceived himself to be a competent, up-to-date practitioner and clearly identified the inherent value and importance of making these changes, Dr Smith felt compelled to make them. In addition, although he had low confidence in the quality of his initial asthma guidelines, he possessed a strong sense of efficacy to modify these guidelines, given his long track record of high achievement and commitment to professional development.

Performance phase—enacting the plan and gathering data

To execute his plan, Dr Smith developed a timeline of specific activities that would guide his reading and consultation behaviours. He decided that the best course of action was to have a solid knowledge base of the key issues before speaking with colleagues. He spent the first 2 weeks reviewing the essential documents and taking notes on the key themes that have to be addressed (self-monitoring). Upon reviewing the proposed guidelines, he initiated contact with colleagues and organized several working lunches to facilitate discussion and analysis. However, during these meetings, many of his older colleagues doubted the utility of these new approaches. They also told Dr Smith that he was wasting his time. He recorded their perceptions as well as his own feelings about the meeting (self-monitoring). Feeling frustrated at what transpired, he engaged in self-talk to keep himself focused and motivated. Interestingly, one of his more knowledgeable colleagues about current practices was quite enthusiastic about the potential impact of these guidelines. Given that this colleague's perspective was consistent with his own goals for his practice, he set up times to speak with him on an individual basis to look more closely at his implementation strategy.

Performance commentary

Although the performance phase in this example extended over a relatively long time period, it serves to illustrate the importance of strategic thinking and self-monitoring. Rather than being reactive and waiting for external factors to motivate him to act, Dr Smith enlisted various self-control tactics (time management and self-talk) to direct his own activities and to support his initiatives to change practice. However, in this phase, it is not simply employing strategies to accomplish one's goal that matters, but also gathering data about how effective the strategies were in attaining one's goals. By self-recording his actions and those of others, Dr Smith will have data to adequately self-evaluate in the next phase of the cyclical loop.

Self-reflection—determining success and need for adaptation

After analysing data from the asthma guidelines and meeting notes from consultations with colleagues, Dr Smith was able to develop an asthma protocol that aligned with the required guidelines and his individual practice. Thus, he concluded that his investigative plan was successful because he attained his forethought goal of establishing a new asthma guideline plan (self-evaluation). He attributed the success of his plan to the many different tactics that he employed to gather information, as well as his use of self-control strategies to keep focused on the task at hand. However, after engaging in this type of reflection, he also realized that he needed to shift his goal from development to implementation. Dr Smith felt confident in his capability to implement the new guidelines but realized that he had to develop new goals and a set of strategies to ensure successful implementation (next forethought phase of the loop).

Self-reflection commentary

Dr Smith relied on information gathered during the performance phase to help him evaluate the success of his plan and to determine how he needed to proceed. Because he concluded that his plan was viable, he needed to take the necessary steps to implement the new guidelines. Thus, during the next phase of the cyclical regulatory feedback loop, Dr Smith elected to implement these protocols within a month (goal) and to conduct professional development training for his staff over the course of three nights (strategic plan). In addition he decided to use the first month as a pilot phase whereby he would track the success of the programme through formal assessment procedures (questionnaires to be completed by patients, staff and colleagues). This data would further his self-evaluation and reflection of the appropriateness and quality of the new guidelines.

Conceptual advantages of feedback loop

One of the key advantages of the cyclical account of SRL is that it integrates motivation, metacognitive, and strategic processes within a single interpretative framework. Ultimately, this integration of distinct, albeit related, processes allows one to address several key questions that are of interest to medical educators—see fig. 40.2.

Another advantage of the three-phase cyclical model of SRL is the emphasis on forethought (*before*) phase processes. Unlike approaches that focus primarily on self-reflection, a cyclical account provides a basis for distinguishing proactive from passive or reactive learners. Proactive learners are those who self-initiate or develop strategic plans in an a priori manner in order to attain

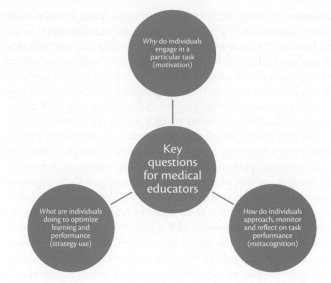

Figure 40.2 Key guiding questions for medical educators.

well-defined goals; whereas reactive learners typically begin to think about their approaches to learning after the fact in a post-hoc fashion. This distinction is particularly relevant to medical education because it is likely that some students and professionals only become vigilant about their performance upon receiving negative feedback regarding high-stakes outcomes, such as failing an exam. This is not to say that reactive regulation is maladaptive or that it will not prompt one to engage in subsequent cycles of learning. Rather, reactive regulators tend to be inefficient in their learning and often struggle to sustain their motivation because of ill-defined performance standards and poor awareness about how to improve.

The cyclical feedback model has also been shown to be a useful approach for developing applied intervention programmes in diverse domains and skill areas; including academic skills and management of chronic illness such as asthma and heart problems (Bonner et al. 2002; Butler 1998; Clark 2013; Cleary et al. 2008; Graham and Harris 2009). Although all these intervention programs do not directly incorporate each of the components of Zimmerman's feedback model, nor were they all social-cognitive in nature, they all emphasize the importance of teaching learners how to engage in recursive cycles of regulatory thinking and action as they attempt to improve. Given that there is a strong literature demonstrating the empirical advantages of these self-regulation interventions across diverse contexts (Cleary et al. 2006; Schunk and Swartz 1993; Zimmerman and Kitsantas 1996, 2002), we believe this type of framework has great potential for addressing emergent issues in medical education.

Relation between self-regulation processes and medical education

Over the past decade, medical education researchers have examined many concepts, such as self-assessment, self-monitoring, metacognition, self-directed learning and reflective practice; all of which are related to various components of the three-phase cyclical model (Brydges and Butler 2012). Self-assessment, also referred to as calibration, involves the extent to which beliefs about one's capabilities to perform an activity match one's actual performance of that activity (Colthart et al. 2008; Dornan 2008; Eva and Regehr 2005; Ward et al. 2002). Self-assessment is important because it relates to performance and underscores individuals' understanding of their own abilities as well as the nature and demands of the tasks that they are being asked to perform. Although the accuracy of these judgements relates to several regulatory processes as defined in the cyclical loop (e.g. task analysis, self-evaluation), self-assessment is relatively narrow in scope because it primarily examines the accuracy of individual's predictive or postdictive judgements. Metacognition, which is related to self-assessment, pertains to individuals' knowledge of themselves and the task, as well as their skills in controlling their cognition in order to guide behaviour (Flavell 1979; Veenman et al. 2003). Some key metacognitive skills include planning (forethought), monitoring (performance), and evaluation (reflection); processes which mirror the phase dimensions of the cyclical loop. Thus, even though self-assessment and metacognition overlap, metacognition can be considered a broader construct because it involves several other cognitive skills. That said, most theorists would argue that metacognitive processes are subsumed under the broader label of SRL (Zimmerman 1995). SRL models tend to go beyond a traditional metacognitive framework by highlighting the role of motivational beliefs, the importance of contextual and environmental factors and the interactive influence of affect, environment, and cognition.

Another important area in medical education is reflective practice. Reflective practice is the process by which a physician engages in some type of critical self analysis in order to learn from their experiences and to develop a more robust understanding of their own behaviours and how such behaviours impact themselves and others (Mann et al. 2009). A key goal of reflection is to enable physicians to achieve and maintain control over their experience (Mann et al. 2009). The reflective practice literature in medical education is consistent with the self-reflection phase of the cyclical feedback loop. However, the subprocesses underlying reflective practice in medical contexts are often not well defined and tend to give less attention to the forethought and performance dimensions of SRL models. Thus, reflective practice is consistent with some aspects of the model discussed in this chapter, but again is much narrower in scope.

Finally, self-directed learning (SDL) is a fairly well-researched construct that has been used in medical education. SDL has been defined as 'a process in which individuals take the initiative, with or without the help from others, in diagnosing their learning needs, formulating goals, identifying human and material resources, choosing and implementing appropriate learning strategies, and evaluating learning outcomes' (Knowles 1975, p. 18). Moreover, in the problem-based learning (PBL) literature within medical education, developing skills for SDL is often touted as a primary outcome of such instructional approaches. Clearly, there is a connection between SDL and SRL; a link that has been explicitly made in the literature (Zimmerman and Lebeau 2000). However, some have argued that SDL is a broader concept, referring to both the design features of the learning environment that can provide opportunities for self-direction, as well as characteristics of the learner; whereas SRL models typically refer to the latter (Brydges and Butler 2012; Loyens et al. 2008). Regardless of how one defines SDL or SRL, some have called for more cross-fertilization between the two literatures (Zimmerman and Lebeau

2000). We would certainly agree with this recommendation, as we suspect that medical education researchers often do not employ comprehensive and integrative approaches to theory application in their research paradigms.

Emergent SRL themes relevant to medical education

The SRL concepts presented in this chapter are in line with emerging research in medical education and offer some fruitful ideas for extending and refining this research and professional practice. Here we briefly outline four SRL research-to-practice ideas that have been established in educational psychology circles and that are clearly relevant to medical education (fig.40.3). Although there is a literature base in medical education that relates to these research-to-practice ideas, one needs to underscore that these principles have not been studied extensively and thus the extent to which they generalise to medical contexts must be explored and verified.

Multi-phase self-regulation training is more effective than narrower self-regulation interventions

Researchers across several disciplines have demonstrated that training individuals to engage in multi-phase self-regulation processes leads to greater motivation (e.g. self-efficacy), self-regulation (e.g. strategy use, self-evaluation), and achievement outcomes, than when they receive single-phase training (i.e. either before, during or after) or no training at all (Borkowski et al. 1988; Cleary et al. 2006; Schunk and Ertmer 1999; Schunk and Swartz 1993; Zimmerman and Kitsantas 1996, 1997). In other words, individuals tend to perform at a higher level when they learn how to integrate and concurrently use multiple regulatory phase processes, such as goal-setting (forethought), self-monitoring (performance), and attributions (self-reflection), rather than a more narrow set of processes when performing a task.

To illustrate the importance of multiphase training of motor skills, Cleary et al. (2006) randomly assigned 50 college students identified as novice basketball players, to one of three experimental groups or a control group. The experimental groups were closely linked to the three phase dimensions of Zimmerman's cyclical feedback loop. Thus, participants assigned to a one-phase condition received training in forethought processes only (i.e. setting process goals). Those assigned to a two-phase condition were provided forethought and performance instruction (i.e. self-recording), whereas the three-phase participants received training in forethought, performance, and self-reflection phase processes.

A key finding from this study was that the three-phase and two-phase groups displayed significantly better free-throw shooting skill during practice and at post-test than all other groups, even though the multiphase training groups shot significantly *fewer*

| Multi-phase self-regulation training is more effective than narrower self-regulation interventions |
| Effective SRL interventions employ contextualised and task-specific strategies |
| Motivation is a skill that can be improved |
| Strategic reflective thinking promotes adaptation and improvement |

Figure 40.3 SRL research-to-practice ideas.

free-throws during the practice sessions. The multiphase participants took fewer practice shots than other groups because they were trained to devote more time and attention to monitoring their use of the shooting strategy during practice. Similar to the case scenario of Dr Smith, the cyclical feedback model predicts that people will be better able to adapt their behaviours or establish new goals and strategies to improve future performance when they have access to self-monitored information about their strategic behaviours (Zimmerman 2000).

Medical education researchers have now begun to examine self-regulatory processes in context as well as the effects of single and to a lesser degree multiple 'regulatory' processes on performance outcomes (Brydges et al. 2009; Kennedy et al. 2009; Mouton et al. 2010). For example, in one study, researchers experimentally examined the effects of an autonomy-supportive context and goal-setting intervention on the suturing skills of students (Brydges et al. 2009). From our perspective, the extent to which researchers continue to evaluate the effects of multiple self-regulatory processes on clinical skills and overall professional practice will greatly aid in the eventual development of applied intervention programmes that incorporate such processes.

Effective SRL interventions employ contextualized and task-specific strategies

Although SRL appears to have some stable dimensions, there is an emerging literature showing that an individual's motivational beliefs and regulatory behaviours vary across situational demands and characteristics (Bandura 1997; Cleary and Chen 2009; Eva 2003; Eva et al. 1998; Kennedy et al. 2009). Within medical education, studies have shown the impact of instructional environments and contextual features on students' clinical skills and regulatory processes (Kennedy et al. 2009; Eva 2003; Eva et al. 1998). For example, researchers have demonstrated that medical trainers perceive intense pressure to act independently in their clinical activities because of factors occurring within themselves as well as the environment and context (Kennedy et al. 2009). Other researchers have shown that physician diagnostic skills are impacted by the context of the clinical encounter; that is, things other than the patient's presenting history and physical examination impact their decision making. For example, two patients can present with the same concerns and have the same underlying diagnosis, yet the physician may not arrive at the same diagnosis and treatment (Durning et al. 2010a, b; Eva 2003; Eva et al. 1998).

Beyond acknowledging the importance of context, most self-regulation intervention programs involve training in both SRL processes (goal setting, self-monitoring) and task-specific strategies (e.g. use of concept maps to learn science) (Butler 1998; Cleary et al. 2008; Graham and Harris 2009). While there is much overlap in the regulatory processes (e.g., goal-setting, monitoring, self-reflection) that are emphasized in applied SRL intervention programs, these interventions tend to vary based on the specific content areas and the strategies linked to these areas. For example, although the regulatory processes emphasized in a science-focused intervention in high school contexts (Cleary et al. 2008) and a writing intervention for elementary school students (Graham and Harris 2009) are quite similar, the science-based intervention involved instruction in the use of concept maps and mnemonic devices to learn course material whereas the writing intervention emphasized instruction using a five- or six-step procedure for effective writing. Providing

contextualized and task-specific strategy instruction is a key element of almost all SRL intervention programmes.

From our perspective, in order for self-regulation interventions to be relevant to medical education, it is essential that these processes be taught 'in context' or in relation to the specific tasks of interest. Of equal or perhaps greater importance is that learners be taught distinct learning strategies for each signature activity, particularly when the activities vary in scope and demands. For example, the strategies that one needs to employ to take a psychiatric history are much different from the strategies needed to perform minimally invasive surgery.

Motivation is a skill that can be improved

In medical education, a number of students, residents and practising physicians not only struggle to demonstrate benchmark proficiencies but also exhibit a poor level of awareness of their deficiencies (Eva and Regehr 2005). From a regulatory perspective, when students do not understand why they struggle or even if they are struggling, their motivation to reflect on and improve their performance will also suffer. The cyclical feedback model is important, in part, because it clearly distinguishes an individual's *will* or *motivation* to engage in learning from their regulatory *skills*. From a social-cognitive perspective, motivation is a goal-directed activity that is initiated and sustained (Zimmerman 2008a). Some of the potential origins of motivation are outlined in fig. 40.4.

In medical education, there are several instructional approaches that can influence students' motivation beliefs and behaviours. For example, research has shown that students who were taught in PBL educational contexts for 2 years reported greater regulation, independence, and general motivation than those who were educated in traditional learning environments (White 2007). Although impressive, future research should devote greater attention to quantitatively and qualitatively measuring key motivation processes, such as self-efficacy, interest, and goal orientation (Artino et al. 2010, 2011, 2012; Artino 2012). Teaching evidence-based medicine (EBM) may also serve as a foundation for studying and applying motivation principles. For example, to build learner self-efficacy of their mastery of EBM principles, the EBM process is typically broken down into component phases (ask, acquire, appraise, apply) and the learners engage in tasks that enable them to master each of the phases before putting them all together (Straus et al. 2005). This is critical because mastery experiences are the most powerful influence on the confidence that individuals develop about performing specific tasks.

Self-regulatory processes, including goal-setting and causal attributions, also have motivational properties. In general, goals tend to produce the greatest levels of motivation when they are specific; personally generated; focused on process; and are hierarchically structured (i.e. both short- and long-term; Zimmerman 2008a).

Motivation evolves primarily from individuals'

- Self-perceptions of their competencies and skills (i.e. self-efficacy; Pajares and Urdan 2006)
- Interest when engaged in a task (i.e. task interest; Eccles and Wigfield 2002)
- Perception of the importance of an activity (i.e. perceived instrumentality; Zimmerman 2000)
- Personal or professional goals (i.e. goal orientation; Pintrich 2000)

Figure 40.4 Key sources of motivation.

The importance of goals has been clearly established in educational psychology, with process goals emerging as a critical topic in medical education research (Bandura 1997; Brydges et al. 2009; Cleary and Sandars 2011; Zimmerman 2008a). In terms of causal attributions, when individuals perceive that the reasons for their performance on a particular activity are due to internal, controllable and unstable or non-fixed factors, they tend to exhibit the most adaptive motivation and performance profiles.

A key implication from motivation research is that to enhance student motivation, it is important to not only enhance their sense of efficacy to perform and interest in (and perception of the value of) a task but to also help them focus on the process of learning before and following learning. The importance of motivation interventions in medical education is further underscored when considering the disproportionate level of burnout and depression in medical students and physicians relative to the general public; a phenomenon that can lead to high levels of disengagement from learning (Artino et al. 2010, 2011, 2012; Dyrbye et al. 2010; Goebert et al. 2009).

Strategic reflective thinking promotes adaptation and improvement

All learners at one time or another perform at a level that is below their personal expectations—e.g. by failing an exam. Although this can cause distress for high-achieving learners, failure or suboptimal performance can become more problematic when learners perceive these outcomes in maladaptive ways. Attribution researchers have shown that how learners think about failure has important implications regarding their affect, motivation, and subsequent strategic behaviours (Borkowski et al. 1988; Hall et al. 2006). One of the most consistent findings to emerge has been that learners who attribute poor performance or failure to *controllable* factors, such as effort and strategy use, tend to exhibit the most desirable motivation and achievement profiles.

Attribution researchers have also emphasized the importance of reinterpreting failure as a positive and potentially control-enhancing experience (Hall et al. 2006). Thus, for learners who exhibit suboptimal performance, it may be helpful for supervisors to help them identify the link between how they learn and how they perform; as well as to restructure their thinking about the meaning of their failure experience. For example, learners can be encouraged to perceive poor performance as an opportunity for growth or a sign that a skill has not yet been mastered. Furthermore, when learners attribute poor performance to uncontrollable factors, such as instructor difficulty or task difficulty, it is important to validate that these factors might be true in certain cases but that such 'hard to change' factors are less important because they do not prescribe a path to success.

Adaptive, strategic thinking, however, is not simply confined to self-reflective thoughts and reactions (attributions). Highly regulated individuals are also strategic in their planning and goal setting prior to learning and during learning—e.g. by monitoring their use of a strategy when learning to suture. To our knowledge, there are few studies that directly examine the quality of students' regulatory and strategic thinking as they perform specific clinical tasks. A fruitful line of research is to examine these beliefs and behavioural patterns more clearly, through the use of contextualised assessment approaches, such as direct observations, think alouds or micro-analytic interviews (Cleary 2011; Durning et al. 2011a; Zimmerman 2008b).

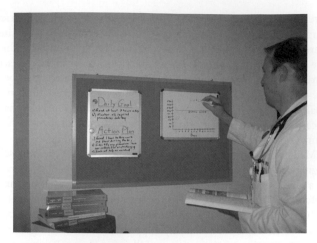

Figure 40.5 Dynamic use of goal-setting and self-monitoring as part of clinical practice.

Broader implications of self-regulation for medical education

In addition to these specific research-to-practice principles, SRL can inform the field of medical education in broader ways. Here we outline several broad implications of the cyclical model of SRL to medical professionals and educators (fig. 40.5).

Nurturing the environment–person reciprocal exchange

There has been increased interest in studying SRL and other related constructs, such as self-assessment, in medical contexts (Brydges and Butler 2012; Durning et al. 2011a). SRL is thought to be affected by a host of contextual variables including the physical features of a classroom; instructional methodology; type and nature of social agents (e.g. instructors, supervisors or peers); and even more granular contextual variables, such as the specific activities and tasks that medical trainees are expected to perform. Thus, a great advantage of social-cognitive theoretical accounts of SRL is the recognition that although the environment impacts students, students can also proactively influence and modify the environments in which they learn and perform. From our perspective, a key issue involves the tactics that medical educators need to use to address both sides of this reciprocal relationship. How can medical educators create learning environments that foster positive, adaptive SRL in students, and conversely how can students be empowered to skillfully navigate and manage these contexts, regardless of their quality? Simply arranging a context in a particular way to foster independence and self-directed behaviours does not necessarily ensure that students will be able to skillfully cope with and handle this level of autonomy. A few important issues to consider include the following:

- How can one provide process-oriented feedback to students that promotes adaptive and strategic reflection?

- What is the quantity and quality of practice opportunities needed by students to help them learn how to use content-specific strategies and regulatory strategies?

- How does one structure learning activities at all levels of medical training to promote self-efficacy and intrinsic interest?

◆ How can remedial activities or self-regulated 'coaching' be provided to students to help them address their individual learning or performance challenges?

Relevance of cyclical SRL models to medical education theory and practice

An important research-to-practice recommendation involves the development and implementation of multiphase self-regulation interventions that help individuals think about their skill development and learning in recursive ways. In a sense, the multiphase, cyclical nature of SRL parallels the nonlinearity and complexity that exists in medical education, as evidenced in continuing medical education (CME) and lifelong learning initiatives. Further, in medical education, there are theoretical paradigms and instructional approaches that speak to a 'process' approach to understanding behaviour. Although different in origin, purpose, and key underlying assumptions, a theory of the dissemination of innovation (Rogers 2003), which has been used to frame thinking about CME, shares some features of the cyclical and process-oriented framework illustrated in the three-phase cyclical model of SRL (Zimmerman 2000).

Consider the scenario of Dr Smith, our primary care internist, to make this comparison. There are five stages in the process of adopting a change in one's practice (Rogers 2003). In the first stage, *awareness*, Dr Smith is initially exposed to the asthma guidelines but has not gathered much information about them. During this stage, Dr Smith has not yet been inspired to find more information because he has yet to see a need (motivation). The second stage is *interest*, which describes Dr Smith's awakening motivation to look a bit closer at the guidelines and to seek additional information. This interest is most often driven by the need to solve a problem, usually represented in a patient case. The notion of interest and so-called *task value* is an important motivational construct that can (and should) be explored further in medical education contexts (Artino et al. 2010, 2011). The third critical stage of the adopting change process is *evaluation*, in which Dr Smith takes the concept of the guidelines and weighs the advantages and disadvantages of using them. He must decide whether to adopt or reject the guidelines—but research demonstrates that this is an individualistic stage, depending heavily on the physician's experiences, priorities, peers and environment (Bleakley et al. 2012; Brydges and Butler 2012). In a general sense, these first three phases correspond to the 'before' or forethought phase of the cyclical model because they collectively involve preparatory activities and motivational dispositions that one would display prior to implementing any change.

The fourth stage, *trial* or *implementation*, would entail Dr Smith's initial attempts to actually use the guidelines. These initial efforts would typically be exploratory because Dr Smith would be seeking evidence regarding whether this change will be more trouble than it is worth. The 'seeking evidence' component of this phase is similar to the performance aspect of the three-phase SRL model in that learners implement the use of strategies (self-control) and attempt to gather self-monitored or externally-provided information about their skills and performance. The final stage in the theory of change (Rogers 2003) is *adoption*. In this phase, Dr Smith would attempt to draw conclusions regarding the benefits and costs of implementation of the guidelines. If Dr Smith perceived that there was a strong benefit to making this change and that he felt confident in doing so, it is likely that he would adopt this practice. This last phase is akin to the self-reflection phase of the three-phase cyclical model (Zimmerman, 2000), particularly regarding self-evaluation and making adaptive inferences.

The general level of correspondence between the SRL model and the five-phase model of dissemination of innovations illustrates that the concept of a 'process-oriented feedback loop' is not a completely foreign concept to medical educators. However, we believe that the three-phase cyclical model is so attractive and potentially applicable to medical practice because it explicitly defines all of the subprocesses within each of these phases and thus allows one to directly measure and improve such processes.

SRL theory as a broad explanatory framework

Another implication of SRL theory is that it can provide a broader framework in which to embed narrower aspects of regulatory functioning, such as self-assessment, metacognition and self-reflective practice. SRL theory can help put into perspective the intense focus in medical education research on the 'accuracy' of self-assessment. The three-phase model reminds us that regardless of accuracy, these self-judgements of gaps in skill or knowledge are critical drivers of SRL activities.

In addition, it may be useful to stop lamenting the inaccuracy of self-assessment because poor self-judgements or predictions may not be the end of the story. In fact, it may represent the starting point from which to develop effective interventions. We know that self-assessment and self-regulation are both types of *teachable* skills (Bembenutty et al. 2013; Bol et al. 2010; Zimmerman and Schunk 2011). Although the self-assessment literature is mixed regarding the effectiveness of assessment accuracy training, there are volumes of data demonstrating that forethought, performance, and self-reflection processes are malleable and teachable but and that such processes improve performance across multiple domains (Zimmerman and Schunk 2011).

SRL theory across the medical education developmental spectrum

Preclinical education

The three-phase model of SRL has important implications for all learners. In undergraduate education, traditional instructional paradigms often do not directly seek to enhance student regulation and problem-solving skills. This is interesting, given that this phase of medical education often involves didactic or classroom-based instruction, the ground on which much SRL research is based. Part of the reason SRL may be less important in the early years of medical school is the structured nature of most curricula and educational experiences. Undergraduate schedules are packed with required courses and activities that leave little need (or room) for independent decision making on what topics to study. In a sense, SRL is not needed to map out one's course schedule and programme of activities. However, even in this structured setting, learners need to draw on self-regulatory skills that are essential for managing multiple demands, optimizing learning, and overcoming failure or challenges.

Clinical education

The importance of SRL skills becomes most pronounced when individuals face challenges, such as when the use of a study strategy no longer works or when students transition from preclinical to clinical education. Difficulty transitioning from the preclinical to the clinical environment often occurs when learners try to use strategies that are effective in lecture-based curricula but not in the clinical context (Cartier et al. 2001; Woods et al. 2011). In this phase of training, most learning takes place in authentic contexts with real patients. This learning becomes central during residency training.

Case scenario—Dr Brown

Consider the case scenario of Dr Brown, a thoracic surgery resident, who was delighted to enter the final year of her programme. Despite her excitement, she was feeling intimidated by the intensity of the clinical environment and the high expectations she observed in her interactions with attendings and senior residents (self-monitoring). Although she had done well in her surgery clerkship and general surgery rotation, she was aware that she had much to learn about the technical aspects of thoracic surgery (metacognitive monitoring). Fortunately, the hospital had a well-equipped simulation centre and a systematic curriculum for the residents. In order to accomplish her goal of mastering thoracic surgery, Dr Brown planned to spend at least three nights refining her surgical skills 'after-hours' in the simulation centre (strategic planning).

In order to ensure that she had sufficient time to spend in the simulation room, she planned to do her required readings on the other nights in which she was free (self-control or time management). During one particular session in the simulation centre, Dr Brown become concerned because she realized that she was making mistakes and was not sure how to correct them, due to the absence of feedback (metacognitive monitoring). Unfortunately, when her attending began to encourage her to take a greater role in procedures, Dr Brown struggled with a sense of inadequacy and unpreparedness because she was not able to get the feedback and information needed to correct her mistakes (poor self-efficacy).

Dr Brown—SRL commentary

Dr Brown's decisions about regulating her learning were somewhat adaptive and were driven by many factors. However, the less structured environment of the residency programme and her poor skills and self-efficacy in initiating contact with her attendings served as barriers to learning. This situation was not easy for Dr Brown, because in such ambiguous performance situations it was difficult for her to determine whether she 'measured up' in comparison with her peers and, more importantly, to clearly understand the expectations of her attendings. Although this situation is different from the demands of coursework, the process of SRL is the same. That is, the extent to which individuals will become masters of their learning is largely determined by the extent to which they engage in effective forethought, performance, and self-reflection.

Arguably, it is when a physician is fully autonomous that effective SRL skills become most important. Because so much of what a physician learns in training becomes rapidly obsolete, a practising physician must learn about new developments throughout their lives. Much of this learning is driven by the specific problems that individual physicians encounter on a daily basis. Ironically, minimal research has been devoted to examining how practising physicians use SRL.

Self-regulated and externally regulated learning

The three-phase model of SRL focuses primarily on the 'self' as the driver and initiator of learning. However, one must recognize that there are often numerous and powerful external forces that seek to define the goals of learning for the individual; in a sense, to supplant the *self* in SRL with an external mandate. Much of the literature involves efforts to push innovations into practice (continuing education, innovation dissemination, academic detailing) (Damschroder et al. 2009). Studies examine the efficacy of interventions at various levels (individual education, information resources, facilitating initial adoption or consolidating changes) in producing change but tend to focus on looking at the problem from a 'group' or 'systems' level rather than from an individual perspective.

In the example of Dr Smith, this external force was the health system in which he works. Other forces include professional societies, state laws, pharmaceutical companies, patient advocacy groups, public health organizations, pundits, and politicians. Indeed, a potentially strong barrier to promoting SRL is the din of competing voices telling the student or individual physician what they ought to learn—regardless of their own, self-identified gaps and priorities. From our perspective, these external forces are not inherently problematic unless students or professionals are unable to infuse these expectations into their own forethought, performance, and reflection phase processes.

Research implications and future directions

Of primary importance is to identify how well findings from SRL research with school age populations and those within higher education translate to medical education practice. Because motivation and SRL tend to be contextualized constructs, it is probable that medical education tasks and activities place unique demands on students, and thus the nature of intervention programmes in medical education should reflect that. From our perspective, one of the most important lines of research, which is actually quite broad in nature, involves the development of situation-specific SRL interventions that are tailored to each of the different phases of medical education.

SRL in its purest form is an individualistic activity—no two people need to acquire exactly the same skills or knowledge at the same time. Thus, SRL research might benefit from an idiographic approach to research (examining the dynamics of the process within the individual and treating individual differences as important data) rather than solely the more traditional nomothetic approach (examining the process across a group of people and treating individual differences as 'error variance'). The use of rigorous case study designs or single participant designs is particularly important when evaluating how SRL unfolds in medical contexts or examining effects of interventions on regulatory processes and behaviours .

The practical and applied emphases of medical care would prompt a need for SRL research to push the endpoint of studies beyond just individual behaviour (the learning part) to actual behaviour and practice changes (implementing the learning part). Such research is more difficult to do and is distinct from many SRL studies that rely on decontextualized and broad measures of regulation, such as self-report questionnaires. Extending outcomes to actual behaviour requires a more comprehensive assessment approach as well as more complex study designs, such as mixed methods approaches.

Much of the existing medical education research that relates to SRL has focused on self-assessment, particularly the accuracy of self-assessment. However, we need to move beyond this focus on accuracy to a broader study of the dynamics of how self-assessment functions within the larger context of SRL. Furthermore, we believe that medical education research on SRL needs to expand its focus beyond undergraduate education into graduate education and continuous professional development. Clearly, examining SRL in students is both important and convenient (in terms of a captive audience), but the learning contexts in medical schools may be limited and prevent a clear examination of how SRL is used to guide behaviour in clinical practice environments. The need for sophisticated SRL skills is perhaps most salient in these independent clinical practice environments, and it is within this phase of physician development that we should examine how SRL might influence learning and performance.

Conclusions

◆ SRL is a dynamic, cyclical process that often varies across situations and settings. Researchers and practitioners need to study and apply this concept in a highly contextualized manner.

◆ Effective SRL instruction involves an integration of motivation, metacognition, and strategic processes. This instruction should enable individuals to strategically prepare, engage, and reflect on their performance on a relevant task or activity.

◆ Although SRL is applicable to all developmental phases of medical education, this process becomes most essential when challenges, obstacles, and shifts in task complexity occur, regardless of the particular phase of training

◆ Although components of SRL have been studied in medical education in recent years, much greater attention needs to be devoted to examining how this process underlies many emergent issues in medical education.

Disclaimer

The views expressed in this chapter are those of the authors and do not necessarily reflect the views of the Uniformed Services University, the United States Air Force, the United States Navy, the Department of Defense, or other federal agencies.

References

Artino, A.R. (2012) Academic self-efficacy: From educational theory to instructional practice. *Perspect Med Educ.* 1: 76–85

Artino, A.R., Hemmer, P.A., and Durning, S. J. (2011) Using self-regulated learning theory to understand the beliefs, emotions, and behaviors of struggling medical students. *Acad Med.* 86: S35–S38.

Artino, A.R., La Rochelle, J.S., and Durning, S.J. (2010) Second-year medical students' motivational beliefs, emotions, and achievement. *Med Educ.* 44: 1203–1212

Artino, A.R., Dong, T., DeZee, K.J., et al. (2012) Achievement-goal structures and self-regulated learning: Relationships and changes in medical school. *Acad Med.* 87: 1375–1381

Bandura, A. (1986) *Social foundations of thought and action: A social cognitive theory*. Englewood Cliffs, NJ: Prentice Hall

Bandura, A. (1997) *Self-efficacy: The Exercise of Control*. New York: W.H. Freeman

Bandura, A. (2001) Social cognitive theory: An agentic perspective. *Ann Rev Psychol.* 52, 1–29.

Bembenutty, H., Cleary, T. J., and Kitsantas, A. (2013) *Applications of Self-Regulated Learning across Diverse Disciplines: A Tribute to Barry J. Zimmerman*. Charlotte NC: Information Age Publishing

Bleakley, A., Bligh, J., and Brice, J. (2012) *Medical Education for the Future: Identity, Power and Location*. New York: Springer

Boekaerts, M., Pintrich, P. R., and Zeidner, M. (eds) (2000) *Handbook of Self-regulation*. San Diego, CA: Academic Press

Bol, L., Riggs, R., Hacker, D. J., Dickerson, D., and Nunnery, J. (2010) The calibration accuracy of middle school students in math classes. *J Res Educ.* 21: 81–96

Bong, M. (2005) Within-grade changes in Korean girls' motivation and perceptions of the learning environment across domains and achievement levels. *J Educ Psychol.* 97(4): 656–672

Bonner, S., Zimmerman, B.J., Evans, D., Irigoyen, M., Resnick, D., and Mellins, R.B. (2002) An individualized intervention to improve asthma management among urban Latino and African-American families. *J Asthma.* 39(2): 167–179

Borkowski, J.G., Weyhing, R.S., and Carr, M. (1988) Effects of attributional retraining on strategy-based reading comprehension in learning-disabled students. *J Educ Psychol.* 80(1): 46–53

Brydges, R., and Butler, D. (2012) A reflective analysis of medical education research on self-regulation in learning and practice, *Med Educ.* 46: 71–79

Brydges, R., Carnahan, H., Safir, O., and Dubrowski, A. (2009) How effective is self-guided learning of clinical technical skills? It's all about process. *Med Educ.* 43: 507–515

Butler, D. (1998) The strategic content learning approach to promoting self-regulated learning: A report of three studies. *J Educ Psychol.* 90: 682–697

Cartier S., Plante A., and Tardif J. (2001) Learning by reading: Description of learning strategies of students involved in a problem-based learning program. http://eric.ed.gov/PDFS/ED452511.pdf Accessed 8 May 2013

Carver, C.S. (2004) Self-regulation of action and affect. In R. F. Baumeister and K. D. Vohs (eds) *Handbook of Self-regulation: Theory, Research, and Applications* (pp. 13–39). New York: Guilford Press

Clark, N.M. (2013) The use of self-regulation intervention in managing chronic disease. To appear in H. Bembenutty, T. J. Cleary, and A. Kitsantas (eds) *Applications of Self-Regulated Learning across Diverse Disciplines: A Tribute to Barry J. Zimmerman*. in press

Cleary T.J. (2011) Emergence of self-regulated learning microanalysis: Historical overview, essential features, and implications for research and practice. In B. J. Zimmerman and D. H. Schunk (eds) *Handbook of Self-Regulation of Learning and Performance* (pp. 329–345). New York, NY: Routledge

Cleary, T.J., and Chen, P. (2009) Self-regulation, motivation, and math achievement in middle school: Variations across grade level and math context. *J School Psychol.* 47(5): 291–314

Cleary, T.J., and Sandars, J. (2011) *Self-regulatory skills and clinical performance: a pilot study*. *Med Teach.* 33: e368–e374

Cleary, T.J., Zimmerman, B. J., and Keating, T. (2006) Training physical education students to self-regulate during basketball free-throw practice. *Res Q Exerc Sport.* 77: 251–262

Cleary, T.J., Platten, P., and Nelson, A. (2008) Effectiveness of the self-regulation empowerment program (SREP) with urban high school youth: An initial investigation. *J Adv Acad.* 20: 70–107

Colthart, I., Bagnall, G., Evans, A., et al. (2008) The effectiveness of self assessment on the identification of learner needs, learner activity, and impact on clinical practice: BEME Guide n. 10. *Med Teach.* 30: 124–145

Damschroder, L.J., Aron, D.C., Keith, R.E., Kirsh, S.R., Alexander, J.A., and Lowery, J.C. (2009) Fostering implementation of health services research findings into practice: a consolidated framework for advancing implementation science *Implement Sci.* 4: 50

Dornan, T. (2008) Self-assessment in CPD: lessons from the UK undergraduate and postgraduate education domains. *J Cont Educ Health Prof.* 28: 32–37

Durning, S.J., and Artino, A.R. (2011) Situativity theory: A perspective on how participants and the environment interact. *Med Teach.* 33: 1–12

Durning, S.J., Artino, A.R., Pangaro, L.N., van der Vleuten, C.P.M., and Schuwirth, L.W.T. (2010a) Reframing context in the clinical encounter: Implications for research and training in medical education. *Acad Med.* 85: 894–901

Durning S.J., Artino A.R., Boulet J., et al. (2010b) Contrasting the views of participants in the same encounter: are they the same? *Med Educ.* 44: 953–961

Durning, S.J., Cleary, T.J., Sandars, J.E., Hemmer, P.A., Kokotailo, P.K., and Artino, A.R. (2011a) Viewing 'strugglers' through a different lens: How a self-regulated learning perspective can help medical educators with assessment and remediation. *Acad Med.* 86: 488–495

Durning S.J., Artino, A.R., Pangaro L.N., van der Vleuten C., and Schuwirth L. (2011b) Context and clinical reasoning: understanding the situation from the perspective of the expert's voice. *Med Educ.* 45: 927–938

Durning S.J., Artino A.R., Boulet J., Dorrance K., van der Vleuten C., and Schuwirth L. (2012) The impact of selected contextual factors on experts' clinical reasoning performance. *Adv Health Sci Educ.* 17: 65–79

Dyrbye, L.N., Thomas, M.R., Power, D.V., et al. (2010) Burnout and serious thoughts of dropping out of medical school: a multi-institutional study. *Acad Med.* 85: 94–102

Eccles, J.S., and Wigfield, A. (2002) Motivational beliefs, values, and goals. *Ann Rev Psychol.* 53: 109–132

Epstein, R.M., Siegel, D.J., and Silberman, J. (2008) Self-monitoring in clinical practice: a challenge for medical educators. *J Cont Educ Health Prof.* 28: 5-1

Ericsson, K.A. (2006) The influence of experience and deliberate practice on the development of superior expert performance. In K.A. Ericsson, N. Charness, P.J. Feltovich and R.R. Hoffman (eds) *The Cambridge Handbook of Expertise and Expert Performance* (pp. 683–704). New York: Cambridge University Press

Eva, K.W. (2003) On the generality of specificity. *Med Educ.* 37: 587–588

Eva, K.W., Neville A.J., and Norman, G.R. (1998) Exploring the etiology of content specificity: factors influencing analogic transfer and problem solving. *Acad Med.* 73: S1–S5

Eva, K.W., and Regehr, G. (2005) Self-assessment in the health professions: a reformulation and research agenda. *Acad Med.* 80: S46–S54

Flavell, J.H. (1979) Metacognition and cognitive monitoring. *Am Psychol.* 34: 906–911

Frellsen, S.L., Baker, E.A., Papp, K.K., and Durning, S.J. (2008) Medical school policies regarding struggling medical students during the internal medicine clerkships: Results of a national survey. *Acad Med.* 83: 876–881

Glenberg, A.M. (2011) Positions in the mirror are closer than they appear. *Perspect Psychol Sci.* 6: 408–410

Goebert, D., Thompson, D., Takeshita, J., et al. (2009) Depressive symptoms in medical students and residents: A multischool study. *Acad Med.* 84: 236–241

Graham, S., and Harris, K. R. (2009) Almost 30 years of writing research: Making sense of it all with The Wrath of Khan. *Learning Disabilities Res Pract.* 24(2): 58–68

Greenburg, D.L., Durning, S.J., Cohen, D.L., Cruess, D., and Jackson, J.L. (2007) Identifying medical students likely to exhibit poor professionalism and knowledge during internship. *J Gen Intern Med.* 22: 1711–1717

Hadwin, A.F., Winne, P.H., Stockley, D.B., Nesbit, J.C., and Woszczyna, C. (2001) Context moderates students' self-reports about how they study. *J Educ Psychol.* 93: 477–487

Hall, N.C., Perry, R.P., Chipperfield, J.G., Clifton, R.A., and Haynes, T.L. (2006) Enhancing primary and secondary control in achievement settings through writing based attributional retraining. *J Soc Clin Psychol.* 25(4): 361–391

Institute of Medicine (2000) *To Err is Human: Building a Safer Health System.* Washington, DC: Institute of Medicine

Kennedy, T.J., Regehr, G., Baker, G.R., and Lingard, L.A. (2009) 'It's a cultural expectation...' the pressure on medical trainees to work independently in clinical practice. *Med Educ.* 43: 645–653

Knowles, M.S. (1975) *Self-directed Learning: A Guide for Learners and Teachers.* New York: Association Press

Li, S.-T.T., Paternniti, D.A., Co, J.P.T., and West, D.C. (2010) Successful self-directed lifelong learning in medicine: a conceptual model derived from qualitative analysis of a national survey of pediatric residents. *Acad Med.* 85: 1229–1236

Loyens, S.M.M., Magda, J., and Rikers, R.M.J.P. (2008) Self-directed learning in problem-based learning and its relationships with self-regulated learning. *Educ Psychol Rev.* 20: 411–427

Mace, F.C., Belfiore, P.J., and Hutchinson, J.M. (2001) Operant theory and research on self-regulation. In B. J. Zimmerman and D. H. Schunk (eds) *Self-regulated Learning and Academic Achievement: Theoretical Perspectives* (pp. 39–66) (2nd edn). Mahwah, NJ: Lawrence Erlbaum Associates

Mann, K., Gordon, J., and MacLeod, A. (2009) Reflection and reflective practice in health professions education: a systematic review. *Adv Health Sci Educ Theory Pract.* 14: 595–621

Mouton, C.-A.E., Regehr, G., Lingard, L., Merritt, C., and MacRae, H. (2010) Slowing down to stay out of trouble in the operating room: remaining attentive in automaticity. *Acad Med.* 85: 1571–1577

Norman, G. (2005) Research in clinical reasoning: past history and current trends. *Med Educ.* 39: 418–427

Pajares, F., and Urdan, T. (eds) (2006) *Self-efficacy Beliefs of Adolescents.* Greenwich, CT: Information Age Publishing

Pintrich, P.R. (2000) The role of goal orientation in self-regulated learning. In M. Boekaerts, P. R. Pintrich, and M. Zeidner (eds) *Handbook of Self-regulation* (pp. 451–502). San Diego, CA: Academic Press

Puustinen, M., and Pulkkinen, L. (2001) Models of self-regulated learning: A review. *Scand J Educ Res.* 45: 269–286

Rogers, E.M. (2003) *Diffusion of Innovations.* 5th edn. New York, NY: Free Press

Schunk, D.H., and Ertmer, P.A. (1999) Self-regulatory processes during computer skill acquisition: Goal and self-evaluative influences. *J Educ Psychol.* 91: 251–260

Schunk, D.H., and Swartz, C.W. (1993) Goals and progress feedback: Effects on self-efficacy and writing' achievement. *Contemp Educ Psychol.* 18(3): 337–354

Schunk, D.H., Pintrich, P.R., and Meece, J.L. (2008) *Motivation in Education: Theory, Research, and Applications.* 3rd edn. Upper Saddle River, NJ: Pearson Prentice Hall

Slotnick, H.B. (2001) How doctors learn: education and learning across the medical-school-to-practice trajectory. *Acad Med.* 76: 1013–1026

Straus, S.E., Richardson, W.S., Glasziou, P., and Haynes, R.B. (2005) *Evidence-Based Medicine: How to Practice and Teach EBM.* 3rd edn. Edinburgh: Churchill Livingstone.

Veenman, M.V.J., Prins, F.J., and Verheij, J. (2003) Learning styles: Self-reports versus thinking aloud measures. *Br J Educ Psychol.* 73: 357–372

Vohs, K.D., and Baumeister R.F. (2004) Understanding self-regulation: An introduction. In R. F. Baumeister and K. D. Vohs (eds) *Handbook of Self-regulation: Theory, Research, and Applications* (pp. 1–12). New York: Guilford Press

Ward, M., Gruppen, L.D., and Regehr, G. (2002) Measuring self-assessment: Current state of the art. *Adv Health Sci Educ.* 7: 63–80

White, C.B. (2007) Smoothing out transitions: How pedagogy influences medical students' achievement of self-regulated learning goals. *Adv Health Sci Educ.* 12: 279–297

White, C.B., and Gruppen, L.D. (2007) *Self-regulated learning in medical education* (Vol. 21). Edinburgh: Association for the Study of Medical Education

Winne, P.H. (2001) Self-regulated learning viewed from models of information processing. In B. J. Zimmerman and D. H. Schunk (eds) *Self-regulated Learning and Academic Achievement: Theoretical Perspectives.* 2nd edn (pp. 153–190). Mahwah, NJ: Lawrence Erlbaum Associates

Winne, P.H., and Jamieson-Noel, D.L. (2002) Exploring students' calibration of self-reports about study tactics and achievement. *Contemp Educ Psychol.* 28: 259–276

Woods, N.N., Mylopoulos, M., and Brydges, R. (2011) Informal self-regulated learning on a surgical rotation: uncovering student experiences in context. *Adv Health Sci Educ Theory Pract.* 16: 643–653

Zimmerman, B.J. (1995) Self-regulation involves more than metacognition: A social cognitive perspective. *Educ Psychol.* 30: 217–221

Zimmerman, B.J. (2000) Attaining self-regulation: A social cognitive perspective. In M. Boekaerts, P.R. Pintrich, and M. Zeidner (eds) *Handbook of Self-regulation* (pp. 13–39). San Diego, CA: Academic Press

Zimmerman, B.J. (2008a) Goal setting: A key proactive source of academic self-regulation. In D.H. Schunk and B.J. Zimmerman (eds) *Motivation and Self-regulated Learning: Theory, Research, and Applications* (pp. 267–296). New York: Lawrence Erlbaum Associates

Zimmerman, B.J. (2008b) Investigating self-regulation and motivation: Historical background, methodological developments, and future prospects. *Am Educ Res J.* 45(1): 166–183

Zimmerman, B.J. and Kitsantas, A. (1996) Self-regulated learning of a motoric skill: The role of goal setting and self-monitoring. *J Appl Sport Psychol.* 8(1): 60–75

Zimmerman, B.J., and Kitsantas, A. (1997) Developmental phases in self-regulation: Shifting from process goals to outcome goals. *J Educ Psychol.* 89(1): 29–36

Zimmerman, B.J., and Kitsantas, A. (2002) Acquiring writing revision and self-regulatory skill through observation and emulation. *J Educ Psychol.* 94(4): 660–668

Zimmerman, B.J., and Lebeau, R.B. (2000) A commentary on self-directed learning. In D.H. Evensen and C.E. Hmelo (eds) *Problem-based Learning: A Research Perspective on Learning Interactions* (pp. 299–313). Mahwah, NJ: Lawrence Erlbaum Associates

Zimmerman, B.J. and Schunk, D.H. (eds) (2001) *Self-regulated Learning and Academic Achievement: Theoretical Perspectives.* 2nd edn. Mahwah, NJ: Lawrence Erlbaum Associates

Zimmerman, B.J. and Schunk, D.H. (2008) Motivation: An essential dimension of self-regulated learning. In B.J. Zimmerman and D.H. Schunk (eds) *Motivation and Self-regulated Learning: Theory, Research, and Applications* (pp. 1–30). New York: Taylor and Francis

Zimmerman, B.J. and Schunk, D.H. (eds) (2011) *Handbook of Self-regulation of Learning and Performance.* New York: Routledge

CHAPTER 41

Formative assessment

Diana F. Wood

Formative assessment tools in the workplace facilitate reflection and professional development, enabling the bringing out into the open of those deficiencies that the individual may not have been aware of, or would rather have kept hidden.

Tim Swanwick

Reproduced from Swanwick T, 'Work based assessment in general practice: three dimensions and three challenges', Work Based Learning in Primary Care, 1, 2, p. 99, © Radcliffe Publishing, 2006, with permission

Introduction

The past three decades have seen a great expansion in the literature on assessment, reflecting the complexity of its many functions. Early debate focused around the contrast between assessment as a means of determining the accountability of an educational institution and its learning programmes versus the assessment of progress for individual students, their teachers and curricula—the aptly named 'double duty' (Boud 2000). These positions have been to some extent encapsulated in the familiar categories of 'summative' and 'formative' assessment, commonly described as 'assessment of learning' and 'assessment for learning', respectively. Simplistically, summative assessment measures the achievement of learning goals at the end of a course or programme of study whereas formative assessment provides feedback to learners about their progress. By extrapolation, summative assessments have been seen as providing 'hard' evidence of learning and of achievement of institutional aims whereas formative assessments have come to be regarded as a 'soft' means of assisting student learning. If we accept that all assessments are fundamentally linked to learning then this simple division becomes unsatisfactory. In a programmed approach, summative and formative assessments should be linked in a way that places the enhancement of student learning at its centre.

Many authors have identified the numerous roles of assessment (Brown et al 1997, p. 11). In general, assessment functions fall into three groups: assessment to measure achievement (assessment of learning), assessment to encourage student learning (assessment for learning) and assessment for quality assurance and standards (fig. 41.1). A list of the functions of assessment might include:

- measurement of student learning
- awarding grades
- summarizing individual student achievement
- indicating readiness to progress
- satisfying external regulators
- motivating students to learn
- provision of feedback
- diagnosis of specific misunderstandings
- focusing and directing student learning
- helping students learn more effectively
- informing curriculum development
- promoting staff development
- contributing to education quality assurance.

Superficially, the first group might be assigned to summative assessment, the second group to formative assessment, and the final group to institutional goals and accountability. However, closer inspection reveals that although some forms of assessment are more closely linked with accountability and others more directly with student learning, these are not clear distinctions. For example, detailed feedback on students' performance in summative assessments collected for the purposes of monitoring achievement leading to graduation is rarely given to students. However, preparing for and taking a summative assessment can enhance learning and aid knowledge retention (Rohrer and Pashler 2010). Furthermore, grades in intermediate summative assessments may be used by students to focus their future learning; and analysis of summative results should be considered at faculty and institutional levels to establish areas of curriculum weakness or the need for faculty development. Conversely, teachers will form a view on students' performance and knowledge following formative assessments, and external accrediting organizations are interested in the full range of assessments offered in a teaching programme and their effects on student learning (GMC 2009; QAA 2011).

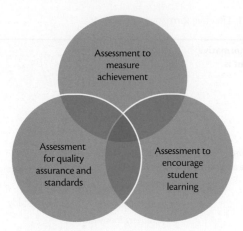

Figure 41.1 Assessment functions.

It is acknowledged that assessment drives the curriculum (Newble and Jaeger 1983; Ramsden 1992, p. 187). Assessment also influences student opinion, such that students will use the weighting of assessments to rank the importance of various curriculum components and therefore the study time allocated to each. The concept of the 'hidden curriculum' has been widely accepted as an explanation of student behaviour when faced with their assessment programme within a crowded curriculum (Snyder 1971). In essence, students behave strategically, adopting their learning style to meet the needs of the assessment, rejecting deep learning methods in favour of the memorization often required to pass a particular examination. Less widely discussed has been Snyder's further observation of the role of the faculty in driving students to behave in this strategic fashion by poor design of assessment programmes. Deep learning includes understanding and interpretation of material (Entwistle and Entwistle 1991) and good assessment programmes should foster the development of a deep approach, ensuring both understanding and the creation of conceptual frameworks, rather than memorization of facts. Both formative and summative assessments should be developed alongside a teaching programme and not added on at the end to test 'what the students have learned'.

Assessment not only drives the curriculum, it also drives learning (Gibbs 1992; Rust 2002). In order for an assessment programme to achieve its goals and to have positive effects on learning then improving the quality of all assessments, whether formative or summative, must be undertaken. van der Vleuten (1996) describes five characteristics of an assessment, each of which is of equal importance and should be considered: reliability, validity, educational impact, cost, and acceptability. A well-designed series of formative assessments should have high validity and acceptability, low cost, and make a major contribution to the educational impact of an overall assessment programme. Formative and summative assessments are two sides of the same activity; in a good assessment programme both fulfil all the roles of assessment to a greater or lesser extent. The main difference between the two is the amount and nature of feedback generated and the way in which this information is used.

Feedback is central to the debate about the impact of assessment on learning. Both formative and summative assessments produce feedback, each with a different focus, but both relevant to the three main assessment function groups described earlier.

Generally speaking, summative assessment produces largely quantitative data including the grades, progression rates, graduation and other data used by institutions to inform quality assurance procedures and their external regulators. Formative assessment tends to generate qualitative data of more frequent and ongoing value to individual students, their teachers and the curriculum design team.

Much of the literature relating to formative assessment derives from the general educational arena, including the school, further and higher education sectors. This chapter focuses on these general principles of formative assessment and their translation into medical education.

Formative assessment and its impact on learning

Bell and Cowie (2001) describe two types of formative assessment—that involving regular planned assessment tasks ('planned formative assessment') and more informal, ad-hoc activities ('interactive formative assessment'). Formative assessment offering regular feedback is not a new construct. For generations, traditional university education involved the production of weekly assignments with one-to-one tutorial supervision and immediate feedback. The implications of modern resource constraints and increased student numbers have been noted as part of the reason for the decline in this informal interactive formative assessment (Gibbs and Simpson 2004).

Definitions of formal planned formative assessment are characterized by the link to learning and curriculum development, although this has not always been recognized explicitly in practice. Thus 'formative evaluation' was described by Bloom et al (1971, p. 117) as '. . . evaluation which all who are involved—student, teacher, curriculum maker—would welcome because they find it so useful in helping them to improve what they wish to do'. Sadler's definition of formative assessment (Sadler 1989) goes to the heart of the problem when assessment is not linked to learning and curriculum:

> Formative assessment is concerned with how judgements about the quality of student responses (performances, pieces or works) can be used to shape and improve the student's competence by short-circuiting the randomness and inefficiency of trial–and-error learning.

In an influential review, Black and Wiliam provided a definition of formative assessment which is widely recognized to describe assessment that directly aids learning by the provision of feedback. It encompasses '. . . all those activities undertaken by teachers, and/or by their students, which provide information to be used as feedback to modify the teaching and learning activities in which they are engaged' (Black and Wiliam 1998a). Crucially, formative assessment should be an active process involving both teacher and student, in which the evidence from assessment is used to adapt teaching to meet student needs (Black and Wiliam 1998b).

These definitions were formulated within the context of general school education. Clearly, the learning environment plays an important part in the provision of effective formative assessment. In schools most learning takes place within a classroom setting where there is a high level of teacher–student interaction. In higher education settings students are expected to perform more independent learning and, for the reasons noted, contact time is tending to become more limited. Self-directed learning outside the classroom setting is fundamental in higher education and this activity is intimately involved with the concept of the hidden (or informal) curriculum (Hafferty 1998; Atherton 2011). Students use a wide range of learning methods and materials in addition to those provided formally (Zhang et al. 2011). The context of the learning environment thus influences the nature and efficacy of formative assessments (Joughin 2004) and must be considered in the design of formative assessment programmes.

More recently Black and Wiliam (2009) have refined their definition to include five strategies crucial to formative assessment:

- 'Clarifying and sharing learning intentions and criteria for success'

- 'Engineering effective classroom discussions and other learning tasks that elicit evidence of student understanding'

- 'Providing feedback that moves learners forward'

- 'Activating students as instructional resources for one another'

- 'Activating students as the owners of their own learning'.

These strategies encompass wider activities than classroom questioning and feedback and have more direct applicability to the higher education sector. In particular, the importance of students' understanding the criteria for success is stressed, a factor recognized as an important feature of higher education programmes (GMC 2009, p. 48; QAA 2006, p. 5) and featuring routinely in the UK National Student Survey (2012). The desirability of students acting as resources for each other and encouraging students to be the owners of their own learning also resonate with the features of adult learning (Knowles 1980), accepted as an important theory of learning in higher education and widely used in medical education (Kaufman and Mann 2010).

The features of effective formative assessment are drawn from a range of criteria are shown in table 41.1.

The most important characteristic of formative assessment is its potential to enhance learning although the reported effect sizes vary and have recently been brought into question (Bennett 2011). This critique reflects the lack of uniformity of research studies which include widely differing sets of learners and educational environments and a variable nature and quality of feedback delivered. The theoretical reason for any observed enhancement of learning is uncertain but most authors agree that a developed theory of formative assessment should have an emphasis on constructivism and reflect understanding of the cognitive effects of learning through feedback (Yorke 2003). A number of the other features of formative assessment shown in table 41.1 are consistent with the development of deep learning. Gibbs (1992) reviewed the characteristics of courses associated with deep and surface learning. Features of deep learning, including intrinsic motivation for learning, active learning and interaction with others, can be fostered by a programme of formative assessment. A further way in which formative assessment can enhance learning is that it encourages students to spend time on a particular area of study, the 'time on task' principle (Chickering and Gamson 1987). The available evidence suggests that there is a direct relationship between time allocated to a subject, student 'time on task' and student achievement (Gibbs and Simpson 2004). Students focus their study time onto assessed tasks (Gibbs 2010) suggesting that a planned programme of formative assessment can benefit learning directly.

Table 41.1 Effective formative assessment

Effective formative assessment is	active
	a dynamic interaction
	ongoing and frequent
	embedded in the curriculum
	non-judgemental
	non-threatening
For students, formative assessment	is developmental
	encourages deep learning and understanding
	provides detailed feedback
	ensures time is spent in necessary study
	is positively motivational
	promotes self-directed learning
	allows students to demonstrate understanding
	raises self-esteem
	encourages collaborative learning
	identifies insecurities
	offers opportunities for remediation
For teachers, formative assessment	facilitates detailed feedback
	promotes self-directed learning
	identifies students in difficulty
	fosters varied teaching methods
	develops teaching skills
For the curriculum, formative assessment	should be aligned with summative assessment
	provides ongoing evaluation of teaching and learning
	gives timely identification of challenging subject areas
	offers ongoing quality assurance
For the institution, formative assessment	provides evidence of achievement of learning outcomes
	demonstrates plurality of assessment methodologies
	suggests areas for staff development
	contributes to high quality summative outcomes

Reproduced from 'Learning-oriented assessment: conceptual bases and practical implications', David Carless, *Innovations in Education and Teaching International*, 44, 1, Copyright 2007 Taylor & Francis, reprinted by permission of Taylor & Francis Ltd.

Frequent formative testing has been associated with subsequently improved scores in summative assessments (Bangert-Drowns et al. 1991). Formative assessment can also be designed to enhance student productivity in learning. For example, revision for repeated MCQ tests may encourage a surface approach to learning with memorization, but appropriately designed tasks will lead the student to higher productivity with effective deep learning strategies (Macdonald 2002).

The importance of formative assessment as a means by which learning can be enhanced has been further developed by the concept of learning-orientated assessment (Carless 2007, 2009). Learning-orientated assessment identifies the importance of making assessment tasks into learning tasks, of gaining student involvement in assessment and giving appropriate feedback, as follows (Carless 2007):

- 'Principle 1: Assessment tasks should be designed to stimulate sound learning practices amongst students'.

- 'Principle 2: Assessment should involve students actively in engaging with criteria, quality, their own and/or peers' performance'.

- 'Principle 3: Feedback should be timely and forward-looking so as to support current and future student learning'.

Learning-orientated assessment thus forms a conceptual basis in which learning, rather than the measurement of achievement, is placed centrally in an assessment programme. The principles are consistent with Black and Wiliam's (2009) definition and together form the basis for a programme of learner-centred formative assessments.

Formative assessment can play a major role in the acquisition of lifelong learning skills by helping students to self-regulate their learning activities and become more autonomous learners. Teachers should be motivated by the promotion of learning skills in their students and by the dynamic interaction fostered by formative assessment in a challenging yet supportive environment. Overall, consideration of the effects of formative assessment on students and teachers suggests that it should be a positive experience for both groups.

Feedback in formative assessment

Feedback is central to the concept of formative assessment, providing the route by which assessment becomes a tool for learning. It encourages student and teacher to work together to improve the student's understanding of a subject and, when provided in a non-judgemental and open fashion, allows the student to feel more confident in discussing their difficulties and planning better approaches to learning. Feedback is positively correlated with student achievement and is the single most important determinant of learning (Hattie 1987); although it is also clear that the quality of the feedback is vital. Poor quality feedback may have no effect or even may be detrimental (Black and Wiliam 1998a). Effective, constructive feedback can enhance the learning experience and develop learner self-regulation, whereas destructive feedback can have profoundly negative effects on learning (Kluger and DeNisi 1996).

Effective feedback

Feedback describes an interaction between the teacher giving the feedback and the student receiving it (Hattie and Jaeger 1998), crucially both activities requiring a specific skill set that needs to be learned. Feedback is usually defined as addressing the 'gap' between a student's current level of knowledge or skill and the desired goal, with effective feedback only being achieved when the student takes action to narrow the gap (Ramprasad 1983; Sadler 1989; Rushton 2005). To do this, students must be aware of the educational goals and able and empowered to take the necessary action to achieve them.

Theoretically, this process encompasses a constructivist approach, in which the student identifies and builds upon prior knowledge. Vygotsky's 'zone of proximal development' (ZPD) defines the region between the student's current problem-solving ability and their being able to solve more complex problems given suitable guidance by a more skilled person (Vygotsky 1978). This leads to an upwards spiral of improved learning as the student

and teacher return to further feedback at a later date, building on knowledge and thereby adjusting the ZPD. This 'social constructivism' in which students' internal learning processes are enhanced by external guidance, is echoed in Kolb's work on experiential learning (Kolb 1984). The dynamic collaboration between teacher and student, in which educational goals are constantly being identified and modified, is at the heart of effective feedback (Rust et al 2005). If formative assessment becomes only a means by which information is transmitted from teacher to student then the student may struggle to understand without the opportunity for discussion and elaboration. Furthermore, such a one-way procedure fails to recognize the importance of students' beliefs and their level of self esteem (Nicol and Macfarlane-Dick 2006). An effective feedback process requires students to take an active role and to develop skills of self-regulation (Butler and Winne 1995). It should be specific, non-judgemental, behavioural and descriptive and provided within a supportive educational environment close to the time of the learning experience.

These principles provide a framework within which the student can move towards learner self-regulation. They clarify the teacher's role in providing information to the student about their performance and also, importantly, about what is expected of them and how to recognize the gap between current and expected attainment (O'Donovan et al 2001).

The principles of formative assessment apply to all forms of assessed work. Thus, in practical terms, simply giving a grade for written work or making a comment ('excellent'; 'disappointing') is not helpful in itself, whereas a description of why the work is good or bad and offering suggestions for improvement helps student understanding. In the SOLO taxonomy (structure of observed learning outcome), Biggs and Collis (1982) described a hierarchy of responses in students' work that is not content specific and can be summarized as follows:

- Prestructural: use of irrelevant information or no meaningful response.

- Unistructural: answer focuses on one relevant aspect only.

- Multistructural: answer focuses on several relevant features but they are not coordinated together.

- Relational: the several parts are integrated into a coherent whole: details are linked to conclusions: meaning is understood.

- Extended abstract: answer generalizes the structure beyond the information given: higher order principles are used to bring in a new and broader set of issues.

Understanding and implementing SOLO, or other similar frameworks, allows the teacher to develop structure in their feedback practice by identifying different levels of achievement clearly and this assists students in developing the higher orders associated with deep learning. Well structured and constructive feedback given in this way is thus more conducive to learning than simple judgemental statements.

At the end of a feedback discussion, the teacher should check that the student has understood the feedback they have been given, that their interpretation of the feedback is correct and that they have made sensible plans to address the issues raised. A student's perception of feedback may not reflect the teacher's intentions and time spent checking will identify any discrepancies between the two (Sender Liberman et al. 2005).

Teacher perspectives on formative assessment

Many of the features of formative assessment could equally be ascribed to good teaching itself and the literature from school environments highlights the use of frequent feedback in the daily teaching and learning process, such that for many it is seen as an intrinsic part of their work. Teachers in higher education may have to be more explicit by setting time for formative assessment tasks, but it is clear that training for teachers in both school and higher education sectors can improve their ability to enhance student learning through formative assessment (Gibbs and Coffey 2004; Mitchell 2006).

The expertise of individual teachers and their differing levels of skill and experience, particularly in giving feedback, are important features in the development of learner-centred assessment. Teachers in training at any level, be they undergraduates in education faculties or experienced practitioners undertaking continuing professional development, are influenced by their own prior experience of feedback and assessment. This may have a profound influence on the way in which they accept the need to develop skills for feedback and formative assessment and the speed with which they do so.

In its simplest form, any piece of student work can be reviewed by a teacher, evaluated against the expected standard and judged, either by the award of a grade or by a qualitative piece of feedback. Clearly, the characteristics that the teacher brings to this process have a profound effect on the quality of the assessment process. Sadler (1998) identified six important characteristics that 'highly competent' teachers possess in their approach to formative assessment, which can be summarized as follows:

- knowledge
- attitudes towards teaching and towards learners
- skill in devising assessment tasks
- understanding of appropriate standards and expectations of student performance
- experience in the use of judgements for the assessment task
- expertise in giving effective feedback.

Subject knowledge is fundamental to the teaching and learning process and takes many forms. The teacher should understand the accuracy of factual content and also possess an ability to evaluate students' responses in terms of their full or partial correctness within a certain context. Furthermore the teacher's personal experience might indicate whether it is better to perform a task one way or another. Competent teachers have a positive attitude towards teaching, are empathic towards their students and are motivated by evidence of student learning and improvement. They demonstrate skill in devising a range of assessment tasks that will foster deep learning and understanding, and they involve the students by explaining the goals of the assessment and encouraging them to design assessment tasks themselves. Coupled with this, they understand the standards and assessment criteria and use their experience to formulate appropriate expectations of student performance in relationship to the level of the curriculum and previous student activity. This draws on past experience and requires teachers to be conscientious in their approach to assessment—they themselves may learn new things from student work but need to be able to conceptualize these within an overall framework for judgement. Finally, competent teachers are expert in giving effective feedback and are reflective about their own role in the process.

In any faculty, the level of expertise will vary between teachers. Given the importance of formative assessment as a means to foster deep learning, self-regulation and lifelong learning skills, it is important that at institutional level suitable staff development programmes are made available for teachers and that there is a good system for education quality assurance in place, including peer review and appraisal of teaching skills. For many teachers the development of constructive feedback skills is seen as the most important aspect of their professional development (Hewson and Little 1998).

Student perspectives on formative assessment

Formative assessment is a two-way process, a dynamic interaction between the teacher and the student centred around effective feedback. At its most basic, this involves educating students about the aims of the assessment process and ensuring their clear understanding of what is expected of them in order to succeed. However, if formative assessment is to fulfil its major role as a driver of learning then a greater level of student engagement with the process itself is required. Ultimately, formative assessment should be a means by which students improve their performance and develop themselves as self-directed, motivated learners with high levels of self-regulation. In essence, self-regulated learners are aware of their own knowledge, beliefs and cognitive skills and they use these to interpret external feedback effectively by monitoring their learning behaviours (and adapting these where necessary), generating their own internal feedback mechanisms and managing learning resources effectively (Butler and Winne 1995). Nicol and Macfarlane Dick (2006) developed a model to demonstrate the way in which the external outcomes, required for an assessed task, are linked to internal outcomes, such as motivation and understanding, by feedback provided as part of the formative assessment process. Evidence from the literature suggests that students with a higher level of self-regulation are more effective learners, demonstrating greater resourcefulness, persistence, and success.

Once students become engaged with their assessment programme as a means to improve learning, there are opportunities to further enhance the role of formative assessment. Self-assessment and peer-assessment can help students to evaluate their own and other's work in a meaningful way, particularly with respect to closing the gap identified by effective feedback. Self-assessment requires students to understand the assessment criteria (even being involved in their development where appropriate) and to develop judgement skills with which to review their own work. Peer-assessment enables students to review and consider the value of work produced by others at the same level of learning as themselves. Such procedures enable students to understand the purpose of assessments, to review their own work critically, to act as an assessor by reviewing other students' work and to give and receive feedback to and from their peers, all of which assist the development of self-regulation skills. Furthermore, peer assessment helps students recognize good work and to develop the skills of self-assessment and reflection that are essential to becoming lifelong learners (Orsmond 2004; Carless et al. 2006).

Introduction of a system of self- and peer-assessment requires excellent communication between student and teacher in order for the student to understand the assessment criteria and develop their judgement and feedback skills. This process in itself is valuable in developing the student-teacher relationship. Initially self- and peer-assessment may be daunting to students and inaccurate judgements of their own and others' abilities may be problematic. While most studies demonstrate a reasonable correlation between grades awarded by students and those by teachers (Orsmond 2004), it is clear that both under-rating and over-rating themselves and others is a problem for students (Boud and Falchikov 1995; Gordon 1991). Furthermore, this rating behaviour appears to be linked to achievement, such that, in general, low achieving students tend to mark themselves and others generously while high achievers are over critical of their own work although they apply criteria effectively to work of their peers (Boud and Falchikov 1995; Ward et al. 2002; Langendyk 2006). Interpretation of the results of studies on self- and peer assessment is difficult due to the wide range of variables present in the process (by its very nature) and to the level at which these have or have not been taken into account in experimental and quasi-experimental studies. However, two main conclusions can be drawn. First, student demographics, their level of achievement and, crucially, the amount of training and experience in assessment they have, affects both their accuracy of judgement and the development of positive attitudes towards the process. Second, the central role of effective, non-judgemental feedback is demonstrated (Topping 2010).

Curriculum design with formative assessment

A well designed programme of formative assessment should be a positive experience for students and teachers. Students should learn more effectively, develop higher levels of autonomy and self-regulation and gain better outcomes in terms of their learning and overall success—all of which should be motivational for teaching staff. The central importance of linking teaching with assessment was suggested by Martinez and Lipson (1989): 'We envision a new generation of assessment products that are instructionally useful—products in which testing and teaching complement and reinforce each other'. The social constructivist model described earlier is designed to harness the power of the assessment process for learning and it implies that everything in the curriculum, including the intended learning outcomes, the teaching and learning methods and the assessment procedures are fully integrated (Shepard 2000). 'Constructive alignment' of the curriculum (Biggs 2003) ensures that students construct meaning through relevant learning activities, that teachers create a suitable learning environment that supports the learning activities and that the assessments facilitate learning by being explicitly linked to the intended learning outcomes. For constructive alignment to occur within a teaching institution, assessment components should be internally coherent (Gitomer and Duschl 2007) such that formative assessments are planned strategically alongside summative assessments, and both are embedded in curriculum design and review. A programmatic approach to assessment should develop the need for assessment to meet its three main aims (assessment of learning, assessment for learning and assessment for quality assurance and standards) in a coherent structure that is fit for purpose (Schuwirth and van der Vleuten 2011; van der Vleuten et al. 2012).

In order to embed an assessment programme successfully into the curriculum, a number of key features need to be considered. First, staff involved in curriculum planning must be clear about the overall aims of the curriculum, the explicit intended learning outcomes for each component module of the course, and how they can be assessed. Second, within that plan, the educational goals and nature (formative or summative) of each assessment must be made clear, and these should be linked to the expertise of the student and their expected performance at each level of the course. It is useful to consider this process within a framework for learning, of which the most well recognized, is Bloom's taxonomy (Bloom 1965). This describes the development of expertise in terms of the progressive complexity of handling information, ranging from basic knowledge retention through comprehension, analysis, application, synthesis, and evaluation; the higher orders indicating understanding, integration of knowledge and deep learning. Assessments placed at different times within a curriculum should reflect this progression and their formats must be varied according to what is being assessed and when. Third, the assessment programme as a whole should be blueprinted against the curriculum to ensure that the assessments are mapped against the learning outcomes (Wass et al. 2007). Careful blueprinting will ensure that content is widely and appropriately sampled, that context specificity is accounted for, that the assessment method is appropriate to the intended learning outcomes and that a degree of triangulation between differing formats is included in the programme. Finally, the module design should show clearly how evaluation of teaching, learning, and assessment will be performed both for quality assurance purposes and to allow future development of the teaching programme.

To ensure that module design incorporates assessment, feedback, and evaluation, an iterative process of review and modification of curriculum content, learning outcomes, and assessment practice should be undertaken. The aims of the teaching module are translated into learning outcomes and linked with assessment criteria in an interactive fashion, taking into account the level of student attainment expected at a particular point in the curriculum. Having delivered the module and performed the assessment as designed, evaluation of the module includes a review of the teaching methods and the appropriateness of the learning outcomes and assessments used. This format for curriculum design facilitates the development of embedded assessment which can be blueprinted against curriculum content and teaching methodologies. The explicit linkage of the assessment programme to the design and evaluation of the module and to the curriculum as a whole also ensures that evaluation of the assessment process itself will occur (Fowell et al. 1999). Furthermore, careful codesign of curriculum and assessment means that the measurement characteristic of formative assessment is not lost, and full consideration can be given to its performance in terms of reliability, validity, and educational impact.

Formative assessment for educational institutions

Educational institutions have numerous lines of accountability including students, parents, academic and non-academic staff, external regulators, professional bodies, and local and national government departments. At institutional level, assessment forms an important part of the process of accountability to the external world and, as discussed earlier, whether assessment's primary purpose should be for accountability or for the enhancement of student learning has been the source of much debate. Both formative and summative assessments play a major role in accountability and are inextricably linked; a programme of formative assessment and feedback designed to enhance student learning will be undermined and ultimately will fail if summative assessments inhibit the process by demanding different learning and teaching skills. Conversely, if the main role of assessment is to enhance student learning, then appropriate alignment of summative assessments alongside the formative programme should be reflected in better student learning and improved institutional outcomes. Institutions should aim to collect information systematically from all forms of assessment to close the assessment loop—in other words to learn from the data generated by their assessment programmes in order to inform decisions about future curriculum, teaching, and learning and staff development activities. This requires all members of the institution, not just students and teachers but also administrators and other non-academic staff, to engage with the assessment process as part of a community of learning (Walvoord 2010). This change, from viewing assessment as a separate activity within an institution to one that is central to the organization as part of a programme of continuous improvement, has been labelled transformative assessment (Angelo 1999). Wehlburg (2008) describes assessments that form part of a transformational process; they can be summarized as being:

* appropriate and focused on the mission statement of the institution and desired outcomes of the faculty or department

* meaningful, such that data gathered from assessments are used to inform curriculum decisions and focus on areas needing change

* sustainable and established as part of an institution's routine cycle of work

* flexible, allowing future modification and forming part of an upward spiral of quality and achievement

* used for improvement such that data collected are used to enhance the quality of student learning rather than just stored as part of the institutional record.

In order for an institution to transform itself into a learning community, a number of changes to its overall culture may have to occur, including the development of trust between all its members, building motivation by identifying shared goals for learning and assessment, developing a collective understanding of new concepts and creating a list of guidelines by which the institution as a whole will promote learning by assessment (Angelo 1999). This process requires strong academic leadership and willingness on behalf of the organization to promote assessment for learning and to facilitate the necessary training of staff and students and the ongoing professional development required for its implementation and sustainability.

Formative assessment in medical education

Medical education is scrutinized at all stages in order to provide evidence to external regulators and the general public that medical students, doctors in training, and experienced clinicians become and remain competent. A large number of stakeholders have an interest in medical education including the students and trainees, teaching staff, university medical schools and other educational institutions, health service employers, external regulators and the public at large. While regulators and the public increasingly desire summative evidence of achievement and competence, the arguments made previously in favour of a constructively aligned programme of formative and summative assessment leading to enhanced learning and increased quality equally apply to undergraduate, postgraduate, and continuing medical education. Lifelong learning is an important feature of a career in medicine and the development of skills including deep learning, self-assessment, reflection, and self-regulation as a learner, all promoted by formative assessment, are essential for life in 'the learning society' (Boud 2000) and specifically for medical students and doctors to develop their careers in clinical learning environments.

The advent of outcomes-based medical education has facilitated the production of clearly defined assessments which are varied in nature and designed to be appropriate to the educational domain being assessed. For example, the UK General Medical Council divides its learning outcomes for undergraduates into three groups, Doctor as Scientist, Doctor as Practitioner, and Doctor as Professional (GMC 2009), roughly equivalent to the familiar testing domains of knowledge, skills, attitudes and professional behaviour. A range of testing formats is thus required to fulfil the assessment needs of undergraduate and postgraduate medical education. All assessment formats have a set of common criteria (Norcini et al 2011), irrespective of their use in a formative or summative fashion; in summary, they should:

* be reliable, valid, feasible, fair and beneficial to learning

* have content and form that are aligned with their purpose and desired outcomes

* reflect broad sampling to achieve an accurate representation of ability to account for content specificity

* be constructed according to clearly defined standards and derived using systematic and credible methods.

Teaching and learning for medical students and trainees takes place in a wide range of educational environments demanding different teaching methodologies, with the focus generally moving from an emphasis on lectures, laboratory demonstrations, and small group or problem-based learning in the earlier years to experiential learning and simulation, complemented by self-directed study in the senior student and postgraduate trainee curricula. The choice of assessment format should reflect the teaching and learning. Formative assessment techniques can be applied to all areas of medical education—see table 41.2.

The ability of formative assessment to identify students with difficulties and thus providing opportunities for early remediation is important and can provide a basis for academic guidance interviews or other supportive interventions (Denison et al. 2006). Entry to medical school requires students to have achieved excellent grades in school exit examinations, previous higher degrees or medical school selection assessments. Despite new students being motivated and academically capable, a small number go on to early failure and for some this disastrous situation results in internal demotivation and a cycle of further failure. The learning styles that students develop to produce exceptional performance in secondary school examinations may be part of the reason for their failure in university (Sayer et al. 2002). Many students have learned previously in

Table 41.2 Applications of formative assessment techniques

Formative assessment techniques can be applied to all areas of medical education including assessment of:

◆ Knowledge

◆ Competence—clinical, communication, and practical skills in real and simulated settings

◆ Experiential learning—in hospital clinical placements, general practice, community placements

◆ Portfolio learning

A complete formative assessment may include differing test formats, this triangulation allowing teachers to give a more global assessment of student performance.

didactic teaching environments, often becoming expert at memorizing facts rather than using deep approaches to learning. As medical students, they are exposed to different teaching and learning methods from entry to the course, aimed at fostering deep learning and understanding. These include small group, problem-based learning, or problem-solving exercises. Students may find these challenges daunting. A well-designed programme of formative assessment helps them to understand their learning goals and the ways in which these might be achieved. Specific instruction in how to utilize feedback and develop skills of self- and peer-assessment should be delivered in order to maximize their gain from the process. Ideally, this should take the form of a curriculum programme about formative assessment and feedback—a single lecture will not provide sufficient time or indicate the nature and importance of the topic. Inclusion of early formative assessment, during which teachers model good feedback practice within a learning group, is more likely to be educationally valuable (Henderson et al, 2005) (fig. 41.2). However, even with education about the process itself, the size of the shift in student attitudes needed to embrace a fully formative assessment system that encourages them to make judgements about their own performance and that of their peers should not be underestimated (Altahawi et al, 2012).

A number of effective techniques for formative assessment in the early student years, both in large and small group settings, have been described and the evidence suggests that students find formative assessments valuable, for example in the basic biomedical sciences (Carroll 1995; Vaz et al. 1996; Stead 2005), progress testing (Oldham 2007), paper-based assessment of clinical knowledge (Hill et al. 1994), and, in early years, problem-based learning (Rolfe and McPherson 1995). On-line quizzes have been shown to be effective as a means of delivering formative assessment with improved subsequent performance for some students (Kibble 2007; Dobson 2008), although student views on computer-assisted learning and testing are varied (Vogel and Wood 2002; Rudland et al. 2011) and concerns about 'cheating', by way of online access to learning materials, persist.

Clinical education begins in medical school and lasts throughout a doctor's working life. A competency-based approach to medical education encompasses all forms of clinical teaching and learning, including simulated settings for both basic and complex skills learning and other experiential learning in clinical settings. The development of expertise depends on regular assessment and feedback, and competency-based learning demands a range of assessments, all of which should be formative to the extent they facilitate

further learning and development (Wass et al. 2007; Epstein 2007; Holmboe et al. 2010). In a well aligned curriculum summative assessments within the programme, designed to assure competence for medical practice, may also provide feedback to the learner.

Much of the research into feedback in medical education comes from the field of teaching competence in communication skills and these principles have been carried forward into other experiential and reflective learning environments (Ende 1983; Pendleton et al. 1984; Neher et al. 1992; Silverman et al. 1996; Roy Chowdhury and Kalu 2004; Kurtz et al. 2005; Mohanna et al. 2011). The principles of formative assessment with constructive feedback for experiential learning in medicine are the same as in other disciplines. It should be ongoing, frequent, non-judgemental and informal and offer students the availability of regular interaction with their teachers, motivating and encouraging them towards deep learning (Wood 2010).

The development of increasingly sophisticated simulation-based teaching should not detract from learning in clinical settings, either hospital-based placements (student clerkships and trainee workplace-based learning) or in general practice and community settings. Programmes of formative assessment using a wide range of different assessment formats are well established for clinical students and trainees, including: objective structured clinical exams, mini-clinical evaluation exercises (see fig. 41.2) and direct observation of procedural skills, direct observation of consultation, debriefing, portfolios, 360-degree feedback, and combinations of formats aimed at offering a more holistic approach to the process (McKinley et al. 2000; Elizondo-Montemayor 2004; Higgins et al. 2004; Alves de Lima et al. 2005; Daelmans et al. 2005; Driessen et al. 2005; Gray et al. 2008; Rudolph et al. 2008). Observation-based formative assessments are central to clinical education but it is clear that the learners' perceptions of and reactions to feedback within the formative process are often negative. Learners report a lack of feedback or feedback that it is poorly delivered or unfair. Sometimes they become defensive, particularly to feedback from other professionals such as nurses and paramedical staff (Higgins et al. 2004). Student satisfaction is higher when feedback is simply positive, irrespective of the positive effects of constructive criticism on future performance (Boehler et al. 2006). Furthermore, the learner's emotional state and self-assessment of their own performance affects the way in which feedback is perceived, such that if the teacher's feedback is in conflict with the learner's view (even if the teacher is more positive), the learner is less likely to accept it and may remain resistant to constructive formative feedback in future assessments. This phenomenon may also affect teachers when two-way evaluation is practised between learners and senior faculty (Watling and Lingard 2012). In other circumstances students may feel inhibited from seeking feedback if the specific learning climate is thought to be hostile or indifferent. It is important that student and trainee views on feedback are sought and acted upon, not only because students can be helped to elicit feedback, but also to foster a feedback culture within the institution (Archer 2010; Milan et al. 2011).

Conclusions

◆ Formative assessment, or assessment for learning, should play an important part in teaching and learning programmes at all stages.

mini-Clinical Evaluation Exercise (mini-CEX) for Core Medical Training

mini-CEX is a directly *observed* trainee/patient interaction primarily designed to assess clinical and communication skills.

1. **Setting for assessment (eg. ward round, outpatients etc) and brief summary of case**

2. **Please comment on what was done well and areas for improvement. Please note constructive feedback is required in order for this assessment to be valid, and aim to identify areas for learning and reflection.**

Consultation and communication skills	
Physical Examination	
Clinical Judgement	
Organisation/Efficiency	

3. **Agreed action plan**

4. **Based on this observation please rate the level of overall competence the trainee has shown:**

Rating	Description
☐ Below level expected during Foundation Programme	Demonstrates basic consultation skills resulting in incomplete history and/or examination findings. Shows limited clinical judgement following encounter
☐ Performed at the level expected at completion of Foundation Programme / early Core Training	Demonstrates sound consultation skills resulting in adequate history and/or examination findings. Shows basic clinical judgement following encounter
☐ Performed at the level expected on completion of Core Training / early Higher Training	Demonstrates good consultation skills resulting in a sound history, and/or examination findings. Shows solid clinical judgement following encounter consistent with early higher training
☐ Performed at level expected during Higher Training	Demonstrates excellent and timely consultation skills resulting in a comprehensive history and/or examination findings a complex or difficult situation. Shows good clinical judgement following encounter

Figure 41.2 Formative assessment in action in medical education: min-CEX assessment report form for the UK Joint Royal Colleges of Physicians Training Board. Reproduced with permission from BMJ Learning.

♦ Formative assessment demands time and commitment from teachers and students alike and requires both groups to develop, practise, and maintain new educational skills.

♦ Institutional commitment is essential to foster an environment in which frequent, ongoing and effective formative assessment is given priority within a learning culture.

♦ Used effectively within a programme in which all assessments are aligned fully with teaching, learning, curriculum development and faculty training, the benefits offered by formative assessment for the development of skills necessary for lifelong learning should have a major impact on the quality of medical education, ultimately leading to better patient care.

References

Altahawi, F., Sisk, B., Poloskey, S., Hicks, C., and Dannefer, E.F. (2012) Student perspectives on assessment: Experience in a competency-based portfolio system. *Med Teach.* 34: 221–225

Alves de Lima, A., Henquin, R., Thierer, J., et al. (2005) A qualitative study of the impact on learning of the miniclinical evaluation exercise in postgraduate training. *Med Teach.* 27: 46–52

Angelo, T.A. (1999) Doing assessment as if learning matters most. *AAHE Bull.* 51: 3–6

Archer, J.C. (2010) State of the science in health professional education: effective feedback. *Med Educ.* 44: 101–108

Atherton, J.S. (2011) Managing the hidden curriculum. *Doceo; Hidden Curriculum.* [Online] http://www.doceo.co.uk/tools/hidden.htm Accessed 8 March 2013

Bangert-Drowns, R.L., Kulik, J.A., and Kulik, C.C. (1991) Effects of frequent classroom testing. *J Educ Res.* 85: 89–99

Bell, B. and Cowie, B. (2001) The characteristics of formative assessment in science education. *Sci Educ.* 85: 536–553

Bennett, R.E. (2011) Formative assessment: a critical review. *Assess Educ Principles, Policy Pract.* 18: 5–25

Biggs, J.B. (2003) *Teaching for Quality Learning at University.* 2nd edn. Buckingham: Open University Press/SRHE

Biggs, J.B. and Collis, K.F. (1982) *Evaluating the quality of learning: the SOLO taxonomy.* New York: Academic Press

Black, P. and Wiliam, D. (1998a) Assessment and classroom learning. *Assess Educ.* 5: 7–74

Black, P. and Wiliam, D. (1998b) Inside the black box: raising standards through classroom assessment. *PhiDeltaKappa International.* Phi Delta Kappan 80, No. 2 139–144, 146–148

Black, P. and Wiliam, D. (2009) Developing the theory of formative assessment. *Educ Assess Eval Accountability.* 21: 5–31

Bloom, B.S. (1965) *Taxonomy of Educational Objectives.* London: Longman

B.S., Bloom, J.T. Hastings, and G.F. Madaus (eds) (1971) *Handbook on the Formative and Summative Evaluation of Student Learning.* New York: McGraw Hill

Boehler, M.L., Rogers, D.A., Schwind, C.J. et al. (2006) An investigation of medical student reactions to feedback: a randomised controlled trial. *Med Educ.* 40: 746–749

Boud, D. (2000) Sustainable assessment: rethinking assessment for the learning society. *Studies Cont Educ.* 22: 151–167

Boud, D. and Falchikov, N. (1995) What does research tell us about self-assessment? In D. Boud (ed.) *Enhancing Learning through Self Assessment* (pp. 155–166). London: Kogan Page

Brown, G., Bull, J., and Pendlebury, M. (1997) *Assessing Student Learning in Higher Education.* London: Routledge

Butler, D.L. and Winne, P.H. (1995) Feedback and self-regulated learning: a theoretical synthesis. *Rev Educ Res.* 65: 245–281

Carless, D. (2007) Learning-orientated assessment: conceptual bases and practical implications. *Innovations in Education and Teaching International.* 44: 57–66

Carless, D. (2009) Learning-orientated assessment: principles, practice and a project. In L.H. Meyer, S. Davidson, R. Anderson, et al. (eds) *Tertiary*

Assessment and Higher Education Student Outcomes: Policy, Practice and Research (pp. 79–90). Wellington, New Zealand: Ako Aotearoa

Carless, D., Joughin, G. Ngar-Fun, L., et al (2006) A conceptual framework for learning-oriented assessment. In D. Carless, G. Joughin, L. Ngar-Fun, et al. (eds) *How Assessment Supports Learning: Learning-orientated assessment in action* (pp. 7–15). Hong Kong: Hong Kong University Press

Carroll, M. (1995) Formative assessment workshops: feedback sessions for large classes. *Biochem Educ.* 23: 65–67

Chickering, A.W. and Gamson, Z.F. (1987) Seven principles for good practice in undergraduate education. *AAHE Bulletin.* [Online] www.aahea.org/aahea/articles/sevenprinciples1987.htm Accessed 12 March 2013

Daelmans, H.E.M., Hoogenboom, R.J.I., Scherpbier, A.J.J.A., Stehouwer, C.D.A., and van der Vleuten, C.P.M. (2005) Effects of an in-training assessment programme on supervision of and feedback on competencies in an undergraduate Internal Medicine clerkship. *Med Teach.* 27: 158–163

Denison, A.R., Currie, A.E., Laing, M.R., and Heys, S.D. (2006) Good for them or good for us? The role of academic guidance interviews. *Med Educ.* 40: 1188–1191

Dobson, J.L. (2008) The use of formative online quizzes to enhance class preparation and scores on summative exams. *Adv Physiol Educ.* 32: 297–302

Driessen, E., van der Vleuten, C., Schuwirth, L., Van Tartwijk, J., and Vermunt, J. (2005) The use of qualitative research criteria for portfolio assessment as an alternative to reliability evaluation: a case study. *Med Educ.* 39: 214–220

Elizondo-Montemayor, L.L. (2004) How we assess students using an holistic standardized assessment system. *Med Teach.* 26: 400–402

Ende, J. (1983) Feedback in clinical medical education. *JAMA.* 250: 777–781

Entwistle, N.J. and Entwistle, A.C. (1991) Forms of understanding for degree examinations: the pupil experience and its implications. *Higher Educ.* 22: 205–227

Epstein, R.M. (2007) Assessment in medical education. *N Engl J Med.* 356: 387–396

Fowell, S.L., Southgate, L.J., and Bligh, J.G. (1999) Evaluating assessment: the missing link? *Med Educ.* 33: 276–281

Gibbs, G. (1992) *Improving the Quality of Student Learning*. Bristol: TES

Gibbs, G. (2010) Using assessment to support student learning. Leeds Met Press. [Online] http://www.leedsmet.ac.uk/staff/files/100317_36641_Formative_Assessment3Blue_WEB.pdf Accessed 12 March 2013

Gibbs, G. and Coffey, M (2004) The impact of training of university teachers on their teaching skills, their approach to teaching and the approach to learning of their students. *Active Learn Higher Educ.* 5: 87–100

Gibbs, G. and Simpson, C. (2004) Conditions under which assessment supports students' learning. *Learn Teach Higher Educ.* 1: 3–30

Gitomer, D.H. and Duschl, R.A. (2007) Establishing multilevel coherence in assessment. *Yearbook of the National Society for the Study of Education.* 106: 288–320

GMC (2009) *Tomorrow's Doctors*. London: GMC

Gordon, M. (1991) A review of the validity and accuracy of self-assessments in health professions training. *Acad Med.* 66: 762–769

Gray, C.S., Hildreth, A.J., Fisher, C., et al. (2008) Towards a formative assessment of classroom competencies (FACCs) for postgraduate medical trainees. *BMC Med Educ.* 8: 61

Hafferty, F. (1998) Beyond curriculum reform: confronting medicine's hidden curriculum. *Acad Med.* 73: 403–407

Hattie, J.A. (1987) Identifying the salient factors of a model of student learning: a synthesis of meta-analyses. *Int J Educ Res.* 11: 187–212

Hattie, J. and Jaeger, R. (1998) Assessment and classroom learning: a deductive approach. *Assess Educ Principles, Policy and Practice.* 5: 111–122

Henderson, P., Ferguson-Smith, A.C., and Johnson, M.H. (2005) Developing essential professional skills: a framework for teaching and learning about feedback. *BMC Med Educ.* 5: 11

Hewson, M.G. and Little, M.L. (1998) Giving feedback in medical education: verification of recommended techniques. *J Gen Intern Med.* 13: 111–116

Higgins, R.S.D., Bridges, J., Burke, J.M., et al (2004) Implementing the ACGME general competencies in a cardiothoracic surgery residency program using 360-degree feedback. *Ann Thorac Surg.* 77: 12–17

Hill, D.A., Guinea, A.I., and McCarthy, W.H. (1994) Formative assessment: a student perspective. *Med Educ.* 28: 394–399

Holmboe, E.S., Sherbino, J., Long, D.M., Swing, S.R., and Frank, J.R. (2010) The role of assessment in competency-based medical education. *Med Teach.* 32: 676–682

Kaufman, D.M. and Mann, K.V. (2010) Teaching and learning in medical education: how theory can inform practice. In T. Swanwick (ed.) *Understanding Medical Education* (pp. 16–36). Oxford: Wiley-Blackwell

Kibble, J. (2007) Use of unsupervised online quizzes as formative assessment in a medical physiology course: effects of incentives on student participation and performance. *Adv Physiol Educ* 31: 253–260

Kluger, A.N. and DeNisi, A. (1996) The effects of feedback interventions on performance: A historical review, a meta-analysis, and a preliminary feedback intervention theory. *Psychol Bull.* 119: 254–284

Knowles, M.S. (1980) *The Modern Practice of Adult Education: from pedagogy to andragogy.* 2nd edn. New York: Cambridge Books

Kolb, D.A. (1984) *Experiential Learning. Experience as the Source of Learning and Development.* New Jersey: Prentice Hall

Kurtz, S., Silverman, J., and Draper, J. (2005) *Teaching and Learning Communication Skills in Medicine.* Oxford: Radcliffe Publishing Ltd, pp. 123–129

Langendyk, V. (2006) Not knowing that they do not know: self-assessment accuracy of third-year medical students. *Med Educ.* 40: 173–179

Macdonald, J. (2002) Getting it together and being put on the spot: synopsis, motivation and examination. *Studies Higher Educ.* 27: 329–338

Martinez, M.E. and Lipson, J.I. (1989) Assessment for learning. *Educ Leadership.* 46: 73–75

McKinley, R.K., Fraser, R.C., van der Vleuten, C., and Hastings, A.M. (2000) Formative assessment of the consultation performance of medical students in the setting of general practice using a modified version of the Leicester Assessment Package. *Med Educ.* 34: 573–579

Milan, F.B., Dyche, L., and Fletcher, J. (2011) 'How am I doing?' Teaching medical students to elicit feedback during their clerkships. *Med Teach.* 33: 904–910

Mitchell, J. (2006) Formative assessment and beginning teachers: ready or not? *Scottish Educ Rev.* 38: 186–200

Mohanna, K., Cottrell, E., Wall, D. and Chambers, R. (2011) Giving effective feedback. In K. Mohanna, E.. Cottrell, E. Wall and R. Chambers (eds) *Teaching Made Easy: a manual for health professionals.* Chapter 13. Oxford: Radcliffe Publishing

National Student Survey (2012) [Online] http://www.thestudentsurvey.com/ Accessed 8 March 2013

Neher, J.O., Gordon, K., Meyer, B., and Stevens, N. (1992) A five-step 'microskills' model of clinical teaching. *J Am Board Fam Pract.* 5: 419–424

Newble, D.I., and Jaeger, K. (1983) The effect of assessments and examinations on the learning of medical students. *Med Educ.* 17: 165–171

Nicol, D.J. and Macfarlane-Dick, D. (2006) Formative assessment and self-regulated learning: a model and seven principles of good feedback practice. *Studies Higher Educ.* 31: 199–218

Norcini, J., Anderson, B., Bollela, V., et al (2011) Criteria for good assessment: consensus statement and recommendations from the Ottawa 2010 Conference. *Med Teach.* 33: 206–214

O'Donovan, B., Price, M., and Rust, C. (2001) The student experience of criterion-referenced assessment. *Innovations in Education and Teaching International.* 38: 74–85

Oldham, J. (2007) Formative assessment for progress tests of applied medical knowledge: the role of the student. From the REAP International Online Conference on Assessment Design for Learner Responsibility, 29–31 May, 2007. [Online] http://www.reap.ac.uk/reap/reap07/Portals/2/CSL/feast%20of%20case%20studies/Formative_assessment_for_progress_tests_of_applied_medical_knowledge.pdf Accessed 12 March 2013

Orsmond, P. (2004) Self-and peer-assessment: guidance on practice in the biosciences. In S. Maw, J. Wilson, and H. Sears (eds) *Teaching Bioscience Enhancing Learning Series.* Leeds: The Higher Education Centre for Bioscience. [Online] http://www.bioscience.heacademy.ac.uk/ftp/teachingguides/fulltext.pdf Accessed 24 July 2012

Pendleton, D., Schofield, T., Tate, P., and Havelock, P. (1984) *The Consultation: an Approach to Learning and Teaching*. Oxford: Oxford University Press

Quality Assurance Agency for Higher Education (2006) Code of Practice for the Assurance of Academic Quality Standards in Higher Education. Section 6 Assessment of Students. [Online] http://www.qaa.ac.uk/Publications/InformationAndGuidance/Documents/COP_AOS.pdf. Accessed 24 July 2012

Quality Assurance Agency for Higher Education (2011) UK Quality Code for Higher Education. [Online] http://www.qaa.ac.uk/Publications/InformationAndGuidance/Pages/quality-code-A6.aspx Accessed 24 July 2012

Ramaprasad, A. (1983) On the definition of feedback. *Behav Sci.* 28: 4–13

Ramsden, P. (1992) *Learning to Teach in Higher Education*. London: Routledge

Rohrer, D. and Pashler, H. (2010) Recent research on human learning challenges conventional instructional strategies. *Educ Res.* 39: 406–412

Rolfe, I. and McPherson, J. (1995) Formative assessment: how am I doing? *Lancet.* 345: 837–839

Roy Chowdhury, R. and Kalu, G. (2004) Learning to give feedback in medical education. *Obstetrician and Gynaecologist.* 6: 243–247

Rudland, J. R., Schwartz, P., and Ali, A. (2011) Moving a formative test from a paper-based to a computer-based format. A student viewpoint. *Med Teach.* 33: 738–743

Rudolph, J.W., Simon, R., Raemer, D.B., and Eppich, W.J. (2008) Debriefing as formative assessment: closing performance gaps in medical education. *Acad Emerg Med.* 15: 1010–1016

Rushton, A. (2005) Formative assessment: a key to deep learning? *Med Teach.* 27: 509–513

Rust, C. (2002) The impact of assessment on student learning: how can research literature practically help to inform the development of departmental assessment strategies? *Active Learn Higher Educ.* 3: 145–158

Rust, C., O'Donovan, B., and Price, M. (2005) A social constructivist assessment process model: how the research literature shows us this could be best practice. *Assess Eval Higher Educ.* 30: 231–240

Sadler, D.R. (1989) Formative assessment and the design of instructional systems. *Instruct Sci.* 18: 119–144

Sadler, D.R. (1998) Formative assessment: revisiting the territory. *Assess Educ.* 5: 77–84

Sayer, M., Chaput de Saintonge, M., Evans, D., and Wood D.F. (2002) Support for students with academic difficulties. *Med Educ.* 36: 643–650

Schuwirth, L.W. and van der Vleuten, C.P. (2011) Programmatic assessment: from assessment of learning to assessment for learning. *Med Teach.* 33: 478–485

Sender Liberman, A., Liberman, M., Steinert, Y., McLeod, P., and Meterissian, S. (2005) Surgery residents and attending surgeons have different perceptions of feedback. *Med Teach.* 27: 470–472

Shepard, L.A. (2000) The role of assessment in a learning culture. *Educ Res.* 29: 4–14

Silverman, J.D., Draper, J., and Kurtz, S.M. (1996) The Calgary–Cambridge approach to communication skills teaching. 1. Agenda-led outcome—based analysis of the consultation. *Educ Gen Pract.* 7: 288–299

Snyder, B.R. (1971) *The Hidden Curriculum*. New York: Alfred A Knopf

Stead, D.R. (2005) A review of the one-minute paper. *Active Learning in Higher Education.* 6: 118–131

Swanwick, T. (2003) Work based assessment in general practice: three dimensions and three challenges. *Work Based Learning in Primary Care.* 1(2): 99

Topping, K.J. (2010) Methodological quandaries in studying process and outcomes in peer assessment. *Learn Instruct.* 20: 339–343

van der Vleuten, C. (1996) The assessment of professional competence: developments, research and practical implications. *Adv Health Sci Educ.* 1: 41–67

van der Vleuten, C.P.M., Schuwirth, L.W.T., Driessen, E.W., et al (2012) A model for programmatic assessment fit for purpose. *Med Teach.* 34: 205–214

Vaz, M., Avadhany, S.T., and Rao, B.S. (1996) Student perspectives on the role of formative assessment in physiology. *Med Teach.* 18: 324–326

Vogel, M. and Wood, D.F. (2002) Love it or hate it? Medical student attitudes to computer assisted learning. *Med Educ.* 36: 214–215

Vygotsky, L.S. (1978) *Mind in Society: The Development of Higher Psychological Processes*. Cambridge MA: Harvard University Press

Walvoord, B.E. (2010) *Assessment Clear and Simple: a Practical Guide for Institutions, Departments, and General Education*. San Francisco: Jossey-Bass

Ward, M. Gruppen, L., and Regehr, G. (2002) Measuring self-assessment: current state of the art. *Adv Health Sci Educ.* 7: 63–80

Wass, V., Bowden, R. and Jackson, N. (2007) The principles of assessment design. In N. Jackson, A. Jamieson, and A. Khan (eds) *Assessment in Medical Education and Training: a Practical Guide* (pp. 11–26). Oxford: Radcliffe Publishing Ltd

Watling, C.J. and Lingard, L. (2012) Toward meaningful evaluation of medical trainees: the influence of participants' perceptions of the process. *Adv Health Sci Educ.* 17: 183–194

Wehlburg, C.M. (2008) *Promoting Integrated and Transformative Assessment: a Deeper Focus on Student Learning*. San Francisco: Jossey-Bass

Wood, D.F. (2010) Formative Assessment. In T. Swanwick, (ed) *Understanding Medical Education* (pp. 259–270). Oxford: Wiley-Blackwell

Yorke, M. (2003) Formative assessment in higher education: Moves towards theory and the enhancement of pedagogic practice. *Higher Educ.* 45: 477–501

Zhang, J., Peterson, R.F., and Ozolins, I.Z. (2011) Student approaches for learning in medicine: what does it tell us about the informal curriculum? *BMC Med Educ.* 11: 87.

CHAPTER 42

Technology enhanced assessment in medical education

Zubair Amin

> Examination, like fire, is a good servant but a bad master.
>
> Thomas Huxley
>
> Reproduced from *British Medical Journal*, Starling EH,
> 'Medical education in England: The Overloaded Curriculum and
> the Incubus of the Examination System', 2, p. 258, Copyright 1918,
> with permission from BMJ Publishing Group Ltd.

Introduction

The purpose of this chapter is to provide an overview of the use of technology in assessment in medical education, especially in high stakes summative examinations. The dominant theme is how educators can judiciously and optimally use technology to enhance assessment in medical education. Although much of the works cited here relate to undergraduate medical education, the basic tenets can be applied to postgraduate and continuing medical education. The term examinee is used as a generic descriptor of a learner, test-taker, student or trainee.

While technology has contributed significantly towards the management of assessment processes such as question banking, blueprinting, test administration, statistical analysis, and reporting, the primary focus of this chapter is on the use of technology in assessment in medical education from the perspective of a medical teacher—who is more likely to be concerned with how technologies can strengthen and broaden the competencies tested in examinations. Thus, the major discussions are related to educational and clinical innovations (machines, processes, or a hybrid; with or without human interactions) that have the potential to assist and enhance assessment.

Nature of technology in healthcare and medical education

Physicians, students, and patients interact with technology in an increasingly intimate manner (Amin et al. 2011). As working professionals in a healthcare or educational institute, our interactions with technology can be conceptualized into three somewhat overlapping dimensions: technology that we use in personal and everyday life such as computers, mobile computing devices and smart phones; technologies that we use predominantly in the process of delivering healthcare such as Electronic Medical Records (EMR), digital image processing and archiving systems; and technologies that support various educational functions such as e-portfolio, PowerPoint, and a range of learning management systems (see fig. 42.1).

Although from a user perspective the main reason for owning a piece of technology may not include healthcare, the influence of technology on healthcare delivery should not be underestimated. According to recent published data, the ownership of mobile telecommunication devices has reached a level previously thought to be unachievable (The Economist 2012). For practicing physicians, it is commonplace now to encounter patients who walk into consultation rooms with extensive research on their condition. Similarly, patients or accompanying family members now bring images of their clinical conditions or audio-video recordings of clinical events such as seizures or gait. Face-to-face consultations are being supplemented by emails or internet-based consultations. Although not so common as with the above examples, patients may now request caregivers to provide a video or an audio recording of the clinical encounters. In clinical rounds, instant access to guidelines, patient-management information, and other supporting materials has opened up an entirely new way in which doctors and clinical educators interact with the students and trainees (Honeybourne et al. 2006; Pluye et al. 2005). Ubiquitous availability of desktops, laptops, and other mobile devices has revolutionized the way students perform their assigned works. Student presentations, projects, clinical reports, and portfolios are now supported by online research. In many hospitals, students are given limited access to clinical databases including patients' past and present medical records, laboratory reports, and radiological images. Emergence of myriad simulation technologies in healthcare education is not only

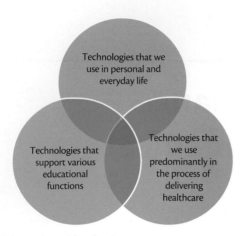

Figure 42.1 Interactions with technology.

influencing the curriculum but also how we assess our students, and what we assess (Dauphinee 2012). It is increasingly indefensible now to allow a trainee to perform a technical procedure, such as a chest tube insertion, in a patient without first undergoing training in a simulator and subsequently assessed to be competent in the said procedure (Ziv et al. 2003).

Technology is now ubiquitous in healthcare and education; its influence is pervasive, relentless, and expanding (Ellaway and Masters 2008; Amin et al. 2011). Technology has allowed students pursue learning in an entirely new way; and in the process is blurring the distinction between information provider (i.e. teachers) and information recipients (i.e. students). As healthcare is becoming more intertwined with technologies, our responsibility as informed assessors should be to capture trainees' performance within the context of their practice (Amin et al. 2011). Failure to do so would undermine the very purpose of assessment in medical education.

Defining technology

Technology is a complex construct where a unified definition is difficult to achieve because of the versatility of its nature, usages, and an incredibly diverse range of applications that are often context specific. The National Center for Biotechnology Information (NCBI) defines technology as 'the application of scientific knowledge to practical purposes in any field. It includes methods, techniques, and instrumentation.' (National Center for Biotechnology Information). Therefore, in defining technologies we should include methods, techniques, and instruments which might coexist and interact with each other in a seamless manner. A smart instrument employs significant methods or processes in order to achieve its intended purpose; however, the nature and magnitude of this interplay can be highly variable. A pelvic trainer without built-in feedback is an example of an instrument or a device that pretty much depends on human interactions as processes. Harvey, a cardiac examination simulator (Jones et al. 1997), which provides pre-recorded cardiac sounds, pulse waves, blood pressure, and other physical examination findings, is an example of a machine with some degree of processing power but without any built-in feedback mechanism or interaction. An example of more advanced technology in medical education would include an anesthesia manikin, which combines machines

with significant processing power (Grenvik and Schaefer 2004). Such advanced machines are able to change the output based on users' input and provide real-time feedbacks to users. Many such intelligent devices have an automated scoring system to assess users' level of competency. Similarly, technologies used in healthcare include a diverse range of machines and processes that interact with human beings in a complex way that can be static or dynamic (Issenberg et al. 2005). It is necessary to recognize this diverse scope of technologies in education and healthcare, so that they can be applied appropriately to assessment in medical education.

Recent history

The use of technology in assessment parallels the availability and acceptability of computer technology in general. In the beginning, the use of technology in assessment was largely confined to management of large-scale testing, especially its administration (Pellegrino and Quellmalz 2010). Computer technology allowed speedier data handling, faster transport of test materials, automated scoring, larger storage of data and a secure environment (Norcini and McKinley 2007). The primary reason for early adoption was efficiency—computer technology facilitated the migration from paper-and-pencil assessment to more efficient and speedier computer-based multisite assessment. This is still true today as most adoptions of computer-based testing are from national and international licensing examinations (e.g. United States Medical Licensing Examinations) and, to a lesser degree, other specialty examinations (e.g. online tests administered by specialty and subspecialty boards). Logistics requirements, costs associated with initial set-up and subsequent maintenance, and efforts needed for the development of a robust examination system still remain as major obstacles to wider adoption of computer-based testing in most medical schools around the world.

Further technological advancement in assessment came when educational features and priorities merged with technological progress. For examples, test authoring tools allow question setters to manage the entire life-cycle of question development—from writing questions to sorting, storing, and administration (Questionmark 2012). Web-based platforms allow the question writing and review process to be carried out collaboratively from

Table 42.1 Examples of applications of computer technology in assessment

Technology	Illustrated benefits
Test authoring	Multisite collaboration and review
Storage and banking	Sharing of resources with other institutions
Question paper development	Blueprinting with specified criteria such as content coverage, difficulty and weightage
Automated marking	Reduction of human errors
Statistical analyses and data reporting	Item statistics such as difficulty and discriminatory indices and reliability
Post examination quality review	Flagging of questions for moderation and creating equivalent examination papers
Plagiarism detection	Quantitative analysis of originality of the work

multiple locations while maintaining necessary security. Provided that the question bank is sufficiently large and well-maintained, it is possible to generate an examination paper based on a defined blueprint. Web-based banking of questions allows many medical schools to form partnerships with like-minded institutes to develop and maintain shared question banks (table 42.1). An example of shared resources is the IDEAL Consortium (International Database for Enhanced Assessments and Learning) which pools questions from various medical schools and shares among the partners (IDEAL Consortium 2009).

Plagiarism detection software provides an analysis of whether a submitted assessment work is authentic or plagiarized (Dahl 2007). Such software can compare submitted works with other published works, online materials, and even prior submissions from the same or other students, and generate a statistical report on originality (Dahl 2007). Examples of assessments in medical education that are in need of plagiarism detection include patient write-ups, open book examinations, projects, and portfolios.

More recent advances in the use of technology in assessment were made possible with improved programming, greater processing power of computers, more widespread availability of technology, and perhaps more importantly, an ongoing collaboration between educators and technologists (Pellegrino and Quellmalz 2010). Examples include introduction of interactive test formats, adaptive testing, automated feedback to the test-takers, and incorporation of audio, video and other multimedia materials in the assessment. Computer adaptive testing (CAT) is based on examinees' response history and an underlying measurement model of proficiency (Quellmalz and Pellegrino 2009). This is a dynamic examination format that changes the question difficulty based on the answers provided. For example, if the examinee continues to answer questions correctly, the difficulty of the questions gets progressively higher and vice-versa. As the CAT allows test configuration based on examinees' prior response and level of sophistication, it can potentially reduce the time needed for the test. Medical schools planning to use CAT for summative examinations need to have robust psychometric support to determine the test sequence and end-point proficiency required to attain a certain grade.

It would be erroneous to think that technological advancements in assessment are limited to test administration and more efficient and intelligent data handling. While logistical efficiencies and cost-reduction were the primary drivers for early development of technologies, recent advances offer more exciting opportunities for educators to expand the horizon of assessment to both 'probe and promote a broad spectrum of human learning advocated in various policy reports' (Quellmalz and Pellegrino 2009). Simulation allows us to broaden the scope of domains to be tested in an assessment to include important, but previously neglected, facets of physician competencies (Issenberg et al. 1999, Issenberg and Scalese 2007; Norcini and McKinley 2007). Technological advances also allow us to test patient safety, team work, and interprofessional collaboration with more authenticity than conventional examinations (Amin et al. 2011; Boulet 2008b). In the future we can expect technological advancements to bring more realistic assessments into clinical medicine; there could be an opportunity to assess candidates through a direct measurement of patient outcomes (Dauphinee 2012; Issenberg et al. 1999).

Benefits of using technology in assessment

There are many potential benefits of using technology in assessment in medical education (Issenberg et al. 1999; Gordon et al. 2001; Ziv et al. 2003).

Assessment of broader domains of competencies

One of the arguments for using technology in assessment is that it allows educators to assess domains of physicians' competence that could not be tested before (Amin et al. 2011). In conventional paper-and-pencil tests and traditional examinations with real patients, many essential skills that are germane to physicians' performance are neglected. For example, emergency situations, acute care, patient safety, and team work are either under-assessed or assessed in an artificial manner. Simulation technology allows medical teachers to assess these competencies in a more realistic way with greater efficiency (Issenberg et al. 1999; McGaghie and Issenberg 2009). Simulation can provide an experience that gets closer to practice and can be used for high stakes and rare but important clinical events that are critical for safe care (Gordon et al. 2001; Boulet 2008b). It is now possible to assess the operative performance of a surgeon from the telemetric data generated by the manipulation of a scalpel (Fried et al. 2004). An examinee's clinical decision making ability and performance can be assessed using high fidelity manikins that can detect examinee's adherence to or variance from protocols (Boulet et al. 2003).

Improvement of learning through feedback

Feedback has a powerful influence on learning (Hattie and Timperley 2007). In line with best practice in assessment (Norcini et al. 2011), feedback should be a key consideration while designing and implementing an assessment using technology. For example, simulation technology can create a safe and learner-centric environment where the mistakes are forgiven and feedback is immediate (Gordon et al. 2001; Issenberg et al. 2005; Boulet 2008a). As the focus of attention is the examinee, the feedback can be provided more easily and with more attention to the examinees' needs. In online examinations, it is straightforward to provide online feedback to the examinees. The beneficial effects of such feedback on learning and skills acquisition cannot be overstated (Veloski et al. 2006).

Assessment of performance

Measuring performance—what students actually do with real patients in real environments and how their actions impact on patient care—is the ultimate goal of assessment (Dauphinee 2012; Shapiro et al. 2004). Technology can support a move towards assessment at the level of performance (McGaghie and Issenberg 2009). For example, auditing clinical databases and patient outcomes can be used to monitor progress and maintenance of competence among practitioners; team-based performance can be monitored from a remote location; quality assurance parameters such as patient safety and adverse events can be tracked longitudinally to assess individual as well as team performance. Besides the outcome measures, process measures such as adherence to and deviation from guidelines can be assessed. Despite the attractiveness and desirability of assessing performance using patient data, this has remained largely an unexplored territory because of multiple confounding factors that can influence the data collected and

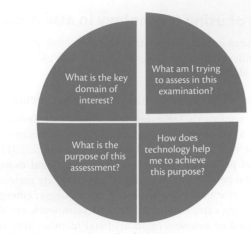

Figure 42.2 Assessment using technologies.

also logistical complexities inherent to measuring such complex constructs (Norcini 2005).

Educational and psychometric considerations

The general principles that are used to make an assessment robust are equally applicable to situations when technologies are used in assessment. Consideration of technology should come only after proper thought is given to fundamental assessment principles.

Validity

Validity is the foremost consideration in assessment (Norcini et al. 2011). This is especially so in assessment using technologies where the main purpose of the assessment may become obscured by inappropriate incorporation of technologies. The questions to ask are outlined in fig. 42.2.

Let us consider two examples where technologies might actually threaten the robustness of assessment.

In a computer-based assessment using digital animation, examinees were asked to determine the relationship between cardiac nerve conduction and cardiac cycle. Examinees were given different levels of block in the conduction pathway and asked to draw the changes in the cardiac cycle as a result of the block in the pathway. The manipulation of the images required significant manual dexterity. Thus, in reality, the test was actually assessing examinees' ability in two separate domains: their knowledge of cardiac nerve conduction and their skill in image manipulation. Although the main objective of the assessment was to assess examinees' knowledge, the measurement data obtained got contaminated by an irrelevant factor. Of course, if the purpose of the test were to assess examinees' knowledge and dexterity concurrently, then the validity of the examination would be preserved.

In a skills-based assessment, examinees were asked to take a history, perform a focused clinical examination, and review laboratory findings. Examinees were required to summarise their findings and deliberations in text using a predefined format on a computer. The time allocated for the task was 20 minutes, out of which 15 minutes were allocated to history taking, physical examination, and review of laboratory results. The remaining

5 minutes were for writing onto a computer. This was an unobserved station. The marking was based solely on the examinees' note of the encounter. During the post-examination review it was revealed that a large number of examinees failed because they could not complete the note on time. Moreover, some examinees, whose first language was not English, performed poorly. In this scenario, the major purpose of assessment—to find out the examinees' ability to take history, perform physical examination, and interpret laboratory data—was overshadowed by extraneous factors such as language proficiency and ability to type quickly and accurately.

Create and support learning

One of the key functions of assessment is to support learning (Norcini et al. 2011). As a guiding principle, in every assessment using technology it is imperative that assessors explore opportunities to improve learning and provide feedback to the examinees (Veloski et al. 2006). The form of feedback should include, in addition to grades or a pass/fail decision, developmental information such as strong and weak areas of performance in the test, advice on remediation, and recommendations for further study (Hattie and Timperley 2007).

There are various ways feedback can be provided. Format, timing, nature, and quantity of information provided would depend on the examination. For example, in a written assessment, such as a multiple choice question (MCQ) or extended matching question (EMQ) exam, it is fairly easy to provide explanations to the answers at the end of the test based on automatic scoring of examinees' responses. In progressive patient management problems, it is also best practice to provide feedback to examinees at the end. In summative, high stake examinations, for logistic reasons, the feedback can be provided at the completion of the examination either individually or with the group. The information provided to the examinees should include a correct or model response and an explanation as to why incorrect responses were wrong. If the test is formative, the information might include advice and guidance on their readiness to progress into summative assessment (e Assessment: Guide to Effective Practice 2007).

The level of feedback provided by the test system to the student may consist of (e-Assessment: Guide to Effective Practice 2007):

- the overall result only
- the score for the whole assessment, with sub-scores or results for sub-sections of assessment
- the score for individual items
- feedback on correct responses together with reasons or explanations, and
- hints for further study and reference to relevant learning materials or information sources.

The opportunity to create learning is one of the strongest reasons to support simulation (Issenberg et al. 1999). In simulation-based assessments it is comparatively easy to identify examinees' strengths and weaknesses and provide remedial guidance wherever needed. It is recommended that in such examinations the marking template includes itemized scores, as opposed to just a global score, in order to capture test-takers' deficiencies in specific domains. Also, written qualitative comments captured during the examination are invaluable in specifying exact weaknesses.

Technology also allows those responsible for providing education to receive feedback (Quellmalz and Pellegrino 2009). Information that can be useful to educators includes the pattern of students' responses including their strengths and weaknesses, the time taken to complete the test, recurring patterns of deficiencies across the test-takers, performance of a particular test-item such as its ability to differentiate better performing students from the poorly performing ones.

Cost and practicality

There are concerns about the cost of some technological innovations used in assessment (Vargas et al. 2007). Technological devices can be costly to obtain and maintain even for resource rich institutions. Moreover, the rapid turnover of technology can add unforeseen burdens to already overstretched budgets (Greenhalgh 2001). However, alternatives to costly technologies can be deployed during the assessment without compromising the authenticity of the test.

Let us consider the following example. In an examination, the expected task for the candidate is to examine the respiratory system. Although, there are chest examination manikins available, they can be costly, they tend to portray the findings in a standardized manner, and the quality of reproduction is not that good. In such situations, it might be useful to use real or simulated patients. Conversely, suppose the task is to perform a respiratory examination in a patient with an underlying pneumothorax. It is neither feasible to have a real patient in the examination nor it is easy to get a manikin that can faithfully reproduce the examination findings especially the crucial percussion note. In such a situation, an audio recording of an abnormal percussion note can be provided to the student supplemented by a simulated patient. This would reduce the cost of examination significantly without comprising the fidelity of the scenario.

Higher cost does not necessarily mean better quality of assessment. Sometimes, if the technology is used inappropriately it might even compromise the quality of the assessment. In situations when there are several options available, the decision regarding choice of particular gadgets should be based on the need of the assessment rather than availability of technological devices.

Applications of technology in written assessments

Written examination is still the dominant mode of assessment in medical education—because of its relative ease of development and implementation, fairly standardized marking scheme, and efficiency in assessing a large body of information in a relatively short period of time (Norcini and McKinley 2007; Schuwirth and Vleuten 2003). It is unsurprising that many early technological innovations in assessment were related to written assessments, particularly the use of technology in computerized MCQs (Pellegrino and Quellmalz 2010).

Written examinations commonly consist of one of several formats such as closed-ended MCQs and EMQs; semistructured open-ended questions such as short answer questions (SAQ) and modified essay questions (MEQ); or more open-ended ones such as the long essay questions (Schuwirth and Vleuten 2003; Amin et al. 2006). There are concerns regarding the overuse of testing using only MCQs (Pellegrino and Quellmalz 2010) where overstandardization of questions may lead to simple, structured problems that 'tap fact retrieval and the use of algorithmic solution procedures' (Pellegrino and Quellmalz 2010). Furthermore, they may not probe students' understanding of complex, authentic clinical problems (Schuwirth and Vleuten 2003). Technological advances allow modifications of written examinations to extend the capabilities of testing: clinical vignettes with multimedia can be created to enable better assessment of clinical reasoning (Botezatu et al. 2010; Pellegrino et al. 2001).

Multiple choice questions

Standard MCQs are static, text-rich questions with occasional incorporation of images, audio-visual materials, and other non-clinical or clinical materials. One of the major advantages of using technologies in MCQ is to increase the level of fidelity of the scenarios through judicious incorporation of multimedia (Dillon et al. 2004). In addition to multimedia, the fidelity of the question in portraying a real-life clinical situation also depends on the level of details provided in the clinical scenario and whether the information is given to the examinees in interpreted or undigested form (Dillon et al. 2004).

The following examples illustrate the concept of levels of fidelity. A brief clinical scenario with interpreted information could be 'A 24-year-old male presented to the emergency room with acute onset of respiratory distress'. A more challenging version with partially undigested information could be 'A 24-year-old male presented to the emergency room with breathing difficulties. On examination, his heart rate is 96/minute, respiratory rate is 32/minute, and oxygen saturation is 93% while breathing on room air. On examination, he has intercostal and subcostal retraction'. However, even in this scenario a critical piece of information, retraction, is provided as an interpreted version. A higher fidelity MCQ would add a short video where an examinee needs to recognize the findings from the video and conclude them as signs of respiratory distress.

Let us construct few MCQs with increasing level of fidelity and sophistication—see box 42.1.

Typically, assessment of this clinical scenario, recognizing a patient with acute respiratory distress and arriving at preliminary working diagnosis, would need a simulated patient as it is unrealistic to have a real patient with acute respiratory distress in an examination. In many cases, this important scenario might not be tested because of logistic difficulties. Technology allows us to overcome these logistic difficulties (fig. 42.3).

Modified essay questions (MEQ)

The MEQ was originally developed in the 1960s to test the clinical reasoning and decision making abilities of candidates (Lim et al. 2007; Knox 1989). In its early versions, MEQs were administered as paper-and-pencil tests which appeared as a booklet. The MEQ would begin with a clinical situation, generally a patient's presenting problem, followed by any number of questions related to the scenario. Space was provided for the examinees to write in their response. Once they answered a question they would move to the next page which would contain more information about the same patient. More questions would be asked and answers sought until examinees reached the final page (Knox 1989; Lim et al. 2007). In the process of answering the MEQ, the examinees would follow the typical steps of a consultation, i.e., presenting problem, history taking, physical examination, refining the initial differential diagnoses, ordering investigations, formulation of a management plan and communication (Lim et al. 2007). As one of the defining

---

Box 42.1 MCQs with increasing level of fidelity and sophistication

Basic format:

Domain to be tested: Recognizing the primary underlying disease condition in a child with acute respiratory distress.

A 6-year-old girl presented to the emergency medicine department with complaints of shortness of breath, cough, and runny nose for 2 days. Thrice in the last 6 months she had similar episodes for which she was seen. She was given cough medicine on these occasions. Today, on examination, her respiratory rate is 44 breaths/minute associated with subcostal retraction. She has prolonged expiration with wheezes in both lung fields.

What is the most likely diagnosis?

a) Foreign body aspiration

b) Bronchiolitis

c) Pneumonia

d) Bronchial asthma

e) Croup

(Correct answer: d)

Features: Pertinent information is provided to the students in an interpreted format. Students do not need further interpretation of clinical examination findings.

Intermediate format:

Domain to be tested: Interpreting the history and physical examination findings of a child with acute respiratory distress and identifying the most likely cause.

A 6-year-old girl presented to the emergency medicine department with complaints of shortness of breath, cough, and runny nose for 2 days. Thrice in the last 6 months she had similar episodes for which she was seen in the emergency room. She was given cough medicine on these occasions. Inspection of her chest showed following findings <insert a video clip of a patient with tachypnoea and retractions>. Auscultation of the lung revealed the following <insert an audio clip of a patient with prolonged expiration and expiratory wheezes>.

What is the most likely diagnosis?

(Same option list and correct answer)

Features: Pertinent information is provided to the students in undigested format. Students need to interpret the clinical examination findings from the audio and video clip.

Advanced format:

Domain to be tested: Interpreting the history and physical examination findings of a patient with acute respiratory distress, evaluating the response to the therapy, and deciding on the most likely cause.

A 6 year old girl presented to the emergency medicine department with complaints of shortness of breath, cough, and runny nose for 2 days.

Click here for past medical history.

Click here for her vital parameters.

Click here for chest inspection.

Click here for lung auscultation.

Click here for lung auscultation after administration of β-2 agonist.

What is the most likely diagnosis?

(Same option list)

Features: Only the presenting history is provided to the students. Students need to ask for further information and interpret the examination findings on their own. Showing an audio clip after the administration of β-2 agonist would make the scenario more challenging.

- Determine the domains to be tested first.
- Use audio and video clips only if they add value to the scenarios.
- Pilot the questions to ensure clarity and software compatibility.
- Delete patient identification data from the clips.
- Use audios and videos sparingly as they take up a lot of bandwidth and may slow down the computer.

Figure 42.3 Tips for using audio or video clips in MCQs.

features of MEQs is the realistic portrayal of the consultation where information is available sequentially, it is essential that information provided in subsequent questions did not provide clues to earlier questions (Lim et al. 2007; Knox 1989). Thus, once the examinees committed to a particular question they could not go back to earlier sections.

Later adaptations of paper-and-pencil based MEQs include presentation of patient problems on a screen via electronic media (such as PowerPoint). All examinees sit in the examination hall, the clinical scenario is shown using PowerPoint simultaneously to all examinees followed by one or several questions. Examinees answer the questions using paper-and-pencil within a specified allocated time. Once they finish answering the questions, the computer projects new information. Examinees are not allowed to review the earlier slides. The advantages of using computer projection include better and consistent image quality and the ability to include sound clips and videos. However, the disadvantage is that all examinees need to answer individual questions within the predetermined time regardless of their ability and inherent individual variations.

Computer-based MEQs allow sequential presentation of information to the examinees who can answer the questions at their own pace. They allow incorporation of multimedia in the test and may have a mix of open and closed questions (Lim et al. 2007). Although in general education there have been developments in computerized marking of open response questions based on semantic analysis (Quellmalz and Pellegrino 2009), in reality, even the correct response to a question can be variable in terms of variations in spelling, grammatical constructs or use of abbreviations. In high stakes examinations with a manageable number of students it is perhaps easier to mark the open-ended questions manually with the aid of marking template.

Let us return to the patient with acute shortness of breath and develop a sequential MEQ (box 42.2).

There are logistical considerations that need to be addressed before implementing computer-based MEQs in high stake examinations. For example, simultaneous running of many high quality videos may slow or overwhelm the IT system. This can be partially alleviated by creating multiple versions of the same question paper so that only a limited number of examinees are likely to view the videos simultaneously. Other important logistical considerations include examination security, verification of the personal identity of the examinees, back-up of data in case of system failure, and dealing with malfunction of computers at individual examinees' level.

Here are some tips on developing computer aided MEQs:

- Use MEQs sparingly for selected high impact topics.
- Reserve MEQs to assess depth of knowledge, as opposed to breadth of knowledge.

Box 42.2 Developing an MEQ

A 3-year-old girl presented to the emergency medicine department with complaints of shortness of breath, cough, and runny nose for 2 days. Thrice in the last 6 months she had similar episodes for which she was seen in the emergency room. She was given cough medicine on each occasion.

Question 1: What are the top two most likely differential diagnoses that you would consider at this point?
Model answers: Asthma or bronchiolitis.

Question 2: What are the vital parameters you would like to measure immediately? Name up to four.
Model answers: Temperature, heart rate, respiratory rate, and oxygen saturation. No mark is given for blood pressure.

Question 3: This video shows the patient in the emergency room. (Insert a video clip with patient with respiratory distress.) What are the pertinent positive findings in this patient?
Model answers: distressed patient, tachypnoea, use of accessory muscles of respiration, and subcostal and intercostal retractions.

Question 4: At triage, her vital parameters are as follow: temperature 36.6 °C, heart rate 132/minute, respiratory rate 48/minute, and oxygen saturation 88% on room air. Based on the findings, what would be the expected PaO_2 in an arterial blood sample of this patient?

a. 20–40 mmHg

b. 40–60 mmHg

c. 60–80 mmHg

d. 80–100 mmHg

e. 100–120 mmHg

Correct answer: b

Comments: It is not possible to ask this last question in paper-and-pencil tests as the information provided in Question 4 gives the answer to Question 2. Also, it is possible to have a mixture of short, open-ended questions and MCQs.

Question 5: You inform your consultant of the patient's history including the vital parameters. You also mention that you believe that the patient is hypoxic. The consultant agrees.

What are the two immediate therapeutic measures that you would like to provide?
Model answers: give oxygen and nebulized β-2 agonist.

Comment: The section provides the correct answer to the earlier question. This would prevent students for being penalized repeatedly for the same mistake.

- Include a mixture of short open-ended and restrictive response questions.

- Provide clues or answers to earlier questions to avoid examinees getting penalized repeatedly for the same mistakes.

- Do not use too many videos or high-intensity imageries which may use up the available bandwidth.

- Allow students to practise sample questions before the actual examination.

Virtual patients (VPs)

VPs are online, interactive simulations of patient encounters (Huwendiek et al. 2009). VPs can be defined as a 'specific type of computer program that simulates real-life clinical scenarios; learners emulate the roles of healthcare providers to obtain a history, conduct a physical exam, and make diagnostic and therapeutic decisions' (Cook and Triola 2009). A distinguishing feature of VPs is the responsiveness of the case to examinee's inputs—i.e. the case unfolds depending on the choices made (Ellaway et al. 2008). This differentiates VPs from other question formats such as complex, scenario-based MCQs, MEQs, simulated patients or simulations where the case presentation remains indifferent to user inputs.

Early efforts in using VPs in medical education were limited to learning and occasional formative assessments and self-assessments (Poulton and Balasubramaniam 2011; Cook and Triola 2009). In learning and formative assessments VPs have shown to improve clinical reasoning amongst learners (Cook and Triola 2009). Experience of VPs in high-stakes, summative examinations is limited. The attractiveness of VPs in summative examinations, as compared to static paper-and-pencil cases (Huwendiek et al. 2009), includes portrayal of more realistic clinical encounters; assessment of higher-order cognitive functions such as problem-solving and decision making skills; assessment of medical errors (Ziv et al. 2005); and emergency medical conditions (Poulton and Balasubramaniam 2011).

VPs are occasionally used in summative examinations to test clinical reasoning (Cook and Triola 2009)—where examinees' choice of responses would provide information about their ability to take a rational and efficient history, perform physical examination, order cost-effective laboratory tests, and develop a coherent management plan. As clinical reasoning is highly context specific, the answers provided by the examinees need to be marked or graded on a scale (as opposed to dichotomous correct and incorrect responses) by a content expert. This makes the marking scheme of VPs in a high-stakes examination inherently difficult. VPs are also costly to develop and maintain (Huang et al. 2007). Alternative written examination formats that can potentially assess clinical reasoning include context-rich MCQs (Schuwirth and Vleuten 2003), script concordance tests (Charlin et al. 2000), and key features questions (Page et al. 1995).

The design and complexity of VPs is variable (Ellaway et al. 2008; Cook and Triola 2009). They may be in string-of-pearls or branching formats. The string-of-pearl design is a linear model of a patient's story where information is presented sequentially in small chunks. Each chunk of information has a predetermined endpoint (Huwendiek et al. 2009). Question format can be either close-ended as in MCQs or open-ended as in MEQs. In the branching format, the flow of the case depends on the response chosen by the students. Students can select from any number of branching alternatives with

several different end-points (Huwendiek et al. 2009). Further variations in the design may include how the information is provided to the students and the nature of materials. For example, information about laboratory results can be given to the students or be made available to students if they ask for it. Figure 42.4 shows some features of VPs in assessment.

| Assessment of clinical reasoning |
| More realistic portrayal of patient cases and scenarios |
| Dynamic, interactive, and flexible format |
| Incorporation of multimedia and |
| Opportunity to assess conditions that are difficult to test with real patients |

Figure 42.4 Features of VPs in assessment.

E-portfolio

An e-portfolio is a web-based collection of evidence and materials assembled by the examinee under the guidance of a faculty mentor over the course of time. An e-portfolio can be student-led or teacher-led, or a combination of both. Although the e-portfolio enjoys a high degree of face validity (Davis and Ponnamperuma 2010), the use of e-portfolios for high-stake summative examinations is limited because of concerns related to validity, reliability, and practicality (Buckley et al. 2009; Roberts et al. 2002). The e-portfolio has been used more successfully in continuous personal and professional development and recertification and remediation of physicians or trainees (Wilkinson et al. 2002).

The following are the advantages of e-portfolios over paper-and-pencil portfolios:

- Flexibility: the e-portfolio can be customized by students to reflect their creativity, context, and the purpose of the assessment.

- Multimedia materials: the e-portfolio allows trainees to include multimedia materials such as audio or video clips of interactions with patients.

- Storage: a paper-and-pencil portfolio requires large storage space.

- Portability: in e-portfolios data can be entered, reviewed, edited, and maintained from any computer.

- Navigability: paper-and-pencil portfolios tend to be bulky and difficult to navigate; the e-portfolio allows easy navigation.

- Varying degrees of audience access: the e-portfolio system can be customized to permit varying degrees of access to the assessor.

Applications of technology in performance assessment

There are two somewhat distinct uses of technologies in assessment of performance:

1. The use of simulators and simulation in the assessment of clinical skills, and

2. The use of patient outcome data in the assessment of performance in the workplace.

Simulators and simulation

Simulation is likely to be best used in assessing

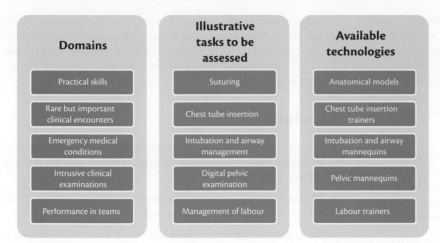

Figure 42.5 Simulation in assessment.

- ◆ students' competency in the management of emergency conditions
- ◆ students' competency in practical skills such as suturing
- ◆ students' competency in clinical skills that intrude on patient privacy such as pelvic examination
- ◆ team performance in important scenarios such as labour management (Amin et al., 2011, Issenberg et al., 2005).

Figure 42.5 gives some examples of the use of simulation in assessment.

There are several challenges in using simulation in assessment that need to be taken into consideration (Boulet and Murray 2010). First, unlike real patient encounters where variations are the norm, simulation tends to portray the clinical scenarios in a fixed and unvarying manner. These attributes might be useful for early stages of clinical training with focus on the acquisition of basic skills; however, in later clinical training when students are expected to deal with real patients, too much standardization may actually undermine the reality of encounters and invalidate the assessment (Amin 2012). Secondly, there is an emerging consensus that simplification and overt standardization that frequently accompany simulators compromise the actual clinical reality which can be messy and unpredictable (Kneebone 2009a; Kneebone 2009b). A viable alternative is hybrid simulation that combines unpredictability and complexity with standardized tasks. Examples of hybrid technologies include pioneering works on patient-focused simulation where inanimate simulators are combined with real actors so that the trainees need to overcome unpredictability and uncertainties that are typical of clinical work (Kneebone et al. 2005; Kneebone 2003). Finally, the scoring, grading, and determination of pass/fail criteria for performance-based assessment using simulation is challenging and an area of much needed research. The scoring of examinee's performance using simulation can consist of explicit processes such as checklists, implicit process such as rating scales, and explicit outcomes such as the status of the patient after the encounter (Boulet and Murray 2010). In a checklist based scoring system, the content experts, typically in conjunction with assessment experts, determine the key steps that an examinee needs to perform before they can be certified as competent. Although, use of this kind of checklist improves the reliability of marking, the development of the checklist itself is prone to many potential errors including missing key steps of performance in the checklist,

introducing non-critical items, skewed marking where unimportant tasks get more marks than important tasks, and a lack of clarity in defining the tasks (Boulet and Murray 2010). Implicit rating scales depend on the experts' judgment of the examinee's performance and typically have a graded marking scheme. As the marking of this type of scale depends on subjective judgments of the examiners, a shared understanding of expected level of competencies and thorough examiners briefings are imperative. In explicit outcome-based scoring, the examinee's performance in a given scenario depends on achieving a desired outcome in the patient's status (e.g., improvement of oxygenation, heart rate, and blood pressure following a sudden desaturation of an anaesthetized patient). However, this would depend on the manikin's ability to response realistically to the candidate's management (Boulet and Murray 2010). Also, determining the exact end-point of patient outcome that would corroborate an expected performance can be challenging as this depends on, among other factors, content experts' opinions.

Although simulation technologies provide us with many exciting opportunities with regards to assessment of physician competencies, they are unsuitable for the assessment of every clinical task. There are inherent limitations that examiners need to keep in mind before incorporating simulation technologies in assessment (Boulet 2008b; Amin et al. 2011). A fundamental step that determines the success is to define the purpose of the assessment for the group of examinees and to choose real patients, simulated patients, simulators, other technological innovations, or a combination based on the needs.

Information technology (IT)

A potential application of technologies in assessment could be the use of IT to link patient outcome data to individual, team, or institutional performance (Norcini et al. 2011; Dauphinee 2012). IT can allow us to link a variety of patient outcome data (e.g. patient satisfaction surveys, length of stay or complication rates) to a particular physician or a healthcare provider group and allow us to draw valid conclusions about the performance of the individual or group. In many clinical settings these data are already in existence, but there is no efficient way to link the data to the individual physician or group and isolate the effect of physician mediated interventions from other variables that might coexist.

The level of evidence supporting the use of patient and healthcare data in assessing physician performance is variable. For certain measures, such as patient satisfaction, the data is fairly robust and method feasible. Other measures that could be used to assess performance include: process of care (e.g. referral of patients to smoking cessation clinics), adherence to standard practice protocols (e.g. completion of immunizations on schedule) and patient outcomes (e.g. blood pressure control).

However, considerable research is needed to answer several critical questions before we can recommend widespread usage of such data in high stakes summative situations (Norcini et al. 2011). These questions include: what aspects of patient care are most appropriate to measure, what outcomes physician is directly responsible for, how many patients are needed for reproducible results, and how to account for confounding factors.

Let us consider the following example. A hospital-based multidisciplinary clinic wanted to use patient data as a measurement of individual physicians' performance. The clinic decided to focus on the HbA1c level of all diabetes patients at the clinic. The clinic compiled the HbA1c levels of all patients registered at the clinic and compared the results with national targets. However, the potential confounding factors in this exercise that need to be reconciled before making any meaningful interpretations are many. For example, the assessors will need to know whether the patient profile of the clinic is comparable to the national norm; how to isolate the effect of care from one individual physician from that of the group; and the minimum number of patients that individual doctors need to see for the sampling to be adequate.

This area also needs a change of mind-set among policy makers so that assessment in medical education is shifted away from being solely focused on the performance of an individual in isolation to an approach that includes the performance of an individual within a team.

Faculty training

Faculty training is key to successful incorporation of technologies in assessment. Technology is by nature ever-changing. Ongoing faculty orientation, training, and refresher courses are imperative to help keep up to date with the emerging technologies (Jeffries 2005).

Curriculum integration

Curriculum integration is another prerequisite for successful implementation of technologies in medical education assessment (Issenberg et al. 2005). Students and faculty must not view the technology as an add-on element to the curriculum. For example, if the intention is to assess team performance in a trauma patient, students must be given opportunity for repeated practice during curriculum time and this specific competency must be part of the core curriculum (Issenberg et al. 2005). It is also recommended that that technology should be integrated in a spiral manner within the curriculum.

Privacy and patient safety

Technological innovations are double-edged swords; they offer unparalleled opportunities to capture data from a variety of sources but open up possibilities of misuse of data. Anyone involved in assessment including patients, standardized patients, examinees, examiners, and faculty administrators, can be a potential victim of misuse of data. Assessment policies should include guidelines on the type of data to be collected, who can access the data and for what purpose and any restrictions of data usage (Pellegrino andQuellmalz 2010).

Conclusions

◆ Medical teachers should incorporate available technologies in healthcare and education to strengthen and broaden the range of competencies tested.

◆ The basic principles governing good assessment apply to technology-enhanced assessment as well.

◆ Preserving the validity of the test is one of most critical elements that should be taken into account while incorporating technologies in assessment.

◆ Technology can simplify assessment tasks and bring efficiency into the entire lifecycle of assessment administration.

◆ Both written- and performance-based assessment can benefit from judicious use of technologies.

References

Amin, Z. (2012) Purposeful assessment. *Med Educ.* 46: 4–7.

Amin, Z., Boulet, J.R., Cook, D.A., et al. (2011) Technology-enabled assessment of health professions education: Consensus statement and recommendations from the Ottawa 2010 conference. *Med Teach.* 33: 364–369

Amin, Z., Chong, Y.S. and Khoo, H. E. (2006) *Practical Guide to Medical Student Assessment*. Singapore: World Scientific Publishing Company.

Botezatu, M., Hult, H., Tessma, M. K. and Fors, U.G.H. (2010) Virtual patient simulation for learning and assessment: Superior results in comparison with regular course exams. *Med Teach.* 32: 845–850

Boulet, J. (2008a) Teaching to test or testing to teach? *Med Educ.* 42: 952–953

Boulet, J.R. (2008b) Summative assessment in medicine: the promise of simulation for high-stakes evaluation. *Acad Emerg Med.* 15: 1017–1024

Boulet, J.R. and Murray, D.J. (2010) Simulation-based assessment in anesthesiology: requirements for practical implementation. *Anesthesiology.* 112: 1041–1052

Boulet, J.R., Murray, D., Kras, J., et al. (2003) Reliability and validity of a simulation-based acute care skills assessment for medical students and residents. *Anesthesiology.* 99: 1270–1280

Buckley, S., Coleman, J., Davison, I., et al. (2009) The educational effects of portfolios on undergraduate student learning: a Best Evidence Medical Education (BEME) systematic review. BEME Guide No. 11. *Med Teach.* 31: 282–298

Charlin, B., Roy, L., Brailovsky, C., Goulet, F. and van der Vleuten, C. (2000) The script concordance test: a tool to assess the reflective clinician. *Teach Learn Med.* 12: 189–195

Cook, D.A. and Triola, M.M. (2009) Virtual patients: a critical literature review and proposed next steps. *Med Educ.* 43: 303–311

Dahl, S. (2007) Turnitin®. *Active Learn Higher Educ.* 8: 173–191

Dauphinee, W.D. (2012) Educators must consider patient outcomes when assessing the impact of clinical training. *Med Educ.* 46: 13–20

Davis, M.H. and Ponnamperuma, G.G. (2010) Examiner perceptions of a portfolio assessment process. *Med Teach.* 32: e211–e215

Dillon, G.F., Boulet, J.R., Hawkins, R.E. and Swanson, D.B. (2004) Simulations in the United States Medical Licensing Examination™ (USMLE™). *Quality and Safety in Health Care.* 13: i41–i45 e-Assessment: Guide to Effective Practice (2007) Qualifications and Curriculum Development Authority. London: Department of Education

Economist, The. (2012) Platform wars: a history of personal computing. *The Economist*. London: The Economist Newspaper Limited.

Ellaway, R. and Masters, K. (2008) AMEE Guide 32: e-Learning in medical education Part 1: Learning, teaching and assessment. *Med Teach*. 30(5): 455–473.

Ellaway, R., Poulton, T., Fors, U., McGee, J.B. and Albright, S. (2008) Building a virtual patient commons. *Med Teach*. 30: 170–174

Fried, G.M., Feldman, L.S., Vassiliou, M.C., et al. (2004) Proving the value of simulation in laparoscopic surgery. *Ann Surg* 240: 518–528

Gordon, J.A., Wilkerson, W.M., Shaffer, D.W. and Armstrong, E.G. (2001) 'Practicing' Medicine without risk: students' and educators' responses to high-fidelity patient simulation. *Acad Med*. 76: 469–472

Greenhalgh, T. (2001) Computer assisted learning in undergraduate medical education. *BMJ*. 322: 40–44

Grenvik, A. and Schaefer, J. (2004) From Resusci-Anne to Sim-Man: The evolution of simulators in medicine. *Crit Care Med*. 32: S56–S57

Hattie, J. and Timperley, H. (2007) The power of feedback. *Rev Educ Res*. 77: 81–112

Honeybourne, C., Sutton, S., and Ward, L. (2006) Knowledge in the Palm of your hands: PDAs in the clinical setting. *Health Information and Libraries Journal*. 23(1): 51–59

Huang, G., Reynolds, R. and Candler, C. (2007) Virtual patient simulation at U.S. and Canadian medical schools. *Acad Med*. 82: 446–451

Huwendiek, S., De leng, B.A., Zary, N., et al. (2009) Towards a typology of virtual patients. *Med Teach*. 31: 743–748

IDEAL Consortium (International Database for Enhanced Assessments and Learning) (2009) [Online]. http://temporary.idealmed.org/wp Accessed 14 March 2013

Issenberg, B.S. and Scalese, R.J. (2007) Best evidence on high-fidelity simulation: what clinical teachers need to know. *Clin Teach*. 4(2): 73–77.

Issenberg, S.B., McGaghie, W.C., Hart, I.R., et al. (1999) Simulation technology for health care professional skills training and assessment. *JAMA*. 282: 861–866

Issenberg, B.S., McGaghie, W.C., Petrusa, E.R., Lee Gordon, D. and Scalese, R.J. (2005) Features and uses of high-fidelity medical simulations that lead to effective learning: a BEME systematic review. *Med Teach*. 27: 10–28

Jeffries, P.R. (2005) A frame work for designing, implementing, and evaluating simulations used as teaching strategies in nursing. *Nursing Education Perspectives*. 26: 96–103

Jones, J.S., Hunt, S.J., Carlson, S.A. and Seamon, J.P. (1997) Assessing bedside cardiologic examination skills using 'Harvey', a cardiology patient simulator. *Acad Emerg Med*. 4: 980–985

Kneebone, R. (2003) Simulation in surgical training: educational issues and practical implications. *Med Educ*. 37: 267–277

Kneebone, R. (2009a) Perspective: simulation and transformational change: the paradox of expertise. *Acad Med*. 84: 954–957

Kneebone, R.L. (2009b) Practice, rehearsal, and performance. *JAMA*. 302: 1336–1338

Kneebone, R.L., Kidd, J., Nestel, D., et al. (2005) Blurring the boundaries: scenario-based simulation in a clinical setting. *Med Educ*. 39: 580–587

Knox, J.D.E. (1989) What is…a modified essay question? *Med Teach*. 11: 51–57

Lim, E.C.-H., Seet, R.C.-S., Oh, V.M.S., et al. (2007) Computer-based testing of the modified essay question: the Singapore experience. *Med Teach*. 29: e261–e268

McGaghie, W.C. and Issenberg, S. (2009) Simulations in assessment In Downing, S.M. and Yudkowsky, R. (eds) *Assessment in Health Profession Education* (pp. 245–268).New York: Routledge

National Center for Biotechnology Information. *Medical Subject Headings* [Online]. Available: http://www.ncbi.nlm.nih.gov/mesh/68013672 Accessed 20th Dec 2011

Norcini, J.J. (2005) Current perspectives in assessment: the assessment of performance at work. *Med Educ*. 39: 880–889

Norcini, J.J., Anderson, B., Bollela, V., et al. (2011) Criteria for good assessment: consensus statement and recommendations from the Ottawa 2010 Conference. *Med Teach*. 33: 206–214

Norcini, J.J. and McKinley, D.W. (2007) Assessment methods in medical education. *Teach Teach Educ*. 23: 239–250

Page, G., Bordage, G. and Allen, T. (1995) Developing key-feature problems and examinations to assess clinical decision-making skills. *Acad Med*. 70: 194–201

Pellegrino, J.W., Chudwosky, N. and Glaser, R. (eds.) (2001) *Knowing What Students Know: the science and design of educational assessment*. Washington DC: Board of Testing and Assessment, Center for Education, Division of Behavioral and Social Sciences and Education, National Academy Press

Pellegrino, J.W. and Quellmalz, E.S. (2010) Perspectives on the integration of technology and assessment. *J Res Technol Educ*. 43: 119–134

Pluye, P., Grad, R.M., Dunikowski, L.G., and Stephenson, R. (2005) Impact of clinical information-retrieval technology on physicians: a literature review of quantitative, qualitative and mixed methods studies. *Int J Medl Informatics*. 74(9): 745–768

Poulton, T. and Balasubramaniam, C. (2011) Virtual patients: a year of change. *Med Teach*. 33: 933–937

Quellmalz, E.S. and Pellegrino, J.W. (2009) Technology and testing. *Science*. 323: 75–79

Questionmark. (2012) http://www.questionmark.com/us/index.aspx Accessed 31 January 2012

Roberts, C., Newble, D.I. and O'Rourke, A.J. (2002) Portfolio-based assessments in medical education: are they valid and reliable for summative purposes? *Med Educ*. 36: 899–900.

Schuwirth, L.W.T. and van der Vleuten, C.P.M. (2003) Written assessment. *BMJ*. 326: 643–645

Shapiro, M.J., Morey, J.C., Small, S.D., et al. (2004) Simulation based teamwork training for emergency department staff: does it improve clinical team performance when added to an existing didactic teamwork curriculum? *Quality and Safety in Health Care*. 13: 417–421

Vargas, A.L., Boulet, J.R., Errichetti, A., et al. (2007) Developing performance-based medical school assessment programs in resource-limited environments. *Med Teach*. 29: 192–198

Veloski, J., Boex, J.R., Grasberger, M.J., Evans, A. and Wolfson, D.B. (2006) Systematic review of the literature on assessment, feedback and physicians' clinical performance: BEME Guide No. 7. *Med Teach*. 28: 117–128

Wilkinson, T.J., Challis, M., Hobma, S.O., et al. (2002) The use of portfolios for assessment of the competence and performance of doctors in practice. *Med Educ*. 36, 918–924.

Ziv, A., Ben-David, S. and Ziv, M. (2005) Simulation based medical education: an opportunity to learn from errors. *Med Teach*. 27: 193–199

Ziv, A., Wolpe, P. R., Small, S. D. and Glick, S. (2003) Simulation-based medical education: an ethical imperative. *Acad Med*. 78, 783–788

CHAPTER 43

Assessing professionalism

Richard Hays

Mere examining corporations which have done practically nothing for medical education, and are chiefly engaged in extracting fees from students, should be allowed to retire into obscurity.

James Barr

Reproduced from *British Medical Journal*, James Barr, 2, p. 157, Copyright 1912, with permission from BMJ Publishing Group Ltd.

Background

Over the last 20 years professionalism has emerged as an important domain in undergraduate and postgraduate medical curricula. Prior to this, the teaching and assessment of medical students and postgraduate trainees were dominated by biomedical science and traditional clinical apprenticeships. These are still essential, because medical practice is the application of medical science in an evidence-based manner. For example, medical graduates need a strong platform in the foundation sciences as these are fields with an expanding knowledge base, including new and evolving areas such as immunology and molecular genetics. Medical education has responded to the challenge of how to fit more learning into less time through pedagogical developments such as problem based learning, which uses small group learning, curriculum integration and increased learner responsibility.

The resulting debates about gaps in curricula and in graduates' knowledge—for example, concerning anatomy, pathology, and prescribing—feature prominently in the media. However, medical education providers are under pressure to consider other aspects of medical practice. Contemporary 'good medical practice' is defined more broadly in terms of roles such as 'professional' and 'manager'; medical councils in most jurisdictions have produced clear documentation on this (Frank et al. 1996; General Medical Council 2006; Royal College of Physicians of Canada 1996; Accreditation Committee on Graduate Medical Education 2012; Australian Medical Council 2010a, b)). More emphasis is now placed on the need for doctors to understand people, value diversity, interpret complex information from different perspectives, take a more holistic view of health, and help patients make choices. They must also understand society and the health system through which they have to guide their patients. Further, medical graduates, and therefore students, must behave like a professional and make decisions that reflect consideration of common ethical and legal issues.

Professionalism is now regarded as something that can be taught and learned in basic medical education (Swick, 1999; Saultz, 2007; General Medical Council 2008; World Federation of Medical Education 2003), and any concerns about the professional behaviour of individual students are expected to be identified and corrected before graduation. While regulation remains an important strategy in achieving society's expectations about professionalism (Cohen, 2006; Irvine, 2007), medical education is expected to play a substantial role in preventing further instances of catastrophic failure of professionalism, such as occurred in the Bristol Royal Infirmary case (Bristol Royal Infirmary Inquiry 2001; Casali and Day 2010; The Shipman Inquiry 2006). The expectations on medical educators and students have therefore increased substantially.

This increased focus on professionalism concerns more than what to include in the curriculum; it also raises questions of how to assess whether learners have acquired the expected professional knowledge and skills and demonstrate the expected behaviours. This expanded assessment role is more complex, because the professionalism domain is different from other domains. This chapter attempts to cover the key issues relevant to the assessment of professionalism, at a time when there are still many unanswered questions about how best to do this.

What is meant by professionalism?

A detailed description of professionalism is the topic of another chapter, but here it is worth reflecting briefly on what should be considered within this domain. There is no universally agreed definition of professionalism in medicine. Its underpinnings lie in philosophy, as attributed to greats such as Hippocrates, Aristotle, and Socrates. It is interesting that many of the early physicians were as much philosopher as healer, and many appeared to function at the boundaries of religious beliefs. This is unsurprising at a time when most medical practice concerned dealing with serious illness or injury, often resulting in death. While the knowledge base has expanded substantially and human intervention is now more effective, uncertainty is still common, intervention is not always successful and all humans eventually die, so the contemporary aura of a modern doctor still includes a somewhat mystical dimension. Much of the success of a doctor lies in effective communication and therapeutic relationships; poor communication is found in a high proportion of complaints (Katz et al. 2007) To these ingredients may be added complex relationships, power imbalances, ethics, morality, social justice, and more contemporary issues such as rationing, use of technology and the relative values of evidence-based and non-evidence-based practice. Further, the more recent concerns about the effect on patient safety of poor leadership and poor teamwork (Dupree et al. 2011) have become part of the broader agenda of professionalism. The combination of these issues varies between cultures and nations, due to differences in health and legal systems, such that the same behaviours can be regarded quite differently, depending on the location (Ho et al. 2011; Worthington and Hays 2012). It is difficult to separate individual characteristics and professional behaviours from these broader societal issues (Martimianakis et al. 2009), and so these differences must be reflected in the curriculum of any particular medical school.

Broadening of medical curricula is thought to provide a more appropriate preparation for modern practice, but the development of professionalism as a vertical curriculum domain has proved challenging. It is relatively easy to include lectures and seminars on components of professionalism, but the impact of this may be limited. For the more clinically experiential part of programs, learners should observe professionalism in action through role modelling and specific incorporation of professionalism into clinical case discussions. Professionalism used to be regarded as a small proportion (say 5–10%) of the curriculum, but greater prominence is now placed on this domain in documents such as *Tomorrows' Doctors* (General Medical Council 2009), where it forms one of only three domains and is highly integrated with other domains. One of the perennial questions about professionalism is whether it is about attitudes or behaviours. The most likely answer is both, but attitudes are much more difficult to measure.

The development of professionalism: from proto- to mature professionalism

Until recently it was assumed that professionalism developed as medical students became immersed in clinical contexts. It is reasonable to assume that most learners in medicine are academically strong and motivated to become competent professionals. They are likely to commence with a sense of altruism. Their understanding of medical careers may, however, be limited to personal interactions with doctors and the portrayal of medicine in film and TV. The latter rarely reflect reality, as the media is more interested in the unusual and sensational. Hence, attributes such as being clever can appear to be more important than being compassionate. Doctors save lives in every dramatic episode, despite sometimes being poor communicators and role models.

Furthermore, experiences as a medical learner are not always positive, with increasing evidence that bullying by senior clinicians, teaching by intimidation and uncaring behaviour remain common (Crutcher et al. 2011. It is common for students to cope poorly with the suffering or death of patients, and to develop an emotional shield that improves coping skills but that can make them appear callous (Rentmeester 2007). These experiences form part of the hidden curriculum (Hodges and Kuper 2012). It is possible for some medical learners to commence with a limited understanding of what professionalism means, be exposed to poor role models,

and become inured to human suffering. It should therefore be no surprise that learners need guidance on what is appropriate. The development of professionalism is now much better understood. Hilton describes the stages of development, from early proto-professionalism to mature professionalism (Hilton and Slotnick 2005; Hilton and Southgate 2007)), providing guidance on what should be expected of medical students and postgraduate trainees as they gain experience.

Measuring and selecting for professionalism amongst candidates for medical school: can we prevent poor professionalism?

Selection of medical students remains a controversial topic. Medical schools receive many more applications than they can accept. Selection processes are therefore about choosing the best from a pool of applicants that have strong academic ability and high motivation; typically measures of academic performance and personal qualities are combined. The former is relatively simple, as applicants have come through recognized academic pathways and have objective scores that predict future academic performance, at least in the first half of medical programmes (Wilkinson et al. 2011; Donnon et al. 2007). In addition, some jurisdictions require medical schools to use specific entrance examinations open to all applicants; this is particularly common for graduate entry schools, where applicants must take the Medical Colleges Admissions Test (MCAT) or Graduate Australian Medical Schools Admissions Test (GAMSAT) (Association of American Medical Colleges 2011; Australian Council for Education Research 2011).

The latter is more complex, because personal qualities include a range of attributes, including components of professionalism, such as interpersonal skills, understanding of roles and capacity for teamwork. While their consideration in selection addresses community concerns about how the profession communicates with patients, they are difficult to measure. Tests for 'aptitude' to practise medicine are often combined with academic tests, such as Undergraduate Medical Admissions Test (UMAT), UK Clinical Aptitude Test (UKCAT) (Wright and Bradley, 2010), and Health Professions Admission Test (HPAT) (Australian Council for Education Research 2012). These tests are controversial, as there is debate over what they measure and only limited evidence that results predict performance in medical school or later (Coates 2008; Prideaux et al. 2011; Poole et al. 2012) . Personal statements and testimonials are often collected at application, but there is little evidence of their reliability or validity. Interviews are widely used to assess interpersonal skills and awareness of broader health issues, and there is modest evidence that interview performance, particularly using the 'multiple mini-interview' approach, can predict academic performance in the senior years of medical school and postgraduate training (Eva et al. 2009). However, it would appear that interview performance does not necessarily detect certain personality traits which, although uncommon, are difficult to manage in learners. Perhaps unsurprisingly, these assessments often do not correlate well with either each other or with academic measures. The measurement of potential professionalism prior to commencing medical education is therefore no easier than measuring professionalism during training or later practice.

Contemporary issues in professionalism

While it is tempting to view professionalism as a stable construct, with its roots in the times of early philosophers, the societal values that underpin our understanding of professionalism evolve over time. Relatively few doctors live and work in monocultural communities; instead, most doctors must deal respectfully with the health beliefs of different ethnic and religious communities, even when these differ from their own. To do otherwise would be regarded as poor professionalism. This more recent aspect of professionalism is known as cultural competence (Ho 2011), and is perhaps dependent on underlying, deeply ingrained attitudes.

One example of changing culture is the effect of emerging communications technology, where development is well ahead of legal and ethical frameworks. It is now easy to rapidly transmit messages that are electronically dated and recorded for the long term on multiple computers, and therefore impossible to retract or amend. It is easy to react instantly to situations in an emotionally reflexive manner, using words that are at best unwise, and at worst offensive or defamatory. It is also now common for medical students and graduates to carry several mobile communication devices and to almost constantly access messages, emails and websites. Some social commentators have described this as a form of 'technology-induced attention deficit hyperactivity disorder'. Is this now normal or acceptable behaviour? Further, some students invite their teachers to be friends on social networking sites, but accepting such invitations can expose staff to inappropriate information. What responsibilities do staff members have to respond to information that they access via social networks? Younger faculty members may deal with this risky situation better because they are more familiar with the new media (Chretien et al. 2011; Guseh et al. 2009). Better guidance on email and social networking etiquette is now available (Snyder 2011; Australian Medical Association Council of Doctors In Training 2010), but this is still an emerging area in professionalism.

Much has also been written about the millennium generation and generation Y (White and Kiegalde 2011; Borges et al. 2010), to which most learners in undergraduate education and specialty training now belong. In comparison to the 'baby boomers', the generation to which most senior clinicians belong, current students and recent graduates are said to be more self-focused, more likely to read the fine print and debate rules, and more interested in achieving a better work–life balance. This may mean a different sense of duty, such that long hours are avoided unless well paid or compensated by time off. As a result, defined shifts are preferred and continuing care is shared by multiple teams of doctors who infrequently interact personally. This has the potential to fragment care, as was seen initially with the introduction in the UK of the European Working Time Directive (Garvin et al. 2008). While reducing the number of hours worked should result in less fatigue and (hopefully) fewer errors, this work pattern requires many more workers and excellent communication between interprofessional teams. Much is still not known about these changes in social norms, but these contemporary aspects of professionalism should be considered in assessment.

Why measure professionalism

The simplest reason for assessing professionalism relates to the great aphorism: 'Learners respect what we inspect' (Norcini, after Cohen, personal communication). There is little point in including professionalism in the curriculum unless professionalism is assessed. Professionalism concerns in medical students are common, and often associated with poor academic performance (Hays et al. 2011). On the other hand, high academic achievement does not necessarily mean sound professionalism (West et al. 2007), so assessments need to be broad enough to assess all curriculum domains. There is also community pressure to prevent the graduation of problem doctors, based on the proven association between reports of problem behaviours in students and subsequent poor professionalism in doctors (Papadakis et al. 2004). This suggests that the quality and safety of healthcare could be improved through early intervention.

In this context early intervention includes teaching, assessment, and remediation or disciplinary action. The more permissive approach, where problem behaviours were regarded as high spirits or normal for certain specialties, is no longer acceptable. All students regardless of age should understand that they are expected to behave as junior members of the profession from the start of their course. How professionalism is viewed may evolve through the course—attendance, confidentiality, and respect for peers, patients, and teachers are expected from the start, but dress code on campus may be more relaxed than on clinical settings. Some medical schools now require a signed mutual contract between students and the school to provide an agreed baseline—for example the Medical Students Charter developed jointly by UK medical schools and the British Medical Students Association in the UK and incorporated in part in the GMC's monograph 'Student Fitness to Practice' (General Medical Council, 2008).

Remediation and disciplinary action

Even with the increasing consensus on the need to foster professionalism as an important curriculum domain, there is little point in measuring professionalism unless something is done with the information. This means that there should be consequences for those whose professionalism is measured. For the majority of learners, the consequences will be an affirmation that learners are on track to becoming clinicians who demonstrate appropriate professionalism. For a minority of learners—those who demonstrate problem behaviours—the consequences should be primarily remediation. As with other domains of a curriculum, the main purpose of assessment is to guide learning. Learners may simply need to receive feedback about concerns, allowing for correction as part of professional development that raises self-awareness and fosters change as maturity develops.

Reality may however not match this theoretical approach. Remediation for behaviour problems may be more difficult than for knowledge deficits, which is itself difficult (Pell, 2012; Hays, 2012). It is common for doctors with poor professionalism to appear to have little insight or capacity for change (Hays et al. 2002a). Two recent systematic reviews of the effect of workplace based assessment on doctors' performance showed relatively few studies had even addressed the topic of measuring professionalism (Miller and

Archer 2010; Overeem et al. 2007). Only multisource feedback resulted in any evidence of behaviour change. The reasons for this weak effect are not clear, although it is known that changing attitudes is difficult. Should remediation fail, taking disciplinary action is also difficult. University procedures for managing poor professional behaviour are generally not designed for the more serious breaches of professionalism that may be found in a small minority. Students facing potentially high-stakes disciplinary procedures will often involve lawyers and attempt to exploit procedural errors or mismatches in the wording of school and university regulations. It may be preferable to combine a non-adversarial, formative approach in most professionalism breaches, reserving the more adversarial disciplinary procedures for students exhibiting serious breaches and poor insight, such that severe sanction or even expulsion is under consideration. However, there is a grey zone between minor and major breaches, and getting the balance right is difficult.

Why is professionalism difficult to measure?

One characteristic that almost all aspects of professionalism share is that they are not easy to assess. The literature often refers to such terms as 'measuring the hard to measure' when discussing the assessment of professionalism; this is for several reasons. The first is that some aspects of professionalism relate to attitudes, which are not as readily observable as behaviours. For example, an individual may have a prejudice against a particular ethnic, religious, or age group of people with whom they have to deal professionally. These attitudes are most evident when expressed openly in front of others, but can also be evident through being dismissive to people against whom there is a prejudice. The latter is more measurable than the former, but is something that can be downplayed as being the incorrect perception of a person who is easily offended. On the other hand, it may be acceptable to have a prejudice as long as it does not influence behaviour, such that there would be no negative effect on health outcomes, no complaints to investigate and therefore no problems to assess. This pragmatic position is controversial as not everybody would agree that attitudes are unimportant.

Even harder to detect is what may be called institutionalized bias, where there may be no obvious biased behaviours, but a particular group receives different treatment. One example of this is the debate in Australia about lower rates of coronary procedures performed in Aboriginal peoples (Bradshaw et al. 2009). There is more than one possible interpretation, such as Aboriginal people not wanting the intervention, perhaps due to not understanding the choices or a clash of cultural beliefs. Another interpretation is that the services are less available in rural and remote communities, similar to the postcode lottery concept reported in the UK, where access to certain services (e.g. cancer treatment) is worse in health facilities that serve deprived populations (Graham et al. 2010). Another more worrying interpretation is that doctors make decisions, either consciously or unconsciously, to offer interventions less often on the grounds that certain populations do not merit expensive interventions.

Second, the assessment of professional behaviours is one of the major points of differentiation between competence (shows how) and performance (does) (Miller 1990). For this reason the concept of performance domains—based on what learners are expected to do in the workplace—has been suggested as an alternative to competence domains (Hays et al. 2002b). This shifts the emphasis for teaching and assessing professionalism to the workplace. For example, observing behaviour amidst the routine of the workplace is more important than observing behaviours under controlled conditions, because it is difficult to sustain good behaviour over time in a busy environment without allowing the 'real' person to shine through. On the other hand, workplace-based assessment is not necessarily valued by learners, because it can appear to be a tick-box exercise (Bindal et al. 2011).

Third, many people with poor attitudes that might result in behaviour problems have sufficient self-awareness to avoid displaying the behaviours when they could be observed; self-evaluation requires external benchmarks and guidance (Hays, 1990). This means that poor professionalism is more difficult to capture; complaints can be dismissed as one person's word against another's or just a personality clash. Similar complaints from several different people are often necessary before a problem is realized. Those with poor professionalism and little insight are much easier to assess because multiple complaints are more likely and less is done to mask what are not regarded as problems by perpetrators.

Fourth, there are often strong correlations between scores for professionalism and those for other curriculum domains. While it is tempting to think that better professionalism is associated with better knowledge and skills, a more likely interpretation is that there can be a strong halo effect in clinical assessment (Haurani et al. 2007), particularly with the increasing trend to assess clinical and professional skills together (Ponton-Carss et al. 2011). Hence, clinicians may overrate the professionalism of academically strong students.

A related issue is that clinical teachers may be reluctant to make adverse assessments on students unless they demonstrate extreme behaviours and are clear outliers. The amount of direct contact between students and more senior clinical teachers is often limited, and the chances are low that poor professional behaviours will be observed by a single observer, particularly on multiple occasions. Many people will feel that they should not make negative assessments unless they are certain, as such a negative assessment could have serious repercussions. Nobody feels comfortable recording information that might impede the career of a learner. Instead, the decision to make a negative comment is deferred in the hope that others will notice. This, however, is flawed thinking, as it is possible for a learner to provoke concerns about professionalism with clinical teachers in every clinical rotation, but for those making progress decisions to know nothing of this. This tendency to under-report poor professionalism must be addressed in teacher training.

Finally, peer assessment poses significant challenges in all curriculum areas, but particularly in the domain of professionalism. Learners may be more honest in low-stakes than high-stakes assessment and may need substantial engagement to accept and participate effectively in peer assessment practices (Arnold, 2007). Hence educational programmes should teach and assess professionalism in partnership with learners to a greater extent than with other curriculum domains.

Principles of assessing professionalism
Overview

While academics await the results of the research that promises to make clearer what and how to measure, educators must do their best now, based on the current evidence. Many available

1. Professionalism should be assessed early in programmes

2. Professionalism should be assessed often and throughout programmes

3. Professionalism should be assessed from multiple perspectives

4. Professionalism should be assessed by multiple methods, both quantitative and qualitative, including a wide range of written and clinical assessment methods

5. Professionalism should be assessed, wherever possible, in workplace settings

6. Professionalism should be assessed both formatively and summatively.

Figure 43.1 Principles in assessing professionalism.

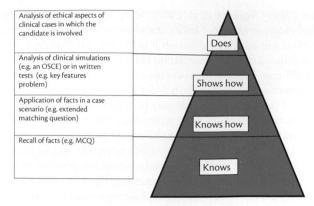

Figure 43.2 Assessment of professionalism according to assessment levels.
Adapted from Miller G., 'The assessment of clinical skills/competence/performance', Academic Medicine, 65, 9, S63–67, copyright 1990 with permission from Wolters Kluwer.

assessments can and should be used, rather than waiting for new methods (Lynch et al. 2004) Professionalism should be assessed often, commencing early in courses, and should use multiple methods to gain multiple perspectives across knowledge, skills, and behaviours in both campus and workplace settings. Assessment should be primarily formative, to guide and reward appropriate development. These principles are summarized in fig. 43.1 and build on a generic approach to developing sound assessment practices and an overview of current practice (Newble et al. 1994; Anderson et al. 2011). The steps described in this generic approach reflect the context of professionalism and are listed in the sequence that is most appropriate to follow; they should help educators determine what, how and when to assess professionalism.

Because professionalism is not a single construct, but rather one that includes a range of knowledge, skills, and attitudes related to health law, ethics, societal values, relationships and codes of conduct, it is essential to be precise about what is to be assessed on each occasion. For example, medical learners will almost certainly be expected to learn some facts and principles about how to behave professionally. However, not all knowledge is the same: in professionalism there are two categories.

The first is that which all graduates should know in order to make the right decisions about how to behave professionally. This is often called working knowledge, and it can be assessed by methods that test recall of factual knowledge. This concept is illustrated in Miller's Pyramid, a useful framework for considering levels of assessment (Miller 1990) (see fig. 43.2).

For example, we could use a multiple choice question, such as that in box 43.1. This question category has limited use beyond the early years of a course, where facts are taught as a precursor to application: this approach is used less often in integrated curricula. The approach may however be more useful in a formative assessment, where the aim is to provide a depth indicator to guide student learning.

The second category of knowledge is that which does not need to be carried at the forefront of memory, but is accessible through a simple search of a book or on-line resource. Learners will need to know enough to work out what and where to search. This form of knowledge can be assessed by methods that define a task, allow candidates time to access materials, and then respond. There are several related assessment methods for such a task, in most cases developed to match problem-based learning curricula, such as the triple jump or 'seen case' exercises, which are commonly used in problem-based learning curricula; an example is provided in box 43.2.

Box 43.1 A sample MCQ testing simple recall

The desire to first do no harm to patients is enshrined in medical ethics. Which one the following terms best describes this principle?

A. Non-maleficence

B. Munificence

C. Benevolence

D. Non-malfeasance

E. Beneficence

Box 43.2 A sample exercise testing application of knowledge

1. (available on the intranet at 9 am)
   The following case scenario forms the basis of a question in this afternoon's written examination.

   A 13-year-old girl makes an appointment as a new patient to see a GP in an after-hours cooperative, telling reception that she has a sore throat. Once with the doctor, she requests a prescription for oral contraceptives. She says that she is in a sexual relationship with her boyfriend, aged 18. She is on her own.

   Your tasks are, as follows:

   A. Analyse the situation to identify the ethical dilemma.

   B. You have 4 hours research the background to the case and identify the information necessary to answer further questions in this afternoon's examination.

2. (available in invigilated session at 1 pm)

   C. What is the ethical dilemma described in the case scenario? Describe the components of the ethical dilemma that should be considered.

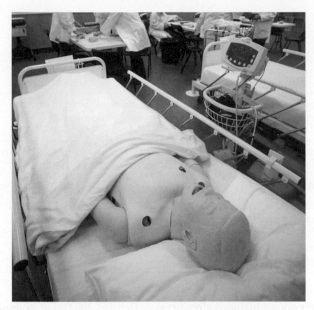

Figure 43.3 Simulation can be used to used to assess some aspects of professionalism.
Reproduced with permission from Bond University.

More senior learners should be assessed on their ability to understand and apply knowledge. This can be achieved in higher level written assessments, but is more suited to the observation of professional behaviours in simulated or workplace encounters (fig. 43.3). Examples include scenarios that require candidates to seek patient consent for a procedure or to communicate concern about a colleague to a senior member of staff. For students about to graduate, it may be more appropriate to ask them to identify and analyse an ethical aspect of a patient interaction in which they are a participant.

Hence, the decisions about what to assess and how to assess are more complex than many may think. This overview has worked through from what to how, and the same process should be done for the entire assessment. The steps in developing assessments are now described.

Table 43.1 The hierarchical nature of learning outcomes

Level of intended learning outcome	Descriptor
Graduate	Demonstrates professional and ethical behaviours in clinical practice as listed in graduate outcomes of the national medical council
End of year/phase	Demonstrates respect for the beliefs of patients from diverse ethnic and religious groups
End of module	Can apply analytical frameworks to resolve ethical dilemmas involving potential conflict between ethical, moral and legal positions
End of week	Knows the difference between ethical, moral and legal positions on common health dilemmas

Step 1: Define what is to be tested: identify the problems and tasks that the learner should be able to perform

The best place to commence defining individual assessments is the intended learning outcomes of the course. This is outcomes-based learning, where the curriculum is based on clear and measurable outcomes that are appropriate for each stage that is being assessed (Harden et al. 1999). It is important for curriculum design, delivery, and assessment to be aligned, as this rewards learners who learn the planned curriculum, rather than those who are diverted by a hidden curriculum. Learning outcomes may be at different levels. A hierarchy of outcomes is demonstrated in table 43.1. Lower level outcomes are relatively easily transformed into individual assessment items and are a good place to start.

The learning outcomes should reflect curriculum domains, which are conceptual groupings of curriculum content that are meaningful to learners and teachers. The traditional way of defining curriculum domains reflects the original approach from 40 years ago—knowledge, skills, and attitudes—which are relatively discrete groups that are assessed using different methods. A more contemporary approach regards curriculum domains as integrated, reflecting the reality that knowledge, skills and attitudes are interrelated. For example, domains may reflect roles, such as 'scholar and scientist', 'practitioner', and 'professional', as used by the General Medical Council in the UK (General Medical Council 2009), or the broader model of roles adopted in Canada. Another approach is used in Australia, with content groups such as 'scientific basis of medicine', 'health and society', 'clinical skills', and 'professionalism' (Australian Medical Council 2010). With these integrated approaches, curriculum domains can be assessed by several different methods.

Putting aside a for a moment the effect of how the domains are organized, a curriculum is likely to have hundreds, if not thousands, of intended learning outcomes, each of which has the potential to become an assessment task. The initial task in assessing professionalism is to develop some of those learning outcomes into assessment items. This is easier if learning outcomes are well designed, clear and measurable. For example, if a learning outcome states 'accepts responsibility for actions', an assessment item writer knows where to start—by writing a case scenario in which a candidate demonstrates correct knowledge that responsibility should be accepted. It does not matter at this stage how the particular case scenarios will be adapted to methods: it may become clear only later in the process whether a particular item will become a multiple choice question (MCQ), a short answer question, an objective structured clinical exam (OSCE) station or a workplace-based assessment.

Step 2: Prepare a blueprint to guide the selection of problems and tasks that are to be assessed

The process detailed in the preceding sections needs to be repeated many times in order to compile a bank of items for assessing professionalism. Ideally, a bank has many more items than are necessary for a single assessment episode, with more than one item for each learning outcome and a total number in the thousands for the whole curriculum. This provides plenty of choice when setting examination papers and allows examiners to choose different items for primary, deferred and re-sit examinations; ideally, these

Table 43.2 A simple assessment blueprint

	Scholar and scientist	Practitioner	Professional
Knowledge	MCQ: identifies specific peripheral nerve injury	EMQ :determines likely chest pain aetiology from scenarios	MCQ: analyses ethical principles
History taking and synthesis	OSCE: gains accurate history from patient with diabetes	Workplace: gains accurate histories from a series of real patients in Mini-CEX assessments	OSCE: deals respectfully with simulated patient from ethnic minority
Formulate management	EMQ: interprets test results and chooses appropriate management plans	OSCE: interpretation of findings in patient with acute chest pain	Short answer question: generates options for reporting suspected child abuse
Examination skills		OSCE station:measures blood pressure accurately	Workplace: appropriate use of chaperones for sensitive examinations
Evidence-based practice	MCQ: interprets trial data	Case presentation: correctly identifies and appraises evidence for a patient with a common clinical condition subject to contemporary debate	Workplace: Demonstrates appropriate decision making in complex scenario involving ethical and legal dimensions

should be set together, as this facilitates equivalence of standards. The larger the item bank, the less worrying are leaks about individual items. An unfortunate but unintended consequence of assessment to inform progress decisions in medical education is gaming. There are websites on which candidates submit memorized items and their attempts at correct answers. Learners sometimes focus on studying past papers rather than what is in the curriculum. There are also reports of learners deliberately missing primary examinations so that they can hear what was in them before the re-sit or deferred examination, hoping that there will be significant overlap and so an opportunity to obtain a higher score. There is a need for tight examination security to minimize the success of gaming and to ensure fairness. This is a substantial challenge to most institutions, as many learners do not regard such behaviours as serious.

Once the bank has been established, it needs to be organized into a blueprint, or document that demonstrates the relationship between curriculum domains and the bank of items. This ensures alignment of the curriculum to its assessment. A blueprint looks like a two dimensional table, as illustrated in table 43.2, which cross tabulates curriculum domains by specific tasks expected of candidates. A third dimension might be an overlay that ensures that assessment items are assessed across age groups, males and females, and ethnic groups and social classes.

EMQ, extended matching question; MCQ, multiple choice question; OSCE, objective structured clinical exam.The point of this organization is that it guides both item writing and selection. For item writing, it is clear when looking at the blueprint where there may be either too many items or no items. When selecting items for examinations, the blueprint makes it easier for the sample of items to reflect the curriculum. For example, if 20% of a curriculum covers professionalism, then it can be seen first that there are sufficient items available to assess professionalism, and second that 20% of the items do assess professionalism.

Step 3: Select the test methods that are most appropriate to assess the blueprinted problems

With the blueprint populated, it now becomes clearer how items should be developed according to selected assessment methods (Jha et al. 2007; Veloski et al. 2005). While it is tempting and probably necessary to develop new methods of assessing professionalism,

many sound methods already exist (Deirdre, 2004). For example, an item on 'demonstrates respect for patients with diverse backgrounds' is most appropriately assessed by observing the candidate deal with a genuine patient from a minority background, ideally in the workplace. This however may be difficult to arrange in a way that is standardized and able to be compared across candidates, so the most likely method would be a standardized interview with a simulated patient in an OSCE—which now more commonly includes stations specifically designed to test professionalism (Srinivasan et al. 2004).

Step 4: Develop test items to populate the blueprint

Larger numbers of assessment items are now developed for the chosen methods, according to their particular characteristics. For example, an MCQ may be based on either a simple, direct question or a case scenario that is followed by a question. The addition of a case scenario provides context and can help to elevate the assessment from simple knowledge to applied knowledge and can promote integrated assessment in an integrated curriculum (Hays et al. 2009). On the other hand, it increases reading time, reducing the total number of sampled learning outcomes. Further, adding only relevant information can cue candidates to the correct answer and adding irrelevant information can be confusing. Much depends on the skill of the item writer.

Assessment items are best developed by small teams of teachers, so that the wording can be checked to reduce ambiguity, the answer can be verified and the item calibrated for the level of the candidate. For integrated assessment the small team of item writers should include representatives from different contexts. For example, a question on ethics in a clinical context should ideally be written jointly by an ethicist and clinicians from different specialties, as this increases the accuracy of the content and the relevance of the question to the real world.

It is common for a single learning objective to be developed into more than one assessment item. For example, two similar MCQs could be developed, one more appropriate for assessing simple knowledge in junior medical students, the other more embellished and integrated into clinical practice and so more appropriate for a senior student. The bank would need a database field for level of student to ensure that the appropriate item is available for the right level of candidate. Further, it may be possible to develop both a written simulation (a key feature problem) and a clinical simulation (an OSCE station) from the same scenario. Again the bank would have to flag the items that share the assessment of a single outcome to ensure that only one of these was selected for a given examination. This multiple item writing approach is an efficient way of increasing the number of items in a bank.

The process of writing items is never ending. While individual items can be reused a number of times, and probably should be as part of examination quality assurance, new items should be developed every year to reflect knew knowledge. Questions that are reused should be checked at least every 2 years to ensure currency. Older items should be retired, even if they are still correct; retired items are ideal for formative assessment, where security is not a concern.

The resource intensive nature of maintaining fresh, high quality item banks has resulted in some schools sharing items. Most of these sharing arrangements are informal collaborations conducted at low cost, usually within nations or common jurisdictions, as this increases the relevance of all questions to member schools that work towards a common outcomes framework. Other assessment banks are international, such as the International Database for Enhanced Assessment and Learning (IDEAL) Consortium and International Foundations of Medicine (IFOM) (International Database for Enhanced Assessment and Learning 2012; National Board of Medical Examiners 2012); the former is a lower-cost, non-commercial collaboration while the latter is a higher-cost professional service run by the National Board of Medical Examiners. There are, however, pitfalls in using international banks in professionalism, as the nature of professionalism and the underlying professional, legal and societal frameworks differ across national boundaries and many of these questions may be contextually or factually inaccurate for medical schools outside the country in which the question was written (Worthington and Hays 2012).

Step 5: Select the assessment tasks from the blueprint

The setting of an examination paper should involve a process of random selection of assessment items from a bank, according to the assessment blueprint, the format, the number of items, and the weighting of the curriculum themes. For example, an end-of-year test might be intended to equally assess three curriculum themes, one of which is professionalism. A decision is then made about how professionalism will be assessed: for the sake of this example it is decided to place 80% of the professionalism assessment into workplace-based assessment and in 2 of 16 OSCE stations. This leaves 20% of the theme to be assessed in written assessment, in this example mostly as part of two scenario-based questions in a short answer questions paper and 10 questions in scenario-based MCQs. This inclusion of professionalism questions across a range of methods sends a clear message to learners that professionalism is important, but focuses the questions on integrated, clinical scenario-based questions that measure competence and performance.

Ideally, there will be many more than 10 MCQs on professionalism available in the assessment bank, so items are selected from the available bank according to the assessment blueprint. In the case of a curriculum theme for professionalism, the blueprint may indicate that about 33% of the questions are each on medical ethics, professional behaviour and resource allocation. A computerized assessment system will randomly select the desired number of questions according to database fields, but this can also be done manually. It is best to initially select more than the desired number of questions (say 10–15% more), as the examination paper must be reviewed carefully for errors and then the standard must be set; it is common for a few questions to be removed, leaving about the right number.

Assessment can only ever be based on a sample of the large number of intended learning outcomes. Much of the art of assessment lies in balancing under- and over-assessing. Under-assessment may risk not measuring sufficiently the requirements of a sound graduate, while over-assessment may encourage learners to focus on assessment rather than learning. The better the sample matches the learning outcomes and the theme weighting of the planned curriculum, the easier it is to have less assessment. For example, consider two medical schools in the same nation. School A always sets two 180-question MCQ papers (with no clinical stems) and a four-station OSCE. School B sets a single 120-question MCQ papers (with clinical stems) and a 16-station OSCE. Students at these two schools receive different messages. At school A, students may interpret the assessment as encouraging factual learning and poor attendance at clinical placements in the weeks prior to examinations. At school B, students are more likely to see that learning from patients is best and so remain in their clinical placements for longer. These two examination approaches differ in their assessment utility (Van der Vleuten 1996): both should achieve high reliability coefficients, but differ in validity and educational impact.

Step 6: Set the standard for each assessment

Standard setting is now regarded as an essential step in increasing the precision of assessment. There are several approaches, each with characteristics that suit particular methods. Detailed presentation of methods is beyond the scope of this chapter, but can be found elsewhere (Norcini 2003; Van der Vleuten 1996). Most combine a degree of prospective consensus on how candidates should perform with some retrospective view of examination performance. From the perspective of assessing professionalism, it is essential that a group of teachers, including clinicians and ethicists, agree on the correct answer and the standard expected of candidates at the particular level (e.g. junior medical student, senior medical student, or postgraduate trainee). This not a simple process, as different groups may arrive at different standards, and it is possible for examiners at different medical schools to set different standards on identical assessment items and tests (Boursicot et al. 2006). Further, criterion-referenced assessment often results in a different passing score for each examination. There is still as much art as science in standard setting in the context of professionalism.

Step 7: Administer the tests

This is a largely logistic exercise, where the assessment team prints sufficient copies of the examination papers, engages invigilators, supervises candidates, collects the score sheets, and enters results. Written examinations, which are commonly used in ethics and professionalism, require substantial marking time and resources. For workplace-based assessment, several ratings may be required from clinicians, who need to be trained.

Step 8: Manage scores to produce results

The scores of most interest are those in the borderline group, because all assessment scores include a margin for error, and further assessment, sometimes after a period of remediation, may be required before a candidate is passed with confidence. Of particular concern are borderline candidates who just manage to get a pass on a re-sit examination but continue to demonstrate poor or borderline performance in assessments (Pell et al. 2012).

Step 9: Make decisions based on the results

For all kinds of assessment it is essential that there are clear, consistent processes for making decisions and that there is congruence between regulations at all levels where decisions can be made and/or appealed against. For medical schools, this means alignment of school, faculty, and whole of university regulations, such that the rules that guide decisions made in medical schools are consistent with those of the whole institution; without this, student appeals are likely to be successful. While this congruence is important for all decisions based on assessment results, it is of particular importance where decisions are made on the grounds of poor professionalism. In an ideal world, students with poor professionalism would fail their examinations, but in many cases students with professional problems perform well enough in tests of knowledge and skills for total performance to be judged as a pass. Much depends on how the rules of progression are written, including whether and how compensation is allowed across domains. It is possible to make progression rules apply greater weight to professionalism, such as making professionalism assessments hurdles (as long as these rules are supported by institutional regulations). Candidates will often appeal against adverse decisions, and appeals may be upheld only on the grounds of incorrect process or lack of congruence between rules at different levels.

Methods more suitable for assessing professionalism

Many assessment methods are not particularly suitable for assessing professionalism because they assess either theoretical knowledge or, at best, what happens in simulations. While it is possible and indeed sound, to use appropriately designed MCQs, structured short answer, and OSCEs to assess professionalism, more emphasis should be placed on measuring what happens in the workplace, where basic knowledge and conceptual frameworks must be applied and appropriate behaviours demonstrated. There are some recently developed simulated tasks that show promise (Stewart et al. 2010), but effort is being placed in developing evidence-based, workplace-based assessments. So far, however, most workplace-based assessment methods appear much more effective for formative than summative assessments (Mitchell et al. 2011) and so care must be taken in making high-stakes decisions based on a narrow sample of workplace-based assessments.

Workplace-based assessments

In-training assessments

In-training assessments came into prominence after research showed that about 12 ratings by peers produced a reliable assessment of the performance of clinicians (Ramsey et al. 1996) It made no difference whether the raters were chosen by person being rated or allocated centrally. This has led to many variations on the theme, but the consistency is that learners are subject to ratings by their clinical teachers. The scores are added up to inform a decision about the learner's performance. In some cases the score forms a hurdle which may prevent progress to formal written and clinical examinations; in others scores are combined with other examination scores, but in many cases they are used only as formative assessment, because it is difficult to collect enough in-training assessments forms to achieve a valid, reliable result.

Multisource feedback

This is a variation on in-training assessments, whereby ratings are sought deliberately, using the same questions, from a range of people with whom the learner has contact during work (Wood et al. 2006). These may include clinical teachers, peers, patients, and other health professional, administrative, and technical staff, each of whom has professional contact with the learner. It is a variant of the 360-degree evaluations used in management training, and is based on the premise that self-awareness is improved by formal feedback from those with whom we work, regardless of their place in the organizational structure. The feedback from multiple perspectives can produce interesting and valid information that is useful for reflection by learners. For example, a clinical teacher might think that an individual has excellent relationships with other staff, whereas those staff members report that the individual is dismissive of their contributions and rude to nurses. Multisource feedback may be more appropriate when used formatively (Campbell et al. 2011).

Self-evaluation

In self-evaluation learners think about and complete an assessment of their own performance, and then compare personal views with those of teachers, peers, patients, and other health workers. It is common for individuals to be unaware of how they are perceived by others, and discussion about differences can facilitate self-awareness, an important component of emotional intelligence (Goleman 1996). Self-assessment is interesting but not always reliable. There is evidence that self-assessment is more honest and accurate when the results are used formatively rather than summatively, and less accurate when made by poorer performers (Lipsett et al. 2011).

Reflection

Reflection is a topical issue. The concept is broad and spans a range of methods. One method requires individuals to think about their own performance, with or without external feedback. This thinking is then written down, forming a commentary on lessons learned and implications for future personal development. Another, and perhaps the most commonly used, method requires learners to reflect on what can be learned from a discussion trigger. In medical professionalism, the trigger is commonly a written clinical case report based on a patient that the learner has encountered. Many patients present professional challenges alongside their clinical problems and learners are asked to identify these issues and comment on what this means for their own learning. For example, a young adult with cerebral palsy that has resulted in a physical disability is undergoing surgical treatment of an orthopaedic complication. This person is cared for by middle-aged parents who devote considerable time and effort to the task, and yet are anxious about care when they can no longer provide it. The young adult wants greater autonomy, but independent living requires substantial funding for life. The learner will be expected to identify and discuss the ethical issues and comment on what kind of healthcare they believe should be provided.

The role of reflection in assessment is controversial. Many believe that reflection is more effective when personal, honest and private; while others believe that it is essential to be open about personal opinions and beliefs. Assessment, particularly summative assessment, can influence candidate behaviour. For example, there are reports of gaming by candidates, who make up personal experiences for reflection, download from an online bank of reflective essays, or simply follow a reflection formula that is available on some web sites (Hays and Gay 2011).

Other workplace-based assessment methods

It is possible to critically appraise almost any documentation that a learner might contribute to clinical records (Papadakis and Loeser 2006). This includes looking at the quality of interprofessional communication, looking for evidence of respect and collegiality. Such appraisals can be performed by learners or their teachers, again potentially finding triggers for discussion and reflection. These are. however. time-consuming tasks that are difficult to use in summative assessment and so far do not show strong evidence of effectiveness in formative assessment (Overeem et al. 2007). More recent developments include analysis of videotaped surgical procedures, which show promise as a means of tracking development in surgical residents (Larsen et al. 2005).

Learning portfolios

Much has been written about learning portfolios (Buckley et al. 2009). Here a learning portfolio is defined as a receptacle (folder, box, or electronic device), in which anything that aids learning can be placed. As such it is actually not an assessment method, but a format for gathering a range of different assessments. Portfolios appear more appropriate to formative assessment, but they are used increasingly in summative assessment. Some portfolios contain two sections in order to meet the dual requirements of formative and summative assessment—one for personal information used only by the learner and one to be submitted for formal assessment. Portfolios demonstrate the same advantages and challenges of their individual components—they can provide valuable information that guides the development of learners, but they can also distort behaviours and are prone to gaming.

Common pitfalls in assessing professionalism

It is worth highlighting the pitfalls commonly encountered in assessing professionalism.

Trying to use formative information in a summative manner

The best evidence for using assessments of professionalism is for formative assessment, although there is still limited evidence that formative assessment produces meaningful long-term change (Overeem et al. 2007). The temptation is strong to use summative assessment of professionalism, largely because this is now regarded as such a key part of being a medical practitioner. However, the best advice in this regard is to be cautious when using measures of professionalism in making high-stakes decisions. Extreme behaviours will generally be obvious and also generally agreed by panels to be unacceptable, but the situation is less clear for behaviours that can always be blamed on one-off situations, personality clashes, personal stress or immaturity. The most effective way of making such decisions more valid and reliable is to collect information from multiple sources, using multiple methods. Congruence of information from different sources can send a powerful message

that is more likely to survive panel discussions, including those in appeal processes.

Undervaluing or overvaluing experience and judgement capacity

Using clinicians to assess the professional behaviour of learners is valid, efficient, and likely to have educational impact through role modelling by people that learners aspire to become. On the other hand, this requires the clinicians to make sometimes complex judgements about the behaviours that they observe in learners under their supervision. Several things can go wrong here, primarily affecting reliability, but also diminishing other aspects of utility. Some concerning behaviours might not be much different from those of more experienced clinicians (Ainsworth and Szauter, 2006), blurring the threshold for reporting. More experienced clinicians who see their learners often will make better judgements, yet learners are not often in frequent contact with experienced clinicians over prolonged periods. Contributing factors include the effect of shorter working hours on clinical team rosters (Garvin et al. 2008), the expansion of medical education requiring almost every clinician to teach and assess, including the less experienced and the unwilling, and the tendency for more junior staff to provide clinical supervision. It is common for clinicians to under-report concerns about learners; they may be anxious that they have not seen enough of the learner to be sure, they may worry that they have had a personality clash or that they could inadvertently harm careers. Training may be necessary for all clinicians in the workplace, including more junior clinicians, to support reporting (at least in a descriptive sense) of concerning behaviours.

Failure to provide sufficient qualitative information about potential breaches

It is common for reports of potentially unprofessional behaviour to be described poorly, often with just a brief condemning judgment, such as 'arrogant and rude to patients'. This kind of statement provides too little information and may be open to challenge as 'merely an opinion'. A better approach is for clinical teachers to describe in detail both the behaviours and their impact on the learning environment or the patient experience, For example, it is better to state:

> During a ward round the student asked rather aggressive questions of a patient and criticized her for having been a smoker. He suggested in the patient's presence that she was less deserving of expensive treatments because the disease was largely self-inflicted. The patient was upset and I had to go to considerable effort to reassure her that we would do our best to treat the cancer, regardless of her smoking history. After the ward round I advised the student that this behaviour was inappropriate, and likely to worsen the patient's anxiety and perhaps even affect recovery. However, he showed no remorse and defended his position on the grounds that demand was outstripping resources and that doctors will soon have to make these decisions. This lack of insight makes even more serious his earlier breach of professionalism. This discussion also derailed the normal learning about lung cancer in which his fellow students would normally participate.

This kind of report, particularly by a senior clinician, makes it easier for education managers to make defensible decisions about whether or not to intervene. Professionalism includes complex competencies that require expert professional judgement, often based on qualitative, rather than quantitative data. Hence, credibility, transferability, dependability, and confirmability are just as important as the utility index (reliability, validity, educational impact) that is applied to quantitative assessment methods. This example may be serious enough to warrant immediate intervention, while repeated episodes of less serious breaches build a robust case that facilitates both detailed feedback and potential disciplinary action. The complexity surrounding the assessment of professionalism is summarized well in a recent review (Hodges et al. 2011). The authors state 'the results presented here reveal several different ways of thinking about professionalism that can lead towards a multi-dimensional, multi-paradigmatic approach to assessing professionalism at different levels: individual, inter-personal, societal-institutional'. The review recommends substantial research into how to assess meaningfully the professional behaviour of medical students and graduates.

Adding together scores in breach of measurement theory

Because workplace-based assessments of professionalism commonly produce qualitative rather than quantitative information, there are potential problems when educators try to add a rating for professionalism to scores from other assessments. It is worthwhile considering measurement theory, which dictates what and how scores can be added together. For example, a score of 4 on a 5 point Likert scale is not necessarily 80% and cannot easily be added to a score for an MCQ paper to produce an overall score. It is sometimes better to regard categorical data as a hurdle that must be cleared before interval numerical scores are combined (Foulkes et al. 1994). One recent concept is to consider 'profile analysis' rather than overall scores, but its use in medical education is not yet well understood. As learners and lawyers become more knowledgeable about fine print, it is possible to lose an appeal based on inappropriate combination of scores producing a borderline fail score.

Unclear or inconsistent assessment practices and rules of progression

Another feature of appeals by candidates against adverse assessments is that they focus on the processes by which decisions are reached. As a rule, appeals cannot overturn judgements by a clinical teacher in the workplace, so long as it is detailed—that is regarded as the expertise of the clinical teacher. However, a candidate may be allowed to be retested or even to proceed to the next stage if the judgement was made by a clinical teacher who can be shown to be poorly trained, inexperienced, to have used the wrong form at the wrong time or to have failed to inform the candidate about their concerns in a timely manner. It is essential that the clinical teacher and the education office follow the written assessment procedures to the letter. Further, it is essential that assessment procedures are either consistent with the regulations of the broader institution or covered by special institutional regulations. For example, it is common for a medical school to limit the number of re-sits or fails that a student is permitted during a course, whereas the university as a whole may not. Furthermore, it is essential that those making the decisions about progress do not include either the individual who made the failing rating (if on the committee, this person should declare a conflict of interest and withdraw) or any person sitting in judgement at an appeal (such as the dean). It is therefore essential that assessment regulations are carefully written, describe in detail the process of how decisions are made and are checked many times before being made available to students and staff—they are public

documents. Finally, the quality and quantity of evidence may be challenged, so it is important to formally document everything and to consider having all conversations with learners exhibiting unprofessional behaviours witnessed by an observer, Failure to comply strictly with process and governance will result in appeals overturning decisions, either at the broader institutional level or external appeal boards.

Conclusions

- Professionalism is now a more overt and substantial component of medical curricula.

- Learners will focus more on the professionalism domain of a curriculum if it is assessed.

- Because professionalism is made up of knowledge, skills, attitudes, and behaviours, the domain should be assessed by multiple methods and from multiple perspectives.

- The assessment of professionalism should include assessment of performance in the clinical workplace, as this more closely reflects likely performance after graduation.

- One of the most significant challenges in assessing professionalism is dealing with learners with strengths in knowledge and skills, but weaknesses in professional behaviours.

References

Ainsworth, M.A. and Szauter, K.M. (2006) Medical student professionalism: are we developing the right behaviours? A comparison of professional lapses by students and physicians. *Acad Med.* 81: S83–S86

Anderson, B., Bollela, V., Burch, V., et al. (2011) Criteria for good assessment. *Med Teach.* 33(3): 206–214

Arnold, L., Shue, C.K., Kalishman, S. et al. (2007). Can there be a single system for peer assessment of professionalism among medical students? A multi-institutional study. *Acad Med.* 82: 578–586

Association of American Medical Colleges (2011) Medical College Admission Test. https://www.aamc.org/students/applying/mcat/ Accessed 11 March 2013 Australian Council for Education Research. Graduate Australian Medical School Admissions test. http://www.acer.edu.au/tests/gamsat Accessed 11 March 2013

Australian Council for Education Research. Health Professions Admission test. http://www.acer.edu.au/tests/hpat-ireland Accessed 11 March 2013

Australian Council for Education Research. Undergraduate Medical Admission test. http://www.acer.edu.au/tests/umat Accessed 11 March 2013

Australian Medical Association Council of Doctors-in-training; New Zealand Medical Association Doctors-in-training Council, New Zealand Medical Students' Assoc. and the Australian Medical Students' Assoc. *Social Media and the Medical Profession. A guide to online professionalism for medical practitioners and medical students* (Nov 2010). https://ama.com.au/social-media-and-medical-profession Accessed 11 March 2013

Australian Medical Council (2010a) Standards for Assessment and Accreditation of Medical Schools by the Australian Medical Council 2010. http://www.amc.org.au/images/Medschool/accreditation-standards-medical-schools-2010.pdf Accessed 11 March 2013

Australian Medical Council (2010b) Good medical practice: A code of conduct for doctors in Australia. ACT http://www.amc.org.au/index.php/about/good-medical-practice Accessed 11 March 2013

Barr, J. (1912) President's Address, delivered at the eightieth annual meeting of the British Medical Association. *BMJ.* 2: 157

Bindal, T., Wall, D., and Goodyear, H.M. (2011). Trainee doctors' views on workplace-based assessments: Are they just a tick box exercise? *Med Teach.* 33: 919–927

Borges, N.J., Manuel, R.S., Elam, C.L., and Jones, B.J. (2010) Differences in motives between Millennial and Generation X medical students. *Med Educ.* 44: 570–576

Boursicot, K.A.M., Roberts, T.E., and Pell, G. (2006) Standard setting for clinical competence at graduation from medical schools: A comparison of passing scores from five medical schools. *Adv Hlth Sci Educ.* 11: 173–183

Bradshaw, P.J., Alfonso, H.S., Finn, J.C., Owen, J., and Thompson, P.L. (2009) Coronary heart disease events in Aboriginal Australians: incidence in an urban population. *Med J Aust.* 190(10): 583–586

Bristol Royal Infirmary Inquiry (2001) Inquiry into the management of care of children undergoing complex heart surgery at the Bristol Royal Infirmary. http://www.bristol-inquiry.org.uk Accessed 11 March 2013

Buckley, S., Coleman, J., Davison, I., et al. (2009) The educational effects of portfolios on undergraduate student learning: a Best Evidence Medical Education (BEME) systematic review. BEME Guide No.11. *Med Teach.* 31: 282–298

Campbell, J.L., Roberts, M., Wright, C., et al. (2011) Factors associated with variability in the assessment of UK doctors' professionalism: analysis of survey results. *BMJ.* 343: d6212

Casali, G.L. and Day, G.E. (2010) Treating an unhealthy organisational culture: the implications of the Bundaberg Hospital Inquiry for managerial ethical decision making. *Aust Hlth Rev.* 34 (1): 73–79

Chretien KC, Farnan JM, Greyson ST, Kind T (2011) To friend or not to friend? Social networking and faculty perceptions of online professionalism. *Acad Med.* 86: 1545–1550

Coates, H. (2008) Establishing the criterion validity of the Graduate Medical School Admissions Test (GAMSAT) *Med Educ.* 42(10): 999–1006

Cohen, J.J. (2006) Professionalism in medical education, an American perspective: from evidence to accountability. *Med Educ.* 4: 607–617

Crutcher, R.A., Szafran, O., Woloschuk, W., Chatur, F., and Hansen, C. (2011) Family medicine graduates' perceptions of intimidation, harassment, and discrimination during residency training. *BMC Med Educ.* 11: 88

Deirdre, C., Lynch, D.C., Patricia, M., Surdyk, P.M., and Eiser, A.R. (2004) Assessing professionalism: a review of the literature. *Med Teach.* 26(4): 366–373

Donnon, T., Paolucci, E.O., and Violato, C. (2007) The predictive validity of the MCAT for medical school performance and medical board licensing examinations: a meta-analysis of the published research. *Acad Med.* 2(1): 100–106

Dupree, E., Anderson, R., McEvoy, M.D., and Brodman, M. (2011) Professionalism: a necessary ingredient in a culture of safety. *Jt Comm J Qual Patient Saf.* 37(10): 447–455

Eva, K.W., Reiter, H.I., Trinh, K., Wasi, P., Rosenfeld, J., and Norman, G.R. (2009) Predictive validity of the multiple mini-interview for selecting medical trainees. *Med Educ.* 43(8): 767–775

Foulkes, J. Bandaranayake, R., Hays, R.B., et al. (1994) Combining components of assessment. In D. Newble, R. Wakeford, and B. Jolly (eds) *The Certification and Recertification of Doctors: issues in the assessment of competence* (pp. 134–150). Cambridge, UK: Cambridge University Press

Frank, J.R., Jabbour, M., Tugwell, P., et al. (1996) Skills for the new millennium: report of the societal needs working group, CanMEDS 2000 Project. *Ann Roy Coll Phy Surg Can.* 29: 206–216

Garvin, J.T., McLaughlin, R., and Kerin, M.J. (2008) A pilot project of European working time directive compliant rosters in a university teaching hospital. *The Surg.* 6: 88–93

General Medical Council (2008) Medical Students Professional values and fitness to practice. http://www.gmc-uk.org/publications/index.asp Accessed 11 March 2013

General Medical Council (2009) Tomorrow's Doctors. http://www.gmc-uk.org/publications/index.asp Accessed 11 March 2013

General Medical Council. Good Medical Practice. 2001 Edition. http://www.gmc-uk.org/guidance/good_medical_practice/index.asp Accessed 11 March 2013

Goleman, D. (1996) *Working With Emotional Intelligence.* London: Bloomsbury Publishing. http://books.google.com.au/books?id=AcJ7dwsnWiIC&printsec=frontcover&source=gbs_ge_summary_r&cad=0#v=onepage&q&f=false Accessed 11 March 2013

Graham, J., Guglani, S., Elyan, S., Falk, S., Braybrooke, J., and Roques, T. (2010) Return of the postcode lottery. *BMJ.* 341: c7389

Guseh, J.S. 2nd, Brendel, R.W., and Brendel, D.H. (2009) Medical professionalism in the age of online social networking. *J Med Ethics.* 35(9): 584–586

Haurani, M.J., Rubinfeld, I., et al. (2007) Are the communication and professionalism competencies the new critical values in a resident's global evaluation process? *J Surg Educ.* 64(6): 351–356

Harden, R.M., Crosby, J.R., Davis, M.H., et al. (1999) *Outcomes Based Education.* Dundee: AMEE

Hays, R.B. (1990) Self-evaluation of videotaped consultations (1990) *Teach Learn Med.* 2: 232–236

Hays, R.B. (2012) Remediation and reassessment in undergraduate medical school examinations. *Med Teach.* 34(2): 91–92

Hays, R.B. and Gay, S. (2011) Reflection or 'pre-flection': what are we actually measuring. *Med Educ.* 45: 116–118

Hays, R.B., Jolly, B.J., Caldon, L.J.M., et al. (2002a) Is insight important? Measuring the capacity to change. *Med Educ.* 36: 965–971

Hays, R.B., Davies, H.A., Beard, J., et al. (2002b) Selecting performance assessment methods for experienced physicians. *Med Educ.* 36: 910–917

Hays, R.B., Coventry, P., Wilcock, D., and Hartley, K. (2009) Short and long multiple choice question stems in a primary care oriented undergraduate medical curriculum. *Educ Primary Care.* 20: 173–177

Hays, R.B., Lawson, M., and Gray, C. (2011) Problems presented by medical students seeking support: A possible intervention framework. *Med Teach.* 33(2): 161–164

Hilton, S. and Slotnick, H.B. (2005) Proto-professionalism: how professionalization occurs across the continuum of medical education. *Med Educ.* 39: 58–65

Hilton, S. and Southgate, L. (2007) Professionalism in medical education. *Teach Teach Educ.* 23: 265–279

Ho, M.J., Yu, K.H., Hirsh, D., Huang, T.S., and Yang, P.C. (2011) Does one size fit all? Building a framework for medical professionalism. *Acad Med.* 86(11): 1407–1414

Hodges, B.D. and Kuper, A. (2012) Theory and practice in the design and conduct of graduate medical education. *Acad Med.* 87(1): 25–33

Hodges, B.D., Ginsburg, S., Cruess, R., et al. (2011) Assessment of professionalism: Recommendations from the Ottawa 2010 Conference. *Med Teach.* 33: 354–363

International Database for Enhancement of Assessment and Learning (2012) Overview Document. http://www.idealmed.org Accessed 11 March 2013

Irvine, D.H. (2007) Everyone is entitled to a good doctor. *Med J Aust.* 186: 256–261

Jha, V., Bekker, H.L., Duffy, S.R.G., and Roberts, T.E. (2007) A systematic review of studies assessing and facilitating attitudes towards professionalism in medicine. *Med Educ.* 41: 822–829

Katz, J.N., Kessler, C.L., O'Connell, A., and Levine, S.A. (2007) Professionalism and evolving concepts of quality. *J Gen Intern Med.* 22: 137–139

Larsen, J.L., Williams, R.G., Ketchum, J., Boehler, M.L., and Dunnington, G.L. (2005) Feasibility, reliability, and validity of an operative performance rating system for evaluating surgery residents. *Surgery.* 138: 640–647

Liaison Committee on Medical Education (2012) Functions and structure of a medical School, May 2012. http://www.lcme.org/standard.htm Accessed March 2013

Lipsett, P.A., Harris, I., and Downing, S. (2011) Resident self-other assessor agreement: influence of assessor, competency and performance level. *Arch Surg.* 146: 901–906

Lynch, D.C., Surdyk, P.M., and Eiser, A.R. (2004) Assessing professionalism: a review of the literature. *Med Teach.* 26(4): 366–373

Martimianakis, M.A., Maniate, J.M., and Hodges, B.D. (2009) Sociological interpretations of professionalism. *Med Educ.* 43: 829–837

Miller, A. and Archer, J. (2010) Impact of workplace-based assessment on doctors' education and performance. *BMJ.* 341: c5064

Miller, G. (1990) The assessment of clinical skills/competence/performance. *Acad Med.* 65: S63–S67

Mitchell, C., Bhat, S., Herbert, A., and Baker, P. (2011) Workplace-based assessments of junior doctors: do scores predict training difficulties? *Med Educ.* 45: 1190–1198

National Board of Medical Examiners (2012) International Foundations of Medicine Program Overview. http://www.nbme.org/Schools/iFoM/index.html Accessed 11 March 2013

Newble, D. Dauphinee, D., Dawson-Saunders, B., et al. (1994) Guidelines for the development of effective and efficient procedures for the assessment of clinical competence. In: D. Newble, B. Jolly, and R. Wakeford (eds) *The Certification and Recertification of Doctors: Issues in the Assessment of Clinical Competence.*(pp. 69–91). Cambridge: Cambridge University Press

Norcini, J.J. (2003) Setting standards on educational tests *Med Educ.* 37: 464–469

Overeem, K., Faber, M.J., Arah, O.A., et al. (2007) Doctor performance assessment in daily practise: does it help or not? A systematic review. *Med Educ.* 41: 1039–1049

Papadakis, M. and Loeser, H. (2006) Using clinical incident reports and longitudinal observations to assess professionalism. In D. Stern (ed.) *Measuring Medical Professionalism* (pp. 159–174). Oxford: Oxford University Press

Papadakis, M., Hodgson, C.S., Teherani, A., and Kohatsu, N.D. (2004) Unprofessional behaviour in medical school is associated with subsequent disciplinary action by a state medical board. *Acad Med.* 79: 244–249

Pell, G., Fuller, R., Matthew, M., and Roberts, T. (2012) Is short term remediation after OSCE failure sustained? A retrospective analysis of the longitudinal attainment of underperforming students in OSCE assessments, *Med Teach.* 34(2): 146–150

Ponton-Carss, A., Hutchinson, C., and Violato, C. (2011) Assessment of communication, professionalism and surgical skills in an objective structured performance-related examination (OSPRE): a psychometric study. *Am J Surg.* 202: 433–440

Poole, P., Shulruf, B., Rudland, J., and Wilkinson, T. (2012) Comparison of UMAT scores and GPA in prediction of performance in medical school: a national study. *Med Educ.* 46(2): 163–171

Prideaux, D., Roberts, C., Eva, K., et al. (2011) Assessment for selection for the health care professions and specialty training: consensus statement and recommendations from the Ottawa 2010 Conference. *Med Teach.* 33(3): 215–223

Ramsey, P.G., Carline, J.D., Blank, L.L., and Wenrich, M.D. (1996) Feasibility of hospital-based use of peer ratings to evaluate the performances of practicing physicians. *Acad Med.* 71(4): 364–370

Rentmeester, C.A. (2007) Should a good healthcare professional be (at least a little) callous? *J Med Philos.* 32: 43–64

Royal College of Physicians and Surgeons of Canada. CanMEDS Competency Framework (1996) http://rcpsc.medical.org/canmeds/index.php Accessed 11 March 2013

Saultz, J.W. (2007) Are we serious about teaching professionalism in medicine? *Acad Med.* 82: 574–586

Snyder, L. (2011) Online professionalism: social media, social contracts, trust, and medicine. *J Clin Ethics.* 22(2): 173–175

Srinivasan, M., Litzelman, D., Seshadri, R., et al (2004) Developing an OSTE to address lapses in learners' professional behaviour and an instrument to code educators' responses. *Acad Med.* 79: 888–896

Stewart, M., Kennedy, N., and Cuene-Grandidier, H. (2010) Undergraduate interprofessional education using high fidelity paediatric simulation. *Clin Teach.* 7: 90–96

Swick, H.M., Szenas, P., Danoff, D., and Whitcomb, M. (1999) Teaching professionalism in undergraduate medical education, *JAMA.* 282: 830–832

Shipman Inquiry (2003) *The Shipman Inquiry: First Report.* London: The Stationery Office

United Kingdom Clinical Aptitude Test Consortium. United Kingdom Clinical Aptitude Test. www.ukcat.ac.uk Accessed 21 March 2013

van der Vleuten, C.P.M. (1996) The assessment of professional competence: developments, research and practical implications. *Adv Hlth Sci Educ.* 1: 41–67

Veloski, J.J., Fields, S.K., Boex, J.R., and Blank, L.L. (2005) Measuring professionalism: a review of studies with instruments reported in the literature between 1982 and 2002. *Acad Med.* 80: 366–370

West, C.P., Huntington, J.L., Huschka, M.M., et al. (2007) A prospective study of the relationship between medical knowledge and professionalism among internal medicine residents. *Acad Med.* 82: 587–591

White, G. and Kiegalde, D. (2011) Gen Y learners: just how concerned should we be? *Clin Teach.* 8: 263–266

Wilkinson, D., Zhang, J., and Parker, M. (2011) Predictive validity of the Undergraduate Medicine and Health Sciences Admission Test for medical students' academic performance. *Med J Aust.* 194(7): 341–344

Wood, L., Hassell, A., Whitehouse, A., Bullock, A., and Wall, D. (2006) A literature review of multi-course feedback systems within and without healthcare services, leading to 10 tips for their successful design. *Med Teach.* 28: 185–191

World Federation for Medical Education (2003) Basic Medical Education. WFME Global Standards for Quality Improvement. http://www.saidem.org.ar/docs/Normas/WFME.%20Global%20standards%20for%20quality%20improvement.pdf Accessed 11 March 2013

Worthington, R. and Hays, R.B. (2012) Addressing unprofessional behaviours. *Clin Teach.* 9(2): 71–74

Wright, S.R. and Bradley, P.M. (2010) Has the UK Clinical Aptitude Test improved medical student selection? *Med Educ.* 44: 1069–1076

CHAPTER 44

Assessment in the context of relicensure

W. Dale Dauphinee

From the start, the aim of revalidation has been to enable doctors to show that they are up to date and fit to practise, and to encourage improvement through meaningful reflection based on evidence drawn from practice.

Graeme Catto

Introduction

The current concept of assessment for relicensure has been influenced by many developments that originated in the medical measurement and regulatory communities. The improvement in methods of assessment for undergraduate medical education and clinical postgraduate training led to significant progress at the conceptual and applied levels in the late 20th century (Norman 2002). More recently, insights have included increased focus on assessment in the practice phase of the physician career. For example, follow-up studies have described the lack of impact from many continuing education programs on the practice of medicine (Davis 1998) and showed that physician's self-assessment skills are weak (Davis et al. 2006). In the last decade, new models of assessment in clinical postgraduate medical training have widened the scope of assessment activities to practice-based and system-oriented skills (Leach 2004). Furthermore, frameworks about optimal medical educational activities, often based on expert opinion or on the 'out of clinical context' views of educational theorists, were being increasingly challenged (Norman 1999). An important change in educational thinking was the recognition that the optimal results for learning occurred when the objectives of the assessment plan and the curricular plan match. This shift was accompanied by the need to define the expected level of performance from trainees and students in behavioural terms, and the realization of the advantage of assessing their performance in more authentic clinical settings (van der Vleuten and Schuwirth 2005). In fact, recent discussions have moved this perspective further, and the concept of assessment *for learning* has been discussed and even promoted in a recent consensus statement (Schuwirth et al. 2011). After the concept of content specificity was recognized as an important factor in planning the

assessment of clinical performance (Schmidt et al. 1990), another critical insight emerged in the 1990s. In order for various performing professionals to achieve optimal expertise, repeated and deliberative practice was required (Erricson 2004). These findings were subsequently applied to learning for practising physicians wherein both valid feedback and peer support are required for best results (Sargeant et al. 2008). An associated development was the wider acceptance of the concept of the validity argument approach to the interpretation of the results of assessment instruments (Kane 1992; Clauser et al. 2008, p. 12). The argument approach required three dimensions to be considered when deciding if assessment results had been interpreted validly: evaluation (what was the quality of the performance observed on a test or assessment); generalizability (what was the performance on this test versus other tests of similar content), and extrapolation (what can be inferred for the performance in actual or future practice). The latter perspective was a crucial change in thinking because it addressed whether the interpretation of results are 'verified' in terms of impact on patients' outcomes, the ultimate beneficiary of the physician's practice activities. Hence, validation is about establishing the impact on the patients in respect to both clinical and social outcomes. These developments will serve as the underpinning for this analysis of assessment for relicensure.

What about the licensure side of the issue? Have there been similar insights? The answer is yes but rather than incremental change, the new reality of relicensure and revalidation, particularly in the United Kingdom, has been framed by dramatic political events of the late 1990s and anchored in legislative actions (Department of Health 2008). Specifically, as Smith (1998 p. 917) observed, the comfortable world of self-regulation and licensure was badly shaken by two events. The Royal Bristol Infirmary Inquiry (2001) and the Shipman cases were to 'change all'.

Rebuilding the licensure system: building in better accountability and quality improvement

To better appreciate the significance of the upheaval in the UK, a review of the bases of licensure is needed. The historical evolution of medical licensure was reviewed in detail by Dauphinee (2002, p. 837). This summary outlines that the origins of physician licensure can be traced back to ancient times, but with the development of modern licensure in the 19th century, certain operational and legal features became established. These include the fact that while principles and ethical practices could be proclaimed, it was only with the coming of legal precedents and legislated mandates that licensure became functional by virtue of having its legal responsibilities defined and the limits of its actionable steps against underperforming doctors established. Through new legislation or other existing legal frameworks, an authority can be legally recognized and thereby consider and adjudicate on professional matters. This evolution is reflected in the recent recharging of the mandates of regulatory authorities in the UK. Since the status of profession implies both a contract with society and accountability to society (Irvine 2006), licensure provides the legal framework by which physicians can and are accountable to society for the privilege of practising as a physician.

The manner in which this is accomplished can vary. In western society, self-regulation emerged with the creation of the General Medical Council (GMC) in 1858 (Irvine 2006), and later with the development of state medical acts in the 1870s in the USA (Stevens 1971, p. 32). Specifically, licensure responsibility was assigned to profession-based self-regulatory bodies that were regulated in their scope of jurisdiction and actions by legislation. In turn, the medical regulatory bodies were expected to protect the public and provide guidance and standards for the profession (Irvine 2006). That implies two roles: accountability to the public and guidance for improvement for the profession. By the mid-20th century, these notions of self-regulation and licensure were well established and remained so until the end of that century.

Events of the mid-1990s demonstrated the need for clearer lines of accountability and evidence of good practice performance. While there were serious failures at many institutions, in public health monitoring, and at the GMC, the Bristol Royal Infirmary Inquiry led to major changes in the regulation of health professions. In the case of medicine, they led to the idea of enforcement of quality assurance through relicensure and revalidation, as outlined by the Report of the Chief Medical Officer (Donaldson 2007). Those developmental steps would include the need to create numerous instruments and processes to produce feasible, reliable and valid results on which relicensure and recertification decisions could be made. Underlying the approach was the need for performance assessment for relicensure, and a clear extension of the principle of guidance to the professions.

Will this approach work? In their 2002 review of Relicensure, Recertification and Practice-Based Assessment, Cunnington and Southgate (2002, p. 884) pointed out that the measurement of outcomes through maintenance of competency activities is difficult from administrative, scientific and political points of view. Their concern was based on the persistence of emphasis on the existing approach to continuing medical education and the lack of evidence of significant impact. They identified examples of documenting maintenance of competence activities in real practice settings, but asked if maintenance of competence activities would provide sufficient evidence to justify restriction of licensing privileges? Would it win support with a concerned public as an effective approach to revalidation–relicensure? Given the new legislative actions emerging in the UK and in other jurisdictions internationally, will the new frameworks adequately define and impose accountability terms on the regulators that will eliminate many of the political and jurisdictional concerns of Cunnington and Southgate? If so, is there evidence from the measurement literature to answer their scientific concerns about validity and effectiveness?

Definitions, goals, and inclusion criteria for citation

What is relicensure? Given the current societal context, relicensure is a process by which an individual or public agency renews, reactivates, or reinstates a prior or existing license to either practise a profession or execute a collective societal function, such as operating a hospital or nursing home. For this discussion, relicensure is being defined as the obligatory process of evaluating the professional knowledge, skills, and actions of a physician by a regulatory authority or legally recognized certifying agency. It is assumed that to achieve its intent and to be publically accountable, the full cycle of the relicensure process should be organized so as to be executed in an integrated, deliberative, and recurrent manner, based on an assessment of each physician's practice, in order to make a determination of that physician's suitability to practise.

This chapter will examine the current state of relicensure assessment in the contexts of public accountability and a continuous quality improvement system. It will focus on both the issues and challenges to be addressed, and the actual execution of relicensure and revalidation assessment processes. Finally, the local context of any individual physician's work will be considered in order to validate the process in terms of its contextual applications and thus decision about relicensure.

A review of potential assessment methods must be conducted within an integrated learning and assessment system. Integration of assessment and learning has been one of the assessment lessons of the last two decades. Hence, the chapter will consider assessment tools used within models or frameworks and systems (Bordage 2009). What are the optimal models or frameworks for which evidence exists that the outputs lead to the anticipated outcomes? That question will define the first consideration in selecting articles or sources as illustrative examples for this analysis.

Second, the inclusion criteria for citing possible methods or systems of assessment for this review were current literature published in peer-reviewed journals or grey literature prepared by independent authors, or internally generated documents from regulatory authorities or certifying bodies that, in turn, were approved by the executive board or a legally defined oversight agency. The search of original literature was limited to English, although articles or reviews that summarize or quote existing literature, meeting the same criteria, will be used for languages other than English. In addition, cited articles must demonstrate evidence that the outcome indicators or assessment instruments have achieved reliability, feasibility, discrimination, evidence of long-term validity, and applicability to the physician population under review. All articles considered, whether qualitatively or quantitatively oriented, must include analyses that any effect identified is not due to chance, error, or biased selection of the population sample. The intent is to identify examples of best practice in a rapidly changing field (Dauphinee 2012b).

In considering best practice, there are established standards in high stakes testing that are relevant for relicensure. This is true In North America where high-stakes testing and assessment in medicine and other arenas have been under scrutiny, especially by the courts. The joint American Educational Research Association, American Psychological Association, and National Council on Measurement in Education standards for educational and psychological testing are examples (1999a, b). For relicensure and revalidation, the GMC has set out guiding principles (General Medical Council 2010b). Standards and predefined criteria for best practice must be applied to any practice-based assessment tools being considered.

Consideration of an underlying assumption: the quality improvement cycle

Following revision of regulatory legislation, a second set of developments was needed for more effective relicensure. That was the clarification of the underlying principles and best practices in quality improvement processes as applied to the practicing physician. A basic concept upon which physician relicensure is built is the quality improvement cycle (Berwick 1996). Similarly, within a legislative or regulatory framework, the quality improvement cycle implies an afferent loop of feedback to inform and guide improvement (International Association of Medical Regulatory Authorities 2012). However, quality improvement evidence can also inform any practice improvement programme, through the relicensure assessment programme's feedback loop, even if all relicensure requirements are met. Thus, relicensure offers two potential benefits. One is for the stakeholders and accountability processes whereby it not only helps meet the implied social contract, but also provides valid and reliable feedback to all professions implicated in patient care. Thereby, it enables the practitioner to engage in continuous quality improvement (CQI) for better patient care.

The intent to apply CQI as a model for relicensure requires evidence of its successful application. It is new to relicensure. While long-term outcome studies for revalidation exist (Hawkins and Weiss 2011), aside from the use of total quality management frameworks in the information technology industry and in International Organization for Standardization ISO 9000 (Tari 2005), what has been CQI's impact in healthcare quality? Chassin and Loeb (2011) at the Joint Commission in the USA reviewed the 50-year history and the current status of on-going quality improvement. Disregarding short-term quality improvement, such as hand-washing, they concluded that systematic and sustained quality improvement has been a much more difficult journey. As more agencies move forward in relicensure as a CQI process, it is imperative to learn from their ongoing experiences. This analysis will describe the road that is being taken along with the steps and milestones, but will reserve the final conclusion of success to the point at which

relicensure produces evidence of impacts that are sustained and documented.

Progress in performance assessment in medicine

The first decade of the 21st century has been associated with a major interest on what has become known as workplace-based assessment (WPBA). The key notion behind WPBA is the direct observation of physicians in realistic settings (Norcini, 2005). Much of this development has taken place around postgraduate training assessment procedures. Good examples are the development of the mini-clinical exercise (mini-CEX) (Norcini et al. 2003) and the multisource peer assessment tool (mini-PAT) (Archer et al. 2008). These are isolated sets of observations made in the context of a candidate demonstrating a clinical skill during an 'out of context' period of observation or in quasi-testing situations. Developments in the field of recertification of specialists in the USA under the sponsorship of the member boards of the American Board of Medical Specialties, have contributed many examples of empirical work that attempt to assess performance more closely to what the physician does every day in medical practice. Other counties have now developed similar maintenance of performance programs, but in some cases it has been through the specialty boards (the USA) or specialty colleges (the UK, Canada, and Australasia) and in some cases through medical regulatory authorities, as in Canada or Australia (Dauphinee 2012b).

Recent progress in programme assessment has emphasized long-term or predictive validity, and the need to assess clinical performance against the outcomes of care. The key concept is the distinction between patient outcomes and clinical outputs or clinical activities of the physician (Dauphinee 2012a). The most popular and well-documented framework for approaching the impact of any activity is the Logic Model (Kellogg Foundation 2004). It is based on the model of assessing impacts over time as well as outcomes, versus assessing activities or processes or outputs. In this model inputs lead to activities; which lead to outputs; which lead to outcomes; which lead to impacts (Dauphinee 2012a).

The critical notions for using the logic model are that inputs and activities are planned actions or work, and that outputs through to impacts are the intended results over time with the measurement of impact addressing the ultimate goal. Using a clinical example, the inputs might be investments in physician training. Physician activities might be undertaking courses and creating a new practice activity (e.g. a new protocol) for postmyocardial infarction. Outputs might be improved by prescribing a hypertension treatment. Initial outcomes might be documenting if patients are following the protocol with follow-up of prescription use. An intermediate outcome might be improved blood pressure control. Long-term outcomes or impacts might be sustained blood pressure control and return to normal activities. This approach is becoming increasingly used and recommended (Perrin 2006). Further, it offers an important measure of validity for any assessment process by asking if the practice processes (inputs and activities and outputs), as planned work in practice, have led to the attainment of intended outcomes and impacts over time. These links illustrate an important concept—the need for evidence of impact(s)—as we begin an analysis of assessment methods in relicensure.

Similarly, the logic model offers a sequence of steps that are necessary to ensure that the issue of validity of an assessment programme or instrument is addressed. The validity of any interpretation of the assessment results, must be carried out with a view to three possible perspectives: was the process properly executed; to whom is the result generalizable; to whom can the result be extrapolated (Kane 1992, Clauser et al. 2008) These same questions must be asked of any assessment process or instrument that is to be used in relicensure processes: was it done properly; to which population of physicians is the result to be applied; and is the result extractable to the future intended use? In short, is the panel's interpretation of the results of a relicensure assessment appropriate and suitable in anticipating each physician's future performance?

Before delving into the analyses of assessment for relicensure, a brief reference should be made on the current state of assessment from two perspectives: recent research and criteria for good assessment. Two recent consensus statements from the 2010 Ottawa Conference have dealt with these matters and offer insights into the current foci of assessment research (Schuwirth et al. 2011) and the criteria for good assessment (Norcini et al. 2011). Additionally, readers are referred to other chapters on specific aspects of assessment for more detailed discussion of current practice.

Establishing the bases of the relicensure assessment process

For every undertaking there needs to be a vision and a mission before goals and strategies are defined. Building on the UK experience of the last 15 years, the relicensure vision can be easily identified. At the height of the Royal Bristol Infirmary Inquiry, under the leadership of Sir Donald Irvine (2006), the GMC issued its first guide for *Good Medical Practice*. It was a critically important development as it offered a framework for good practice and established the first descriptions of what good quality practice should entail. *Good Medical Practice* was a pathway with clear signposts that characterized and enunciated behaviours which could serve as points of reference as well as floors of expected performance. Revisions have expanded on these themes and on the criteria of good practice (General Medical Council 2012a). *Good Medical Practice* is the starting point. Later, the publication of the Chief Medical Officer's paper further refined the process and its expected impacts (Donaldson 2007). The ensuing Health and Social Care Act 2008 (Department of Health 2008) built on the Chief Medical Officer's Report by defining the mission, goals and scope of *Good Medical Practice* in law. The act also defined the limitations and scope of the various agencies' and authorities' responsibilities in the processes. It defined the new legal bases of licensure, relicensure, and revalidation. Society had re-established its contract with the profession in the UK.

For this discussion, the examples of models or systems of assessment for relicensure must be operational or in the course of being evaluated. There are many variations on the model of maintenance of competence or revalidation that assess hours or courses of continuing medical education or lifelong learning programs (Merkur et al. 2008). These typically do not involve a formal and direct measure of performance and will not be considered in this review. This review focuses on practice-based frameworks or systems for relicensure. Further, in keeping with the assumption that the basic framework is the quality improvement cycle (Berwick 1989); the relicensure model must include or have identified the means for peer-support or mentoring to assist the physician during or after the process (Archer 2010). Given these criteria, the search for potential model systems will be limited to the GMC model and the framework used by member boards of the American Board of Medical Specialists (ABMS). In some cases, elements of the cited examples exist in regions within the Netherlands, Canada, and Australasia.

Existing or evolving practice-based frameworks for relicensure assessment

While the longest evolution of assessment for revalidation and recertification has taken place in the USA, recent developments in the UK offer an appropriate blueprint for a system; even though it is still evolving and undergoing validity studies (General Medical Council 2011b, Royal College of Surgeons of England 2010). How do the basic elements of ABMS and UK approaches compare?

First, the UK system has a clearly defined governance structure that oversees the assessment processes for both the general relicensure and recertification standards across an integrated system for England, Wales, Scotland, and Northern Ireland (General Medical Council 2012b). The GMC, to which the UK Revalidation Programme Board reports, sits at the top. Each of the regions has a Revalidation Delivery Board. The UK Revalidation Delivery Board and the UK Communications Board ensure continuity and common communications processes. Second, the actual application of the assessment processes is being built on *Good Medical Practice*. The legislated requirements, the planning documents, the implementation steps, and the pathfinder pilots of all processes and assessment tools are impressive and readily available on-line for outsiders. The intraprofessional communication, through the various support services of the many partners like the GMC, the royal colleges, the NHS and the Department of Health suggest that previously determined best practices in implementation are being followed (General Medical Council 2012b). The GMC revalidation programme plan has four phases: developmental, implementation, roll-out and long term delivery, revision and on-going management (General Medical Council 2012a, b).

From the doctor's point of view, the basic structural and functional model under national legislation has two limbs: a re-licensure limb and a recertification limb. The initial basic processes involve gathering and accumulating the supporting information which then must be appraised and, for which a 'responsible officer', is named to handle the file (Department of Health 2009). For the relicensure limb, the GMC is the authority under which the review proceeds and the recommendations are made. In the case of a Royal College or a Specialty Faculty, each must offer a specialty specific enquiry within which the process is conducted. The model includes identifying the 'responsible officer' (Department of Health 2009). In this case the decision panel reports back to the appointed responsible officer after the assessment is completed and a decision is made. Several features are to be noted: the process is obligatory and follows a cycle of assessment and feedback with a peer appointed to oversee the process. Further, there is an integration and thus accompanying peer-support system via appraisal and clinical governance with institutions, the NHS regions and the Academy of Royal Medical Colleges that can offer support (Shaw et al. 2007). While the UK model is following a plan that uses current best practices, it is a work in progress, and progress must be assessed in terms of outcomes and impact on the public. It must be empirically informed and guided. This cascade of pilots and revisions follows the principles of CQI. The framework is well described in the GMC's guidelines (General Medical Council 2010a).

The four domains that are the foundation for relicensure assessment in the UK include attributes that flow from *Good Medical Practice* (General Medical Council 2011). They frame the basic scope of performance to be deconstructed and reconstructed as indicators or measures of basic performance attributes that validly and reliably assess those domains of each practitioner's practice situation. They are:

* Domain 1: knowledge, skills and performance
* Domain 2: safety and quality
* Domain 3: communication, partnership and team work
* Domain 4: maintaining trust.

Thus the scope of the development programme needed to create measures and indicators of practitioner performance for each domain of the relicensure and revalidation approach in the UK has been a huge undertaking. Fortunately, there have also been significant insights from recertification work over the decades in the Specialty Boards in the USA (Dauphinee 1999) and for the Maintenance of Competence of the American Board of Medical Specialists (2009). The ABMS's approach is not required of all certificate holders and it is exclusive to the specialty side of the accountability framework. All specialists who were certified before 1990 are exempted (Levinson et al. 2010). All subsequent certificate holders are required to undergo recertification. As expected, the uptake of recertification by the so called grand-parented specialists is low (Levinson and Holmboe 2011). Governance-wise, the ABMS sets the rules for Board membership that includes the basic model of requirements for recertification, but each Board can implement its programme within the requirements. Compliance by Boards is reported through the ABMS but is less regulated than in the UK system. Regarding relicensure, it should be noted that studies were conducted by the Federation of State Medical Boards on the need for relicensure processes in the USA (Federation of State Medical Boards 2010). These would have had to be carried out at the state level as basic licensure is a state function. Based on that report, relicensure, as a first step in the licensing accountability process in the USA, has been accepted in principle and a final decision has been made to proceed (Federation of State Medical Boards 2011). It too will need to be developed in an iterative, empirically based manner, but work in recertification certainly will be of benefit and integrated into state relicensure programmes.

What are some key issues and developments in the ABMS recertification system that could assist planners and evaluators on the assessment side of relicensure? Of particular interest for the GMC is graduate clinical training linkage. The American Accreditation Council for Graduate Medical Education (ACGME) has also developed standards for assessing competency that are entirely complementary to ABMS framework (Leach 2004). Holmboe (2008) offers an example of an integrated ABMS and ACGME competency framework that addresses the six competencies:

* systems-based practice
* practice-based learning and improvement
* patient care

* medical knowledge
* professionalism
* interpersonal and communication skills.

Clearly, within the ACGME framework, tools or techniques exist at the ABIM that overlap in their potential contributions to assess these competencies for clinical trainees (Holmboe 2008).

* medical record and quality improvement projects
* evidence-based practice logs or outcome data
* assessment of medical knowledge
* multisource feedback, including professional behaviours
* clinical simulations, including procedures.

As can be seen, to meet the target competencies to meet the ABMS recertification categories, just as the GMC model requires the deconstruction of its basic domain attributes, a Board must deconstruct the broad competencies into assessment elements and reconstruct a set of assessment tools within which the Maintenance of Competence programme will operate. The tools cited by Holmboe can be adapted for practitioners. Consider the ABMS framework. There are four broad-based components (American Board of Medical Specialties 2009), for which instruments must be developed and assessed. The categories are:

* Part 1: Evidence of professionalism or by professional standing from a licensing authority or confirmation of institutional standing.
* Part 2: Evidence of life-long learning and self-assessment on approved courses or modules.
* Part 3: Cognitive assessment by specialty designed on-line or open book examination.
* Part 4: Evaluation of performance in practice by specialty approved practice improvement programmes or modules, or by participation in approved external practice improvement programmes and/or case log improvement programmes.

From an evaluative point of view, Parts 3 and 4 require assessment tools, as opposed to documentation and a peer-based binary check-off of 'met or not met' against preset standards for Parts 1 and 2. Part 2 includes preset standards for continuous professional development (CPD) courses similar to the UK approach (Academy of Medical Royal Colleges 2012). Part 3 and methods of cognitive assessment will be considered later. For Part 4, two broad categories of well-studied assessment tools exist for evaluating performance for relicensure. They are individual self-administered practice-based improvement tools (PBITs), such as the American Board of Internal Medicine's Practice Improvement Modules (Duffy et al. 2008), and specialty-based practice assessment programmes (SPAPs) (American Board of Surgery 2012). While PBITs can be carried out on an individual practice by an individual physician, the SPAPs are databases with standards that can be populated, for example, with case or procedural data from a surgeon's files using a standardized grid by clinical disorder or procedure. Comparison performance scores are generated. Their common features are: an on-line programme or specialty based programme that has been standardized and validated is available by disease or practice activities; using these programmes, the physician or surgeon inserts actual data and results against which a judgement is made based on specified outcomes or indicators by peers or against specified standards; and then a practice improvement plan is generated. In turn, these results are submitted to the certifying body review by peers. From these assessments, an intervention plan is developed that could be remedial for skills based issues or quality improvement based on outcomes and indicators.

Five of the AMBS specialties illustrate the various approaches to the Part 4 requirements: the American Board of Family Medicine (2008 and Bazemore et al, 2010); the American Board of Internal Medicine (2012a, b); the American Board of Surgery (2012), American Board of Pediatrics (Miles 2009); and the American Board of Emergency Medicine (2012). Some Boards have numerous subspecialties under their programmes. While many of the PBIT or modules are disease or procedurally oriented, there are modules that focus on team care or communication capabilities (American Board of Internal Medicine 2012b), information science management or cultural competencies (American Board of Family Medicine 2009). However, it is to be appreciated that recertification is specialty based in the USA, as application of revalidation at the basic licensure level is still evolving.

Other international frameworks in evolution

On the international scene, there are specific points of development. None are as close to an integrated, systematic, national approach as the American or UK ones. Developments in Canada have not moved as quickly as one might have expected given that they were the creators of the Enhancement Model which incorporates the integrated concept of monitoring to enhance performance (Dauphinee 1999). Follow-up studies on the previously established multisource feedback in Alberta (Violato et al. 2008) on the random office visits in Ontario (Norton et al. 2004) and on the impact of remediation for under-performing doctors in Quebec (Goulet et al. 2007) are encouraging and are guiding the iterative development of integrated systems. In fact, some Canadian leaders in the quality area have chided their colleagues for resting on their laurels and failing to verify impact with follow-up evidence (Levinson 2008). With a decentralized provincial distribution of the legal responsibility for health, Canada has not been able to promote concerted action independent of its national associations' focus on maintenance of competence and their 'outputs' of declarations of intent to change. Australia has been fraught with quality issues (Burton 2005) and the responsibility for revalidation at the specialty level is even more divided than Canada (Newble et al. 1999), but that may be changing. The federal government's move to creating a national physician registry with common credentialing assessment standards may be evidence of shifts to come (Medical Board of Australia 2012).

Consider the evidence level: moving closer to the reality of actual practice

What possible tools are available and how does one decide which to use? One issue is the level of demonstrated performance—from the 'ability to perform', to 'can perform', to 'what is actually done' in reality (Miller 1990). In addition, the instrument developer must consider the levels of evidence for any change, such as Kirkpatrick's four levels (Dauphinee, 2012a), wherein the definitions of levels of evidence range from a practitioner 'considering change' to the actual implementation of change and measuring its outcomes. Thus the evaluation of a revalidation programme's impact must include measures of follow-up and assessment of performance that move beyond the intention to improve to assessing the actual implementation of change and documenting the outcomes and long-term impact.

Returning to the WPBA framework can its tools be considered for use in relicensure? As Norcini and Burch (2007) have summarized, WPBAs are primarily intended for formative assessments in clinical training, or perhaps in diagnostic settings for candidates who have been found to clinically underperform. Crossly and Jolly (2012) have noted the need for careful analyses of results around WPBA scores and scoring keys in any summative assessment. They have also captured a major validity principle within their title, 'Making sense of worked based assessment: ask the right question, in the right way, about the right thing of the right people'.

In summary, instruments that are being considered within any framework must be evaluated for each application in which they are used (Streiner and Norman 2009, p. 9). Interestingly, because relicensure assessments may not be designed to capture the basis of performance shortcomings, the WPBA processes may be well suited for formative assessment or other diagnostic activities amongst under-performers. The following WPBA tools are listed as possible options that have been proven acceptable, feasible, reliable and valid in certain formative settings (Norcini and Burch 2007).

◆ mini-clinical examination exercise (Mini-CEX)

◆ case-based discussions

◆ procedure-based assessments or direct observation of procedural skills (DOPS)

◆ clinical encounter cards

◆ clinical work sampling

◆ blinded patient encounters.

Examples of measurement instruments for practice-based performance

As noted, the ABMS model represents the deconstruction of competencies into levels of performance and then developing measures that reflect what various specialists do in practice. Bearing in mind the various GMC domains needed for revalidation and relicensure, the reconstruction of the domains by the royal colleges and the GMC must cover all four domains using practice-based instruments or indicators of practitioner performance. One principle in the UK is that the GMC system is to be based on local appraisals from each practitioner's workplace. The second principle is that each practitioner must demonstrate that they are up-to-date and fit to practise. Fit to practise in the UK refers to all aspects whereas fit to practise in the North American context often refers to physical and mental wellbeing. The basic expectations are that each practitioner will meet the values as defined by *Good Medical Practice* (General Medical Council 2011a) in an on-going manner, using the following processes.

◆ Maintain a portfolio of supporting information directly derived from the practice which must address the principles of good medical practice.

◆ Have an annual appraisal conducted on the portfolio.

◆ Appoint a Responsible Officer to ensure that all these steps are taken and that the appraisal is carried out as per the guidelines.

◆ Obtain information from the institutional clinical governance system where the practitioner works.

◆ Gather recommendations from the Responsible Officer for the GMC—usually every 5 years.

In turn, six types of supporting information must be documented (General Medical Council 2010c):

◆ CPD (e.g. Academy of Medical Colleges, 2012)

◆ quality improvement activities

◆ significant clinical events

◆ feedback from colleagues

◆ feedback from patients (where applicable)

◆ complaints and compliments.

The standards and evidence needed to support these requirements, including feedback tools, are being or have been piloted and studied by the Academy of Royal Colleges. The following bodies offer examples that illustrate the approach as well as expected supporting information.

1. Royal College of Physicians, London (2009a and 2009b)

2. Royal College of Surgeons of England (2010 and 2011)

3. Royal College of General Practitioners (2011)

4. Faculty of Occupational Medicine (2011).

These cited programmes require a considerable degree of infrastructure to support their execution and that will permit reliable, fair and valid results. For regulators or institutions with limited resources but who wish to offer revalidation programmes, there are alternatives, but care must be taken to consider feasibility and acceptability as well as the needed measurement properties in order to obtain valid results and ultimate impacts.

Use of examinations in assessment for relicensure

In 2000, the ABMS moved to require an assessment of cognitive aspects of practice as one pillar in its recertification programme. The elements needed for an assessment of cognitive and problem-solving aspects of practice are similar to any other assessment of knowledge or cognitive functions. Fundamentally, the basic written methods remain: every question should begin with an introductory stimulus (i.e. a clinical scenario), which requires a constructed response (e.g. short answer questions); or selected response in either true–false format or best answer format (e.g. multiple choice questions); or a hybrid format of case clusters to assess on-going clinical decision-making (e.g. key features) (Hawkins and Swanson 2008, p. 43). Such formats can be delivered on-line if the number of candidates makes it fiscally feasible. Newer technical approaches can both shorten testing time and improve test comparability via adaptive testing and multistage testing methods, but require significant technical support. Then there are the questions of whether to score by the case or by item and how best to set passing standards (Norcini and Guille 2002, p. 811).

Much of the developmental work in high-stakes certification and recertification examinations was carried out in the USA where the numbers of takers are of a magnitude that is sixfold greater than the UK or 10–12-fold greater than Canada and Australasia, respectively.

This has three consequences: loss of costing scalability; specific issues with reliability as the size of cohorts of takers decreases; and significant problems with tiny subspecialties around reliability and standard setting (General Medical Council 2010d). These are all manageable, but precautionary steps should be exercised. Smaller bodies could consider the sharing of item banks and staff overhead, or subcontracting for materials with other bodies. Then the challenges are content and context issues, as illness patterns and support systems vary between countries. Further, within any testing format, use of written assessments raises other considerations. Do the examinations need to be proctored? Can they be delivered on-site to the candidate? How is content adjusted for practice setting? And what about subspecialists; do they take the core examination? If examinations are contemplated, the valid sampling of the practice knowledge and cognitive domains is a critical issue for each discipline. On the positive side, there is evidence that if carefully constructed, recertification examinations are predictive of practice performance (Tamblyn et al. 1998, Holmboe et al. 2008).

Specific challenges in relicensure assessment

Critical importance of scoring for relicensure purposes

In considering the use of any tool, either new or used elsewhere, the issue of valid and effective scoring elements is a primary concern. There are two issues to be considered. First, how is the score to be used? The tool or test must be evaluated to assure that both the clinical content and clinical context are linked to the intended area of concern and that the performance measures are direct measures of the expected attributes. Even so, the scoring key and rubric (guidelines for the scorers) for clinical observations must be as explicit as possible so that misclassifications by scorers are minimized (Baldwin et al. 2009). Second, to ensure that the scoring measures of any practice appraisal are validated in every use, the developers have clear responsibilities. The scoring format should have been nurtured with target groups and refined iteratively and assessed in real circumstances. The scoring results should then have been reviewed in light of that interpretative framework. To ensure content and context validity, the cases or processes used need to have been reviewed and have included direct measures of performance or behavior, as is realistically possible. Have the scoring keys functioned well in all expected settings? Explanations of required standards are provided in the AERA-APA-NCME standards (1999a, p. 54). While sampling of domains is an issue in the traditional summative examinations, the GMC and ABMS approaches do offer alternatives to sample practice activities fairly.

Making and defending decisions

Chapter 36 deals with standard setting. Typically, in medical education, standard setting deals with medical student and postgraduate trainee promotion decisions and is particularly important in high-stakes exit examinations such as medical school finals or licensing examinations. In assessment for relicensure, which should be thought about as either an appraisal or promotion decision, the same principles apply but there is an added responsibility. The 'to promote' or 'not to promote' decision, has two aspects: how to make the decision and how to validate the interpretation of the assessment results. But what if there should be four separate assessment components? How should the four component scores be combined into a single score? Is weighting of components needed? These issues have been considered elsewhere and examples of best practice recommendations exist (Norcini and Guille 2002, p. 829). Whatever is decided about how the decision process is to be executed, best practice should be followed with experienced psychometric advice. The main point is that there must be a documented approach approved in advance, with clear descriptions of what components are to be considered, how they are to be weighted, or not weighted, and how the component scores are to be assembled and the total score calculated. Only then does the final decision-making panel set the standard for a successful performance. To repeat, the processes must be established in advance, clearly state how the panel proceeded, be readily available for the candidates, and followed by the decision-making panel. The decisions arising from any assessment must be recorded, including discussion of all unusual circumstances or unexpected influences that occur during the administration of the assessment processes. These points must be included in the record for the committee or panel.

A second issue in making the final decision for a successful or unsuccessful performance in a relicensure assessment is the interpretation placed on the scores and observations of performance. In relicensure, the use of Kane's validity argument approach to interpretation of final scores is recommended (Clauser et al. 2008, p. 12). There are three reasons why. One relates to careful evaluation of the appraisal process and resulting scores. The second is a key step in relicensure as it deals with the generalization that is being made from the doctor's score(s) in relation to the content and context of the assessment tools versus that doctor's practice make-up and location. Do they match? Third, the nature of relicensure means extrapolating to the physician's future performance based on the present score. Is there evidence to support the committee's interpretation into the future? The principle to be followed is that there has been an explicit discussion of each failure so that the committee's interpretation of the score is clear and justified.

Measurement issues of particular concern in relicensure assessment:

There are basic issues which an assessment system must consider when using measurement tools for relicensure. This review is not a 'how to do it' document, but certain issues must be explicitly considered in the design. They can be tracked with a check-off list by the administrative staff to ensure that they are considered in the design and piloting studies. They are shown in fig. 44.1.

- ◆ Establishing scoring validity
- ◆ Deciding when to use holistic ratings versus check-off scoring for disease or procedure based measures (Pangaro and Holmboe 2007, p. 28)
- ◆ Considering attribution confounders hidden within scores due to institutional and team activities versus the candidate's activities.
- ◆ Considering options for future sequenced assessments and 'drilling down' for feedback on underperformers

Figure 44.1 Measurement issues of particular concern.

Due process

Due process is now widely accepted when making high-stakes decisions such as who qualifies or who gets promoted. The principle must be followed to avoid challenges and successful appeals. The basic principle is that the person under review has the right to the last word before any negative decision is made. That means that the candidate must be informed that, based on the information available, the panel is tending toward a negative decision. The candidate, who should have full access to all information under review, can speak last and offer their views of the situation in terms of how it might impact on the final decision. Readers are referred to (Taylor et al 1995; O'Brien 1986).

Delivering the results

How should the final results be delivered to the candidate? For students and trainees, this is usually predetermined by local custom or by national processes, as in national licensing examinations. In the relicensure situation, it is an exit assessment but also a formative assessment due to the quality improvement loop. The insertion of a responsible officer in the UK system is crucial during the assembling of the data and submission. Even assuming that most physicians will be relicensed, there will likely be key points of feedback on specific deficits or emerging practice guidelines that are identified as potential benefit to their patients. Such findings must be organized and sufficiently clear that the physician is able to act on them—preferably with a knowledgeable and qualified peer. The form and clarity of this feedback are crucial. Thus, the use of global scores must be accompanied by breakdown results that match the assessment blueprint (Newble et al. 1994).

Risks

Challenges and appeals

The possibility of an appeal is always a risk. There are four principles that can minimize or prevent appeals and unnecessary challenges are outlined in fig. 44.2.

Notions of evidence and nature of proof required

The body of law under which most quasi-organizations (such as regulatory authorities) operate is often known as administrative law. The two basic principles of administrative law are 'hear the other side', as in due process or natural justice, and 'no person can judge a case in which he or she is a party or has an interest' (Duhaime 2012). These basic rules are then supplemented by each authority's own rules and regulations. Other legal precedents from prior decisions may apply

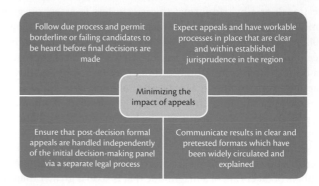

Figure 44.2 Minimizing the impact of appeals.

and form distinct bodies of law within administrative law, depending on the jurisdiction. However, the UK situation raises a specific set of legal issues. There are clinical issues that can be raised in a physician's relicensure hearing wherein licensure could be denied, but findings could be used against the same physician in other legal proceedings. This is the issue of discoverability of evidence. For example, does the Health and Social Care Act (2008) or other GMC legislation specifically protect both the process and the assessors from being involved in further legal actions? The outside world of law must be anticipated and managed as possible risks for the sake of the organization, its assessors, and the physicians under review.

Four questions should be considered by any authority developing and executing a relicensure, revalidation or recertification process, based on jurisdictional law and the legislative mandate for the acting authority. These questions are outlined in fig. 44.3. All procedures must be aligned with the local law.

Where are we, what is missing, and where are we going next?

Assessment in the context of relicensure is a massive undertaking for not only the profession, but for the whole health and medical enterprise. Healthcare in an era of international travel, of ageing populations, of increasing prevalence of chronic illness, and of advanced and expensive interventions is under public scrutiny and concern over sustainability (Dauphinee 2012a). The consideration

---

1. Is any evidence arising from relicensure assessments discoverable in other legal proceedings?

2. To deny relicensure, what are the legislatively defined mandates and what are the limitations on the authority in executing the relicensure process?

3. For each jurisdiction and each authority, what is the quality of evidentiary proof required for denial of licensure?

4. If the quality of evidence and proof needed is different, does it limit the interpretation of findings should the assessors' staff be subpoenaed elsewhere?

Figure 44.3 Four legal questions to be considered by any authority developing a relicensure process.

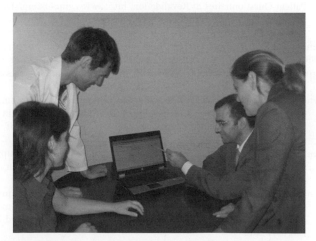

Figure 44.4 Future steps—integrating real-time prescribing information with physician continuous quality improvement, relicensure and system improvement research.

---

of assessment for relicensure fits into the broader context of societal accountability and society's concern over economic sustainability. While there are prior events leading to a legislated and centralized programme of processes for the closer scrutiny of the professions within the health field, it must be recognized that wherever revalidation is taking place, the technical and psychometric infrastructures that are being assembled are often new or untried in certain situations. The intent is to derive evidence and inform the quality improvement cycle. It must be recognized that relicensure has the potential to improve outcomes and impacts. The keyword is 'potential'. Thus all procedures must be formulated within the framework of measurably improved outcomes, impacts and safety by reducing errors and omissions in performance.

Whatever the ultimate outcome of these dramatic changes, revisions and new tools will emerge. The nature of the quality improvement process, and of the potential lessons from outcomes and impacts research, as well as legal challenges, will hopefully improve the processes. However, there is another implication. The application of clinical effectiveness and quality assurance and improvement at the institutional level will complement and maybe even subsume aspects of relicensure in time. Institutional accrediting bodies like the Joint Commission in the USA and the NHS and GMC leadership are aware of these joint opportunities and will be ready to embrace unforeseen opportunities for better quality and improved patient safety. Assessing for individual relicensure and/or recertification is only the beginning. Accountability, in the name of effective and sustainable care will require evidence of effectiveness at the institutional and the individual levels (fig. 44.4).

Conclusions

- The validity of all high-stakes assessments, like relicensure, must be established with each use and in each setting. Validity does not lie in the test, but in each use and its interpretation.

- The notion of licensure provides the legal framework by which physicians are accountable to society for the privilege of practising as a physician

- The form and clarity of this feedback are crucial. Thus, the use of global scores must be accompanied by breakdown results that match the assessment blueprint.

- In keeping with the assumption that the basic framework is the quality improvement cycle, the relicensure model must include or have identified the means for peer-support or mentoring to assist the physician during or after the process.

- Be clear about due process or natural justice. The basic principle is that the person under review has the right to the last word before any negative decision is made.

References

Academy of Medical Royal Colleges (2012) Standards and Criteria for CPD Activities. A Framework for Accreditation. January 2012. http://www.aomrc.org.uk. Accessed 27 February 2012

American Board of Emergency Medicine (2012) Maintenance of Certification—Part IV—Performance in Practice. http://theabem.org/moc/part4.aspx. Accessed 13 February 2012

American Board of Family Medicine (2009) Cultural Competency Method in Medicine Module (MIMM). http://www.theabfm.org/news/2009/ccmimm.aspx. Accessed 13 February 2012

American Board of Internal Medicine (2012a) MOC Part 4 Requirements. http://abim.org/MOC/part4.apsx. Accessed 29 January 2012

American Board of Internal Medicine (2012b) Communication—Primary Care Practice Improvement Module (PIM). http://wwwabim.org/moc/earning-points/productinfo-demo-ordering.aspx.communication-primary-care#60. A. Accessed 13 February 2012

American Board of Medical Specialties (2009) Standards for ABMS MOC© (Parts 1–4) Program. http://www.abms.org/News_and_Events/Media_Newsroom.pdf/Standards_for_ABMS_MOC_Approved_3_16_09.pdf Accessed 22 February 2012

American Board of Surgery (2012) Examination and MOC requirements. http://www.absurgery.org/default.jsp?exam_mocreqs Accessed 27 March 2013

American Educational Research Association-American Psychological Association-National Council on Measurement in Education (1999a) Chapter 4. Scales, Norms and Score Compatibility and Chapter 5. Test Administration, Scoring and Reporting. In: *The Standards for Educational and Psychological and Testing*. Washington, DC: AERA Publications, pp. 49–66

American Educational Research Association-American Psychological Association-National Council on Measurement in Education (1999b) Chapter 12. Psychological Testing and Assessment. In: *The Standards for Educational and Psychological and Testing*. Washington, DC: AERA Publications, pp. 119–134

Archer J., Norcini J., Southgate L., Heard S., and Davies H. (2008) mini-PAT (Peer Assessment Tool): A Valid Component of a National Assessment Programme in the UK? *Adv Health Sci Educ*. 13: 191–192

Archer, J.C. (2010) State of science in health profession education: effective feedback. *Med Educ*. 44: 101–108

Baldwin, S.G., Harik, P., Keller, L.A., Clauser, B.E., Baldwin, P., and Rebbecchi, T.A. (2009) Assessing the impact of modification to the documentation component's scoring rubric and rater training on USMLE integrated clinical encounter scores. *Acad Med*. 84(10): S97–S100

Bazemore, A.W., Xierali, I.M., Petterson, S.M., et al. (2010) American Board of Family Medicine (ABFM) Maintenance of certification: Variation in the Self-Assessment Modules within the 2006 Cohort. *J Am Board Fam Med*. 23(1): 49–58

Berwick, D. (1996) Primer on leading improvement systems. *BMJ*. 312: 619–622

Berwick, D.M. (1989) Continuous improvement as an ideal in health care. *N Engl JMed*. 320: 53–56

Bordage, G. (2009) Conceptual frameworks to illuminate and magnify. *Med Educ*. 43: 312–319

Burton, B. (2005) Queensland report on deaths recommends sweeping changes. *BMJ*. 331: 70

Catto, G. (2005) GMC and the future of revalidation: Building on the GMC's achievements. *BMJ*. 330: 1205

Chassin M.R. and Loeb, J.M. (2011) The ongoing quality improvement journey: next stop, high reliability. *Health Affairs*. 30(4): 559–568

Clauser, B.E., Margolis, M.J., and Swanson, D.B. (2008) Issues in validity and reliability for assessments in medical education. In: E.S. Holmboe and R.E, Hawkins (eds) *Practical Guide to the Evaluation of Clinical Competence* (pp. 10–23). Philadelphia, PA: Mosby, Elsevier.

Crossly, J. and Jolly, B. (2012) Making sense of work-based assessment: ask the right questions, in the right way, about the right things, of the right people. *Med Educ*. 46: 28–37

Cunnington, J. and Southgate, L. (2002) Relicensure, recertification and practiced–based assessment. In: G. Norman, C. Van der Vleuten, and D. Newble (eds) *International Handbook of Research in Medical Education* (pp. 883–912). Editors, D. Dordrecht: Kluwer Academic Publishers

Dauphinee, W.D. (1999) Revalidation of doctors in Canada. *BMJ*. 319: 1183–1190

Dauphinee, W.D. (2002) Licensure and certification. In: G. Norman, C. Van der Vleuten, and D. Newble (eds) *International Handbook of Research in Medical Education*(pp. 837–843). Dordrecht: Kluwer Academic Publishers

Dauphinee W.D. (2012a) Educators must consider patient outcomes when assessing the impact of clinical training. *Med Educ*. 46: 13–20

Dauphinee, W.D. (2012b). Best practices and lessons learned in the recertification and revalidation of physicians. An international view. In: W. McGaghie (ed.) *Best Practices in Medical Education*. Abingdon: Radcliffe Publishing, Ltd, in press

Davis, D.A. (1998) Does CME work? An analysis of the effect of educational activities on physician performance or health care outcomes. *Int J Psychiatry Med*. 28: 21–39

Davis, D.A., Mazmanian, P.E., Fortis, M., Harrison, R.V., Thorpe, K.E., and Perrier L. (2006) Accuracy of Physician Self-assessment compared with observed measures of competence. A systematic review. *JAMA*. 296(9): 1094–1102

Department of Health (2008) Health and Social Care Act 2008. Chapter 14. London: Department of Health. http://www.legislation.gov.uk/ukpga/2008/14/contents Accessed 27 March 2013

Department of Health (2009) The framework for responsible officers and their duties relating to the medical profession. http://webarchive.nationalarchives.gov.uk/+/www.dh.gov.uk/en/Consultations/Closedconsultations/DH_104587 Accessed 27 March 2013

Donaldson, L. (2007) Medical revalidation—principles and next steps. Response of the Chief Medical Officer for England's Working Group. First published: 21 July 2008. http://www.dh.gov.uk/prod_consum<dh_digitalassets/@dh@en/documwnts/digitaassewt/dh_086431_pdf

Duffy, F.D., Lynn, L., Didura, H., et al. (2008) Self-assessment of practice performance: development of the ABIM Practice Improvement Modules (PIM™). *J Cont EducHealth Prof*. 28(1): 38–46

Duhaime's Legal Dictionary (2012) Administrative Law Definition. http://www.duhaime.org/LegalDictionary/AdministrativeLaw.aspx Accessed 10 February 2012

Erricson, K.A. (2004) Deliberate practice and the acquisition and maintenance of expert performance in Medicine and related fields. *Acad Med*. 10: S1–S12

Faculty of Occupational Medicine (2011) CPD and revalidation. Latest updates. http://www.facoccmed.ac.uk/cpd/reval.jsp Accessed 27 February 2012

Federation of State Medical Boards (2010) Report of the Board of Directors. Maintenance of Licensure. http://fsmb.org/pdf/mol-board-report-1003.pdf Accessed 27 March 2013

Federation of State Medical Boards (2011) Report to the Board of Directors. Report of the Maintenance of Licensure Implementation Group. http://wwwfsmb.org/pdf/mol_impact_analysis_reoprt.pdf Accessed 24 March 2013

General Medical Council (2010a) Revalidation: the way ahead. Annex 2—Specialties and General Practice Frameworks. London: GMC

General Medical Council (2010b) Revalidation. The way ahead. Annex 3: GMC Principles, Criteria and Key Indicators for Colleague and Patient Questionnaires in Revalidation. http://www.gmc-uk.org/static/documents/content/Revalidation_way_ahead_annex3.pdf Accessed 13 February 2012

General Medical Council (2010c) Supporting information for appraisal and revalidation. http://www.gmc-uk/static/documents/content/supporting_information_for_appraisal_and_revaliadtion.pdf. Accessed 24 March 2013

General Medical Council (2010d) Reliability issues in the assessment of small cohorts. Supplementary Guidance. http://www.gmc-uk.org?reliability_issues_in_the_assessment_of_small_cohorts_0410.pdf_48904895.pdf Accessed 24 March 2013

General Medical Council (2012a) Good Medical Practice Framework. http://www.gmc-uk.org/GMP_framework_for_appraisal_and_revalidation.pdf.41326960.pdf Accessed 24 March 2013

General Medical Council (2012b) UK Revalidation Programme. Programme Brief. Version 1.0, 15 February 2011. http://www.gmc-uk.org/Item4_revalidation_delivery_progress_report.pdf_48128724.pdf Accessed 28 February 2013

Goulet, F., Gagnon, R., and Gingras, M.-E. (2007) Influence of remedial professional development programs for poorly performing physicians. *J Cont Educ Health Prof*. 27(1): 42–48

Hawkins, R.E. and Swanson, D.B. (2008) Using written examinations to assess medical knowledge and its application. In: E.S. Holmboe and R.E. Hawkins (eds) *Practical Guide to the Evaluation of Clinical Competence* (pp. 42–59). Philadelphia, PA: Mosby, Elsevier.

Hawkins, R.E. and Weiss, K.B. (2011) Building the evidence base in support of the American Board of Medical Specialties' Maintenance of Competence. *Acad Med.* 86(1): 6–7

Holmboe, E.S. (2008) Assessment of the practicing physician: challenges and opportunities. *J Cont Med Educ Health Prof.* 28(S1): S4–S10

Holmboe, E.S., Meechan, T.P., Tate, J.P., Ho, S.-Y., Starkey, K.S., and Lipner, R.S. (2008) Association between maintenance of certification examination scores and quality of care for medicare beneficiaries. *Arch Intern Med.* 168(13): 1396–1403

International Association of Medical Regulatory Authorities (2012) Purpose and goals. http://iamra.com/about.asp Accessed 9 February 2012

Irvine, D. (2006) A short history of the General Medical Council. *Med Educ.* 40: 202–211

Kane, M. (1992) An argument based approach to validation. *Psychometr Bull.* 112: 527–535

Kellogg Foundation (2004) *Logic Model Development Guide. Using Logic Models to Bring Together Planning, Education and Action.* Battle Creek, MI:W. K. Kellogg Foundation

Leach, D.C. (2004) Model for graduate medical education: shifting from process to outcomes. A progress report from the Accreditation Council for Graduate Medical Education. *Med Educ.* 281: 12–14

Levinson, W. (2008) Revalidation of physicians in Canada. Are we passing the test? *CMAJ.* 179(10): 979–980

Levinson, W. and Holmboe, E. (2011) Maintenance of certification in internal medicine. *Arch Intern Med.* 171(2): 174–176

Levinson, W., King, T.E. Jr, Goldman, L., Goroll, A.H., and Kessler, B. 2010. American Board of Internal Medicine Maintenance of Certification Program. *N Engl J Med.* 362: 948–952

Medical Board of Australia (2012) Types of Medical Registration. http://medicalboard.gov.au/Registration/Types.aspx Accessed 23 March 2013

Merkur, S., Mossialos, E., Long, M., and McKee, M. (2008) Physician revalidation in Europe. *Clin Med.* 8(4): 371–376

Miles, P.V. (2009) Maintenance of Certification. The Role of the American Board of Pediatrics in Improving Children's Health. *Pediatr Clin N Am.* 56: 987–994

Miller, G.E. (1990) The Assessment of clinical skills/competence/performance. *Acad Med.* 65: S63–S67

Newble, D., Dawson-Saunders, B., Dauphinee, W.D., et al. (1994) Guidelines for assessing clinical competence. *Teach Learn Med.* 6(3): 213–220

Newble, D., Paget, N., and McLaren, B. (1999) Revalidation in Australia and New Zealand: approach of the Royal Australasian College of Physicians. *BMJ.* 39: 1185–1188

Norcini, J.J.(2005) The assessment of performance at work. *Med Educ.* 39: 80–89

Norcini, J. and Burch, V. (2007) Workplace-based assessment as an educational tool: AMEE Guide No. 31. *Med Teach.* 29: 855–871

Norcini, J. and Guille, R. 2002. Combining Tests and Setting Standards. In: G. Norman, C. van der Vleuten and D. Newble (eds) *International Handbook of Research in Medical Education* (pp. 829–834). Dordrecht: Kluwer Academic Publishers

Norcini, J., Anderson, B., Bollela, V., et al. 2011. Criteria for good assessment: Consensus statement and recommendations from the Ottawa 2010 Conference. *Medl Teach.* 33: 206–214

Norcini, J.J., Blank, L.L., Duffy, D., and Fortna, G.S. (2003) The Mini-CEX. A method for assessing clinical skills. *Ann Intern Med.* 138(6): 476–481

Norman, G. (2002) Research in medical education: three decades of progress. *BMJ.* 324: 1560–1562

Norman, G.R. (1999) The adult learner: a mythical species. *Acad Med.* 74(8): 886–889

Norton, P.G., Ginsburg, L.S., Dunn, E., Beckett, R., and Faulkner, D. (2004) Educational interventions to improve practice of nonspecialty

physicians who are identified in need of peer review. *J Cont Educ Health Prof.* 24: 244–252

O'Brien, T.L. (1986) Legal trends affecting the validity of credentialing examinations. *Eval Health Prof.* 9: 171–185

Pangaro, L. and Holmboe, E.S. (2007) Evaluation Forms and Global Rating Scales. In: E.S. Holmboe and R.E. Hawkins (eds) *Practical Guide to the Evaluation of Clinical Competence* (pp. 24–39). Philadelphia, PA: Mosby, Elsevier.

Perrin, B. (2006) *Moving from Outputs to Outcomes: Practical Advice from Governments around the world. IBM center for The Business of Government.* http://siteresources.worldbank.org/CDINTRANET/Resources/Perrinreport.pdf. Accessed 23 February 2012

Royal Bristol Inquiry (2001) Learning from Bristol: the report of the inquiry into children's heart surgery at the Royal Bristol Infirmary 1984–1995. London: The Stationary Office.

Royal College of General Practitioners (2011) Guide to Revalidation for GPs. http://regp.org.uk/revalidation-and-cpd/in/media/files/Revalidation-and-CPD/guide%2040%20Revalidation%20v70.ashk Accessed 24 March 2013

Royal College of Physicians of London (2009a) Revalidation tools. http://rcplondon.ac.uk/projects/revalidation-tools-support-and-training. Accessed 24 March 2013

Royal College of Physicians of London (2009b) Revalidation questionnaires. http://www.rcplondon.ac-uk/resources/colleagues-and-pattient-feedback-questionnaires. Accessed 24 March 2013

Royal College of Surgeons of England (2010) Revalidation. Guidance on supporting information for surgeons involved in Pathfinder Pilots. http://www.rcseng.ac.uk/publications/docs/revalidation-guidance-on-supporting-information-for-surgeons-involved-in-pathfinder-pilots Accessed 24 March 2013

Royal College of Surgeons of England (2011) Guidance on Supporting Information for Revalidation for Surgery. http://rcseng.aac.uk/surgeons/working/docs/guidance-for-revalidation-supporting-information. Accessed 24 March 2013

Sargeant, J, Mann, K., van der Vleuten, C., and Metsemakers, J. (2008) directed self-assessment: practice and feedback within a social context. *J Cont Educ Health Prof.* 28(1): 47–54

Schmidt, H.G., Norman, G.R., and Boshuizen, H.P. (1990) A cognitive perspective in medical expertise: theory and implications. *Acad Med.* 65: 611–621

Schuwirth, L., Colliver, J., Gruppen, L., et al. (2011) Research in assessment: Consensus statement and recommendations from the Ottawa 21010 Conference. *Med Teach.* 33: 224–233

Shaw, K., Mackillop, L., and Armitage, M. 2007. Revalidation, appraisal and clinical governance. *Clin Governance: Int J.* 12(3): 170–177

Smith, R. (1998) All changed, changed utterly. *BMJ.* 316: 1917–1918

Streiner, D.L. and Norman, G. (2008) Health measurement scales: a practical guide to their development and use. 4th edn. Chapter 2: Basic Concepts (pp. 5–15). Oxford: Oxford University Press

Stevens, R. (1971) From colonial times to the Civil War. The first two hundred and fifty years. In: *American Medicine and the Public Interest* (pp. 9–33). New Haven and London: Yale University Press

Tamblyn, R., Abramhamowicz, M., Brailovsky, C., et al. 1998. Association between licensing examination scores and resources use and quality of care in primary care. *JAMA.* 280(11): 989–996

Tari, J.J. (2005) Components of successful total quality management. *The TQM Magazine.* 17(2): 182–194

Taylor, M.S., Tracy, K.B., Renard, M.K., Harrison, J.K., and Carroll, SJ. (1995) Due process in performance appraisal: a quasi-experiment in procedural justice. *Administrative Science Quarterly.* 40(3): 495–523

van der Vleuten, C.P.M. and Schuwirth L.W.T. (2005) Assessing professional competence: from methods to programs. *Med Educ.* 39: 309–317

Violato, C., Lockyer, J.M., and Fidler, H. (2008) Changes in performance: a five year longitudinal study of participants in a multi-source feedback programmes. *Med Educ.* 42: 1007–1013

CHAPTER 45

Objective structured clinical examinations

Susan Humphrey-Murto, Claire Touchie, and Sydney Smee

Student assessment is often described as "the tail that wags the dog" of medical education. It is seen as the single strongest determinant of what students actually learn (as opposed to what they are taught) and is considered to be uniquely powerful as a tool for manipulating the whole education process.

Stella Lowry

Reproduced from *British Medical Journal*, Lowry S, 'Assessment of students', 306, pp. 51–54, Copyright 1993, with permission from BMJ Publishing Group Ltd.

Introduction

The objective structured clinical examination (OSCE) is a performance-based test and was developed to assess clinical performance. The concept of a performance-based test is not new. Demonstrating one's ability to drive a car or swim 25 metres are examples where individuals must demonstrate their skills under direct observation of an examiner in order to acquire a license or move to the next swimming level. The OSCE is a format wherein examinees demonstrate their skills in a simulated setting, most commonly with individuals who have been trained to portray a patient problem in a consistent manner. Several other forms of simulation for assessment exist and are discussed in other chapters of this textbook. Because the OSCE uses simulation, it can be highly structured and standardized for use in summative assessments.

The following chapter is divided in two parts. The first outlines the background of the OSCE and reviews the theoretical underpinning and literature that supports the validity of this format. The second part is a practical 'how to' guide to running an OSCE for first time administrators, although it should also serve as a quality assurance tool for those already conducting OSCEs.

Background

Miller (1990, pp. S63–S67) proposed a framework, or pyramid, for clinical assessment consisting of four levels; knows, knows how, shows how, and does. Assessing examinees' knowledge (knows) or application of knowledge (knows how) are not sufficient for assessing clinical skills. The OSCE is a point-in-time performance assessment

tool for assessing 'shows how'. Workplace assessment strategies focus on the 'does', based on actual performance over time.

Harden et al. (1975, pp. 447–451) introduced the OSCE in the mid-1970s to overcome perceived deficiencies of the traditional oral clinical examination; including lack of direct observation of clinical skills, limited sampling, and the problem of rater bias. The OSCE is a circuit of stations that examinees move through in a coordinated fashion (fig. 45.1). Examinees are observed at each station as they complete a clinical task and are scored according to pre-set criteria. History taking, physical examination, test interpretation, procedural skills, management, and communication skills can all be assessed, along with other skills. The OSCE ensures direct observation of a relatively large sample of clinical skills that are scored by multiple raters according to standardized scoring sheets. The OSCE has become the gold standard for performance assessment.

By the mid-1990s the OSCE was a widely used form of assessment in many jurisdictions including the United Kingdom, the United States, Canada, and Australia. Initially designed to assess students in the final year of medical school (Harden 1975), the OSCE format is also used as an approach to assess postgraduate trainees, and for high-stakes licensure and certification examinations (Reznick 1996; Grand'Maison 1996; Boulet 2009).

Formative and summative OSCEs

The OSCE is a format for formative and summative purposes. As a teaching tool, the OSCE is used to provide direct observation

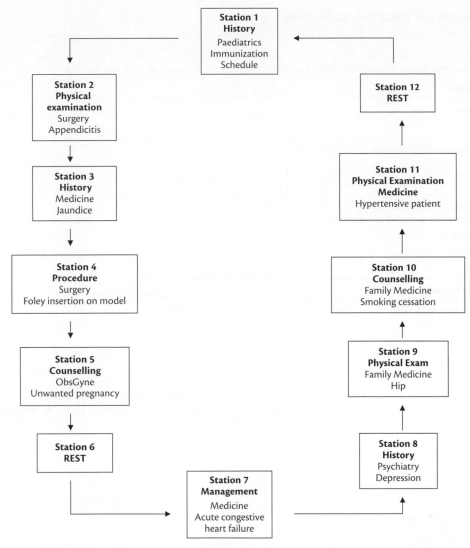

Figure 45.1 Sample of a 10-station OSCE with rest stations.
This figure was published in *A Practical Guide for Medical Teachers*, JA Dent and RM Harden, Copyright Elsevier 2009.

and feedback on history taking, physical examination, and doctor–patient relationship skills (Brazeau 2002). OSCEs are also used for teaching skills that vary from managing prescription errors (Varkey 2007), learning and practising how to provide feedback (Cushing 2011) to directing one's own continuing professional development (Arnold and Walmsley 2008). The OSCE is also useful for assessing various skills including: surgical skills (Martin 1997; Friedlich 2002); patient-management skills such as handoffs, telephone management, and note writing (Williams 2011); and patient safety (Wagner 2009). The team-observed structural clinical examination (TOSCE) measures interprofessional collaboration (Hall 2011). Another innovative use of the OSCE format is the integrated procedural performance instrument (IPPI), a sophisticated approach that uses standardized patients (SPs), in conjunction with bench models and manikins, to encourage a patient-centred approach to procedural skills (Kneebone 2006). The multiple mini-interview (MMI) is also an adaptation of the OSCE format. This tool is used for the selection of medical students and assesses non-cognitive domains such as moral reasoning, communication skills, and the ability to collaborate (Eva 2004).

When an OSCE is used for formative purposes, feedback can be provided verbally, in the form of review of the checklist or through review of videotapes, during or after the examination. Immediate feedback by physician examiners after each OSCE station has been found to improve student skills in stations of similar content (Hodder 1989; Khan 1997). Feedback can also be provided by non-experts, such as senior medical students (Reiter 2004; Moineau 2011).

Standardized patients (SPs)

The development of SPs was essential to the development of the OSCE. In general, a SP is a person who has been carefully trained to take on the characteristics of a real patient in order to produce a consistent and realistic portrayal (Barrows 1968). If abnormal physical findings are desired, the recruitment process is more difficult as it may be difficult to reproduce the findings consistently. Attempts have been made to overcome some of these challenges with technology. Verma et al. (2011, pp. e388–396) used modified stethoscopes that play abnormal auscultatory findings. Wendling et al. (2011, pp. 384–388) used virtual standardized patients to add consistency to the portrayal of abnormal findings with some success.

Table 45.1 Abbreviated examiner checklist and communication rating scale

Examinee Instructions
John Smith, 59 years old, presents to your office complaining of jaundice. In the next 5 minutes, obtain a focused and relevant history.

Done/asked satisfactorily

1. Elicits onset/duration

2. Elicits progression

3. Elicits associated symptoms—dark urine
  - abdominal pain
  - colour of stool
  - fever

4. Elicits risk factors—previous exposure to hepatitis
  - recent blood transfusion
  - intravenous drug use
  - foreign travel

5. Elicits an alcohol use history

6. Conducts a review of systems—skin
  - weight loss
  - change in appetite

7. Elicits medication history

Total = /15

Communication skills	1. Poor	2. Fair	3. Good	4. Very Good	5. Excellent
1. Interpersonal skills: ◆ listens carefully ◆ treats patient as an equal					
2. Interviewing skills: ◆ organized ◆ uses words patient can understand ◆ does not interrupt, allows patient to explain					
3. Patient education: ◆ provides clear, complete information ◆ encourages patient to ask questions ◆ confirms patient's understanding/opinion					
4. Response to emotional issues: ◆ recognizes and discusses emotional issues ◆ controls own emotional state					

Communication skills total = /20

Scoring instruments

To generate an examinee score for each station, there must be scoring instruments to capture rater judgements. Commonly, checklists and/or global rating scales are used (table 45.1). Checklists are usually station-dependent with multiple items representing what the examinee is expected to demonstrate. Rating scales tend to be station-independent scales that measure general areas of competence such as organization, communication, and rapport; behaviours that are not well captured on a binary checklist. Global rating scales capture holistic judgements of examinees' overall performance, which may not be fully represented by the checklist.

Checklists have some advantages. They are useful when assessing structured tasks, when recording specific actions, when assessing junior trainees, and when limited time is available for training raters. Exhaustive checklists are not necessary. Checklist length depends upon the clinical task, the time allowed, and who is scoring. For example, if SPs are scoring by recall, then the number of items becomes important as too many items may reduce SP accuracy. Vu and her colleagues (1992, pp. 99–104) suggest checklists should have 10–20 items for optimal accuracy. Item structure also matters. They noted poorer recording accuracy when a checklist item included more than one piece of information (e.g. 'the student tested patient orientation to time, place, and person'). They also found SP raters demonstrated a similar loss of accuracy if the item required them to indicate not only if the item was performed, but if it was performed correctly. Checklists should be concrete guides to raters. For example, 'examines the abdomen' is a general item that might better be separated into a series of items like 'inspects the abdomen', 'auscultates the abdomen', 'lightly palpates all four quadrants', and so on. This approach focuses the judgement of the rater.

Checklists have potential disadvantages. Longer checklists deconstruct patient interactions inappropriately and therefore may not capture more expert performance (Hodges 1999). Global ratings can produce scores with reliabilities equal to or greater than those for checklist scores and better distinguish between different levels of expertise (Cunnington 1997; Hodges 1999; Regehr 1999). The belief is that experts gather more focused information while novices collect extensive data, increasing their checklist scores without improving diagnostic accuracy.

Rating scales allow examiners to rate the quality of an action, and are better suited to assessing skills such as communication skills where a binary score may not reflect the range of skill demonstrated. They can be used to score skills across different cases. Rating scales are generally comprised of items with three to seven points with descriptive anchors to define some or all the points on the item. The items might be aspects of a skill, for instance aspects of history taking, or the items might reflect clinical skills more broadly with items for history taking, physical assessment, communication, or providing a follow-up plan. As rating scales are generally not case-specific, station development requires less effort. A number of different scales have been developed for communication (Yudkowsky 2009; Schirmer 2005) and for minor surgical skills (Martin 1997).

Rating scales also present some problems. Rating scales allow more range for individual judgement and they are cognitively harder for assessors to score—so more examiner training is important. Further, it is not always clear what heuristic each examiner uses for rating (Smee, 2007). As with any scoring instrument, more items on a rating scale will positively influence score reliability. However, too many items forces assessors to deconstruct performance similarly to a checklist and increases the time needed for scoring.

Combinations of checklists and rating scales (table 45.1) can work quite well. Checklists that identify key components of what is being assessed in a station combined with rating scale items that represent the more qualitative aspects of the interaction can produce valid and reliable scores. Regardless of the scoring format selected, the instruments should be reviewed by clinical experts to ensure that they are appropriate to the level of training; that items are task-based; and that expected performance is observable. They should also be evidence-based so far as is possible and reflect best practice guidelines.

When different scoring instruments are used within one station, calculating the final mark for the station requires a decision on the relative weights for the rating scale and the checklist. For example, communication rating scales may be included on all history taking and counselling stations and be worth 20–50% of the station mark.

Differentially weighting items within a scoring instrument; that is, making certain items worth more than others, has little impact on score reliability and is generally not encouraged (van der Vleuten and Swanson 1990; Russell and Hubley 2005). However, studies suggest that only scoring critical actions or using items of greater importance in a checklist may improve score reliability. This approach helps separate examinees who are ready to perform critical aspects of a skill from those who have mastered only limited steps (Kahraman 2008; Payne 2008).

The addition of a written component after each patient encounter that asks examinees to summarize their clinical findings, provide a differential diagnosis and suggest a management plan allows for some assessment of an examinee's ability to synthesize the information they elicited from the patient (Boulet 2004; Clauser 2008).

Raters

Who should act as raters in the OSCE is the subject of some debate. Physicians, non-physician personnel, and SPs are used as raters in formative and summative examinations. Physicians may be more qualified to understand the logical sequencing of questions in history taking stations and the technical adequacy of physical examination manoeuvres but they are a limited resource, especially for large scale OSCEs. Multiple studies have demonstrated that non-physician raters can be used, including standardized patients (SP), trained paramedical assessors and student peers (van der Vleuten et al. 1989; Humphrey-Murto et al. 2005; Chenot 2007; Moineau 2011). Many studies have examined the inter-rater reliability of SPs and shown proportion agreement rates that range from fair to excellent (0.37 to 0.92) (Tamblyn 1991; Vu 1992; De Champlain et al. 1997). Inter-rater reliability of physician raters has been shown to be similar (Stillman et al. 1991a; Touchie 2010). A study by Pangaro et al. (1997, pp. 1008–1011) provides validity evidence for SP scoring accuracy in a study that blinded SPs to standardized examinees trained to achieve preset scores. In another study non-physician raters were found to be as accurate at completing checklists as physicians but showed poor agreement on a global rating scale (Humphrey-Murto et al. 2005). Boulet et al. (2002, pp. 85–97) showed good comparability of scores between SP recorders and physician raters. However, Martin et al. (1996, pp.170–175) compared scores from observing physicians, observing SPs and SPs scoring by recall. The most accurate scores (based on a preset gold standard) were provided by physicians (Martin et al. 1996).

Rater training is important for ensuring score reliability. Raters who are too lenient (doves) or too severe (hawks) introduce unwanted variability to OSCE scores. However, the impact of training appears to vary with rater background. Van der Vleuten et al. (1989, pp. 290–296) compared training to no training in lay persons, medical students and physician raters. When comparing accuracy of scoring, this study suggested that training is least needed and least effective for the physician group, more needed and effective for the medical students, and most needed and effective for the lay group.

Of note, studies have shown that the use of multiple raters per station has a marginal effect on score reliability (van der Vleuten and Swanson 1990). If more raters are available, increasing the number of stations with a single rater increases reliability far more than does two raters per station. (Swanson and Norcini 1989; Govaerts 2002)

Ultimately, the purpose of an examination and local feasibility considerations will frame how each institution determines who should score for any specific OSCE.

Setting standards for an OSCE

A detailed account of standard setting can be found in McKinley and Norcini's chapter. A brief discussion of the standard setting

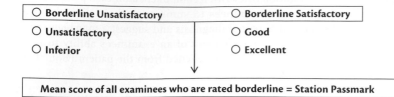

Overall, did the examinee meet the needs of the patient?

- ○ Borderline Unsatisfactory
- ○ Unsatisfactory
- ○ Inferior

- ○ Borderline Satisfactory
- ○ Good
- ○ Excellent

Mean score of all examinees who are rated borderline = Station Passmark

Figure 45.2 Example of global rating for borderline group standard setting.

for a performance examination such as an OSCE is offered here because of its importance. No consensus exists on the most appropriate standard setting method for the OSCE and many procedures can be used such as the Angoff, Ebel, Hofstee, and contrasting group methods (Norcini 1994; Cusimano 1996; Boulet 2003a). The modified borderline group and the borderline regression methods can also be used (Dauphinee 1997; Humphrey-Murto and McFadyen 2002; Wood 2006). Decisions as to which is most appropriate for a given examination depends on who is rating and whether the standard setting judgement will be based on test items, the whole test or examinee performance (Downing 2006).

The modified borderline group method, which depends upon physician raters, is described here as it is an easily implemented and widely used approach. For this method, multiple physician examiners identify borderline performances by completing a global rating at the end of each encounter. The examiner responds to a question such as 'Overall, did the examinee meet the needs of the patient?' Rating scale categories range through some version of inferior, poor, borderline unsatisfactory, borderline satisfactory, good, and excellent. These judgements are translated into station pass marks by taking the mean score of all those rated as borderline (fig. 45.2). The pass mark for the entire OSCE is the sum of the cut scores for each station, often reflected as a percentage score (Dauphinee 1997). This method has been successfully used in high-stakes examinations with over 2000 examinees as well as in smaller examinations with as few as 60 examinees (Dauphinee 1997; Wilkinson 2001; Humphrey-Murto and McFadyen 2002; Cusimano and Rothman 2004). A risk with smaller scale examinations is that the number of examinees identified as borderline is small and thus the cut score is less reliable. A similar method, called the borderline regression method, incorporates a linear regression approach allowing the cut score to be set using the scores from all examinees, and not just a subset. This method appears to have less statistical error and can be done with a simple linear regression analysis (Wood 2006).

Validity

Validity of scores is always relative to the purpose of the assessment, the population being assessed and the context (Petrusa 2002; Hodges 2003). Evidence of validity begins with the examination blueprint. A blueprint should be developed by content experts and medical educators who agree that the cases chosen are representative of the course objectives or domains to be tested (Boulet 2003b). Consideration must be given to the population being tested (e.g. clinical clerks or residents), the content that should be tested, the clinical skills (e.g. history taking, physical examination, and patient management) and the degree of authenticity required for the given context. For example, some fragmentation of the skills

being assessed for second year medical students may be acceptable whereas more realistic and comprehensive situations are needed for the valid assessment of more advanced learners. Valid scores may be achieved from assessing a medical student's ability to examine the chest in a 10-minute station whereas achieving valid scores for a resident would require the more authentic demonstration of an integrated approach to the patient with chest pain, including the history, physical examination, and management plan (Ruesseler 2010; Hatala 2011).

To achieve valid scores, an OSCE must have a sufficient number of stations to counteract the effect of case specificity. Case specificity is a well-documented phenomenon wherein examinee performance on one case is a poor predictor of performance on other cases (van der Vleuten and Swanson 1990). How many stations are enough depends on the purpose of the examination. For formative examinations, case specificity and score reliability are of lesser importance. For summative high-stakes examinations sampling enough of the content domain is essential for a valid interpretation of the scores. Studies suggest that to obtain an acceptable reliability estimate, 10 stations or more are needed (van der Vleuten and Swanson 1990; Brannick 2011). Determining the length of the stations depends primarily on the OSCE's purpose and the skills being tested (van der Vleuten and Swanson 1990). OSCEs run best when all stations are the same length. For any given period of time, the challenge is to provide sufficient time for each task while maximizing the number of stations to ensure the broadest possible sampling of the competence.

For valid interpretation of OSCE scores, station scores should be correlated to some degree indicating internal consistency, meaning they are assessing aspects of the same construct of competency. Internal consistency, which is one measure of score reliability, is most often reported with an alpha coefficient. Alpha coefficients are calculated on the number of stations (across-station) or on the number of items in a checklist of a particular station (across-items). In a meta-analysis of over 150 studies, Brannick et al. (2011, pp. 1181–1189) reported mean estimates for across-station reliability of 0.66 (95% confidence interval 0.62–0.70) and for across-items reliability of 0.78 (95% confidence intervals of 0.73–0.95). Across-item reliability estimates may be best suited for within-station analyses. As a single rater completes all the items, the reliability is not based on independent judgements and therefore may over-estimate the true reliability of the OSCE scores. Therefore, across-station reliabilities are more valid indicators of internal consistency.

Score reliability can also be estimated with generalizability coefficients. Error variances can be calculated for the raters, SPs and other influencing factors such as examination track or site. These variances may help to detect problems with the examination or with the station. For example, van der Vleuten and Swanson (1990, pp. 58–76) used a generalizability study to show that different SPs playing the same role at the same site, although contributing to the error variance, did not significantly affect score reliability. They concluded that minimizing error variances and achieving reproducible scores requires a 'large' number of cases and testing time. Practically speaking, this means 10 or more stations (Vu 1992; Boulet 2003b).

Item total score correlations (ITC) contribute to item analysis and may provide further evidence of validity. For an OSCE, the ITC is the correlation of a station score to the total OSCE score. In general, a station ITC of less than 0.2 indicates a potential problem with the station. Station ITCs exceeding 0.8 suggest redundant content across stations (Downing and Haladyna 2004).

OSCEs are thought to measure something more than knowledge or simple decision making. Validity evidence for this interpretation of OSCE scores is supported by studies that show low correlation with written assessment scores (divergent evidence) and stronger correlations with other forms of performance assessment (convergent evidence). An example of this kind of evidence is provided in a review by Williams (2004, pp. 215–222) that reported low correlations (0–0.16) between OSCE scores and written examination scores and somewhat stronger correlations (0.27–0.42) between OSCE scores and residency supervisors' ratings. This evidence supports the difference in the two constructs being assessed (i.e. knowledge versus skill). However, the OSCE scores are only moderately correlated with the supervisor ratings. The lack of stronger correlations between scores from two performance assessments may have been due to differences between a point-in-time assessment and a workplace assessment. In addition, the general lack of direct observation and poor reliability seen with in-training assessments may have been a factor.

Whether OSCEs can predict how a physician will perform in practice is a question that several researchers have attempted to answer. Studies of practice outcomes have shown that better performing candidates on an OSCE demonstrate improved hypertensive care and antibiotic prescribing in practice (Tamblyn 2010; Cadieux 2011). Studies of the communication components of a national OSCE used for licensing purposes have indicated a positive relationship between higher OSCE scores and better outcomes (Wenghofer 2009), including fewer complaints against physicians (Tamblyn 2007).

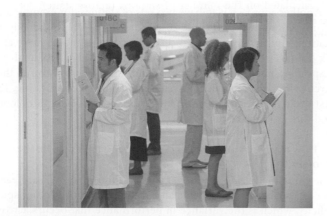

Figure 45.3 An OSCE in action—candidates about to enter their stations. Reproduced with permission of the Medical Council of Canada © (2012).

Test security

Breaches of security are a concern when OSCEs assess large cohorts that require the re-use of stations over several days or when stations are banked for re-use over time (fig. 45.3). Some studies have found little to no evidence of examinees being advantaged by prior knowledge of an OSCE (e.g., Niehaus et al. 1996; Swartz 1993). In a study where OSCE stations were re-used over 4 days, scores increased over time but only for stations where feedback was provided (Khan 1997). Two other studies that looked at OSCEs where security breaches or collusion were known to have occurred (Wilkinson 2003; Furman 1997) also found no significant advantage for test takers. However, de Champlain et al. (2000: pp. S109–S111) showed that when examinees were given access to checklists, scores did increase.

Swygert et al. (2010, pp. 1506–1510) observed mean score increases for repeat takers on the United States Medical Licensing Examination Step 2 Clinical Skills examination on total examination score, but no significant score increases for those examinees who encountered repeat stations. One early study (Cohen et al. 1993) also found a significant upward trend in scores for stations used repeatedly over time. Conversely, test takers may be disadvantaged as three studies (Stillman 1991b; Schoonheim-Klein et al. 2008; Boulet 2009) found station scores decreased with re-use.

Two general interpretations that can be drawn from the research to date are that foreknowledge of the OSCE content is not sufficient to allow for significant changes in one's clinical performance and that such knowledge may even be detrimental to clinical performance. While these studies suggest no significant concern about re-use of stations in summative settings, the potential advantage or disadvantage to those whose performance is close to the pass mark and for whom even a small change in performance may change their result is still unclear.

Practical considerations

For any OSCE to provide a valid assessment of clinical skills, substantial effort is required. This section lays out important practical steps to running an OSCE that generates sufficiently valid scores for summative decisions. Two important underlying assumptions of this section are that any institution planning an OSCE is planning on running it more than once and that the OSCE is being run at a single site. The first assumption is made because OSCEs become more cost effective as a case bank is developed and a team gains expertise. The second assumption is made to limit the scope of this section (although OSCEs can be run quite successfully at multiple sites).

Six questions

Formulating the answers to the following six questions will provide you with a framework that supports the planning, development, budgeting and administering of an OSCE.

1. What is the purpose of the assessment?

Is an OSCE the right test format? An OSCE is a poor choice for assessing knowledge domains as it does not sample widely enough and there are better, more cost effective formats such as multiple choice questions. Is the purpose formative, or will results be used for decision making, such as pass/fail? For a formative OSCE,

Table 45.2 Sample of partial examination blueprint (four stations)

Problem	Discipline	History taking	Physical exam	Procedural skills	Patient education/ management	Diagnosis
30 y/o woman, abdominal pain, appendicitis	Surgery		X			X
6 months old, vomiting (parent only)	Paediatrics	X				
50 y/o male, hypertensive, poor adherence with medication	Medicine	X			X	
80 y/o woman in emergency room with dehydration, requires intravenous fluids	Emergency medicine			X	X	

the validity of the content and the nature of the feedback is more important than high score reliability. For a summative OSCE, defensibly valid interpretation of scores is critical and more attention must be paid to all aspects of station development. A summative OSCE must have a sufficient number of stations (usually 10 or more) with well-designed scoring instruments that are congruent with the OSCE's purpose. Likewise, the patient training must ensure a high level of standardization and the raters must be well oriented to their scoring tasks.

2. What is the performance standard?

A statement of the standard of the performance being assessed will define all decisions that follow, such as the level of difficulty of clinical presentations and the format of scoring instruments. A performance standard may be as simple as the statement 'Trainees are expected to demonstrate the clinical skills and judgement of an acceptably competent end of third year clinical clerk'.

3. What domain is being assessed?

An examination blueprint is essential to planning any examination and should reflect training objectives. Individuals familiar with the training programme should be part of this process and should guide the selection of content areas and skills to be sampled. For example, the blueprint for a general undergraduate medical OSCE would identify the skills students should have mastered for their level of training, such as history taking, physical examination techniques, basic patient management, counselling, communication skills, and procedural skills. Then specific domains of practice to be covered, such as internal medicine, surgery, psychiatry, obstetrics, paediatrics, family medicine, and emergency medicine would be identified (table 45.2). Another approach would be to determine common clinical presentations from across different body systems that define the practice domain.

4. Who are the raters?

Possible raters for an OSCE include SPs scoring by recall after each encounter, pairs of SPs alternating between one scoring by observation and the other simulating, physicians scoring by observation, and less common but worth considering, non-physicians with relevant expertise scoring by observation. Who should score depends on the purpose of the OSCE and the amount of time available for training the raters. Formative OSCEs with patient-based feedback put the emphasis on training the SPs to provide good feedback. When a higher level of clinical expertise

is being assessed, then the clinical expertise of the raters is likely an issue. Regardless of who scores and/or provides feedback, they require some form of training.

5. How long should stations be?

The length of the station depends on the purpose of the examination and the nature of what is being assessed. Short stations (5–10 minutes) allow for greater sampling and therefore will generate more reliable scores within a reasonable testing time. Tasks for short stations must be quite defined, e.g. 'examine the left knee'. Longer stations allow for more complex problems to be presented. Having fewer, longer stations maximizes learning relative to the selected patient problems, especially if trainees receive feedback on their performance.

Usually all OSCE stations are the same length of time so that examinees circulate on a fixed schedule. Any administrator who has run stations of varying lengths can attest to the significant risk this poses. If stations really must be of differing lengths, there are a few considerations to keep in mind. First, station times should all be in some multiple of each other. If some stations are ten minutes long, then the longer stations should be 20 minutes long. A circuit of 10-minute stations can have a branch in it for a longer station where there are two rooms for one station in the circuit used for a 20-minute station. The multiple rooms allow for staggered entries and exits from the long station and test takers continue moving around the circuit efficiently. However, be warned, if you have problems on the day of the OSCE they will occur here.

Another approach is to have two sets of stations; for example six 10-minute stations and three 20-minute stations with the longer stations running in two parallel circuits. In this model there are six test takers in each type of station and they will complete their respective circuits at the same time and can then cross over to the circuit they have not yet completed. In 120 minutes of testing, 12 test takers will complete nine OSCE stations; six 10-minutes long and three 20-minutes long.

6. How many stations are needed to adequately sample the domain?

The short answer is as many as one can afford. As discussed earlier, performance assessments all have to contend with case specificity, which is the variance in performance that occurs across different stations. Practically speaking, 10–20 stations are commonly used.

Table 45.3 Tasks and timeline

Task	Suggested time required prior to OSCE	Comments
Design OSCE Logistics: location, number of tracks required, reserve space early Plan for: staff, equipment and models	10–12 months	Develop blueprint by committee
Create budget	10–12 months	
Recruit case authors	4–6 months prior	Earlier if possible
Station writing workshop	4–6 months	
Determine how to set the pass mark	4–6 months	
Edit and review cases—finalize	4–6 months	Ideally this works starts as soon as workshop is over, pilot test
Recruit raters/faculty to examine Determine training needs	3–4 months	
Recruit trainers, standardized patients (SPs) and support staff	2–3 months	Start earlier if possible
Logistics: site to finalize details of location, number and location of rooms for OSCE, flow of candidates ◆ equipment and models ◆ signalling system (heard in all rooms?)	2–3 months	Rooms for orientation/registration of examinees, SPs, raters Rooms for lunch/breaks Sign out location Confirm parking and catering
Train SPs	5–8 weeks	
Provide examinees with specific information	3 weeks	
Print mark sheets, make signs	2 weeks	Earlier if possible
Remind everyone of date Have spares (raters, SPs, support staff) ready to attend on the day of examination	1 week	For physician raters contact administrative assistants
Exam day planning includes: ◆ Diagram of station layout ◆ Information sheets for all participants ◆ Registration set-up and process ◆ Timing process & signals ◆ Collection process for mark sheets ◆ Sign out process	Start as early as possible—this work occurs over time and there are often unexpected snags	
Adminster the OSCE	DATE	
Process and analyse results		Depends on many variables
Report results	DATE	
Post-exam review: feedback on cases and process, pass marks and pass rates Consider changes to stations	2–4 weeks post exam	Important to document especially if annual event
Respond to appeals	Specify deadline for making an appeal	Assumes high stakes, summative assessment

Tasks and timeline

Once the initial design decisions highlighted previously have been made, then the tasks, timelines and costs can be determined. If the results suggest your OSCE is not feasible, then return to the initial standardized specifications to see which ones can be modified so that the limits defined by the resources can be met. An overview of the tasks with an ideal timeline is shown in table 45.3.

Cost

OSCE design has a significant impact on cost. Costs vary greatly because the number of stations and other specifications determine the number of SPs, raters and staff required (Reznick et al. 1993). Whether or not faculty members volunteer to write cases, set standards, or examine are all significant factors. Keep in mind that the cost of creating an OSCE remains much the same regardless of the number of examinees. For example, administering an

OSCE twice in one day costs only a little more but assesses twice as many test takers.

Another significant cost driver is station development. Reuse of stations saves time and money. Considerations when reusing stations are keeping the content of each test form secure, having a sufficient mix of new and reused content, and having a plan for managing a growing item bank. Either give careful consideration to how station documents are formatted, to key word tagging, and to version control, or choose an item banking software.

The people who make the OSCE happen; like the SPs, the support staff and the raters, are usually paid. SPs may be volunteers or paid employees. While volunteers may be recruited for a small OSCE, working with a programme that recruits and trains SPs is valuable for large scale OSCEs (Ker 2005; Vargas 2007). Many institutions do have such programmes. Paying SPs allows the institution to demand regular attendance and a higher standard of performance. Likewise, raters may or may not be volunteers. When planning and budgeting, allow extra time during the OSCE for SPs, support staff and raters to have periodic rests, especially for SPs in physically demanding stations.

A 10-station OSCE run over one evening that assesses 160 examinees at a Canadian university costs approximately $60, 000. If raters are reimbursed, the cost increases substantially. To accommodate this many examinees, the OSCE is run across seven simultaneous tracks and administered twice. In addition, rest stations are added to each track to increase capacity (fig. 45.1). An evening administration takes advantage of clinic space which may be available free of charge.

Station writing

An OSCE station is a test item, a training guide, and an administrative primer. There are many users: examinees, raters, SPs, SP trainers, and OSCE coordinators. Other users may include the staff person who edits and formats the material for various uses, including creating the mark sheets, and the programmer who prepares the scoring application.

An OSCE station has four main components:

* the stem or task assignment for the examinee

* the scoring instruments

* the SP training materials and

* materials and prop specifications.

Stations should be written by content experts with knowledge of the trainees to be tested and an understanding of the performance standard. Provide the station authors with the domain and skill to be tested. Encourage authors to base the station on an actual patient they have seen. This strategy increases authenticity and facilitates the writing task.

Stem

Instructions to examinees must be clear and concise. Use a standardized format; for instance, provide the patient's name, age, presenting complaint(s), and the setting (e.g. clinic or ward) for all stations. The stem must clearly state the task; for example, 'Complete a focused physical examination in a patient with suspected congestive heart failure. You have 8 minutes to complete this station' or, for higher level testing, the stem can simply say, 'In the next 20 minutes assess the patient and respond to their concerns'. The importance of clarity cannot be overstated. Having a colleague review the stem and outline their approach to the task can quickly identify an ambiguous or poorly constructed stem.

The use of language in the stem is important. If the information is from a clinical source (e.g. a chart, a paramedic, or a consultant's report) then use medical jargon. If the information is from the patient or family member, use layperson's terms. Eva and colleagues (2010) have shown that language influences how clinicians judge information and therefore congruence between the language in the stem and the source of the information creates a more valid and realistic simulation.

Scoring instruments

Given the information in the stem, what actions should be taken by the examinee? The answers to this question are the foundation of the scoring instrument. The most common scoring formats are checklists and rating scales, as discussed earlier. For an example see table 45.1.

SP training materials

Basic information for SP recruitment and training begins with gender and age range; sometimes body type and race also matter. In general, SPs need to understand the clinical presentation from the patient's perspective, in the language that a patient uses to describe the problem. Training information focuses on the pertinent positives and on the most critical pertinent negatives.

Training information provides responses to checklist items and guidelines to standardize responses to both expected and unexpected examinee behaviours. As much as possible, the patient's behaviour and affect in terms of body language, verbal tone, and pace is described. Describe symptoms to be simulated in patient terms. For example, describe a loss of range of motion by how it impacts daily living or intermittent symptoms as coming and going. Frame timelines relative to seeing the doctor; for example 'my headache started six hours ago', not 'my headache started at 2 am in the morning'. SPs can adjust their presentation to the actual time of day during the OSCE.

Training information must be detailed enough to ensure the consistency of each SP across candidates, and the consistency across multiple SPs portraying the same role. Include all relevant data from the presenting complaint and history of the present illness, past medical history, medication, family history, and social history. Guidance on how much information the SP should share in response to common open-ended questions is helpful. Finally, identify specific questions that the SP must ask, including instructions as to when they should be asked. Unnecessary details like the names of family members should be avoided. Examples of SP scripts can be found in OSCE reference books or on the internet.

Materials and props

The supporting props and materials needed may be minimal. However, clarifying if props (e.g. intravenous stand or radiograph) or make-up are necessary is critical information for the OSCE coordinator. A simple list of necessary equipment is likely all that is required for a physical examination station. However, a detailed outline of how equipment is to be presented to each examinee for stations where models, technical equipment, and simulators are being used is necessary. Case authors should provide these details as well as any props at the time the station is being developed.

Station writing process

While anyone can develop a case on their own, when multiple cases are required, or when case writers are new to the process, a workshop approach works well. At its simplest, a workshop means bringing a small group of clinicians together, providing them with common instructions and examples and then letting them write while in the same room as their colleagues. For new authors, an example of a previous station (if available) is especially important as most who have not had experience developing OSCEs fail to include the amount of detail required to guarantee standardization. The workshop approach also allows authors to consult and advise each other, thereby providing a preliminary review of the stations.

Recruit content experts with some knowledge of the trainees to be tested and their required skill level. Provide the content experts with a specific skill or task level and domain of practice to be assessed ahead of the workshop and ask them to look through their patient cases for ones that could be the basis for such a station.

As a first step, authors should be oriented to the components of a case and told the skill (e.g. physical examination) and the domain (e.g. internal medicine) to be assessed. Second, the authors should define the purpose of their station; for example: 'to assess an examinee's ability to complete an appropriate physical examination of a patient with congestive heart failure'. Third, they should write the stem. After writing the stem, a colleague should be asked to interpret the instructions to ensure clarity. After establishing the stem, the station author should develop the scoring instruments. Only after these steps are completed should an author begin writing the training information for SPs.

Once the station is written, it should reviewed to identify any difficulties with the instructions or scoring instruments. Other checks are whether the length of the station is appropriate and whether the SP information is sufficient. If possible, having a SP and/or a SP trainer review the content is also useful and may identify important questions to be answered before training begins.

Following the workshop, support staff edit and format the content. Then, the stations should be reviewed and finalized by a committee of station authors. However, the reality is often that one or two individuals do most of the editing.

SP recruitment and training

SPs come from different walks of life and bring different skills to the task. Word of mouth and articles in local newsletters are helpful recruitment strategies. Holding information sessions with short intake interviews of interested individuals is useful, especially when a large number of SPs are needed. When individuals are well matched to a role and the skills expected of them, training is shorter and OSCE performance is more consistent.

SPs have to match the demographics of the role and should be at or above the educational level of the patient role. An interest in the work, confidence, a sense of humour, and a willingness to act are other desirable characteristics. Applicants with rigid ideas, particularly about physicians, those who are shy, overly extroverted, or physically unable to do a role due to frailness or limited hearing

(for example), are not suitable. Of note, a study by Peitzman (2001, p. 383) suggests caution when recruiting individuals as more than half of the SPs applying to serve in a high-stakes examination were found to have easily detectable incidental physical findings which could have inappropriately affected examinee's diagnostic thinking. Humphrey-Murto et al. (2009, pp. 521–525) and Carson et al. (2010, pp. 1772–1776) found that students examining female SPs outperformed students examining male SPs portraying the same patient problem. Keeping SP gender the same for a case is an important consideration.

After SPs are matched to a role, they should receive the training information and be given time to review it before practice begins. During training sessions the trainer's role is to highlight critical aspects of the role, answer questions, and ensure a strong emphasis on role playing and feedback.

If physical simulation is involved, teaching SPs how to simulate the symptoms starts with helping them understand their normal and then understanding how to adjust it. For example, to teach simulation of shortness of breath, the trainer asks the SP to count their respirations while breathing normally for a minute. Then the trainer asks them to increase their rate to that required for the role, say 20–22 per minute. Then the SPs are asked to practise speaking with the kind of pauses created by shortness of breath, and lastly, they need to be coached to not hyperventilate.

SPs must practise the role. Talking about it is not sufficient. Simulating is a performance skill and to do it well takes practice and feedback, especially when several SPs are learning the same role. In this latter instance, the SPs should be trained together as much as possible so they learn from each other and adjust their performance accordingly.

Ideally, a physician will observe the SPs prior to the examination for quality assurance. How long it takes to train SPs doing the same role varies from 30 minutes to 15 hours depending on the complexity of the case and the experience of the SPs. If SPs are scoring or providing feedback then training times are longer.

Rater recruitment and orientation

Raters can be faculty clinicians or senior trainees, depending on the examination. SPs or trained observers have also been used to complete checklists and global rating scales. Using physician examiners has several advantages. There is increased validity in having a member of the profession examine; standard setting can be completed using a borderline group method; and immediate feedback can be provided to examinees. Disadvantages include difficulty in finding available faculty and the costs incurred if they are remunerated. For formative OSCEs, training SPs to score and provide feedback can be a powerful approach to teaching basic clinical interviewing and physical examination techniques. SPs can also be trained to record consistently for summative decisions (Boulet 2009).

At a minimum, rater training consists of a short introduction to the purpose of the examination, a basic review of the scoring instruments and tasks, plus guidance regarding what (if any) feedback is being provided. More extensive training that is case-specific is always better but often unrealistic in terms of the time available with the raters. If SPs are recording, then more training is required regarding what to observe in examinees. Of note, rater recruitment should be done weeks or months in advance of the examination but the orientation is best completed just preceding the examination to ensure attendance and recall by all raters.

OSCE administration

Detailed plans should be made for everyone's arrival and where they should sign in. Back-up plans for missing raters, SPs or support staff are important. Set-up includes all of the following: signage, registration desks, rooms, and audiovisual equipment for orientations, mark sheets or computers for each station, hand sanitizer, hospital gowns, and drapes and props. Orientation sessions for raters and examinees can occur simultaneously. Having a reliable means for timing is critical. Buzzers or bells can signal the beginning and end of stations. Leaving 1 or 2 minutes in between stations allows the examinees to move to the next station and read the stems. If feedback is to be provided, a different signal such as an intermittent buzzer can be used. Timing sheets should be prepared ahead of time and verification that the signal can be heard in all rooms is essential.

Ensure there is appropriate catering and access to washrooms. Lastly, have a process for logging irregularities during the OSCE so that there is good documentation for lessons learned and potential appeals.

Processing mark sheets

How mark sheets are processed varies with the scale of the OSCE and the resources available. For all but the smallest OSCE, some form of scanning and automated scoring is desirable. Whatever approach is used, analyse thoughtfully where mistakes could occur in the process and establish procedures to prevent such events. You will also need to decide how to deal with missing data to ensure consistency in resolving this problem. Work with an analyst so that the set-up of the data files is appropriate for test and item analyses, as well as for making pass/fail judgements. Automate as much as is feasible. Also, consider how to track information about items and examinees over time. Basic analyses can be done in software like Excel and there is a range of item banking applications available.

Reporting results

Long before you run the OSCE, decide what will be reported and to whom. Will there only be individual reports to examinees? Or only the pass/fail decision? Will there be feedback on how they performed by station? By station type? Relative to other examinees? Will there be a report to the institution? Knowing what will be reported creates the framework for formatting data and shapes the scoring analyses.

Appeals

Clarify what grounds for appeal are acceptable and what responses to complaints are appropriate. For instance, for a high stakes OSCE with a heavy investment in station development, the only grounds for appeal may be administrative error that disadvantages an examinee or a group of examinees. If the problem is localized to a station, or portion of a station, then one solution is to remove the invalid component and assess pass/fail standing on the remaining examination. If there is error and it cannot be localized, then the examination may be invalid and reassessment will be required.

Conclusions

◆ The OSCE is a performance-based examination format that can be used for formative or summative purposes. It allows for direct observation of a relatively large sample of clinical skills that are scored by multiple raters using standardised scoring sheets. Many authors consider it the gold standard for performance assessment.

◆ Standardized or simulated patients are essential to the OSCE. They are able to provide realistic portrayals of real patients, thus increasing the authenticity of this form of simulation.

◆ Checklists are usually station-specific and are useful for assessing structured tasks and assessing more junior trainees. Rating scales tend to be station-independent and measure general areas of competence. Global rating scales produce reliable scores and better distinguish experts from novices.

◆ Raters can be physicians, standardized patients or trained paramedical personnel. The choice will depend on the purpose of the examination and local resources. Rater training requirements are usually greater for non-physicians and when rating scales are used.

◆ Running an OSCE requires substantial effort and planning. When done well, it can provide invaluable assessment data on individual examinees, provide an opportunity for direct observation and feedback, and examination results can inform future curricular development.

Acknowledgement

We would like to acknowledge the support of the Academy for Innovation in Medical Education, University of Ottawa and its founder, the late Dr Meridith Marks (1962–2012).

References

Arnold, R.C., and Walmsley, A.D. (2008) The use of the OSCE in postgraduate education. *Eur Educ Dent Educ.* 12: 126–130

Barrows, H.S. (1968) Simulated patients in medical teaching. *Can Med Ass J.* 98: 674–676

Boulet, J.R., McKinley, D.W., Norcini, J.J., and Whelan, G.P. (2002) Assessing the comparability of standardized patient and physician evaluations of clinical skills. *Adv Health Sci Educ Theory Pract.* 7: 85–97

Boulet, J.R., De Champlain, A.F., and McKinley, D.W. (2003a) Setting defensible performance standards on OSCEs and standardized patient examinations. *Med Teach.* 25: 245–249

Boulet, J.R., McKinley, D.W., Whelan, G.P., and Hambleton, R.K. (2003b) Quality assurance methods for performance-based assessments. *Adv Health Sci Educ Theory Pract.* 8: 27–47

Boulet, J.R., Rebbecchi, T.A., Denton, E.C., McKinley, D.W., and Whelan, G.P. (2004) Assessing the written communication skills of medical school graduates. *Adv Health Sci Educ Theory Pract.* 9: 47–60

Boulet, J.R., Smee, S.M., Dillon, G.F., and Gimpel, J.R. (2009) The use of standardized patient assessments for certification and licensure decisions. *Simul Healthcare.* 4: 35–42

Brannick, M.T., Erol-Korkmaz, H.T., and Prewett, M. (2011) A systematic review of the reliability of objective structured clinical examination scores, *Med Educ.* 45: 1181–1189.

Brazeau, C., Boyd, L., and Crosson, J. (2002) Changing an existing OSCE to a teaching tool: the making of a teaching OSCE. *Acad Med.* 77: 932

Cadieux, G., Abrahamowicz, M., Dauphinee, D., and Tamblyn, R. (2011) Are physicians with better clinical skills on licensing examinations less likely to prescribe antibiotics for viral respiratory infections in ambulatory care settings? *Med Care.* 49: 156–165

Carson, J.A., Peets, A., Grant, V., and McLaughlin, K. (2010) The effect of gender interactions on students' physical examination ratings in objective structured clinical examination stations. *Acad. Med.* 85: 1772–1776

Chenot, J.F., Simmenroth-Nayda, A., Koch, A. et al. (2007) Can student tutors act as examiners in an objective structured clinical examination? *Med Educ.* 41: 1032–1038

Clarke, R.M. (2009) Criterion-referencing: the baby and the bathwater. *BMJ.* [Online] http://www.bmj.com/content/338/bmj.b690/reply# bmj_el_209927?sid=c01598e6-7fa7-4552-bbff-d3bc10847fd9 Accessed 11 March 2013

Clauser, B.E., Harik, P., Margolis, M.J., Mee, J., Swygert, K., and Rebbecchi, T. (2008) The generalizability of documentation scores from the USMLE Step 2 Clinical Skills examination. *Acad Med.* 83(10 Suppl): S41–S44

Cohen, R., Rothman, A.I., Ross, J., and Poldre, P. (1993) Impact of repeated use of objective structured clinical examination stations. *Acad Med.* 68(10 Suppl): S73–S75

Cunnington, J.P., Hanna, E., Turnhbull, J., Kaigas, T.B., and Norman, G.R. (1997) Defensible assessment of the competency of the practicing physician. *Acad Med.* 72: 9–12

Cushing, A., Abbott, S., Lothian, D., Hall, A., and Westwood, O.M. (2011) Peer feedback as an aid to learning—what do we want? Feedback. When do we want it? Now! *Med Teach.* 33: e105–e112

Cusimano, M.D. (1996) Standard setting in medical education. *Acad Med.* 71(10 Suppl): S112–S120

Cusimano, M.D. and Rothman, A.I. (2004) Consistency of standards and stability of pass/fail decisions with examinee-based standard-setting methods in a small-scale objective structured clinical examination. *Acad Med.* 79(10 Suppl): S25–S27

Dauphinee, W.D., Blackmore, D.E., Smee, S., Rothman, A.I., and Reznick, R. (1997) judgments of physician examiners in setting the standards for a national multi-center high stakes OSCE. *Adv Health Sci Educ Theory Pract.* 2: 201–211

De Champlain, A.F., Margolis, M.J., King, A., and Klass, D.J. (1997) Standardized patients' accuracy in recording examinees' behaviors using checklists. *Acad Med.* 72(10 Suppl): S85–S87

De Champlain, A.F., Macmillan, M.K., Margolis, M.J., Klass, D.J., Lewis, E., and Ahearn, S. (2000) Modeling the effects of a test security breach on a large-scale standardized patient examination with a sample of international medical graduates. *Acad Med.* 75(10 Suppl): S109–S111

Downing, S.M. and Haladyna, T.M. (2004) Validity threats: overcoming interference with proposed interpretations of assessment data. *Med Educ.* 38: 327–333

Downing, S.M., Tekian, A., and Yudkowsky, R. (2006) Procedures for establishing defensible absolute passing scores on performance examinations in health professions education. *Teach Learn Med.* 18: 50–57

Eva, K.W., Rosenfeld, J., Reiter, H.I., and Norman, G.R. (2004) An admissions OSCE: the multiple mini-interview. *Med Educ.* 38: 314–326

Eva, K.W., Wood, T.J., Riddle, J., Touchie, C., and Bordage, G. (2010) How clinical features are presented matters to weaker diagnosticians. *Med Educ.* 44: 775–785

Friedlich, M., Wood, T., Regehr, G., Hurst, C., and Shamji, F. (2002) Structured assessment of minor surgical skills (SAMSS) for clinical clerks. *Acad Med.* 77(10 Suppl): S39–S41

Furman, G.E., Colliver, J.A., Galofre, A., Reaka, M.A., Robbs, R.S., and King, A. (1997) The effect of formal feedback sessions on test security for a clinical practice examination using standardized patients. *Adv Health Sci Educ Theory Pract.* 2: 3–7

Govaerts, M.J., van der Vleuten, C.P., and Schuwirth, L.W. (2002) Optimizing the reproducibility of a performance-based assessment test in midwifery education. *Adv Health Sci Educ Theory Pract.* 7: 133–145

Grand'Maison, P., Brailovsky, C.A., and Lescop, J. (1996) Content validity of the Quebec licensing examination (OSCE). Assessed by practising physicians. *CanFam Physician Medecin de famille canadien.* 42: 254–259

Hall, P., Marshall, D., Weaver, L., Boyle, A., and Taniguchi, A. (2011) A method to enhance student teams in palliative care: piloting the McMaster-Ottawa Team Observed Structured Clinical Encounter. *J Palliative Med.* 14: 744–750

Harden, R.M., Stevenson, M., Downie, W.W., and Wilson, G.M. (1975) Assessment of clinical competence using objective structured examination. *BMJ.* 1: 447–451

Hatala, R., Marr, S., Cuncic, C., and Bacchus, C.M. (2011) Modification of an OSCE format to enhance patient continuity in a high-stakes assessment of clinical performance. *BMC Med Educ.* 11: 23

Hodder, R.V., Rivington, R.N., Calcutt, L.E., and Hart, I.R. (1989) The effectiveness of immediate feedback during the objective structured clinical examination. *Med Educ.* 23: 184–188

Hodges, B. (2003) Validity and the OSCE. *Med Teach.* 25: 250–254

Hodges, B., Regehr, G., McNaughton, N., Tiberius, R., and Hanson, M. (1999) OSCE checklists do not capture increasing levels of expertise. *Acad Med.* 74: 1129–1134

Humphrey-Murto, S. and MacFadyen, J.C. (2002) Standard setting: a comparison of case-author and modified borderline-group methods in a small-scale OSCE. *Acad Med.* 77: 729–732

Humphrey-Murto, S., Smee, S., Touchie, C., Wood, T.J., and Blackmore, D.E. (2005) A comparison of physician examiners and trained assessors in a high-stakes OSCE setting. *Acad Med.* 80 (10 Suppl): S59–S62

Humphrey-Murto, S., Touchie, C., Wood, T.J., and Smee, S. (2009) Does the gender of the standardised patient influence candidate performance in an objective structured clinical examination? *Med Educ.* 43: 521–525

Kahraman, N., Clauser, B.E., and Margolis, M.J. (2008) A comparison of alternative item weighting strategies on the data gathering component of a clinical skills performance assessment. *Acad Med.* 83(10 Suppl): S72–S75

Ker, J.S., Dowie, A., Dowell, J. et al. (2005) Twelve tips for developing and maintaining a simulated patient bank. *Med Teach.* 27: 4–9

Khan, J., Rooney, K., Prosciak, C., Javadpoor, A., and Rooney, P.J. (1997) Effect of immediate feedback on performance on subsequent stations during an objective structured clinical examination. *Educ Health.* 20: 351–357

Kneebone, R., Nestel, D., Yadollahi, F., et al. (2006) Assessing procedural skills in context: exploring the feasibility of an integrated procedural performance instrument (IPPI). *Med Educ.* 40: 1105–1114

Martin, J.A., Regehr, G., Reznick, R., et al. (1997) Objective structured assessment of technical skill (OSATS) for surgical residents. *Br J Surg.* 84: 273–278

Martin, J.A., Reznick, R.K., Rothman, A., Tamblyn, R.M., and Regehr, G. (1996) Who should rate candidates in an objective structured clinical examination? *Acad Med.* 71: 170–175

Miller, G.E. (1990) The assessment of clinical skills/competence/performance. *Acad Med.* 65(9 Suppl): S63–S67

Moineau, G., Power, B., Pion, A.M., Wood, T.J., and Humphrey-Murto, S. (2011) Comparison of student examiner to faculty examiner scoring and feedback in an OSCE. *Med Educ.* 45: 183–191

Niehaus, A.H., DaRosa, D.A., Markwell, S.J., and Folse, R. (1996) Is test security a concern when OSCE stations are repeated across clerkship rotations? *Acad Med.* 71: 287–289

Norcini, J.J. (1994) Research on standards for professional licensure and certification examinations. *Eval Health Prof.* 17: 160–177

Pangaro, L.N., Worth-Dickstein, H., Macmillan, M.K., Klass, D.J., and Shatzer, J.H. (1997) Performance of 'standardized examinees' in a standardized-patient examination of clinical skills. *Acad Med.* 72: 1008–1011

Payne, N.J., Bradley, E.B., and Heald, E.B., et al. (2008) Sharpening the eye of the OSCE with critical action analysis. *Acad Med.* 83: 900–905

Peitzman, S.J. (2001) Physical diagnosis findings among persons applying to work as standardized patients. *Acad Med.* 76: 383

Petrusa, E.R. (2002) Clinical performance assessments. In: D. Newble, G.R. Norman, and C. van der Vleuten (eds) *International Handbook of Research in Medical Education* (pp. 678–693). Norwell: Kluwer Academic Publishers

Regehr, G., Freeman, R., Hodges, B. and Russell, L. (1999) Assessing the generalizability of OSCE measures across content domains. *Acad Med.* 74: 1320–1322

Reiter, H.I., Rosenfeld, J., Nandagopal, K., and Eva, K.W. (2004) Do clinical clerks provide candidates with adequate formative assessment during Objective Structured Clinical Examinations? *Adv Health Sci Educ Theory Pract.* 9: 189–199

Reznick, R.K., Smee, S., Baumber, J.S., et al. (1993) Guidelines for estimating the real cost of an objective structured clinical examination. *Acad Med.* 68(7): 513–517

Reznick, R.K., Blackmore, D., Dauphinee, W.D., Rothman, A.I., and Smee, S. (1996) Large-scale high-stakes testing with an OSCE: report from the Medical Council of Canada. *Acad Med.* 71(1 Suppl): S19–S21

Ruesseler, M., Weinlich, M., Byhahn, C., et al (2010) Increased authenticity in practical assessment using emergency case OSCE stations. *Adv Health Sci Educ Theory Pract.* 15: 81–95

Russell, L.B. and Hubley, A.M. (2005) Importance ratings and weighting: old concerns and new perspectives. *Int J Testing.* 5: 105–130

Schirmer, J.M., Maatsch, L., Lang, F., et al. (2005) Assessing communication competence: a review of current tools. *Fam Med.* 37: 184–192

Schoonheim-Klein, M., Muijtjens, A., Habets, L., et al. (2008) On the reliability of a dental OSCE, using SEM: effect of different days. *Eur J Dent Educ.* 12: 131–137

Smee, S.M. (2007) Comparing scoring instruments for the performance assessment of professional competencies, PhD thesis, University of Ottawa

Stillman, P., Swanson, D., Regan, M.B., et al. (1991a) Assessment of clinical skills of residents utilizing standardized patients. A follow-up study and recommendations for application. *Ann Intern Med.* 114: 393–401

Stillman, P.L., Haley, H.L., Sutnick, A.I., et al. (1991b) Is test security an issue in a multistation clinical assessment? A preliminary study. *Acad Med.* 66(9 Suppl): S25–S27

Swanson, D. and Norcini, J. (1989) Factors influencing the reproducibility of tests using standardized patients. *TeachLearn Med.* 1: 158–166

Swartz, M.H., Colliver, J.A., Cohen, D.S., and Barrows, H.S. (1993) The effect of deliberate, excessive violations of test security on performance on a standardized-patient examination. *Acad Med.* 68(10 Suppl): S76–S78

Swygert, K.A., Balog, K.P., and Jobe, A. (2010) The impact of repeat information on examinee performance for a large-scale standardized-patient examination. *Acad Med.* 85: 1506–1510

Tamblyn, R., Abrahamowicz, M., Dauphinee, D., et al. (2007) Physician scores on a national clinical skills examination as predictors of complaints to medical regulatory authorities. *JAMA.* 298: 993–1001

Tamblyn, R., Abrahamowicz, M., Dauphinee, D., et al. (2010) Influence of physicians' management and communication ability on patients' persistence with antihypertensive medication. *Arch Intern Med.* 170: 1064–1072

Tamblyn, R.M., Klass, D.J., Schnabl, G.K., and Kopelow, M.L. (1991) The accuracy of standardized patient presentation. *Med Educ.* 25: 100–109

Touchie, C., Humphrey-Murto, S., Ainslie, M., Myers, K., and Wood, T.J. (2010) Two models of raters in a structured oral examination: does it make a difference? *Adv Health Sci Educ Theory Pract.* 15: 97–108

van der Vleuten, C.P.M. and Swanson, D.B. (1990) Assessment of clinical skills with standardized patients: State of the art. *Teach Learn Med.* 2: 58–76

van der Vleuten, C.P., van Luyk, S.J., van Ballegooijen, A.M., and Swanson, D.B. (1989) Training and experience of examiners. *Med Educ.* 23: 290–296

Vargas, A.L., Boulet, J.R., Errichetti, A., van Zanten, M., Lopez, M.J., and Reta, A.M. (2007) Developing performance-based medical school assessment programs in resource-limited environments. *Med Teach.* 29: 192–198

Varkey, P. and Natt, N. (2007) The objective structured clinical examination as an educational tool in patient safety. *J Comm J Qual Patient Saf.* 33: 48–53

Verma, A., Bhatt, H., Booton, P., and Kneebone, R. (2011) The Ventriloscope (R) as an innovative tool for assessing clinical examination skills: appraisal of a novel method of simulating auscultatory findings. *Med Teach.* 33: e388–e396

Vu, N.V., Marcy, M.M., Colliver, J.A., Verhulst, S.J., Travis, T.A., and Barrows, H.S. (1992) Standardized (simulated) patients' accuracy in recording clinical performance check-list items. *Med Educ.* 26: 99–104

Wagner, D.P., Hoppe, R.B., and Lee, C.P. (2009) The patient safety OSCE for PGY-1 residents: a centralized response to the challenge of culture change. *Teach Learn Med.* 21: 8–14

Wendling, A.L., Halan, S., Tighe, P., Le, L., Euliano, T., and Lok, B. (2011) Virtual humans versus standardized patients: which lead residents to more correct diagnoses? *Acad Med.* 86: 384–388

Wenghofer, E., Klass, D., Abrahamowicz, M., et al. (2009) Doctor scores on national qualifying examinations predict quality of care in future practice. *Med Educ.* 43: 1166–1173

Wilkinson, T.J., Fontaine, S., and Egan, T. (2003) Was a breach of examination security unfair in an objective structured clinical examination? A critical incident. *Med Teach.* 25: 42–46

Wilkinson, T.J., Newble, D.I., and Frampton, C.M. (2001) Standard setting in an objective structured clinical examination: use of global ratings of borderline performance to determine the passing score. *Med Educ.* 35: 1043–1049

Williams, R., Miler, R., Shah, B., et al. (2011) Observing handoffs and telephone management in GI fellowship training. *Am J Gastroenterol.* 106: 1410–1414

Williams, R.G. (2004) Have standardized patient examinations stood the test of time and experience? *Teach Learn Med.* 16: 215–222

Wood, T.J., Humphrey-Murto, S.M., and Norman, G.R. (2006) Standard setting in a small scale OSCE: a comparison of the Modified Borderline-Group Method and the Borderline Regression Method. *Adv Health Sci Educ Theory Pract.* 11: 115–122

Yudkowsky, R. (2009) Performance tests. In: S.M. Downing, and R. Yudkowsky, (eds) *Assessment in Health Professions Education* (pp. 223–226). New York: Routledge

CHAPTER 46

Workplace based assessment

Gominda Ponnamperuma

In order to build up a picture of an individual doctor's performance, it is helpful to make multiple 'snapshot' assessments of different real clinical problems encountered in the workplace.

Robert Clarke

Reproduced from Clarke R, 'Foundation programme assessments in general practice', Education for Primary Care, 17, p. 291, © Radcliffe Publishing, 2006, with permission

Introduction

Workplace-based assessment (WBA) refers to a broad category of examinations conducted using the *resources* available in the candidate's *workplace*, during the course of their usual work schedule. The resources include patients, clinical supervisors, equipment (e.g. intravenous cannulae), peers (i.e. fellow trainees), and other healthcare professionals (e.g. nurses). The workplace includes clinics, wards, surgical theatres, laboratories and even the community, in which the doctors carry out their day-to-day professional duties.

There are two basic categories of WBA:

1. Assessment based on observation—these use 'assessment forms', filled-in by the assessors (ranging from clinical supervisors to patients), to collect data about the candidate in the workplace. They can be further divided into two sub-categories depending on the number of observations or assessor–assessee encounters necessary per assessment form:

    a. Rating based on a single observation or assessor–assessee encounter; e.g. mini-clinical evaluation exercise (mini-CEX), direct observation of procedural skills (DOPS), case-based discussion (CBD).

    b. Rating based on multiple observations or several assessor–assessee encounters; e.g. mini-peer assessment tool (mini-PAT), patient surveys. These are also called multisource feedback (MSF).

2. Assessment based on accumulation and documentation of evidence—these provide a structured framework for a repository that collates evidence for achievement of curricular competencies or learning outcomes; e.g. logbooks.

Figure 46.1 illustrates this classification.

This chapter first discusses the educational rationale of WBA, and the basic tools used in WBA. Then, the key features of the individual WBA instruments are considered. Finally, the utility of the WBA instruments is evaluated and some specific issues related to WBA are discussed.

The educational rationale

All assessment can be conceptualized into four levels: knows, knows how, shows how, and does (Miller 1990). The lower two levels assess knowledge. The lowest level assesses recall of knowledge (knows), while the second level assesses application of knowledge (knows how). The next two levels assess behaviour. 'Shows how' assesses 'simulated' behaviour, while 'does' assesses 'naturalistic, real-life, practice-based' performance. WBA represents the 'does' level.

Miller (1990) argues that to determine the ability of a candidate, one has to assess all four levels, as each level provides a distinct aspect of candidate ability. Notwithstanding the importance of all four levels, the 'does' level or real-life performance denotes the ultimate aim of learning.

Studies have shown that there is a 'skill loss' when one moves from 'shows how' to 'does' level (Rethans et al. 1991; Kopelow et al. 1992). So, unless trainees are assessed at 'does' level this loss of ability cannot be accounted for. Hence, to certify that a healthcare professional is fit-for-practice, the unique blend of knowledge, skills, and attitudes that goes into the performance in the workplace needs to be assessed.

WBA tools

Before discussing the assessment instruments used in WBA, it is important to understand the basic tools used within the assessment instruments or forms. An assessment form can comprise two basic tools: checklists and ratings scales.

Checklists

The purpose of a checklist is to record whether the steps of a procedure (e.g. venepuncture) or an event (e.g. taking informed consent)

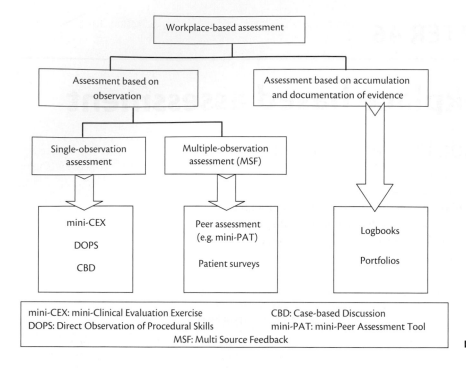

mini-CEX: mini-Clinical Evaluation Exercise   CBD: Case-based Discussion
DOPS: Direct Observation of Procedural Skills   mini-PAT: mini-Peer Assessment Tool
                        MSF: Multi Source Feedback

Figure 46.1 Workplace-based assessment.

have been followed. It does not assess the quality to which each step is carried out. So, it is a 'yes/no' decision that the assessors record by ticking or encircling the checklist item corresponding to a given step of a procedure.

Rating scales

The purpose of a rating scale is to grade the *quality* to which the steps of a procedure or event take place. Rating scales may have a variable number of rating points ranging typically from 3 to 11, with one end of the scale representing low performance and the other high performance. Each rating point (e.g. '3' in a 5-point scale) or each cluster of adjacent rating points (e.g. '9' and '10' in a 10-point scale) may have a label, such as 'average' or 'excellent'. Further, each label may have an 'anchoring descriptor' that describes the trainee performance required to achieve a given rating point; e.g. a descriptor for 'excellent' may be 'performs all the steps of the procedure, in correct sequence without any external help'. The configuration of rating points, labels and descriptors is called 'rating rubrics'. The assessors are required to select the most appropriate rating point that fits the trainee performance.

An assessment form may have one or more rating scales, each assessing the trainee performance on a competency such as clinical skills or communication skills. In addition, there may be a global rating scale that assesses the trainee's overall performance; i.e. did the candidate combine all the competencies into a single act? Evidence indicates that global ratings are more valid and reliable than checklists (Hodges and McIlroy 2003; Goff et al. 2002; Norman 2005).

The nature of judgement in WBA requires the assessor to record the occurrence, quality, and/or fitness related to the behaviour under assessment (Norcini 2010). The first (i.e. occurrence of behaviour) can be recorded using a checklist. The second (i.e. quality of behaviour), as a rule, should be recorded using rating scale(s).

The third (i.e. fitness-to-practise at a given level of training) can be recorded using either checklists or rating scales, depending on whether a simple 'yes/no' decision or a graded decision is required; e.g. descriptors of a three-point scale that assesses 'fitness-to-practise' may be: fit to practise independently; fit to practise with the supervisor out-of-site; fit to practise with the supervisor on-site.

WBA assessment instruments

A description of the commonly used WBA instruments based on the key questions that one should ask regarding any assessment (Harden 1979) now follows.

Assessment based on observation: rating based on a single observation

Mini-CEX

The mini-CEX assesses the trainee's ability to take a brief, focused history or to carry out the relevant physical examination of a patient that they may encounter during their routine training.

What

What is assessed by any assessment can be broadly divided into *competencies* and *content*. These constitute the two basic dimensions of an assessment blueprint (Hamdy 2006).

The mini-CEX assesses competencies such as: history taking; physical examination; communication skills; clinical reasoning; professionalism; and organizational ability. In addition, there is an opportunity to assess the overall ability of the trainee through a global rating.

Norcini et al. (2003) observe that the content of mini-CEX includes: *presenting complaints* such as abdominal or chest pain; and *disease conditions* such as arthritis or asthma. In addition, the mini-CEX can focus on a *body system* (e.g. cardiovascular system). If so, it is commoner and perhaps more feasible, given the time constraints, to assess only a part rather than the entire body system; e.g. auscultating the heart instead of examining the cardiovascular system.

Why

To answer this question more comprehensively, it is useful to look at the history of mini-CEX. In 1972, when the American Board of Internal Medicine (ABIM) abandoned its oral examination, it requested its programme directors to conduct an examination called clinical evaluation exercise (CEX). The CEX involved taking a full history and carrying out a full physical examination of a single patient to reach diagnostic and therapeutic conclusions (Norcini et al. 2003). The trainee was observed and assessed by a single assessor, and the examination took 2 hours (Day et al. 1990). The time that the CEX consumed per encounter was thus too long to be repeated frequently. Hence, the CEX was essentially a 'structured, observed long case' (Ponnamperuma et al. 2009). Soon the ABIM realized that this assessment was not generalizable as it was dependent on a single patient encounter with a single examiner; i.e. the examination could not provide a reasonable estimate about the trainee performance, beyond the encounter assessed (Noel et al. 1992; Kroboth et al. 1992). This led to the introduction of mini-CEX, which essentially was the traditional CEX, but with the ability to sample the trainee performance more widely, mainly due to the shorter time span it consumes. This makes the mini-CEX capable of being carried out many times, with more patient encounters, with different examiners, and more frequently. So, the answer to the question 'why mini-CEX' is to assess the trainees' clinical ability in the workplace, based on many patient encounters, by many examiners, over a long period of time.

How

The mini-CEX assesses trainees on a brief clinical encounter lasting around 15 to 20 minutes (Norcini et al. 2003). The trainee at the end of the encounter summarizes the findings and outlines the next steps of management. An examiner observes and scores the trainee performance using a structured assessment form. A further 5 minutes is spent giving feedback to the trainee by the trainer/examiner, based on the observations made. The patient and the timing of assessment are decided by the trainee or trainer (Norcini 2010).

The rating scale used is a Likert type scale. In the original version of the mini-CEX, developed for the ABIM, the trainer rates the trainee on each of the competencies detailed under 'what', using a nine-point scale. On this scale, the ratings 1 to 3 are labelled as 'unsatisfactory', 4 to 6 as 'satisfactory', and 7 to 9 as 'superior'. Each label accompanies a specific descriptor that details the behaviour expected of a trainee (Norcini et al. 1995).

Each competency on which a candidate is assessed is explicitly described in terms of the expected positive behaviour (i.e. the best possible behaviour). For example, the mini-CEX in the UK Foundation Programme describes 'history taking' as 'facilitates patient telling their story; effectively uses appropriate questions to obtain accurate, adequate information; responds appropriately to verbal and non-verbal cues' (The Foundation Programme 2012).

There is also space to record if a competency has not been observed by the trainer during a given encounter. Trainees are advised to complete on average four to six forms per year. The ratings for individual competencies are then aggregated across encounters to obtain an aggregate score for a given competency of a trainee (Norcini et al. 1995).

Apart from the numerical ratings, there is space to record qualitative feedback. For example, in the UK Foundation Programme, the trainer could fill-in the boxes on 'anything especially good',

'suggestions for development', and 'agreed action'. The form also has specific boxes to record the clinical setting, clinical problem category, focus of the clinical encounter, complexity of the problem, and the number of times the trainee has seen the patient. Finally, there are boxes to document assessor and assessee information, and certain logistical considerations, such as the time spent on the encounter.

Where

A variety of settings such as inpatient, outpatient, accident and emergency department, or any other relevant setting, can be used (Norcini et al. 1995). Though there is no evidence as yet, 'any other setting' could be interpreted to include even 'community settings'. If one expands the scope of 'where', there are also reports that mini-CEX has been used successfully both in the undergraduate (Kogan et al. 2002, 2003; Driessen et al. 2012) and postgraduate (Norcini et al. 1995; Holmboe et al. 2004a) settings. Wilkinson et al. (2008), however, have shown through a significantly higher mean inpatient than outpatient rating that the setting may have an effect on the ratings.

When

The mini-CEX should be performed throughout the year. If four to six encounters are completed (Norcini 2010), it is advisable to perform them with adequate spacing between encounters, as this provides the trainee sufficient time to improve their performance based on the feedback of the previous encounter. Further, such spacing can sample the trainee performance throughout the year, rather than during a certain part of the year.

By whom

Given the type of judgements necessary to fill-in the mini-CEX form, it is obvious, that the assessor needs to possess superior technical skills. Thus, depending on the stage of training of the trainee, the assessor should be either at a higher stage of training or a person who has completed training (fig. 46.2). For example, when trainees are at the lowest stage of training, the assessors can be consultants, general practitioners (GPs), senior trainees, or middle grade doctors. However, there is evidence that the ratings given by the consultants are lower than those given by the residents (Torre et al. 2007; Kogan et al. 2003). In light of this finding, two guidelines for selecting assessors can be recommended. First, each candidate needs to maintain a healthy balance of assessors, representing various levels of experience. Second, all the trainers, irrespective of their experience, should be trained in using the mini-CEX. Not

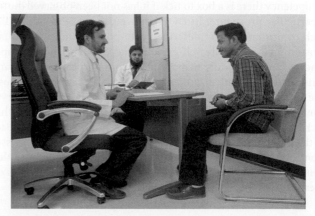

Figure 46.2 Workplace based assessment in action.

only should they be trained in assessment, they should also be trained in giving feedback (Holmboe et al. 2004b).

DOPS

DOPS is designed to assess the ability to perform practical procedures. Various disciplines have named this type of assessment differently. In surgical specialties it is called procedure-based assessment (PBA) (Thornton et al. 2003; Burt et al. 2003), and in obstetrics and gynaecology it is called objective structured assessment of technical skills (OSATS) (Goff et al. 2000, 2002; Swift and Carter 2006).

What

The procedures such as venepuncture or lumbar puncture on which the trainees need to be assessed are usually pre-identified by the relevant curricula. For example, the Royal College of Paediatrics and Child Health has identified 28 practical procedures that the trainees should complete (RCPCH 2011). Similarly, The Foundation Programme (2012) in the UK has listed 15 procedures. Wilkinson et al. (2008) note, however, that the procedures, though widely variable, do not have a significant impact on the assessment result. These procedures are the *content* of assessment. The criteria on which the observations are made when assessing each of these procedures are the competencies. For example, the procedures of the UK Foundation Programme (2012) are judged on a variety of competencies, from demonstrating understanding of indications to the actual technique of the procedure.

Why

This assessment has been developed to assess the procedural skills of the trainee through direct observation (Wragg et al. 2003) and to provide feedback on those skills.

How

Since DOPS is a variation of mini-CEX (Norcini, 2010), how the assessment is conducted is similar to that described under mini-CEX. In most instances, it is trainee-driven in that the trainee decides the timing and the procedure to be assessed. The trainees, however, are required to select the procedures recommended by the curriculum. The time spent for a single DOPS encounter, depends on the procedure. In a study by Wilkinson et al. (2008), the time taken for a DOPS encounter ranged from 1 to 75 minutes, with a median of 5 minutes. The feedback time was approximately 20 to 30% of the time taken for the procedure.

Each of the competencies assessed in the UK Foundation Programme (2012) is rated on a six-point scale, categorized and labelled to represent different levels of ability. Also, for a given competency there is a box to tick if it has not been observed during a particular procedure. In DOPS, however, unlike in mini-CEX, each competency is not described with positive indicators. Since most competencies are self-explanatory, only the three competencies, 'post procedure management, communication skills, and consideration of patient/professionalism', are described with positive indicators. When collating the decisions of individual observations, the numerical ratings are averaged for a given trainee within each competency. Apart from the numerical ratings, there is space in the DOPS assessment form to document assessor and assessee identification details, the clinical setting, and the procedure that is assessed. There is also a box to record qualitative comments on 'areas of strength and any suggested development'.

Where

The settings in which DOPS can be performed are: ward; accident and emergency department; outpatient department; general practice surgery; and specialty clinics.

When

Similar to mini-CEX, it is recommended to space DOPS appropriately so that this gives sufficient time for the trainee to improve their performance before the next DOPS encounter. Certain programmes recommend that the trainees be assessed frequently throughout the year (Norcini 2010). Wilkinson et al. (2008) have found that two to three encounters per year are sufficient.

By whom

Given that both mini-CEX and DOPS assess technical abilities, the assessor qualities required for DOPS are similar to those for mini-CEX. However, apart from the assessors mentioned under mini-CEX, DOPS also uses nurses, depending on their familiarity with the skill that is being assessed (RCPCH 2011; Norcini 2010).

CBD

Similar to the original version of chart-stimulated recall (CSR) developed by Maatsch et al. (1983) for the American Board of Emergency Medicine, CBD assesses trainee performance based on the patients that they have clerked, treated, and followed up.

What

In the UK Foundation Programme (2012), CBD assesses candidates on a wide variety of conditions. The competencies assessed are: medical record keeping; clinical assessment; investigation and referrals; treatment; follow-up and future planning; and professionalism.

Why

Although the content of assessment may change from specialty to specialty, the competencies assessed, by and large, remain the same across specialties: e.g. reasoning, application of knowledge, and decision making (Norcini 2010).

How

Like the previous assessment instruments, this also is mainly trainee driven, as the trainee decides the timing. However, it is up to the assessor to select one or two records randomly from the records that the trainee has collected. Based on the record(s), usually a particular aspect of management, such as patient investigations or ethical issues, is selected. Then the assessor explores by questioning the reasons as to why the trainee managed the patient in a given way, and rates the candidate on a multitude of competencies, similar to those described under 'what'. On average, a CBD encounter takes around 15 minutes with a further 5 minutes for feedback (Norcini 2010). As with other WBA, ratings per candidate are averaged per competency.

Where

The setting, to an extent, depends on the specialty. For example, in obstetrics, CBD is performed in the antenatal clinic, antenatal ward, labour ward, postnatal ward, and assessment unit (RCOG, 2012), whereas in the UK Foundation Programme (2012), CBD is carried out in a wide variety of settings.

When

In the UK Foundation Programme, the trainees are advised to complete four to six encounters per year (Norcini 2010). As with other instruments these should be appropriately spaced so that they capture performance over the year.

By whom

Like in mini-CEX, CBD is assessed by consultants, senior trainees, and middle grade doctors—depending on the candidate's stage of training (Norcini 2010).

Assessment based on observation: rating based on multiple observations

Previously known as 360-degree assessment (Whitehouse et al. 2002), this category of assessment as a group is now known as MSF. MSF collects information about the trainee from many sources. These sources can be divided into two groups: healthcare professionals (e.g. doctors and nurses); and patients that the trainee meets during their practice. Since the competencies on which the healthcare workers and patients can comment are different it is customary to collect data from the healthcare workers using the same instrument, while different instruments are used for patients. Hence, this chapter considers the former as peer assessment (PA) and the latter as patient surveys separately.

Peer assessment (mini-PAT)

There is a plethora of instruments used to collect data from healthcare workers. To name a few:

- Physician Achievement Review—PAR (Violato et al. 1997)

- Team Observation Form of the Royal College of Obstetricians and Gynaecologists (RCOG 2012)

- mini-Peer Assessment Tool—mini-PAT (Archer et al. 2008)

- SPRAT—Sheffield Peer Review Assessment Tool (Archer et al. 2005)

- Team Assessment of Behaviours—TAB (Whitehouse et al. 2007), used by the College of Physicians and Surgeons of Alberta , Canada (Lockyer 2003), and

- Appraisal and Assessment Instrument—AAI (Geeraerts and Hoofwijk 2006; Overeem et al. 2010), used in the Netherlands, is of particular interest as this is a method entirely based on qualitative information (Overeem et al. 2010).

Since all these instruments cannot be described individually, mini-PAT is described as a prototype.

What

The assessment *content*, not only for mini-PAT, but for any MSF instrument, is selected from the routine situations, during which the assessors interact with trainees. The *competencies*, though widely vary, are mostly based on soft skills (e.g. relationship with colleagues) with a few technical competencies (e.g. ability to diagnose a patient). Mini-PAT used in the UK Foundation Programme (2012) uses *Good Medical Practice* of the General Medical Council (GMC) as the competency framework (GMC 2006). Hence, the competencies that mini-PAT assesses are: good clinical care; maintaining good medical practice; teaching and training, appraising and assessing; relationship with patients; and working with colleagues.

Why

Unlike the technical skills, soft skills such as humanistic qualities cannot be assessed validly and reliably, entirely by the clinical supervisors. First, this is due to the inadequate contact time between the assessor and the assessee. Second, since the contact time is low, the trainee can fake certain desirable behaviours in the presence of the supervisor. Such artificial maintenance of behaviour is not possible all the time; i.e. when working with other healthcare workers. Third, certain skills are best judged by certain categories of personnel. For example, 'willingness and effectiveness when teaching/learning colleagues' is best assessed by those who learn from the trainee.

How

The competencies in the mini-PAT are further broken down into 15 items. They are assessed using the same six-point rating scale used in the DOPS. However, the competencies are not explained with positive indicators as in the other WBA instruments. The same scale is used to record the global rating of the assessor. As in the other instruments there is a box to tick if the assessor cannot comment on a given item. Finally, the assessors indicate, by marking 'yes' or 'no', whether they have any concerns about the doctor's probity and health, which are the other two broad aspects that the *Good Medical Practice* framework (GMC 2006) addresses. The trainees nominate eight assessors each year. The assessors send the filled-in forms to a central office, where they are collated. In addition, the trainees assess themselves on the same scale. Assessment data are aggregated by the competencies, and the processed results are sent to the supervisor. During a formal feedback session, the overall results are communicated to the trainee. Thus, the anonymity of the individual raters is maintained.

Where

The assessors can fill-in the forms at leisure, either in their office or at home. However, the assessment needs to be based on the professional contact that the assessor had with the trainee. MSF has been used in undergraduate (Arnold et al. 1981, Small et al. 1993), postgraduate (Whitehouse et al. 2002), and continuing professional development (Sargeant et al. 2005) settings.

When

The Foundation Programme (2012) recommends that a set number of forms be completed for each trainee per year (Davis et al. 2009b). These forms, unlike those in previously discussed instruments, need not be spaced out. They could be administered at the same time, preferably towards the end of the year, so that the assessors are given sufficient contact time, before they assess the trainee.

By whom

The assessors are consultants, senior trainees and middle grade doctors, GPs, nurses, or allied health personnel (Norcini 2010).

Patient surveys

Patient surveys, being a part of MSF, have similarities with mini-PAT. However, the patients generally have fewer encounters with the doctor than the peers do. Since ratings based on fewer encounters may be less valid and reliable, patient surveys usually require more assessors.

What

The content assessed is similar to that of mini-PAT. The broad competencies assessed are generally the same as in mini-PAT, as most patient questionnaires in the UK (Campbell et al. 2008) are based on the *Good Medical Practice* competencies (GMC 2006). However, the emphasis is more towards non-technical competencies, as the patients do not have the knowhow to assess technical skills.

Why

As discussed under mini-PAT patients are in the best position to assess certain competencies such as empathy and communication skills.

How

Patient surveys contain a variable number of items to collect quantitative and qualitative data using various rating scales and free text questions respectively. For example, the Consultation and Relational Empathy (CARE) form (Mercer et al. 2004, 2005), piloted with GPs in the UK, has 10 items to be rated on a five-point scale. Similarly, the patient survey piloted by Campbell et al. (2008) has 18 items, out of which nine require ratings on a Likert scale, while the others require 'yes/no' answers, free text or contextual data. However, the patient survey developed by the Joint Royal College of Physicians Training Board (JRCPTB) has all free text items (JRCPTB 2012). Trainees are advised by the JRCPTB to agree with the supervisor about the timing and the logistics of the survey. Once the time period of the survey is decided the trainees are advised to distribute questionnaires to 30 consecutive patients that they see (although the number of questionnaires required per trainee is 20, to allow for variability in the response rate the trainees are advised to distribute 30 questionnaires). Patients can opt not to fill in a questionnaire. If they do consent, however, they need to complete the questionnaire before they leave the premises. Patients can stay anonymous by delivering the completed questionnaire to another healthcare professional such as a nurse. At the end of each day, the trainee should return the completed questionnaires under sealed cover to a named consultant. Once 20 questionnaires are returned the trainee is supposed to book a meeting with the supervisor. The supervisor should then collate the information from the completed questionnaires and discuss the results with the trainee.

Where

Although the trainees can distribute questionnaires in any setting, it is usually done in outpatient settings.

When

Trainees are advised to administer the questionnaire consecutively over an agreed period of time, during a year. This is to preclude the trainee selecting patients who are favourable to them.

By whom

Patients are the sole assessors; and they should be selected for this purpose in an unbiased way, using consecutive sampling.

Differences between single and multiple observation WBAs

The main differences between the single and multiple observation WBA instruments are shown in table 46.1.

Despite these differences, most weaknesses of both categories of assessment are overcome by the same method; i.e. using multiple encounters and assessors. The unreliability of the 'snapshot' assessments in single observation WBA is countered by sampling through multiple such snapshots, using many assessors. The lack of objectivity and vagueness of MSF assessments are countered by

Table 46.1 Differences between the single and multiple observation WBA instruments

Assessment based on a single observation	Assessment based on multiple observations
Uses solitary, brief assessor-trainee encounters	Uses the assessors' knowledge about the trainee during many encounters over a period of time
Assesses both technical and non-technical skills, with perhaps more emphasis on technical knowledge and skills	Mostly concerned with non-technical skills
Requires clinical cases	Clinical cases not needed as the assessors comment on their previous interactions with the trainee
Generally assessed by those who are more experienced and technically proficient than the trainee	Assessors can be more and less experienced or technically proficient than the trainee
Uses structured rating scales with clear descriptors to score objective observations	Uses opinion or perception based questionnaires and these scales may not have descriptors for each rating point
More objective due to the: ◆ proximity of the encounter to the assessment ◆ technical nature of the competencies assessed ◆ assessors, who are more experienced and trained in assessment, being at a higher educational level ◆ utilization of tools that have detailed descriptors	Less objective due to the lack of the features detailed on the left.

collecting information from multiple assessors, who provide information based on multiple situations.

Assessment based on accumulation and documentation of evidence

The two instruments used to accumulate and document evidence are logbooks and portfolios.

Logbooks sequentially record the trainee achievement of various workplace tasks (e.g. procedures). Usually each task is signed-off by a supervisor to attest that the evidence is authentic.

Portfolios are 'a collection of student work, which provides evidence of the achievement of knowledge, skills, appropriate attitudes, and professional growth' (i.e. achievement of learning outcomes or core-competencies) 'through a process of self-reflection over a period of time' (Davis and Ponnamperuma 2009, p. 349).

Basically logbooks and portfolios collect the same evidence. The most significant difference, however, is that portfolio evidence is annotated by the learner's reflection (Davis and Ponnamperuma, 2005). Reflection can be defined as 'deliberate, purposive exploration of experience, undertaken in order to promote learning, personal and professional development, and improvement of practice' (Pee et al. 2002).

Highlighting the key role that reflection plays in portfolio development, Challis (1999) notes that 'the portfolio's purpose is to demonstrate learning, not to chronicle a series of experiences. Learning from experience will only happen once reflection and application of resulting modifications in practice have taken place. It is evidence of how the learning has been, or will be applied that will form the basis of the review or assessment'. Of the various models available for reflection, the cyclical model promoted by Kolb and Fry (Kolb 1984) provides a simple framework to achieve the kind of learning that involves 'modifications in practice' that Challis (1999) refers to.

Since logbooks and portfolios share similar features, both can be considered as the two extremes of the same continuum. The degree to which a logbook differentiates from a portfolio is determined by the extent to which *reflection* has been incorporated into the evidence for learning. Thus, evidence from logbooks is often included in portfolios. Hence, both portfolios and logbooks are discussed together under the broad, inclusive term 'portfolios'.

Portfolios
What

A portfolio is used to show evidence of the trainee's progression towards the achievement of the *competencies* identified by the course. The *content* that is included in the portfolio to show such achievement varies widely (Friedman Ben-David et al. 2001). For example, a postgraduate portfolio could include: curriculum vitae of the learner; results of the WBA instruments discussed previously; case reports of patients; patient presentations; audit and research projects; and any other material that shows evidence for achievement of learning outcomes. Ideally all such evidence should: (a) accompany the learner's reflection: and (b) indicate how they improved practice.

Why

It has been shown that portfolio evidence, when combined with reflection, promotes professional growth not only in achieving technical competencies, but also competencies such as ethics, attitudes and professionalism (Pee et al. 2002).

How

There are five steps in portfolio assessment: collection of evidence; reflection on evidence; evaluation of evidence; defence of evidence; and the assessment decision (Davis and Ponnamperuma, 2009). First, the trainee collects evidence to show progression towards the achievement of competencies. Reflection on such evidence should lead to an improvement of practice, for which fresh evidence should also be provided. Then assessors go through the portfolio to provide an initial assessment. The trainee is next called for an interview, which serves two purposes. First, it provides the examiner the opportunity to explore more on certain less-clear aspects of the portfolio. Second, it provides the trainee with the opportunity to defend their work. Finally, based on both the initial assessment and the interview the final assessment decision is made. The three basic criteria that should govern the final assessment decision are: the strength of evidence on achieving the competencies; the degree to which the competencies have been covered; and the level of reflection on learning.

Where

The portfolio material is collected from the workplace. Portfolios have been used over a decade in undergraduate (Davis et al. 2001), postgraduate (Pitts 1999), and continuing medical education (Mathers et al. 1999) settings.

When

Given the educational rationale of portfolios, the collection of evidence needs to be continuous. The assessment also has to be periodical, and not only at the end of the course. The reason for such continuous assessment is that the feedback provided during regular assessment is vital for the trainee to improve.

By whom

Although portfolio evidence may contain assessment by various stakeholders ranging from consultants to patients, the overall portfolio should be assessed by a senior panel of examiners who are well trained in portfolio assessment. Apart from the 'external' examiners, there is a longstanding contention that portfolios promote the leaner to be an examiner through self-reflection and self-assessment (Wenzel et al. 1998).

Utility of WBA

The following is a brief analysis of the utility of WBA instruments, using a modified version of the utility criteria, suggested by Van der Vleuten (1996).

Validity

Validity is the extent to which an assessment assesses what it purports to assess. Assessments are designed to assess major competencies that cannot be overtly measured; e.g. clinical reasoning. They are called constructs.

Several studies support the construct validity of mini-CEX. Holmboe et al. (2004b) have shown that mini-CEX could differentiate the abilities of trainees at different stages of training. A similar finding has been reported by Wilkinson et al. (2008) for both mini-CEX and DOPS, and by Beard (2005) for OSATS. Durning et al. (2002) observe that mini-CEX ratings on specific competencies correlated with the monthly faculty ratings on corresponding competencies, while the finding by Boulet et al. (2002) indicates that the mini-CEX ratings on videoed consultations correlated with communication skills ratings. The CSR, the predecessor of CBD, has also produced similar results. In the ABIM recertification programme the CSR pass–fail results and score distributions have been consistent with those of the initial certification (Maatsch et al. 1983). Both Norman et al. (1989) and Solomon et al. (1990) have shown correlations of 0.71 and 0.49 respectively between CSR and oral examination results. The latter study has also shown that the CSR can differentiate different levels of candidate experience. Regarding peer assessment, there is evidence to support face (Lockyer 2003), content (Murphy et al. 2008), consequential (Sargeant et al. 2005), and construct (Ramsey et al. 1989) validity. Portfolios support face (Roberts et al. 2002; Webb et al. 2002), content (Davis et al. 2001), and construct (Ker et al. 2003) validity. However, comparing the portfolios of trainees could be an issue if standardized material has not been prescribed as portfolio content.

Reliability

Reliability is the degree to which an assessment result (or observed score) matches with the true score or the actual candidate ability. The mismatch of the true and observed scores is due to error in the assessment. When the assessment error is small (i.e. when the true and observed scores match closely), the assessment result becomes more reproducible or reliable.

Although the original mini-CEX studies indicate that around 14 raters are needed to achieve a reliability of 0.8 (Norcini et al. 1995; Holmboe et al. 2003), a more recent study has shown that five raters for mini-CEX, and two to three raters for DOPS are sufficient (Wilkinson et al. 2008). This study, however, ultimately recommends eight assessors for mini-CEX, which is also confirmed by other studies (Durning et al. 2002; Kogan et al. 2003). However, Norcini and Burch (2007) argue that if 95% confidence interval is taken as the yardstick, even four raters may be sufficient to produce non-overlapping ratings for mini-CEX. Extra raters may only be necessary for trainees with borderline ratings (Norcini 2010, p. 233). Studies on OSATS have also reported good internal consistency (Martin et al. 1997) and inter-rater reliability (Martin et al. 1997; Beard et al. 2005). With regard to CBD, the CSR has produced reliabilities around 0.7 (Solomon et al. 1990). Pelgrim et al. (2011), based on a literature review, have generalized that 10 single observation encounters are sufficient to achieve acceptable reliability.

Determining the number of assessors required to achieve acceptable reliability for WBA that considers multiple observations per rating effort, however, is not that straightforward. MSF that uses healthcare professionals as assessors requires a variable number of assessors, depending on the type of assessor and the assessment instrument (Swick et al. 2006). Massagli and Carline (2007) report the number of assessors can be as few as five nurses or as many as 23 medical students. Although there are a few studies that achieve high reliability even with eight raters (Lockyer and Violato 2004), in general, the number of raters to achieve acceptable reliability ranges from 11 (Ramsey et al. 1996; Murphy et al. 2009), through 12 (Campbell et al. 2008), to 13 (Wilkinson et al. 2008). With regard to patient surveys, although the JRCPTB (2012) recommends 20 patients per trainee, studies show that this number may range from 36 (Campbell et al. 2008) to 41 (Murphy et al. 2009).

Concerns about the reliability of portfolio assessment have been raised for some time (Roberts et al. 2002; Pitts et al. 2002). There are two schools of thought related to the reliability of portfolios. One school has demonstrated that adequate reliability could be achieved with quantitative methods, if the portfolio material is properly and adequately sampled (O'Sullivan et al. 2004). The other school speculates whether the portfolios should be considered as a qualitative assessment (Driessen et al. 2005, 2012).

Educational impact

Educational impact refers to the ability of an assessment to drive the learner towards desirable learning. Studies have indicated that mini-CEX and related assessment promote deep learning (Alves de Lima et al. 2005) and reflection (Cruess et al. 2006). There is also early work that indicates the diminishing educational benefit of mini-CEX, in the absence of reflective feedback (Soemantri et al. 2012). A systematic review (Miller and Archer 2010), however, reports that only MSF has objective evidence for triggering improvement in practice (Brinkman et al. 2007), although mini-CEX (Malhotra et al. 2008; Weller et al. 2009), DOPS (Morris et al. 2006), and CBD (Bodgener and Tavabie 2011) have subjective evidence for high impact. The impact, however, is dependent upon two factors: specialty and feedback. Surgeons have reported a lesser impact (Lockyer et al. 2003), while family physicians (Sargeant et al. 2003) have experienced a higher educational impact for MSF. The impact also depends on the quality of feedback (Bodgener and Tavabie 2011).

Acceptability

Though some studies indicate favourable acceptability towards mini-CEX (Nair et al. 2008), Wilkinson et al. (2008) report that 46% of the assessors and assessees have commented that the mini-CEX is time consuming. Residents have identified tension between the educational and assessment roles of mini-CEX (Malhotra et al. 2008). In one survey, CBD is singled out as the most acceptable of all WBA assessment instruments, especially to the assessors (Smith et al. 2008). In contrast, Johnson et al. (2011) report that only 13 of the 111 trainees and 2 of the 140 assessors in their study thought that CBD enabled feedback. Though teacher acceptability of portfolio assessment has been favourable (Davis and Ponnamperuma 2010), the student perceptions have been initially poor (Davis et al. 2001). Although there has been a slight improvement of student acceptability subsequently, the time taken for the process is still a major concern (Davis et al. 2009a).

Practicability

Both trainees and trainers have reported that mini-CEX, DOPS, and peer assessment are practicable (Wilkinson et al. 2008). However, they are not without problems. Poor response rates have been an issue that plagues all WBA (Crossley et al. 2005; Wilkinson et al. 2008). On the positive side, an assessment instrument like the mini-CEX has been adapted in many settings, with translations into many languages (Norcini 2010), to assess many related competencies such as professionalism more specifically (Cruess et al. 2006), using many methods of delivery such as the use of mobile technology to deliver the assessment forms (Torre et al. 2007). The same can be said about the practicability of portfolio assessment.

Cost-effectiveness

Though studies are almost non-existent, the widespread use of WBA suggests that the cost is not a particular concern, especially given that it does not require expensive physical resources. If, however, the examiner time is factored into the cost equation, the cost could be high.

Table 46.2 summarizes these findings.

Issues related to WBA

Validity, fairness, and reliability of WBA

The key issue regarding validity is whether the WBA results represent actual workplace practice. A representative sample of workplace assessment material supports content validity, while undermining the threat to 'construct under-representation' (Downing and Haladyna 2004). WBA achieves this through preidentified lists of mini-CEX clinical problems, DOPS procedures,

Table 46.2 Utility of WBA instruments

Assessment instrument	Validity	Reliability	Educational impact	Acceptability	Practicability	Cost-effectiveness
Mini-CEX	Construct validity.	With 4–6 raters per year.	High	Moderate to low—mainly due to the time taken.	Generally good, as they are in widespread use, but poor response rate is a concern.	Their widespread use suggests that they are cost effective, even when assessor time is accounted for.
DOPS	Construct validity.	With 3–5 raters per year.	High			
CBD (mainly for CSR)	Construct validity.	With 4–6 per year.	Low			
Peer assessment e.g. mini-PAT	Face, consequential, and construct validity.	With 8–13 raters per year.	High. Depends on specialty and quality of feedback.	Generally low—due to the high number of forms that needs to be collected.		
Patient surveys	May be.	With 20–40 patients per year.	Not much evidence.			
Portfolios	Face, content, and construct validity.	Adequate reliability possible; needs appropriate criteria.	High if reflection is practised.	Improving, but time taken to document evidence is a concern.		

or CBD case categories. The trainees are encouraged not to repeat a WBA within the same area. They should also ensure that these lists are broadly covered when selecting patients for WBA, preferably according to a blueprint, so that a given clinical area is not over or under sampled.

Fairness is an issue as different trainees take different assessment material. So, it is problematic to compare the results of different trainees. This, to an extent, is addressed by mechanisms such as blueprinting to ensure that all candidates cover the same broad content and competencies. Also there are common guidelines and rating rubrics for the assessors, who, at least in single observation WBA, are trained to use the assessment forms.

Reliability has been a concern, as the unstructured and unstandardized WBA material and the variable quality of examiners pose threats to keeping the assessment error relatively small. Hence, it is questionable whether any WBA result is reproducible, mainly due to case or task specificity (Norman, 2005) of WBA material. These reliability concerns are addressed, to an extent, by the measures discussed previously to mitigate fairness issues.

However, they are mainly overcome by increasing the number of assessment encounters. Hence, assessment decisions should not be based on:

- any single assessment, but on all the assessments within a given WBA instrument
- any single assessment instrument, but on the results of all assessment instruments.

Towards this end a portfolio that collects the results of many assessment forms of many WBA instruments is invaluable.

Crossley and Jolly (2012) argue that to improve validity and reliability, WBA needs refinement along four lines:

- the rating scales should be aligned with the understanding and expectations of the judges
- the judgements (overall ratings) rather than individual objective observations should be used

- assessment should be based on quality of performance rather than on the suitability of the trainee for a particular stage of training and
- assessors who are most suitable should be recruited.

The reliability issues of portfolios could be overcome by considering portfolios as an individualistic form of assessment. Such assessment requires broad and inclusive assessment criteria based on the three basic criteria discussed under portfolios.

Summative versus formative assessment

Although there have been instances where WBA has been used for summative assessment (Davis et al., 2001; Driessen et al. 2012), many prefer WBA to be predominantly formative (Norcini, 2010; Nassrally et al. 2012). The reason for this is that the issues discussed under validity, fairness and reliability preclude its use in high stakes, summative assessment. However, it is customary for most training programmes to stipulate completion of WBA as a mandatory entry requirement for summative assessment. This way WBA, although formative in nature, could still maintain a summative influence.

Enhancing the educational value of WBA

Enhancing the educational value of WBA can be achieved by two inter-related measures: feedback and assessor training.

The need for quality feedback is substantiated by the findings of Johnson et al. (2011), who conclude that both assessors and trainees did not accept that CBD provided adequate feedback. Soemantri et al. (2012) and Bodgener and Tavabie (2011) also acknowledge the importance of feedback.

The importance of assessor training is exposed by the finding that assessors are reluctant to award low ratings (Johnson et al., 2011). Silber et al. (2004) observe that assessors tend to assess only along the dimensions of medical knowledge and interpersonal skills, thereby ignoring other competencies. Similarly, Pulito et al.

(2006) have found that assessors primarily assess cognitive skills and professionalism. To overcome these issues, Davis et al. (2009b) recommend that assessor training should emphasize observation-based assessment.

Conclusions

♦ WBA, when implemented properly, has many benefits.

♦ Validity can be improved by better sampling of assessment material, using an assessment blueprint.

♦ Reliability could be improved by collecting a sufficient number of ratings before assessment decisions are made.

♦ The formative value of WBA should not be compromised in the pursuit of summative requirements.

♦ The major research focus in the coming decade should be on improving rating rubrics, assessor training, and feedback.

♦ The workplace is not a place for complex ratings. The success of WBA depends on keeping it simple.

References

Alves de Lima, A., Henquin, R., Thierer, J., et al. (2005) A qualitative study of the impact on learning of the mini clinical evaluation exercise in postgraduate training. *Med Teach.* 27: 46–52

Archer, J.C., Norcini, J., and Davies, H.A. (2005) Peer review of paediatricians in training using SPRAT. *BMJ.* 330: 1251–1253

Archer, J., Norcini, J., Southgate, L., Heard, S., and Davies, H. (2008) mini-PAT (Peer Assessment Tool): A Valid Component of a National Assessment Programme in the UK? *Adv Health Sci Educ.* 13: 181–192

Arnold, L., Willoughby, L., Calkins, V., and Eberhart, G. (1981) Use of peer evaluation in the assessment of medical students. *Med Educ.* 56, 35–42.

Beard, J.D. (2005) Setting standards for the assessment of operative competence. *European J Vasc Endovasc Surg.* 30: 215–218

Beard, J.D., Jolly, B.C., Newble, D.I., Thomas, W.E., Donnelly, J., and Southgate, L.J. (2005) Assessing the technical skills of surgical trainees. *Br J Surg.* 92: 778–782

Bodgener, S., and Tavabie, A. (2011) Is there a value to case-based discussion? *Educ Prim Care.* 22: 223–228

Boulet, J.A., McKinley, D.W., Norcini, J.J., and Whelan, G.P. (2002) Assessing the comparability of standardised patient and physician evaluations of clinical skills. *Adv Health Sci Educ Theory Pract.* 7: 85–97

Brinkman, W.B., Geraghty, S.R., Lanphear, B.P., et al. (2007) Effect of multisource feedback on resident communication skills and professionalism: a randomized controlled trial. *Arch Pediatr Adolesc Med.* 161: 44–49

Burt, C.G., Chambers, E., Maxted, M., et al. (2003) The evaluation of a new method of operative competence assessment for surgical trainees. *Bull Roy Coll Surg Engl.* 85(5): 152–155

Campbell, J.L., Richards, S.H., Dickens, A., Greco, M., Narayanan, A., and Brearley, S. (2008) Assessing the professional performance of UK doctors: an evaluation of the utility of the General Medical Council patient and colleague questionnaires. *Qual Safety Health Care.* 17: 187–193

Clarke, R. (2006) Foundation programme assessments in general practice. *Educ Prim Care.* 17: 291

Challis, M. (1999) AMEE Medical Education Guide No.11 (revised): Portfolio-based learning and assessment in medical education. *Med Teach.* 21: 370–386

Crossley, J., Eiser, C., and Davies, H. (2005) Children and their parents assessing the doctor–patient interaction: evaluating the feasibility and reliability of SHEFFPAT—a rating system for doctors' communication skills. *Med Educ.* 39: 820–828

Crossley, J., and Jolly, B. (2012) Making sense of work-based assessments: ask the right questions in the right way, about the right things, of the right people. *Med Educ.* 46: 28–37.

Cruess, R., McIlroy, J. H., Cruess, S., Ginsburg, S., and Steinert, Y. (2006) The Professionalism Mini-Evaluation Exercise: a preliminary investigation. *Acad Med.* 81: S74–S78

Davis, M.H., Friedman Ben David, M., Harden, R.M., et al. (2001) Portfolio assessment in medical students' final examinations. *Med Teach.* 23: 357–366

Davis, M.H., and Ponnamperuma, G.G. (2005) Portfolio assessment. *J Vet Med Educ.* 32: 279–284

Davis, M.H., and Ponnamperuma, G.G. (2009) Workplace-based assessment. In J.A. Dent and R.M. Harden (eds.) *A Practical Guide for Medical Teachers* (pp. 349–356). 3rd edn. London: Elsevier Churchill Livingstone

Davis, M.H., and Ponnamperuma, G.G. (2010) Examiner perceptions of a portfolio assessment process. *Med Teach.* 32: e211–e215

Davis, M.H., Ponnamperuma, G.G., and Ker, J.S. (2009a) Student perceptions of a portfolio assessment process. *Med Educ.* 43: 89–98

Davis, M.H., Ponnamperuma, G.G., and Wall, D. (2009b) Work-based assessment. In J.A. Dent and R.M. Harden (eds.) *A Practical Guide for Medical Teachers* (pp. 341–348). 3rd edn. London: Elsevier Churchill Livingstone

Day, S.C., Grosso, L.J., Norcini, J.J., Blank, L.L., Swanson, D.B., and Home, M.H. (1990) Residents' perception of evaluation procedures used by their training programme. *J Gen Intern Med.* 5: 421–426

Downing, S.M. and Haladyna, T.M. (2004) Validity threats: overcoming interference with proposed interpretations of assessment data. *Med Educ.* 38: 327–333

Driessen E.W., Tartwijk, J.V., Govaerts, M., Teunissen P., and Van der Vleuten, C.P.M. (2012) The use of programmatic assessment in the clinical workplace: a Maastricht case report. *Med Teach.* 34: 226–231

Durning, S.J., Cation, L.J., Markert, R.J., and Pangaro, L. N. (2002) Assessing the reliability and validity of the mini-clinical evaluation exercise for internal medicine residency training. *Acad Med.* 77: 900–904

Friedman Ben-David, M., Davis, M.H., Harden, R.M., Howie, P.W., Ker, J., and Pippard, M.J. (2001) AMEE Guide No.24: Portfolios as a method of student assessment. *Med Teach.* 23: 535–551

Geeraerts, G.A.G. and Hoofwijk, H.A. (2006) *Assessing Medical Professionals* [in Dutch]. Houten: Bohn Stafleu van Loghum

GMC (General Medical Council) (2006) *Good Medical Practice.* London: General Medical Council. [Online] (Updated March 2009) http://www.gmc-uk.org/static/documents/content/GMP_0910.pdf Accessed 12 March 2012

Goff, B.A., Lentz, G.M., Lee, D., Houmard, B., and Mandel, L.S. (2000) Development of an objective structured assessment of technical skills for obstetric and gynecology residents. *Obstet Gynecol* 96: 146–150

Goff, B.A., Nielsen, P.E., Lentz, G.M., et al. (2002) Surgical skills assessment: a blinded examination of obstetrics and gynecology residents. *Am J Obstet Gynecol.* 186: 613–617

Hamdy, H. (2006) Blueprinting for the assessment of health care professionals. *Clin Teach.* 3: 175–179

Harden, R.M. (1979) How to…assess students: an overview. *Med Teach.* 1: 65–70

Hodges, B. and McIlroy, J.H. (2003) Analytic global OSCE ratings are sensitive to level of training. *Med Educ.* 37(11): 1012–1016.

Holmboe, E.S., Huot, S., Chung, J., Norcini, J.J., and Hawkins, R.E. (2003) Construct validity of the mini Clinical Evaluation Exercise (Mini-CEX) *Acad Med.* 78: 826–830

Holmboe, E.S., Hawkins, R.E., and Huot, S.J. (2004a) Effects of direct observation of medical residents' clinical competence training: a randomised control trial. *Ann Intern Med.* 140: 874–881

Holmboe, E.S., Yepes, M., Williams, F., and Huot, S.J. (2004b) Feedback and the mini clinical evaluation exercise. *J Gen Intern Med.* 19: 558–561

Johnson, G., Booth, J., Crossley, J., and Wade, W. (2011) Assessing trainees in the workplace: Results of a pilot study. *Clin Med.* 11: 48–53

JRCPTB (Joint Royal College of Physicians Training Board) (2012) Workplace-based assessment. [Online] http://www.jrcptb.org.uk/assessment/Pages/Workplace-Based-Assessment.aspx Accessed 10 March 2012

Ker, J.S., Friedman Ben-David, M., Pippard, M.J., and Davis, M.H. (2003) Determining the construct validity of a tool to assess the reflective ability of final year medical students using portfolio evidence. *Members' Abstracts, Association for the Study of Medical Education (ASME)*, Annual Scientific Meeting, pp. 20–21

Kogan, J.R., Bellini, L.M., and Shea, J.A. (2002) Implementation of the mini-CEX to evaluate medical students' clinical skills. *Acad Med.* 77: 1156–1157

Kogan, J.R., Bellini, L.M., and Shea, J.A. (2003) Feasibility, reliability, and validity of the mini-clinical evaluation exercise (mini-CEX) in a medicine core clerkship. *Acad Med.* 78: S33–S35

Kolb, D.A. (1984) *Experiential Learning.* London: Prentice Hall

Kopelow, M., Schnabl, G., Hassard, T., et al. (1992) Assessing practising physicians in two settings using standardised patients. *Acad Med.* 67: S19–S21

Kroboth, F.J., Hanusa, B.H., Parker, S., et al. (1992) The inter-rater reliability and internal consistency of a clinical evaluation exercise. *J Gen Intern Med.* 7: 174–179

Lockyer, J. (2003) Multisource feedback in the assessment of physician competencies. *J Cont Educ Health Prof.* 23: 4–12

Lockyer, J.M. and Violato, C. (2004) An examination of the appropriateness of using a common peer assessment instrument to assess physician skills across specialties. *Acad Med.* 79: S5–S8

Lockyer, J., Violato, C., and Fidler, H. (2003) Likelihood of change: a study assessing surgeon use of multisource feedback data. *Teach Learn Med.* 15: 168–174

Maatsch, J.L., Huang, R., Downing, S., and Barker, B. (1983) *Predictive validity of medical specialty examinations.* Final report for Grant HS 02038-04, National Center of Health Services Research. Michigan State University, East Lansing, MI: Office of Medical Education and Research and development

Malhotra, S., Hatala, R., and Courneya, C.A. (2008) Internal medicine residents' perceptions of the Mini-Clinical Evaluation Exercise. *Med Teach.* 30: 414–419

Martin, J.A., Regehr, G., Reznick, R., et al. (1997) Objective structured assessment of technical skill (OSATS) for surgical residents. *Br J Surg.* 84: 273–278

Massagli, T.L., and Carline, J.D. (2007) Reliability of a 360-degree evaluation to assess resident competence. *Am J Phys MedRehab.* 86: 845–852

Mathers, N.J., Challis, M.C., Howe, A.C., and Field, N J. (1999) Portfolios in continuing medical education—effective and efficient? *Med Educ.* 33: 521–530

Mercer, S.W., McConnachie, A., Maxwell, M., Heaney, D.H., and Watt, G.C.M. (2005) Relevance and performance of the Consultation and Relational Empathy (CARE) Measure in general practice. *Fam Pract.* 22: 328–334

Mercer, S.W., Watt, G.C.M., Maxwell, M., and Heaney, D.H. (2004) The development and preliminary validation of the Consultation and Relational Empathy (CARE) Measure: An empathy-based consultation process measure. *Fam Pract.* 21: 699–705

Miller, A., and Archer, J. (2010) Impact of workplace based assessment on doctors' education and performance: a systematic review. *BMJ.* 341: 5064

Miller, G. (1990) The assessment of clinical skills/competence/performance. *Acad Med.* 65: S63–S67

Morris, A., Hewitt, J., and Roberts, C.M. (2006) Practical experience of using directly observed procedures, mini clinical evaluation examinations, and peer observation in pre-registration house officer (FY1) trainees. *Postgrad Med J.* 82: 285–288

Murphy, D.J., Bruce, D., and Eva, K.W. (2008) Workplace-based assessment for general practitioners: using stakeholder perception to aid blueprinting of an assessment battery. *Med Educ.* 42: 96–103

Murphy, D.J., Bruce, D.A., Mercer, S.W., and Eva, K.W. (2009) The reliability of workplace-based assessment in postgraduate medical education and training: a national evaluation in general practice in the United Kingdom. *Adv Health Sci Educ Theory Pract.* 14: 219–232

Nair, B.R., Alexander, H.G., McGrath, B.P., et al. (2008) The mini clinical evaluation exercise (mini-CEX) for assessing clinical performance of international medical graduates. *Med J Aust.* 189: 159–161

Nassrally, M.S., Mitchell, E.M., and Bond, J.D.P. (2012) Workplace-based assessments: The emphasis on formative assessment. *Med Teach.* 34: 253

Noel, G.L., Herbers, J.E. Jr., Caplow, M.P., Cooper, G.S., Pangaro, L.N., and Harvey, J. (1992) How well do internal medicine faculty members evaluate the clinical skills of residents? *Ann Intern Med.* 117: 757–765

Norcini, J., and Burch, V. (2007) Workplace-based assessment as an educational tool: AMEE Guide No. 31. *Med Teach.* 29: 855–871

Norcini, J.J. (2010) Workplace assessment. In T. Swanwick (ed.) *Understanding Medical Education: Evidence, Theory and Practice* (pp.232–245). The Association for the Study of Medical Education (ASME) Chichester, UK: John Wiley & Sons Ltd

Norcini, J.J., Blank, L.L., Arnold, G.K., and Kimball, H.R. (1995) The mini-CEX (clinical evaluation exercise): a preliminary investigation. *Ann Intern Med.* 123: 795–799

Norcini, J.J., Blank, L.L., Duffy, F.D., and Fortna, G.S. (2003) The mini-CEX: a method for assessing clinical skills. *Ann Intern Med.* 138: 476–481

Norman, G. (2005) Editorial—checklists vs. ratings, the illusion of objectivity, the demise of skills and the debasement of evidence. *Adv Health Sci Educ Theory Pract.* 10(1): 1–3

Norman, G.R., Davis, D., Painvin, A., Lindsay, E., Rath, D., and Ragbeer, M. (1989) Comprehensive assessment of clinical competence of family/general physicians using multiple measures. In: Proceedings of the 28th Annual Conference on Research in Medical Education. Washington, DC: Association of American Medical Colleges

O'Sullivan, P.S., Reckase, M.D., McClain, T., Savidge, M.A., and Clardy, J.A. (2004) Demonstration of portfolios to assess competency of residents. *Adv Health Sci Educ Theory Pract.* 9: 309–323

Overeem, K., Lombarts, M.J.M.H., Arah, O.A., Klazinga, N.S., Grol, R.P.T.M., and Wollersheim, H.C. (2010) Three methods of multi-source feedback compared: A plea for narrative comments and coworkers' perspectives. *Med Teach.* 32: 141–147

Pee, B., Woodman, T., Fry, H., and Davenport, E. S. (2002) Appraising and assessing reflection in students' writing on a structured worksheet. *Med Educ.* 36: 575–585

Pelgrim, E.A., Kramer, A.W., Mokkink, H.G., van den Elsen, L., Grol, R.P., and Van der Vleuten, C.P. (2011) In-training assessment using direct observation of single-patient encounters: a literature review. *Adv Health Sci Educ Theory Pract.* 16: 131–142

Pitts, J. (1999) Learning portfolios, professional practice and assessment. *Educ Gen Pract.* 10: 423–429

Pitts, J., Colin, C., Thomas, P., and Smith, F. (2002) Enhancing reliability in portfolio assessment: discussions between assessors. *Med Teach.* 24: 197–201

Ponnamperuma, G.G., Karunathilake, I.M., McAleer, S., and Davis, M.H. (2009) The long case and its modifications: a literature review. *Med Educ.* 43: 936–941

Pulito, A.R., Donnelly, M.B., Plymale, M., and Mentzer Jr, R.M. (2006)What do faculty observe of medical students' clinical performance? *Teach Learn Med.* 18: 99–104

Ramsey, P.G., Carline, J.D., Inui, T.S., Larson, E.B., LoGerfo, J.P., and Wenrich, M.D. (1989) Predictive validity of certification by the American Board of Internal Medicine. *Ann Intern Med.* 110: 719–726

Ramsey, P.G., Carline, J.D., Blank, L L., and Wenrich, M.D. (1996) Feasibility of hospital-based use of peer ratings to evaluate the performances of practicing physicians. *Acad Med.* 71: 364–370

RCOG (Royal College of Obstetricians and Gynaecologists) (2012) Education and exams: Mini-CbD Obstetrics. [Online] http://www.rcog.org.uk/education-and-exams/curriculum/advanced+training+skills Accessed 6 March 2012

RCPCH (Royal College of Paediatrics and Child Health) (2011) Directly Observed Procedural Skills (DOPS). [Online] http://www.rcpch.ac.uk/training-examinations-professional-development/quality-training/asset-assessment-services-educatio-4 Accessed 3 March 2012

Rethans, J., Sturmans, F., Drop, R., van der Vleuten, C., and Hobus, P. (1991) Does competence of general practitioners predict their performance?

Comparison between examination setting and actual practice. *BMJ*. 303: 1377–1380

Roberts, C., Newble, D., and O'Rourke, A.J. (2002) Portfolio-based assessments in medical education: are they valid and reliable for summative purposes? *Med Educ*. 36: 899–900

Sargeant, J.M., Mann, K.V., Ferrier, S.N., et al. (2003) Responses of rural family physicians and their colleague and coworker raters to a multi-source feedback process: a pilot study. *Acad Med*. 78: S42–S44

Sargeant, J., Mann, K., and Ferrier, S. (2005) Exploring family physicians' reactions to multisource feedback: perceptions of credibility and usefulness. *Med Educ*. 39: 497–504

Silber, C.G., Nasca T.J., Paskin, D.L., Eiger, G., Robeson, M., and Veloski, J.J. (2004) Do global rating forms enable program directors to assess the ACGME competencies? *Acad Med*. 79: 549–556

Small, P.A., Stevens, B., and Duerson, M. C. (1993) Issues in medical education: basic problems and potential solutions. *Acad Med*. 68: S89–S98

Smith, D., Riley, S., Kazmierczak, A., Aitken, M., Paice, E., and Le Rolland, P. (2008.)*National survey of trainees 2007: summary report*. London: Postgraduate Medical Education and Training Board. http://www.gmc-uk.org/National_Survey_of_Trainees_2007_Summary_Report_20080723_Final.pdf_30376516.pdf Accessed 10 March 2012

Soemantri, D., Dodds A., and McColl, G. (2012) Mini-Clinical Evaluation Exercise (Mini-CEX) as a learning tool: the provision of reflective feedback. In: Proceedings of the 15th Ottawa Conference Assessment of Competence in Medicine and the Healthcare Professions Kuala Lumpur, Malaysia 9–13 March 2012

Solomon, D.J., Reinhart, M.A., Bridgham, R.G., Munger, B.S., and Starnaman, S. (1990) An assessment of an oral examination format for evaluating clinical competence in emergency medicine. *Acad Med*. 65: S43–S44

Swick, S., Hall, S., and Beresin, E. (2006) Assessing ACGME competencies in psychiatry training programmes. *Academic Psychiatry*, 30, 330–350

Swift, S.E., and Carter, J.F. (2006) Institution and validation of an observed structured assessment of technical skills (OSATS) for obstetrics and gynecology residents and faculty. *Am J Obstet Gynecol*. 195: 617–621

The Foundation Programme. (2012) ePortfolio: Assessment and Assessment Tools. [Online] http://www.foundationprogramme.nhs.uk/index.asp?page=home/e-portfolio Accessed 5 March 2012

Thornton, M., Donlon, M., and Beard, J.D. (2003) The operative skills of higher surgical trainees: measuring competence achieved rather than experience undertaken. *Bull Roy Coll Surg Engl*. 85: 190–218

Torre, D.M., Simpson, D.E., Elnicki, D.M., Sebastian, J.L., and Holmboe, E.S. (2007) Feasibility, reliability and user satisfaction with a PDA-based mini-CEX to evaluate the clinical skills of third-year medical students. *Teach Learn Med*. 19: 271–277

Van der Vleuten, C.P.M. (1996) The assessment of professional competence: developments, research and practical implications. *Adv Health Sci Educ Theory Pract*. 1: 41–67

Violato, C., Marini, A., Toews, J., Lockyer, J., and Fidler, H. (1997) Feasibility and psychometric properties of using peers, consulting physicians, co-workers, and patients to assess physicians. *Acad Med*. 72: S82–S84

Webb, C., Endacott, R., Gray, M., et al. (2002) Models of portfolios. *Med Educ*. 36: 897–898

Weller, J.M., Jolly, B., Misur, M.P., et al. (2009) Miniclinical evaluation exercise in anaesthesia training. *Br J Anaesth*. 102: 633–641

Wenzel, L.S., Briggs, K.L., and Puryear, B.L. (1998) Portfolio: authentic assessment in the age of the curriculum revolution. *J Nursing Educ*. 37: 208–212

Whitehouse, A., Hassell, A., Bullock, A., Wood, L., and Wall, D. (2007) 360 degree assessment (multisource feedback) of UK trainee doctors: field testing of Team Assessment of Behaviours (TAB) *Med Teach*. 29: 171–176

Whitehouse, A., Walzman, M., and Wall, D. (2002) Pilot study of 360 degrees assessment of personal skills to inform record of in training assessments for senior house officers. *Hosp Med (Lond)*. 63: 172–175

Wilkinson, J.R., Crossley, J.M.A., Wragg, A., Mills, P., Cowan, G., and Wade, W. (2008) Implementing workplace-based assessment across the medical specialties in the United Kingdom. *Med Educ*. 42: 364–373

Wragg, A., Wade, W., Fuller, G., Cowan, G., and Mills, P. (2003) Assessing the performance of specialist registrars. *Clin Med*. 3: 131–134

Further resources

UK Foundation programme sample WBA forms

The full version of the assessment forms described in this chapter can be downloaded from: http://www.foundationprogramme.nhs.uk/pages/home/curriculum-and-assessment/curriculum2010

CHAPTER 47

Written assessment

Kevin Hayes

> For some years, examination by written papers has been substituted, and practised with apparent success in all the medical classes. This method has the advantage of testing all who undergo the trial with far less consumption of their time; but it cannot be practised so often as some reformers would have it, who forget, or may not know, that the labour and consumption of time in examining the written papers of a large class is enormous, and a most ungrateful task.
>
> Robert Christison

The purpose of written assessment

Undergraduate and postgraduate educational providers have long assessed medical knowledge with written assessments and every reader of this chapter will have extensive experience of a variety of assessment formats. It is only in the last 15 years or so that it has been widely recognized that long-used traditional methods such as essays and true/false multiple choice questions (MCQs) have many intrinsic failings that make them less than ideal methods of assessment. As such there has been a huge shift in assessment to more modern evidence-based methods that provide both a valid and reliable test. Single best answer MCQs (SBAs), extended matching questions (EMQs), and short answer questions (SAQs) are now the predominant formats used in most institutions (Hayes and McCrorie 2010) and these formats, when produced to a high standard, allow contextual and relevant knowledge testing. A number of different question formats are likely to be necessary rather than trying to use one test format for everything—as they all have their advantages and disadvantages (Schuwirth and Van der Vleuten 2004). If you ask questions that encourage rote learning and isolated recall of trivial facts, then that is exactly the type of learning you will encourage (as opposed to the learning of clinically relevant and transferable knowledge that is encouraged by properly constructed written assessments). It is clear that assessment has a significant effect on learning (Newble and Jaeger 1983), and consequential validity is just as important in written formats as any other assessment.

Few would argue with the concept that the purpose of written assessment is to not only make sure that a trainee has acquired the necessary level of knowledge at a given stage of their training, but also to ensure that they are able to apply their knowledge so that they are safe and competent in a range of clinical scenarios. Assessment performance provides trainees with feedback on areas of strength and also areas where development is required. Both formative and summative assessments do this but it is principally an intrinsic aim of former. Assessors similarly gain feedback on the effectiveness of their teaching programmes and with adequate attention to this feedback courses can be continually modified and improved (Goldman et al. 2012).

Written assessment can be used to test basic scientific and clinical knowledge, principles of ethical and legal issues, and interpretation of data and research. It is usually a poor way of assessing clinical skills, communication skills, and workplace-based aspects of professionalism—other formats exist to test these skills. Two fundamental questions for anyone about to devise a written question or whole assessment are: 'What am I truly trying to test?' and 'Is there another way I can or should be testing this?' For example; a SAQ on the theoretical principles of a patient's capacity to give informed consent may be appropriate and valid for a student in the early part of a medical degree, if theoretical knowledge of capacity is the only thing that is to be tested at that stage. If in fact you actually wish to assess their ability to assess a patient's capacity, as is likely later in their course or in the postgraduate sphere, then a written format would be inappropriate. An objective structured clinical examination (OSCE) or workplace based assessment (WPBA) would be a valid option in this situation.

Learning outcomes

Medical curricula are generally large, in both the undergraduate and postgraduate fields, which creates an assessment problem. It is neither possible nor necessarily desirable to test everything. After all, who in any career can claim to know everything? Assessment therefore needs to be driven by the curriculum and if asked 'what should you assess?' then a simple answer would be: the common and important learning outcomes, expressly stated in the curriculum, that are designed to ensure the necessary knowledge, skills and attitudes for a candidate to perform a specific job or duty. Note the emphasis on common and important at the expense of the rare and esoteric—it makes no sense spending disproportionate amounts of time assessing disproportionately unimportant things. Therefore, the curricular learning outcomes should underpin the content of the assessment at all stages of its development. This will ensure that both the assessed and assessors know what is being tested and will also help to avoid the problem where individual examiners decide to assess things of particular interest to them, but which actually may not be in the curriculum.

Blueprinting

Blueprinting the assessment from the curriculum is the first step to ensuring that it is has content validity and covers what it is designed to cover. Blueprinting ensures congruence between content validity, learning outcomes, and learning experiences (Coderre et al. 2009). It is vital that the people who construct the blueprint are intimately involved with delivery of the curriculum and the students or trainees who will be sitting the test. How can other faculty members, unfamiliar with the course and students, be expected to know what questions to pose and at what level to pitch them? A clear blueprint will ensure adequate and appropriate coverage and sampling of the subject areas being tested. Common and core topics will therefore be tested more than rare ones. Table 47.1 is a typical example of a blueprint for a written assessment for a postgraduate examination in obstetrics and gynaecology (clinical application of basic sciences). The simple visual format allows easy identification of curricular coverage.

Assessment criteria and marking schemes

Sometimes these terms are used interchangeably, but they represent distinct concepts. Assessment criteria simply determine which aspects of a particular topic are being assessed while marking schemes build on these criteria and allocate an importance or weighting to each criterion that is being tested. Consider the following written question for postgraduate medicine (box 47.1).

So, what does the question actually want the candidate to answer? This could be answered in a number of ways, from specific hypertension management to wider public health policy and secondary prevention, and the candidate is given no help in deciding what is actually being assessed.

For the marker there is added information to aid their judgements about the question (see box 2).

So, what precisely will a good candidate write a comprehensive, evidence-based argument about? Again this is of little or no help to the examiner either. There is no indication of what is specifically being tested or how important any particular aspect

---

Box 47.1 Sample written question

Critically appraise the long-term management of essential hypertension in a 50-year-old man with no other comorbidities.

(20 marks)

Box 47.2 Marker information

A good candidate will write a comprehensive, evidence-based argument on long-term antihypertensive management. A maximum of 20 marks may be awarded.

Table 47.1 Sample blueprint

	Anatomy	Physiology	Endocrinology	Biochemistry	Embryology	Genetics	Pharmacology	Pathology
Antenatal period		x			x	x	x	
Labour	X	x					x	
Postpartum			x					X
Maternal medicine		x		x			x	X
Menstrual problems	X	x						X
Subfertility			x	x		x		
Malignancy	X					x	x	X
Urogynaecology	X	x					x	
Early pregnancy			x	x	x	x		
Sexual/reproductive health			x	x			x	
Surgical procedures	X	x		x			x	X

(x = topic and domain to be tested)

Box 47.3 Assessment criteria and a marking scheme

Critically appraise the long-term management of essential hypertension in a 50-year-old man with no other comorbidities in relation to:

A. Commonly used first-line antihypertensive agents in current national guidance (8 marks)

B. Evidence pertaining to long-term aims of treatment (6 marks)

C. Cost-effectiveness (4 marks)

D. Patient acceptance of lifelong treatment (2 marks)

Additional information for markers
A good candidate will write a comprehensive, evidence-based argument outlining the pros and cons of long-term antihypertensive management and for each of the sections will be expected to consider:

A. Agents x, y, and z, as per national guidelines—individual drug efficacy, racial variations, side effects, contraindications, and interactions (2 marks for each drug described and 2 marks for clarity of argument)

B. The long-term observational data on reductions in morbidity and mortality including methodological pros and cons of seminal studies in this field (4 marks for correct data and 2 marks for clarity of argument)

C. A definition and balanced view of the concept of cost-effectiveness relating this to the management of hypertension (2 marks for general concept and 2 marks for relating appropriately to hypertension)

D. Evidence from patient surveys and psychological studies looking at the positive and negative aspects of long-term medication (1 mark for data and 1 mark for brief critiques of evidence)

---

of antihypertensive management is deemed to be. The question author, writer, and marker have to guess what the other had in mind. Look at the same example with assessment criteria and a marking scheme in box 47.3.

Now it is clear to all parties which aspects of the management of hypertension are being assessed and there is also a clear indication of the relative importance of each area under scrutiny. Which of the examples will result in the best answers from candidates and which will result in fairer marking which is less open to interobserver variation? Assessment schemes and marking criteria provide guidance to candidates and consistency to marking (Hayes and McCrorie 2010).

Reliability and testing time

Reliability is dealt with in detail elsewhere in this textbook, but it applies just as equally to written formats as any other assessment. As a general rule the longer the testing time, the more reliable an assessment will become, as longer assessments allow more sampling. It is therefore evident that a 3-hour MCQ paper with 300 questions will be more reliable than a 3-hour essay paper with six

30-minute questions. As the number of questions decreases, sampling decreases and bias potentially increases for both candidates and markers. We all have areas where we are more and less knowledgeable and if only six areas of a postgraduate curriculum are tested with essays, then by chance a candidate may perform poorly in some areas and appear much less able than is really the case. Equally if only six examiners mark the same set of essays, then it is possible that a group of 'doves' or 'hawks' may predominate and skew the results. If the method changed to 20 SAQs instead, each marked by a different person, then it is likely that reliability will improve.

Which written method you choose should be a balance of one that ensures adequate reliability while being a valid format to test what you truly want. A number of methods are likely to be necessary to achieve this balance (Schuwirth and Van der Vleuten 2005).

Many written formats, especially MCQs, SBA, and EMQs, are therefore attractive as they can test large amounts knowledge and its application in a relatively short space of time and perform highly in measures of reliability. As a general rule with these multiple choice-type methods, testing time beyond 3 hours is unnecessary as there is only a small increase in reliability for a large increased use of resources (Van der Vleuten and Swanson 1990).

Types of written assessment

While much is made of the pros and cons of different formats, they all have some utility and many of the age-old arguments regarding their ability to test certain things is flawed (Schuwirth et al. 2002; Schuwirth and Van der Vleuten 2006). That multiple choice formats test factual knowledge while open-ended question formats test deeper critical thinking is a commonly held concept, but it does not always hold true. It has become increasingly apparent that the quality of question determines what it is able to test and that well-constructed questions of any format can test both factual knowledge and deeper applied critical thinking—depending upon what is being tested (Norman et al. 1987; Schuwirth et al. 2006).

This rest of this section will look at different formats in current use as well as providing practical tips on good practice.

Multiple choice style questions

Multiple choice type questions are the style that readers will probably be most familiar with. They have been used extensively for decades and essentially fall into one of three types: True/false MCQs (T/F MCQs), SBAs and EMQs. They all fall into the closed question format as the answers are apparent in the form of a list of options or a proposed T/F answer (Schuwirth and Van der Vleuten 2005). In recent years the true/false variety has been overtaken by SBAs and EMQs. This section will take a critical look at each type, outlining their pros and cons and also exploring why the aforementioned shift has occurred.

T/F MCQs

T/F MCQs invariably take the form of a lead in stem question or statement followed by three to five proposed 'answers'. The question requires that a candidate make a true or false judgment for each proposition. Box 47.4 is an example of a T/F MCQ testing anatomical knowledge.

We will return to this example shortly.

T/F MCQs are relatively easy to write and mark, most institutions have large banks of questions and they can test large volumes of knowledge in a short period of time. Unfortunately it also true that they are easy to write badly or, most frustratingly for candidates, ambiguously; they tend to reward learning by rote; and they generally stand up to little educational scrutiny—particularly in clinically relevant settings. They are still used by medical schools and postgraduate bodies, and indeed if written well can still be a useful knowledge test in some areas, but their utility is dependent on the context in which they are being used. Let us return to the example in box 47.4. The answers are in box 47.5.

At face value this may be viewed as a good question. It poses a clear question to which the answers are unequivocally true or false. All the proposed answers are plausible and may therefore catch out the candidate whose knowledge is less good. The ultimate question, however, is: what is actually being tested with this question?

If the answer is pure, basic, scientific, anatomical knowledge of the arterial supply of the pelvis, then this is a sound question. T/F MCQs can be a good way of testing basic scientific knowledge, much of which is indeed completely true or false.

But if the answer is clinically relevant anatomy of the pelvic arterial supply, then problems arise. There is no clinical context and this question rewards learning of isolated anatomical facts.

Most medical curricula have moved to promoting learning in a clinical context. A better example in this context might be as shown in box 47.6.

Now the question is written in a clinically relevant format requiring anatomical knowledge of the pelvic arterial supply and is placed in the context of a common surgical procedure. It is no longer enough to remember a list of arterial branches, so relevant learning is rewarded.

Box 47.4 T/F MCQ

Regarding the branches of the anterior division of the internal iliac artery, which of the following is/are direct branches of it?

A. Ovarian artery

B. Pudendal artery

C. Superior rectal artery

D. Superior vesical artery

E. Uterine artery

Box 47.5 T/F MCQ with answers

Regarding the branches of the anterior division of the internal iliac artery, which of the following is/are direct braches of it?

A.	Ovarian artery	F
B.	Pudendal artery	T
C.	Superior rectal artery	F
D.	Superior vesical artery	T
E.	Uterine artery	T

Box 47.6 T/F MCQ in clinical context

A 43-year-old woman is having a total abdominal hysterectomy, with conservation of the ovaries, for persistent heavy periods. During the procedure, which of the following arteries will need to be ligated?

A.	Ovarian artery	F
B.	Pudendal artery	F
C.	Superior vesical artery	F
D.	Uterine artery	T
E.	Vaginal artery	T

Box 47.7 Another T/F MCQ

A 28-year-old woman has a brother with haemophilia A. She is thus known to carry the haemophilia A gene. She would like to have children and so goes to a genetic counsellor with her husband. The following is/are true regarding the genetics of haemophilia A?

A. It is an autosomal recessive condition

B. The gene has an incidence of 1:5000

C. Affected children may have varying clinical severity of disease

D. All male offspring will be clinically affected

E. It is caused by a defect in the *FGR3714885cx* gene region

---

Are all these answers absolutely true/false? Answers B to E certainly are but the purist may argue that some descending branches of the ovarian vessels will need to be ligated where they anastomose with the upper uterine vessels. So is it true or false? Or ambiguous?

Further problems with T/F MCQs

Consider the example for medical students in box 47.7.

This question is set within a good clinical vignette and answers A and D are unequivocally false (the transmission is X-linked recessive). Answer B is problematic because it is likely nobody knows the exact incidence of gene carriage. If most textbooks agree that the incidence is about 1: 4000–5000 does that make it true or false? Is the question stating the incidence in the UK, worldwide, or for the racial origin of this couple (which is not specified)? Bearing in mind that most things in clinical medicine 'may' occur and that nearly all conditions will be of varied severity then answer C surely becomes true as it is so vague—ultimately little knowledge is being tested here. Also given that this is a medical student question and not a high-level specialist question, answer E actually fails the 'who cares?' test—it is an isolated fact irrelevant to the tested candidates.

Anyone who practises clinical medicine is aware that few things are absolutely true or false—this automatically leads to a degree of ambiguity with this style of question. The fact that these questions have a tendency to ambiguity, are often considered 'unfair' by candidates and indeed examiners (McCoubrie 2004), and that they also tend to reward recall of isolated facts (Chandratilake et al. 2011) are the principal reasons they are being replaced by other newer formats. Another problem with this format occurs when a candidate correctly answers 'false' to a question (inevitably roughly 50% of answers will be false). Looking at the previous example they may have correctly answered that this is not an autosomal recessive condition, but do they know that it is X-linked recessive? Correct knowledge is only inferred and not proven.

SBAs

SBAs have become the predominant format for testing clinical knowledge. SBAs generally have the following features:

- A clinical vignette with an appropriate amount of information.

- A clear unambiguous question requiring the candidate to select the single best answer from the option list.

- A list of usually three to five possible answers to the question posed—this list contains the correct answer (the others are distractors).

- The distractors should be a homogeneous set of answers—for example, they should be all tests, all diagnoses, or all drugs depending upon the question posed—they all need to be plausible alternatives to the correct response.

- Many (and potentially all) of the distractors may be correct to some degree but the actual 'correct' answer needs to be significantly 'more correct' than the others.

- All answers should be listed in alphabetical, numerical, or most logical order so that there is no significance to where in the list they are placed.

- A good candidate should be able to answer the question from the scenario, with the options covered.

Clinical vignettes are used as they are a representation of clinically relevant reasoning. Much has been made of whether vignettes should be short, long, or not used in favour of factual statements that are not framed in a clinical context. The studies addressing this (Case et al. 1996) showed no statistical difference in performance but common sense dictates that clinical vignettes presenting facts in an everyday way are a more realistic way of framing questions.

If SBAs are well constructed they should not have any of the following features:

- Questions of the format 'Which of the following is correct?'

- Questions of the format 'All of the following are correct EXCEPT?'

- Negatively phrased questions such as 'Which test/investigation should not be performed?'

Questions phrased as in the list are unfocused; remember, many if not all options may be 'correct' to some degree; what is required is the SBA. Also, asking a candidate to select the incorrect answer or what you should not do is generally backward clinical thinking and should be avoided.

An example of a good SBA is shown in box 47.8.

The question is framed within a realistic vignette and an unambiguous question is posed. All of the proposed answers are plausible and homogeneous, but with reasonable knowledge of this clinical condition, answer A is the best by a considerable margin. Note that many of the tests would also be performed in this context but that option A is the 'most likely' to confirm the diagnosis.

SBAs are an excellent way of testing knowledge within a clinical context as opposed to rewarding factual recall and they also allow for clinical uncertainty (as the most likely response is requested and not an absolute true/false judgement).

SBAs can be used to test most areas of medicine including the basic sciences and like most multiple choice formats allow testing of large amounts of the curriculum in a short period of time. SBAs invariably perform well in terms of reliability per unit of time when psychometrically tested as long as they are well constructed and a large sample is taken.

Box 47.9 shows some more examples of how SBAs can be used to test different areas of a medical curriculum.

Box 47.8 Sample SBA

A 40-year-old previously fit and healthy woman is admitted with right upper quadrant pain. She has a pulse of 90 bpm, temperature of 36.9 and BP = 120/75. She is in pain and abdominal examination elicits some tenderness under the right costal cartilage with no peritonism. Murphy's sign is negative. A clinical diagnosis of biliary colic is made.

Which single investigation will be most helpful in confirming this diagnosis?

A. Abdominal ultrasound

B. C-reactive protein

C. Liver function tests

D. Oesophagogastroduodenoscopy

E. White cell count

Box 47.9 More sample SBAs

A 30-year-old man attends the sexual health clinic for a check up as he has started seeing a new partner. He has no symptoms and his examination is normal. Two days later his *Chlamydia* urine test is positive. All other tests are negative.

What is the most appropriate treatment for his *Chlamydia* infection?

A. Azithromycin

B. Cephalexin

C. Ciprofloxacin

D. Clindamycin

E. Metronidazole

A 70-year-old man is recovering after a laparotomy for a perforated duodenal ulcer. He was recovering well but develops a paralytic ileus.

Which biochemical abnormality is most likely to exacerbate this postoperative complication?

A. Hypocalcaemia

B. Hypochloraemia

C. Hypokalaemia

D. Hyponatraemia

E. Hypomagnesaemia

As can be seen many different areas of a curriculum can be tested and these questions would be considered of good quality from a style and content point of view. To be considered of good quality every question needs to be able to stand up to the following scrutiny:

1. Is there a clear clinical vignette?

2. Is sufficient clinical detail given to answer the question?

3. Is an unambiguous question posed?

4. Are all the options homogeneous?

5. Are all the distractors at minimum plausible?

6. Is there truly only one most likely answer to the question?

7. Is the correct answer significantly more likely than all the others?

8. Can the question be answered with the option list covered?

Question flaws

Flaws can be introduced into any format, but SBAs are particularly vulnerable. They are difficult to write well and certain areas of curricula do not necessarily lend themselves to the format.

Question flaws tend to fall into one of two categories: those associated with the exam-wise candidate and those associated with unnecessary difficulty (Case and Swanson 2002).

Types of question flaws related to the exam-wise candidate

Figure 47.1 demonstrates some question flaws.

Grammatical clues in the vignette and/or question

Grammatical clues in the vignette are demonstrated in box 47.10.

The answer is inadvertently given away in the clinical vignette in box 47.10 by the use of the word 'real'. Little or no knowledge is required to answer this question. The example in box 47.11 is a slightly more subtle but common flaw.

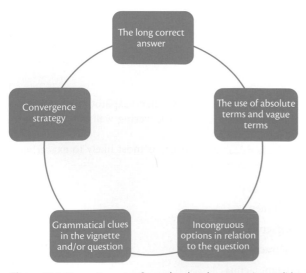

Figure 47.1 Types of question flaws related to the exam-wise candidate.

Box 47.10 More sample SBAs

A 30-year-old man attends his GP describing increasing unprovoked anxiety and a feeling, at times, that the world around him does not feel real.
What term best describe this psychological symptom?

A. Delusions of self worth

B. Derealization

C. Depersonalization

D. Derailment of thought

E. Detachment disorder

Box 47.11 Flawed SBA

A 46-year-old woman is referred to a gastroenterologist with persistent dyspepsia and reflux. Her GP has tried dietary modifications and omeprazole with no benefit.

The most appropriate next investigation to diagnose her symptoms would be an:

A. Barium swallow

B. *Campylobacter* serology

C. CLO breath test

D. CT chest and abdomen

E. Oesophagogastroduodenoscopy

In the example in box 47.11 the inadvertent addition of the word 'an' at the end of the question means the answer must start with a vowel; only answer E does and so must be correct. The use of a plural in the question may also do this: e.g. What are the most appropriate next investigations….?, when not all options have more than one test in them.

Incongruous options in relation to the question

The questions in SBAs should be deliberately focused to make sure that that they are unambiguous. All the options need to be appropriate for any given question. Look at the example in box 47.12.

This question is now narrowed down to an easier choice C, D, or E as it specifically asks for pharmacological interventions. Options A and B can be discounted immediately. The candidates' chances are improved regardless of their knowledge. This flaw usually arises when there are limited possible distractors for the given scenario, so the author puts other things in to fill the gaps. Interestingly, a recent review showed no real change to psychometric performance whether three, four or five answer options were used (Vyas and Supe 2008). Test items should therefore consist of as many options as is feasible given the item content (Tarrant et al. 2009).

Convergence strategy

Consider the question in box 47.13.

At first glance this appears a well-constructed and challenging question. For the exam-wise student, however, it is relatively easy (even with little knowledge). Exam-wise students will ask

Box 47.12 Incongruous options

A 30-year-old woman is admitted to the labour ward at 36 weeks in her first pregnancy. She has a headache and is feeling unwell. Her BP is 190/135 and she has +++ protein on urine dipstick. She has brisk reflexes and clonus and is diagnosed with pre-eclampsia.

What is the most appropriate pharmacological intervention in her immediate management?

A. Central line and HDU care

B. CT scan of the head

C. Magnesium sulphate and labetalol

D. Diazepam and hydralazine

E. Phenytoin and nitroprusside

Box 47.13 Convergence strategy

A 66-year-old man has advanced adenocarcinoma of the lung. He is receiving palliative care. He presents with generalized weakness. After blood tests he is diagnosed with SIADH.

Which biochemical abnormality is most likely to suggest this diagnosis?

A. Hypokalaemia

B. Hyponatraemia

C. Hypernatraemia

D. Hypochloraemia

E. Hypercalcaemia

Box 47.14 Another flawed SBA

A 30-year-old presents to a gynaecologist, saying that she has not had a period for nearly 10 months. She has no clinical symptoms, uses condoms for contraception, and examination is normal. Her hormonal profile is:

BHCG—negative; prolactin 435; FSH = 110; LH = 73; testosterone:SHBG ratio—normal

What is the most likely diagnosis?

A. Anterior pituitary failure

B. Hypothalamic dysfunction

C. Polycystic ovary syndrome

D. Premature ovarian failure

E. Prolactinoma

Box 47.15 Alternative options list

A. Anterior pituitary failure

B. Hypothalamic dysfunction

C. Polycystic ovary syndrome

D. Premature menopause

E. Prolactinoma

Box 47.16 Long correct answer

The National Health Service cervical screening programme has been shown to reduce both the incidence and mortality from cervical cancer. The sensitivity of the primary cytological screening tool is quoted at around 70%.

What is the most appropriate description of sensitivity when applied to this screening test?

A. The proportion of women who have cervical cancer

B. The proportion of women the test ignores without cervical cancer

C. The proportion of women, who actually have the disease, identified as at high risk by the test, picking up cytological dyskaryosis, the essential premalignant prerequisite of cervical cancer.

D. The proportion of women with a positive test who have cervical cancer

E. The proportion of women who have cervical cancer regardless of whether they are screened

themselves the question: 'where do you hide a tree?' The answer is: 'in a forest full of other trees'. So, the correct answer is likely to have most in common with the others. There are three hypo options and only two hyper options so we can discount the hyper options. Of the three hypo options, the natraemia option is also amongst the hyper options. This makes it most likely to be the correct answer. This question would be better if all the options were hypo as they would be more homogeneous.

Another example is shown in box 47.14.

This is more subtle than the example in box 47.13, but again using convergence strategy there are two ovarian diagnoses and two failure diagnoses. The correct answer is most likely to be hidden amongst similar distractors, and the only one that has both features is premature ovarian failure—the correct answer.

Look how this changes with a minor alteration to the list (box 47.15).

Option D is still correct but now the exam-wise candidate is unable to use convergence and can only confidently come to the correct answer if they have the required knowledge.

The long correct answer

Have a look at the example in box 47.16—it should be obvious where the problem lies.

Answer C is so much more detailed and specific than all the others that it just has to be the correct answer. This occurs when the question author makes sure that the correct response is 'absolutely correct' and does not balance the responses by taking as much time on the distracters.

Numerical options can also run into this problem (see box 47.17).

There can only be one correct answer as D is so much more specific than all the other options (at least this flaw can be easily corrected).

Box 47.17 Numerical inconsistencies

Asymptomatic *Chlamydia* carriage has been identified as a major public health issue in the UK. This is particularly true in teenagers.

The proportion of positive *Chlamydia* tests in teenagers attending sexual health clinics in the UK is?

A. 3%

B. 8%

C. 12%

D. 19.4%

E. 26%

Box 47.18 Absolute and vague terms

A 65-year-old man attends the Emergency department with crushing central chest pain and nausea. His ECG shows an inferior ST-elevation myocardial infarction (STEMI). He has long-standing hypertension and type 2 diabetes and takes ramipril and metformin.

The most appropriate statement regarding his acute management is:

A. Acute cardiac catheterization, and angioplasty and stenting may be appropriate

B. Acute thrombolysis is absolutely contraindicated as he has diabetes

C. His antihypertensive medication should never be changed as he has been stable up to now

D. Intravenous diamorphine should always be used for analgesia

E. Tight glycaemic control must be attained immediately

The use of absolute terms and vague terms

Answers that use 'always' or 'never' are always incorrect and never correct! Few things are absolute in medicine, which makes them likely to be wrong. Similarly, when vague terms such as 'possibly', 'may', and 'sometimes' are used they are likely to be correct as most things 'may' happen or be possible (see box 47.18).

Answers B, C, D, and E 'sound' wrong as they are framed in absolute terms, and option A is vague—even with minimal knowledge of the acute management of a myocardial infarction, in what circumstances would acute catheterization with angioplasty and stenting not be appropriate? The use of the word 'may' immediately sounds correct and the others can be discounted.

Flaws related to irrelevant difficulty

Unlike the previous examples, here it is the construction of the question itself that is the problem rather than giving away clues to an exam-wise candidate. Flaws relating to irrelevant difficulty fall into the following categories:

♦ frequency terms used are vague, such as: 'often', 'likely', 'usually' or 'commonly'

♦ the options are long, complicated or double

♦ numerical terms are not used consistently

♦ clinical vignettes are tricky or over-complicated

♦ no clear question is posed.

Box 47.19 demonstrates some of these flaws.

Frequency terms can be vague and it has been shown that even to a group of experts their meaning can vary enormously (Case 1994). Look at the options in box 47.19: How common is commonly? How frequent is frequently? How often is often? How rare is rarely? Depending upon your point of view all or none of these answers could be either right or wrong. It makes the question unanswerable as the candidate has to guess what the examiner means.

Another problem is the use of overlong options (see box 47.20).

As you read those options could you remember the actual question posed? The options are far too long and complicated and they all state several pieces of information about drug classes. The focus of the question is lost in the detail.

Numerical options can be problematic unless carefully considered. They need to be stated consistently and the scale of change through the numbers needs to be in reasonable steps—or some options will look unlikely. Look at the question in box 47.21.

In these options there is a mix of absolute values and ranges. Answer C includes D and E, so they can all be immediately discounted if there is truly only one best answer. This leaves a choice of A or B. The question would be sounder if the options were portrayed as in box 47.22.

It is now a true test of knowledge as long as the correct answer is well agreed in the literature—but what if the agreed rate in the literature is not truly known but thought to be in the range of 20–30%?

Box 47.23 is another example of a problematic question.

While this question is reasonable, there is far too much detail in the vignette, much of which is completely unnecessary to answer the question posed. As a general rule excessive detail in the

Box 47.19 Imprecise terms

A 70-year-old woman is admitted with a left hemiplegia and a diagnosis of a right-sided cerebrovascular accident (CVA) is made. She is admitted to the stroke unit for management.

What is the most appropriate statement regarding the management of her CVA?

A. Acute thrombolysis is frequently the treatment of choice for thrombotic CVA

B. Formal heparinization is often used if thrombolysis is contraindicated

C. Regardless of treatment modality, death in the next few months occurs commonly

D. Surgical management of haemorrhagic CVA is unusual

E. Warfarin is rarely used as a long-term treatment

Box 47.20 Overlong options

A 33-year-old woman is diagnosed with rheumatoid arthritis (RA) and wishes to discuss medication. She is currently on diclofenac and paracetamol regularly but she still has considerable finger and knee joint pain.

What is the most appropriate statement regarding pharmacological control of her RA?

A. Continuing with NSAIDs regularly would be recommended for background relief of symptoms even if other drugs are added to her prescription as long as she remains tolerant of NSAIDs and does not develop any extra-articular manifestations of RA.

B. Methotrexate would be an ideal next drug for her as she clearly has inadequate symptom control with NSAIDs, and its side-effect profile is favourable compared to other disease-modifying agents, as long as she does not wish to conceive

C. Gold or penicillamine are recommended at this stage as they have a long history of successful disease modification as second-line agents and though side effects are common, they can be closely monitored and ameliorated relatively easily

D. High-dose prednisolone is the next appropriate step as this is a potent anti-inflammatory over a longer time period, whose side effects should be manageable as she has no other major medical comorbidities

E. Leflunomide is now recommended at this stage as there is an increasing body of evidence to suggest it results in longer-term disease-free intervals and less use of other disease-modifying drugs

---

Box 47.21 Inconsistent scale

A 24-year-old woman is admitted with lower abdominal pain and pelvic tenderness. She has a temperature of 38.2 and a pulse of 110 bpm. A clinical diagnosis of acute pelvic inflammatory disease (PID) is made. She had a similar episode the year before and is concerned about future fertility.

What is the likelihood of subsequent subfertility following a second episode of PID?

A. <20%

B. 20–30%

C. >50%

D. 75%

E. 90%

Box 47.22 Consistent options

A 24-year-old woman is admitted with lower abdominal pain and pelvic tenderness. She has a temperature of 38.2 and a pulse of 110 bpm. A clinical diagnosis of acute pelvic inflammatory disease (PID) is made. She had a similar episode the year before and is concerned about future fertility.

What is the likelihood of subsequent sub-fertility following a second episode of PID?

A. 10%

B. 20%

C. 30%

D. 40%

E. 50%

Box 47.23 Too much detail

A 60-year-old man with COPD is admitted with increasing shortness of breath. He has been getting worse for 3 days following a 'flu-like' illness and his normal medication is no longer working. He is usually well controlled on beclomethasone 2 puffs b.d., ipratropium 2 puffs b.d. and salbutamol 2 puffs q.d.s. He has a cough productive of green sputum with no haemoptysis and his observations are: respiratory rate = 28 pm, pulse = 100 bpm, BP = 145/90, temperature = 37.6 and SaO_2 = 92% on air. Chest examination reveals widespread wheezes. Cardiovascular and abdominal examinations are unremarkable. He has uncomplicated hypertension for which he takes ramipril. He has an otherwise uneventful medical history. He had a previous appendicectomy aged 18 and a left inguinal hernia repair in the past. He lives with his 62-year-old wife for whom he is a carer due to her chronic rheumatoid arthritis. He hasn't smoked for 15 years and rarely drinks alcohol and is a retired history teacher at a local secondary school.

What is the next most appropriate step in his initial management?

A. Intravenous steroids and salbutamol nebulizers

B. Oral prednisolone and high-flow oxygen therapy

C. Aminophylline and inhaled steroids

D. Intravenous salbutamol and ipratropium nebulizers

E. Adding in montelukast therapy to his current medication

---

vignettes or the use of extra information to try and distract or trick candidates should be avoided (Case 1996).

Eliminating question flaws

Everybody who writes SBA questions will understand how difficult it is to avoid the flaws shown in the boxes. Flaws are common, and two papers in medical and nursing education assessed large numbers of summative questions from high-stakes examinations (Downing 2005; Tarrant and Ware 2008) and both found flaws in up to 35-65% of items. Formal question writing training is vital and specific faculty development has been shown to improve the quality of both MCQs and SAQs (Naeem et al. 2011). Also, no question should ever be used without peer review. Peer review is an excellent way of getting a fresh pair of eyes to look at the questions that have been written and it is particularly helpful for people from outside a speciality to test the questions out. Can the cardiologist answer the psychiatry questions because they have an excellent knowledge of psychiatry; or are the questions flawed and the answers easy to arrive at? Post hoc question analysis will also help to improve or remove questions (Case and Swanson 2002).

EMQs

EMQs are essentially a variation on the SBA question. They have the following characteristics:

- a theme title
- a list of answer options typically ranging from 8 to 20 in number
- between three and five clinical vignettes linked to the original theme.

They are another excellent way of testing clinically relevant knowledge and are considered a context-rich assessment format (Case and Swanson 1993). As they contain longer lists of options under one theme they can be used to test knowledge on different aspects of core areas. SBA type questions are sometimes problematic when it is difficult to find five plausible options for a particular topic, which leads to writing flawed questions. If the topic is still deemed important, then putting the question within an EMQ may be a better alternative. Box 47.24 shows an example of an EMQ.

Clearly option I is the most likely answer for question 1. Once a list of answers has been compiled for a given theme then any number of questions can be written but three to five per theme is the norm.

EMQs can be difficult to write initially and their success depends on the author being able to compose a list of answers that is long enough and plausible enough for some of them to act as distractors. Quite how many options you put in a list for an EMQ is debatable but two studies comparing SBAs and EMQs (Swanson et al. 2006, 2008) found that SBAs using four to five options were psychometrically comparable with EMQs with eight options and that any more than eight was less time efficient with no apparent benefit in terms of item discrimination.

Most of the flaws fall into the same categories as those that affect SBAs. A particular problem with EMQs is heterogeneous lists of options that lead to many of them being implausible and therefore helping candidates by 'narrowing the field'. The question posed also needs to be absolutely clear or the task becomes a guessing game. A question such as 'pair up the statements below with the correct answer' gives no clue as to whether the focus is diagnosis or management. Also, when blueprinting, it is important to take into account curricular coverage, as an EMQ is likely to test up to five questions in one area, whereas five SBAs are likely to test more distinct areas.

Script concordance tests (SCTs)

SCTs are a relatively new tool designed to test whether a trainee's knowledge is adequately organized for clinical action (Charlin et al. 2000). The trainees are tested for the degree of concordance of their actions ('script') with the opinion of a panel of experts. While presented in a written format, the situations are designed to be authentic and to replicate everyday situations that require the candidate to interpret data to inform and make decisions. Each question starts with a short clinical vignette and, as progressive information and data are released, a candidate's reasoning is questioned regarding, diagnosis, investigation and management. No distractors are required and marks can be given to candidates proportional to the degree of expert agreement with their answer. This question format is particularly suited to cases where there is clinical uncertainty (Charlin et al. 2000). These can be challenging to assess and mark in other ways.

An example of a SCT is shown in box 47.25.

A recent study examining construct validity in SCTs (Lubarsky et al. 2011) concluded that the available evidence supports their

---

Box 47.24 Sample EMQ

Theme: Causes of chest pain
Options:

A. Bronchogenic carcinoma

B. Costochondritis

C. Dissecting aortic aneurysm

D. Gastro-oesophageal reflux

E. Lobar pneumonia

F. Stable angina

G. Myocardial infarction

H. Pericarditis

I. Pulmonary embolism

J. Unstable angina

From the list above choose the most appropriate diagnosis for the given clinical scenario. Each option may be used once, more than once or not at all.

1. A 33-year-old woman with a BMI of 35 is 18 weeks pregnant for the first time. She has no significant medical or surgical history. She presents with shortness of breath and left-sided pleuritic pain. On admission, pulse = 110 bpm, BP = 115/75 and temperature = 37°C. Clinical examination is otherwise normal. Her ECG shows a sinus tachycardia only.

2. Further vignettes....

Box 47.25 Sample SCT

A 19-year-old nulliparous woman presents with a 2-month history of intermenstrual and postcoital bleeding in an otherwise regular 28-day cycle. She uses condoms intermittently for contraception.

If you are thinking of…	And you find…	Then this hypothesis (*Chlamydia* cervicitis) becomes….
Chlamydia cervicitis	A normal cervix on speculum examination	1 2 3 4 5

1 = the hypothesis is eliminated
2 = the hypothesis becomes less probable
3 = the information has no effect on the hypothesis
4 = the hypothesis is becoming more probable
5 = it can only be this hypothesis

Progressive information is subsequently released and reasoning is further tested as the case unfolds.

use in terms of testing reasoning in cases of clinical uncertainty but that further work still needs carried out on more far reaching aspects of their validity. Another recent study in emergency medicine in the USA suggested that there was convergent validity with other assessment formats such as the United States Medical Licensing Examination (USMLE) step 2 (Humbert et al. 2011). Early data also supports predictive validity for this test (Brailovsky et al. 2001). Most of the published data reports good reliability scores for SCTs (Charlin et al. 2000; Marie et al. 2005; Carrière et al. 2009; Meterissian 2006).

The available literature appears to support SCTs in terms of validity and reliability in their niche of cases of uncertainty. However, there still needs to be more work done on their overall utility, particularly as the vast majority of work has been done in one centre in Canada. Experts have found them difficult to write and they need an enthusiastic and large panel of experts to check them—this makes marking them labour-intensive to create (Duggan 2007). It would appear that a minimum of 10 experts are required to achieve adequate reliability (Gagnon et al. 2005)—this may be unrealistic or unsustainable in some institutions. There is also the potential for problems with standard setting if experts have varying opinions about individual cases, as is often the case in clinical medicine.

Situational judgement tests (SJTs)

SJTs are another relatively new question format; they have been used in recruitment and university admissions tests, and more latterly in postgraduate selection. They are based on the principle of testing candidates in real-life situations that they will have to face in order to do a particular job. Boxes 47.26 and 47.27 show two examples of SJTs. Note there are two distinct styles where candidates are asked to first rank all of the actions in a given situation and then in the second question to choose the most appropriate actions from a list.

In the context of a Flemish admissions test for dental and medical school, SJTs were found to perform better in a predictive manner than any of their cognitive ability tests and also allowed

---

Box 47.26 Sample SJT

A 65-year-old man comes to see you as he has a tremor in his left hand. On examination he has a resting tremor in both hands (worse on the left) and some cog-wheel rigidity in his left arm. He does not want to see a specialist as he hates hospitals. His father died of Alzheimer's disease and he is terrified in case he should develop a similar illness. He is a bit embarrassed by the tremor but it is not affecting him a great deal—he can do everything that he used to do.

Rank in order the following immediate actions in response to this situation (1 = most appropriate; 5 = least appropriate)

A Advise him to come back to see you in 3 months
B Refer him to a neurologist
C Prescribe a course of levodopa
D Prescribe a course of a dopamine agonist
E Refer him to a physiotherapist

Box 47.27 Sample SJT

You see a 70-year-old man with his wife. He has just been diagnosed with Alzheimer's disease but nobody has told him yet. He has very mild memory loss at the moment. He has a history of anxiety and depression. He doesn't ask you what the problem is but you wonder should you tell him.

Choose the THREE most appropriate actions to take in this situation

A Tell him that he has Alzheimer's disease
B Reassure him that it is just normal ageing
C Arrange another appointment with his wife and ask her if she wants him to be told
D Ask him whether he would like to know the diagnosis
E Arrange another appointment with his wife and tell her the diagnosis

---

a broader range of domains to be tested than with just cognitive tests (Lievens and Coetsier 2002), suggesting that situational tests may be a useful complement to traditional student selection procedures. This view has also been backed up in a two British studies where SJTs were found to be the best individual predictor for selecting GP trainees for postgraduate practice, particularly in combination with clinical problem-solving tests. SJTs were also highly acceptable to candidates (Patterson 2009; Koczwara et al. 2012). SJTs, in the context of personnel selection in non-medical jobs, have been shown to correlate best with the personality traits of emotional stability, conscientiousness, agreeableness, and openness (Cabrera and Nguyen 2001; Lievens and Coetsier 2002) and, if they perform similarly in medical situations, have the potential to help to select for these desirable traits. SJT scores also tend to increase with increasing years of job experience, meaning they may become potentially less discriminatory if used in the later stages of training.

Writing the questions can be difficult and there will often be expert discrepancy about rankings in real clinical scenarios. We still do not know if these tests have any long-term predictive validity in medicine (Sui and Reiter 2009) but work is ongoing in this area and ultimately later job performance will be the most important parameter of their utility (Buyse and Lievens 2011). There is also some concern that the utility of SJTs can be reduced by coaching for assessments (McDaniel et al. 2011).

One advantage of all these types of assessment is that they can be easily machine marked (fig 47.2).

SAQs

SAQs are a popular format for testing knowledge in particularly important topics where several aspects of one area need to be tested. They have the potential to dig deeper into critical thinking and to explore wider aspects of a subject. Box 47.28 shows a sample SAQ for an undergraduate haematology course.

Clearly, the answers will be in free text so a comprehensive marking scheme needs to be written including reasonable alternative answers. These questions are labour intensive to write and mark.

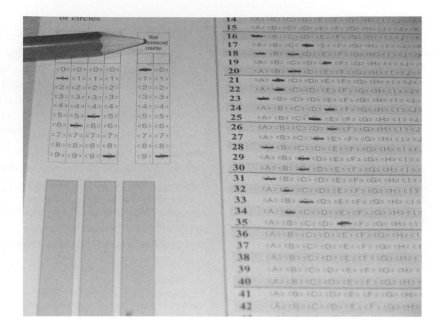

Figure 47.2 An answer sheet.

Box 47.28 Sample SAQ

A 23-year-old man is admitted feeling unwell for the last 3 months. On examination he has firm cervical lymphadenopathy and on direct questioning he states that his glands hurt when he drinks alcohol. You suspect Hodgkin's lymphoma (HL).

A. Name 2 type B symptoms consistent with this diagnosis that should be sought (2 marks)

B. Name the 4 basic histological types of HL that may be found if he has a cervical node biopsy (4 marks)

He is confirmed to have HL and it is confined to his neck and mediastinum on staging.

C. Name the 4 drugs most likely to be used in his initial chemotherapy (4 marks)

He responds well to treatment but at 12 months follow up asks the doctor whether the chemotherapy will affect his chances of having a family

D. State 2 pieces of information he should be given regarding his chemotherapy and future fertility *(4 marks)*

Box 47.29 Vague questions

A 68-year-old man is seen by his family doctor with persistent back pain and fatigue—after investigation he is diagnosed with multiple myeloma.
Question (Q): What tests is his doctor likely to have done? (3 marks)
Answer (A): Blood tests, X-rays and urine tests
Q. What should his doctor do now he has the diagnosis? (2 marks)
A. Explain the diagnosis in a sensitive manner, give him an information leaflet on myeloma
Q. What treatment is he likely to need? (3 marks)
A. Analgesia for back pain, counselling, multidisciplinary support

---

The individual question parts also need to be completely focussed and specific or you will get a huge variety of answers. The example in box 47.29 illustrates this point.

How much does this candidate actually know about myeloma? They have given vague and general answers to poorly written and vague questions. The answers are reasonable responses to the tasks posed. The exam-wise candidate will see an opportunity for easy marks.

SAQs take longer than EMQs and SBAs for candidates to complete so sampling per unit time will reduce with a subsequent reduction in reliability. It is common therefore for a mixture of the formats to be used in any one question paper, so that there is a test of breadth and depth of knowledge.

Essays and modified essay questions (MEQs)

Essays have gradually been replaced with MEQs and the SAQs. Essays were deemed a good way of testing in-depth knowledge on particularly important topics and also allowing room for critical appraisal. It should not be assumed, however, that they will automatically test more critical thinking; quality of the questions is the key, and a study comparing MCQs and MEQs failed to show any benefit in this respect for MEQs (Palmer and Devitt 2007). Essays also take a long time to write, which means sampling and reliability are sacrificed. A 3 hour essay paper will only meaningfully yield five or six questions and even with several papers it is only possible to sample a small part of a curriculum. They are also labour intensive to mark, need detailed marking schemes, and because of the open nature of the style of question,

Box 47.30 Sample essay and MEQ

Essay: Describe the multisystem management of a 30-year-old with progressive chronic renal failure of unknown cause. (20 marks)
MEQ: Describe the multisystem management of a 30-year-old with progressive chronic renal failure of unknown cause. Describe the clinical management in relation to:

A. Optimizing hypertensive control (5 marks)

B. Maintaining haemoglobin concentration (5 marks)

C. Calcium and phosphate metabolism (5 marks)

D. Fluid balance control (5 marks)

they are inevitably open to considerable interpretation, by both candidate and marker. The labour-intensive nature of these question styles is even further magnified if second marking is employed. For these reasons, most institutions have removed them in favour of SAQs or MEQs. Compare the essay and MEQ on the same topic in box 47.30.

The open nature of the essay is more closed and specific in the MEQ—as the topics deemed assessment-worthy are now clear, as are their relative importance in the marking scheme. A candidate could quite reasonably write at length about the psychosocial support in preparing for dialysis, issues around pre-emptive transplantation or the multidisciplinary nature of the care provided in answer to the essay title.

MEQs are therefore a longer version of SAQs, allowing for more free text and in-depth explanation of a topic, but again will be less reliable and more labour intensive than SAQs due to reduced sampling.

Quality assurance (QA)

All assessment needs good evaluation and review as part of the QA process. This starts with author training, extensive question review pretest and is followed by post-test item analysis. Post hoc analysis will assess reliability of the test as a whole, which is usually good if enough sampling has occurred. Cronbach's alpha (Cronbach 1951) is a commonly used method that relies on generalizability theory. It works on the premise that for a perfectly reliable 300-question SBA exam, the statistical performance of any 150 questions (e.g. all odd numbers) will be identical to the remaining 150 questions (evens). A simple comparison of the two subsets will give a score from 0–1. There is no exact value to be reached but for large samples Cronbach's alphas of >0.7–0.8 would be considered acceptable.

Using SBAs as an example, one of the simplest and most effective ways to evaluate each question is to analyse item response rates. Four examples of individual question response rates for some SBAs in a paper sat by 200 candidates are shown in table 47.2. Correct answers are in bold type.

Table 47.2 Item responses

Q 23	A = 18	B = 12	C = 36	D = 28	**E = 106**
Q 39	A = 0	**B = 192**	C = 3	D = 1	E = 4
Q 97	A = 37	B = 43	C = 40	**D = 50**	E = 30
Q 109	A = 74	B = 12	C = 13	**D = 71**	E = 20

For Question 23 this has a good profile. The majority of candidates have answered the question correctly as you would expect for a well-constructed, valid question with a single best answer, and all the options have been selected by a reasonable number of candidates (i.e. they are all plausible). This question would be likely to be used again.

For Question 39 nearly everyone has selected the correct option. This question is either so easy that everyone knows it or so flawed that the answer is given away. This question would need review and either revision or ejection from the bank, unless, in rare circumstances, the question is so fundamental that you are relieved that everyone knows it.

Question 97 is different. This is known as the 'guess-fest'. There are hardly any differences between the response rates for all five options. It is likely that the question is either too difficult for the level of candidate or written in such a way that there is no one single best answer. This question will need a review.

Question 109 may look all right at first glance as all options have been selected by a reasonable number of candidates. However, it is a 'crowd splitter'. The fact that there is no difference in response rates between options A and D suggests that on review you may find that they are indeed equally likely and that there may not be one true single best answer.

Good questions should also be able to discriminate between good and poor candidates. Another QA consideration therefore is whether the individual questions do this. Based on the principle that for any given question, the best performing members of the whole cohort will be much more likely to answer it correctly compared to the worst performing candidates, it is easy to calculate a discrimination index (DI). If you have a large cohort such as the previous example with 200 candidates then you can compare the overall best and worst performing 20% of candidates (20% DI). As your numbers reduce you may have to move to a 33% DI or even 50% if the cohort is quite small (fig. 47.3).

The DI will range from –1 to +1, and the higher the score the more discriminatory. If a DI approaches zero then the question has been non-discriminatory and if it is negative then it is likely the proposed 'correct' answer is in fact incorrect.

Point biserials are another measure of discrimination which look at all the data derived from a question (as opposed to 40% of the total question data in the above 20% DI example) but to a large extent measure a similar concept.

Depending upon human resources, an institution may take a random sample of questions, all of them or just select the worst performing 20% for review. It does not really matter what methods you use, but it is vital that question review is performed to improve your assessment—it is more important that you review and act accordingly rather than the method you use to do so.

$$DI = \frac{\text{Number of correct candidates in top 20\% – number of correct candidates in bottom 20\%}}{\text{Total number of candidates in top group}}$$

Figure 47.3 Discrimination index.

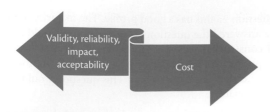

Figure 47.4 Assessment.

Cost and feasibility

Written assessment is relatively cheap to run compared to other formats such as OSCEs. However, good quality written assessment can be labour intensive and the quality is directly proportional to the amount of time and effort put into it. Sharing questions or setting up question banks between institutions is an efficient way of generating large numbers of questions. While there may be concerns over the quality of questions from other institutions or from abroad, it has recently been shown that with good reciprocal collaboration and question review, question performance can be comparable from different sources in the UK and indeed overseas, with minimal need for local adaptation (Freeman et al. 2010). When designing a written test, like all other tests, it is vital to ensure that it is feasible to use in terms of resource and time (McAleer 2009). In most institutions there will always be a trade off between quality and cost (fig. 47.4). Inevitably, it is staff time and availability that will be the single biggest barrier to quality.

Conclusions

- Written assessment is embedded in all medical curricula and is the principal test of *applied* knowledge.

- A variety of question formats within an assessment diet is considered good practice, as all types have advantages and disadvantages.

- SBAs, EMQs, and SAQs are now the predominant formats used worldwide as they have proven validity and reliability if adequate sampling is ensured.

- Question content and quality is much more important than the type of question used (what you ask rather than how you ask).

- Question flaws are common and easy to introduce and reduce the quality of written assessments.

- Institutional investment, question writing training, peer review, and post hoc question analysis are all vital parts of written assessment quality control.

References

Brailovsky, C., Charlin, B., Beausoleil, S., Coté, S., and van der Vleuten, C. (2001) Measurement of clinical reflective capacity early in training as a predictor of clinical reasoning performance at the end of residency: an experimental study on the script concordance test. *Med Educ.* 35(5): 430–436

Buyse, T. and Lievens, F. (2011) Situational judgment tests as a new tool for dental student selection. *J Dent Educ.* 75(6): 743–749

Cabrera, M.A.M. and Nguyen, N.T. (2001) Situational Judgment Tests: A Review of Practice and Constructs Assessed. *Int J Select Assess.* 9: 103–113

Carrière, B., Gagnon, R., Charlin, B., Downing, S., and Bordage, G. (2009) Assessing clinical reasoning in pediatric emergency medicine: validity evidence for a Script Concordance Test. *Ann Emerg Med.* 53(5): 647–652

Case, S.M. (1994) The use of imprecise terms in examination questions. How frequent is frequently? *Acad Med.* 69(Suppl): S4–S6

Case, S.M. and Swanson, D.B. (1993) Extended matching items: a practical alternative to free-response questions. *Teach Learn Med.* 5(2): 107–115

Case, S.M. and Swanson, D.B. (2002) *Constructing written test questions for the basic and clinical sciences*. 3rd edn. Philadelphia: National Board of Medical Examiners, pp. 19–26

Case, S.M., Swanson, D.B., and Becker, D.F. (1996) Verbosity, window dressing and red herrings: do they make a better test item? *Acad Med.* 71: 528–530

Chandratilake, M., Davis, M., and Ponnamperuma, G. (2011) Assessment of medical knowledge: the pros and cons of using true/false multiple choice questions. *Natl Med J Ind.* 4(4): 225–228.

Charlin, B., Roy, L., Brailovsky, C., Goulet, F., and van der Vleuten, C. (2000) The Script Concordance test: a tool to assess the reflective clinician, *Teach Learn Med.* 12(4): 189–195

Christison, R. (1875) President's Address, Delivered at the Forty-Third Annual Meeting of the British Medical Association. *BMJ.* 2: 155

Coderre, S., Woloschuk, W., and McLaughlin, K. (2009) Twelve tips for blueprinting. *Med Teach.* 31(4): 322–324

Cronbach, L. (1951) Coefficient alpha and the internal structure of tests. *Psychometrika.* 16: 297–334

Downing, S.M. (2005) The effects of violating standard item writing principles on tests and students: the consequences of using flawed test items on achievement examinations in medical education. *Adv Health Sci Educ Theory Pract.* 10(2): 133–143

Duggan, P. (2007) Development of a Script Concordance Test using an Electronic Voting System. *J Educ Res Group f Adelaide.* 1(1): 35–41

Freeman, A., Nicholls, A., Ricketts, C., and Coombes, L. (2010) Can we share questions? Performance of questions from different question banks in a single medical school. *Med Teach.* 32(6): 464–466

Gagnon, R., Charlin, B., Coletti, M., et al. (2005) Assessment in the context of uncertainty: how many members are needed on the panel of reference of a script concordance test? *Med Educ.* 39: 284–291

Goldman, E.F., Swayze, S.S., Swinehart, S.E., and Schroth, W.S. (2012) Effecting curricular change through comprehensive course assessment: using structure and process to change outcomes. *Acad Med.* 87(3): 300–307

Hayes, K. and McCrorie, P. (2010) The principles and best practice of question writing for postgraduate examinations. *Best Pract Res Clin Obstet Gynaecol* 24: 783–794

Humbert, AJ., Besinger, B., and Miech, EJ. (2011) Assessing clinical reasoning skills in scenarios of uncertainty: convergent validity for a Script Concordance Test in an emergency medicine clerkship and residency. *Acad Emerg Med.* 18(6): 627–634

Koczwara, A., Patterson, F., Zibarras, L., Kerrin, M., Irish, B., and Wilkinson, M. (2012) Evaluating cognitive ability, knowledge tests and situational judgment tests for postgraduate selection. *Med Educ.* 46(4): 399–408

Lievens, F. and Coetsier, P. (2002) Situational tests in student selection: an examination of predictive validity, adverse impact, and construct validity. *Int J Select Assess.* 10(4): 245–257

Lubarsky, S., Charlin, B., Cook, DA., Chalk, C., and van der Vleuten, CP. (2011) Script concordance testing: a review of published validity evidence. *Med Educ.* 45(4): 329–338

Marie, I., Sibert, L., Roussel, F., Hellot, MF., Lechevallier, J., and Weber, J. (2005) The script concordance test: a new evaluation method of both clinical reasoning and skills in internal medicine. *La Review de Medecine Interne.* 26(6): 501–507

McAleer, S. (2009) Choosing assessment instruments. In J.A. Dent, et al. (eds) *A Practical Guide for Medical Teachers* (pp. 318–324). 3rd edn. London: Elsevier.

McCoubrie, P. (2004) Improving the fairness of multiple-choice questions: a literature review. *Med Teach.* 26(8): 709–712

McDaniel, M.A., Psotka, J., Legree, P.J., Yost, A.P., and Weekley, J.A. (2011) Toward an understanding of situational judgment item validity and group differences. *J Appl Psychol.* 96(2): 327–336

Meterissian, S.H. (2006) A novel method of assessing clinical reasoning in surgical residents. *Surgical Innovation.* 13(2): 115–119

Naeem, N., van der Vleuten, C., and Alfaris, E.A. (2011) Faculty development on item writing substantially improves item quality. *Adv Health Sci Educ Theory Pract.* [Epub], DOI. 10.1007/s10459-011-9315-2

Newble, D.I. and Jaeger, K. (1983) The effect of assessments and examinations on the learning of medical students. *Med Educ.* 17: 165–171

Norman, G.R., Smith, E.K.M., Powles, A.C., Rooney, P.J., Henry, N.L. and Dodd, P.E. (1987) Factors underlying performance on written tests of knowledge. *Med Educ.* 21: 297–304

Palmer, E.J. and Devitt, P.G. (2007) Assessment of higher order cognitive skills in undergraduate education: modified essay or multiple choice questions? Research paper. *BMC Med Educ.* 28: 7–49

Patterson, F., Baron, H., Carr, V., Plint, S., and Lane, P. (2009) Evaluation of three short-listing methodologies for selection into postgraduate training in general practice. *Med* 43(1): 50–57

Schuwirth, L.W.T. and van der Vleuten, C.P.M. (2004) Different written assessment methods: what can be said about their strengths and weaknesses. *Med Educ.* 38(9): 974–979

Schuwirth, L.W.T. and van der Vleuten, C.P.M. (2005) Written assessments. In J.A. Dent, et al. (eds.). *A Practical Guide for Medical Teachers* (pp. 311–322). 2nd edn. London: Elsevier

Schuwirth, L.W.T. and van der Vleuten, C.P.M. (2006) How to design a useful test: The principles of assessment. In *Understanding Medical Education* (p. 6). Edinburgh: Association for the Study of Medical Education

Schuwirth, L.W.T., Southgate, L., Page, G.G., et al. (2002) When enough is enough: a conceptual basis for fair and defensible practice performance assessment. *Med Educ.* 36: 925–930

Schuwirth, L.W.T., van der Vleuten, C.P.M., and Donkers, H.H.L.M. (1996) A closer look at cueing effects in multiple-choice questions. *Med Educ.* 30: 44–49

Siu, E. and Reiter, HI. (2009) Overview: what's worked and what hasn't as a guide towards predictive admissions tool development. *Adv Health Sci Educ Theory Pract.* 14(5): 759–775

Swanson, D.B., Holtzman, K.Z., Allbee, K., and Clauser, B.E. (2006) Psychometric characteristics and response times for content-parallel extended-matching and one-best-answer items in relation to number of options. *Acad Med.* 81(10 Suppl): S52–S55

Swanson, D.B., Holtzman, K.Z., and Allbee, K. (2008) Measurement characteristics of content-parallel single-best-answer and extended-matching questions in relation to number and source of options. *Acad Med.* 83(10 Suppl): S21–S24

Tarrant, M. and Ware, J. (2008) Impact of item-writing flaws in multiple-choice questions on student achievement in high-stakes nursing assessments. *Med Educ.* 42(2): 198–206

Tarrant, M., Ware, J., and Mohammed, A.M. (2009) An assessment of functioning and non-functioning distractors in multiple-choice questions: a descriptive analysis. *BMC Med Educ.* 7: 9–40

Van der Vleuten C.P.M. and Swanson, D.B. (1990) Assessment of clinical skills with standardized patients state of the art. *Teach Learn Med.* 2: 58–76

Vyas, R. and Supe, A. (2008) Multiple choice questions: a literature review on the optimal number of options. *Natl Med J Ind.* 21(3): 130–133

CHAPTER 48

Successful feedback: embedded in the culture

Julian Archer and Joan M. Sargeant

Feedback involves both the giving and receiving, by teachers
and/or learners, and there can be gulfs between these.
John Hattie and Helen Timperley

Introduction

Feedback is 'one of the most important influences on learning and
achievement' (Hattie and Timperley 2007, p. 81). Feedback can
have a profound impact on learning, performance, and behaviours
but it is often not provided; and further, getting the impact right
and avoiding negative outcomes, is not easy for the giver or the
receiver. Feedback comes in many different forms. Ideally, within
an education context, it is specific information provided to a
learner in response to observed performance relative to a standard,
given with the intent to improve subsequent performance (Van De
Ridder et al. 2008). In this chapter, we are referring specifically to
feedback provided by faculty or supervisors in clinical and other
teaching settings, informally or using particular feedback formats
as required by the education programme (e.g. mini-CEX).

However, feedback frequently does not meet all the criteria outlined earlier. Further, feedback is challenging as givers need to
acknowledge the views and needs of the learner and engage the
learner while ensuring the feedback is accurate and offered in a
helpful manner. Learners on the other hand may need to be encouraged to be receptive to feedback that will help them improve.

Feedback in medical education is also challenging as it occurs in
diverse settings: e.g., small groups, examination skills teaching, bedside teaching, advanced operating skills teaching, and emergency
patient care. Additionally, there is a balance to be struck between
protecting professional standards, the needs of the medical student
or doctor but ultimately the rights and safety of the patient. Despite
these challenges, feedback remains as 'the cornerstone of effective
clinical teaching' (Cantillon and Sargeant 2008 p. 1961).

Research shows that providing constructive, focused, relevant
and timely feedback can markedly improve learning and performance, including in medicine (Veloski et al. 2006). In the education literature, Hattie and Timperley (2007, pp. 81–112) reported
a synthesis of a large number of meta-analyses, involving millions
of school pupils, and 6972 effect sizes. They demonstrated that the
typical effect size for 'schooling' (i.e., general classroom instruction

in public education) was 0.40. (i.e. scores improved 40% of a standard deviation). In contrast, individual feedback had on average an
effect size of 0.79 (scores improved 79% of a standard deviation after
feedback). This is impressive, especially when compared to studies in
medical education which show the effect size of lectures and workshops for improving the performance of physicians in practice to be
only 0.07–0.08 (Forsetlund et al. 2009; Grimshaw et al. 2006). Hattie
and Timperley further determined that feedback was variable in its
effect; was most effective when linked to specific activities and learners' goals; and was frequently under-utilized and improperly used.

Seen in this light, direct individual feedback to learners and others can be surprisingly effective in improving performance, and is
sufficient rationale for medical educators to become more adept at
using it effectively.

Getting it right is of central importance. Hattie and Timperley
(2007, pp. 83–84) demonstrated that the average effect sizes of feedback varied considerably between studies and postulated that different types of feedback may have different effects, some working
better than others. Importantly, they identified that multiple factors
influence its effectiveness and that specifically, feedback was most
effective when linked to specific activities and learners' goals, and
was frequently under-utilized and improperly used. Shute (2008,
pp. 153–189) in a further synthesis of the literature identified multiple feedback features and external factors which influence its
effectiveness as a strategy to improve learning. Further, Kluger and
DeNisi (1996, pp. 254–284) found that in a third of the studies they
reviewed, feedback perceived as negative was not seen as accurate or
helpful and actually reduced rather than enhanced performance.

In this chapter we explore the feedback process and the system
and cultural factors influencing it, and propose recommendations
to promote a positive feedback culture. The chapter is divided into
the following sections:

◆ Theoretical perspectives informing feedback

◆ Givers and receivers of feedback

◆ The rules of current feedback models

♦ A re-conceptualization of feedback in medicine as an activity system.

First we discuss the theoretical basis for feedback and propose a theoretical stance that shapes the remainder of the chapter.

Feedback: a theoretical perspective

Feedback is complicated. Indeed what is good feedback is perhaps the first question—how is it successful or effective and how would you know anyway? We will attempt to explore each of these areas but first we are keen to take a theoretical stance. We do this for two reasons: first we have been critical of a lack of theory in the medical feedback literature in the past (Archer 2010), and second we wish to explain the underpinning perspectives and structure that shape this chapter.

Feedback of whatever type is so embedded in clinical practice that we often are not aware that it is there. We often do not label the informal, day-to-day feedback as such. This can be a real problem for educators and for learners. Learners, both students and trainees, complain of rarely receiving feedback (Bing-You et al. 1997; McIlwrick et al. 2006; Sargeant et al. 2010a), while supervisors and clinical educators believe they are giving appropriate feedback. While there is no doubt room for improvement, learners in medical education are often not aware of the feedback they receive.

Medical practice occurs in a multifaceted system and doctors can receive both formal and informal feedback about their performance from many sources—reports, colleagues, patients, managers, as well as family and friends every day. While in this discussion of feedback we will focus on the one-to-one interaction and conversation with the learner, we must not lose sight of the vast experience that doctors bring to medical education in terms of knowledge of feedback from their patient–doctor relationships and even, from their knowledge of physiology and pathophysiology. The following example demonstrates this.

First, think about the consultation with a young depressed person who is struggling following the breakup of her parents' marriage. Ideally, we would hope that the process of recovery begins for this young person at presentation. The doctor has the opportunity, working in collaboration, to provide structured advice to the patient and to refer to a counsellor. As doctors we are most likely to be involved in medication prescription. In this case 2 months later after seeing the practice counsellor regularly, the doctor prescribes her a selective serotonin reuptake inhibitor (SSRI) for ongoing depression.

Six months later the patient returns confused. You discover the SSRI you prescribed has interfered with her antidiuretic hormone (ADH) feedback loop and she has developed hyponatraemia. We all know that feedback loops are an integral part of how we understand physiological regulation and the drive to achieve homeostasis within the human body. We need ADH from our pituitary glands to tell our renal collecting ducts to reabsorb water. If this system fails we cannot concentrate our urine and conserve water. Constant monitoring by the hypothalamus of sodium concentration levels in the blood is required to get the ADH, and therefore fluid levels, right.

So in what way does this clinical scenario help us in our thinking about providing feedback to a junior doctor about whom there have been complaints about unprofessional behaviour, or to a medical student, who having been exceptional for the first 2 years, has

just failed their last two knowledge-based progress tests? Like physiological feedback systems being critical to life, providing feedback to learners is critical to their continued learning and development. As noted in the statistics presented in the Introduction, individualized feedback can have a profound impact on learning. We owe feedback to our learners.

We now move briefly to theories of learning to inform our thinking about feedback and help us to understand the various approaches used (Schunk 2008).

Behavioural scientists understand feedback as a way of reinforcing appropriate and modifying undesirable behaviour (Thorndike 1931). Simply viewed, it is seen as a stimulus–response reaction; i.e. feedback is provided and improvement should result. However, as we can see from some of the evidence presented earlier, it is naïve to consider that feedback will automatically elicit the desired response. Alternatively, while behavioural theories consider feedback as an external influence, cognitive theorists consider the internal mental processes which contribute to learning; e.g. how information is acquired, processed, and stored (Locke and Latham 1990). Learning how these are carried out has led us to understand how best to provide information such as feedback to learners, to enable cognitive processing. For example, providing specific, clear, relevant, timely feedback that is supported by clear standards and understanding of performance expectations, enables learners to more effectively cognitively process and respond to that information.

Constructivists and social theorists provide other lenses on learning. They view learning as taking place in contexts; learners and practitioners construct much of what they learn and understand as a function of their experiences and observations in situations and social interactions (Bandura 1961). They take on feedback, both intended and unintended, from observing and participating in the environment and interactions around them. Messages about what is culturally acceptable and unacceptable, including how to give feedback are internalized.

A fourth group of theorists, humanists, see learning as personal growth and self-actualization and focus upon personal goals and accomplishments. This perspective requires incorporation of the views and perspectives of the individual into the feedback and into developing goals for improvement. Humanist, or person-centred approaches, engage the individual as a partner in the discussion; recipients are not just 'receptacles of feedback' (Aspy and Roebuck 1969; Goodstone and Diamante 1998).

The clinical case of the young woman may be used to illustrate a further point. Clearly, feedback in a physiological biochemical loop is not the same as meeting in an office with a junior doctor to discuss worrying behaviour. However, it helps raise three important principles. First is the idea of continuous feedback. Too often in medical education we think about feedback events and how to do each one better. This is a worthwhile endeavour but not enough. We need to think about feedback as a system in itself that needs to feedback regularly to the recipient. Clearly this is not as regularly as the hypothalamus adjusts ADH levels in response to serum sodium levels but it is a process of regular feedback that has some homogeneity, or at least is clearly linked. Second, is to think about feedback, not in isolation, but as part of a much wider multisystems approach. The ADH feedback loop is not a system in isolation. Other physiological processes impact on it all the time. Similarly, feedback to students and doctors is part of a wider complex system with multiple complex tasks, behaviours, and skills being performed each day. Feedback does not work in isolation from these systems. In the clinical example, prescribing an SSRI, an intervention intended to have a different effect that would rarely affect ADH secretion in most patients, has had a profound unintended consequence. Similarly, we need to understand feedback in medical education and the interventions taking place through the continuum of medical training and practice as potentially healing or harmful. Understanding the potential impact of feedback (remembering that it might not be as intended) is central to success.

So what does this mean for feedback and its educational potential? On returning to the troubled young person we need often to understand the 'causes of the causes'. Why is this patient depressed when many young people experience parental break up, yet cope well? Psychiatrists would look to a biopsychosocial model of understanding the patient as an individual but in a complex world of social conflicts. We advocate a similar approach to feedback conceptualizing feedback as a system—not as a one-to-one activity, but as an activity within the complex system of healthcare.

What theoretical and practical frameworks are there then, that might help us understand and undertake feedback better? We propose that understanding both feedback itself and how it functions within a complex system is central. With this in mind we draw on activity theory as a way of thinking about feedback as an activity within a wider system and culture of healthcare.

Cultural–historical activity theory (CHAT) theorizes that people continually shape, and are shaped, by their social and cultural contexts (Engestrom 1987). It draws on both sociocultural activity and individual behaviour in an analytic approach, which links forms of inquiry from both sociology and psychology.

Engestrom (1999 pp. 19–38) described various inter-relating components within systems. We apply these components to the feedback system as shown in figure 1. Connected across the centre of the triangle is the subject, in this case the feedback receiver, the activity or the feedback itself, the object of feedback which is to bring about positive performance change and the overall outcome of the process which is improved practice and ultimately better patient care. The feedback process is mediated by factors identified at the 3 corners of the triangle, and at the base. The base represents the community, most importantly the feedback givers but also all who make up the healthcare system, such as faculty, practising doctors, managers, patients, nurses and allied health professionals.

Artefacts are mediational means or instruments which influence the feedback activity process—such as forms for recording feedback or student portfolios. The *division of labour* or *roles* refers to both the horizontal division of tasks between the members of the community and to the vertical division of power and status, all of which can influence the culture of feedback. *Rules* refer to the explicit and implicit regulations, norms and conventions that constrain actions and interactions within the activity system (Engestrom 1987). These rules are both explicit in the way feedback is conveyed, and implicit in professional and institutional culture.

Engestrom (1993, pp. 64–103) applied activity theory to understand the consultation in medicine. He analysed the work of a general practitioner within a primary health centre network in Finland. The interview with the patient was the primary activity as the doctor conducted the consultation. Engestrom, by also examining the groups that were seen as part of the community within the medical activity system (the nurses, medical specialists, bureaucrats, and the general public), demonstrated that the division of labour within the constituent groups structured particular interactions between the doctor and patient. The full analysis of the work of the general practitioner during the consultation was adequate only when seen as part of the collective activity system of which the consultation was an element. We argue that the same is true of feedback. While we often see feedback narrowly as an interaction between recipient and giver, using CHAT as a working theory and a structure aids in demonstrating that feedback is part of a much wider complex system. Understanding the influence of the elements of the system upon the feedback process can enable sustainable change in the feedback process.

Actual feedback events are important and important to get right—just like the consultation in Engestrom's example. However, resources on feedback have traditionally focused almost solely on the feedback interaction. We will discuss feedback interactions in detail but first we will start by discussing the wider system itself—placing feedback in context.

Feedback in context

Feedback in medical education takes place within education and healthcare communities, cultures and systems. Because it is so influenced by these contexts, it is difficult and indeed unproductive to think of it as an isolated event. For example, the expectations of the medical profession and the professional messages conveyed influence perceptions of feedback. Freidson (1994) explored the high standards imposed within the medical profession and noted that, although considered a collegial profession, the sharing of constructive feedback between professionals was rarely practised. The expectation is that doctors will be high performers who are self-monitoring. Implicit within that is the notion that collegial feedback is not needed. Kennedy et al. (2004, pp. 386–93) has more recently studied this phenomenon and also the impact that high expectations of competence and performance have upon trainees. They found that doctors in training were reluctant to ask for feedback and that asking was perceived as a sign of weakness, a lack of confidence or competence. Feedback was seen as 'bad', not 'good'.

Another part of our culture is the manner in which much of feedback has traditionally been delivered to learners. A paternalist approach, in which critical or corrective messages are delivered, has been the mainstay of feedback provision. Many doctors now in practice share stories, and even wounds, from such feedback delivered in an unhelpful and damaging manner. Such practices have had a strong influence on the culture of feedback.

Indeed, the professional culture of medicine influences the providing and receiving of feedback in various other ways too. Medicine has followed a traditional hierarchical leadership model. There are some efforts to develop leaders earlier on in doctors' careers but essentially leadership still comes with title and time. This 'top down' model impacts on any espoused feedback model. Take an example from industry where changes in leadership allowed the development of appraisal. It was always conceived that the formal hierarchical structure in organizational management was paramount to the success and growth of any company. But the 1970s witnessed a paradigm shift from 'transactional' to 'transformational' leadership. Transactional leadership involved a leader directing his workforce through control and command strategies. Burns (1978 p. 163) summarizes transformational leadership, as the ability to balance liberty and power by encouraging the empowerment of employees.

This allows and encourages independent practice, thinking and organizational decision making. The change from transactional to transformational leadership led to a flattening out of the management structures within business—opening the way for the development of appraisal systems (Mann 1971). As the 'flattening' progressed further, it ultimately led away from simple downward appraisal models to new more rounded 360-degree approaches to appraisal with feedback going up and down as well as around the pay grades. Without such cultural shifts it is unlikely that such feedback loops would have been possible.

So professional culture is important as this shapes the thinking about who gives and who should receive feedback, about how it is given and what its purpose is. If feedback is seen as a top-down, one-way delivery of corrective information, it shapes the culture, expectations and fears of learners. It can impact unfavourably on relationships within the feedback system. Alternatively, if feedback is viewed as information to help the learner improve, and is offered in a supportive manner which engages the views of the learner, it shapes the culture in a different way.

How then might we respond? In the context of understanding feedback as an activity in a wider system we argue that the whole community involved in giving and receiving feedback is important to getting feedback right. A significant part of this provision comes in understanding who is responsible for what, where the professional 'power' lies, and what impact this power might have on the feedback giving and receiving. Before we explore how to support feedback, we want to discuss what feedback is, in more depth.

Feedback activity

Thinking of feedback as the straightforward transmission of information from a teacher or supervisor to a learner is overly simplistic. Over 40 years ago, Ilgen et al. (1979, pp. 349–71) described feedback as a 'complex and multifaceted cognitive, social and personal activity informed by multiple psychological perspectives'. In spite of this recognition so many years ago, we in medical education still tend to view feedback in a more or less linear, simplistic manner, generally as a one-way delivery of information.

More recent definitions are helpful in moving us along the path to greater understanding and more appropriate use of feedback. Van de Ridder and colleagues (2008, pp. 189–197) propose that feedback is 'specific information about the comparison between a trainee's observed performance and a standard, given with the intent to improve trainee's performance'. Viewing feedback in this manner is especially helpful in medical education where so much of the learning and feedback occurs in clinical and other settings with learners actually 'doing' or 'performing'.

Feedback, to be effective, should follow observation of learners, and formally or informally, communicate information about how the learner is doing. The goal of feedback is to guide further learning and improvement (Epstein and Hunbert 2002). Sometimes though, this goal can appear to be lost, and the learner feels that feedback is solely a criticism of their performance. Focusing on the goal of feedback (i.e. learner improvement) provides both a philosophical and practical stance for providing feedback. If the goal is improvement, then the focus for the provider of the feedback is upon how to provide the feedback in a manner that will best promote learner acceptance and subsequent improvement. Such a perspective can potentially transform traditional perceptions of feedback as 'critique' or 'criticism' to being seen as helpful and enabling.

Providing feedback, then, is critical to helping learners improve. Without it, they report that they do not know how they are doing and do not know what to do to improve (Sargeant et al. 2010a). With feedback from those more experienced, they can see more readily how to improve and what they need to learn and do to get there; feedback speeds up the learning process. In fact, it can be argued, teachers and supervisors are not fulfilling their responsibilities if they fail to give regular and effective feedback. Furthermore, feedback, by informing learners about how they are doing helps them to become more informed and more accurate self-assessors of their own performance and knowledge. Having this occur, within a culture and system which is supportive of

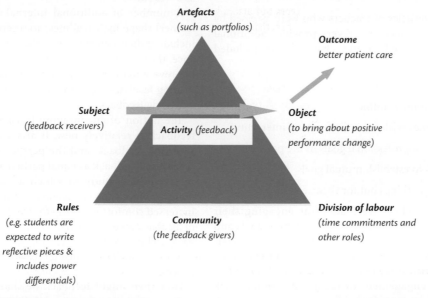

Figure 48.1 A feedback activity system.

Data from Engestrom, Y. (1987). Learning by Expanding: An Activity-theorectical Approach to Developmental Research Helsinki, Finland: Orienta-Konsultit.

learning and improvement, further strengthens the impact of the feedback.

The subject, feedback community and their roles: feedback givers and receivers

As Hattie and Timperley (2007, p. 103) noted 'feedback involves both the giving and receiving, by teachers and/or learners, and there can be gulfs between these'. In this section we will consider the 'givers' and the 'receivers' of feedback (in terms of CHAT: the subject, roles and divisions of labour) and the factors influencing the message. Simply put, frequently the situation is one of a supervisor who is uncomfortable providing feedback and a learner who is uncomfortable receiving feedback. Seen in this light, it is not surprising that constructive feedback is reportedly infrequently shared. For example, supervisors often feel nervous and under equipped to deal with feedback provision especially if it is negative. As a result they often 'fail to fail' learners even when it is appropriate to do so (Dudek and Marks 2005).

Feedback givers

The role of faculty and supervisors as feedback givers is important. Medical education research confirms this importance, with many clinical educators realizing that they need development in this area (Bahar-Ozvaris et al. 2004). They also frequently report feeling ill-prepared to provide feedback, especially feedback seen as negative and unsupported by their education programme in trying to do this effectively. More so, faculty may not recognize the potential of feedback as a developmental tool; they might be unaware of the educational impact of facilitating reflection upon feedback and performance; and might be reluctant to fail the failing student (Dudek and Marks 2005; Menachery et al. 2006). Hence, multiple important and practical factors contribute to a sense of incapacity on the part of faculty; addressing these is central to building their skill and confidence in providing feedback. Understanding rules, roles and responsibilities is important in supporting a successful conversation.

A study of the characteristics of teachers who were assessed by students as being effective feedback givers provides additional insights (Menachery et al. 2006). Positive characteristics included that the faculty:

1. Addressed learners' emotional responses.

2. Were proficient in handling conflict.

3. Asked learners what they wish from the teaching interaction.

4. Had reviewed their own professional goals in the past year.

5. Worked with learners to establish mutual goals.

6. Often let learners figure things out for themselves.

It appears that these teachers were adept at engaging their learners in the feedback conversation, in establishing goals and seeking solutions. Such findings emphasize that success in feedback requires an engaged and active conversation, in which the learner is an active participant, not a passive one. Also noted, informed and sincere engagement of faculty in the feedback process is critical, a finding reinforced by more recent research (Watling et al. 2008).

Effective feedback givers also recognize that performance needs to be observed before feedback can be given. Otherwise, specific and relevant data cannot be shared, and as a result, learners question feedback credibility. This is particularly important when providing feedback on clinical skills and performance (Holmboe and Hawkins 2008; Holmboe et al. 2004). For busy clinicians, observing learners' performance means planning and making time for observation.

An additional skill of effective feedback givers is the ability to promote reflection upon and self-assessment of one's performance and analysis of the feedback—considered by some to be the meta-cognitive skills of feedback (Bing-You and Trowbridge 2009). These activities further enable a feedback conversation between the giver and receiver—feedback is no longer a one-way transmission. Additionally, inquiring as to the learner's goals for the feedback experience and asking them for their self-assessment of how the experience is contributing to meeting those goals can enhance feedback understanding and acceptance (Goodstone and Diamante 1998).

Feedback receivers

A number of studies have documented students' and residents' views that they receive inadequate feedback or feedback lacking in quality and helpfulness (Bing-You et al. 1997; Hewson and Little 1998). While they perceive they are receiving insufficient feedback, their teachers' view may be that they are offering plenty, hence the concept of the gap (Hattie and Timperley 2007; Shute 2008).

Several studies have addressed the feedback seeking and receiving behaviours of medical learners. Teunissen et al. (2009, pp. 910–17) and Nussbaum and Dweck (2008, pp. 599–612) in different types of studies identified two orientations to feedback in learners—a development orientation versus a competence orientation. For the former the need to learn and develop is dominant and learners readily use and even seek out feedback. For the latter orientation, the need to appear competent dominates and hence asking for and even being receptive to feedback is viewed as a weakness.

A number of additional internal influences (i.e. within the learner) shape their readiness to receive, accept and use feedback, including their perceptions of themselves and their own performance, their levels of self-confidence, their motivation to learn and improve, and their emotional reactions to disappointing or disconfirming feedback. All can have a negative impact upon receiving and using feedback.

The notion of encouraging learners to more frequently seek feedback is relatively new. It arises from learners' difficulty in receiving feedback, and the perspective of seeing the giver and receiver of feedback as equal participants in the process. A recent interventional study in which a group of students were formally prepared to seek feedback during their clerkship, showed increased comfort in asking for feedback and increased frequency of feedback received (Milan et al. 2011). Enhancing learners' feedback-seeking skills and creating an environment which supports this are strategies to consider as we seek to improve the feedback process.

How then might feedback be shared and discussed to foster better reception and response? There are a number of types and structures of feedback, which we will highlight next.

The 'rules': current feedback practice and models

Feedback types

The literature summarizes feedback as having either a directive or facilitative function. The old model of directive feedback simply informs the learner of what requires correction. Facilitative feedback, as we advocate, involves the provision of comments and suggestions to support the learner's own revisions. Feedback comes in different structures. It may be as simple as verification ('is it right or wrong?') or be elaborative to support the learner to reach the correct answer. Elaborative or facilitated feedback engages the learner as an active participant in the feedback and improvement process. Shute (2008, pp. 153–189) describes elaborative feedback as breaking down into five types; address the topic, address the response, discuss the particular errors, provide worked errors (by talking through examples of how particular errors could be avoided)and give gentle feedback. Additionally, specific feedback appears to work better than vague and non-specific feedback.

The process of providing constructive feedback that will be accepted and used for improvement is a complex task. Feedback content should be clear, mutually understood, specific and relevant. The feedback process should be timely, interactive, non-judgemental and accompanied by explanation: it should recognize and integrate the recipient's perspectives, foster self-assessment and reflection, and facilitate development of an action plan (Branch and Paranjape 2002; Epstein and Hunbert 2002; Holmboe et al. 2004; Menachery et al. 2006; McIlwrick et al. 2006; Westberg and Jason 2001; Hewson and Little 1998).

Feedback comes from many different sources. The commonest source perhaps is the feedback provided in every day practice through observation and report, the focus of this chapter. Much of this is unstructured and follows interactions between givers and receivers at the bedside or in the classroom. Increasingly such feedback in the clinical setting is becoming more structured through formal workplace-based assessment (WBA) strategies (Norcini and Burch 2008). WBA generally uses standardized formats, allowing a more structured approach to feedback giving (and recording the event). These include:

- capturing learner interactions with patients, such as with the mini-CEX (Holmboe et al. 2004)

- watching and scoring procedures, such as with the direct observation of procedural skills (DOPS) (Wilkinson et al. 2008)

- working with patient notes, such as in case-based discussion (Davies et al. 2009)

- asking colleagues in a systematic way, such as multisource feedback (Archer et al. 2005).

In all these situations, engaging the learner in a discussion about the feedback, which draws upon their self-assessment and perspectives for improvement is the goal, rather than a one-way transmission of information.

An additional source unique to the health professions is feedback directly from patients. Doctors have reported that, in a multisource feedback context, in which patients, medical colleagues and cow-orkers provide formal feedback via questionnaires, they responded most readily to and make the greatest number of practice changes in response to feedback from patients (Sargeant et al. 2005). However, the validity of patient feedback is far from assured as it is currently constructed, as rarely do colleagues and patients agree about doctors' performance even when concerns have been raised (Archer and McAvoy 2011).

Ideally, all feedback is discussed face-to-face with an appropriately prepared feedback giver (Hewson and Little 1998). As noted in the section on 'Feedback givers', supervisors often feel ill-prepared to provide constructive feedback. Providing workshops and faculty development can enhance their skills and degree of comfort. Learning facilitation skills is vital, especially when sharing negative feedback that may elicit a negative emotional response or resistance by the learner. Exploring the learners' emotional reactions and reasons for them can promote acceptance of the feedback and its use for improvement (Goodstone and Diamante 1998). An alternative approach to facilitating feedback is through the use of scaffolding. This may help by providing cues, prompts, hints and partial solutions as well as direct instruction (Hartman 2002). Scaffolding involves motivating, breaking down any task to make it more achievable, providing direction, identifying gaps between performance and desired outcomes, reducing personal risk and helping to define goals. As the name implies, it is called scaffolding as the giver is not meant to become an integral part of the process but something removable over time as the receiver gains knowledge, skills, and confidence.

Timing

A challenge especially within busy clinical practice is being able to give feedback immediately after a procedure, patient interaction, or other performance that has been observed. However, giving feedback immediately after the event, or as close to it as possible, is critical to enhancing its effectiveness (Shute 2008). Students and residents frequently describe receiving feedback too long after the event for it still to be relevant or useful. Evidence suggests that efficacy and the feedback timing may be related to the focus and difficulty of the task (Schroth 1992); doctors, in common with other high achievers, may benefit from delayed feedback when undertaking complex tasks as it is hypothesized that learners are better supported by reducing interruptions (Mason and Bruning 2001). We love to engage with students and doctors as they go through a procedure or consultation but in fact, as high achievers, they are better left to it. How often do we simply 'chip in' to control things or simply to display our own knowledge? Feedback needs to be timely and received 'mindfully' (Bangert-Drowns et al. 1991). That is we should give learners time to think, set the task at the right level to challenge but neither to insult nor overwhelm, and above all be as fair and consistent as we can.

Overall feedback must not be seen as a passive process placed onto the learner who either responds or not. The learner is the focus, the feedback simply a modality. So, as feedback is difficult to get right, and the consequences of getting it wrong can be harmful, there has been a move to provide accessible models to support its delivery. This is the focus of the next section.

The practical models

Feedback is a facilitated and purposeful conversation between the giver and receiver with the goal of enabling feedback acceptance and use for improvement. However, this is a relatively recent conceptualization of feedback. Here, we will briefly review earlier models of providing feedback.

The 'feedback sandwich' is a traditionally used model: it delivers the critical or corrective feedback 'sandwiched' between the positives (Pendleton et al. 1984). It centres on personal protection for the receiver and provider by balancing and even camouflaging the constructive message. However, there is a danger that the receiver is so protected from any critical feedback that it is not perceived and hence the receiver does not seek to make any change. While it is admirable that the giver chooses to balance the feedback with the psychosocial needs of the receiver, ensuring *interactional justice* (Folger and Cropanzano 1998, p. 232), the outcome in terms of positive performance change in response to the feedback cannot be mitigated. Pendleton's rules (1984, pp. 68–71) try to build on the feedback sandwich by introducing a two way conversation, which allows the receiver to respond to feedback first. In a further attempt to transition the feedback exchange from a 'delivery' to a 'conversation' engaging the learner, the ECO model suggests three steps: encouraging an **E**motional response prior to exploring **C**ontent in order to establish **O**utcomes (Bruce and Sargeant 2007). The overall goal of the model is to promote the learner's use of the feedback for improvement, by engaging the learner in self-assessment, reflection, problem-solving, and planning through a series of facilitative questions.

While feedback giving and receiving is complex, there is scientific evidence that points to helpful features of feedback. For example, learners have told us that providing feedback of a general nature, like 'you're doing fine' or 'you have nothing to worry about' is not helpful. Supervisors may offer it because it is easy and they do not want to be seen as critical of learners. Learners describe it as too general and non-specific to help them improve. They would prefer more specific feedback (Sargeant and Mann 2010b). While we argue that one to one interaction is only part of the whole system that needs to support positive feedback it is the core part and needs to be consciously addressed. There are five important elements of effective feedback (van de Ridder et al. 2008). They are summarized in table 48.1.

Supporting feedback through culture and artefacts

Now we have explored the various rules and roles within giving and receiving feedback, consider again being asked to observe a medical student take a history with a patient and report back to you. This time you go with the student and she begins the consultation. Two minutes into the consultation your pager goes off and you leave to take the call, apologizing to the patient as you go. Five minutes later you return to hear the rest of the consultation and retire to your office with the student to discuss the case. During the presentation the phone rings and you take the call; you are brief and excuse yourself, but 2 minutes are lost, in which the student quietly reads their history through and flicks the pages of a small pocket reference book. You then discuss the case with the student. The student is uncertain in areas, but overall is good, and you feed back some positive aspects as well as areas for development. The student hesitates and points out that the areas you highlight as missing or inadequate happened at the bedside while you were absent. You half retreat, but not wanting to miss the 'importance' of your statement you still reinforce the ideas for improvement. The student thanks you and asks if you will complete the online feedback form that the institution requires for the student to complete their portfolio.

You turn to your computer. You watch awkwardly as the 14 various screens of security and boot-up code make slow progress. When you come to log in you are forced to change your password. You then can't remember your password for the university system. You tell the student you have it somewhere and you will complete the form another time. Two weeks later the student emails you and politely asks if you will complete the form as their placement is coming to an end. Does this sound familiar?

Delivering medical training in any healthcare system is challenging. We are pulled between the various roles that any professional position brings. So often we are torn between the immediacy of patient care and the needs of students and doctors in training. We know that, but how often do we think about the impact that the

Table 48.1 Five important elements for effective feedback

Element	Element explained	Working example
Specific information	Feedback information must be specific to the task and not general	'When you spoke to Mrs Jones you appeared distracted and didn't always respond to her answers before moving on' rather than 'you can come across as being rude'
Comparison	Feedback must compare the learner's performance to a specific performance standard so learners can clearly see the gap	'I would expect someone at your level to be able to tie sutures only, so well done' rather than simply 'well done'
Observed performance	The performance of the task must be observed by the individual providing the feedback	If you decide to observe part of a consultation in order to complete a mini-CEX, explain to both the patient and the student/doctor that you will leave at some stage rather than just leaving.
Standard	A standard must be shared or the rationale for the feedback made clear to the learner	'This form gives you a "needs development" score for your cannulation skills. This is because I am asked to score you against someone at finals and you are not there as of yet—but you have 18 months to go'
Intent to improve	Feedback is to be offered in a manner which will enable the learner to improve	'I found that once I could intubate I got a bit overconfident and started to put the blade too far down—losing sight of the cords. I know you can intubate, and wondered if that might have happened to you recently as you said you seem to have lost your touch?'

scenario described earlier may have on individuals? It is likely that we come away from such interactions rationalizing the contribution we make. 'Students have to get used to the realities of medicine', 'I gave her my time and gave feedback when I am busy'; but is this the student's perception and if not what has got in the way of good feedback? In this example let us assume that all other aspects went well in terms of feedback practice, as discussed earlier. What this example shows is the impact of artefacts, the things that inadvertently shape human interactions.

Feedback is often facilitated by various artefacts or instruments, by which it is hoped that feedback will be supported or simply delivered. A critical eye should be cast over such artefacts in order to understand not only how they support feedback in any purported way but also if there are any unintended consequences of their involvement (Fenwick 2011).

In this example interruptions are obvious examples of material things that could get in the way of good feedback practice. Pagers are good examples of everyday materials that are essential to healthcare provision but can become important distractors in feedback and the wider educational experience. Undertaking feedback in real time will always be challenged by such interruptions but making provisions as best as can be achieved can be central to delivering feedback that *matters*. To the recipient the feedback event is important, potentially central to their thinking and even their progression. It is likely to be stressful. As educators we need to think more often about the recipient as the centrepiece of the feedback process. They matter, the feedback matters.

One specific example within this scenario that is worth particular note is that of the information technology (IT). So often in modern training IT systems have been developed to facilitate the provision of feedback as well as its collation. ePortfolios particularly have been developed and advocated as a solution to coordinating and often delivering education for individuals and groups. But where do ePortfolios really sit in the process? In this example, a not unfamiliar one for many, technology use can become the core action rather than simply being part of the process. The information gathered and shared is what feedback is about. This can be helped by systems that store such feedback, collate it over time, and facilitate reflection. However, we need to be careful about what is central and facilitative of the feedback process and what are simply distracters. Another commonly reported aid for the provision and evaluation of feedback is the written clinical encounter card, which tailors feedback to the clinical context and guides faculty and learners through the feedback and improvement process. These are generally completed daily or several times a week by the learner and the faculty and are discussed with the goal of informing improvement (Paukert et al. 2002). Faculty and learners have found this format effective for enhancing feedback, reporting that feedback can be more constructive, timely, and concrete than that received in other, less regular methods (Schum et al. 2003). Such formal strategies are not meant, however, to replace the informal feedback from supervisors and others in clinical settings.

While systems, such as IT systems, can be instrumental in supporting feedback we must always have a critical eye on anything that is in danger of distracting the core business of feedback—recipient and giver working together to positively influence performance. Feedback must be more than simply entering data into a system.

Reconceptualizing feedback: an activity system integrating culture and continuum

As we started by illustrating, all types of feedback can be thought of as taking place in loops geared toward improving learners' development, and as part of wider systems. These feedback loops are not acting in isolation but impact on the wider system and as importantly, the wider system impacts on the feedback.

So we need to reconceptualize feedback as part of a wider healthcare system; influencing healthcare, influenced by healthcare.

The conversation

The limitations of earlier practical models are that they continue to use a rather reductionist approach, and are embedded in the hierarchical paradigm. Later models acknowledge the importance of two-way interactions, but feedback still has largely remained in one direction as an educator-driven process (Molloy 2009). In contrast, those studying feedback are now conceptualizing feedback as a purposeful conversation between the giver and receiver, facilitated by the giver with the goal of engaging the learner and enabling feedback acceptance and use for improvement.

Many factors influence the ability to have such effective feedback conversations. As well as individual factors like supervisor and learner training and preparation for feedback exchange, we will also benefit by returning to the systems and cultural factors which profoundly influence the feedback exchange.

A feedback culture

Building a positive feedback culture is core to the success of helping feedback make a difference. Like all cultures, a feedback culture would give an explicit message about what is acceptable and expected practice. Supporting feedback conversations, which engage the learner and focus on their improvement, sends a different message about what is valued in the culture, than the traditional top-down, one-way delivery of feedback. How can we make this happen? We need to create a culture in which it is safe to give and receive feedback, in which corrective feedback is viewed positively as an opportunity to improve, rather than negatively as painful criticism. Some steps toward this include faculty and supervisors modelling both giving and receiving feedback from each other, their asking for feedback from learners, and explicitly using it for improvement. Encouraging learners to seek out and ask for feedback is another strategy. Setting these expectations as an institution can change the culture.

There are already many opportunities to provide feedback that need not create huge amounts of additional work. For example, we often miss the opportunity to provide robust feedback in summative assessment as we do not see summative tests as part of the educational cycle. Assessment is in danger of being seen as disassociated, becoming an artefact that moves away from learning rather than towards a continuum of life-long learning.

A feedback continuum

We know that performance feedback can improve professional practice but the effects are generally small (Thomson O'Brien et al. 2000). The relative effectiveness appears to be linked to belief in proposed change and when the feedback is delivered intensively.

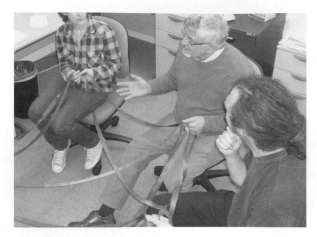

Figure 48.2 A group of people in a feedback conversation.

Therefore facilitation is the cornerstone of feedback success including supporting an appropriate response to negative feedback (Kluger and DeNisi 1996). There is a danger that feedback is seen as a series of unrelated events when, as we have proposed, it should be part of an interactive system.

Figure 48.2 shows a group of people in a feedback conversation. They are linked with ribbons to each other, to other people and other things (such as communities, artefacts, roles, power struggles) that also shape and influence their conversation. It is only by thinking in terms of who has what role, what are the rules of the system, and what artefacts are at play and what impact do they have, that we can start to understand how to develop a culture and continuum of feedback in the workplace for all learners. One way of supporting such a culture is by establishing longer-term professional relationships. The apprenticeship model in western healthcare systems may no longer be sustainable (Dornan 2005)—due to shorter hours and more part-time working. Part of our educational response to this has to be to develop advocate forms of supervision, where supervisors, trainers, and appraisers support individuals over time by bringing together sources of feedback in a meaningful way to provide a profile of and for an individual. This relationship needs protection and while feedback from assessment must go into this facilitative relationship it would be best practice that this learner relationship, be it at medical school, in training, or as part of a revalidation process, should be protected from becoming part of a summative process. Unclear roles of feedback can undermine any system trying to support learners by making the rules unclear about what data is used for.

In order to make any system work effectively there needs to be faculty who are trained and resourced sufficiently to provide the high quality facilitation. The system needs to acknowledge and support those in roles who have a significant proportion of their 'division of labour' dedicated to teaching. We need to work to support learners from the cradle to the grave through powerful systems of facilitated feedback that provide a continuum of learning. In order to do that we need to remember that feedback is a system impacted upon by many factors that need conscious consideration in order to secure the positive impact that we know from the evidence can be achieved to support professional performance and therefore ultimately benefit patient care.

Conclusions

◆ Feedback is not simply the delivery of information to an individual about their performance.

◆ Feedback is better understood as part of a complex system impacted upon and impacting on the wider healthcare system.

◆ Roles, workload and an understanding of communities and artefacts, like IT systems, need to be better understood in order to support not impede effective feedback.

◆ The feedback conversation remains at the heart of effective feedback and should be supported by a trained facilitator to make sure that feedback is specific; follows observation; is standardized and comparative; and has a view to support improvement.

References

Archer, J. (2010) The current state of the science in health professional education: effective feedback. *Med Educ.* 44: 101–108

Archer, J. and McAvoy, P. (2011) Exploring what might undermine the validity of patient and multisource feedback. *Med Educ.* 45(9): 886–893

Archer, J., Norcini, J., and Davies, H.A. (2005) Use of SPRAT for peer review of paediatricians in training. *BMJ.* 330(7502): 1251–1253

Aspy, D. and Roebuck, F. (1969) Our research and our findings. In C.R. Roger (ed.) *Freedom to Learn: a view of what education might become.* (pp. 163–171) Columbus, OH: Charles E Merrill

Bahar-Ozvaris, S., Aslan, D., Sahin-Hodoglugil, N., and Sayek, I. (2004) A faculty development program evaluation: from needs assessment to long-term effects of the teaching skills improvement program. *Teach Learn Med.* 16(4): 368–375

Bandura, A. (1961) Psychotherapy as a learning process. *Psychol Bull.* 58: 143–159

Bangert-Drowns, R.L., Kulik, C.C., Kulik, J.A., and Morgan, M.T. (1991) The instructional effect of feedback in test-like events. *Rev Educ Res.* 61: 213–238

Bing-You, R. and Trowbridge, R.L. (2009) Why medical educators may be failing at feedback. *JAMA.* 302(12): 1330–1331

Bing-You, R., Paterson, J., and Levine, A.M. (1997) Feedback falling on deaf ears: residents' receptivity to feedback tempered by sender credibility. *Med Teach.* 19(1): 40–44

Branch, W.T. and Paranjape, A. (2002) Feedback and reflection: Teaching Methods for clinical settings. *Acad Med.* 77(12): 1185–1188

Bruce, D. and Sargeant, J. (2007) Multi-source feedback. In K. Mohanna and A. Tavabie (eds) *General Practice Specialty Training: Making It Happen* (pp. 135–144). London: RCFP

Burns, J.M. (1978) *Leadership* New York: Harper & Row

Cantillon, P. and Sargeant, J. (2008) Giving feedback in clinical settings. *BMJ.* 337: a1961

Davies, H., Archer, J., Southgate, L., and Norcini, J. (2009) Initial evaluation of the first year of the Foundation Assessment Programme. *Med Educ.* 43(1): 74–81

Dornan, T. (2005) Osler, Flexner, apprenticeship and 'the new medical education'. *J R Soc Med.* 98(3): 91–95

Dudek, N.L. and Marks, M.B. (2005) Failure to fail: the perceptions of clinical supervisors. *Acad Med.* 80(10): S84–S87

Engestrom, Y. (1987) *Learning by Expanding: an activity-theoretical approach to developmental research.* Helsinki, Finland: Orienta-Konsultit

Engestrom, Y. (1993) Developmental studies of work as a testbench of activity theory: the case of primary care medical practice. In S. Chaiklin and J. Lave (eds) *Understanding Practice: Perspectives on Activity and Context* (pp. 64–103). Cambridge UK: Cambridge University Press

Engestrom, Y. (1999) Activity theory and individual and social transformation. In Y. Engestrom, R. Miettinen, and R.L. Punamaki (eds)

Perspectives on Activity Theory (pp. 19–38). Cambridge, UK: Cambridge University Press

Epstein, R.M. and Hunbert, E.M. (2002) Defining and assessing professional competence. *JAMA.* 287: 226–235

Fenwick, T. (2011) Sociomaterial approaches: contributions and issues for educational research. In: T. Fenwick, R. Edwards, and P. Sawchuk (eds) *Emerging Approaches to Educational Research: Tracing the Sociomaterial* (p. 177). Oxford: Routledge

Folger, R. and Cropanzano, R. (1998) Organizational justice and performance evaluation: test and trial metaphors. In: R. Folger and R. Cropanzano (eds) *Organizational Justice and Human Resource Management.* (pp. 108–132) Beverly Hills CA: Sage Publications

Forsetlund, L., Bjørndal, A., Rashidian, A., et al. (2009) Continuing education meetings and workshops: Effects on professional practice and health care outcomes. Vol. 2 *Cochrane Database Syst Rev:* CD003030

Freidson, E. (1994) *Professionalism Reborn: Theory, Prophecy, and Policy.* Chicago: University of Chicago Press

Goodstone, M.S. and Diamante, T. (1998) Organizational use of therapeutic change strengthening multisource feedback systems through interdisciplinary coaching. *Consult Psychol J Pract Res.* 50(3): 152–163

Grimshaw, J., Eccles, M., Thomas, R., et al. (2006) Toward Evidence-Based Quality Improvement. *J Gen Intern Med.* 21(S2): S14–S20

Hartman, H. (2002) Scaffolding and cooperative learning. *Human Learning and Instruction.* New York: City College, University of New York, pp. 23–69

Hattie, J. and Timperley,H. (2007) The power of feedback. *Rev Educ Res.* 77: 81–112

Hewson, M.G. and Little, M.L. (1998) Giving feedback in medical education: verification of recommended techniques. *J Gen Intern Med.* 13(2): 111–116

Holmboe, E.S. and Hawkins, R.E. (2008) *Practical Guide to the Evaluation of Clinical Competence.* Philadelphia, PA: Mosby/Elsevier

Holmboe, E.S., Yepes, M., Williams, F., and Huot, S.J. (2004) Feedback and the mini clinical evaluation exercise. *J Gen Intern Med.* 19: 558–561

Ilgen, D.R., Fisher, C.D., and Taylor, M.S. (1979) Consequences of individual feedback on behavior in organizations. *J Appl Psychol.* 64(4): 349–371

Kennedy, T., Regehr, G., Rosenfield, J., Roberts, S.W., and Lingard, L. (2004) Exploring the gap between knowledge and behavior: a qualitative study of clinical action following an educational intervention. *Acad Med.* 79(5): 386–393

Kluger, A.N. and DeNisi, A. (1996) The effects of feedback intervention on performance: A historical review, a meta-analysis, and a preliminary feedback intervention theory. *Psychol Bull.* 119: 254–284

Locke, E.A. and Latham, G.P. (1990) *A Theory of Goal Setting and Task Performance.* Englewood Cliffs, NJ: Prentice Hall

Mann, F.C. (1971) Studying and creating change: a means to understanding social organisation. In H. Hornstein (ed.) *Social Intervention: A Behavioral Science Approach* (pp. 294–305). New York: Free Press

Mason, B.J. and Bruning, R. (2001) *Providing feedback in computer-based instruction: What the research tells us.* [Online] Center for Instructional Innovation, University of Nebraska-Lincoln. [Online] http://dwb.unl.edu/Edit/MB/MasonBruning.html Accessed 12 March 2013

McIlwrick, J., Nair, B., and Montgomery, G. (2006) 'How am I doing?': Many problems but few solutions related to feedback delivery in undergraduate psychiatry education. *Acad.Med.* 30: 130–135

Menachery, E.P., Knight, A.M., Kolodner, K., and Wright, S.M. (2006) Physician characteristics associated with proficiency in feedback skills. *J Gen Intern Med.* 21: 440–446

Milan, F., Dyche, L., and Fletcher, J. (2011) 'How am I doing?' Teaching Medical Students to elicit feedback during their clerkships. *Med Teach.* 33(11): 904–910

Molloy, E. (2009) Time to pause: giving and receiving feedback in clinical education. In C. Delany and E. Molloy (eds) *Clinical Education in the Health Professions.* 1st edn (p. 304). Sydney: Churchill Livingstone

Norcini, J. and Burch, V. (2008) Workplace-based assessment as an educational tool: AMEE Guide No.31. *Med Teach.* 29(9): 855–871

Nussbaum, A.D. and Dweck C.S. (2008) Defensiveness versus remediation: Self-theories and modes of self-esteem maintenance. *Pers Soc Psychol Bull.* 34: 599–612

Paukert, J.L., Richards, M.L., and Olney, C. (2002) An encounter card system for increasing feedback to students. *Am J Surg.* 183(3): 300–304

Pendleton, D., Schofield, T., and Tate, P. (1984) A method for giving feedback. In D. Pendleton (ed.) *The Consultation: An Approach to Learning and Teaching* (pp. 68–71). Oxford: Oxford University Press

Sargeant, J., Armson, H., Chesluk, B., et al. (2010a) The processes and dimensions of informed self-assessment: a conceptual model. *Acad Med.* 85(7): 1212–1220

Sargeant, J. and Mann, K. (2010b) Feedback in medical education: skills for improving learner performance. In: P. Cantillon, and D. Wood (ed.) *ABC of Learning and Teaching in Medicine* (pp. 29–32). London: Blackwells

Sargeant, J.M., Mann, K., and Ferrier. S. (2005) Exploring family physicians' reactions to multisource feedback: perceptions of credibility and usefulness. *Med Educ.* 39(5): 497–504

Schroth, M.L. (1992) The effects of delay of feedback on a delayed concept formation transfer task. *Contemp Educ Psychol.* 17(1): 78–82

Schum, T.R., Krippendorf, R.L., and Biernat, K.A. (2003) Simple Feedback Notes Enhance Specificity of Feedback to Learners. *Ambul Pediatr.* 3(1): 9–11

Schunk, D.H. (2008) *Learning Theories: An Educational Perspective.* 5th edn. Upper Saddle River NJ: Pearson/Merrill Prentice Hall

Shute, V.J. (2008) Focus on formative feedback. *Rev Educ Res.* 78: 153–189

Teunissen, P.W., Stapel, D.A., van der Vleuten C.M., Scherpbier, A., Boor, K., and Scheele, F. (2009) Who wants feedback? An investigation of the variables influencing residents' feedback-seeking behavior in relation to night shifts. *Acad Med.* 84(7): 910–917

Thomson O'Brien, M.A., Oxman, A.D., Davis, D.A., Haynes, R.B., Freemantle, N., and Harvey, E.L. (2000) Audit and feedback: effects on professional practice and health care outcomes. *Cochrane Database Syst Rev.* CD000259

Thorndike, E.L. (1931) *Human Learning.* New York: Century

Van De Ridder, J.M.M., Stokking, K.M., McGaghie, W.C., and ten Cate, O.T.J. (2008) What is feedback in clinical education? *Med Educ.* 42(2): 189–197

Veloski, J., Boex, J.R., Grasberger, M.J., Evans, A., and Wolfson, D.B. (2006) Systematic review of the literature on assessment, feedback and physicians' clinical performance. *Med Teach.* 28(2): 117–128

Watling, C.J., Kenyon, C.F., Zibrowski, E.M., et al. (2008) Rules of engagement: Residents' Perceptions of the In-training Evaluation Process. *Acad Med.* 83(10 Suppl): 597–600

Westberg, J. and Jason, H. (2001) *Fostering Reflection and Providing Feedback: Helping Others Learn from Experience.* New York: Springer Publications

Wilkinson, J., Crossley, J., Wragg, A., Mills, P., Cowan, G., and Wade, W. (2008) Implementing workplace-based assessment across the medical specialties in the United Kingdom. *Med Educ.* 42: 364–373

PART 9

Quality

CHAPTER 49

Evaluation

John Goldie and Jill Morrison

Nowadays, to appraise a man by his coat needs special
sartorial training, and is at the best perilous.

Michael Foster

Introduction

In education the term evaluation is often used interchangeably with
assessment, particularly in North America. While assessment is
primarily concerned with measurement of student performance,
evaluation is generally understood to refer to the process of obtaining information about an educational programme for subsequent
judgement. Activities which may be evaluated include the teacher's
work with students, a curriculum course, an entire curriculum, or
national programme. This can involve measuring student performance as a source of information, although it requires student testing
both pre- and post-course.

Evaluation is different from research. The main differences are
shown in table 49.1.

However, as we will see, the boundaries between research and
evaluation are increasingly blurred. Evaluation shares many methodological characteristics with research and research is becoming
increasingly politicized and commissioned (Cohen et al. 2000).

Evaluation is an essential part of the educational process. It should
be considered at the planning stage and not left until the curriculum
is up and running. Ideally, it should be part of an on-going cycle of
improvement. As part of their quality assurance procedures medical schools are required to evaluate their curricula. Without proper
evaluation the effectiveness of medical education would be difficult
to establish. Evaluation also contributes to the academic development of an institution and its members (Morrison 2010).

It must be remembered that while evaluation may identify
strengths and weaknesses it cannot correct problems. Managers
and other stakeholders must be committed to acting on the information obtained from evaluation.

History of evaluation

Planned social evaluation has been noted as early as 2200 BCE, with
personnel selection in China (Guba and Lincoln 1981). While evaluations have been chronicled during the last 200 years (Cronbach
et al. 1980; Madaus et al. 1983; Rossi and Freeman 1985), the main

stimulus to the development of modern evaluation practice was
the post- World War II rapid economic growth, particularly in the
USA, and the interventionist role taken by governments in social
policy during the 1960s. With increasing amounts of money being
spent on social programmes there was the growing recognition
that they required proper evaluation and evaluation became mandatory. At the same time there were a growing number of social
science graduates who became interested in policy analysis, survey research, field experiments, and ethnography, and turned their
attention towards evaluation (Shadish et al. 1991).

Educational evaluation is one of the main pillars of the social evaluation field. It is distinct from other areas of evaluation activity as it
has its roots in testing and assessment on one hand and curriculum
and programme evaluation on the other (Kellaghan et al. 2003).
The traditional emphasis on student testing for evaluation was
challenged by Tyler (1949) following his work with the Eight Year
Study, which involved formally appraising the college performance
of students prepared in 'progressive' high schools compared with
students from more conventional schools. He concluded that evaluation should be extended to establish the extent to which students
obtained mastery of the programme's prestated objectives. Tyler's
work, together with that of Bloom (1956) and Taba (1962) led to
the development of the linear, hierarchical, objectives model of
curriculum planning, with its structure of aims-learning experiences–content–organization of learning-evaluation. This 'industrial'
approach to curriculum planning influenced many of the attempts
at curriculum evaluation and the development of formal evaluation strategies (Holt 1981), which often concentrated on comparisons between programmes. Cronbach (1963, p. 675) responding to
the dissatisfaction felt by curriculum development staff, who were
finding little virtue in the existing methods for determining the
effectiveness of their instructional materials, argued that if evaluation was to be of value to curriculum developers it should focus
on the decisions they faced during the development phase. He also
argued that evaluation should deal less with comparisons between
programmes, and more with the degree to which the programme

Table 49.1 Evaluation versus research

	Evaluation	Research
Focus	Program to be evaluated	Theory
Question(s)	Specific to the project	General
Values	Represents multiple value sets Includes data on these values	Value free
Responsibility	To client and stakeholders	Autonomous
Goal	Judgement	Increase scientific knowledge
Interest in generalizability	No	Yes

promoted its desired purpose(s). He also stressed the importance of evaluation in helping refine a course when it was still sufficiently fluid to make changes.

Cronbach's views failed to attract widespread interest outside the field of curriculum developers due to the lack of interest on the part of educators per se (Popham 1988). However, the introduction of mandatory evaluation of educational programmes in the USA in 1965 stimulated activity in the field of educational evaluation. Formal evaluation was also made an essential requirement of all curriculum projects by funding bodies in the UK such as the Schools Council (Kelly 1989). The 1967 essays by Scriven and Stake led to the development of evaluation models in the early 1970s. There was growing belief in the power of evaluation to transform poor educational programmes into highly effective programmes, and of the importance of evaluation results to decision-makers. However, this optimism of the 1970s did not last. Experience showed that most educational decisions of importance, like most important decisions in the field of social policy, continued to be taken in a political, interpersonal milieu, where evidence plays a minor role (Popham 1988). Educational decision-makers typically made their choices without waiting for the 'definitive' results of evaluations. Moreover, when the results were obtained they rarely proved conclusive. With the realization of the political nature of the decision-making process, educational evaluators began to embrace Cronbach's (1980, p. 67) view of the evaluator as an educator, in that he or she should rarely attempt to focus his or her efforts on satisfying a single decision-maker, but should focus those efforts on informing the relevant political community. They also realized that, while many of their attempts at evaluation did not work, some did and, when they worked, programme quality improved to varying degrees. Improvement, even when modest, was recognized to be valuable (Popham 1988).

There has been a 'second boom' in evaluation in recent years (Donaldson and Scriven 2003, p. 56). Evaluation has become more global and has extended beyond large-scale government funded programmes with decentralization of government services. It has also led to the emergence of evaluation as a profession (Picciotto 2011) and the development of new evaluation methods, and new theories of evaluation practice, to address a broader and more diverse range of contexts. This has implications for educational evaluation practice.

Theories of evaluation practice

As evaluation developed, theories evolved which describe and prescribe what evaluators do, or should do, when conducting evaluations. Evaluation theories are largely normative and prescriptive (Chelimsky 1998; Alkin 2004). They are mainly theories of evaluation practice addressing themes such as how to understand the nature of the evaluation (and the object to be evaluated); how to assign value to programmes and their performance; and how to construct and use the knowledge generated by evaluation (Shadish 1998).

Shadish et al. (1991) characterized the development of evaluation theory as a series of stages. The earliest evaluators (e.g. Scriven and Campbell) concentrated on methodology and emphasized the discovery of truth. Reflection on increasing experience, by evaluators such as Wholey, Stake, and Weiss, led to the next stage which focussed on the way evaluation was used and its social utility. Stage 3 theories (e.g. those of Cronbach and Rossi), addressed the integration of inquiry and utility. Shadish et al. (1991) used the following criteria to evaluate the theories:

◆ knowledge—what methods to use to produce credible knowledge?

◆ use—how is knowledge about social programmes used?

◆ valuing—how are value judgements constructed?

◆ practice—how should evaluators practice in 'real world' settings?

◆ social programming—what is the nature of social programmes and their role in social problem solving?

Shadish et al. (1991) found that only those in stage 3 addressed all five criteria. However, they recognized the contributions of the different perspectives to the evolution of theories of practice and argued that evaluators should not follow the same evaluation procedures under all conditions. Alkin and Christie (2004), taking a different perspective, classified the main evaluation theorists according to their orientations towards methods, use and valuing (table 49.2). This helps evaluators understand the fundamental differences and connections between theories which have been built on the dual foundation of accountability and social inquiry.

From 1990, with the publication of Chen's (1990) book *Theory-Driven Evaluations*, there has been a revival in interest among evaluators in Tyler's notion of testing programme theory for evaluative purposes (Donaldson 2007). However, little consensus exists regarding its nomenclature and central features (Donaldson 2003; Rogers 2007). The rubric of theory-driven evaluations consists of many closely related and interchangeable terms—e.g. theories of practice, theory-based evaluation, theory-driven evaluation, realist evaluation, logic models, etc. Coryn et al. (2011, p. 201) provides a useful definition of theory-driven evaluation as 'any evaluation strategy or approach that explicitly integrates and uses stakeholder, social science, some combination of, or other types of theories in conceptualising, designing, conducting, interpreting, and applying an evaluation'. Theory-driven evaluation is increasingly being proposed by evaluation theorists, practitioners, and client organizations as the preferred model for evaluation practice (Coryn et al. 2011).

Programme theory

Programme theory underpins theory-driven evaluation. The elements used to describe a programme theory often include inputs, activities and outputs, which together constitute programme process theory and initial, intermediate, and long-term outcomes, which constitute programme impact theory. Programme theory is often represented as a linear model, however, more contextualized, comprehensive, ecological programme theory models are being proposed (Chen 2005; Rogers 2008).

Donaldson (2007) describes four potential sources of programme theory:

Table 49.2 Classification of the main evaluation theorists according to their orientations towards methods, use and valuing

Methods	Use	
Tyler and other objectives-orientated theories	Stufflebeam	Early theories
	Stufflebeam	
Campbell	Wholey	
Cook	Owen	
Suchman	Provus	
Boruch	Patton	
Rossi	Alkin	
Cronbach	Fetterman	
Weiss	Cousins	
Chen	Preskill	
	King	
Valuing		
	Scriven	
	Stake	
	Eisner	
	House	
	Wolf/Owens	
	MacDonald	
	Guba and Lincoln	
		Later theories

1. Previous theory, often social science theory, and research.

2. Implicit theories of those close to the programme.

3. Observations of the programme in operation.

4. Exploratory research to test critical assumptions in regard to a presumed programme theory.

Patton (2008) favours deductive, inductive or user-orientated approaches, whereas Chen (2005) advocates a stakeholder-orientated approach to programme theory formulation with the evaluator acting as facilitator.

In medical education curriculum development models (e.g. the outcome-based model) could be used as the basis for programme theory.

Programme theory can be used:

1. For needs assessment, programme planning and design, and assessment of the programme's evaluation potential.

2. As a basis for informed decisions about measurement and evaluation methods.

3. To assess the success or failure of a programme's implementation from the validity of the programme's conceptual model.

4. To help provide evidence about how programmes work and how they can be improved.

However, some evaluators argue that there is little need for theory, or at least some forms of theory, in evaluation (Scriven 1998, 2004a, 2004b; Stufflebeam 2001, 2004). Scriven (2004a, b) asserts that it is possible to 'do very good evaluation without getting into evaluation or programme theory'. Stufflebeam (2004, p. 253) questions the feasibility of theory-based evaluation particularly 'given the complexity of variables and interactions involved in running a programme in the complicated, sometimes chaotic conditions of the real world'. He also warns against failed or misrepresented attempts at evaluation being counterproductive for evaluation practice. Coryn et al.'s (2011) review found little empirical evidence to support most evaluation approaches.

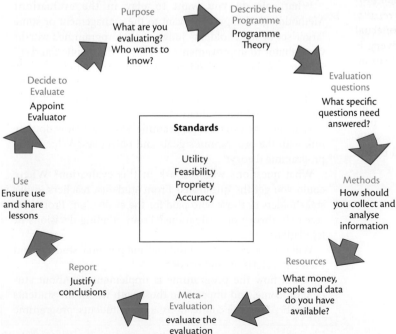

Figure 49.1 Evaluation cycle.

Performing evaluations

Evaluation should be a continuous process leading to on-going improvement (fig. 49.1).

1. Initiation/commissioning

The initial stage of evaluation is where the institutions or individuals responsible for a programme take the decision to evaluate it. Decisions need to be taken on the purpose(s) of the evaluation and who will be responsible for undertaking it. Mark et al. (2000) listed the four main evaluation purposes that have evolved (fig. 49.2).

The potential cost of an evaluation often plays a major role in determining its' scope as the cost will have to be met from the programme budget, or by seeking additional funding. Often those responsible for the implementation of educational programmes view resources committed to evaluation as resources lost. Evaluation should be efficient and produce information of sufficient value to justify the resources spent on it. It can be justified only to the extent that it saves resources and/or adds to the quality of the programme. Hodgkinson, Hurst and Levine (1975, p. 189) first introduced the concept of 'cost-free evaluation' to argue that evaluation can be a means for identifying cost-saving and/or increasing the effectiveness of a programme. Evaluation can help improve productivity and the quality of the programme either through formative recommendations for improvement that results in a better product and/or lower costs, or summative recommendations that result in maintaining or expanding successful, cost-effective educational activities or stopping unsuccessful, costly ones (Worthen et al. 1997).

The cost of not properly evaluating an educational programme should not only be considered in purely financial terms. There may be: personal costs, where the opportunity to enhance stakeholders self-esteem is lost; intellectual costs, with the loss of the opportunity for stakeholder reflection; social and business costs, with the loss of opportunity to discern effective from non effective programmes; ethical costs, with loss of opportunity to detect and challenge unethical practice; and pragmatic costs, the loss of opportunity to detect poor programmes that not only waste resources, but adversely affect the quality of life of students or produce students whose potential is not reached.

The question of whether the evaluator should be internal or external to the programme's development and delivery is also dependent on the purpose(s) and scope of the evaluation. Producing an effective educational evaluation may require skills from many disciplines, for example psychology, sociology, philosophy, statistics, politics, and economics. It is unlikely that an individual member of staff would have the competence to perform all these tasks or an institution would have all these skills in-house. However, this decision may also be influenced by the availability of funding.

> 1. Programme and organizational improvement
> 2. Oversight and compliance
> 3. Assessment of merit and worth
> 4. Knowledge development

Figure 49.2 Purposes of evaluation.

2. Defining the evaluator's role

Evaluation is an inherently value-laden activity. The potential evaluator(s), in deciding whether to accept the position, must reflect on their proposed role(s) and responsibilities. It is at this point that they also decide where, and to whom, their responsibility lies, and on the values which need to be made explicit. This will influence their decision-making process on whether to accept the position. There are a number of situations where evaluation may prove to be of questionable value or even harmful (fig. 49.3). In these circumstances the evaluator must persuade the commissioning body why the evaluation should not be attempted. However, such circumstances are uncommon.

Having accepted the position, the evaluator then needs to reflect on: the political climate and context; the nature of the

> 1. Where the evaluation would produce trivial data
> 2. Where the results would not be used
> 3. Where useful, valid information cannot be produced
> 4. Where evaluation is premature for the stage of the programme
> 5. Where the propriety of the evaluation is questionable e.g. where participants could be threatened or harmed

Figure 49.3 Circumstances where evaluation would be questionable.

Box 49.1 Questions for the evaluator to consider

Why is the evaluation being initiated? Has it been evaluated before? Could the money allocated for evaluation be better spent? Is it worth spending time and money on this evaluation given other things one could do with these resources? Why?

What purposes might the evaluation serve? To measure the effects of the programme? To improve the programme? To influence the decision-makers? To judge its worth? To provide useful information? To explain how an intervention or ones like it work? Why? How will you choose among these purposes?

What role do you want to play in the evaluation? Methodological expert? Servant to the management or some larger set of stakeholders? Judge of the programme's worth? Contributor to improvement? Servant of the 'public interest'? Educator of the client funding the evaluation? Why?

What is the political climate and context surrounding the evaluation? Will any political factors and forces preclude a meaningful and fair evaluation?

What are the essential programme activities? How do they link with the programme's goals and objectives? What is the programme theory?

What questions will you ask in this evaluation? Where could you get the questions? From students, teachers, other stakeholders or those who paid for the evaluation? From past research, theory or evaluations? From pending decisions or legislation?

Will you ask questions about real and potential students and their characteristics and needs?

About how the programme is implemented? About student outcome, and impacts on those with whom the students interact? About the connections among students, programme

(continued)

Box 49.1 (Continued)

implementation, and outcome? About costs and fiscal benefits? Why?

What methods will you use? Why? Will these methods provide good answers to the questions you are asking? How will you measure programme performance?

How do you plan to facilitate the use of the evaluation? Is it your responsibility? Why? How should the results be communicated? Should interim results be reported periodically to users? In the final report should you include an executive summary? Action recommendations? Should oral briefings be used? Should reports of evaluation results be communicated in forms tailored to the specific needs of different stakeholders? Can the results be disseminated through mass-media outlets? Is this desirable?

If you are evaluating an intervention, do you plan to summarize all your results into a final statement about whether the intervention is good or bad? If so, how will you weigh the different criteria to reflect which criteria are more or less important? Is it possible or desirable to construct a different value summary for each stakeholder group?

Can you do all this within time and budget? If not, then what has the highest priority and why?

What is your contingency plan if something goes wrong with any of these matters?

evaluation; the questions to ask; the methodology(s) to be used; the budget available for the evaluation; how the results will be communicated and used; and their contingency plan if things go wrong. The questions in box 49.1 may assist the evaluator with these tasks:

3. Planning the evaluation

Having decided what needs to be done the evaluator has to design an appropriate plan. Rossi and Freeman (1985, p. 190) advocate the 'good enough' rule for choosing evaluation designs:

> The evaluator should choose the best possible design, taking into account practicality and feasibility…the resources available and the expertise of the evaluator.

For each evaluation question or objective it is important to specify:

a. The information required to answer the question or determine if the objective has been achieved.

b. The design(s) to be used to collect information.

c. Source(s) of information.

d. Method(s) to be used to obtain the information.

e. Procedure for data collection—including sampling strategies, who is responsible for collecting data, how and when it will be collected.

f. Analysis procedures.

g. Interpretation procedures.

h. Reporting procedures—report format, content, context, schedule for reporting to potential audience(s).

Dimensions of evaluation

Stake (1976) suggested eight dimensions along which evaluation methods may vary:

1. Formative–summative: This distinction was first made by Scriven (1967). Formative evaluation is undertaken during the course of a programme with a view to adjusting the materials or activities. Summative evaluation is carried out at the end of a programme. In the case of an innovative programme it may be difficult to determine when the end has been reached, and often the length of time allowed before evaluation takes place will depend on the nature of the change.

2. Formal–informal: Informal evaluation is undertaken naturally and spontaneously and is often subjective. Formal evaluation is structured and more objective.

3. Case particular–generalization: Case-particular evaluation studies only one programme and relates the results only to that programme. Generalization may study one or more programmes, but allow results to be related to other programmes of the same type. In practice results may lend themselves to generalization, and the attempt to formulate rules for case study recognizes that generalizing requires greater control, and more regard to setting and context (Holt 1981).

4. Product–process: This distinction mirrors that of the formative–summative dimension. In recent years evaluators have been increasingly seeking information in the additional area of programme impact. Process information is sought on the effectiveness of course materials and activities. Often the materials are examined during both development and implementation. Examination of the implementation of the programme documents what actually happens, and how closely it resembles the stated goals. This information can also be of use in studying outcomes. Outcome information can focus on the short-term or direct effects on participants. The effects on students' learning can be categorized as instructional; e.g. does the programme result in students being able to pass exams? Or nurturant; e.g. does it make a definite change in their personal development? The method of obtaining information on the effects of learning will depend on which category of learning outcome is measured. Impact information looks beyond the immediate results to identify longer-term effects.

5. Descriptive–judgemental: Descriptive studies are carried out purely to secure information. Judgmental studies test results against stated value systems to establish the programme's effectiveness.

6. Preordinate–responsive: This dimension distinguishes between the situation where evaluators know in advance what they are looking for, and one where the evaluator is prepared to look at unexpected events that might come to light as he or she goes along.

7. Holistic–analytic: This dimension marks the boundary between evaluations, which looks at the totality of a programme, from one that looks only at a selection of key characteristics.

8. Internal–external: This separates evaluations using an institution's own staff from those that are designed by, or which require to satisfy, outside agencies.

Approaches to evaluation

The evaluation literature offers a wide variety of alternative approaches to evaluation. These approaches provide multiple options for evaluations. A plethora of evaluation models have been developed that can assist the evaluator in choosing the optimum method(s) for his or her particular evaluation. These range from comprehensive prescriptions to checklists of suggestions and as such are better described as approaches as many do not qualify for the term 'model'. Some of the newer approaches—e.g. empowerment evaluation, participatory evaluation—are more ideologies than methods or theories (Smith 2007). Stufflebeam (2001) offers a detailed critical appraisal of evaluation models for those who wish a more detailed analysis.

With the explosion in the numbers of approaches in recent years, many of which overlap, a number of attempts have been made to categorize the different evaluation approaches. Hansen (2005) proposes that evaluation models fall into six categories. Figure 49.4 lists examples of models in each category.

1. Results models—including goal-attainment and effects models

These are summative evaluation models which focus on the results of a given programme. In the goal attainment model the results are assessed in relation to predetermined goals. In the effects or goal-free evaluation model (Scriven 1974), the evaluator is prepared to look at unexpected events that might come to light as he or she goes along.

2. Explanatory process model

These models focus on the on-going processes. It follows an intervention from its conception to its implementation and its reception among clients and other stakeholders. It is a prospective rather than retrospective evaluation.

3. System model

The orientation of the system model is an analysis of the inputs, structure, process and outcomes in terms of results. The assessment can be based either on comparisons of planned and realized input, structure, process, and results or comparisons with similar programmes judged to be excellent

4. Economic model—including cost-efficiency, cost-effectiveness, and cost–benefit models.

The focus of these models are the assessment of performance, in terms of outputs, effects, or more lasting benefits against the costs of the inputs.

5. Actor model—including client-oriented, stakeholder, and peer review models.

These focus on the evaluation criteria provided by the various interested parties.

6. Programme theory model

This focuses on assessing the validity of the theory on which the programme is built.

Each approach comes with its built-in assumptions about evaluation and emphasizes different aspects of evaluation depending on the priorities and preferences of its author(s). Few come with careful step-by-step instructions that practitioners can follow and most are context specific (Worthen et al. 1997).

4. Data collection

As in the field of medical research, there has long been a tension between the quantitative and qualitative paradigms in evaluation. Quantitative experimental methods dominated early evaluation methodology. However, evaluators soon realized that quantitative methods could not answer all the questions they wished to answer. A range of both quantitative and qualitative methods have been developed and used (fig. 49.5).

Cronbach (1980, 1982) advised evaluators to be eclectic in their choice of methods, avoiding slavish adherence to any particular methods. As a result many evaluators moved toward mixed method designs (Caracelli et al. 1997). However, the tension between advocates of the quantitative and qualitative paradigms has not gone away. It was recently brought to a head by the US Department of Education's 2005 policy, which gives priority in funding to randomized experiments over other methods (Cook et al. 2010; Gargani 2010).

Where both quantitative and qualitative methods are to be used, Shadish (1993) has proposed using critical multiplism to help the evaluator(s) conduct the evaluation. Its central tenet is that when it is not clear which method is most likely to produce results with the least bias, other methods should be used. If these other methods, with different biases, yield similar results it increases confidence in the results obtained. Shadish offers the guidelines shown in fig. 49.6.

Results models
  Tyler's industrial model (Smith and Tyler, 1942)
  Metfessel and Michael (1967)
  Provus's discrepancy model (1973)
  Hammond (1973)
  Kirkpatrick (1994)
  Scriven's goal- free evaluation (1972)
  Case study approach
Explanatory process models
  The CIPP evaluation model (Stufflebeam, 1971b)
  The UCLA evaluation model (Alkin, 1969)
  Provus's discrepancy model (1973)
  Paton's utilization-focused approach (1986)
  Cronbach (1963, 1980)
System models
  Rossi and Freeman 1993
  Lessinger 1970
  PERT (Cook 1966)
Economic models
  Kee (1995)
  Levin (1983)
  Tsang (1997)
Actor models
  Scriven's concerns and checklists (Scriven 1967, 1974, 1984, 1991)
  Educational Connoisseurship (Eisner, 1975, 1991)
  Stake's responsive evaluation framework (1975)
  Paton's utilization-focused approach (1986)
  Parlett and Hamilton's illuminative model (1972)
  Fetterman (1994)
Programme-theory based models
  CDC programme evaluation framework (1999)

Figure 49.4 Examples of models in Hansen's six evaluation model categories

Quantitative methods	Qualitative methods
Experiments	case studies
Surveys	Action research approach
Delphi technique	Naturalistic and
Q-sorts	Ethnographic approaches
Cost-analysis	
Cluster/factor analysis	
Management information system	
Instruments	**Instruments**
Achievement testing	Interviews
Norm referencing	Focus groups
Criterion referencing	Observation
Objectives-referencing	Participant
Domain-referencing	Non-participant
Attitude scales	Diaries/self-reports
Rating scales	Documentary analysis
Questionnaires	

Figure 49.5 Common quantitative and qualitative methods and instruments for evaluation.

Identify the tasks to be done

Identify the different options for performing each task

Identify the strengths, biases, and assumptions associated with each option

When it is not clear which option is the least biased select more than one to reflect different biases, avoid constant biases, and overlook only the least plausible biases

Note convergence of results over options with different biases

Explain differences of results yielded by options with different biases

Publicly defend any decisions to use a single option

Figure 49.6 Shadish's guidelines for employing critical multiplism.

5. Data analysis and interpretation of the findings

Having collected the relevant data, the next stage in evaluation involves its interpretation. This involves both data analysis and interpretation.

Analysis and interpretation of data

Data analysis focuses on organizing and reducing data to allow logical or statistical inferences. Interpretation attaches meaning to organized information enabling conclusions to be drawn. When considering the methods to be used for data analysis and interpretation the evaluator should consider:

1. What methods are appropriate for the questions posed, the method used to collect the data and the data obtained?

2. What methods are most likely to be understood and credible to the audiences receiving the reports?

3. What is the measurement scale of quantitative data and which are the appropriate statistical methods for analysis of such data?

When analysing quantitative data it is important to consider whether to use descriptive and/or inferential statistics. Before moving to inferential statistics, evaluators should carefully explore the data using descriptive statistics to learn about the information that has been obtained. Patton (1987) advocates involving the stakeholder in data analysis at this stage. This helps demystify data analysis and actively involves stakeholder groups. It also helps the evaluator find out what type of information is of most interest to each group and the most effective ways of presenting it. It can also produce further issues and questions that can be addressed at this point.

Inferential statistics are useful for questions concerned with causality or relationships. The evaluator should select the method that matches the measurement scale of data collected and ensures it meets the assumptions of the statistic. It must be remembered that statistics do not establish causality, but merely demonstrate relationships. Statistical findings must be combined with logic and design to establish cause-and-effect. The results need to be interpreted in light of managerial experience e.g. if an experimental design is used and a statistically significant difference between groups found, is the difference enough to be meaningful for decision making? Consideration must be given to these issues at the planning stage and decisions should be taken by client and stakeholder groups rather than the evaluator(s) (Worthen et al. 1997).

For qualitative data the methods of analysis used will be dependent on the method of data collection used e.g. a grounded theory approach may be used to analyse information obtained from interviews whereas content analysis may be used when analysing curricular documentation. Patton (1990) outlines an approach to dealing with the large amount of qualitative data produced by evaluations:

1. Ensure all the data that is required has been collected.

2. Ensure the data is safely stored and backed up/copies made.

3. Organize the data into topics and files.

4. Look for causes, consequences and relationships.

5. Validate the findings—this can involve:

   a. Examinations of rival explanations for the findings

   b. Review of deviant cases

   c. Triangulation—examining the consistency of results from the use of different methods or multiple observers to examine the same phenomenon

   d. Design checks—examining distortions due to design decisions

   e. Look for evaluator reflexivity—reviewing distortions which may have arisen from the evaluator's perspectives or behaviour(s)

   f. Examine the quality of data

   g. Stakeholder reaction to reported data and analyses

   h. Intellectual rigor—how justified are the conclusions?

When both qualitative and quantitative methods are used in the same study, results can be generated that have different implications for the overall conclusion, leading to tension. This may only be resolved after much iteration (Hennigan et al. 1980).

6. Budgeting—cost(s) of evaluation activities

The most obvious cost is the evaluator's time. When the evaluator is internal they will need to be freed from their normal activities to undertake the evaluation. If external, the evaluator's fees will have to be met from the programme budget. They may also require the assistance of various in-house experts whose time would also have to be freed up, or if not available, purchased externally. Other contracted services such as accounting or legal services may also be required. Subcontracts need to be priced as part of budgetary planning. If supplied internally institutions often include these costs in their overhead rates. The evaluator will require administrative and secretarial support throughout, which if not available internally will have to be purchased.

Evaluators can restrict costs by enlisting the services of teachers and other medical staff, administrators, secretarial staff and undergraduate or postgraduate students seeking research experience to assist in the collection and analysis of data. Involving these groups not only helps reduce costs, but also generates interest in the evaluation among stakeholders. However, they may require training and there is a risk of bias if their pre-existing perceptions cause them to alter or distort data to fit these perceptions. The evaluator must provide supervision and monitoring throughout, which may make it less economical than it first appears. Local specialists may be used for data collection to reduce travel costs where data needs to be collected at more than one site.

Time is an important resource. The evaluator must keep the evaluation on course producing good quality data and analysis, while keeping within the proposed timeframe. This involves effective planning. Non-technical, routine tasks may be delegated to less-expensive staff. Knowing when to be ready with results is part of good planning. Limited time can reduce the evaluation's effectiveness as much as a limited budget. If time is an issue the scope of the evaluation may have to be reduced with parts of the evaluation deferred to a later date.

Depending on the methodologies selected, other costs such as purchasing pre-existing evaluation models, questionnaires, attitude or rating scales or other library materials may be incurred. These instruments, however, are often limited by their context dependency. If pre-existing instruments are to be purchased or books or materials ordered, consultation with a librarian or the publisher or author can help estimate costs. Evaluation costs may be reduced by 'piggybacking' on other studies where appropriate. Inexpensive data collection methods may be substituted for situations where precision is less important.

Specialist equipment such as computer hardware or software, video or audio equipment may be required. While many organizations can provide access to computers for data storage and analysis, personal computers or laptops may have to be purchased. If expensive equipment is required it may be cheaper to rent than buy. Specialist software may also be required for statistical or qualitative data analysis. Transcribing of recordings is costly in terms of time (if performed internally) or money (if purchased externally).

Printing and photocopying costs may include preparation of data collection instruments, reports and other documents. Secretarial staff can be helpful in estimating costs. Discussions with other evaluators who have managed similar projects can also be helpful. Costs of printing and duplicating final reports, binding or any special graphics can be checked with book-binding and graphic art companies (Goldie 2010).

Hidden costs
Host organizations (e.g. universities) will have overhead costs such as facilities and utilities. Most will have fixed percentages of a total budget or of salary costs that they charge as an operating overhead. If applying for external funding these costs will have to be built into the funding request. It is important not to include costs already included in the institution's overhead costs when costing an evaluation.

Communication costs including postage and telephone calls will have to be budgeted for. The cost of surveys can be estimated from the sample size. Fixed costs (e.g. monthly telephone bills or broadband subscriptions) can be budgeted for by multiplying the costs per month by the proposed timescale. Variable costs such as long-distance phone calls for particular communications may be estimated based on the context of the evaluation. To reduce costs these may be accessed during times when rates are cheaper.

Routine materials such as paper and pens may be required if not supplied by the commissioning institution. Routine office estimates should be obtained and costs estimated for the duration of the project.

Travel costs may also have to be met. This will be dependent on the amount of fieldwork and the degree of face-to-face contacts required in designing and conducting the evaluation. These can include mileage estimates for meetings, training, observations, data collection, and other activities. Long-distance travel may be required if inspecting similar programmes or disseminating results. This may include airfares, meals and accommodation (Goldie 2010).

Disseminating results may prove costly particularly where the aim is to disseminate them widely. Using the commissioning institutions' media services can prove cheaper than hiring commercial organizations (Goldie 2010).

7. Meta-evaluation

When an evaluation goes wrong it is normally due to the way it has been conducted. This is often due to the political and social contexts in which evaluations take place and the limitations of individual methodologies. Meta-evaluation—i.e. evaluation of evaluations—aims to improve the quality of evaluations and help prevent failed evaluation (Worthen et al. 1997). It evolved early in the first evaluation boom. Several evaluators published proposed guidelines or meta-evaluation criteria: for example Stake (1969), Stufflebeam (1971a), Scriven (1980). However, there was no clear consensus among evaluators until the Joint Committee on Standards for Educational Evaluation publication in 1981. These were revised in 1994 to allow their application beyond the field of education. The standards are commonly agreed characteristics of good evaluation practice and are the benchmark against which evaluations and other meta-evaluation criteria and standards should be judged (Worthen et al. 1997).

Meta-evaluation may be conducted by:

1. The original evaluator—however, there is an inherent risk of bias. This is reduced by using the Joint Committee's Standards (1994).

2. An internal evaluation committee or advisory group.

3. The evaluation consumers—this is limited by the technical competence of such groups.

4. External evaluators—this can increase the credibility of the evaluation particularly if it involves a team of external evaluators.

5. A combination of all these groups.

Meta-evaluation can be formative or summative or both. Formative meta-evaluation aims to improve the evaluation before it is too late. Methods which can be used include: review of research plans by experts and stakeholders; monitoring of the evaluation process by external bodies and independent simultaneous evaluations of the same programme. Summative meta-evaluation can add credibility to final results. Methods include: secondary analyses of collected data; expert review of the findings to determine the validity of the evaluator's interpretations; and including statements in the final report from personnel involved in the programme.

8. Reporting the findings

Evaluators need to report their findings often for a variety of audiences e.g. clients, stakeholders or the wider public. Although reporting mainly involves written reports, it may also involve oral presentations. The reports produced may be for internal or external consumption. Reports may be interim, scheduled or unscheduled, or final. Final reports may be incremental and not necessarily in written form.

Inadequate reporting is perceived by educational administrators and teachers as being a pervasive problem (Newman and Brown 1996). This is often because reporting the findings is often given least reflection by evaluators. A generic structure for writing reports is shown in fig. 49.7.

The results should be produced in an acceptable and comprehensible way. It is important for the evaluator to recognize for which group(s) the particular report is being prepared. It is the

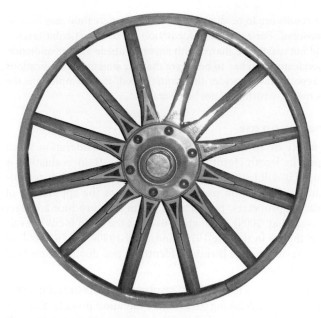

Figure 49.8 The evaluation cycle.

Summary

Introduction

    Aim of evaluation

    Audiences for evaluation report

    Limitations of the evaluation and explanation of disclaimers, if any

    Overview of report contents

Focus of the evaluation

    Description of the evaluation

    Questions or objectives used to focus the study

    Information required for the evaluation

Brief overview of evaluation plan and procedures

Presentation of evaluation results

    Summary of findings

    Interpretation of findings

Conclusions and recommendations

    Criteria and standards used

    Judgements made—strengths and weaknesses

    Recommendations

Minority reports or rejoinders—where those who disagree with the evaluator's judgements, conclusions or recommendations are given the space to share their alternative views

Appendices

    Descriptions of evaluation plan/design, instruments, data analysis, and interpretation

    Detailed tabulations or analyses of quantitative data and transcripts or summaries of qualitative data

    Other information as required

Figure 49.7 Generic format for report writing.

---

evaluator's responsibility to persuade the target audience of the validity and reliability of their results. Circulating a draft to the client and key stakeholders for comment before submitting the report is good practice. It can help correct minor, factual and interpretive errors, increase the number of individuals who read the report carefully and share responsibility for the report's accuracy. This can help motivate groups to use the evaluation findings.

Making recommendations

When reporting evaluation findings evaluators may or may not make recommendations for appropriate actions to be taken (fig. 49.8). In deciding to make recommendations, the evaluator may be limited by the context and operation of legitimate political processes and the possession or absence of required expertise and/or contextual knowledge (Iriti et al. 2005). Iriti et al. (2005) propose nine key variables for evaluators to consider in deciding whether to produce recommendations:

1. The role of the evaluator—nature of her/his relationship with client and evaluation.

2. The use context—the evaluation's purpose(s) in terms of use.

3. The design characteristics of the evaluation—the scope of the evaluation.

4. The quality, strength and clarity of the findings.

5. The evaluator's experience and expertise.

6. Ethical considerations—the evaluator may benefit from recommendations, e.g. recommending further evaluation.

7. Knowledge of costs and trade-offs—need to be aware of, and communicate, costs of potential recommendations.

8. The internal capacity of the programme—does the programme have the capacity to implement the recommendations?

9. The literature in the field of study—can help formulate and support the recommendations.

If the results are to be disseminated more widely they may have to be censored. For example, information about a particular teacher would not usually be shared with anyone outside a select audience. The evaluator also has to be aware that the potential ramifications of a report may go wider than anticipated, for example into the mass media, which may not be desirable.

9. Evaluation use

The utility of an evaluation is of primary consideration when judging its worth (Joint Committee, 1994). If an evaluation is not used it will be judged as ineffective regardless of its technical merits. Evaluation use can be defined as the application of evaluation processes, products or findings to produce an effect (Johnson et al. 2009). Evaluation use was the main focus of evaluation theory in the late 1970s and early 1980s. Alkin and Taut (2003), reviewing the literature identified two distinct aspects of evaluation use:

1. Process use—change that results from the learning that occurs through taking part in the evaluation process. This can involve change in individuals' thinking or behaviours and/or change in programme changes in procedures and culture (Patton 1997).

2. Use of evaluation findings—these are traditionally divided into;

a. Instrumental—where the findings have been used to make decisions or changes

b. Conceptual—indirect and conceptual uses of evaluation to shape the thinking of policy-makers

c. Symbolic—where the evaluation rather than aspects of its findings is used to persuade or convince.

In recent years there has also been recognition and valuing of the intangible influences evaluations have on individuals, programmes, and communities (Kirkhart 2000; Alkin and Taut 2003; Mark and Henry 2004).

Cousins and Leithwood (1986), investigating the factors that contributed to the evaluation use, found two main factors:

1. Characteristics of the evaluation's implementation:This includes the evaluator's credibility, the relevance of the evaluation and its quality. It also includes the quality of communication between the evaluator and stakeholders; the congruence of the findings with decision-maker(s)' expectations and the timeliness of the evaluation.

2. Characteristics of the decision or policy setting:This includes the political climate; the personal characteristics of the decision maker(s); the characteristics of the decision-making process; information required to make the decision and competing information and the user commitment or receptiveness to evaluation.

Shula and Cousins (1997) further recognized the importance of context, including cultural context, for understanding and explaining use. Johnson et al. (2009) added a further category, stakeholder involvement, as empirical research demonstrated that engagement, interaction, and communication between evaluation clients and evaluators is critical to meaningful use. They also added evaluator competence to the evaluation implementation category.

Worthen et al. (1997) make the following suggestions to help evaluators maximize the chance of their evaluation being utilized:

1. Identify the key evaluation issues. Structure the evaluation efforts around the information priorities of the programme decision makers. Involve them and other stakeholders in the conceptualization of the evaluation where possible.

2. Be sensitive to the context. Pay attention to the political climate. Be sensitive to stakeholders' opinions and feelings. Build rapport.

3. Be eclectic in the evaluation approach. Use multiple methods of data collection and analysis. The breadth of data enables the evaluator to reach a wider audience.

4. Present information in a timely fashion. Be punctual with required reports. Provide interim reports.

5. When possible, and appropriate, make recommendations.

The ethics of evaluation

Evaluators face potential ethical problems, for example they have the potential to exercise power over people, which can injure self-esteem, damage reputations, and affect careers. They often come from the same social and educational background as those who sponsor the evaluation, which may be different to that of participants or other stakeholders. They can be engaged in relationships where they are vulnerable to people awarding future work. A consensus code of conduct for evaluation has not been established. This is unsurprising given the various educational backgrounds and professional affiliations of evaluators. As with ethics in medicine a principles-based approach, rather than adherence to external codes, has developed. This promotes individual evaluator's awareness to the values he or she brings to the evaluation and the potential for change in the light of changing knowledge.

Guidance has been provided by a number of organizations. The Joint Committee on Standards for Educational Evaluation (1994) stated that the quality of an evaluation study can be determined by examining its utility, feasibility, propriety, and accuracy. To practise professionally requires the evaluator to practise ethically. The American Evaluation Association (2008) recently restated the following principles to guide evaluators in their professional practice:

1. Systematic inquiry—evaluators should conduct systematic, data-based inquiries about whatever is being evaluated.

2. Competence—evaluators should provide competent performance to stakeholders.

3. Integrity/honesty—evaluators should ensure the honesty and integrity of the entire evaluation process.

4. Respect for people—evaluators should respect the security, dignity, and self-worth of the respondents, participants, clients and other stakeholders with whom they interact.

5. Responsibilities for general and public welfare—evaluators should articulate and take into account the diversity of interests.

Morris's (2011) review of the literature highlighted the importance of the contracting/initiation stage in setting the ethical tone for the evaluation. Evaluation has developed to the point where evaluators are often able to identify the key ethical issues they are likely to encounter. Addressing these matters with stakeholders at the beginning of a project can help prevent serious problems in the later stages—e.g. disputes over distribution of a final report. The ethics of an evaluation, however, are not the sole responsibility of the evaluator(s). Evaluation sponsors, participants and audiences share ethical responsibilities.

Conclusions

◆ Evaluation is an essential part of the educational process. Without proper evaluation the effectiveness of medical education would be difficult to establish.

◆ Evaluation should be planned during the setting up of educational programmes.

◆ Evaluation practice has developed a theoretical basis. Theories, however, are largely normative and prescriptive.

◆ Evaluation often occurs in a political milieu and the evaluator needs to be aware of its influence.

◆ It is important to involve clients and other stakeholders at all stages of the evaluation process.

◆ The budget available often determines the scope of the evaluation.

◆ The methods used to collect data are guided by the questions asked by the evaluator.

◆ The 'good enough' rule should be considered when designing an evaluation.

◆ There are a number of evaluation models which can be used. However, these are often context specific.

◆ In analysing the findings it is important to establish the reliability and validity of the data, concepts which have different meanings to quantitative and qualitative practitioners.

◆ Meta-evaluation improves the quality of evaluations and helps prevent failed evaluation.

◆ Reports, verbal and non-verbal, should be tailored for specific audiences.

◆ The utility of an evaluation is of primary consideration when judging its worth.

◆ It must be remembered that while evaluation may identify strengths and weaknesses it cannot correct problems. This is in the hands of management and other stakeholders.

References

Alkin, M.C. (1969) Evaluation theory development, *Evaluation Comment.* 2: 2–7

Alkin, M.C. (ed.) (2004) *Evaluation Roots.* Thousand Oaks, CA: Sage

Alkin, M.C. and Christie, C.A. (2004) An evaluation theory tree revisited. In: M.C. Alkin (ed.)*Evaluation Roots* (pp.12–68). Thousand Oaks, CA: Sage

Alkin, M.C. and Taut, S.M. (2003) Unbundling evaluation use. *Studies in Educational Evaluation.* 29: 1–12

American Evaluation Association (2008) Guiding Principles for Evaluators. *Am J Eval.* 29(4): 397–398

Bloom, B.S. (1956) *The Taxonomy of Educational Objectives.* London: Longman

Caracelli, V. and Greene, J. (1997) Crafting mixed-method evaluation designs. In: J. Greene, V. Caracelli (eds) *Advances in Mixed-Method Evaluation: The challenges and benefits of integrating diverse paradigms* (pp.19–32). New directions for evaluation. San Francisco: Jossey Bass

Centers for Disease Control (1999) Program evaluation framework. 48(RR11), pp. 1–40. Atlanta GA: CDC

Chelimsky, E. (1998) The role of experience in formulating theories of evaluation practice. *Am J Eval.* 19: 35–55

Chen, H.T. (1990) *Theory-Driven Evaluations.* Newbury Park, CA: Sage

Chen, H.T. (2005) *Practical Program Evaluation: Assessing and improving planning, implementation and effectiveness.* Thousand Oaks, CA: Sage

Cohen L., Manion, L., and Morrison, K. (2000) *Research Methods in Education.* 5th edn. London: Routledge Falmer

Cook, D.L. (1966) *Program Evaluation and Review Techniques, Applications in Education.* Washington, DC: US Office of Education Cooperative Monograph, 17 (OE-12024)

Cook, D.A. (2010) Twelve tips for evaluating educational programs. *Med Teach.* 32(4): 296–301

Cook, T.D., Scriven, M., Coryn, C.L.S., and Evergreen, S.D.H. (2010) Contemporary thinking about causation in evaluation: A dialogue with Tom Cook and Michael Scriven. *Am J Eval.* 31: 105–117

Coryn, C.L., Noakes, L.N., Westine, C.D., and Schroter, D.C. (2011) A Systematic Review of Theory-Driven Evaluation Practice From 1990 to 2009. *Am J Eval.* 32(2): 199–226

Cousins, J.B. and Leithwood, K.A. (1986) Current empirical research on evaluation utilization. *Rev Educ Res.* 56: 331–364

Cronbach, L.J. (1963) Course improvement through evaluation, *Teachers College Record,* 64: 672–683

Cronbach, L.J. (1982) In praise of uncertainty. In: P.H Rossi (ed.) *Standards for Evaluation Practice*(pp. 49–58). San Francisco: Jossey-Bass

Cronbach, L.J., Ambron, S.R., Dornbuch, S.M., et al. (1980) *Towards Reform of Program Evaluation.* San Francisco: Jossey Bass

Donaldson, S.I. (2003) Theory-driven program evaluation in the new millennium. In: S.I. Donaldson and M. Scriven (eds.) *Evaluating Social Programs and Problems: Visions for the New Millennium* (pp.109–141). Mahwah, NJ: Lawrence Erlbaum

Donaldson, S.I. (2007) *Program Theory-Driven Evaluation Science.* New York, NY: Lawrence Erlbaum

Eisner, E.W. (1975) The perceptive eye: toward the reformation of educational evaluation. *Occasional Papers of the Stanford Evaluation Consortium.* Stanford, CA: Stanford University

Eisner, E.W. (1991) Taking a second look: Educational connoisseurship revisited. In: M.W. McLaughlin, D.C Philips (eds) *Evaluation and Education: At Quarter Century,* Ninetieth Yearbook of the National Association for the Study of Education, Part 2 (pp. 169–187). Chicago, IL: University of Chicago Press

Fetterman, D. (1994) Empowerment evaluation. *Eval Pract.* 15(1): 1–15

Gargani, J. (2010) A welcome change from debate to dialogue about causality. *Am J Eval.* 13: 171–172

Goldie, J. (2010) Cost effective evaluation. In: K. Walsh (ed) *Cost Effectiveness in Medical Education* (pp. 101–112). Oxford: Routledge

Guba, E.G. and Lincoln, Y.S. (1981) *Effective Evaluation: Improving the Usefulness of Evaluation Results through Responsive and Naturalistic Approaches.* San Francisco: Jossey-Bass

Iriti, J.E. and Bickel, W.E. (2005) Using recommendations in evaluation: a decision-making framework for evaluators. *Am J Eval.* 26: 464–479

Hammond, R.L. (1973) Evaluation at the local level. In: B.R. Worthen, J.R. Sanders (eds) *Educational Evaluation: Theory and Practice* (pp. 157–169). Belmont, CA: Wordsworth

Hansen, H.F. (2005) Choosing evaluation models: a discussion on evaluation design. *Evaluation.* 11(4): 447–462

Hennigan, K.M., Flay, B.R., and Cook, T.D. (1980) 'Give me the facts': some suggestions for using social science knowledge in national policy making. In: R.F. Kidd, M.J. Saks (eds) *Advances in Applied Social Psychology* (vol 1, pp. 113–147). Hillsdale, NJ: Lawrence Erlbaum

Hodgkinson H., Hurst, J., and Levine, H. (1975) *Improving and Assessing Performance: Evaluation in Higher Education.* Berkeley, CA: University of California Center for Research and Development in Higher Education

Holt, M. (1981) *Evaluating the Evaluators.* Sevenoaks: Hodder & Stoughton

Johnson, K., Greenseid, L.O., Toal, S.A., King, J.A., Lawrenz, F., and Volkov, B. (2009) Research on Evaluation Use: A Review of the Empirical Literature from 1986 to 2005. *Am J Eval.* 30(3): 377–410

Joint Committee on Standards for Educational Evaluation (1994) *The Program Evaluations Standards* 2nd ed. Thousand Oaks, CA: Sage

Kellaghan, T., Stufflebeam, D.L., and Wingate, L.A. (2003) *Handbook of Educational Evaluation.* Dordrecht, Netherlands: Kluwer

Kelly, A.V. (1989) *The Curriculum: Theory and Practice.* 3rd edn. London: Paul Chapman Publishing

Kee, J. E. (1995) Benefit-cost analysis in program evaluation. In: J. S. Wholey, H. P. Hatry, K. E. Newcomer (eds), *Handbook of Practical Program Evaluation* (pp. 456–488). San Francisco: Jossey-Bass

Kirkhart, K.E. (2000) Reconceptualising evaluation use: An integrated theory of influence. *New Directions for Evaluation.* 88: 5–23

Kirkpatrick, D.L. (1994) *Evaluating Training Programs.* San Francisco: Berrett-Koehler Publishers

Lessinger, L.M. (1970) *Every Kid a Winner: Accountability in Education.* New York: Simon and Schuster

Levin, H.M. (1983) *Cost-effectiveness: A Primer. New Perspectives in Evaluation.* 4: Newbury Park, CA: Sage

Madaus, G.F., Scriven, M.S., and Stufflebeam, D.L. (1983) *Evaluation Models: Viewpoints on Educational and Human Services Evaluation.* Boston: Klewer-Nijhoff

Mark, M.M., Henry, G.T., and Julnes, G. (2000) *Evaluation: an integrative framework for understanding, guiding, and improving policies and programs.* San Francisco, CA: Jossey-Bass

Mark, M.M. and Henry, G.T. (2004) The mechanisms and outcomes of evaluation influence. *Evaluation.* 10: 35–57

Metfessel, N.S. and Michael, W.B. (1967) A paradigm involving multiple criterion measures for the evaluation of the effectiveness of school programs, *Educ Psychol Measurement.* 27: 931–943

Morris, M. (2011) The good, the bad and the evaluator: 25 years of AJE Ethics. *Am J Eval.* 32(1): 134–151

Morrison, J. (2010) Evaluation. In: P, Cantillon and D. Wood (eds) *ABC of Medical Education*(pp. 15–19). 2nd edn. London: BMJ Publications

Newman, D.L. and Brown, R.D. (1996) *Applied Ethics for Program Evaluation.* Beverly Hills, CA: Sage

Parlett, M. and Hamilton, D. (1972) Evaluation as illumination: a new approach to the study of innovatory programs. In: G.V. Glass (ed.) (1976) *Evaluation Studies Review Annual* (Vol. 1 pp. 140–158). Beverly Hills, CA: Sage

Patton, M.Q. (1986) *Utilization-focused Evaluation.* 2nd edn. Beverly Hills, CA: Sage

Patton, M.Q. (1987) *How to use Qualitative Methods in Evaluation.* Newbury Park, CA: Sage

Patton, M.Q. (1990) *Qualitative Evaluation and Research Methods.* 2nd edn. Newbury Park, CA: Sage

Patton, M.Q. (1997) *Utilization-focussed Evaluation.* Thousand Oaks, CA: Sage

Patton, M.Q. (2008) *Utilization-focussed Evaluation.* 4th edn. Thousand Oaks, CA: Sage

Piccioto, R. (2011) The logic of evaluation professionalism. *Evaluation.* 17(2): 165–180

Popham, W.J. (1988) *Educational Evaluation.* 2nd edn. Englewood Cliffs, NJ: Prentice Hall

Provus, M.M. (1973) Evaluation of ongoing programs in the public school system. In: B.R. Worthen, J.R. Sanders (eds) *Educational Evaluation: Theory and Practice* (pp. 170–217). Belmont, CA: Wadsworth

Rogers, P.J. (2007) Theory-based evaluation: Reflections ten years on. In: S. Mathieson (ed.) *Enduring Issues in Evaluation: The 20th anniversary of the collaboration between NDE and AEA.* New Directions for Evaluation, No 114, San Francisco, CA: Jossey-Bass, pp.63–67

Rogers, P.J. (2008) Using programme theory to evaluate complicated and complex aspects of intervention. *Evaluation.* 14: 29–48

Rossi, P.H. and Freeman, H.E. (1985) *Evaluation: A Systematic Approach.* 3rd edn. Beverly Hills, CA: Sage

Rossi, P.H. and Freeman, H.E. (1993) *Evaluation: A Systematic Approach.* Newbury Park:CA: Sage

Scriven, M. (1967) The methodology of evaluation. In: R.W. Tyler, R.M. Gagne, M. Scriven (eds) *Perspectives of Curriculum Evaluation,* American Educational Research Association Monograph Series on Evaluation 1. Chicago: Rand McNally, pp. 39–83

Scriven, M. (1974) Goal-free evaluation. In: E.R. House (ed.) *School Evaluation: The Politics and Process* (pp. 319–328). Berkeley, CA: McCutchin

Scriven, M. (1980) *The Logic of Evaluation.* Inverness, CA: Edgepress

Scriven, M. (1984) Evaluation ideologies. In: R.F Connor, D.G. Altman, C. Jackson (eds) *Evaluation Studies Review Annual* (Vol. 9 pp. 49–80). Beverly Hills, CA: Sage

Scriven, M. (1991) Key evaluation checklist. In: M. Scriven, *Evaluation Thesaurus.* 4th edn. Beverly Hills, CA: Sage, p. 204

Scriven, M. (1998) Minimalist theory: The least practice requires. *Am J Eval.* 19: 57–70

Scriven, M. (2004a) *Practical Program Evaluation: A checklist approach.* Claremont Graduate: University Annual Professional Workshop Series

Scriven, M. (2004b) *EvalTalk posting.* April 26 https://listserv.ua.edu/archives/evaltalk.html Accessed 26 March 2013

Shadish, W.R., Cook, T.D., and Leviton, L.C. (1991) *Foundations of Program Evaluation: Theories of Practice.* Newbury Park, CA: Sage

Shadish, W.R. (1993) Critical multiplism: A research strategy and its attendant tactics. In: L. Sechrest (ed.) *Program Evaluation: A Pluralistic Enterprise.* New Directions for Program Evaluation, No 60 (pp. 13–57), San Francisco: Jossey-Bass

Shadish, W.R. (1998) Evaluation theory is who we are. *Am J Eval.* 19(1): 1–19

Shula, L.M. and Cousins, J.B. (1997) Evaluation use: Theory, research, and practice since 1986. *Eval Pract.* 18: 195–208

Smith, N.L. (2007) Empowerment evaluation as evaluation ideology. *Am J Eval.* 28(2): 169–178

Smith, E.R. and Tyler, R.W. (1942) *Appraising and Recording Student Progress.* New York: Harper and Row

Stake, R.E. (1967) The countenance of educational evaluation. *Teachers College Record.* 68: 523–539

Stake, R.E. (1969) Evaluation design, instrumentation, data-collection and analysis of data. In: J.L. Davis (ed.) *Educational Evaluation.* Columbus, OH: State Superintendent of Public Instruction

Stake, R.E. (1975) *Program Evaluation, Particularly Responsive Evaluation,* Occasional paper No. 5 Kalamazoo: Western Michigan University Evaluation Center

Stake, R.E. (1976) *Evaluating Educational Programmes: the Need and the Response.* Menlo Park, CA: CERI/OECD

Stufflebeam, D.L. (1971a) The relevance of the CIPP evaluation model for educational accountability. *J Res Devel Educ.* 5: 19–25

Stufflebeam, D.L. (1971b) *Educational Evaluation and Decision Making.* Itasca, IL: F.E. Peacock

Stufflebeam, D.L. (ed.) (2001) *Evaluation Models.* New Directions for Evaluation, No 89. San Francisco, CA: Jossey-Bass

Stufflebeam, D.L. (2004) The 21st-centuary CIPP model: origins, development, and use. In: M.C. Alkin (ed.) *Evaluation Roots* (pp. 245–266). Thousand Oaks, CA: Sage

Taba, H. (1962) *Curriculum Development: Theory and Practice.* New York: Harcourt, Bracc and World

Tsang, M. C. (1997) Cost analysis for improved educational policymaking and evaluation. *Educ Eval Policy Anal.* 19(4): 318–324

Tyler, R.W. (1949) *Basic Principles of Curriculum and Instruction.* Chicago, IL: University of Chicago Press

Worthen, B.L., Sanders, J.R., and Fitzpatrick, J.L. (1997) *Program Evaluation: Alternative Approaches and Practical Guidelines.* 2nd edn. New York: Longman

CHAPTER 50

Continuous quality improvement

Jan Kleijnen, Diana Dolmans,
Jos Willems, and Hans van Hout

Teaching staff, being the carriers of education, should be
seen as the instigators and primary actors and pillars of
quality management.

Hans van Hout

Reproduced from Van Hout, H. 2006 Kwaliteitszorg in het HO: nog veel werk
aan de winkel. [Quality assurance in higher education: much remains to be done].
In: H. van Hout, G. ten Dam, M. Mirande, C. Terlouw and J. Willems, eds. 2006.
Vernieuwing in het hoger onderwijs. Onderwijskundig handboek [Innovation in
higher education. Education handbook]. Assen, The Netherlands: Van Gorcum,
pp. 215–228, with permission from Van Gorcum.

Introduction

In the last part of the 20th century higher education saw a massive
rise in student numbers, causing an increase in public spending on
higher education, followed by a major redirection of government
policy from detailed national legislation, to more autonomy for the
institutions (Harvey and Newton 2007). These developments were
accompanied by calls for increased public accountability, resulting
in the creation of statutory systems of external quality management.
In response to this, many universities stepped up their efforts in the
development and implementation of internal quality management,
which encompasses all activities and processes deliberately organized to design, assure, evaluate, and improve the quality of teaching
and learning. However, doubts have been raised as to the effectiveness of internal quality management. Some argue that it increases
bureaucracy and hinders professionals in delivering education.
Others argue that it does promote continuous improvement. So far
there is no substantive empirical evidence on this issue.

The aim of this chapter is to explore the effectiveness of internal
quality management within teaching departments from the perspective of teaching staff. They are the professionals who develop
the educational programmes, deliver them, and supervise and assess
the students. As Van Hout (2006, p. 224) claims, teaching staff are
not just stakeholders that might be involved in quality management:
'Teaching staff, being the carriers of education, should be seen as
the instigators and primary actors and pillars of quality management'. Teachers' perceptions of the effectiveness of internal quality
management may depend on how they view quality. Does quality

mean that the educational programme has to meet certain basic
standards or does it mean continuous improvement? This question
could also be asked with regard to departments, but at departmental level it can only be answered if there is a shared view of quality, the objectives of education and the aims of the department. In
other words the answer depends on the organizational values that
are preferred within a specific department and the degree to which
these values are integrated in day-to-day practice (Van Kemenade
and Van Schaik 2006).

The effectiveness of quality management might also depend on
how quality management is interpreted. When there is one shared
vision with regard to quality management, it can be confined to
straightforward evaluations and improvements, but when different
starting points and perspectives are accepted as legitimate, a more
complex and more formalized system of quality management may be
required with consultations and agreements and with clear rules and
procedures. Such a system may have bureaucratic tendencies and
may be regarded as cumbersome (Van Kemenade and Van Schaik
2006). In such cases 'tension may arise between educational quality
and the quality of quality management' (Van Hout 2006, p. 223).

This chapter addresses the effectiveness of internal quality management within teaching departments from the perspective of the
teaching staff. First, it focuses on teachers' conceptions of quality.
Do teaching staff see quality as meeting basic requirements or as
continuous improvement of education? Second, it deals with teachers' perceptions of quality management within their department.
In the eyes of the teachers, do departments pay sufficient attention
to the relevant aspects of quality and do they undertake enough

quality management activities? This part also pays attention to the effectiveness of internal quality management in the eyes of teaching staff. Third, the chapter explores teachers' preferred organizational values within the context of their teaching departments, and which values teachers perceive to be current in their department. The final section relates to whether an understanding of teachers' conceptions and perceptions can contribute to answering the question as to why quality management is more effective in some departments than in others.

Quality in higher education

Defining quality is an intricate endeavour. Harvey and Green (1993, pp. 10–11) call quality 'a slippery concept', 'no easier even to describe and discuss than deliver in practice' (after Gibson 1986). The definition may vary according to the interests and priorities of different stakeholders and in different situations. Judgements of the quality of education and the effectiveness of quality management are strongly affected by the conceptions of those making the judgements, including teaching staff. How people conceive of the quality of higher education depends on their answers to the following questions: '… what is the purpose of a university? What are the right things for the university to do to achieve its purpose? What are the right ways of doing them?' And 'how can we…do better towards achieving our purposes' (Houston 2008, p. 68). Quality is thus a 'highly contested concept' (Tam 2001, p. 47). It may be the subject of a power struggle (Tam 2001; Barnett 2003) or 'a matter of negotiating between all parties concerned' (Vroeijenstijn 1995, p. 14).

Harvey and Green (1993) elaborated the idea of a wide range of views on quality from different angles, and their classification of concepts is widely used (EUA 2006; Parri 2006; Newton 2007). Based on the tenets of the quality movement in the 20th century, quality is described in seven different ways, the first three of which are product or result oriented:

1. Quality is an *apodictic and universal entity*, which is well-nigh impossible to define but has originality, uniqueness, and invested efforts as its vital ingredients.

2. Quality is *conforming to a set of minimum standards*.

3. Quality is *excellence*, based on high standards that have to be exceeded (Harvey and Green, 1993, p. 12).

In the following views the production process is central:

4. Quality is *perfection* (zero defects). This concept embraces a philosophy of prevention rather than inspection.

5. Quality is *fitness for purpose*, depending on the specifications of teaching staff, or *fitness for use*, depending on the expectations of students and the professional field.

6. Quality is *value for money*: do students, the government, taxpayers, and the business community receive value for money?

7. The last concept describes quality as *transformation*. This concept is rooted in the notions of fundamental change and innovation, of enhancement of students' knowledge, abilities and skills and of the empowerment of participants.

Are teachers aware of this variety of quality concepts? Despite the manifold definitions, many authors distinguish two broad categories, one focused on the accountability process, the other focused on improvement (Harvey and Green 1993; Sallis 2002; EUA 2006).

Harvey and Green (1993), describing the seven concepts of quality, also identify two conceptions of quality. The first one is based on absolutes: quality is self-evident or based on more or less absolute and accepted standards or thresholds, which '…have to be exceeded to obtain a quality rating' (Harvey and Green 1993, p. 10). These standards may be professional or academic, minimal, or of a high level to attain excellence. The focus is on results and external accountability. The second conception 'is relative to the processes that result in the desired outcomes' (Harvey and Green 1993, p. 10). The focus is not on how objectives can be attained as effectively as possible but on whether transformation or improvement and qualitative change can be achieved. Sallis (2002) also distinguishes two types of conceptions of quality: procedural quality, with key descriptors relating to proving, approving, and reporting of service standards, and transformational quality, focusing on the customer: improving rather than proving, and aspiring to excellence, even when not yet meeting it (Sallis, 2002, pp. 14–15). A third example of the two distinct conceptions is presented in the final report of the Quality Culture Project of the European University Association (EUA 2006), which investigated the quality culture in European universities by means of discussions with network representatives of these institutes. Starting from a list of nine quality definitions, project participants identified ample evidence of two quality approaches: a standards-based approach and an approach focused primarily on the processes of development, implementation, and improvement. 'Quality is an on-going exercise; it is not a state that is reached once and for all but one that needs to be pursued continuously' (EUA 2006, p. 10).

Research on conceptions of quality

Apart from the EUA report, based on experts' opinions (EUA 2006), there has not been a great deal of research into conceptions of the quality of teaching. Using an indirect approach, Cartwright (2007) conducted in-depth interviews with six academics about their perceptions of the national quality agenda of the Quality Assurance Agency in the UK. The interviewees described the agenda as a system 'in which the language of quality has been high-jacked' and which is characterized by a 'tick-box approach', 'imposition of control by increasingly intrusive management, the emergence of a blame culture and being forced to jump through irrelevant hoops' (Cartwright 2007, p. 296). Cartwright concluded: 'All my interviewees believed in "quality" and had personal and professional commitment to the idea that their students were entitled to a "quality" academic experience' (Cartwright 2007, p. 295). Nevertheless, this study did not clarify teachers' conceptions of quality.

In interviews with 20 university lecturers about their perceptions of quality initiatives of universities in the UK, Lomas (2007) found that the lecturers perceived the quality initiatives as relating to consumers' perspectives, as quality assurance and control, as concentrating on process rather than content, as striving for standardization and for conformity instead of diversity. They expressed a preference for a 'hands-off' approach as regards their professionalism and for more time for research, reading scientific literature and preparing educational materials. A postal survey by Watty (2006) asked 231 academics from 39 Australian universities which of four of Harvey and Green's concepts (1993) ('fitness for purpose', 'value for money', 'excellence', and 'transformation') were currently being promoted in their departments and which they thought should be promoted. For the current situation, 'fitness for purpose' and 'value for money' received high ratings and the lowest rating was for 'transformation'. However, transformation scored highest among the concepts the respondents thought should be promoted. All these studies suggest that teaching staff have a preference for improvement and transformation, whereas in practice quality tends to be focused on compliance with standards. Empirical data are, however, scarce.

In a quantitative survey among 266 teaching staff from 18 departments of applied sciences in the Netherlands, Kleijnen et al. (2011a) found that teachers within higher education mainly perceive quality as an enrichment of the student's learning process and as improvement of the department and the academic processes. This conception of quality scores higher than compliance with minimum criteria and other imposed criteria, external accountability and the desire to secure a prominent position in league tables.

Overall, teachers see quality more as a process of *enhancement and improvement* than as a *compliance and accountability* tool. These two conceptions, however, are not mutually independent; they show a moderate positive correlation. They cannot be considered as the opposite ends of one continuum (Harvey and Newton 2007, p. 232). In complementary qualitative interviews of senior staff from three teaching departments with an effective and three with a less effective quality management it also appeared that the respondents within both kinds of departments think that quality implies that the department must focus on continuous improvement and innovation (Kleijnen 2012). External standards and regulations play a part here and focus direction, but focusing on standards is not in itself enough. The standards must be interpreted and given substance by the department. This view prevails within all departments, but receives greater emphasis within the more effective ones.

Conclusions

It can be concluded that teachers perceive quality first and foremost as an enhancement of the possibilities and opportunities for students, and as an improvement of the department, rather than as a compliance tool to satisfy standards and external accountability. This conclusion seems heartening since some authors argue that departments are more concerned about meeting basic standards, compliance and external accountability than about improvement and enhancement of teaching and learning (Sallis 2002; Harvey and Newton 2007). *Enhancement and improvement*, however, appears to be the core idea of quality, which is alive in the minds of the teaching staff, both overall and in all investigated departments. *Compliance and accountability* may fulfil necessary functions for the organization but continuous improvement approves to be the key driver of quality (Huisman and Currie 2004; Harvey and Newton 2007). This fits in with the idea that without continuous improvement, 'compliance and accountability' will be reduced to 'feeding the beast' of bureaucracy (Newton 2000, p. 153). While the negative connotations of quality in the literature (buzzword, lack of trust in professionals, bureaucracy), and the resistance to quality still may exist (Spencer-Matthews 2001; Sallis 2002; EUA 2010), research demonstrates that they are not the dominant voice of the teachers.

Quality management and its effectiveness

It is assumed that the judgement of teaching staff of the effectiveness of quality management depends not only on their conceptions of quality but also on the operation of internal quality management. The term internal quality management is used here with reference to all quality-related activities for which the initiative and responsibility lie with the institution (Vanhoof and Van Petegem 2007). Within teaching departments it comprises all activities and processes that are deliberately carried out to design, assure, assess, and improve the quality of teaching and learning, including human factors. Internal quality management also includes external focus, communication with external partners and insight into consumers' expectations (Westerheijden 1999; Harvey and Newton 2004).

In the 20th century, quality management evolved in an additive process of overlapping stages (Garvin 1988; Brundrett and Rhodes 2011). The first stage is 'quality inspection' with a focus on products, defect tracking during and after the manufacturing process and statistical methods of measuring and specifying tolerance limits. The second stage focuses on 'quality engineering' or 'quality control' and concentrates on the design of products, based on a list of specifications to avoid or minimize defects. The third stage focuses on 'quality assurance' and working processes, with more consideration of motivational aspects of work, such as communication, organization, and training. Industry and organizations are aware of the importance of customers' expectations and emphasize the importance of documentation, standards, and auditing. Total quality management (TQM) is mostly seen as the final phase of the quality management process. The purpose of TQM is to avoid a one-sided approach to quality management by ensuring that quality management is an integral part of the work process and not a separate entity for which management is responsible. TQM is based on research, facts and evidence (Grant et al. 2004; Harvey and Newton 2007) and it pays systematic and comprehensive attention to all relevant aspects. Quality management focuses on continuous improvement, using methodical proceedings rooted in the Deming cycle (plan, do, check, act), and on involvement of all relevant organizational levels, from strategic management to grassroots teaching staff. It implies changing mind-sets, organizational culture and external communication with consumers, suppliers, and other external partners. Transparency and communication are essential to maintain external focus and internal participation (Garvin 1988, Lewis and Smith 1994; Sallis 2002; Sahney et al. 2004; Brundrett and Rhodes 2011).

The wheel in fig. 50.1 represents the central quality-management activities of the plan, do, check, act Deming-cycle. They are geared to continuous improvement and secured by standardizing processes. Nevertheless the figure should be interpreted cautiously—the various participants may have different views on the direction of improvement. In addition the process of improvement is not a

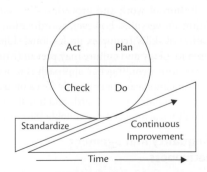

Figure 50.1 The plan, do, check, act cycle.
Reproduced from Outsidethesquaresolutions, with permission.

steady one. We often see iterative processes of steps forward and relapses. The figure represents standardizing the processes as a means to guarantee continuity of improvement.

The comprehensive aspects of education subjected to quality management are usually described as inputs or requirements, processes, and outputs or results (Owlia and Aspinwall 1996; Cave et al. 1997; Van Damme 2004; Sahney et al. 2004). Inputs include financial, physical, and human resources, such as staff quantity and quality, the competencies of enrolling students and facilities. Processes comprise technical and professional variables, such as the goals of teaching and learning, the design and delivery of programmes, or the creation of an educational organization. Processes also comprise soft process or relational variables, such as trustworthiness of teaching staff, accessibility, friendliness, or credible communication (Parasuraman et al. 1991). Output factors include pass/fail rates and competency levels of graduates but also indirect factors, such as career opportunities for alumni and impact on the labour market (Vroeijenstijn 1995; Van Damme 2004). In some way quality management has to take account of all these elements, for example the European Foundation for Quality Management and its Dutch partner INK do so by including steering processes, primary and supportive processes, results and evaluations of results and processes of improvement and innovation in their management models (INK 2008).

The concept of TQM has been widely embraced in higher education (Lewis 1994; Owlia and Aspinwall 1996; Sallis 2002; Venkatraman 2007) and heavily criticized (Zbaracki 1998; Hoecht 2006; Koch 2003). It has been embraced because of a supposed match between the principles of TQM and the nature of higher education on important issues: both emphasize service to students, staff, and other customers on the one hand and active engagement and collaboration of the same groups on the other. Both want to meet their needs and expectations. The importance of transformation processes is recognized, as well as problem-solving and decision-making based on facts and analysis. Both are based on respect for people, confidence in professional competencies, and students' motivations and ambitions (Lewis and Smith, 1994). TQM has been criticized because of its emphasis on the customer. There are, indeed, many ambiguities in higher education: Who is the customer? What is the product of education? And what are the requirements that higher education must meet (Newton 2007)? The requirements and views of the various customer and stakeholder groups do not always coincide—they often collide (Sallis 2002, p. 22). In addition, it is contended that affinity of TQM and higher education can especially be found in the principles of TQM but less in its techniques and tools (Owlia and Aspinwall 1996; Westerheijden 1999, p. 240). Industry may focus on Mintzberg's (1983) coordination mechanisms of 'direct supervision', 'standardisation of work and procedures' or 'standardisation of output'. Within universities, however, coordination mechanisms of 'standardization of skills' (complex professional skills and knowledge) and shared ideology and culture may prevail (Mintzberg 1983; Marx 1986). Therefore a contingency approach is most appropriate. TQM in higher education cannot primarily focus on quality control, standardization, compliance to standards and transfer of procedures. Focussing on quality learning is more suitable (Sitkin et al. 1994).

Research on quality management and its effectiveness

There is no general agreement on the wisdom of dedicating significant time and energy to internal quality management. According to Zbaracki (1998) and Ahaus (2006), ardent advocates of quality management frequently resort to a rhetoric that claims success. Experiences with mounds of paperwork, however, often result in a growing belief that quality management stifles rather than boosts quality. The aforementioned rhetoric of advocates spawns equally impassioned counter-rhetoric from opponents (Ahaus 2006). Most professionals and researchers, however, are well aware of the ambivalences of quality management (e.g. Brennan and Shah 2000; Newton 2000, 2002; Harvey and Newton 2004; Milliken and Colohan 2004), and research has moved from the question 'whether quality assurance systems and procedures are developed and in existence' to their real impact on quality (Stensaker 2007, p. 59). Initial over-enthusiasm has faded and quality management has become a 'maturing field'. The emphasis in research has shifted to the impact of quality management on educational improvement. Nevertheless, evidence-based quality management is still in its infancy (Ahaus 2006; Stensaker 2007).

Many negative effects have been reported, mostly based on interviews or discussion groups and case studies but sometimes also from small surveys among teaching staff. Newton (2000, 2002) conducted extensive qualitative research, including focus group interviews with front-line academics, revealing perceptions of increasing bureaucracy, a rise of standardization and control, and a shift of power from the departments to central level, 'linked to a withdrawal of the trust accorded to the academic community' (Newton 2002, p. 41). Various researchers found that staff experienced loss of ownership and pride as well as reduced individual professional responsibility and accountability, effects that were perceived as impeding new developments and innovation, discouraging young academics and withdrawing creative energy from senior staff who cooperated reluctantly (Newton 2002; Findlow 2008). Staff perceived a tendency to emphasize measurable aspects of quality, tick-box items that were easy to identify irrespective of their relevance, while relevant issues were being neglected. It was concluded that organizations may over-analyse whether things are being done well, while failing to analyse whether the right things are being done (Koch 2003; Cartwright 2007).

Other authors have pointed to positive effects of quality management, although empirical evidence remains scarce. They claim that quality management can emphasize responsibility and break through prevailing internal orientations, that it subjects activities to critical review from outside and that it leads to more attention to the teaching function of departments and the teaching methods used (Brennan and Shah 2000; Huisman and Currie 2004; Stensaker 2007; Westerheijden et al. 2007). Furthermore, they claim a reinforcement of the organization: students are empowered when their perspectives are taken into consideration, institutions are stimulated to underpin their decisions by more transparent information (Brennan and Shah 2000) and there is 'a constraint on arbitrary power' (Huisman and Currie 2004, p. 531). Finally, quality management and transparency may raise public trust in the organization: 'trust is built on verification and grows as a spiral' (Lanarès 2008, p. 4).

Kleijnen et al. (2011b) found that teaching staff were neutral about the degree to which sufficient quality management activities were conducted within departments but were positive about attention paid to relevant quality aspects within departments. Furthermore, faculty were positive about the effects of quality management in terms of improvement but its effects in terms of

Table 50.1 Internal quality management: differences between effective and less effective departments

Departments with the most effective quality management	Departments with the least effective quality management
Clear, quality objectives for the study programme, a clear, common vision	Unclear quality objectives
Reflection upon the results of evaluations, considering the results of related evaluations	Insufficient reflection upon the evaluations
Evaluations lead to improvements in plans Practicable annual plans or policies	Little relationship between evaluations and measures of improvement Little operational annual plans or policies
Implementation of improvements/innovations is monitored Completed PDCA cycle	Inadequate monitoring PDCA cycle incomplete
Commitment and active participation of most staff	Limited commitment, little active participation Support is dependent on pressure from management and external standards
Quality management is a structural element of the usual work/tasks of all staff Bureaucratic paperwork is limited	Quality management is too complicated and mostly a matter for quality management staff Quality management is mostly just consigned to paper
Clear responsibilities; a sense of shared responsibilities. It is clear who monitors this	Pushing responsibilities aside Unclear as to who monitors this
Effective formal and informal communication Consultations held to arrive at consensus	Inadequate formal and informal communication

PDCA, plan, do, check, act.

control scored poorly. Faculty indicated that quality management enhances both their work and educational quality within their departments. Another finding relates to differences between departments. Departments vary substantially in perceptions of faculty. Departments perform quality management activities to different degrees and differ in the amount of attention paid to quality. Perception of improvement as an effect of quality management also shows considerable variations across departments. Finally, the findings demonstrated that the 'perceived improvement' effect of quality management is strongly associated with the perceived amount of quality management activities conducted within the department and the attention that is being paid to quality aspects.

The results of qualitative interviews in three teaching departments with effective quality management and three with less effective quality management indicate that in almost all departments various quality instruments are regularly applied (Kleijnen, 2012). Most departments work with policy plans or annual plans, consultative meetings regarding vision and policy, procedures and criteria for designing and carrying out programmes and assessment, evaluations amongst students, teaching staff and the external working field, and job performance or assessment interviews. There is often a person whose job it is to focus on quality management. Furthermore, within most departments, teaching staff are more or less familiar with the existence of quality management and the instruments deployed.

There are nevertheless big differences between the effective and less effective teaching departments (table 50.1). In the case of effective departments, the policy plans, procedures, criteria and other instruments are based on clear quality objectives for the study programme. Evaluations frequently lead to a structured reflection and analysis, considering related evaluations as well; to feasible plans for improvements; and to communication and feedback. In these departments the teaching staff may not be just familiar with quality management

and intentions to improve, but they may also demonstrate commitment and active participation. Responsibilities are clear and communication is organized efficiently. Committees work with short reports and linking pins ensure a smooth transfer of information. Differences of opinion lead to discussions focused on obtaining consensus and often also to sessions of mutual consult or training. Discussions are taken seriously and lead to concrete policy decisions.

In the case of departments with the least effective quality management, on the other hand, the quality objectives are unclear. The system exists mostly on paper and the support of teaching staff depends upon the pressure exerted by the management. Quality management is something that exists outside, rather than forms part of, day-to-day work. There is little coherence between evaluations, and the plan, do, check, act cycle is not monitored. In these departments responsibility for quality management is pushed onto quality management portfolio holders. Too much is planned, and too little systematically carried out.

How are the effects of internal quality management perceived? In the case of effective teaching departments, improvements are based not solely on low or high scores from written questionnaires but also on in-depth analysis and fundamental insights into the strengths and weaknesses of the curriculum (table 50.2). In addition respondents mention effects of improving processes of learning, a more active involvement of students and the external professional working field and sometimes of higher achievement levels amongst graduates. In these departments, quality management leads to satisfied students who receive timely and adequate responses to their questions. They see that their opinions count. This results in an improved atmosphere, which directly benefits education. Finally, according to the respondents, quality management also contributes to greater compliance with external standards and expectations.

In the case of the less-effective departments, the respondents have doubts about the effectiveness of quality management.

Table 50.2 Effectiveness and effects of quality management: differences between effective and less effective departments

Departments with the most effective quality management	Departments with the least effective quality management
Innovation of the curriculum	Only a limited improvement to the curriculum
In-depth analysis of strengths and weaknesses of the curriculum	In-depth analysis is lacking but there is some understanding of the deficiencies
Improvement of learning processes and of the achievement level amongst graduates	Hardly any improvements in learning processes
Active involvement of students and the external professional working field	Little involvement of students and external working field
Good communication with students, fast feedback	Insufficient feedback to students
The study programme meets external standards	Meeting external standards not cited as an effect

Improvements in the curriculum or in the learning processes are limited. Nevertheless, even in the case of the less-effective departments, people recognize some positive effects (Kleijnen, 2012).

Conclusions

Overall, departments pay sufficient *attention to the* relevant *quality aspects* of education, but engage only to a moderate degree in organized *quality management activities*. Quality aspects are frequently evaluated but the evaluations do not always result in improvements. There are considerable differences between the departments. In some departments, quality management is characterized by clear quality objectives, by reflection and discussion on improvements, and by decisions whose implementation is monitored. Here, quality management is embedded within the practice of teaching staff and management. It is not too complicated and everybody is involved. In other departments, quality management activities, if implemented, are not integrated into practice but mostly just consigned to paper.

As to the effectiveness of quality management, teaching staff perceive more improvement effects from internal quality management than from the effects of control. However, these perceptions of improvement vary significantly across the teaching departments. Some departments do well while others perform poorly, even within the same institution. This seems to confirm the observation by Knight and Trowler (2000) that departments are not powerless in the face of institutional, national and international developments. Departments have freedom in creating their own culture.

Organizational values

In the preceding sections, we saw that judgements of the effectiveness of quality management depend on conceptions of quality, and the way quality management is organized. The literature also assumes that conceptions and perceptions of quality and quality management are embedded in the culture and values of an institution (Harvey and Green 1993; Cameron and Quinn 1999; EUA 2006). Quality management endeavours frequently falter because

they fail to address the specific circumstances of the organization (Sitkin et al. 1994). Successes in one organization are seen as a universal remedy for quality problems plaguing other organizations. Following extensive field research, Cameron and Quinn (1999, pp. 7–8) conclude that quality management strategies frequently fail to meet expectations. In their opinion, organizational culture and values may be the prime factors determining the success of quality management strategies. Values are seen as a core element of culture (Hofstede, 2001). They are desirable motivational goals that touch upon all spheres of life, transcend situations and are the guiding principles by which people can lead their day-to-day lives and by which they assess situations and behaviour (Hitlin and Piliavin 2004).

To classify and examine the organizational values, this chapter adopts the 'competing values framework' of Cameron and Quinn (1999) and Quinn et al. (1996). The framework is a two-dimensional model. The first dimension is related to competition between internal and external orientation, the second deals with the tension between control and flexibility. These two dimensions result in four quadrants, each quadrant representing an ideal type of values (Cameron and Quinn 1999). Thus the framework consists of two control-oriented value orientations: the *rational goal* model or *market* with an external focus and with the main values of planning, efficiency, goal setting, and adherence to agreements; and the *internal process* model or *hierarchy* with an internal focus and the main values of stability, control, measurement, and information management. In addition, the framework comprises two flexibility-oriented organizational values: the *human relations* model or *clan* with an internal focus and with the main values of participation, involvement, cohesion, and openness; and the external *open system* model or *adhocracy* with values such as flexibility, willingness to change, growth, and resource acquisition. Control-oriented organizations cherish their traditions. They adopt strict rules and work methods and attach importance to approved professional skills. Flexibility-oriented organizations value openness and innovation; they create opportunities and take risks.

Although values are guiding principles in life, there is often a gap between the values that people espouse, and what they actually do (Brunsson 1989; Argyris 1990; Cartwright 2007). Therefore, Cameron and Quinn (1999) make a distinction between preferred and current organizational values. They contend that every organization tends to be characterized by one of the four value models, although these are not mutually exclusive. In fact, they are in competition with one another. They also claim that organizational culture influences how people within the organization think about quality and internal quality management. Control-oriented values are supposed to have a positive correlation with the conception of quality as *compliance with standards*, whereas the flexibility-oriented values are supposed to correlate positively with *enhancement and improvement* (Cameron and Quinn, 1999, p. 45). Empirical evidence for this relationship is needed for both preferred and current values.

Research on organizational values

The past 10 years have seen a growing interest in organizational culture and values and their relationships with quality management (EUA 2006, 2010; Gordon and Owen 2008; Lanarès 2008; Harvey and Stensaker 2008), resulting in frequent references to a quality culture. Lanarès (2008) defines quality culture as a subculture of the organizational culture. Several aspects of the quality culture and of organizational values have been researched. The first aspect relates to the organizational culture and organizational values that are characteristic of higher education. Cameron and Freeman (1991) conducted a survey of organizational culture within 334 higher education institutions. No institution was characterized by only one culture. However, the values of the human relations model were found most frequently and the values of the rational goal model occurred least frequently. Berings et al. (2011) performed a pilot study among 28 (sub)organizations of higher education in Belgium (university colleges and universities) and reported similar findings: collective and people oriented organizational values were the most preferred values, followed by values of innovation, coordination, and formalization.

A second aspect of research into organizational culture and values concerns their relationship with individual and organizational barriers to the implementation of quality management and change. Values that are preferred are often blocked by defence mechanisms and structural barriers like faulty communication channels, large hierarchical distances or financial constraints (Harvey 2007; EUA 2010). Mundet Hiern et al. (2006) analysed the perceptions of middle managers and found that the following barriers impeded organizational change: lack of trust due to labour instability, dissatisfaction with the result of actions, and faulty communication channels due to large hierarchical distances. These barriers induced concealment of facts by convenient but deceptive speech and refraining from expressing ideas that were seen as deviant from the ideas of management or the majority. Cruickshank (2003, pp. 1161–1162) conducted a literature review and found the following barriers: negative attitudes towards 'the application of TQM within universities', 'scepticism for management fads', a culture that nurtures, recognizes and rewards individual accomplishments more than group, organizational or community achievements, and resistance to external interference and the introduction of new management techniques.

The impact on the organization is a third aspect of organizational values that has been researched. It is often stated that quality is fostered by communication, participation, a combination of top-down and bottom-up interaction (Ehlers 2009) and other values related to a learning organization, such as responsibility, empowerment, and reflection (Lanarès 2008). Cameron and Freeman (1991, p. 45) found that *human relations* cultures scored highest on students' educational and personal satisfaction, faculty satisfaction, and organizational health, and *open system* cultures scored highest on students' academic and career development, professional development of staff, and system openness. Berings (2009, p. 13) found that current collective values and people-oriented values, and values of innovation (i.e. the flexibility-oriented values), but also system values, were significantly positively related with student and employee satisfaction.

In a survey of teaching staff within Dutch universities of applied sciences, Kleijnen et al. (2009) focused on the four competing values of Cameron and Quinn (1999). The results showed that there are significant differences as to the desirability of the four values: the flexibility-oriented *human relations* and *open system values* are much more preferred than the control-oriented *internal process* and *rational goal values*. At the same time, however, all four organizational values are only moderately experienced in practice, which results in large gaps between the preferred values and the values

that are current in practice. These gaps indicate dissatisfaction and they are larger for the flexible than for the control oriented values. Finally, the results showed that there is little variation between the departments as to the preferred values, but that the current values and the gaps between current and preferred values vary significantly between departments.

Similar findings were found in qualitative research (Kleijnen 2012). These results revealed that the respondents within all teaching departments, including the most and least effective ones, have a substantial preference for the flexible *human relations* and, to a somewhat lesser degree, for the *open system values*. Within most departments the control-oriented *rational goal* and *internal process values* are mentioned as well. The preference for these control-oriented values, however, is rarely the dominant preference.

In contrast to the preferred values, the teaching departments differ substantially from each other in the values that are actually realized in practice (table 50.3). In the case of the effective departments, the preferred organizational values and especially the *human relations* values are often put into practice. Teaching staff here work together, feel jointly responsible, inspire each other and feel involved both with each other and with the department. There is a safe climate, which stimulates reflection, mutual criticism and appraisal. People are allowed to make mistakes, and differences in opinion lead to discussion and learning. There is lot of informal communication and little hierarchy. Important values of the *open system model* are also made concrete within effective departments. The respondents indicate that teaching staff try to excel and take pleasure in developing. They contribute actively to improvement and innovation. Teaching staff are externally oriented and willing and able to represent the department, to express its vision and to follow developments in working practice and to translate them into educational content.

Within the less effective departments there is a clear gap between the *human relations* and *open system values* deemed preferable and the values that are implemented in practice. There is no habit of addressing each other directly with criticisms and the external orientation is limited. In all departments *rational goal* and *internal process values* are less dominant and, in the case of the less effective departments, they are mentioned mostly in terms of complaints—e.g. that in policy formation too few choices are made, that ambitions are unrealistic or that staff members frequently wish to backtrack on agreements.

Conclusions

Within departments with an effective quality management, the preferred organizational values are actually being put into practice. Teaching staff collaborate, there is a good collegiate atmosphere and a good relationship with students. Teaching staff and fellow workers are perceived as being open to criticism. Furthermore, they are perceived as having an outward vision and a willingness to change and innovate. In addition they are also more goal oriented and show a higher responsibility for results.

Organizational culture may contain elements that are beneficial or detrimental to organizational change. Because the existing academic culture is often valued within the organization, it is recommended that quality management should be implemented and developed 'within the framework of the existing culture, rather than going to war with it' (Cruickshank 2003, p. 1165). Vettori and Lueger (2011, p. 53) expressed the same view in a different way: 'A successful

Table 50.3 Current organizational values: differences between effective and less effective departments

Departments with the most effective quality management	Departments with the least effective quality management
Human relations values (frequently mentioned)	
Collaboration, feeling of joint responsibility, inspiring each other, involvement with each other and with the department	Little collaboration, little involvement with each other
	Poor school atmosphere
Good collegiate atmosphere, togetherness, work satisfaction, a good atmosphere for students	Little communication and openness, feeling of insecurity
Open to criticism, vulnerability, holding each other accountable, constructive criticism, praise for each other, trust and integrity	Sub-groups, no direct contact between people on the issue of performance
	People often talk about each other instead of to each other
Short communication lines, proximity, informal contacts	Insufficient critical self reflection
Difference in opinion leads to discussion and learning, openness to good examples, being a learning organization	Decisions are taken, or are perceived to be taken, at the top
Teaching staff support students, connection with young people, willingness to talk with students	
Self reflection	
Little hierarchical etiquette, values and culture grow from the ground up	
Open system values (less frequently mentioned)	
Dynamic	Little willingness to take steps
Willingness to take steps to continually improve	Proposals for improvements are treated with suspicion
Enthusiasm, desire to excel, to distinguish oneself, to have pleasure in learning from experiences, addressing issues	Dominant internal orientation
External orientation	
Willing and able to represent the department externally, to present the vision	
Balance between stability and change	
Rational goal values (seldom mentioned)	
Making and carrying out agreements, goal-oriented, responsibility for results	Abandoning existing agreements. Agreements are mostly left on paper
Making choices, realistic ambitions	Pushing responsibilities to one side
	Plans for improvement regarded as unachievable
Internal process values (seldom mentioned)	
Strong organisation, clear tasks, authorities, responsibilities, transparency of decision-taking	Weak organization
	Less effective decision-taking

Q[uality] A[ssurance] system is not built *for* the organisation, but *from* the organisation'. It has to be built in the context of the culture that people are living in and that is a part of their identity (Harvey and Stensaker 2008). Consequently, it is always necessary to study the organizational culture of institutes and departments in higher education, when quality management is introduced.

Relationships between variables

The literature frequently underlines the importance of organizational culture for the success or failure of quality management (Harvey and Green 1993; Cameron and Quinn 1999; Kezar and Eckel 2002; Van Kemenade et al. 2008). It is expected that the conception of quality as *compliance to standards and accountability* shows a positive correlation with the control-oriented values. The conception of quality as *enhancement and improvement* is expected to correlate positively with the flexibility-oriented values (Cameron and Quinn 1999; Brundrett and Rhodes 2011). The results of some studies are in line with expectations, although the relationships are not strong (Kleijnen et al. 2011a; Kleijnen 2012). In these studies it was also found that staff members' conceptions of quality and of

preferred values are virtually the same within all departments. The differences between effective and less effective departments, however, are related to their perceptions of current practice. Quality management is perceived as effective if it is systematically implemented in the departments and if the preferred organizational values are experienced in day-to-day practice. Figure 50.2 illustrates this connection. These findings are in line with the claims of Harvey and Green (1993), Cameron and Quinn (1999) and Kezar and Eckel (2002): an organizational culture within which the *human relations values* and the *open system values* are made dominant in practice provides a good seedbed for quality. Such an organizational culture has to a large degree the character of a learning organization (Sitkin et al. 1994; Lanarès 2008). Nevertheless, in practice, all too often a gap is experienced between preferred and current values, between the *espoused theory* and the *theory in practice* (Brunsson 1989; Argyris 1990). In these circumstances quality management can hardly be effective.

Conclusions

In all researched departments teachers prefer the flexible organizational values and cherish the conception of quality as *enhancement*

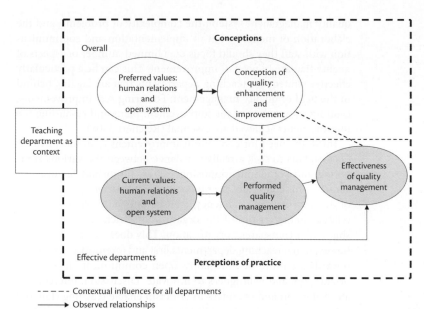

Figure 50.2 Empirical framework: conceptions and perceptions, environmental influences and observed relationships.

and improvement. Therefore these preferences and conceptions can hardly explain the variation of *quality management activities* and their perceived effectiveness over the departments.

Practice, however, offers a better explanation for the differences between departments. Quality management is more effective in departments where, according to teaching staff, quality management is performed systematically, as part of day to day practice, and flexible organizational values are put into practice. Within these departments, the flexibility-oriented organizational values and the characteristics of systematic quality management seem to be mutually supportive, a conclusion that finds support in the literature in which it is argued that quality management and organizational values should be aligned (Kezar and Eckel 2002, Harvey and Stensaker 2008).

Three dilemmas

'Compliance and accountability' or 'enhancement and improvement'?

As a result of the introduction of external quality management systems, internal quality management frequently focuses on compliance with standards and accountability to management and external agencies. Some authors argue that compliance with standards can have quality enhancing effects (Huisman and Currie 2004; Vanhoof and Van Petegem 2007). It can broaden the scope of interest, stimulate internal quality assurance processes and legitimize the results of internal and external evaluations and the resulting quality claims of schools and individual teachers, which are also made transparent. Other authors have argued, on the other hand, that emphasis on standards may give rise to a tendency to 'focus on the mechanistic implementation of recommendations' (Quinn and Boughey 2009, p. 263), especially when external quality management and accreditation are linked to the funding of the programme. This may result in a legalistic approach to internal quality management in which exceeding standards or innovation are not the primary concerns.

In contrast to these misgivings and despite teachers and staff preferring the conception of *enhancement and improvement* as the key driver of quality, this chapter shows that the two conceptions of *compliance and accountability* and *enhancement and improvement* are moderately positively correlated and should not be characterized as the opposite ends of a continuum. Provided the standards leave room for professional interpretation by teaching staff, they are frequently accepted and used as they are meant to be used, i.e. to guide the implementation of internal quality assurance activities (ENQA 2005, p. 13). *Compliance and accountability* and *enhancement and improvement* are not mutually exclusive but characteristics that can support each other.

Focus on flexible organizational values or on creating a balance between the flexible and the control-oriented organizational values?

The second discussion bears on the issue of seeking a balance between the different organizational values or placing special emphasis on some values (Cameron and Quinn 1999; Berings 2001; Lanarès 2008). Each department should have strategies to cope with organizational ambivalences and competing values, and tensions between competing values should be regulated. Overemphasizing certain values may have detrimental effects: *human relations* values may turn into extreme permissiveness and individualism and relentless discussion; *open system* values may lead to disastrous experimentation, ad hoc decisions, opportunism without principles, and chaos; *rational goal* values may foster callous pressure for achievement; and *internal process* values may end in stagnation, rigid behaviour, and cynicism (Quinn et al. 1996).

This chapter demonstrates that teaching staff prefer the flexibility-oriented *human relations* and *open system* values over the control-oriented *rational goal* and *internal process* values. It also indicates that in the departments where the flexible organizational values are put into practice teachers perceive internal quality management as more effective. In order to enhance the effectiveness of internal quality management, priority should be given to putting the flexibility-oriented values into practice. They create a flow that not only stimulates continuous improvement but also acceptance of the related process control.

Focus on quality management or creating a quality culture?

The third discussion regards the relationship between management and culture (Vettori et al. 2007). From a management perspective,

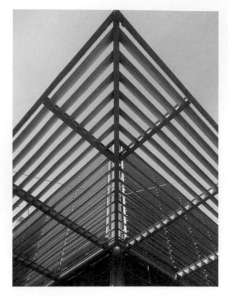

Figure 50.3 Quality culture: ambition and collaboration in an open structure. Reproduced with permission from Maril Donders.

internal quality management is characterized by clear quality objectives, a well-organized process with explicit responsibilities, established criteria and standards, tangible aims of evaluation, clearly defined institutional data, and systematic methods of data gathering and analysis (Harvey and Newton 2004). As a consequence, quality management entails the control of management over internal and external developments and seems mainly based on control-oriented values, such as achieving the planned targets.

In this chapter, however, it is argued that departments with an effective quality management are characterized by a culture of external orientation, openness to criticism, reflection, innovation, and a willingness to collaborate. Flexible organizational values are perceived as a fertile feeding ground for quality and quality management. They foster an atmosphere of inspiring, mobilizing, valuing, and reflecting (INK 2008). Improvement of education depends not only on the systematic performance of quality management activities, but also on a flexible organizational culture in current practice (fig. 50.3).

Implications for practice

First, quality management and ideas about improvement of education should not be imposed, but linked up with the prevailing conceptions among teaching staff of quality as *enhancement and improvement* and with their preferences for flexible organizational values. Management has a steering task, but should also encourage teachers *themselves* to formulate and discuss the preferred transformations for their students, and the improvements they would like to implement in their departments. Management should refrain from focusing primarily, and exclusively, on compliance with standards, but should examine the degree to which management and teaching staff can coordinate their objectives, shaping them in a systematic and consistent manner (Van Hout 2006).

Second, quality management activities should be incorporated into the normal work of teaching staff and excessive paperwork avoided. Quality management should not be too complicated. Management should take care of the comprehensiveness of the

quality management system, the complexity of problems, and the elaboration of methods, but in implementation and communication with staff they should focus on a limited number of aspects of quality that are in need of improvement. This can be a particularly effective strategy for teaching departments that are lagging behind in the field of quality management. Fostering real improvements, cautious monitoring of the improvement plans and rewarding the improvements achieved are essential (Reichert 2008).

Third, the need for continuous improvement is an incentive for departments to seek a realistic balance between the various competing and sometimes opposing values. Important features for assuring this continuity are *rational goal* and *internal process values* of decision making, efficiency, transparency and continuity, and related characteristics of the organization, such as stable leadership and a transparent organization. This does not alter the fact, however, that teaching departments first and foremost should work towards a culture of collegiality, open communication, external orientation, and willingness to innovate. Discussion, intercollegiate evaluation and openness to criticism enable teaching staff and management to reinforce each other's efforts. These flexible *human relations* and *open system values* may well be the salient issues in quality management in present-day higher education.

Conclusions

♦ Continuous improvement should be the most important aim of internal quality assurance, although standards and control are also useful as long as they are not too detailed and prescriptive.

♦ Most departments engage only to a moderate degree in organized *quality management activities.*

♦ Internal quality assurance has more chances to result in continuous improvement if internal quality assurance activities are carried out systematically, but above all if there is an organizational culture characterised by flexible organizational values in which teaching staff collaborate, communicate well, are open to criticism and feel little threatened by it, have an external orientation, and have a willingness to innovate.

♦ More time and effort should be put into implementing actions for improvement instead of carrying out too many evaluations that do not result in continuous improvement.

Acknowledgements

This text is based on: Kleijnen, J. 2012. Internal quality management and organisational values in higher education. Conceptions and perceptions of teaching staff. Maastricht, The Netherlands: Maastricht University; Unpublished thesis.

References

Ahaus, K. (2006) *Kwaliteit uit waardering [Quality through appraisal]. Inaugural address held at the Faculty of Management and Organization of the University of Groningen on acceptance of his appointment to the endowed chair of Quality Management at the Management Science department on Tuesday 4 April 2006.* Groningen: Rijksuniversiteit Groningen: Faculteit Bedrijfskunde

Argyris, C. (1990) *Overcoming Organizational Defenses. Facilitating Organizational Learning.* Boston, London: Allyn and Bacon

Barnett, R. (2003) *Beyond All Reason: living with ideology within the university*. Buckingham: The Society for Research into Higher Education and Open University Press

Berings, D. (2001) *Omgaan met concurrerende waarden als voorwaarde tot de ontwikkeling van integrale kwaliteitszorg in het hogescholenonderwijs in Vlaanderen*, proefschrift *[Coping with competing values as a prerequisite for developing integral quality management within university colleges in Flanders, dissertation]*. Brussels, Belgium: EHSAL

Berings, D. (2009) Reflection on quality culture as a substantial element of quality management in higher education. *Paper presented at the 4th European Quality Assurance Forum*. Copenhagen, Denmark 19–21 November 2009

Berings, D., Beerten, Z, Hulpiau, V. and Verhesschen, P. (2011) Quality culture in higher education: from theory to practice. In: EUA. 2011. *Building bridges: making sense of quality assurance in European, national and institutional contexts. A selection of papers from the 5th European Quality Assurance Forum*. Lyon, France 18–20 November 2010. Brussels, Belgium: EUA, pp. 38–49

Brennan, J. and Shah, T. (2000) Quality assessment and institutional change: experiences from 14 countries. *Higher Educ.* 40(3): 331–349

Brundrett, M. and Rhodes, C. (2011) *Leadership for Quality and Accountability in Education*. London and New York: Routledge

Brunsson, N. (1989) *The Organization of Hypocrisy. Talk, Decisions and Actions in Organizations*. Chichester, New York: John Wiley & Sons Inc.

Cameron, K.S. and Freeman, S.J. (1991) Cultural congruence, strength, and type: relationships to effectiveness. *Res Organis Change Devel.* 5(1): 23–58

Cameron, K.S. and Quinn, R.E. (1999) *Diagnosing and Changing Organizational Culture. Based on the Competing Values Framework*. Reading, MA: Addison-Wesley

Cartwright, M.J. (2007) The rhetoric and reality of 'quality' in higher education. An investigation into staff perceptions of quality in post-1992 universities. *Qual Assur Educ.* 15(3): 287–301

Cave, M., Hanney, S., Henkel, M., and Kogan, M. (1997) *The Use of Performance Indicators in Higher Education. The challenge of the quality movement*. 3rd edn. London: Jessica Kingsley Publishers

Cruickshank, M. (2003) Total quality management in the higher education sector: a literature review from an international and Australian perspective. *TQM Business Excellence.* 14(10): 1159–1167

Ehlers, U.D. (2009) Understanding quality culture. *Qual Assur Educ.* 12(4): 343–363

ENQA, European Network for Quality Assurance in Higher Education (2005) *Standards and guidelines for quality assurance in the European higher education area*. Brussels, Belgium: ENQA. [Online] http://www.enqa.eu/files/ENQA%20Bergen%20Report.pdf Accessed 13 March 2013

EUA, European University Association (2006) *Quality Culture in European Universities: a Bottom-up Approach. Report on the three rounds of the Quality Culture Project 2002-2006*. Brussels, Belgium: EUA

EUA, European University Association (2010) *Examining Quality Culture: part I—Quality assurance processes in higher education institutions*. Brussels, Belgium: EUA

Findlow, S. (2008) Accountability and innovation in higher education: a disabling tension? *Studies Higher Educ.* 33(3): 313–329

Garvin, D.A. (1988) *Managing Quality. The strategic and competitive edge*. New York, London: The Free Press

Gibson, A. (1986) Inspecting education. In G.C. Moodie (ed.) *Standards and Criteria in Higher Education* (pp. 128–135). Milton Keynes: SRHE and Open University Press

Gordon, G. and Owen, C. (2008) *Cultures of Quality Enhancement: a short overview of the literature for higher education policy makers and practitioners*. [Online] www.enhancementthemes.ac.uk Accessed 13 March 2013

Grant, D., Mergen, E., and Widrick, S. (2004) A comparative analysis of quality management in US and international universities. *Total Qual Manage.* 15(4): 423–438

Harvey, L. (2007) Quality culture, quality assurance and impact. Overview of discussions. In: EUA. 2007. *Embedding quality culture in higher education.*

A selection of papers from the 1st European Forum for Quality Assurance, München, Germany 23–25 November 2006. EUA, Brussels, pp. 81–84

Harvey, L. and Green, D. (1993) Defining quality. *Assess Eval Higher Educ.* 18(1): 9–34

Harvey, L. and Newton, J. (2004) Transforming quality evaluation. *Qual Higher Educ.* 10(2): 149–165

Harvey, L. and Newton, J. (2007) Transforming quality evaluation: moving on. In D.F. Westerheijden, B. Stensaker, and M.J. Rosa (eds) *Quality Assurance in Higher Education. Trends in Regulation, Translation and Transformation* (pp. 225–245). Dordrecht, The Netherlands: Springer

Harvey, L. and Stensaker, B. (2008) Quality culture: understandings, boundaries and linkages. *Eur J Educ.* 43(4): 427–442

Hitlin, S. and Piliavin, J.A. (2004) Values: reviving a dormant concept. *Ann Rev Sociol.* 30: 359–393

Hoecht, A. (2006) Quality assurance in UK higher education: issues of trust, control, professional autonomy and accountability. *Higher Educ.* 51(4): 541–563

Hofstede, G. (2001) *Culture's Consequences: Comparing Values, Behaviors, Institutions and Organizations Across Nations*. 2nd edn. Thousand Oaks, CA: Sage

Houston, D. (2008) Rethinking quality and improvement in higher education. *Qual Assur Educ.* 16(1): 61–79

Huisman, J. and Currie, J. (2004) Accountability in higher education: Bridge over troubled water? *Higher Educ.* 48(4): 529–551

INK (2008) *Introductie. Inhoud en toepassing van het INK-managementmodel [Introduction. Theory and practice of the INK management model]*. Zaltbommel: INK

Kezar, A. and Eckel, P.D. (2002) The effect of institutional culture on change strategies in higher education. Universal principles or culturally responsive concepts? *Higher Educ.* 73(4): 435–460

Kleijnen, J., Dolmans, D., Willems, J., Muijtjens, A., and Van Hout, J. (2009) Organisational values in higher education: perceptions and preferences of staff. *Qual Higher Educ.* 15(3): 233–249

Kleijnen, J., Dolmans, D., Willems, J., and Van Hout, J. (2011a) Teachers' conceptions of quality and organisational values in higher education: compliance or enhancement? *Assess Eval Higher Educ* DOI:10.1080/02602938.2011.611590. [Online] http://dx.doi.org/10.1080/02602938.2011.611590 Accessed 13 March 2013

Kleijnen, J., Dolmans, D., Willems. J., and Van Hout, J. (2011b) Does internal quality management contribute to more control or to improvement of higher education? A survey on faculty's perceptions. *Qual Assur Educ.* 19(2): 141–155

Kleijnen, J. (2012) *Internal quality management and organisational values in higher education. Conceptions and perceptions of teaching staff*. Maastricht, The Netherlands: Maastricht University; Unpublished thesis

Knight, P.T. and Trowler, P.R. (2000) Department-level cultures and the improvement of learning and teaching, *Studies Higher Educ.* 25(1): 69–83

Koch, J.V. (2003) TQM: why is its impact in higher education so small? *TQM Mag.* 15(5): 325–333

Lanarès, J. (2008) Developing a quality culture. In E. Froment, J. Purser and L. Wilson (eds) *EUA Bologna Handbook* (pp. 1–27). Berlin: Raabe Verlag

Lewis, R.G. and Smith, D.H. (1994) *Total Quality in Higher Education*. Delray Beach Florida: St. Lucie Press

Lomas, L. (2007) Zen, motorcycle maintenances and quality in higher education. *Qual Assur Educ.* 15(4): 402–412

Marx, E.C.H. (1986) Universitaire organisatie in ontwikkeling [Academic organisation under development]. In P. Frissen, P.M.Th. Van Hoewijk, and J.F.M.J. van Hout (eds) *De universiteit: een adequate onderwijsorganisatie [The university: an adequate education organisation]* (pp. 56–80). Utrecht: het Spectrum BV.

Milliken, J. and Colohan, G. (2004) Quality or control? Management in higher education. *J Higher Educ Policy Manage.* 26(3): 381–391

Mintzberg, H. (1983) *Structure in Fives: Designing Effective Organizations*. 2nd edn. Englewood Cliffs, NJ, USA: Prentice Hall

Mundet Hiern, J., Suñé Torrents, A., Sallán Leyes, J.M., and Fernández Alarcón, V. 2006. The impact of defensive barriers on organizational performance and learning. *Management Avenir.* 2(8) 27–37

Newton, J. (2000) Feeding the beast or improving quality? Academics' perceptions of quality assurance and quality monitoring. *Qual Higher Educ.* 6(2): 153–163

Newton, J. (2002) Views from below: academics coping with quality. *Qual Higher Educ.* 8(1): 39–61

Newton, J. (2007) What is quality? In: EUA. 2007. *Embedding quality culture in higher education. A selection of papers from the 1st European Forum for Quality Assurance.* München, Germany 23–25 November 2006. Brussels, Belgium: EUA, pp. 14–20

Owlia, M.S. and Aspinwall, E.A. (1996) Quality in higher education. *Total Qual Manage.* 7(2): 161–171

Parasuraman, A., Berry, L.L., and Zeithaml, V.A. (1991) Refinement and reassessment of the Servqual scale. *J Retailing.* 67(4): 420–450

Parri, J. (2006) Quality in higher education. *Vadyba/Management.* 2(11): 107–111

Quinn, L. and Boughey, C. (2009) A case study of an institutional audit. *Qual Higher Educ.* 15(2): 263–278

Quinn, R.E., Faerman, S.R., Thompson, M.P., and McGrath, M.R. (1996) *Becoming a master manager: A competency framework.* 2nd edn. New York: John Wiley & Sons Inc.

Reichert, S. (2008) Looking back—looking forward: quality assurance and the Bologna process. In: EUA. 2008. *Implementing and using quality assurance: strategy and practice, a selection of papers from the 2nd European Quality Assurance Forum.* Rome, Italy 15–17 November 2007. Brussels, Belgium: EUA, pp. 5–10

Sahney, S., Banwet, D.K., and Karunes, S. (2004) Conceptualizing total quality management in higher education. *TQM Mag.* 16(2): 145–159

Sallis, E. (2002) *Total Quality Management in Education.* 3rd edn. London: Kogan Page

Sitkin, S.B., Sutcliffe, K.M., and Schroeder, R.G. (1994) Distinguishing control from learning in Total Quality Management: a contingency perspective. *Acad Manage Rev.* 18(3): 537–564

Spencer-Matthews, S. (2001) Enforced cultural change in academe. A practical case study: implementing quality management systems in higher education. *Assess Eval Higher Educ.* 26(1): 51–59

Stensaker, B. (2007) Impact of quality processes. In: EUA. 2007 *Embedding quality culture in higher education. A selection of papers from the 1st European Forum for Quality Assurance*, München, Germany 23–25 November 2006. Brussels, Belgium: EUA, pp. 59–62

Tam, M. (2001) Measuring quality and performance in higher education. *Qual Higher Educ.* 7(1): 47–54

Van Damme, D. (2004) Standards and indicators in institutional and programme accreditation in higher education: a conceptual framework and a proposal. In L. Vlasceanu and L.C. Barrows (eds) *Indicators for Institutional And Programme Accreditation in Higher/Tertiary Education* (pp. 127–159). Bucharest: UNESCO-CEPES

Vanhoof, J. and Van Petegem, P. (2007) Matching internal and external evaluation in an era of accountability and school development: Lessons from a Flemish perspective. *Studies Educ Eval.* 22(2): 101–119

Van Hout, H. (2006) Kwaliteitszorg in het HO: nog veel werk aan de winkel. [Quality assurance in higher education: much remains to be done]. In: H. van Hout, G. ten Dam, M. Mirande, C. Terlouw, and J. Willems (eds) *Vernieuwing in het hoger onderwijs. Onderwijskundig handboek* [*Innovation in higher education. Education handbook*] (pp. 215–228). Assen, The Netherlands: Van Gorcum

Van Kemenade, E. and Van Schaik, M. (2006) Interne kwaliteitszorg, van ambacht naar visie [Internal quality assurance, from craft to vision]. In: H. van Hout, G. ten Dam, M. Mirande, C. Terlouw, and J. Willems (eds) *Vernieuwing in het hoger onderwijs. Onderwijskundig handboek* [*Innovation in higher education. Education handbook*] (pp. 229–244). Assen, The Netherlands: Van Gorcum

Van Kemenade, E, Pupius, M., and Hardjono, T.D. (2008) More value to defining quality, *Qual Higher Educ.* 14(2): 175–185

Venkatraman, S. (2007) A framework for implementing TQM in higher education programs, *Qual Assur Educ.* 15(1): 92–112

Vettori, O., Lueger, M., and Knassmüller, M. (2007) Dealing with ambivalences—strategic options for nurturing a quality culture in teaching and learning. In: EUA. 2007. *Embedding quality culture in higher education. A selection of papers from the 1st European Forum for Quality Assurance.* München, Germany 23–25 November 2006. Brussels, Belgium: EUA, pp. 11–13

Vettori, O. and Lueger, M. (2011) No short cuts in quality assurance—Theses from a sense-making perspective. In: EUA. 2011. *Building bridges: making sense of quality assurance in European, national and institutional contexts. A selection of papers from the 5th European Quality Assurance Forum.* Lyon, France 18–20 November 2010. Brussels, Belgium: EUA, pp. 50–55

Vroeijenstijn, A.I. (1995) *Improvement and Accountability, Navigating Between Scylla and Charybdis. Guide for external quality assessment in Higher Education.* London and Bristol, PA: Jessica Kingsley Publishers

Watty, K. (2006) Want to know about quality in higher education? Ask an academic. *Qual Higher Educ.* 12(3): 291–301

Westerheijden, D.F. (1999) Where are the quantum jumps in quality assurance? Developments of a decade of research on a heavy particle. *High Educ.* 38(2): 233–254

Westerheijden, D.F., Hulpiau, V., and Waeytens, K. (2007) From design and implementation to impact of quality assurance: an overview of some studies into what impacts improvement. *Tertiary Educ Manage.* 13(4): 295–316

Zbaracki, M.J. (1998) The rhetoric and reality of total quality management. *Admin Sci Q.* 43(3): 602–636

CHAPTER 51

Cost and value in medical education

Kieran Walsh

The education is so expensive that none enter upon the study except the sons of men of independent fortune.

John Banks

Cost and value in medical education

At its core the cost-value or cost effectiveness of medical education depends on a few concepts. These are the cost of medical education, its effectiveness or value and the degree of effectiveness or value considering the cost. If we are to know anything about cost and value in medical education, then what we know must be built on firm foundations of facts about cost and value or effectiveness.

The UK spend on medical education is approximately £4.8 billion (Department of Health 2010). This includes undergraduate, postgraduate, and continuing professional development, and spans medical, nursing and allied healthcare professional education; but even taking this into account, it is still an enormous sum. It is likely that £1 billion is spent in the UK on undergraduate medical education alone. In Western Europe the estimated average spend per medical graduate is $400 000—this contrasts with the spend in the United States of $497 000 per graduate and that of China with a remarkably low spend of $14 000 per graduate (Frenk et al. 2010). At this point, however, further delving into figures reveals few enlightening results. We do not know how much of the expenditure on healthcare professional education is spent on problem-based learning or interprofessional learning, or even on assessment in medical education. We do not know how much is spent on online learning, simulation, or face to face education. One of the foundation stones of cost and value in medical education is that of cost itself, but unfortunately we have insufficient knowledge of its size or depth.

Another foundation stone upon which we can build up this chapter is the issue of value or effectiveness. What do we know about what is valuable or effective in medical education and how do we know this? Thankfully, this part of the foundation is somewhat firmer. Researchers and evaluators within medical education have over many years built up an ever stronger evidence base and conceptual framework upon which medical education can be based. Medical education need no longer be empirical—the literature that has blossomed over the past 40 years points clearly as to what works and what does not within medical education. To take just one example—assessment—we know that, for assessment to be of value, it must be valid, reliable, feasible, and acceptable to the learner and it must have a positive impact on the learner (Norcini et al. 2011). Similar summary statements could be made about what constitutes value in e-learning or undergraduate medical education or simulation. What we know to be of value in medical education is based not just on the best available evidence from whatever form of study but also on an increasingly robust conceptual framework that underpins medical education. The evidence base is not yet complete, nor will it ever be, but we know that it is considerably stronger than it was.

However, when we grasp for what is likely to constitute cost-effectiveness or a cost-value proposition within medical education, then unfortunately we find only shadows. There are few or no systemic reviews of cost and value in medical education and precious few evaluation or research studies that look at cost (Walsh 2010a). We do not know whether medical education in the UK as it currently exists offers good value for money or poor value for money—the research has not yet been done. No approach is inherently cost effective—rather it is cost effective in the context of what other approaches are available. Without a strong evidence base then estimating the relative cost-effectiveness of an intervention is speculation. We simply do not know where we lie on table 51.1.

Research is needed but this will take time and, with healthcare throughout the world facing an economic crisis, time is not on our side. Medical education cannot be protected from budgetary cuts that may be imposed on healthcare spending. While we are waiting for research to come up with a clear answer, then we must look at first principles in education and examine what components of medical education truly add value. The next section takes this approach to look in detail at cost and value in medical education in the contexts of simulation, e-learning, and finally assessment.

Table 51.1 Cost and value in medical education

	Low value	High value
High cost		The present
Low cost	The past	The future?

Simulation: cost and value

Simulation may be defined as 'the reproduction of all or some aspect of a job or task' (Ker et al. 2010: p. 61). The purpose of simulation is to help the healthcare professional learn by practising and sometimes self-testing in an authentic environment that is safe for learners and patients. Simulation can help the learning of knowledge, skills, and behaviours. The star of simulation has been on an inexorable rise over the past 10 years and not all the drivers for simulation have been purely educational. Non-educational drivers include shortened working hours for doctors in training, the need to ensure patient safety as much as is feasible and the fact that doctors are increasingly working in teams rather than as individuals.

Shortened working hours mean that modern doctors in training have less time to see the range of case scenarios that were seen by their predecessors. This is especially true of out of hours and emergency care. Simulation enables doctors in training to practise their skills in controlled environments where their learning can be planned rather than incidental (Issenberg et al. 2005). Equally, in the modern world, junior doctors must learn without compromising patient care. It is no longer acceptable for doctors or other healthcare professionals to practise on patients when alternative modes of learning are available.

The last driver to simulation as a means of education is the changed working practices of doctors. The single-handed practitioner in primary or secondary care is becoming a creature of the past—nearly all doctors now work in teams, and simulation centres are an effective way for team members to train and test their skills in high-fidelity and contextualized simulated environments (Ostergaard et al. 2004).

The cost of simulation

Simulation can be expensive. Ker et al. (2010, pp. 61–71) divide the costs of simulation into two categories—obvious costs and hidden costs. According to Ker et al. (2010 p. 64) 'the most obvious cost associated with simulation is that of purchasing the simulator hardware itself, some of which may be highly specialised'. The purchase may be as simple as buying a manikin or as complex as procuring a state of the art simulated resuscitation room. Regardless of this, the simulation will have to take place in a building, which will have associated cost, and there is also the hardware required for video and audio recording and storage. The technology available to support simulation is growing rapidly, but costs are growing at an equally rapid rate. Mobile simulators, however, may be purchased at a much lower cost (Kneebone et al. 2010).

Simulation centres do not run themselves—they need dedicated staff to ensure that they are managed as effectively and efficiently as possible. Staff will include facilitators, simulated patients (be they real or actors), audiovisual and technology support staff, as well as managerial, administrative, and secretarial support teams

(Zendejas et al. 2012). Some will work full time in the centre, some part time, and some will only work fixed or occasional sessions, but all need to be paid or have their time compensated for. All staff will need to learn about education when they start and continue to update their knowledge and skills as they develop expertise in simulation. Time and resources will thus need to be dedicated to faculty development (Dieckmann et al. 2008).

Content specific expertise is not sufficient to be an effective facilitator in simulation—health professionals need tailored education to help them develop their facilitation skills. The most important stakeholder involved in simulation that incurs costs is of course the learner. Learners' off-the-job time must be accounted for and if learners have to travel to the simulation centre then travel costs, and sometimes accommodation and subsistence costs, must be accounted for.

In the enthusiasm of setting up a simulation centre, the hidden costs of simulation are often forgotten about (Ker et al. 2010). Simulators can break down or wear out or get damaged accidentally—the maintenance, repair, and replacement costs must not be overlooked. Some simulation companies will offer insurance with their products, but it is well to read the fine print before making your purchase. Consumables (everything from syringes to paper forms) will also require a section of a simulation centre's budget. Another commonly neglected cost is the scenarios upon which simulations are to be based. These scenarios need to be written, reviewed, and continually updated. They need to fit in with rest of the curriculum and ideally should be based on real-life events that occurred in the learner's own institution. Ultimately, simulation is only as effective as the scenarios upon which it is based.

What works in simulation?

Bearman et al. in their chapter (Chapter 16) gives a comprehensive account of simulation in medical education and it would be redundant to reproduce this content here. However, a very short reprise is probably worthwhile. According to Ker et al. (2010 p. 63) the 'evidence base for the effectiveness of simulation training in healthcare is both limited and sporadic'. However, we do know that elements within the simulation black box that consistently facilitate learning include:

◆ 'providing feedback,

◆ allowing repetitive practice

◆ integrating the use of simulation events within a curricular programme

◆ providing a range of difficulties and scenarios and

◆ defining learning outcomes' (Ker et al. 2010, p. 63; Issenberg et al. 2005).

How can simulation add to the value proposition of medical education?

Unfortunately, there are no systematic reviews on the cost-effectiveness of simulation and few original articles. There is little hard evidence on whether particular forms of simulation might add more value at the same or reduced costs. However, there are some straightforward guidance points that are likely to apply to cost and value in simulation (fig. 51.1).

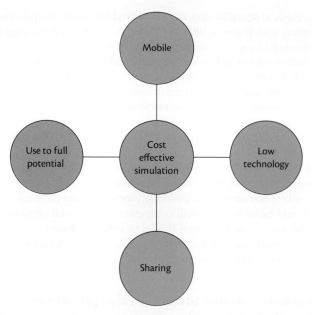

Figure 51.1 Cost-effective simulation.

First, there is an important adage that simulation in medical education should only be as high fidelity as it needs to be. State of the art simulation centres can be very tempting, but purchasers should look hard at what learning outcomes they are trying to achieve and how the facilities will help them achieve them. It is unlikely to be cost effective to purchase a cardiothoracic surgery simulation laboratory if your hospital rarely undertakes this form of surgery. Statements like this seem so obvious as to be hardly worth saying, but there are anecdotal reports of medical education institutions in developed countries and emerging economies purchasing simulation equipment that was not subsequently used or that was not used to its maximum capacity. Certain specialties, such as general practice or psychiatry, do not need high-fidelity, high-cost simulation environments to help their doctors learn—an effective simulation can take place with a room, a table, some chairs, and some well-scripted scenarios.

Second, it is likely to be a cost-inefficient practice to fail to get maximum use out of a simulation centre or to use it for the wrong purpose. There is nothing inherently wrong with a resuscitation expert using a simulation centre to teach the dose of adrenaline—it is, however, likely to be a very inefficient way of achieving a learning outcome. It would be far cheaper and quicker to achieve this outcome by means of a lecture or by recommending reading materials. Simulation centres are better for learning skills—be they procedural skills or team-working skills—and it is better to use them for this purpose.

Third, if simulation centres are to be used to enable mandatory training then it is probably best to standardize this training so that when a health professional has done simulation training in one centre then his or her certificate of completion becomes common currency at neighbouring institutions that he or she might work in also. Asking healthcare professionals to do slightly different versions of the same course, simply because they have changed institutions, is likely to be inefficient and cost-inefficient practice.

Fourth, sharing scenarios between different centres is likely to be a good way of controlling costs and at the same time maintaining

quality. High-quality simulation scenarios are valuable but take time to develop, and so it is best to ensure that efforts in writing the simulation scenarios are spread as widely as possible.

Fifth, although mobile simulation is still in its infancy it has the potential to result in major savings (Kneebone et al. 2010). Mobile simulators are easily transported and can enable elements of immersive simulations to 'be provided within a lightweight, low-cost and self-contained setting, which is portable and can therefore be accessed by a wide range of clinicians' (Kneebone et al. 2010, p. 65). The cost of transporting the simulator to the health professionals is likely to be much lower than that of transporting the health professionals to the simulator.

Finally, medical educators are to get full the best possible return from their investment in simulation centres, then these centres should be open to learners as often and for as long as is feasible. Simulation rooms lying unused during working hours are unlikely to be delivering maximum return. There is an argument that simulation centres should be open outside of office hours (like a gym) to enable more usage.

Apart from this further research is needed. In simulation the facilitator:learner ratio is high but there is little research to show us the optimal facilitator:learner ratio—it may be that similar learning outcomes may be achieved with a lower ratio. The traditional apprenticeship model of medical training did not require simulation and its associated costs, but this model took time and was not always efficient. It may be that more use of simulation will enable shorter and more efficient training times—but this will remain speculation until the research is done. Much simulation is based on critical incidents or near misses that occurred in the learners' institution, and has as its specific outcome improved patient safety; if simulation does 'work' and improves patient safety, then the costs of simulation will be easily saved as a result of shorter hospital admissions, fewer readmissions, and less litigation. According to Ker et al. (2010, p. 68):

> although the evidence for effectiveness of simulation training in reducing such costs is not currently available, there is no other high reliability profession which has waited for such evidence before adopting simulation into training programmes because the cost of failure is simply too high.

E-learning: cost and value

E-learning is the use of electronic technology to enhance the education of healthcare professionals (Walsh and Dillner 2003) (fig. 51.2). According to Sandars (2010a, p. 41), the:

> 'traditional vision of e-learning is to provide multimedia educational content that can engage the learner. This content is assembled as training packages that can be offered to the learner using a wide variety of technology, from websites, podcasts, CD ROMs and a range of mobile devices, including Personal Digital Assistants (PDA's) and mobile phones.

However, web 2.0 technologies can also enable a wide variety of user-created content that can facilitate medical education—this can include blogs, wikis, and discussion fora (Sandars and Schroter 2007).

In a relatively short space of time an enormous quantity of medical education resources has been made available via the internet—the main challenge to the learners and their guides is to signpost content that is of high quality according to a number of agreed

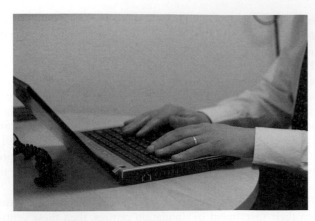

Figure 51.2 E-learning.

criteria. These criteria might be traditional ones: one how up-to-date or evidence based the content is; and also more modern ones that examine to what degree the online learning makes the most of the functionality enabled by the internet (such as interactivity and multimedia).

The costs of e-learning

The costs of e-learning in medical education can be divided into provider costs and learner costs.

The provider is the individual or institution that creates the online learning resource and makes it available. The costs depend on the degree of complexity in the resource and as such may be very high or very low. The cost of producing a short and simple text-based learning resource is likely to be a fraction of that of producing a simulation-based, immersive and interactive, multimedia programme (Johnson et al. 2006).

Regardless of the production costs there will also be the costs of hosting, updating, and maintaining the content, and providing site support and administration. As with any other educational intervention, there is the cost of curriculum development, content creation, assessment, and evaluation. E-learning content (whether commercial or not) is likely to require marketing resources to let learners know about it and it is as well to cost this from the outset.

The costs to the learner are commonly forgotten about completely. Both providers and learners may talk about learning resources being freely available on the internet, but of course they are not really free at all. Learners or the learners' institution will have to pay for hardware, software, internet connection (now almost ubiquitously broadband—in the Western world at least), and electricity, as well as libraries or computer-aided learning rooms where the learning can take place. All this will need to be rented or bought, but regardless of that, depreciation costs also need to be considered. There is also the learners' time that they spend on training when their day to day work will still have to be covered.

What makes for effective e-learning in medical education?

First of all, there is evidence that e-learning is effective compared to no intervention and the evidence is strongest for the outcomes of knowledge and skills, but less so for health professionals' improved performance (Cook et al. 2008). It is perhaps not surprising that any medical education intervention should be better than no intervention, and it also a sobering thought considering the massive enthusiasm for e-learning over the past decade.

According to Cook and McDonald (2008, p. 5), 'e-learning is a tool that, when designed appropriately, can be used to meet worthy educational goals' but it is questionable as to whether it represents 'a fundamental advance in educational methodology'. According to Sandars (2010a, p. 46) 'there has been little work that compares the effectiveness between different approaches of e-learning interventions'.

However, if e-learning is like most other educational methodologies, then what makes these methodologies work is also likely to make e-learning work. So ideally, for e-learning to be effective, it should be learner-centred, competency-based, and curriculum-driven and the content itself should be evidence-based, up to date, and comprehensive. Ultimately, it should deliver education that is consistent with the principles of adult learning theory (Zigmont et al. 2011).

How can e-learning add to the value proposition of medical education?

As with other forms of medical education, there are no systematic reviews on the cost effectiveness of e-learning in medical education. There are few original research studies in this field. Two studies give a positive account as to the cost effectiveness of videoconferencing in healthcare professional education (Allen et al. 2003; Miller et al. 2008). Another study has demonstrated increased applied knowledge, problem-solving skills, and self-reported improved practice amongst users of interactive, multimedia learning modules for a very low cost per user (Walsh et al. 2010). Outside of the field of healthcare, there is a multiplicity of reports of the cost effectiveness of e-learning interventions (Broadbent 2002). To what degree their conclusions can be extrapolated to medical education is subject to debate.

In the absence of definitive research findings, we are once again left to draw guidelines to maximize the cost effectiveness of e-learning from first principles.

One of the unique features of medical education is its scalability. Typically, for a fixed investment cost, an online learning resource can be made available to almost limitless numbers of learners at negligible extra cost (the more users, the higher the hosting costs but these increased costs are usually minimal) (fig. 51.3). Thus the more users of an e-learning resource, the lower the cost per individual learner. In order to enable high usage then sufficient attention should be paid to usability and accessibility of e-learning resources (Sandars 2010b).

Adequate thought should also be paid to marketing the e-learning resource. Marketing is often dismissed as something only relevant to commercial providers of e-learning but public providers would do well to learn lessons from their commercial counterparts.

As with simulation, it is important that the degree of functionality and sophistication of an online learning is only sufficient to achieve the planned learning outcomes—and no more. The cost of producing e-learning medical education resources often relates to the complexity of their instructional design and the degree of multimedia within them. If multimedia is used then it is well that it is used for its optimal purposes—there is little to be gained from multimedia presentations of experts giving short accounts to camera, when the same accounts could be given just as effectively and with less expense using text. When multimedia is used it is best for

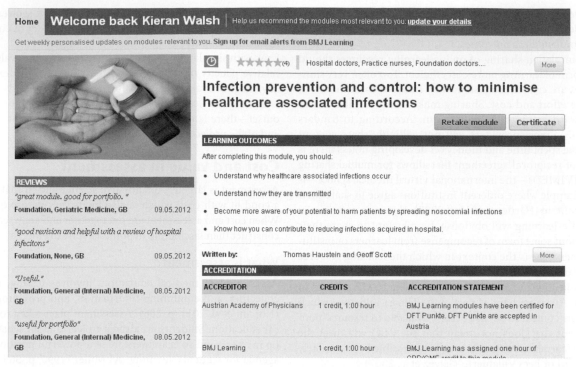

Figure 51.3 E-learning.
Reproduced with permission of BMJ Learning.

it to capture education that cannot be delivered in another way—so multimedia resources that feature filmed simulations aimed at changing behaviours, or that feature patients or carers adding conviction and humanity to the learning and enabling changed attitudes amongst learners, are more likely to represent money well spent (Walsh and Donnelly 2008).

Even then considered thought should be given to the format of the multimedia—audio is less expensive than video but can be very effective at achieving certain outcomes (Morant et al. 2009).

Web 2.0 is another case in point (Sandars and Haythornthwaite 2007). The costs of creating or using online programs that enable learners to discuss their learning needs with others in real-time or asynchronously are likely be minimal, but the outcomes in terms of learning may be significant: a learner may get a timely and accurate answer to the specific question that they have via this medium.

Point of care decision tools that enable a learner to get an immediate answer to their question as and when they need it are likely to be cost and time efficient as well. This just-in-time learning gives an immediate return to the learner—an additional benefit is that the learner gets an added reinforcement by hopefully putting the learning into action for the benefit of his or her patient without delay (Fiks 2011).

Another key feature of e-learning is its credentials as an easier and simpler method of distant learning. E-learning enables medical education providers to strike a line through the travel, accommodation, and subsistence costs of both learners and educators. Time of work should be shorter and classroom and print costs also saved by this mode of learning. All these statements are true and thus real savings can be made with e-learning initiatives, but only if providers make a decision to ensure that these advantages and savings are deliberately enabled. If e-learners have to travel to

a central learning point to do the learning, if learning resources are too enthusiastically printed out, if class rooms must be booked, then many potential savings will be lost. Perhaps one of the most efficient methods of e-learning is mobile learning—learning via an electronic mobile device (Desai et al. 2011). The strategic direction of e-learning development should encourage this mode of learning—rather than forcing e-learning to fit in with traditional methods of education.

If we are to make maximum use of e-learning then medical educators will need to ensure that it complements rather than reproduces or competes with education in other formats (such as face to face medical education). All too often educators hear anecdotal reports of learners being asked to complete a learning resource online on say the diagnosis chronic obstructive pulmonary disease (COPD) and then subsequently attending a lecture on the diagnosis of COPD. This is likely to represent poor use of inevitably limited resources—far better for the learners to study the subject beforehand online and then have a short face to face discussion with the peers and a tutor on continuing unanswered questions that they may have. Any new form of technology is disruptive and it is inevitable that it a time will come when it will replace old ways of doing things—foresight will result in an evolutionary rather than a revolutionary approach to change that results in truly blended learning solutions (Shaw et al. 2011).

A recent approach to further the efficiency and cost effectiveness of e-learning has been to use the interactivity of the online environment to personalize the learning experience to the needs of the learner. A study by Schroter et al. (2011, p. 35) showed that a diabetes needs assessment tool, that enabled learners to assess their learning needs online and then signalled what learning resources would help them meet their needs, was acceptable to learners and was effective and may have helped learners achieve their learning goals more quickly (Schroter et al. 2011). Further research is needed to confirm these outcomes.

As with simulation sharing of online learning resources should make this form of learning more cost efficient. Too often very similar resources are created from scratch by different institutions—at considerable effort and cost. Sharing makes sense but it is not as straightforward as might initially seem. According to Sandars (2010a, p. 45), 'most providers will not willingly share content that they have spent time and money on developing unless there is some form of reciprocal agreement that allows for mutual sharing of content'. IVIMEDs—the international virtual medical school—is one good example where different institutions agree to share their e-learning content (Harden and Hart 2002). However, commercial providers of e-learning will obviously be reluctant to share their content without some form of recompense from learners or institutions. Another issue is the context in which the learning resource is hosted or used. A reusable learning object (RLO) developed for GP trainees in England may be made available to GP trainees in sub-Saharan Africa perhaps as part of the Hinari initiative (which enables online content to be made freely available in resource-poor countries), but that does not mean that the RLO will meet the needs of the learner in Africa, or even be accessible by or remotely relevant to him or her (Villafuerte-Gálvez et al. 2007).

Another problem thrown up by the ever growing multiplicity of learning providers is lack of interoperability between different systems. So a learner may complete a learning resource that is captured on one portfolio hosting system but will be lost to them if that is not the portfolio that they normally use. The issue of interoperability between different portfolios is not straightforward either—for a learning resource to be hosted or recognized by different systems requires import–export functionality between the two systems that works seamlessly—it is no good a provider claiming that they can export learning resources if no one can import them. SCORM (Sharable Content Object Reference Model)—a system of standards in online learning—is one way of overcoming this, but it is a system with variable take up (Zary et al. 2009). Interoperability between systems would also overcome the commonly reported problem of doctors in training doing a learning module on, say fire safety, at the start of their training post in one hospital and then being required to do the same module 6 months later in a neighbouring hospital whether they have started a new post—simply because the different institutions' informational technology infrastructures fail to recognize each other.

Many healthcare institutions use e-learning to provide mandatory training for their staff—commonly as part of their induction and often on non-clinical topics such as better manual handling or safe handover. This enables institutions to track and record their staff's compliance with safety training and is likely to represent a cost efficient use of e-learning (Yassi et al. 2009).

Such learning may also deliver a return on investment to institutions: many insurance companies offer discounts on premiums to institutions that can prove that staff members have completed learning resources on problems that are a common reason for claims from these companies. The amount of such discounts may be greater than the cost of producing the online learning resource (Bleetman et al. 2011). In some cases the costs for medical education are transferred from the employing institution to the learner—for example, the learning may take place in the learner's home, on the learner's computer and during non-work time. However, learners often claim such hidden and often forgotten expenses from their study leave budgets and so the transfer of costs is likely to be only temporary.

As with simulation, this is a rich area for further evaluation. The relative paucity of studies makes it virtually virgin territory. The advantage of evaluating e-learning resources from this perspective is that the costs can usually be well-defined and captured from the outset—there is no excuse for not returning to these costs at the end of the project with evaluation in mind.

Cost and value in assessment

Assessment is largely a quantitative science and in that regard it is a good fit with cost, which is also by its very nature quantitative. When cost and assessment are put together and analysed as a single construct then fascinating hypotheses start to emerge.

What is assessment?

Assessment in medical education 'involves testing, measuring, collecting, and combining information, and providing feedback' (Norcini et al. 2011, p. 206). Assessment plays a key role in medical education. Students are driven to learn about what will come up in exams and so examiners are in a powerful position to set the agenda for students' learning. As Miller (1990, p. S63) succinctly put it 'assessment drives learning'.

What are the costs of assessment?

The costs of assessment vary widely depending on what is being assessed, what formats are being used to do the assessment, as well as who is being assessed, and who is doing the assessment.

The first two variables—what is being assessed and what formats are being used to do the assessment—are closely related. Broadly, assessment within medical education can and should measure applied knowledge, problem-solving skills, attitudes, and behaviours (or performance) (Crossley et al. 2002). To get what medical educators ultimately want to achieve—competent and safe healthcare professionals—then all of these are required (it is difficult to imagine an expert with a poor knowledge base).

Ideally, the format of the assessment should be a good fit with what is being assessed. So applied knowledge can often be assessed using a written or online text-based multiple choice exam (be the format single best answer or extended matching question). Behaviours, however, are best measured in the real-life setting or in environments that are as close to it as we can reproduce. So multi-source feedback from colleagues in the workplace are is one way of assessing behaviours of fully qualified healthcare professionals and objective structured clinical exams (OSCEs) are a way of assessing simulated behaviours amongst medical students (Norcini 2005a).

Many assessment methods will allow inferences to be drawn within a variety of different domains; an OSCE, for example, may measure applied knowledge and attitudes. These different domains of competence (and formats for assessing them) have resulted in a blossoming of a variety of different assessment tools. These include: written multiple choice questions, 360 degree appraisal tools, direct observation of procedural skills; there are simply too many to mention here.

They all bring with them different costs—for each individual method the costs will need to be worked out by doing the cost–value analysis. The costs of running an OSCE for example might include the costs of planning, facilities, materials, catering, real patients or actors, manikins, administrative staff, technical staff, collating and processing results, and training everyone involved (including the examiners and students).

However, regardless of the format of the assessment, two core costs will always have to be accounted for—these are the costs of the examiners and of the candidates. Their salaries, travel, accommodation, and subsistence will have to be paid for.

What makes for effective or accurate assessment?

Much progress has been made in defining criteria that make for best practice in assessment. Good assessment is assessment that is valid, reproducible, fair, feasible, acceptable, that has a positive effect of the overall educational experience and that has a catalytic effect on students' learning (van der Vleuten 1996).

High validity implies that there is clear evidence that shows that the inferences drawn from results of a test can be relied upon when the test is used for a particular purpose (that is, the test measures what it is supposed to measure). High reproducibility means that if a test were to be repeated under the same circumstances then the results of the test would be the same. Fairness or equivalence means that the same assessment will deliver roughly the same results when used on different groups of learners or at different times. Feasibility means that the test is practical—that it can be done within the educational institution. Acceptable means that the assessment and the inferences drawn from the results are credible amongst candidates and examiners. An example of a positive effect on the educational experience would be when an examination that encourages students to work hard to become safe, competent, and patient-centred healthcare professionals. A strong catalytic effect on students' learning results in an environment where the results of tests encourage appropriate learning that further drives up standards in a continuous virtual circle of quality improvement.

These criteria can be applied to any assessment but they can be given different weighting in different forms of assessment. So for example, a formative end of month examination on safe prescribing for medical students should encourage them to improve their prescribing skills, but the test itself need not have particularly high levels of reproducibility. Another important point is that best practice in assessment should not be viewed in isolation: an assessment may tick all the boxes but if it does not fit properly with the rest of the curriculum then it will not work. A curriculum may be reformed but if the assessment is not reformed along with the curriculum then the students will simply follow the old curriculum with a view to passing their exams (Newble 1998).

Finally, we should remember that assessment in medical education is highly domain specific; this means that performance on one test is by no means predictive of performance on other tests (Schuwirth et al. 2002).

How can we add to the value proposition of assessment within medical education?

As we have seen in the previous section a good assessment is valid, reproducible, fair, feasible, and acceptable, that has a positive effect of the overall educational experience, and that has a catalytic effect on students' learning.

Feasibility relates to how practical the test is, but of course feasibility is a relative concept. Feasibility is closely related to cost—ultimately most assessment methods will be feasible if there is sufficient funding (Walsh 2011a). So the value proposition in assessment can be seen as a balance between cost or feasibility on one side and all the other criteria of good assessment on the other. We can, for example, improve validity but it will likely drive up costs; conversely, we can try to save costs but this may affect reproducibility.

Schuwirth and van der Vleuten (2010, pp. 94–100) examine cost and value in assessment from the premise that we can improve the value of assessment by eliminating examples of cost inefficiencies in practice.

Examining validity balancing it against cost is a good place to start. With regards to validity, research has shown that what we test is more important than the format used in the assessment (Norman et al. 1996). Researchers in assessment have often developed increasingly complicated assessment methods that add considerably to the cost but only a small amount to the validity—as what is being tested is more important than the format. Doing a test in a high-fidelity simulation centre is a good example—it will certainly be expensive but may not necessarily add to validity (it depends on what is being assessed). Similarly, in written tests much work has been done comparing multiple choice questions (MCQs) to free text answer questions. If the different question types assess the same content, then the difference between the two will not be great; however, the cost of marking free text answer questions will be much greater, as MCQs can be machine-marked.

Improving the reproducibility of an assessment, although another important goal will have inevitable effects on costs. Once again there will be a balance between reproducibility and cost to be found and the challenge for assessors is to find the optimal balance point. In OSCEs many examining authorities specify that there should be two examiners per station; but the added benefit of having two examiners is in fact minimal (Van der Vleuten and Swanson 1990). Having two examiners, however, doubles the cost. As competence is domain specific it is likely that more gain will be had from adding more stations to an OSCE—as the sampling of competence that the candidate undergoes will be wider.

Sharing assessment questions between different institutions is another logical way to control costs. Constructing, reviewing, and standardizing questions for high-stakes summative examinations takes time and it can be difficult to motivate faculty to write such questions when there is much competition for their time and there is little academic kudos associated with question writing. Many institutions, however, do successfully share their questions (Muijtjens et al. 2008). For such sharing to work—a number of barriers have to be overcome: copyright and intellectual property may need to be ascertained to confirm that questions can be used outside of their originating institution, and the issue of context also needs to be addressed. A question that is relevant to students in one region or country may be completely irrelevant in another. Such questions can be localized, and it is generally easier and more time efficient to modify an existing question than to start with a blank sheet of paper. This collaborative approach to question production can obviously only work where there is a collaborative relationship between educational institutions or consortia of such institutions; competition between institutions is likely to render cooperation of this kind unworkable.

Intelligent use of sequential testing may be another way of improving the cost-effectiveness of examinations (Cookson et al. 2011). Cookson et al. (2011, pp. 741–747) looked at whether, in an OSCE, the performance in the first part of the exam could predict performance overall. They found that performance in the first stage was predictive of performance in the second stage and thus that significant savings could be made by sequential design. Sequential testing may also save on the costs of administrative staff required to run an exam and also may result in less wear and tear on equipment and less use of consumables (such as Venflons)—particularly in OSCEs (Walsh 2011b).

Schuwirth and van der Vleuten (2010, pp. 94–100) cite the issue of too many resit possibilities as another problem that can cause cost inefficiencies. Allowing a resit opportunity after a reasonable time period, in which the candidate who has failed the first sitting of the exam has had a chance to revise and remediate, is only fair. Re-sits by their very nature are only created for a small number of students (for example 5% of those who sat the first exam) and yet the cost of creating a written resit exam is largely the same as the cost of creating a written exam for a large number of students. Also, resits inevitably increase the likelihood of candidates passing by chance alone (much like clinical tests in medicine, the more tests that you do, the more likely you are to get a positive result). So limiting the number and frequency of resit opportunities should help control costs and reduce the possibility of candidates passing by chance.

Workplace-based assessment is a powerful tool to drive learning amongst junior doctors in training (Norcini and Burch 2007). However, a major issue with its implementation is its feasibility or cost. Both assessors and learners have to find time to do the assessments. There have been anecdotal reports that in some institutions the assessment becomes a simple tick box exercise, with nearly everyone passing. There needs to be more research to find out the optimal number and frequency of these assessments, which will balance cost with effectiveness.

For fully qualified family doctors or hospital specialists the focus of assessment shifts from assessment of knowledge and skills and observed simulated or actual behaviours to actual performance and clinical outcomes (Cohen and Rhydderch 2010). Here, much work needs to be to first develop effective assessments—before even thinking about cost-effective assessments. Assessments of the process of care and the outcomes of care are two basic ways to do this, but both are fraught with potential sources of error. Ensuring that adequate numbers of outcomes are assessed will improve reproducibility but will drive up costs—as will effective measures to adjust for case mix and confounding factors (Crossley and Davies 2005). Once again only pilot studies will find the optimal balance between cost or feasibility and the other criteria that make for good assessment.

The ideal assessment would score highly on all criteria but this would be prohibitively expensive and is simply not necessary for all types of assessments. Formative assessment, for example, should score highly on validity, on positive effects on candidates' studying and on a catalytic effect on education generally but reproducibility is less important. So the time and effort and ultimately cost that is spent on achieving high levels of reproducibility in formative assessment is likely to be wasteful; far better to spend the time and cost on developing formative assessment that will have a positive overall effect on education at the institution (Norcini et al. 2011).

Assessment of a doctor whose performance has given rise to concern has been the subject of much debate (Williams 2006). An assessment in this circumstance must be fair, valid, and reproducible—not least because a flawed assessment may give rise to a legal challenge. However, if the assessment can be used to measure a

doctor's performance and at the same time to enable more targeted remediation towards areas where the doctor needs to improve then the assessment should result in a more tailored and personalized intervention (that as a result may be less expensive). In this context the positive effect of the assessment on a doctor's learning is important and has the potential to speed up the remediation process and save costs. Although assessment in a doctor with performance difficulties and their subsequent remediation will have associated costs, these costs should also be considered in the context of the costs of not assessing doctors in difficulties or not attempting remediation. Not doing these things could result in catastrophic error, with resultant malpractice costs in a failing doctor continuing to practise, or the loss of many years of potentially good practice for a doctor with temporary and remediable difficulties. No form of assessment or education is cost efficient or cost inefficient in itself, but rather its cost and efficiency must be considered in the context of alternatives.

Similarly, in undergraduate medical education, assessment has the potential to have indirect but important effects on overall educational costs. One way to control costs in undergraduate medical education is to reduce the attrition rate of students. According to Finucane and McCrorie (2010, p. 11), 'between 5% and 15% of medical school entrants withdraw or are excluded from courses before graduation, at significant cost to the students, their medical schools and to society'.

Attrition rates will never reach zero (nor do we want them to) but the closer they get to 5% the smaller the loss to the students and the medical school. If students leave medical school in their first year, then the loss is fairly modest; but if they reach their last year or so and never qualify as a doctor then the loss will be significant. Students leave medicine for a variety of reasons: some change their minds about becoming doctors, some are expelled for unprofessional behaviour and some repeatedly fail their exams (O'Neill et al. 2011). If a student drops out after failing an invalid assessment, then it is a double tragedy and another strong reason to consider a range of factors when examining the cost and value of various forms of assessment.

Setting standards for assessments in medical education is another area of controversy, Setting standards can take considerable time and effort—all of which adds up in terms of cost (Norcini 2003; Cusimano 1996). As a consequence it is best that efforts to ensure that standards are credible (they can never be perfect) and are as efficient as possible. It is beyond the scope of this section to describe the different types of standards and the methods for arriving at them; however, a few specific points can be made. Relative standards are less used nowadays as the results that they deliver rely upon the performance of the particular cohort of candidates (which of course varies from sitting to sitting). In their defence, relative standards are quick and easy to arrive at and standard setters generally need little explanation or education on what they are supposed to do. However, many would argue nowadays that the balance between cost and outcomes is weighs against going for cheap and easy relative methods. Absolute standards are undoubtedly more time consuming and costly to develop but there are ways of streamlining their development. For example, applying the Angoff or Ebel methods to an OSCE could result in different standards being applied to all the items in a checklist at an individual OSCE station (Norcini 2005b). It is far more efficient to apply methods at the level of the station only. Regardless of the method used to create standards, the standard setters will have to meet and the cost of such meetings is likely to contribute to the majority of costs in standard setting. It is therefore best to ensure that the number of meetings is kept to a minimum, that only the minimum required number of standard setters is present and that everyone is briefed beforehand so that they know the exact task that they are being asked to carry out.

The next steps

Most studies of medical education rarely cite the costs of different medical education approaches or interventions. Considering the cost of medical education, this is a remarkable state of affairs. It is difficult to think of a pharmaceutical or medical device company bringing a new product or innovation to market without hard evidence of its effectiveness and cost effectiveness, and increasingly any return on investment that it may bring back into the health service. Any yet in medical education, innovations happen continually and are adopted widely without evidence of their cost effectiveness and sustainability (Walsh 2010b). Instead, we tend to see serial innovators who have moved on to their next innovation before proving the long-term value of the current task in hand (Sarason 1990).

There is also a tendency in the medical education research literature to publish only the results of successful projects or innovations. Only rarely in this literature do we read of new developments that failed to live up to initial expectations, or that simply failed. The medical research community has faced similar dilemmas for many years with many blaming the pharmaceutical industry for failing to adequately prove the cost-effectiveness of its new products or more seriously for suppressing the results of research that fail to show its product in a good light (Lexchin 2011).

Medical education researchers are unlikely to have similar financial conflicts of interest but not all conflicts of interest are financial in nature—occasionally researchers will have built their careers and reputations on certain hypotheses, which can ultimately become self-fulfilling. Perhaps a start could be made if innovators in medical education could commit to costing their innovations and publishing these costs when writing up the results of their evaluations. No method within medical education is cost effective in itself—rather it is only cost effective in comparison to what else is available. So researchers and editors and publishers should also commit to publishing the costs of innovations in the context of the cost of current best practice.

All these suggestions may seem frightening to certain medical educationalists who might foresee economists poring over spreadsheets of what is spent on education within their institutions and deciding what can be crossed through with a red pen. We should not be defensive in this regard—a cost-effective option does not necessarily equal a cheap option—in fact it may be that to get to an optimal balance of cost and outcomes we may have to spend more (Walsh 2010c).

Certainly, more research is needed into the cost and value of medical education (Calvert 2010). Randomized controlled trials of different educational interventions are one way to do such research; however, there are conflicting views on the usefulness of these types of trials within the medical education research paradigm (Baernstein et al. 2007; Norman 2003).

At present it is unclear to what degree current problems with randomized controlled trials of medical education research may be compounded by adding the extra factor of cost into the equation. Epidemiological studies, such as cohort studies, may be an alternative but these inevitably incur problems of case mix and confounding factors (Calvert 2010). The outcomes of prognostic modelling research may enable educational researchers to compare the outcomes of different approaches in medical education and following on from this the cost effectiveness of different approaches (Harrell et al. 1996; Moons et al. 2009). Regardless of the precise research models used, certain key principles will have to be taken into account. Prospective educational research involving undergraduate or postgraduate learners should not be undertaken without considering ethical review (Cate 2009).

In cost-effectiveness research there will be a danger that those students who receive perhaps the less expensive educational intervention may be at an educational disadvantage as a result. More seriously, their patients may also be at a disadvantage. There will also be a need for the medical educational research community to review the skills that they currently have and consider what additional skills they may need to learn or co-opt in order to do research in this area. Cost-effectiveness researchers from clinical medicine or health economists may be able to offer valuable insights into this emerging field.

To do such research properly then extra funding will be required—existing staff with their existing duties can only be stretched so far (Parry et al. 2008) There may, however, be conflicting forces that operate in funding environments for medical education that could fail to incentivize educators from taking up the results of research or a more cost-effective approach. An example might be graduate entry schemes for medical school (Charlton and Sihota 2011). In graduate entry students typically do a shorter course (lasting 4 years); this shorter course will be less expensive to students and society but universities may be reluctant to establish them as the savings will result in a loss of funding to the university (Finucane and McCrorie 2010).

A cost and value analysis of spend within a medical educational institution may conclude that the institution is under-spending and should spend more. Equally, it may conclude that the spend is correct but that more can be achieved with the spend. If costs do need to be contained, then it is best for medical educators to develop an evidence-based approach to cost containment—rather than have a non-evidence-based framework imposed upon them. What is least likely to work is an approach where educators say we need to continue to spend what we always have without clear justification of need. In a world where the cost of a graduate medical education varies more than 10-fold between certain countries, this approach is unlikely to be credible or sustainable (Walsh 2012). A vital first step in the process is to capture all the investments that are required to produce educational outputs (fig. 51.4).

Ultimately, convincing arguments as to the cost effectiveness of medical education and its potential to deliver return on investment should persuade payers to invest more rather than less in medical education (Walsh 2011c).

Conclusions

◆ Medical education is expensive.

◆ Great progress has been made in working out what is effective in medical education (even though clearly much work still needs to be done).

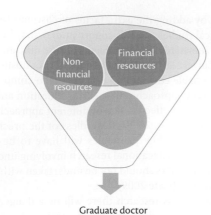

Figure 51.4 Capturing investments.

♦ There is little hard data on what might constitute cost effectiveness in medical education.

♦ Ideal forms of medical education will be low cost and high impact.

♦ Much research is needed before we will be able to say what these ideal forms of medical education will be.

References

Allen, M., Sargeant, J., Mann, K. et al. (2003) Videoconferencing for practice-based small-group continuing medical education: feasibility, acceptability, effectiveness, and cost. *J Contin Educ Health Prof*. 23(1): 38–47

Baernstein, A., Liss, H.K., Carney, P.A., and Elmore, J.G. (2007) Trends in study methods used in undergraduate medical education research, 1969–2007. *JAMA*. 298(9): 1038–1045

Banks, J. (1890) Preliminary medical education and the medical curriculum. *BMJ*. 2: 1213

Bleetman, A., Sanusi, S., Dale, T., and Brace, S. (2011) Human factors and error prevention in emergency medicine. *Emerg Med J*. 29(5): 389–393

Broadbent, B. (2002) *ABCs of E-Learning*. San Francisco, CA: Jossey-Bass/Pfeiffer

Calvert, M. (2010). Research into cost effectiveness in medical education. In: K. Walsh (ed.) *Cost Effectiveness in Medical Education*. Abingdon: Radcliffe, pp. 121–129

Cate, O. (2009) Why the ethics of medical education research differs from that of medical research. *Med Educ*. 7: 608–610

Charlton, R. and Sihota, J. (2011) Challenges & opportunities—graduate entry medicine (GEM). *Ir Med J*. 104(1): 25–26

Cohen, D. and Rhydderch, M. (2010) Making an objective assessment of a colleague's performance. *Clin Teach*. 7(3): 171–174

Cook, D.A. and McDonald, F.S. (2008) E-learning: is there anything special about the 'E'? *Perspect Biol Med*. 51(1): 5–21

Cook, D.A., Levinson, A.J., Garside, S., et al. (2008) Internet-based learning in the health professions: a meta-analysis. *JAMA*. 300(10): 1181–1196

Cookson, J., Crossley, J., Fagan, G., McKendree, J., and Mohsen, A. (2011) A final clinical examination using a sequential design to improve cost-effectiveness. *Med Educ*. 45(7): 741–747

Crossley, J. andDavies, H. (2005) Doctors' consultations with children and their parents: a model of competencies, outcomes and confounding influences. *Med Educ*. 39(8): 807–819

Crossley, J., Humphries, G., and Jolly, B. (2002) Assessing health professionals. *Med Educ*. 36: 800–804

Cusimano, M.D. (1996) Standard setting in medical education. *Acad Med*. 71(10 Suppl): S112–S120

Department of Health (2010) Liberating the NHS: developing the healthcare workforce. 20 December 2010. http://www.dh.gov.uk/en/Consultations/Liveconsultations/DH_122590 Accessed 13 March 2013

Desai, T., Christiano, C., and Ferris, M. (2011) Understanding the mobile internet to develop the next generation of online medical teaching tools. *J Am Med Inform Assoc*. 18(6): 875–878

Dieckmann, P., Rall, M., and Sadler, C. (2008) What competence do simulation instructors need? *Minerva Anaesthesiol*. 74: 277–281

Fiks, A.G. (2011) Designing computerized decision support that works for clinicians and families. *Curr Probl Pediatr Adolesc Health Care*. 41(3): 60–88

Finucane, P. and McCrorie, P. (2010) Cost-effective undergraduate medical education. In: K. Walsh (ed.) *Cost Effectiveness in Medical Education*(pp. 5–13). Abingdon: Radcliffe

Frenk, J., Chen, L., Bhutta, Z.A., et al. (2010) Health professionals for a new century: transforming education to strengthen health systems in an interdependent world. *Lancet*. 376(9756): 1923–1958

Harden, R.M. and Hart, I.R. (2002) An international virtual medical school (IVIMEDS): the future for medical education? *Med Teach*. 24(3): 261–267

Harrell, F.E., Lee, K.L., and Mark, D.B. (1996) Multivariable prognostic models: issues in developing models, evaluating assumptions and adequacy, and measuring and reducing errors. *Stat Med*. 15: 361–387

Issenberg, S.B., McGaghie, W.C., Petrusa, E.R., Gordon, D.L., and Scalese, R.J. (2005) Features and uses of high-fidelity medical simulations that lead to effective learning: a BEME systematic review. *Med Teach*. 27(1): 10–28

Johnson, J., Dutton, S., Briffa, E., and Black, D.C. (2006) Broadband learning for doctors. *BMJ*. 332(7555): 1403–1404

Ker, J., Hogg, G., and Mann, N. (2010). Cost effective simulation. In: K. Walsh (ed.) *Cost Effectiveness in Medical Education* (pp. 61–71). Abingdon: Radcliffe

Kneebone, R., Arora, S., King, D., et al. (2010) Distributed simulation—accessible immersive training. *Med Teach*. 32(1): 65–70

Lexchin, J. (2011) Those who have the gold make the evidence: how the pharmaceutical industry biases the outcomes of clinical trials of medications. *Sci Eng Ethics*.18(2): 247–261

Miller, G. (1990) The assessment of clinical skills/competence/performance. *Acad Med*. 65(9): S63–S67

Miller, P.A., Huijbregts, M., French, E., et al. (2008) Videoconferencing a stroke assessment training workshop: effectiveness, acceptability, and cost. *J Contin Educ Health Prof*. 28(4): 256–269

Moons, K.G.M., Royston, P., Vergouwe Y., Grobbee, D.E., and Altman, D.G. (2009) Prognosis and prognostic research: what, why, and how? *BMJ*. 338: b375

Morant, H., McDermott, C., Sivanathan, R., and Walsh, K. (2009) User response to audio (podcast) elearning modules. *Med Teach*. 31(11): 1041

Muijtjens, A.M.M., Schuwirth, L.W.T., Cohen-Schotanus, J., Thoben, A.J.N.M., and Van der Vleuten, C.P.M. (2008) Benchmarking by cross-institutional comparison of student achievement in a progress test. *Med Educ*.42(1): 82–88

Newble, D. (1998) Assessment. In: B. Jolly and L. Rees (eds) *Medical Education in the Millennium* (pp. 131–142). 1st edn. Oxford: Oxford University Press

Norcini, J. (2003) Setting standards on educational tests. *Med Educ*. 37(5): 464–469

Norcini, J. (2005a) Current perspectives in assessment: The assessment of performance at work. *Med Educ*. 39: 880–889

Norcini, J. (2005b) Standard setting. In: R. Harden and J. Dent (eds). *A Practical Guide for Medical Teachers* (pp. 293–301). London: Churchill Livingstone

Norcini, J. and Burch, V. (2007) Workplace-based assessment as an educational tool. *Med Teach*. 29: 855–871

Norcini, J., Anderson, B., Bollela, V., et al. (2011) Criteria for good assessment: Consensus statement and recommendations from the Ottawa 2010 Conference. *Med Teach*. 33: 206–214

Norman, G. (2003) RCT = results confounded and trivial: the perils of grand educational experiments. *Med Educ.* 37: 582–584

Norman, G., Swanson, D., and Case, S. (1996) Conceptual and methodology issues in studies comparing assessment formats, issues in comparing item formats. *Teach Learn Med.* 8(4): 208–216

O'Neill, L.D., Wallstedt, B., Eika, B., and Hartvigsen, J. (2011) Factors associated with dropout in medical education: a literature review. *Med Educ.* 45(5): 440–454

Ostergaard, H.T., Ostergaard, D., and Lippert, A. (2004) Implementation of team training in medical education in Denmark. *Qual Safety Health Care.* 13(S1): i91–i95

Parry, J., Mathers, J., Thomas, H., Lilford, R., Stevens, A., and Spurgeon, P. (2008) More students, less capacity? An assessment of the competing demands on academic medical staff. *Med Educ.* 42(12): 1155–1165

Sandars, J. (2010a). Cost effective e-learning. In: K. Walsh (ed.) *Cost Effectiveness in Medical Education* (pp. 40–47). Abingdon: Radcliffe

Sandars, J (2010b). The importance of usability testing to allow e-learning to reach its potential for medical education. *Educ Prim Care.* 21(1): 6–8

Sandars, J. and Haythornthwaite, C. (2007) New horizons in medical education: ecological and Web 2.0 perspectives. *Med Teach.* 29(4): 307–310

Sandars, J. and Schroter, S. (2007) Web 2.0 technologies for undergraduate and postgraduate medical education: an online survey. *Postgrad Med J.* 83(986): 759–762

Sarason, S.B. (1990) *The Predictable Failure of Educational Reform.* San Francisco, CA: Jossey-Bass

Schroter, S., Jenkins, R.D., Playle, R.A., et al. (2011) Evaluation of an online interactive Diabetes Needs Assessment Tool (DNAT) versus online self-directed learning: a randomised controlled trial. *BMC Med Educ.* 11: 35

Schuwirth, L. and van der Vleuten, C. (2010) Cost-effective assessment. In: K. Walsh (ed.) *Cost Effectiveness in Medical Education*, (pp. 94–100). Abingdon: Radcliffe

Schuwirth, L.W., Southgate, L., Page, G.G., et al. (2002) When enough is enough: a conceptual basis for fair and defensible practice performance assessment. *Med Educ.* 36(10): 925–930

Shaw, T., Long, A., Chopra, S., and Kerfoot, B.P. (2011) Impact on clinical behavior of face-to-face continuing medical education blended with online spaced education: a randomized controlled trial. *J Contin Educ Health Prof.* 31(2): 103–108

van der Vleuten, C. (1996) The assessment of professional competence: Developments, research and practical implications. *Adv Health Sci Educ.* 1: 41–67

Van der Vleuten, C.P.M. and Swanson, D. (1990) Assessment of clinical skills with standardized patients: State of the art. *Teach Learn Medic.* 2(2): 58–76

Villafuerte-Gálvez, J., Curioso, W.H., and Gayoso, O. (2007) Biomedical journals and global poverty: is HINARI a step backwards? *PLoS Med.* 4(6): e220

Walsh, K. (ed.) (2010a) *Cost Effectiveness in Medical Education.* Abingdon: Radcliffe

Walsh, K. (2010b) 'This thorough, tedious, expensive and disappointing study…'. *Med Educ.* 44(11): 1151

Walsh, K. (2010c). Cost effectiveness in medical education: conclusion and next steps. In: K. Walsh (ed.) *Cost Effectiveness in Medical Education* (pp. 130–134). Abingdon: Radcliffe

Walsh, K (2011a). Cost in assessment—important to examinees who are paying to sit and governments who are paying to set. *Med Teach.* 33(7): 592

Walsh, K (2011b). Sequential testing: costs and cost savings may be greater. *Med Educ.* 45(12): 1262

Walsh, K (2011c). Incremental cost benefit of an innovation. *Med Teach.* 33(8): 687

Walsh, K. (2012) Medical education: what the West could learn from Africa. *Med Educ.* 46(3): 336

Walsh, K. and Dillner, L. (2003) Launching BMJ Learning. *BMJ.* 327: 1064

Walsh, K. and Donnelly, A. (2008) Constructing a multimedia resource for managing Clostridium difficile: feedback on effectiveness. *Med Educ.* 42(11): 1119–1120

Walsh, K., Rutherford, A., Richardson, J., and Moore, P. (2010) NICE medical education modules: an analysis of cost-effectiveness. *Educ Prim Care.* 21(6): 396–398

Williams, B.W. (2006) The prevalence and special educational requirements of dyscompetent physicians. *J Contin Educ Health Prof.* 26(3): 173–191

Yassi, A., Bryce, E.A., Maultsaid, D., Lauscher, H.N., and Zhao, K. (2009) The impact of requiring completion of an online infection control course on health professionals' intentions to comply with infection control guidelines: A comparative study. *Can J Infect Dis Med Microbiol.* 20(1): 15–19

Zary, N., Hege, I., Heid, J., Woodham, L., Donkers, J., and Kononowicz, A.A. (2009) Enabling interoperability, accessibility and reusability of virtual patients across Europe—design and implementation. *Stud Health Technol Inform.* 150: 826–830

Zendejas, B., Wang, A.T., Brydges, R., Hamstra, S.J., and Cook, D.A. (2012). Cost: The missing outcome in simulation-based medical education research: A systematic review. *Surgery.* 153(2): 160–176

Zigmont, J.J., Kappus, L.J., and Sudikoff, S.N. (2011) Theoretical foundations of learning through simulation. *Semin Perinatol.* 35(2): 47–51

Further reading

Belfield, C.R. and Brown, C.A. (2002) How cost-effective are lectures? A review of the experimental evidence. In: H.M. Levin and P.J. McEwan (eds) *Cost-Effectiveness and Educational Policy.* AEFA Handbook. Larchmont NJ: Eye on Education

Brown, C.A., Belfield, C.R., and Field, S. (2001). A review of the cost-effectiveness of continuing professional development for the health professions. *BMJ.* 324: 652–655

Finucane, P., Shannon, W., and McGrath, D. (2009) The financial costs of delivering problem-based learning in a new, graduate-entry medical programme. *Med Educ.* 43: 594–598 (doi:10.1111/j.1365–2923.2009.03373.x)

Mansouri, M. and Lockyer, J. (2007) A meta-analysis of continuing medical education effectiveness. *J Contin Educ Health Prof.* 27(1): 6–15

PART 10

Research and scholarship

CHAPTER 52

Theoretical perspectives in medical education research

Jan Illing

Just as there is no one way to understand why, for instance, a culture has formed in a certain way, many lenses can be applied to a problem, each focusing on a different aspect of it. For example, to study doctor-nurse interactions on medical wards, various theories can provide insights into different aspects of hospital and ward cultures.

Reeves et al.

Introduction

The purpose of this chapter is to introduce the reader to the range of different theoretical perspectives (also called philosophical stances) that underlie the assumptions about the creation of knowledge from research (Guba and Lincoln 2005). Many researchers new to medical education who have medical training arrive in medical education research having been exposed to the scientific method and its *positivist* stance in relation to knowledge creation, and with little awareness of other theoretical perspectives. The problem that then can arise is that this worldview becomes the default position and is used to assess the quality of medical education research, sometimes inappropriately. Much concern has focused on whether it is appropriate to study the social world using the same methods and perspectives as are used in the natural sciences.

Science aims to explain phenomena by using methods and procedures that are repeatable, to generate conclusions that are predictive. Research that is able to predict or to make statements about populations on the basis of findings generalized from samples is considered to produce a superior form of knowledge and acquires status. In the past this approach was also considered appropriate and desirable for the study of the social world. However, from the 1970s the debate over the appropriateness of the scientific method for research in the social world has gained momentum. The methods used to study the objects of the natural world did not fit easily with the study focus of people in the social world. The debate gathered further momentum after Kuhn (1970) wrote about the need for a paradigm shift, recognizing the limitations of positivism. The development of differing theoretical perspectives signalled a move away from the acceptance of the scientific method and positivism as the ideal approach for research in the social world, other perspectives gained support. Guba and Lincoln (2005) discuss five main perspectives under the headings: positivist, post-positivist, constructivist, critical theory, and participatory action research (Guba and Lincoln, 2005).

Questions about the nature of reality and the researcher's access to it need to be read against the backdrop of dominant ideas of the time and how this has developed and changed from when the scientific method was first devised by Bacon.

Using research to discover truth

Learning about the natural and social world can be classified into three broad categories: experience, reasoning and research (Mouly 1978). The categories are not mutually exclusive—they overlap a great deal (fig. 52.1) Cohen et al. (2007). Research is a combination of both experience and reasoning and has been the most successful approach to the creation of knowledge.

Medical education research has absorbed a range of competing views of the social world from the positivist (and post-positivist) paradigm as well as from the new paradigms which include constructivism, critical theory, and participatory action research. The range of perspectives differs in the assumptions they make about social reality and researcher access to it.

Assumptions about social reality

Cohen et al. (2007 pp. 7–9) suggested that there are broadly two conceptions of social reality: objectivism and subjectivism. Objectivism assumes that social phenomena have an existence that is independent of social actors and subjectivism (also referred to as constructionism). Bryman (2008) asserts that social phenomena are subjective, individual, and changing.

Ontological assumptions

Ontological assumptions are concerned with the social phenomenon being examined and whether what is being studied is assumed to have an objective reality. These questions come from the philosophical nominalist-realist debate; nominalism considers the social world to be subjective and dependent on individual cognition, the realist view holds that objects have an independent existence outside that of the individual cognitions (Cohen et al. 2007).

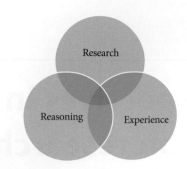

Figure 52.1 Learning about the natural and social world.
Data from Cohen, L., Manion, L. and Morrison, K. (2007) Research methods in education, Routledge, London.

Epistemological assumptions

Epistemological assumptions are concerned with the bases of knowledge, how knowledge is acquired, and its form and nature. Where the researcher positions him or herself in this debate influences how research and knowledge are identified. The answer to the epistemological question (the nature of the relationship between the researcher and what is to be known) is dependent on the answer to the ontological question. For example, if reality is assumed to be real (independent of any cognition), then what can be known about it can be independent of any relationship between the researcher and the subject of enquiry, and knowledge can be said to be objective and attempts to access it will be made as objectively as research methods allow—like in the natural sciences (this is the positivist perspective). Those who view reality as subjective, take the view that there are multiple perspectives and the researcher, and others involved in the research, may have a perspective that may or may not be shared with others. This type of knowledge is personal and unique and these researchers take an antipositivist stance.

Burrell and Morgan (1979) identify two further assumptions: first, *determinism* and *voluntarism*, which concerns human nature and the environment. The issue here is whether people respond predictably to their environment (determinism) or whether they have complete free will in producing their own environments (voluntarism). A researcher who views the social world (like the natural world) as having an external reality that is objective would attempt to use methods to control environments and remove bias in order to focus on the relationships under investigation. Second, Burrell and Morgan identified an assumption focused on procedures and methods designed to discover laws, termed *nomothetic*, as opposed to a focus on the subjective nature of the social world which uncovers individual cases and finds explanations, termed *idiographic*. This dichotomy is helpful in identifying and clarifying how different assumptions have implications for the type of study that is conducted.

Theoretic grand theories and explanatory middle-range theories

Theories are important in research as they set assumptions about the type of knowledge produced and the rational. Theoretical perspectives are also *grand theories* that operate at an abstract level. Grand theories do not direct the researcher in terms of how to collect data; they can be challenging and difficult to test with real data (Merton 1967). *Middle-range* theories fall between grand theories and the research data, and attempt to explain a limited aspect of social life. Middle-range theories, rather than grand theories, are more likely to guide research as middle-range theories are not as remote—they are closer to data observations (Bryman 2008).

Deductive and inductive theory

Deductive and inductive theory stem from deductive and inductive reasoning. Deductive reasoning is based on Aristotle's formal logic based on syllogism. This, at the most basic level, starts from a self-evident a priori premise, which is followed by a more minor premise, providing an example of the evidence and a conclusion. An example would be as follows: an a priori premise is that all flowers have petals; a minor premise would be that roses have petals; the conclusion would be that roses are therefore flowers. The logic moves from the general to the particular and the assumption underlying the syllogism is that a valid conclusion can result from a valid premise. The weakness of syllogisms is that they are limited as they do not relate to observation or to experience. Bacon was critical of deductive reasoning involving preconceived ideas which could bias the conclusions (Cohen et al. 2007). Bacon proposed inductive reasoning, involving the study of a number of different cases that would then lead to a hypothesis and later to a generalization. Mouly (1978) suggested Bacon's argument was that, if you collect sufficient data, relationships in the data would start to be apparent to an observant researcher. Bacon's inductive approach was later followed by a deductive–inductive approach where the researcher moves back and forth from the data to hypothesis and from hypothesis to implications (Cohen et al. 2007). This formed the basis of deductive and inductive theory. Deductive theory is the most common approach to examining the relationship between theory and research. In deductive theory the researcher starts from the point of what is already known, deriving hypotheses from it which then drive the research. Hypotheses are identified and tested using a specific research method and findings are then found to support, disprove or revise the theory. At this level theory is middle-range.

Inductive theory starts from the data and refers the research findings back to an established theory. An example here would be as follows: a study on medical graduate preparedness for practice reports a lack of preparedness to start work as a junior doctor in areas that are best learned on the job (e.g. managing time, managing workload, dealing with acute scenarios, prescribing, and managing paperwork). The medical graduates who were less prepared report insufficient opportunity to practice skills on-the-job. This finding of needing more training on-the-job feeds back into a body of work about apprenticeship learning and the importance of learning from doing in the workplace (Lave and Wenger 1991). Lave and Wenger's work highlighted the role of the novice in a peripheral but legitimate role, but as the role became more central the demands of the role moved from being merely an observer to one involving more participation in the tasks required as a doctor. Thus the research findings were referred back to an established theory.

Thus there are competing views about knowledge. The traditional (positivist) view holds that the social world is essentially the same as the world of the natural sciences and the researcher's focus should be on identifying patterns and rules that determine individual and social behaviour. This contrasts with the interpretative view that the social world requires a different approach as people act differently to molecules and in a more complex way.

Positivism

Positivism has been the dominant perspective in the natural sciences dating back to the Enlightenment in the eighteenth century.

Auguste Compte is considered to be the founder of positivism, although Francis Bacon was noted to use the scientific method in empirical science. Ludwig Wittenstein is credited with the *verification principle*, a central tenet of positivism that focuses on verifying statements using the *scientific method* to test them.

The term positivism is derived from the phrase 'something that is posited'—i.e. it is firmly grounded in science, rather than supposition. Compte's positivism seeks patterns, regular relations, facts, rules, and laws that are identified using the scientific methods of observation, experimentation, and comparison. Positivism approaches theory in both deductive and inductive ways. The purpose of theory is to generate hypotheses that can be tested. This will enable rules and laws to be supported, refuted or refined by further rounds of data collection and refinements of hypothesis.

The ontology of positivism is realism, where reality is assumed to exist and the aim is to explain the social world (as well as natural world) in terms of laws, often using cause and effect. Positivism shares two aspects of realism: a belief that there is a 'reality' that exists separately from our interpretation of it; and a belief that we can use the same types of approaches to access 'reality' as we do when studying the natural sciences. While this is comprehensible in the natural sciences (e.g. gravity will continue to operate without our knowledge of it) this belief in a 'true' reality in the social world becomes more complex when we have multiple players. Empirical realism asserts that by using appropriate research methods reality can be accessed and understood—often referred to as naive realism (Denzin and Lincoln 2005).

The epistemology of positivism is objectivism, maintaining that an objective view of the social world can be achieved. Positivism upholds the view that there are 'facts' that can be accurately collected about the social world which are independent of individual views. With good research methods researchers can access the facts without influencing and changing them.

Positivist methodology is often concerned with cause and effect; it is usually deductive; and it aims to be predictive. The approach frequently involves using a hypothesis to test a theory. Research design follows the scientific method to ensure that the bias and values of the researcher do not affect the data.

The scientific method involves a series of steps, which can result in the identifying of new problems to research (fig. 52.2).

The methods are reported in detail to enable other researchers to repeat the study and to show that the results can be replicated by others. The methods used are largely quantitative, involving experimental research design. Often the relationships examined are focused on cause and effect, achieved by focusing on specified variables in advance and anticipating and controlling unwanted effects from other variables often using a design such as randomization, which allocates subjects to one or more arms of a study. The randomization process assumes that differences between individuals are evenly distributed and are unlikely to be found in one arm of the study, so that any uncontrolled effects are dispersed.

Causation cannot be observed, but is inferred from repeated experiments reporting the same findings. The method aims to exclude all other possible causes. Statistics are used to control for

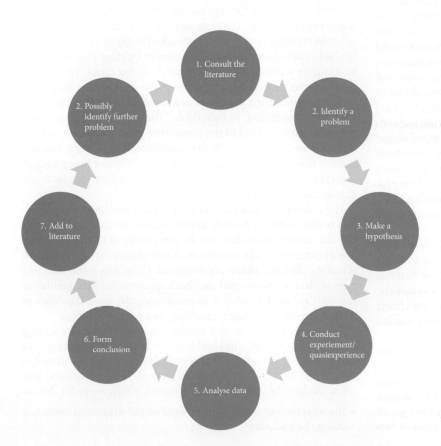

Figure 52.2 The scientific method.

Table 52.1 Criteria to assess the quality of research

Objectivity	The researcher or research design has not influenced findings
Internal validity	Findings fit well with reality
External validity	Findings are generalizable
Reliability	Findings are stable

unexpected events. The quality of research is assessed by the criteria shown in table 52.1.

The results are generally presented using statistics to illustrate that any differences are beyond mere chance and to draw inferences that extend beyond the sample studied to a larger but similar population. The use of statistics implies assumptions about the homogeneity of the population—that like is being compared with like.

Knowledge is generated by identifying facts that then lead to the development of rules or laws. New knowledge builds on old and by this process knowledge is increased and extended. Values are excluded by the epistemological position (the aim is to be objective and access uncontaminated value-free data). Values would need to be removed or controlled for to exclude any potential bias. Ethical concerns are something that is applied to the research, to ensure it meets the expected ethical standard (rather than ethics being internal to the study design). Research is a specialist activity conducted by experts with status. The aim is to understand how best to design a study that controls for unwanted confounding effects, leaving the outcome measure as pure as possible.

The strengths of positivist research lies in the control and limitation of variables and the ability to generalize from the study sample to a larger population of people—who are the same but who are not in the study. The questions answered by positivists are defined with a limited set of measurable outcomes. The research questions tend to focus on asking is A is better or more than B in a quantified manner, rather than seeking to understand the qualitative details of A and B in order to make recommendations for change.

Criticisms from other perspectives argue that scientific knowledge assumes a higher status on the basis that it is objective and accurate. Antipositivists also argue that the type of questions answered are limited and lack depth. Latterly, the word positivism has acquired negative connotations signifying criticism of the philosophy and associated methods (e.g. randomized controlled trials; RCTs) that are often viewed as superficial and inappropriate in the social world.

Evidence-based medicine is based almost exclusively on positivist research. The Cochrane reviews grade research on the methods used—qualitative methods are not featured. Even the best methods have to be re-screened for quality to be considered in a systematic review of literature. This process implies (even if it is not clearly stated) that knowledge that is produced using the scientific method is of a higher quality.

An example of a positivist philosophy in medical education research is a study by Warnecke et al. (2011). Warnecke et al. conducted an RCT to determine whether the practice of mindfulness reduced stress in medical students. The study used an RCT design. The difference between the intervention group and control group was measured on a validated stress scale. Statistical analysis was conducted to identify if the differences were greater than would be expected by chance. Conclusions refer to how the intervention could be used with the wider population of medical students.

Postpositivism

Post-positivism followed as a result of disillusionment with positivism. There was a realization that the scientific method was not perfect and that outputs were often theoretical, rather than observed, and that they provided only a perspective rather than a truth. In the natural sciences Heisenberg reported that the act of observing subatomic particles changed them, making it impossible to determine both their position and momentum. Popper (1902–1994) introduced the principle of *falsification*, putting the emphasis on attempting to falsify a theory rather than proving it was correct and recognizing that theories could never be proven, only disproven (Popper 1934).

In 1962 Kuhn (1922–1996) published a monograph in which he argued about the objectivity and value neutrality of the scientific method. He questioned the adequacy of the paradigm and called for a paradigm shift away from the way scientists viewed reality. Kuhn built on many of his ideas following the work of Fleck (Bryant and Charmaz 2007) who considered that facts did not exist independently in an external reality but instead were constructed by the scientists. Kuhn's argument highlighted that the narrow perspective of positivism could stifle innovation by viewing only certain types of knowledge as legitimate. Kuhn's work critiqued positivism and helped establish the postpositivist perspective which was less absolute and allowed for more uncertainty in seeking an approximation of truth rather than an absolute.

In addition, there was awareness that the researcher or research method could change the experimental effect. The Hawthorne effect is one example of this. The term was coined by Landsberger (1958) when he reported factory workers worked better as a result of being studied rather than due to the changes in lighting that were used to stimulate a change in productivity. A similar effect was the recognition that patients who are given a non-active tablet may show improvement in their condition as a result of belief that they have been given something to help them. 'The placebo effect' as it was termed is usually dated to the pioneering paper published in 1955 on 'The Powerful Placebo' by the anaesthesiologist Henry Beecher. Both of these examples illustrate how the process of being studied (observed) or being involved in research (intervention effect) can change the object under investigation.

The ontology of postpositivism is critical realism as it was felt that reality could not be truly known. Access to reality is imperfect due the human researcher and the complexity of the social world. The epistemology, like positivism, is still objectivist, as objectivity is still the ideal but claims are tempered. Collecting more than one type of data is encouraged and both quantitative and qualitative methods are used. Quality is assessed using the same standards as positivist research (validity, reliability, and generalizability).

Knowledge is built up in a similar way to positivism by adding new knowledge to old—like building new blocks upon existing ones and generating knowledge that is probably true. Post-positivism is less certain about accessing reality (compared to positivism) and acknowledges the difficulties in this regard, which are partly due to:

◆ the weakness of the human researcher (all aspects of influence cannot be excluded)

♦ the fact that all research methods are not perfect

♦ the fact that measuring what there is to be measured is imprecise.

Like positivism, the aim is to exclude values that are viewed as introducing bias from the researcher, who may value a particular viewpoint over another and thus change the data that is to be collected.

Although there is less certainty with postpositivism, the criticisms from other perspectives are similar; arguments abound about the objectivity and accuracy of study data and about the higher value placed on this type of research by journals.

An example of research conducted in the post-positive perspective is Durning et al. 2011. The study explored the influence of context on diagnostic and therapeutic clinical reasoning. The study does not report which grand theory was drawn on (common when drawing from the positivisms), data were analysed using the constant comparative approach from grounded theory, and attempts were made to generalize beyond the data to a model that would explain the influences on clinical reasoning.

Constructivism

Constructivism as described by Guba and Lincoln (1994) is a broad perspective embracing interpretative, phenomenological and hermeneutic frameworks (Crotty 2003; Denzin and Lincoln 2005; Schwandt 1994; Burr 2003).

Constructivism is the view that knowledge is not discovered but is socially constructed. The world and its objects have meaning that is created from the social world. It is argued that social realities are constructed (positivists also agree on this). However, where constructivists disagree with positivists is that they maintain that all meaningful reality is socially constructed. For example, a bench has a real existence, even if we do not perceive it as a bench and something we can sit on. According to constructivists the object exists but is only perceived as a bench when our consciousness recognizes it as a bench. The bench is constructed through our social and cultural life and informs us about how we see objects and the sense and meaning we give to them. Culture influences how we perceive objects—for example the exaggerated story that the Inuit perceive 50 different types of snow (in reality it is only about 12), provides nonetheless a useful example of how an important experience in daily life may change how an object (in this case snow) is perceived. The assumption here is that the ability to detect differences in the type of snow is culturally driven and serves a purpose in that culture. This is not shared in other cultures that experience snow infrequently. We learn about the natural world and social world throughout our lives and learn to interpret our experience in a combined way as part of the human world. Schwandt (1994) identifies a form of constructivism whereby the individual's own mind constructs meaning (perhaps like finding one's own meaning in abstract art) and another form of constructionism whereby the culture of the society the individual belongs to constructs the meaning.

The ontology of constructivism, the assumptions that are made about social reality, is relativism, meaning reality depends on individual perspectives, which all differ. People could therefore have differing sets of knowledge due to subjectivity, even when experiencing the same phenomena. Let us look at attending a scientific meeting and how this can be subjectively experienced. A student attends their first scientific meeting as a novice, and on hearing the plenary tries to relate it to what they have heard and assimilate it within their existing knowledge. As they are new to the field, much of the argument presented is accepted. An expert in the field listens attentively, notes the nuances in the plenary, checks this against their prior knowledge, asks for further clarification, and then ponders on how the plenary has revised their understanding of the subject. Both heard the same information but have different perspectives and interpretations on what was said. Both generate different meaning from the same information.

Constructions can change over time and become more informed, as in the progression from novice to expert, but the expert does not develop knowledge that is true, only more informed. This philosophical stance is quite different from the positivist and postpositivist, where there is still a basic view that at least a proximal truth can be achieved.

Research for the constructivist is about identifying more constructs. Returning to the previous example, this could be by gaining the conference delegates' views on the plenary. How it is understood, listened to and thought about, will depend on the individual receiving the information.

The epistemological question that asks about the theory of knowledge and its nature is 'how do I know what I know?' The answer is that reality is subjective. Unlike positivism, the researcher and object of study are assumed to be related. The knowledge created from the research is seen as a new construct created from the data, but also seen and filtered through the eyes of the researcher. Constructivists recognize the part the researcher plays in seeing what there is to be seen in the data, but seeing it from the perspective of the researcher. The positivists do their utmost to remove the bias that the researcher brings or at least diluting it so that it no longer reflects the perspective of one researcher. Guba and Lincoln (1989) suggest the enquiry method listens to the perspective of both the researcher and research object to form a new construction and the optimum process for this is via what is termed the 'hermeneutic–dialectic', which is a process of comparing and contrasting different constructions to achieve a consensus. Guba and Lincoln (1989) state that the researcher cannot and should not be separated from the research participant and that the aim is to achieve a reconstruction which includes the researcher in this process.

Quality is assessed using two sets of criteria. The first set is similar to those used to judge quality in positivist research and is grouped under the heading of *trustworthiness*, which Bryman (2008) reports as being made up of four components:

1. *Credibility* parallels internal validity; if there can be multiple accounts of social reality, does the account provided by the researcher have credibility and is it acceptable to others? To check that this is the case, researchers often present the analysis of their findings back to the study participants who then comment on the findings as being a fair reflection of the data or not, a process called *respondent validation*. Gaining another perspective can be achieved via *triangulation*. Triangulation involves using more than one method to collect data or more than one source of data; it is a method used to cross check data and also to gain more than one perspective.

2. *Transferability* parallels external validity, and is concerned with whether the findings can be used to help explain or understand something similar but in another context (positivists use the term generalizable).

3. *Dependability* parallels reliability, but Bryman, quoting the work of Guba and Lincoln, suggests they use it as a way of auditing the research process, such that another researcher could examine the research records of all phases of a study, to ensure that the proper procedures were followed. For example, by examining

   ♦ How the participants were recruited to the study

   ♦ The interview questions used

   ♦ How the analysis was conducted and the data was interpreted and

   ♦ Whether the conclusions drawn did come from the study data.

This auditing is rarely conducted, Bryman (2008 p. 379) noted that it would be a demanding task as qualitative researchers collect so much data (Belk et al. 1988).

4. *Conformability* parallels objectivity. While objectivity is not seen as realistic, *conformability* is an attempt to remove obvious researcher bias in the form of personal views that would influence and change the data collected (Bryman 2008).

In addition to the criteria of trustworthiness, Guba and Lincoln also proposed a second set of criteria that together make up authenticity. These are

   ♦ fairness (all voices are represented in the data collected)

   ♦ ontological authenticity (the research helps people to understand the environment that they are living in and influenced by)

   ♦ educative authenticity (the research leads to better understanding of others within their social setting)

   ♦ catalytic authenticity (the research provides a stimulus for action)

   ♦ tactical authenticity (the research empowers people to act).

Bryman comments that the second set of criteria have not been influential. The second set has some commonality with critical theory, and participatory research (which is concerned with empowering people to act).

Knowledge is built up from new constructions with the aim of a achieving a relative consensus. Multiple constructions can coexist and be of equal weight (e.g. supervisor and trainee views on a new intervention). Values have a central role. The role of the researcher is recognized in shaping the research and interpreting the findings and directions of the outputs. Like values, the role of ethics is built into the research and the researcher is expected to consider ethics throughout. As with critical theory, the expectation is that study participants are fully informed about the study prior to taking part. The researcher takes on the role of facilitator or sometimes participant. The researcher's task is to identify the constructs from the participants and produce new constructions from the data.

Constructivism holds the view that the social world is a social construction and we cannot go beyond constructions. As a result there are no objective or factual constructions, only subjective ones. This is in contrast to the positivists who aim to strip out the subjectivity with the experimental method.

For Pawson and Tilly (1997) the weakness of constructivism is its lack of ambition and hesitation in commenting beyond the sample studied—something which positivism aims to achieve. They quote from Guba and Lincoln: 'Evaluation data derived from constructivist inquiry have neither special status nor legitimation; they represent simply another construction to be taken into account in the move towards consensus' (Guba and Lincoln, (1989, p. 45) reported in Pawson and Tilly (1997, p. 21)). Pawson and Tilly report that many researchers would be disappointed to hear that they are presenting just another version, with no legitimacy and limited scope. 'Phenomena can be understood only within the context in which they are studied; findings from one context cannot be generalised to another; neither problems nor their solutions can be generalised from one setting to another' (Guba and Lincoln (1989, p. 45) reported in Pawson and Tilly (1997,p. 22)). Pawson and Tilly suggest that the pendulum has swung too far and constructivists have failed to recognize that many structures are similar from context to context. Stripping out the context so that findings can be generalized from one setting to another is an aim of positivist research, but not so with constructivist research, which describes the context and aims to provide the understanding from the findings.

An example of a study using the constructivist perspective is Ginsburg and Lingard (2011). The authors report on a qualitative study involving clinical decision-making in medical students. The methods involved 30 interviews and the findings were reported using constructivist grounded theory.

Critical theory

Critical theory is concerned with critiquing the social world and bringing about change. There are a range of perspectives that are associated with critical theory. Two of the main perspectives are feminist and Marxist perspectives, both are concerned with inequalities, which they seek to address. Areas which critical theorists have focused on include: gender, disability, sexuality, ethnicity, and social class.

Feminist research views science as incomplete and reflecting a male-dominated and distorted view of the social world. There are a range of feminist perspectives; Tong (1989) identifies seven forms:

> No short list could be exhaustive, but many, although by no means all, feminist theories are able to identify their approach as essentially liberal, Marxist, radical, psychoanalytic, socialist, existentialist, or postmodern.

> Tong, 1989, p. 1

There is agreement among feminist perspectives that women have been marginalized by society, and that this marginalization is reflected in research practice. Feminist perspectives maintain that there is a male view of science that is narrow and limits understanding of the social world. Positivism is seen as being linked to the male dominated view of science which aims to remove potential researcher influences. Similar to constructivist approaches, feminist ones maintain that researcher influence cannot be removed and that objectivity is not possible.

Marxist analysis identified that the industrial revolution did not bring equal benefits to all. Capitalism was seen to benefit the middle and upper classes but not the working classes. The Marxist perspective does not accept the status quo and seeks to challenge and bring about change in favour of weaker groups in society. Marx maintained that economic forces influence thinking and those with the economic power also hold the intellectual power. The ruling classes dominated with their ideas. For Marx the solution was for the weaker groups in society to revolt and emancipate themselves.

Kuper and Hodges (2011) highlight these issues in terms of medicine in the USA, where the rise of the medical profession was brought about through capitalist-derived wealth and resulted in the Flexner report (1910) that brought about the closure of all but the elite medical schools. Class issues remain a concern in medicine. In the UK, for example, medical training is dominated by the middle and upper social groups (Secretary of State for Education 2004).

The ontology of critical theory (the form and nature of reality) is historical realism. Reality is shaped over time by a society that reflects economic and political factors as well as gender, culture, and ethical issues, which have become 'set' and reflect a status quo. The epistemology of critical theory (the nature of the relationship between researcher and what is to be known) is transactional and subjectivist. The researchers, their values (and relevant others) link them to the object of the research. The knowledge produced by the research reflects the values of the researchers. The role of values is central to the research—they are key to shaping the research outputs. The aim is to empower the powerless and give them a voice that will be listened to by more powerful and dominant groups.

Methods require the researchers to identify a problem of inequality and to seek to change it through research. The knowledge created from critical theory is made up of historical and structural insights that transform over time. Change happens as new research provides more insight into the area of study. Generalizations are made when the social demographics and contexts are similar.

Ethical considerations are embedded into the research rather than being something that is applied externally to it. Critical theorists focus on being open with participants to ensure they are fully informed about the research.

The critical theorist researcher takes on the role of an intellectual who sees the inequality in a situation and seeks to redress it by informing others about the injustices and is seeking to facilitate change. The researchers and their values are driving the research—this is in contrast to the positivist aim, which is to remove the researchers from a position of influence. The researcher aims to make the participant more aware of power differentials or injustices and to initiate a change using the research. Researchers need to be aware of social issues and structures and uphold the values of empowerment and altruism.

Critical theory, like constructivism, is in conflict with positivism over whether objectivity can be achieved, and also the place of values in research. Clearly, values influence what research is seen as worthy of study in both perspectives, but critical theory aims to empower the weaker groups and bring change in this way. The positivists may want to address the issues of the powerless in a different way.

Critical theorists seek to understand and bring about social change by redressing the balance. Oliver (1998) highlights this conflict between positivism and critical theory:

> Health research about impairment and disability is dominated by positivist theories...[but]...disabled people are beginning to influence scientific research. This influence poses difficulties for positivist research in questioning one of its bedrocks: the notion of objectivity
>
> Oliver, 1998, p. 1446.

Oliver goes on to report on the bias in favour of funding for positivist research. Despite the Peckham report claiming that the NHS 'is attaching increasing importance to seeking out and acting upon the views of its users on the coverage and delivery of the services it provides' (Peckham 1995 cited in Oliver 1998, p. 1446), healthcare systems continue to spend the vast majority of their funding on positivist research.

The impact of critical theory has often been to raise awareness of a problem and support and empower a group to gain power and through campaigns to bring about improvements. In medical education this has been reflected in policies to support students from lower socioeconomic groups getting into medical school and in policies to ensure students with a disability or other 'protected characteristics' are not discriminated against (protected characteristics include age, disability, sex, gender reassignment, pregnancy and maternity, race, sexual orientation, religion or belief, and marriage and civil partnership status) (Equality Act 2010).

Participatory action research

Participatory action research (PAR) is action research that involves the participants as both subjects of the research and also as co-researchers. PAR is based on the work of Kurt Lewin who proposed that inferences about human behaviour are more likely to be valid if those participating in the research are involved in both developing and testing the research. The popularity of PAR is partly due to disappointment with the implementation of research findings. The lack of implementation of findings is partly due to the problem of researchers completing the research but then requiring another group to respond and implement the research findings. PAR involves the research participants as researchers as well as participants. Heron and Reason (1997) were responsible for PAR being added to Guba and Lincoln's (2005) list of the major paradigms.

The ontology of PAR is subjective-objective: participation forms the reality; experience informs understanding and meaning. The epistemology of PAR involves the participant in the knowing in four ways (see table 52.2).

Each form of knowing can be autonomous, but some forms of knowing are interdependent.

Heron and Reason (1997) argue PAR has two principles:

◆ that the research is grounded in the researcher's experiential knowledge, and

◆ that the research participants have a right to participate in research that is about them.

In this way both researchers and participants are coinvestigators and co-study participants. Knowledge is built up by involving the participants who are expected to implement the findings. The focus is on creating knowledge that is of relevance to an issue for the

Table 52.2 Involving the participant in the knowing in four ways

Experiential knowing	By direct feedback from living in and experiencing the social world
Presentational knowing	Via rehearsal processes and the creation of new practices as symbolized in art, dance, theatre, and writing
Propositional knowing	Knowing in conceptual terms that something is the case, e.g. factual knowledge or theoretical knowledge
Practical knowing	Knowing how to do something, knowledge in action

study participants (who will implement the findings). Values and ethics are embedded in the research and, as co-investigators; participants are fully informed about the study.

The PAR researcher is in the role of coinvestigator and facilitator of the research. The power balance is more equal and participants are experts in having knowledge about the problem and ideas about solutions that are likely to work. The PAR researcher works with the research participants who can also shape the direction of the research. This is in contrast to the positivist researcher who controls all aspects of the research design, data collection, and analysis and 'stands apart' from the participant in an attempt to be neutral and in order to avoid influencing data collection.

Heron and Reason (1997) argue that PAR is closer to critical theory than to constructivism as, like critical enquiry, it seeks to empower the study participant and achieve practical change by involving participants. The aim of constructivism is to seek understanding and build new constructions; PAR is committed to receiving input from the study participants who are committed to the outputs generated from the study.

Criticisms of PAR include concerns about the validity and reliability of the methods used (which are seen as subjective and biased). Other critiques comment on the lack of an end date for the research, which can have much iteration as is necessary until the issue is resolved.

An example of a study using PAR—was conducted by Tolhurst et al. (2012) to explore gender equality in health internationally. The study reports using a feminist participatory action research methodology. The authors reported working with over 200 participants from 15 countries. The study used seminars to debate issues. The authors report that the purpose of using PAR was to achieve social change.

Changes in perspective: the example of grounded theory

> Within the last decade, the borders and boundary lines between these paradigms and perspectives have begun to blur. As Lincoln and Guba observe the 'pedigrees' of various paradigms are themselves beginning to 'interbreed'.
>
> Denzin and Lincoln 2005, p. 184

In 2005 Guba and Lincoln reported a blurring of genres, in both perspectives and research methods. However, the philosophical assumptions about reality are not easily combined (Illing 2010) as their assumptions about reality and objectivity are in conflict. The positivists (and post-positivists) assume that there is a 'real' reality and that data collected about it can be objective. However, the antipositivists (constructivists, critical theorists, and participatory action researchers) assume that there is no 'real' reality but multiple realities and that access to these realities is subjective. These two positions are not easily combined; either there is a 'real' reality or there is not, and access to it cannot be both subjective and objective. Despite these conflicting positions boundaries have started to move. Two examples illustrate first how a methodology was moved from postpositivism into constructivism, and second how postpositivism and constructivism have been combined.

The first example focuses on grounded theory, which has become one of the most popular approaches in qualitative research (Glaser and Strauss 1967). Although qualitative research is generally considered to be located in a different perspective to quantitative research, the origins of grounded theory are within the postpositivist paradigm (Guba and Lincoln 1994; Glaser and Strauss 1967; Harris 2002). Grounded theory was developed by Glaser and Strauss (1967) as an inductive approach, building from the specific to the generic—largely without a priori assumptions (Bryant and Charmaz 2007). Haig (1995) criticized Glaser and Strauss for not raising awareness of potential problems with inductive theories, which generalize and form conclusions on what has been seen in the data without raising awareness of what could have been seen outside the data. Bryant and Charmaz (2007 p. 45) illustrate this point with an example about swans. A researcher counting swans may observe only white swans, the black ones having been present before the study started, or afterwards. The researcher is likely to conclude that all swans are white. There is no certainty that generalizing from observations provides a conclusion that is valid in a range of different circumstances.

Another approach is abductive reasoning, which Bryant and Charmaz explain(2007, p. 46):

> The logic of abductive [theory] entails studying individual cases inductively and discerning a surprising finding and then asking how theory could account for it. The researcher subsequently puts all these possible theories to test by gathering more data to ascertain the most plausible explanation. Abductive reasoning resides at the core of grounded theory logic: it links empirical observation with imaginative interpretation, but does so by seeking theoretical accountability through returning to the empirical world.

Glaser studied at Columbia University where he was trained in positivistic methodology and mid-range theory. He worked with Larzarsfeld and Merton and brought epistemological assumptions from positivism and postpositivism, treating qualitative data much like the analysis of variables in quantitative data (Bryant and Charmaz 2007). Strauss studied at the University of Chicago and brought symbolic interactionism to the partnership with Glaser. Strauss brought a focus on process and meaning to research following the influences of Blumer. Grounded theory emerged in the 1960s against a background of quantitative and postpositivism dominance. Qualitative research was clearly considered weaker, less scientific, and subjective. Grounded theory was an attempt to make the approach to qualitative study more systematic, transparent, and repeatable, thus matching the approaches and standards of quantitative research by using similar terms to justify its scientific approach. The process of constant comparison (each incident in the data was compared with other incidents for similarities and differences in order to classify data) was seen as a process that supported objective analysis of data. Grounded theory made some of the processes of analysing the data visible and repeatable, an important concept in quantitative approaches.

Against this backdrop Glaser and Strauss applied the criteria in use for postpositive quantitative studies, where objectivity was desirable, and access to a 'true' reality was thought possible although difficult, due to imperfect methods and the human researcher. The ontology was critical realism as reality could not be truly 'known'. The epistemology, like positivism is still objectivist.

Bryant and Charmaz (2007) identify that in Strauss's earlier work *Mirrors and Masks* (1959) Strauss was aware that people's perspective's shaped how they viewed objects, a view which emerged again in later work (Strauss and Corbin 1997). The writings of Berger and Luckmann (1966) and Garfinkel (1967) challenged the positivist perspective, arguing that people constructed their own realities. Bryant and Charmaz (2007) viewed the positivist stance as a weakness and repositioned grounded theory within social constructivism.

Postpositivism assumes that researchers can collect and analyse data objectively. Glaser and Strauss (1967) made strong truth claims, which put the researcher in the role of expert, without reflecting on the role of the researcher and how they construct and reconstruct reality by starting with their own personal perspective and understanding and then constructing a new meaning from the data collected. Glaser did not acknowledge that the researchers themselves brought their own lens to the collection and analysis of data by determining what is *seen* in the data. Glaser maintained that the important concepts would emerge from the researcher's analysis, but failed to recognize the role of the researcher in this by recognizing that the experience and personal perspective of the researcher will influence what is seen and understood in the data.

Changes in perspective: the example of *realistic evaluation*

Smith and Hodkinson (2005) discuss the combining of perspectives: the ontology of realism and the epistemology of constructivism.

The former (the ontology of realism) means that there is a real world out there independent of our interest in or knowledge of that world. The latter (the epistemology of constructivism) means that we can never know for sure whether we have depicted reality as it actually is. Although the line of argument varies, those who combine perspectives 'assert a belief in a real world independent of our knowledge while also making it clear that our knowledge of this metacognition is quite fallible' (Leary, 1884, p. 918 quoted in Smith and Hodkinson 2005, p. 918).

Pawson and Tilly (1997 p. 24) serve to illustrate this point having combined a realist ontology with pluralist epistemology: 'one can imagine the attractions of a perspective which combines the rigour of experimentation with the practical nous on policy making of the pragmatists, with the empathy for the views of the stakeholders of the constructivist'.

The thesis of Pawson and Tilly, termed realistic evaluation, focuses on identifying the context that an intervention occurs in and the mechanism or trigger that is employed to produce the desired outcome. This involves analysing the context in which an intervention does or does not produce the intended outcome and identifying what it is about the context that has led to the outcome. An example of this would be exploring the context in which an intervention on workplace bullying works and identifying that the intervention only works when the organization's leaders are involved and are supportive. The actual trigger to reducing bullying would depend on the intervention, but this could involve psychological changes in staff that lead to better self awareness of acceptable and unacceptable behaviours and to changes in behaviour that support staff wellbeing. This approach is rapidly gaining traction and has been used to conduct qualitative systematic reviews which aim to make generalizable findings from in-depth analysis of the themes and patterns within contexts and mechanisms that are necessary to achieve desired outcomes. This approach moves towards making generalizable statements. Pawson and Tilly argue that 'realism has sought to position itself as a model of scientific explanation which avoids the traditional epistemological poles of positivism

and relativism' (p. 55). They feel that 'realism's key feature is its stress on the mechanics of explanation, and its attempt to show that usage of such explanatory strategies can lead to a progressive body of scientific knowledge' (p. 55).

They argue that most social science experiments are *sucessionist* (e.g. that the explanation is linear, X educational intervention influences Y employment), but that experiments in the natural sciences follow *generative* logic (e.g. how things change, the action of a mechanism between X and Y that brings about the change). The latter offers more explanatory power when dealing with complex interventions such as those in the field of medical education.

Bhaskar (1989) describes critical realism and encourages the social scientist to uncover the structures that govern events:

> critical realism which I have expounded conceives the world as being structured, differentiated and changing. It is opposed to empiricism, pragmatism and idealism alike. Critical realists do not deny the reality of events and discourses; on the contrary, they insist upon them. But they hold that we will only be able to understand—and so change— the social world if we identify the structures at work that generate those events or discourses (p. 2).

Pawson and Tilly outline the need to uncover and identify patterns and structures from qualitative research and to use these patterns to generalize from one context to others. They emphasize the need to empower the qualitative research and constructivist perspectives to move beyond the local sample to making generalizations from the identified structures that are common to studies. For example, rather than focusing on the findings of a small study exploring the experiences of new doctors in their first post, realistic evaluation seeks to identify the contexts and structures of their work.

Different types of knowing

Different theoretical perspectives make different assumptions about reality and our access to it (fig. 52.3). Raising awareness of our own assumptions can be useful, as often these assumptions influence the way we do research; the role of the researcher; the values and ethics of research; and how we write about the knowledge produced. To illustrate how the different theoretical perspectives contribute a different kind of 'knowledge' and how each perspective influences the research that is conducted I will briefly exemplify how each

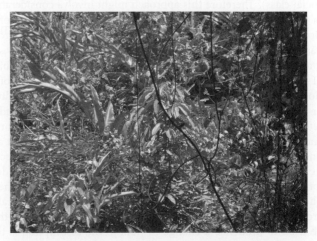

Figure 52.3 Fighting your way through the jungle of research perspectives!

theoretical perspective might approach a study about professionalism. Each perspective will have different assumptions about how to access data and how to use and understand the data that is collected.

The postpositivists (including any remaining positivists) might be concerned with identifying professionalism and might assume professionalism was something that could be measured by identifying its constructs (this assumes that professionalism is a real entity and that the researcher's influence about what it is and how it can be measured can be removed and made neutral). The professionalism measurements might be used to show that some people are more professional than others, and to identify people who might be predicted to be unprofessional in the future. The assumption is that people respond predictably and mechanistically to their environment (determinism) and the methodology will attempt to identify an objective reality, mainly using quantitative methods to identify rules or trends in the data (nomothetic approach) (Morgan 1979, in Cohen et al. 2007).

Constructivists might want to identify what a certain group perceived as professional and whether other individuals agreed (possibly taking different views from different grades and from differing medical specialties). The researchers might analyse the data and try to identify a new construct that would provide a deeper understanding about how people view and understand professionalism. The researcher would be aware that their own subjectivity, background and experience would influence what data was *seen*. Those who are familiar with issues of professionalism might think about the context, the development of professionalism and how it might change from novice to expert and from role to role and about the role of personal values. This awareness of *themes* might influence the questions asked and what is then *seen* in the data. The findings are the result of questions asked and answers received and then interpreted by the researcher who creates a new construction of professionalism. The assumption is that people have free will in responding to and producing their own environment (voluntarism)—unlike determinism (see earlier) where people are viewed more as the product of their environment. The methodology will seek to identify individual views and explanations rather than general views, and is more likely to use a qualitative approach (idiographic approach) (Cohen et al. 2007).

The critical theorist is concerned with critiquing the social world and bringing about change (areas critical theorists have focused on include: gender, disability, sexuality, ethnicity, and social class). Therefore this approach might involve consideration of who is valued more and who is perceived to be more professional. The approach might possibly argue that the dominant group has defined the concept of professionalism (the epistemology sets it apart from positivism, as the researcher has a link to the object of study). It is possible that one group may appear less professional. An example might be doctors trained in a different culture or older doctors (in the UK both groups are over-represented in referrals to the National Clinical Assessment Service for performance concerns (NCAS 2009)). The aim might be to highlight any unequal treatment, ensure equality of opportunity and access to relevant training to support the professionalism of these doctors, or to challenge the system that may be biased against them. The research starts with the intention of empowering the weaker group and through research highlights inequalities which can then be used to influence a change in policy. The assumption is that people respond predictably to their environment—in this case an environment of oppression from the dominant group (determinism). The methodology might seek to identify rules or trends that illustrate the limitations and restrictions imposed on these doctors. (nomothetic approach). By highlighting potential inequalities in the system, the research might seek to empower and bring about justice for the oppressed or weaker group. From the PAR perspective the researcher might work with a group of doctors to improve a particular problem associated with professionalism (ontology is subjective-objective, the participant forms the reality). The doctors will help to identify the problem and work with the researcher on the research (the participants have free will in responding to their environment—*voluntarism*). The solution might be personal to the group (idiographic), who keep working with the researcher until a satisfactory solution has been agreed and implemented.

In each of the examples cited earlier, the research is placed in a different position. The positivists try to remove researcher influence from the study to reduce bias. The other perspectives use the researcher in the role of facilitator to bring about a new understanding via the creation of new constructs, or to empower study participants to improve their position or support them reaching a solution to a problem. Each perspective contributes a different type of 'knowing' and asks different questions.

The examples described in this chapter highlight that each perspective creates a different type of knowledge and often this depends on the research question and purpose of the research. Researchers need to be aware of their assumptions, and what the consequences of those assumptions are for the interpretation of their findings.

Conclusions

This chapter has explored different theoretical perspectives that underlie the creation of knowledge:

- The positivist perspective assumes that there is an actual reality independent of our cognitions and that with careful research design access to it can be achieved. This perspective attempts to identify relationships between variables and where possible make predictive statements about a wider population than the one studied.

- Constructivists view the social world differently—they maintain that access to the social world is subjective and that there are multiple views and perspectives of reality. Constructivist research is interested in accessing these individual views. Unlike the positivist paradigm, there is more emphasis on the influence of the human researcher who cannot be removed or made neutral. Instead the researcher is acknowledged and used in the co-creation of new knowledge that is constructed from the meaning-making between the researcher and the data.

- Critical theorists start with a different purpose—they aim to bring about empowerment or justice for a weaker group, and use research to achieve this.

- Participatory action research involves participants in all stages of the research—this keeps the research relevant and focused on the needs of the study participants. The outcomes are ultimately more likely to be implemented by the study participants.

- Having an understanding of what each perspective is aiming to achieve can enhance understanding and appreciation of all types of research (rather than viewing one approach as superior to others).

Acknowledgements

I would like to thank Dr Bryan Burford, Dr Jane Margetts, and Mr Paul Crampton for their helpful comments and suggestions on this chapter.

References

Beecher, H.K. (1955) The powerful placebo. *JAMA*. 159: 1602–1606

Belk, R.W., Sherry, J.F., and Wallendorf, M. (1988) A naturalistic inquiry into buyer and seller behavior at a swap meet. *J Consumer Res*. 14: 449–470

Berger, P. and Luckmann, T. (1966) *The Social Construction of Reality: A Treatise in the Sociology of Knowledge*. New York: Anchor

Bhaskar, R.A., (1989) *Reclaiming Reality: A Critical Introduction to Contemporary Philosophy*. London: Verso

Bryant, A. and Charmaz, K. (2007) *The Sage Handbook of Grounded Theory*. London: Sage

Bryman, A. (2008) *Social Research Methods*. Oxford: Oxford University Press

Burr, V. (2003) *Social Constructionism*. Falmer: Routledge

Burrell, G. and Morgan, G. (1979) *Sociological Paradigms and Organisational Analysis*. London: Heinemann Educational

Cohen, L., Manion, L., and Morrison, K. (2007) *Research Methods in Education*. London: Routledge

Crotty, M. (2003) *The Foundations of Social Research: meaning and perspective in the research process*. London: Sage

Denzin, D.K. and Lincoln, Y.S. (2005) *Handbook of Qualitative Research*. 3rd edn. Thousand Oaks, CA: Sage

Durning, S., Artino, A.R., Pangaro, L., van der Vleuten, C.P., and Schuwirth, L. (2011) Context and clinical reasoning: understanding the perspective of the expert's voice. *Med Educ*. 45: 927–938

Equality Act (2010) The National Archives. [Online] http://www.legislation.gov.uk/ukpga/2010/15 Accessed 22 March 2013

Fleck, L. (1935) In T.J. Trenn and R.K. Merton (eds) *The Genesis and Development of a Scientific Fact*. Chicago: University of Chicago

Flexner, A. (1910) *Medical Education in the United States and Canada*. New York: The Carnegie Foundation

Garfinkel, H. (1967) *Studies in Ethnomethodology*. Englewood Cliffs, NJ: Prentice-Hall

Ginsburg, S. and Lingard, L. (2011) 'Is that normal?' Pre-clerkship students' approaches to professional dilemmas. *Med Educ*. 45: 362–371

Glaser, B. G., and Strauss, A. L. (1967) The discovery of grounded theory: Strategies for qualitative research. Chicago: Aldine.

Guba, E.G. and Lincoln, Y.S. (1994) Competing paradigms in qualitative research. In: In D. K. Denzin and Y. S. Lincoln (eds) *Handbook of Qualitative Research* (pp. 105–117). Thousand Oaks, CA: Sage

Guba, E. G., and Lincoln, Y. S. (2005) Paradigmatic controversies, contradictions, and emerging influences. In N.K. Denzin and Y.S. Lincoln (eds) The SAGE handbook of qualitative research. 3rd edn (pp. 191–215). Thousand Oaks, CA: Sage.

Guba, Y. and Lincoln, E. (1989) *Fourth Generation*. London: Sage

Haig, B.D. (1995) *Grounded Theory as Scientific Method*. Philosophy of Education. [Online] http://www.ed.uiuc.edu/EPS/PES-Yearbook/95_docs/haig.html

Harris I (2002) In: G.R. Norman, C. van der Vleuten, and D. Newble, (eds) *International Handbook of Research in Medical Education* (pp. 711–755). London: Kluwer Academic

Heron, J. and Reason, R. (1997) A participatory inquiry paradigm. *Qual Inq*. 3: 274–294

Illing, J. (2010) Thinking about research: frameworks, ethics and scholarship. In: T. Swanwick (ed.) *Understand Medical Education: evidence, theory and practice* (pp. 283–300). London: Wiley Blackwell

Kuhn, T.S. (1962) *The Structure of Scientific Revolutions*. Chicago, IL: University of Chicago Press

Kuhn, T.S. (1970) *The Structure of Scientific Revolutions*. 2nd edn. Chicago, IL: University of Chicago Press,.

Kuper, A. and Hodges, B. (2011) Medical education in an interprofessional context. In T. Dornan, K. Mann, A. Scherpbier, and J. Spencer (eds) *Medical Education: Theory and Practice* (pp. 39–50). Oxford: Churchill Livingstone Elsevier

Landsberger, H. A. (1958) *Hawthorne Revisited*. Ithaca: Cornell University

Lave, J. and Wenger, E. (1991) *Situated Learning. Legitimate Peripheral Participation*. Cambridge: University of Cambridge Press

Merton, R. (1967) *Social Theory and Social Structure*. New York: Free Press

Mouly, G.J. (1978) *Educational Research: The Art and Science of Investigation*. Boston, MA: Allyn & Bacon (cited in Cohen et al. 2007)

National Clinical Assessment Service (2009) *NCAS casework: the first eight years*. London: NPSA.

Oliver, M. (1998) Theories of disability in health practice and research. *BMJ*. 317: 1446–1449

Pawson, R. and Tilley, N. (1997) *Realistic Evaluation*. London: Sage Publications

Peckham, M. (1995) Foreword. In: *Consumers and research in the NHS*. Leeds: Department of Health

Popper, K. (1934) *The Logic of Scientific Discovery* (1992 edition). London: Routledge

Schwandt, T.A. (1994) Constructivist, interpretivist approaches to human inquiry. In D.K. Denzin and Y.S. Lincoln (eds) *Handbook of Qualitative Research* (pp. 118–137). Thousand Oaks, CA: Sage

Secretary of State for Education (2004) *Medical schools: delivering the doctors of the future*. London: Department for Education and Skills

Smith, J.K. and Hodkinson, P (2005) Relativism, criteria and politics. In N.K. Denzin and Y.S. Lincoln (eds) *The SAGE Handbook of Qualitative Research* (3rd edn, pp. 191–215). Thousand Oaks, CA: Sage

Strauss, A. (1959) *Mirrors and Masks*. New York: Free Press

Strauss, A. and Corbin, J.M. (1997) *Grounded Theory in Practice*. Thousand Oaks, CA: Sage

Tolhurst, R., Leach, B., Price, J., et al. (2012) Intersectionality and gender mainstreaming in international health: Using a feminist participatory action research process to analyse voices and debates from the global south and north. *Soc Sci Med*. 74: 1825–1832

Tong, R. (1995) *Feminist Thought: A Comprehensive Introduction*. London: Routledge

Warnecke, E., Quinn, S., Ogden, K., Towle, N., and Nelson, M. R. (2011) A randomised controlled trial of the effects of mindfulness practice on medical student stress levels. *Med Educ*. 45: 381–388

CHAPTER 53

Quantitative research methods in medical education

Tyrone Donnon

Rigorously designed research into the effectiveness
of education is needed to attract research funding, to
provide generalisable results, and to elevate the profile of
educational research within the medical profession

Linda Hutchinson

Reproduced from *British Medical Journal*, Hutchinson, L., 'Evaluating and
Researching the Effectiveness of Educational Interventions, 318, p. 1267,
Copyright 1999 , with permission from BMJ Publishing Group Ltd.

Introduction

Medical education research draws on a history of quantification
espoused by the physical sciences and more recently framed by
researchers in the education and psychological disciplines of the
late 19th and 20th centuries. A tradition of experimental research
design in education achieved a period of heightened interest in the
1920s with the work of psychologists such as Edward Thorndike.
The evolution of quantitative research in medical education stems
from researchers' interest in using a systematic empirical methodology to investigate and develop models, theories and hypotheses
related to educational phenomena. In particular, the use of measurements as a form of empirical observations and being able to
investigate relationships between variables using descriptive and
inferential statistics is central to quantitative research design.

In general, quantitative methods in medical education can be
grouped into one of two sets of research designs: (1) observational
studies that focus on describing the situation, and, (2) experimental studies that investigate the effects related to a manipulated variable commonly referred to as the educational intervention. Unlike
clinical research, where specific trials are used to study the influence of say medications in enhancing patient outcomes, the focus
of medical education experimental research is to study the influence of educational initiatives that might lead to improved learner
outcomes (and that may in turn have an influence on patient care—
even though this latter effect is notoriously difficult to prove).

Medical education researchers explore research problems from
a variety of approaches. As outlined by Norman (2002), since 1970
medical education has benefited from a more rigorous expectation of
evidence-based research that will inform practice. In a review of the
medical education research published in three journals during 2004–
2005, Todres et al. (2007) found that most of the research articles
used observational or survey designs (69%) and only a fraction used
experimental designs where participants were randomized into intervention and control groups (3%). The medical education community
has been challenged to expand the rigor and breadth of the studies
across the continuum of medical education (Whitcomb 2002).

The major issue faced by researchers, however, is that unlike
in clinical trials it is impossible to blind teachers and students
to the interventions provided, while at the same time expecting
participants not to educate themselves during the study period.
Correspondingly, most educational studies demonstrate statistically significant changes to participants' learning outcomes within
a specific research time period and contextual setting. However, in
most cases it is not reasonable to expect direct connections between
an educational intervention offered in medical school and what
physicians do in their actual practice—due to the long time frame
involved and the potential for physicians to be affected by a range
of different factors unrelated to their undergraduate education.

The use of disciplined, scientific inquiry to investigate medical education research questions is the hallmark of quantitative
research methods. The quantitative methodology includes elements of both deductive and inductive reasoning with the rigor of
experimental design to create a research approach to understanding what is viable and what has general implications for medical
education practice. An important feature of the scientific approach
to quantitative research design, however, is that the methods and
statistical analyses identified are expected to be described in reproducible detail—to allow for other researchers in the field to critique
and potentially verify findings through research of their own.

Clarifying the research question

In clarifying the medical education research question, the
researcher correspondingly defines the research design. As with
any research endeavour, the premise of the study should be situated

within a theoretical framework based on pre-existing literature and research. Although much current research in medical education is done on an ad hoc basis, generally research should be conducted in a sequential manner using a programmatic approach (Bordage 2007). Ultimately, the research question should be framed to reflect existing research and theory and delineated by the researcher to reflect how the present study will address a gap in our understanding of the topic in question.

Independent and dependent variables

In quantitative research, the variables of interest can be categorized into:

* *Independent variables* (IVs) that include general demographic characteristics of study participants (e.g. sex, age, year of programme) or the manipulated variable of interest (e.g. inquiry-based learning, virtual reality trainers) and

* *Dependent variables* (DVs) that provide the researcher with measures of change to participants' learning outcomes as a result of a medical education intervention. These dependent measures can be provided by the participant in the form of test scores on written exams or through the completion of self-reported surveys or questionnaires. Alternatively, observation of participants' behaviours or performances can be obtained from examiners.

The results obtained on the DV are, in essence, 'dependent' on the manipulated or IV of interest. For example, a participant's 'deep' approach to learning (DV) may be dependent on an inquiry-based programme (IV) that promotes students' motivation to learn (Donnon and Hecker 2008).

In the process of identifying the DVs and IVs, it is important that the researcher can provide a clear or operational definition of each of the variables of interest. Although the use of the variable 'sex' to define whether a participant is either a man or woman is obvious, the clarification of DVs (e.g. a 50 item multiple choice question (MCQ) exam used to assess diagnostic and clinical reasoning skills) or IVs (e.g. use of case-based learning) will be expected to be explicit and to allow others to duplicate findings in subsequent research.

Instrumentation: importance of reliability and validity in educational measurement

The success of any research project is based, in part, on the quality of the dependent measures used to assess the independent variable of interest (educational intervention). A researcher's ability to demonstrate the benefits of any medical education intervention will be influenced greatly by the quality of the measures or instruments used (fig. 53.1). There are two principal psychometric characteristics necessary for any quantitative research design:

* reliability—a measure of the consistency of the responses or performance assessed and

* validity—an interpretation of a measure that supports the evidence and theoretical constructs being assessed.

Reliability

The most commonly reported estimate of reliability reported in medical education research is the internal consistency of a single measurement instrument administered to a sample of participants on any one occasion (Hopkins 1998). In general, an internal consistency coefficient of the measure such as Cronbach's alpha (α) is reported that can range from no reliability ($\alpha = 0.00$) to perfect reliability ($\alpha = 1.00$). The reliability of an instrument reflects how well the items measure the constructs of interest (e.g. knowledge, skills, or attitudes) consistently from person to person. For example, a reliable instrument is able to differentiate consistently between participants' abilities in diagnosis, investigation and management—across items or performance assessments (thereby reducing errors in measurement). In terms of accuracy, the greater the reliability coefficient the smaller the standard error of measurement and the closer the instrument or assessment tool approaches a person's true score on each of these clinical domain measures.

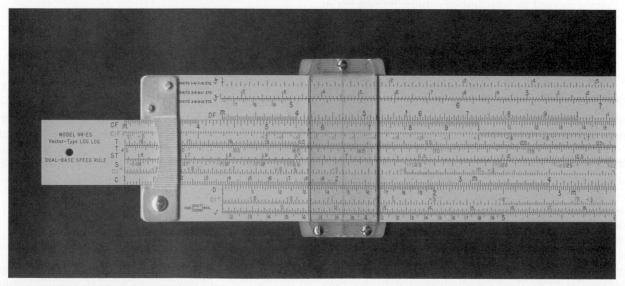

Figure 53.1 Assessment instruments used must be precise.
Reproduced with permission from Eric Marcotte, PhD (www.sliderule.ca).

Validity

The quality of any instrument or assessment tool used in medical education research is also based on the validity of the constructs or domains being measured. For example, an instrument may be found to have high reliability, in that it measures differences consistently between persons' knowledge of the basic sciences, but may not be relevant to a study that has a primary focus on differentiating between participants' clinical-reasoning skills. There are three types of validity that should be considered in the selection of measurements in medical education research: content, criterion and construct validity.

Content validity refers to the degree that the measures used have sampled representatively from the construct or domain of interest. This type of validity is typically outlined in a table of specifications or blueprint.

Criterion-related validity is used in research designs when an instrument is evaluated in comparison with another standard criterion measure. In predictive validity studies, the scores on a measure are compared in reference to a future assessment on a related criterion variable of interest. Similarly, the concurrent validity of an instrument can be compared within a study to another standard criterion measure either immediately or relatively close to the same time. In both predictive and concurrent validity analyses, the strength of the relationship between the dependent measures and the criterion scores are usually reported using correlation coefficients.

Construct validity is based on understanding a collection of related behaviors that are associated in a meaningful or theoretical way to the measure of a construct. Convergent validity examines the degree to which the construct is similar to (converges on) other conceptualizations that it theoretically should be similar to. Divergent (discriminant) validity examines the degree to which the construct is not similar to (diverges from) other conceptualizations that it theoretically should not be similar to.

Observational research designs

The observational research design is commonly use in quantitative studies that are focused on investigating existing phenomena in medical education. They can be categorized into one of three study design groups:

- survey
- correlational and
- causal-comparative.

As illustrated in table 53.1, there are a variety of research design derivations that can be generated within each group.

Survey research designs

Surveys in quantitative research are primarily focused on the collection of descriptive data from a group of individuals about their perceptions of and attitudes to variables of interest. The purpose of this approach is to collect information about the current state of affairs in relation to the research question. There are two general categories of survey research design where participants agree to: (1) complete a questionnaire or (2) answer questions posed in an interview (Fowler 2009). There are advantages and disadvantages to both methods. Unlike interviews, the purpose of a survey is to produce statistics or quantitative descriptions that reflect the perceptions of the population being studied.

As in any research design, the participants in a study define a sample taken from a much larger population of individuals that by definition have similar personal (e.g. sex, age, ethnic background) or educational (e.g. 2nd year medical students) characteristics. For example, a sample of participants selected from one medical school may be representative of students from other schools thus allowing the findings to be generalized. There are some survey research designs that look for changes in variables over time.

In medical education, many survey research designs look for changes in students' learning outcomes after an educational event has occurred. The introduction of a new curriculum or approach to teaching may result in changes in survey responses. Surveys may also help inform how various components of a curriculum are perceived by students. For example, a study might look at the reasons why medical students may or may not select a rural clerkship placement. It might be helpful for the medical school to know that medical students are less concerned about the clinical experiences they will receive than about the practical implications of relocating to a rural community (Donnon et al. 2009).

Correlation research designs

Correlation research focuses on the direction and degree of relationships between two (or more) variables of interest (based on observations of existing conditions). Similar to survey research, in that the researcher establishes a process for the collection of data, correlation studies tend to focus on determining if there is a positive (or negative) relationship between variables and to what degree can we quantify this association (Gay et al. 2009). The most commonly used statistical test used to measure the relationship between two variables is known as the Pearson product moment correlation coefficient (r) or simply the correlation coefficient. The value of a correlation coefficient can vary from $r = +1.00$ (indicating a perfect and positive or direct relationship between the two variables) to $r = -1.00$ (indicating a perfect, but negative or indirect relationship). In general, there tends to be modest relationships between quantifiable variables in education, such as students' scores on achievement, competency and performance tests.

The primary purpose of correlation research is to investigate the relationship between quantifiable variables—either concurrently or predictively. In a study of the admission criteria used for medical school, for example, we determined that applicants' undergraduate grade point average (uGPA) correlated significantly with the physical and biological sciences subtests on the Medical College Admission Test (MCAT) at $r = 0.31$ and 0.24 ($p < 0.01$), respectively (Donnon and Violato 2006). Once into medical school, however, we found that students' initial uGPA was a better predictor of how they would perform on their academic achievement tests in the first ($r = 0.43$, $p < 0.01$) and second ($r = 0.38$, $p < 0.01$) preclinical years.

In correlation design studies there should be a rationale for the relationships between concurrent or predicted variables that are founded on observed experiences or more typically, existing research or theoretical frameworks.

Causal-comparative research designs

In causal-comparative research design, the researcher focuses on being able to make comparisons between groups on dependent measures (e.g. applied knowledge) that show that the IV of interest

Table 53.1 Observational research designs and internal validity concerns

Research Designs	Existing population	Independent variable	Independent variable of interest	Dependent variable(s)	Statistics reported	Internal validity concerns — Historical changes	Participant growth	Pretesting	Measurements Used	Regression to mean	Sample discrepancy	participant attrition	Internal Interactions
Survey													
Sample survey	A					–	–	0	0	0	0	–	0
Follow-up surveys	A					–	–	–	–	–	(+)	+	(+)
Correlational													
Relationship between variables	A					–	–	(+)	(+)	(+)	(+)	–	(+)
Predictive relationship	A					–	–	–	–	–	(+)	+	(+)
Causal-comparative													
Retrospective causal-comparative (cause ← effect)	A B					–	–	–	+	–	–	–	–
Prospective causal-comparative (cause → effect)	A B					–	–	–	+	–	(+)	+	–

Symbols: = Independent variable of interest

= Bar chart frequencies

= Analysis of variance between groups

= Dependent variable measure

= Correlation between variables

Internal validity concerns: – = Factor not controlled for

+ = Factor controlled for

( ) = Factor controlled for, as not relevant

(e.g. educational initiative) makes a difference. The research design in causal-comparative research focuses on determining the cause or variable that might explain differences between groups of students after the fact or *ex post facto*. In essence, the effect of the educational phenomenon the researcher has observed and the potential cause for it has already occurred. Although cause–effect comparisons may be explored following this type of study, without control of the independent variables that is provided in experimental research studies, conclusions drawn will be open to debate.

For example, a medical education researcher may observe that students at one medical school tend to perform better in their clinical years than a similar group of students from another medical school at the same hospital. The researcher may hypothesize that the reason for the different results is the different clinical skills education provided at the students' medical schools. Although a retrospective research design in causal-comparative studies (a cause is investigated after an effect is identified) is the most common approach used by researchers, the prospective causal-comparative design allows the researcher to investigate if a potential cause results in a subsequent effect (this tends, however, to take much more time and effort).

Experimental research designs

Experimental research designs allow the researcher to test hypotheses by investigating the cause and effect relationship between variables. An experimental study in medical education, however, is different from an observation study in one crucial way: the researcher is actively involved in the provision of the educational intervention or experimental variable (the independent variable thought to make a difference to participants' learning outcomes).

In most types of medical education research, the manipulated or intervention variable is related to one of the following:

♦ curriculum (e.g. implementing a problem-based curriculum)

♦ teaching (e.g. investigating the use of small group teaching) or

♦ assessment (e.g. introducing an objective structured clinical exam (OSCE) format to test both clinical and nonclinical skill development).

Although there can be more than one independent variable, for simplicity we will focus our discussion on medical education experimental studies that examine a single manipulated or IV. In addition, the research design classically described as the randomized controlled trial (RCT) will not be referred to further—as this form of research works well in clinical research but not so well in educational research (Hill 1952). Pure RCT research designs are impractical in medical education research (for example both the teacher and learner know the type of intervention they are receiving, and preventing individuals from educating themselves during the study is not realistic). Therefore, in this chapter where the emphasis is on enhancing the educational components related to curriculum, teaching, and assessment the term experimental research designs is used.

Threats to internal and external validity

As with any type of research, there are both internal and external factors that have the potential to influence the validity of the

research findings in experimental research. The more rigorous the research design used to investigate the effectiveness of interventions however, the more likely it is that the researcher can control for confounding factors. The internal validity of an experimental study is based on the ability of the researcher to demonstrate that the results in the dependent measures are modified only by the independent variable introduced to the participants. The external validity of the study refers to the extent to which the findings of the experiment can be generalized to other persons and contexts.

Based on the work of Campbell and Stanley (1963), the following descriptions of the potential risks to internal validity in experimental research designs are provided (see fig. 53.2):

1. *Historical changes*: During the intervention or before critical testing periods, unexpected events may influence the DVs of interest. Although associated with studies that have lengthy interventions or long times between testing periods, sudden events such as healthcare labour disputes or financial cuts to educational programmes can have a detrimental effect on participants. In general, this can be controlled for if a control group that experiences the same historical or unexpected events is used in the research design.

2. *Participant growth*: During the intervention or before critical testing periods, participants become more informed, experienced, or motivated to learn. Commonly associated with studies that have lengthy interventions or time between testing periods, participants in educational research cannot be asked to restrain from becoming more educated about topics of interest. In most cases, participant growth can be controlled for if a comparison or control group is used and, in very long studies, if regular testing is incorporated into the research design.

3. *Pretesting influences*: In some research designs, the use of a pretest may have an influence on participants' expectations for an educational intervention and may thus prepare them for the post-test to follow. Sensitizing participants to the anticipated content has the potential to inflate the effectiveness of an educational intervention in that it allows them to think a priori

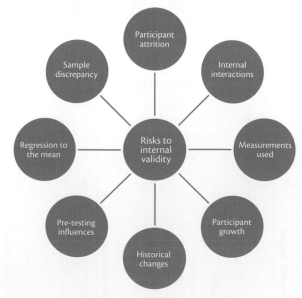

Figure 53.2 Risks to internal validity in experimental research design.

about (and act upon) their pre-existing knowledge, skills and attitudes. Pretesting risks to internal validity can be controlled for if a comparison or control group receives the same pre-/post-testing protocols.

4. *Measurements used*: Unreliable or invalid instruments or alterations in the pre- and post-testing instruments used result in the inability to measure desired changes in the participants' learning. While the internal consistency or reliability of the measures used is important, the validity of the measures is essential if the researcher is going to be able to draw conclusions about the effectiveness of the educational intervention. When possible it is preferable to use existing measures or instruments that have been shown to have strong psychometric characteristics when tested with similar participants and in comparable contextual settings. The development of new measures may be required if none are available for the purposes of a study, but the quality of the findings will be dependent on how well the measures assess the anticipated educational benefits of the intervention.

5. *Regression to the mean*: Participants who perform extremely well or badly on pretests tend to regress to the mean on subsequent testing. Regression to the mean may be controlled for if the participants are randomized to an intervention or control group, or matched with individuals in a comparison group.

6. *Sample discrepancy*: When participants in the intervention and control groups have different characteristics, discrepancies on key measurement variables may result. This can be most problematic when the researcher needs to select from existing groups in different classrooms or from a previous programme year or even from students in another institution. When randomization is not possible, it is important for the researcher to take into consideration the characteristics of the participants (e.g. sex, age, year of programme, ability levels) to allow for matching with a selected non-intervention group, to ensure that valid comparisons can be made between groups.

7. *Participant attrition*: Participants may decide to leave the study, altering the total numbers in the intervention or control groups. This occurs most commonly in the intervention group when the participant's motivation wanes or the effort to continue infringes on other commitments. Although it is important to collect the demographic information of participants when using any type of research design, in studies that have high attrition rates the researcher should be able to identify if there are certain characteristics of participants who drop out of the study.

8. *Internal interactions*: Combined effects of sample discrepancies with historical changes, pre-testing with interventions, attrition with participant growth, and the other concerns to internal validity previously discussed may lead to uninterpretable findings and invalid results. Therefore, the more rigorous the experimental research design used the less likely each of the internal validity concerns will influence the researcher's ability to make reliable and valid inferences about the results of the medical education intervention.

Problems with external validity in experimental studies may limit researchers' ability to generalize their findings to other groups (population validity) and contextual settings (ecological validity). Bracht and Glass (1968) described these sources of invalidity as 'generalizability limitations'. For example, pretesting itself may influence the participants in ways that may restrict how an intervention works with other groups that are not pretested. The researcher also needs to be aware of any other effects that may result from educational influences being provided outside of the study intervention. For example participants can be motivated simply by knowing they are part of a study.

Steps in experimental research

As in other research studies, there are a set of steps that the researcher should follow in the medical education experimental process:

1. Defining the research question and, if relevant, the specific objectives of the study.

2. Identifying the appropriate research design.

3. Implementing the educational intervention.

4. Collecting and analysing the data.

5. Extrapolating from the findings to defensible conclusions.

Although the purpose of the study can also be postulated in the form of a research statement or a hypothesis, the researcher needs to stipulate the anticipated causal relationship between the IV (the educational intervention) and corresponding DVs (the learning effects) of interest. The strength of the experimental process is that the researcher has the ability to manipulate the educational intervention, select the participants involved, regulate internal and external factors, and choose how best to measure the intervention effect.

We can categorize experimental studies that identify a single manipulated variable of interest as follows:

◆ pre-experimental

◆ quasi-experimental and

◆ true experimental (table 53.2).

Other than the ability to manipulate the intervention itself, the distinguishing features between these experimental designs is the ability to assign or randomize participants into groups, identify a comparison or control group, implement pretesting measures, and analyse data in an optimal manner. Although each of the following categories of experimental designs have advantages based on the research question being tested, the more rigorous the experimental design the more control the researcher has regarding threats to internal and external validity. Therefore the real strength of experimental designs is that the researcher takes into consideration the influence of extraneous factors that may influence the dependent variables and limit the generalizability of the effect that the independent variable has in learners or contexts beyond the experimental study itself.

Pre-experimental

Pre-experimental research designs are typically used as a preliminary step in understanding how a medical education intervention may influence participants' learning outcomes. For example, a pilot study may show that the use of an interactive teaching module on the cardiovascular system enhances a group of medical students' understanding of cardiology. However, this probably does not add

Table 53.2 Experimental research designs and internal validity concerns

Research designs		Groups	Randomization	Pretest (DV)	Intervention (IV)	Posttest (DV)	Statistics reported	Internal validity concerns							
								Historical changes	Participant growth	Pretesting	Measurements Used	Regression to mean	Sample discrepancy	Participant attrition	Internal Interactions
Pre-experimental															
One-shot case study design		1			(IV)	(DV)	(chart)	−	−	0	0	0	0	−	0
One-group, pretest and post-test design		1		(DV)	(IV)	(DV)	(chart)	−	−	−	−	(?)	0	+	0
Static group comparison design 1		2	(random)	(DV)	(IV)	(DV)	(chart)	+	(?)	0	+	+	0	−	−
Quasiexperimental															
Non-equivalent comparison group design		1		(DV)	(IV)	(DV)	(chart)	+	+	+	+	(?)	+	+	−
		2		(DV)		(DV)									
Time series design		1		(DV)	(IV)	(DV)	(chart)	−	+	+	(?)	+	0	+	0
Counterbalanced design		1		(DV)	(IV)	(DV)	(chart)	+	+	+	+	+	+	+	(?)
		2		(DV)	(IV)	(DV)									
True experimental															
Pretest and post-test, control group design		1	(dice)	(DV)	(IV)	(DV)	(chart)	+	+	+	+	+	+	+	+
		2	(dice)	(DV)		(DV)									

Research designs

Research designs	Groups	Randomization	Pretest (DV)	Intervention (IV)	Posttest (DV)	Statistics reported	Internal validity concerns							
							Historical changes	Participant growth	Pretesting	Measurements Used	Regression to mean	Sample discrepancy	Participant attrition	Internal Interactions
Post-test only, control group design	1	(dice)		(cards)	(curve)	(graph)	+	+	0	0	0	+	–	+
	2	(dice)			(curve)									
Solomon four group design	1	(dice)	(curve)	(cards)	(curve)	(graph)	+	+	+	+	+	+	+	+
	2	(dice)	(curve)		(curve)									
	3	(dice)		(cards)	(curve)									
	4	(dice)			(curve)									

Symbols:

(cards) = Intervention (independent variable)

(curve) = Pretest or post-test (dependent variable)

(dice) = Random assignment of participants to groups

Internal validity concerns:– = Factor controlled for, as as not relevant

( ) = Factor controlled for

+ = Factor controlled for

(?) = Factor may not be controlled for

a great deal to our knowledge of medical education (it is unsurprising that an educational intervention has some effect). It is important to keep in mind that the strength of experimental research designs are in the ability of the researcher to make contrasts before and after the implementation of an educational intervention or with a comparison group of study participants.

One-shot case study design

As illustrated in table 53.2, the *one-shot case study* design is the most basic approach to the experimental process, in that the introduction of an educational intervention results in scores on a post-test measure of performance. This single group design is commonly used in medical education research but has the least control over internal invalidity concerns.

One-group, pretest, and post-test design

As the name aptly defines, the *one-group, pre-test and post-test design* compares a single group's test scores before and after an educational intervention. The pretest reflects a baseline measure (DV) of the expected learning outcome that will be influenced by the introduction of the educational intervention. For example, if the purpose of intervention is to enhance students' communication skills the dependent measure could be scores on a pre- and post-test OSCE station where students are expected to take a history from a standardized patient. This design overcomes some internal validity concerns such as participant attrition (i.e. the researcher completes the analysis on only those students that have both pretest and post-test scores). However, the pretest sensitizes the learners and has an educational effect in its own right.

Static group comparison design

In this pre-experimental research design, the effectiveness of a medical education intervention is compared to a static group that follows a traditional approach to educating the students (note that it is generally not acceptable for the static group not to receive anything at all). Therefore, the groups are compared on educational post-test measures to see whether the intervention is as good, better or worse than the current approach. Although there are only two groups shown in table 53.2, any number of groups may be incorporated into the static group comparison design. In this case, the addition of modifications to the medical education intervention (e.g. increased intensity or duration) could also be explored as a way to better understand how to maximize the benefits of an intervention.

Quasiexperimental

The medical education researcher usually has access to a continuous flow of students; this allows for studies to be conducted on a variety of curriculum, teaching, and assessment initiatives. Nevertheless, in this setting it is often not possible to assign participants to specific experimental groups and the research must instead use 'naturally' occurring clusters of students (Cook and Campbell 1979). There are a variety of quasiexperimental research designs that have been used in education research; however, the three basic designs described next reflect important considerations when using pre-established groups or 'convenience samples' of participants.

Non-equivalent comparison group design

In general, the most commonly used pragmatic experimental design is the *non-equivalent comparison group design*. While most medical education researchers have the ability to establish pre-

test and post-test protocols, the identification of intervention and comparison groups are often based on the use of existing classes of students. Therefore the researcher will identify and match intact classes of participants to be either the intervention or comparison groups. For example, a medical school may allow a study where team-based learning activities are introduced as a way to enhance collaboration between students in a pre-clinical course. Using the 10 small group sessions scheduled for the course, the researcher may designate half of the groups to the team based learning activities while the other half would receive the traditional small group assignment. While this design addresses many of the internal validity concerns, the non-randomization of groups does not address the issue of regression to the mean or the internal interactions that may occur between sample discrepancy, historical changes, participant growth, and pre-testing. The researcher should make every effort to use similar groups for the purposes of comparison; however, if between group differences are anticipated due to another variable (e.g. sex, age, or pre-existing levels of achievement) then an analysis of covariance can be taken into consideration.

Time series design

When there is an expectation of change over a period of time with the use of a single-group design (whether short- or long-term), the *time-series design* allows the researcher to introduce regular measures of progress throughout the duration of the experimental study. Without a comparison or control group to deal with the internal validity concern of historical change, the researcher can consider using a number of repeated pretest and post-test measures as a way to isolate the effectiveness of an intervention once it has been implemented. The use of repeated pretesting measures provides the researcher with a baseline of participants' progress with respect to the dependent measures of interest. For example, medical students may demonstrate small and steady improvements on regular pretesting scores related to patient interviewing skills during the first half of an academic year. With the introduction of a communication medical skills initiative, post-testing may show significant growth initially ($p < 0.05$) with subsequent small and steady non-significant progress until the end of the second half of the year. When using a series of pre- and post-testing with any one particular study group, it is important that consideration is given to the intervals scheduled between testing periods. As students are constantly being exposed to new ideas and experiences that are beyond the intervention being studied, historical changes are a serious concern to internal validity (as participants cannot be experimentally isolated as happens in a science laboratory).

Counterbalanced design

In a counterbalanced design, each of the groups identified will be provided with the same educational interventions but in a different crossover sequence. The number of groups included in this design should reflect the corresponding number of interventions. However, the order the groups receive the interventions is not so much a concern for these existing groups. Without the ability to randomly select students into their respective groups, it is important for the researcher to obtain a pre-test baseline measure of the participants' abilities before the interventions begin (Langhan et al. 2009). As shown in table 53.2, the interventions provided in the counterbalanced design are different (illustrated by the size of the intervention symbol) in that the medical educational intervention may be of greater duration, intensity, or approach to the teaching and learning process. In this example, we see on the first post-testing that the distribution of participants' scores on the dependent measure is greater (more to the right) for the larger intervention symbol than for the smaller intervention symbol. After the interventions are crossed over during the second phase of the study, the final post-testing scores are now realigned—showing no significant differences between the groups after both of the interventions had been completed by the two groups. Although any number of groups can complete any equal number of interventions in this type of research design, the time duration between testing combined with the interaction effect that can occur between educational interventions may influence the effectiveness of any one intervention.

True experimental

Most of the *true experimental* research designs are able to control for all of internal validity concerns. The most important difference between true and the other medical education experimental designs is that in true designs the researcher is able to randomize the participants into intervention and control groups. Nevertheless, it is important to understand that while random *assignment* of participants is essential for the creation of a control group, the *selection* of individuals from a population of interest is limited by their willingness to voluntarily agree to participate in the study. Another important feature of the true experimental design is that the randomization process allows for the generation of 'true' control groups and not the comparison groups found in pre- and quasiexperimental research designs (or for that matter, in observational study designs).

Pretest and post-test, control group design

As indicated earlier in the non-equivalent comparison group design, the *pretest and post-test, control group design* is the most commonly accepted true experimental design used in medical education research. In this study design there is at least one intervention and one control group that are both pre- and post-tested and individuals are assigned randomly by the researcher to be a participant in one group or the other. Although sample size should always be a concern in any type of research study, this design can be modified to include any number of intervention or control groups and to incorporate additional pre- or post-testing measures. Nevertheless, it is important to understand that the use of a pretest and post-test, control group design does not guarantee that other extraneous variables will have an influence on the reliability and validity of your findings.

Post-test only, control group design

As implied by the name, the *post-test only, control group design* uses randomization to assign participants into intervention and control groups but limits testing on the dependent measure to a post-test. The absence of a pretest overcomes concerns related to informing or sensitizing participants to the anticipated intervention and post-testing measures to follow. The post-test only design is most effective in short-term studies where the expectation is that the 'drop-out' rate will be low (less than 10% from any one group). In long-term studies where attrition rates may be high or there is a chance that an extraneous variable may have influenced either group's ability initially, then the pre-test and post-test control group design should be considered instead.

Solomon four group design

The *Solomon four group design* combines the randomized groups assigned in the pretest and post-test only groups, with those of the post-test only groups to address concerns related to the effects of testing and the interaction effects of pre-testing and intervention. This four group design introduced by Solomon (1949 pp. 137–150) has the benefit of increasing the generalizability of the results by analysing all combinations of pretest and post-test dependent measures as an estimate of the main effects of the intervention. This approach involves a two by two (2×2) factorial analysis of variance (or covariance in the event that the interactive effects of pretesting are different), with the main effect of the intervention crossed with the main effect of pretesting. In essence, a pretesting and intervention interaction effect is reported if the pretested intervention group was to score differently on the post-test (potentially higher, as this group was sensitized a priori) to the non-pretested intervention group. Although this allows the researcher to make better inferences about the effectiveness of the intervention, the finding of a sufficient number of participants to achieve an appropriate sample sizes for each of the four groups may not be practical.

In a true experimental research design, the researcher presides over the sample that participates in the study and controls the selection process through randomization to ensure that all participants have similar chances of being in the intervention or control groups. As in all experimental designs, researchers also identify the measurements used to collect data about the effects of the intervention. It is the selection of participants from a single pool of learners and the ability to apply different interventions or programmes to participants with similar characteristics that permit true experimental research to provide cause-effect results. The essence of experimentation is control, although in many education settings it is not possible to meet stringent control conditions. Ultimately, the selection of the 'ideal' experimental research design is determined by the nature of the research question, access to sufficient numbers of participants, and the contextual setting in which the intervention is to be established (i.e. its duration and intensity).

Suggestions for enhancing the research design

Generally, the main purpose of conducting an experimental study in medical education is to investigate the effect that an intervention has on improving participants' educational outcomes. The ability of the researcher to achieve statistical significance on any or all dependent variables of interest is to some degree within the control of the researcher. In particular, the experimental researcher can influence the 'power' of the study in three ways:

◆ increase the number of participants

◆ manipulate the intervention or independent variable of interest

◆ establish a justifiable critical level of significance.

Meta-analysis research designs in medical education

A meta-analysis is a type of quantitative research design that is used to investigate the effectiveness of interventions across a number of primary studies that use similar educational outcomes. Unlike systematic reviews that provide thematic summaries of the similarities found between studies, a meta-analysis focuses on combining empirical data to derive an effect size estimation of the effectiveness of the intervention. Since the initial use of meta-analysis in psychotherapy (Smith and Glass 1977) and educational research (Glass and Smith 1979), this quantitative approach to summarizing the effectiveness of interventions has gained wide acceptance across many different academic disciplines. With advances in methodological protocols and statistical analyses, meta-analyses are now recognized as an important advance in quantitative research design and have seen an exponential growth in publications across all fields (Cooper and Hedges 2009).

This synthesis of research on a topic in medical education may begin with an exploration of whether there is enough empirical data to combine similar measures from related studies. For example, you may want to study the effectiveness of a type of curriculum module, where measures of students' learning are assessed in comparison with a control group of students. Unfortunately, there are a number of issues that will arise in identifying studies that will meet the inclusion and exclusion criteria you might establish for including a study in your meta-analysis (Stroup et al. 2000).

An example of a meta-analysis is as follows. A standardized assessment measure—the MCAT—was introduced to identify the best candidates for medical schools in the United States and Canada. However, the majority of studies that explored the use of the MCAT and its subtests as a predictive measure of students' performance in the future (i.e. on medical school or board exams) were limited by small sample sizes. In a meta-analysis of the predictive validity of the MCAT, Donnon et al. (2007) showed that as a total score and specific to three of the subtests (verbal reasoning, biological sciences, and physical sciences) the MCAT had small to medium predictive validity effect sizes on medical students' performance during the preclinical and clinical years of medical school. The total MCAT score was found to be better at predicting performance on the US medical licensing exams Step 1 and 2 accounting for 42% of and 21% of the overall variance, respectively. The interpretation of the magnitude of the effect size for linear correlations is based on Cohen's (1988) suggestions of r of 0.10 ($r^2 = 0.01$) as 'small', r of 0.30 ($r^2 = 0.09$) as 'medium', and r of 0.50 ($r^2 = 0.25$) as 'large'.

Conclusions

- Although experimental research represents the most rigorous approach to studying cause and effect relationships, caution must be used in generalizing the findings of a single study beyond the types of participants involved and the context of the study.

- Research designs in medical education can be either observational (e.g. survey, correlation, causal-comparative) or experimental (pre-experimental, quasiexperimental, true-experimental). In each design, an independent variable of interest (e.g. an existing or introduced educational intervention) is investigated using dependent measures.

- The dependent measures of interest need to have strong psychometric characteristics. These are generally defined and reported in terms of their reliability and validity.

- Experimental research designs in medical education allow the researcher to manipulate the educational intervention or independent variable of interest.

- There are three main things that researchers can do to improve the rigor of their research designs: (1) maximize the sample size or number of participants, (2) establish an appropriate significance level criteria (e.g. $p < 0.05$), and (3) modify the education intervention to enhance the anticipated effects.

References

Bordage, G. (2007) Moving the field forward: going beyond quantitative-qualitative. *Acad Med.* 82(10 Suppl): S126–S128

Bracht, G.H. and Glass, G.V. (1968) The external validity of experiments. *Am Educ Res J.* 5: 437–474

Campbell, D.T. and Stanley, J.C. (1963) *Experimental and Quasi-Experimental Designs for Research in Teaching.* Chicago: Rand McNally

Cohen, J. (1988) *Statistical Power Analysis for the Behavioral Sciences.* Hillsdale NJ: Erlbaum

Cook, T.D. and Campbell, D.T. (1979) *Quasi-experimental Design and Analysis for Field Settings.* Chicago: Rand McNally

Cooper, H. and Hedges, L.V. (2009) *The Handbook of Research Synthesis.* New York: Russell Sage Foundation

Donnon, T. and Hecker, K. (2008) Relationship of approaches to learning and academic achievement of undergraduate students from an inquiry based Bachelor of Health Sciences program: A confirmatory factor analysis. *Can J Higher Edu.* 38: 1–19

Donnon, T. and Violato, C. (2006) Medical students' clinical reasoning skills as a function of basic science achievement and clinical competency measures: A structural equation model. *Acad Med.* 81: S120–S123

Donnon, T., Oddone Paolucci, E., and Violato, C. (2007) The predictive validity of the MCAT on medical school performance and medical board licensing examinations: a meta-analysis of the published research. *Acad Med.* 82: 100–106

Donnon, T., Woloschuk, W., and Myhre, D. (2009) Issues related to medical students engagement in rural placements: an exploratory factor analysis of the Integrated Community Clerkship questionnaire. *Can J Rural Med.* 14(3): 105–110

Fowler, Jr., F.J. (2009) *Survey Research Methods, 4th Edition. Applied Social Research Methods Series.* London, UK: Sage Publications

Gay, L.R., Mills, G.E., and Airasian, P.W. (2009) *Educational Research: Competencies for Analysis and Application.* 9th edn. Upper Saddle River: Pearson

Glass, G.V. and Smith, M.L. (1979) Meta-analysis of research on class size and achievement. *Educ Eval Policy Anal.* 1:2–16

Hill, A.B. (1952) The clinical trial. *N Engl J Med.* 247: 113–119

Hopkins, K.D. (1998) *Educational and Psychological Measurement and Evaluation.* 8th edn. Needham Heights, MA: Allyn and Bacon

Hutchinson, L. (1999) Evaluating and researching the effectiveness of educational interventions. *BMJ.* 318: 1267

Langhan, T.S., Rigby, I., Walker, I., Howes, D., Donnon, T., and Lord, J. (2009) Simulation based training in procedural skills improves residents' competence. *Can J Emerg Med.* 11: 535–539

Norman, G. (2002) Research in medical education: three decades of progress. *BMJ.* 324: 1560–1562

Smith, M.L. and Glass, G.V. (1977) Meta-analysis of psychotherapy outcome studies. *Am Psychol.* 12: 752–760

Solomon, R.L. (1949) An extension of control group design. *Psychol Bull.* 46: 137–150

Stroup, D.F., Berlin, J.A., Morton, S.C., et al. (2000) Meta-analysis of observational studies in epidemiology: a proposal for reporting. *JAMA.* 283: 2008–2012

Todres, M., Stephenson, A., and Jones, R. (2007) Medical education research remains the poor relation. *BMJ.* 335: 333–335

Whitcomb, M.E. (2002) Research in medical education: what do we know about the link between what doctors are taught and what they do? *Acad Med.* 77: 1067–1068

Further reading

Cook, D.A. (2012) Randomized controlled trials and meta-analysis in medical education: What role do they play? *Med Teach.* 34(6): 468–473

Ringsted, C., Hodges, B., Scherpbier, A. (2011) 'The research compass': An introduction to research in medical education: AMEE Guide No. 56. *Med Teach.* 33(9): 695–709

Searle, J. and Prideaux, D. (2005) Medical education research: being strategic. *Med Educ.* 39(6): 544–546

Torgerson, CJ. (2002) Educational research and randomised trials. *Med Educ.* 36(11): 1002–1003

Torgerson, CJ. (2002) Researching outcomes of educational interventions. *BMJ.* 324: 1155

CHAPTER 54

Qualitative research in medical education

Patricia McNally

Why do clear thinking clinicians and researchers sometimes apply illogical thought to education?

Jill Morrison

Reproduced from Morrison, J., 'Jill Morrison', Medical Education, 34, 6, p. 491, 2001, with permission from Association for the Study of Medical Education and Wiley

Introduction

The majority of health professionals feel comfortable with quantitative research methods—as these methods are more commonly used in clinical settings. However, qualitative research methods are important in medical education. This chapter outlines the commonly used methods in qualitative medical education research. It explains their theoretical underpinnings, the evidence for their use and gives practical guidance on their application. Specific case studies from the current literature will demonstrate the application of each of the qualitative research approaches outlined.

Qualitative research has its foundation in social sciences, and the humanities—from disciplines such as anthropology, sociology, education, and history (Lingard and Kennedy 2007). The importation of methods from these disciplines into medical education began in the 1980s when more prescriptive theory was called for to complement the dominant paradigm of a controlled experiment.

Some define qualitative methods as the antithesis to quantitative methods (Pope and Mays 2000). Because qualitative research is primarily concerned with the meanings people attach to their experiences of the social world as well as how they make sense of that world, qualitative research attempts to interpret social phenomena through methods such as interviews, focus groups, and observations. Yin referred to different forms of data collection: documents, archival records, interviews, direct observation, participant observation, and physical artefacts (Creswell 1998, p. 123). Lincoln and Guba (1985) propose an alternative paradigm—a 'naturalistic' rather than 'rationalistic' method of inquiry—in which the investigator avoids manipulating research outcomes a priori. They propose that the different assumptions of the two approaches are focused on the nature of reality, subject-oriented interaction and the possibility of generalization.

Introduction to three paradigms: the foundational eras

Biklen (1992) defines a paradigm as a loose collection of logically held together assumptions, concepts, or propositions that orient thinking and research. Lincoln and Guba (1985) and Denzin and Lincoln (2008, 2011) see a paradigm as a systematic set of beliefs and their accompanying methods, which provide a view of the nature of reality. They contend that the history of inquiry can be divided into eras based on people's world view and how to study that world view.

The three major paradigms in the history of social-science inquiry are prepositivist, positivist, and postpositivist (see fig. 54.1).

The prepositivist era ranges over the time of two millennia—from the time of Aristotle (384–322 BCE) to the pre-Hume era (1711–1776)—with science as a passive observer. During this time the researcher was more of a recorder of the event than someone who had any influence either over the structure or the outcome of data collection. It was considered unnatural to intervene in any way because the outcome could then be distorted.

Positivism begins in the 19th century, developed by the philosopher and founding sociologist, August Compte—who formulated the positivist philosophy and was the person who named it. However, it was Hume who was the first to apply this philosophy to actual scientific activities (Lincoln and Guba 1985).

Positivism was seen simply as a way to get to the truth, understand it well enough to predict it, and to control it. The goal of science then, from a positivist view, is to stick to what we can observe and measure. It was different from prepositivism in that the key approach of the scientific method was now the experiment, the attempt to discern natural laws through direct manipulation and observation. Positivism had its greatest impact on the reform of the scientific method—a new rationale for science developed (Lincoln

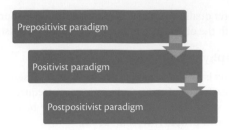

Figure 54.1 Paradigms in the history of social-science inquiry.

and Guba 1985). The idea that observation and measurement is the core of the scientific endeavour came of age.

Postpositivism has basic tenets that are virtually the reverse of those presented in positivism—in fact a wholesale rejection of central tenets of positivism; again, a reaction to the failings of the previous perspective. Naturalist inquiry is a postpositive paradigm. A naturalist inquiry paradigm perceives reality as multiple, constructed, and holistic; the knower and the known are interactive and inseparable. Only time and content-bound working hypotheses are possible; all entities are in a state of mutual, simultaneous shaping so that it is impossible to distinguish causes from effects; all inquiry is value bound. The positivist paradigm, on the other hand, perceives reality as single, fragmentable, and tangible—the knower and the known are independent. Naturalist inquiry focuses on meaning in context and requires a data collection instrument sensitive to underlying meaning when gathering and interpreting data. Humans are best suited for this task when using methods that make use of human sensibilities such as interviewing, observing, and analysing.

While one would think each of these three paradigms would build upon the findings of the previous one, quite the opposite occurred—'paradigm wars' are referred to in much of the literature. Each new era was reactionary to the prior one.

Qualitative research

Lincoln and Guba (1985) indicate that qualitative researchers 'empathize, describe, judge, compare, portray, evoke images, and create for the reader or listener the sense of having been there'. There are four major interpretive paradigms that structure qualitative research:

+ positivist and postpositivist
+ contructivist–interpretive
+ critical (Marxist, emancipatory) and
+ feminist (womanist) poststructural.

These four abstract paradigms each identify the lens through which a researcher can interpret data. The researcher most frequently aligns with the worldview that they identify most with. The researcher makes that alignment based on the systematic set of beliefs that they have been exposed to during their life. Positivist and postpositivist were defined previously. The constructivist–interpretive researcher understands society through their experiences—i.e. their social construct. For example, someone growing up in the south of the United States has a different social construct than a person growing up in the north of the United States. They even call the same war different names. In the north it is referred to as the Civil War and in the south as the War of Northern Aggression—a different social

construct. Most postpositivists are constructivists who believe that we each construct our view of the world based on our own perception of it. The last two paradigms (critical and feminist) posit that the real world makes the material difference of perception and experience as it relates to presenting research findings in terms of race, class, and gender. Therefore the social text, its logic and the inability to ever truly present the lived experience of anyone else becomes a central component of these forms of naturalistic inquiry and must be identified as such by the researcher.

Qualitative research in medical education

So how does all this relate to qualitative research in medical education? For the day to day qualitative researcher, it does not relate. But it would be remiss not to present the rich and varied historical and philosophical framework to this research methodology.

Qualitative researchers study social, relational and experiential phenomena in their natural setting (Lingard and Kennedy 2007). Hence, the naturalist inquiry name. While qualitative inquiry is rather new to medical education, the foundation of the three eras and paradigms listed above is critical. Qualitative research provides insight into the natural setting of that being studied and can do so using a number of different approaches (fig. 54.2). While these approaches may be identified differently by different authors, for this work they are identified as: ethnography, grounded theory, case study, phenomenology, hermeneutics, narrative research and action research. As they are defined, one can begin to see the possibility of overlap between them as well as in their data collection methodologies.

Key features of a qualitative research study design include the sampling framework employed; the data collection methods, types and sources used: and the data analysis methods undertaken. Qualitative research designs more often than not evolve during data collection and analysis (Devers 1999). Therefore it is critical to remember, that the research question is what drives the research approach as well as the data collection methodology.

Too often, researchers new to qualitative methods are more focused on the data collection methodology as opposed to

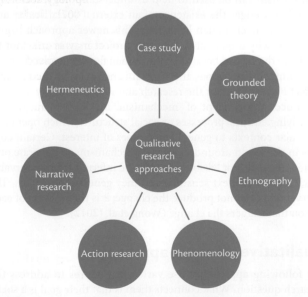

Figure 54.2 Qualitative research approaches.

identification of the appropriate approach for the research question. It is not uncommon to see a researcher determine the outcome for which they are looking and then develop the research methodology to achieve that outcome. In essence, they back into the research as opposed to choosing the appropriate methodology that best fits the research question.

Qualitative research has several recognizable characteristics. It is frequently done in natural settings, usually as part of an observation or analysis of the behaviour of an individual or a group. This observation is then presented with a description rich with both detail and insight into the setting. Kirk and Miller define qualitative research as a 'particular tradition in social science that fundamentally depends on watching people in their own territory, and interacting with them in their own language, on their own terms' (Pope and Mays 2000).

The researcher is separate from that which is observed. Their social construct must be withheld in observing the behaviour of that which is observed. Personal bias of the researcher must always be recognized and identified so that the outcomes of the research are not altered or modified in any way. Most often qualitative research is not designed to be replicated. The same process may be used with another group, but the nature of this methodology does not expect the same outcome as it would with a quantitative research project.

In medical education, the dominant paradigms currently framing qualitative research tend to be postpositivist and constructivist (Lingard and Kennedy2007). The postpositivist paradigm believes that there is an objective reality and that this can be discovered with appropriate research procedures. Constructivism, or social construct, accepts reality and meaning as relative—relative to the researcher's world view and that of the research group.

Somewhere between postpositivism and constructivism, is a newer approach, which is neither qualitative nor quantitative in its research method. Rather it is a way to attempt to understand the why and how of the research—based on the people and the events involved. It is called realism or realistic methods. This newer approach can improve our understandings of reality because the 'real world' constrains the interpretations we can reasonably make of it. Realism can be used to help us understand the social world and acknowledges the existence of an external social reality and its influence over human behaviour. This newer approach begins to look at why a qualitative research project may or may not be able to be duplicated because of the human factors involved. So the environment, the people, their social construct and the research project itself impact on the research and its duplicability. Realism introduces the concept of 'mechanism'. Mechanism means the underlying entities, processes or social structures which operate in particular contexts to generate outcomes of interest. Certain contexts in the world around us trigger mechanisms to generate outcomes. They are not 'visible' but must be inferred from observable data; they are context sensitive and they generate outcomes. The intervention does not produce the change; it is the reaction of each person that triggers the change (Wong et al. (2012).

Qualitative research approaches

The following approaches use varied procedures to address the research question. What connects them is that their goal is a social process, as defined within each methodology, through which they will interpret qualitative data. While each of these approaches can overlap with the other, they all have unique characteristics.

Ethnography

Ethnography is a type of qualitative study that presents a sociocultural interpretation of data. Culture is most frequently defined as the beliefs, values, and attitudes that shape the behavior of a particular group of people (Merriam 2002).

While ethnography has its roots in anthropology, it has become popular in many fields as a form of research (box 54.1). Observation of any group or subculture would fall under this approach. One major influence on ethnography was what was called the 'Chicago School' of sociology. It was named after work carried out at the University of Chicago: the researchers observed specific social groups in that area that had arisen during the 1920s onward: specifically marginal social groups including gamblers, drug addicts, and even jazz musicians (Pope and Mays 2000).

An early example of research in healthcare using the Chicago school ethnographic method would include the observation of tuberculosis patients and staff within sanitoria—including timelines of progress during treatment both for patients and staff (Pope and Mays 2000).

Most would use the written word to articulate what they have observed but a newer form of ethnography, visual ethnography (Schlesser, 2010), has emerged. Visual ethnography uses photographs to chronicle a groups' development or behaviour. While it is unlikely photography would be a preferred ethnographic technique within medical education, it does demonstrate how even with long, historical roots in anthropology, newer techniques can develop.

Each qualitative research method should be appropriate to the research question. Ethnography is perfect for observing a group and their behaviour and for describing systems or processes. Personal bias is always a challenge when reporting back observed behaviour or systems and can therefore become a weakness. Detailed coding and confirmation within the group of data collected could address this challenge. The detail in the coding helps the researcher limit personal bias and present data that is more closely aligned with was observed.

Grounded theory

Grounded theory is the study of experience from the perspective of the person living it. Research in this methodology builds a theory as it goes, as opposed to working with a theoretical hypothesis. Grounded theory was founded by two sociologists, Glaser and Strauss in 1960 to provide a systematic approach to the analysis of qualitative data that would live up to the standards of rigour

---

Box 54.1 Ethnography as a research method

Teaching and learning in morbidity and mortality rounds: an ethnographic study (Kruper et al. 2010).

Kruper et al. (2010) chose ethnography as the approach by which they observed a weekly morbidity and mortality round. The purpose was to explore the teaching and learning process that occurred in rounds in order to better understand their role in and contribution to current medical education. Their method of collecting data included observation followed by focused interviews to further clarify what was observed.

Box 54.2 Grounded theory as a method of qualitative research

Institutional marginalization and student resistance to learning about culture, race and ethnicity (Roberts et al. 2010).

This study explored how contrasting approaches to learning about cultural diversity impacted medical students. Using grounded theory and a thematic analysis the authors found that two potentially competing views were espoused at the two schools.

imposed by the quantitative paradigm. This type of systematic approach would focus on theory generation rather than theory testing, which would present a newer model of investigation for research (Lingard and Kennedy 2007). Glaser and Strauss studied illness and dying and developed grounded theory during those studies. Much of early grounded theory had its foundation in nursing and medical education.

Glaser and Strauss used the term grounded theory to describe the inductive process of coding incidents in the data and identifying analytical categories that emerge from the data. This process involves identifying a theme and attempting to verify, confirm and quantify it by searching the data (Pope and Mays, 2000). The coding is used as a method of searching the data looking for trends as well as repetitive themes that emerge and give insight.

Most grounded theory studies derive their outcomes from interviews and observations—this can work well as a research method in medical education. Lingard and Kennedy identify three elements of grounded theory methodology:

• an iterative study design which include cycles of simultaneous data collection and analysis, in which the results of ongoing data analysis informs subsequent data collection

• a purposeful sampling that compares data looking for that which would confirm, challenge, or expand an emerging theory

• a constant comparison approach that compares data looking for similarities and differences.

Grounded theory examines data as it emerges from the data collection. As stated, this is a strong method for nursing and medical education research. Again the concern of personal bias has to be addressed. In the case shown in box 54.2, thematic analysis supports the grounded theory method and addresses personal bias.

Case study

In many ways, a case study is defined both by what it studies as well as the way in which the data is studied. As with many of the qualitative research methods, the term can be used in a number of different ways and a lack of specificity can obscure the true meaning of a case study. In the true sense of qualitative research, a case study focuses on a single unit for analysis—for example one person, one group, one event, or one organization (Saldana 2011). Therefore a case study is identified as a bounded study—bounded both by time and place—a specific group or event studied for a specific time. The researcher is the primary instrument of data collection and analysis—as with all of the qualitative research methods. The case study is an inductive

investigative study that includes a description rich with details of all events in the case as it is studied. That which is to be studied in a case is chosen with purpose and intent—knowing that it would be bound by time, place and content (box 54.3). Again, as a qualitative method, a case study works well in academic medicine. The researcher must, however, be aware of potential personal bias when describing the case components and identify any bias to the best of their ability. The limitations of a study must also be included when writing up the report. The limitations could be lack of time, inadequate access to participants, or poor support for the research.

The case study allows for analysis of data within a bounded time period ... a definite strength in healthcare research. However, this limit in time can also be a weakness when a longer-term observation is required. When this challenge occurs, it may be better to choose another qualitative methodology.

Box 54.3 Case study as a method of qualitative research

Using a structured clinical coaching program to improve clinical skills training and assessment, as well as teachers' and students' satisfaction (Rego et al. 2009).

This was a case study that looked at a one year programme to observe the development of a Structured Clinical Coaching Programme that was needed to develop explicit learning objectives for both students and clinical tutors. Greater satisfaction was observed by both students and faculty with regard to their clinical skills development; there was also earlier identification of at-risk students.

Phenomenology

As with most methods within qualitative research, phenomenology has its roots in philosophy—in its case a twentieth century school of philosophy associated with Edmund Husserl. Husserl was a German mathematician who began the search for the essential or essence in all things. Phenomenology focuses on the subjective experience of the individual. Although, as presented, all qualitative research is phenomenological in the sense that there is a focus on people's experience, a phenomenological study seeks to understand the essence or structure of a phenomenon (Merriam 2002). The researcher's focus is thus on neither the human subject nor the human world but on the essence of the meaning of this interaction (Merriam 2002). Some qualitative research studies take a phenomenological approach when attempting to come to a deep understanding of how a person experiences an event.

All the common data collection techniques used in qualitative research are used in phenomenology: examples include interviews and participant observations and even analysing literary fiction (box 54.4). However, with this research method, the primary task is the researcher reflecting on the data to capture the essence that makes it what it is. For instance, Saldana gives the example of the study of motherhood as a phenomenon. When attempting to capture the essence of motherhood, commonalities can be gathered: such as 'caretaking responsibilities' or 'protecting one's child'. Another approach could be through themes such as 'Motherhood is' or 'Motherhood means'. This could also be found in literary

> **Box 54.4** Phenomenology as a method of qualitative research
>
> Interprofessional education: a nurse practitioner impacts family medicine residents' smoking cessation counseling experiences (Mitchell et al. 2009).
>
> In this study the researchers used phenomenology to understand how professional students' learning and practice can be affected by a member of another profession—through direct and indirect approaches (direct educator roles and indirect mentoring roles respectively). This study methodology gives true insight into interprofessional education as well as collaboration and its impact on learning in graduate medical education.

fiction, as well as interviews. Much has been written in many different genres about motherhood in society (Saldana, 2011). The data collection and analysis proceeds through the methodology of reduction, the analysis of specific statements and themes, and a search for all possible meanings (Creswell 1998).

Bracketing is critical to the effectiveness of this research methodology. Bracketing is recognizing one's own bias and setting it aside to rely on one's intuition, imagination and universal structure to obtain a picture of the experience (Creswell 1998).

According to Creswell (1998) a phenomenological study may be challenging for the following reasons:

- the researcher requires a solid grounding in the philosophical precepts of phenomenology

- the participants in the study need to be carefully chosen so that they are individuals who have truly experienced the phenomenon

- bracketing personal experiences by the researcher may be difficult

- the researcher needs to decide how and in what way their personal experiences will be introduced into the study.

With its roots in philosophical reflections, phenomenology is used most successfully when there is a need to understand a social phenomenon. One strength phenomenology is that it allows the researcher to go into great details when analysing behaviour.

Hermeneutics

Hermeneutics is more commonly integrated into one of the other methods than used as a method on its own. As a result there are few examples of hermeneutics in the medical educational research literature. The term hermeneutics historically refers to the interpretation of biblical texts or a branch of philosophy concerned with the understanding and interpretation of texts. Hermeneutics assumes that the text remains as written but that its interpretation changes with time and across contexts (Illing 2010). In the domain of qualitative research, Lingard and Kennedy define hermeneutics as using the lived experience of participants as a means to understand their political, historical, and sociocultural contexts (Lingard and Kennedy 2007).

Both grounded theory and narrative analysis are known to include hermeneutics as part of the data analysis. Narrative analysis is conducted within two hermeneutic traditions detailed by Ricoeur: a hermeneutics of faith, which aims to restore meaning to a text, and a hermeneutics of suspicion, which attempts to decode meanings that are disguised within it (Josselson 2004).

Fundamental to this approach of determining meaning is Schleiermacher's idea of the hermeneutic circle in which the understanding of the whole illuminates the parts, which in turn create the whole (Wertz et al. 2011). Lingard and Kennedy describe the hermeneutic circle as a cyclical analysis that moves back and forth between the consideration of the meaning of individual parts and the meaning of the whole text.

This is perhaps the least relevant to medical education as evidenced by the lack of any usage found within the current literature search. Either it is not relevant or too difficult to understand as an applicable method.

Narrative research

Narrative research is, like hermeneutics, a methodology that is imbedded within one of the other qualitative methods (Saldana 2011). Narrative inquiry is a research genre inclusive of a variety of approaches; however, it shares the goal of transforming data from, by, and/or about participants into literary story formats—an approach colloquially labelled 'creative non-fiction'.

We know from adult education theory that adults learn best and have better long-term retention of information when it is presented in story form. Adults think in stories.

There are several methodological approaches to dealing with narrative, according to Merriam et al. (2002). Each approach examines how the story is constructed, what linguistic tools are used and the cultural context of the story. Biographical, psychological, and linguistic approaches are the most commonly used.

Wertz et al. (2011) define narrative researchers as people who read texts for personal, social, and historical conditions that mediate the story. Analysis is aimed at discovering both the themes that unify the story and the disparate voices that carry, comment on, and disrupt the themes.

The authors go on to identify thematic analysis and discourse analysis as the methods by which the whole account of the story becomes known. It is when all these parts are integrated that the whole story is known and meaning can be determined.

Recently, narrative methods have been used to promote the development of both communication skills and empathy in medical students. Narratives, as personal critical reflection, are also used as an educational tool that allows the writer to further identify both what they have learned as well as ongoing gaps in their knowledge. Some medical schools require their students to write reflection papers for each course they attend; frequently for each activity, they are required to write a reflection to identify what exactly was learned.

The narrative form can be used in phenomenology, grounded theory, ethnography and case studies (box 54.5).

> **Box 54.5** Narrative research as a method of qualitative research
>
> Qualitative analysis of medical student impressions of a narrative exercise in the third-year psychiatry clerkship (Garrison et al. 2011).
>
> The researchers used the narrative method to allow students to develop a more holistic approach to patient care. The outcome allowed the students to know the patient in a much fuller and mutually beneficial way which resulted in better communication, understanding and patient outcomes.

The strength of this method is that is results in a deep under-standing of the research subject—as a result of critical reflection. The weaknesses are that often there is insufficient time to gather information and subsequently constraints on sharing all the information gathered.

Action research

Action research has its roots in the social activism of the mid-20th century. It is so rooted in this paradigm that it is frequently referred to as emancipatory research, critical research, feminist research, participatory action research or activist-oriented research. All of these derivatives of action research call for some form of social change—most often attempting to address problems faced by those parts of society that have been marginalized.

Action research is not without its detractors, however. In many of the resources used to define the other qualitative methods, action research is not even listed as a method. One author even describes action research as neither quantitative nor qualitative (Ross 1999).

The prime purpose of action research is to do better things (Pedler 2005). Meyer associates action research in 1946 with Kurt Lewin, a social scientist concerned with intergroup relations and minority problems in the United States (Meyer 2000). Lewin's proposition was that casual inferences about human behaviour are more likely to be valid if the relevant humans participate in building and testing them (Illing 2010). Meyer identifies the three most important elements of action research

♦ participatory character

♦ democratic impulse and

♦ simultaneous contribution to social science and social change.

Action research is conducted with the expressed purpose of not just observing social life, but reflecting on one's own practice or working collaboratively with those self-identified as needing to change their life circumstances through research and action. Therefore the identified participants and researchers work collaboratively to change their social environment through critical reflection (Saldana 2011). The research involves the design, implementation and evaluation of some specific action or event. What makes action research so different from the other qualitative research models is implementation.

As with critical theory, the goal is to critique and challenge, to transform and provide an environment where those with less power learn to develop and become an active part of society. This transformation is best described as perspective transformation. Perspective transformation is the process of becoming critically aware of how and why our assumptions have come to constrain the way we perceive, understand, and feel about our world; changing these structures of habitual expectations to make possible a more inclusive, discriminating, and integrative perspective; and, finally, making choices or otherwise acting upon these new understandings (Mezirow1991). The key component of action research is the 'acting upon', thereby taking the research to the community to effect change.

Participatory action research focuses on the political empowerment of people through participant involvement in the design and implementation of a research project. Collective action, as a result of the investigation, is a crucial component of this type of research (Merriam 2002). Teachers can and do apply this method to improve their classroom environment.

Box 54.6 Action research as a method of qualitative research

Peer-facilitated virtual action learning: reflecting on critical incidents during a pediatric clerkship (Plack et al. 2010).

Action learning facilitates reflection, critical thinking, and learning while solving real-world problems. In this research situation, the researchers used this method to reveal challenges faced by the residents—these challenges were uncovered using critical reflection. With their responses, the authors were able to identify weaknesses in the curriculum and make changes accordingly.

Hart and Bond (1995) selected seven criteria which they felt distinguished action research from other types of research.

Action research:

♦ has an educational function

♦ deals with individuals as members of a social group

♦ is problem focused, context specific and future oriented

♦ involves a change intervention

♦ aims at improvement and involvement

♦ involves a cyclic process, in which research, action, and evaluation are interlinked

♦ is found in a research relationship where those involved are participants in the change process.

The strengths of action research, as with any and all qualitative methods can only be strengths when they are appropriate to the research question. In the article in box 54.6 the researchers wanted to not just study a challenge they were facing, but then make a change based on the outcomes of their study. Action research is the method to be used when a behaviour change is required.

Pope and Mays (2000) noted that action research is gaining credibility in healthcare settings. Action research is frequently used in medical education today to identify concerns about quality (even though it is not always identified as action research—despite meeting all the relevant criteria). A challenge is determined; a group works collaboratively to identify barriers to a solution; works through those barriers; implements a new plan; and measures its effectiveness.

This action research model from Hart and Bond (1995) is an exact representation of a quality review (frequently done in a healthcare environment):

♦ identification of the problem (challenge)

♦ discussion and negotiation between researchers and practitioners

♦ literature review

♦ redefinition of the problem

♦ selection of the research and evaluation methods

♦ implementation of change, data collection and feedback. this can involve revisiting earlier steps.

♦ an overall review of the study—following the 'design, implement, and evaluate' model of action research

♦ dissemination to the group as a whole.

While action research may not be identified as such, it certainly is occurring in the healthcare environment.

Mixed method research

Mixed method research has recently become more popular in medical education. As the name indicates, this method combines the best of both quantitative and qualitative methods and data collection techniques. As with all methods of research, the research question is what should drive the research methodology. Creswell (2003) provides three strategies for the use of mixed method research. They are:

♦ sequential procedures: where the researcher may want to elaborate on the findings of one method with another method

♦ concurrent procedures: where the researcher converges both quantitative and qualitative data to develop a comprehensive analysis of the research question

♦ transformative procedures: where the researcher uses a theoretical lens as an overarching perspective within a design that contains both quantitative and qualitative data.

Mixed methods research is research question-driven, conciliatory and underpins much robust research in education (Maudsley 2011). However, the literature regarding mixed method research use in medical education is fragmented and poorly indexed generally.

Delphi and nominal group technique in health services research

These are amongst the most well-known of the mixed method techniques. They are most often used to build consensus in health services research. Both these methods seek to maximize the benefits of having informed panels consider a problem while minimizing the disadvantages associated with collective decision making (Jones and Hunter 1995).

Jones and Hunter have identified the most effective features of the consensus methods:

♦ anonymity: to avoid dominance by one or more members of the group—a questionnaire is used in Delphi and a private ranking of data in the nominal method

♦ iteration: discussions occur in rounds so as to allow the participants to reconsider their position and change accordingly

♦ controlled feedback: sharing each persons' iterative response

♦ statistical group response: this is where a summary of the group responses is shared in more detail—therefore giving more information.

Bourgeois et al. (2006) identify the uniqueness of the Delphi model as its reliability and its ability to be administered remotely and without direct participant interaction (box 54.7). They also provide

> **Box 54.7** Consensus building models as methods of qualitative research
>
> Needs and priorities of faculty development for medical teachers in India: a Delphi study (Singh et al. 2010).
> This study was the first time faculty were allowed to identify their faculty development needs. A questionnaire was distributed; themes were identified and reviewed by senior teachers. Themes were prioritised after the consensus building occurred, and a faculty development plan informed by faculty needs was developed.

a specific list of steps to achieve an effective process for developing consensus:

1. Identify problem/challenge.
2. Select experts.
3. Administer questionnaire.
4. Evaluate responses.
5. Redistribute questionnaire.
6. Interpret results.
7. Practical application.

This is a good method for consensus building. It allows for all voices to be heard and informed decisions to be made as a result of the consensus building. A weakness could be that those making the decision do not have the requisite knowledge to make an informed decision. If they do not have the appropriate ability to make an informed decision, their decision may not be the right one.

Qualitative research in medical education

Qualitative research can give greater depth and breadth to an inquiry. It can tell us how or why a student or resident is doing or not doing something. It broadens the research field to include qualities that give greater insight to both the research question and the data collection. It attempts to explain a phenomenon, the how and why of something and to build an understanding—with explicit data for support.

Qualitative research is there to explore and develop a hypothesis, whereas quantitative research is structured and aims to confirm a hypothesis. Qualitative research is deductive, quantitative research is inductive. Qualitative describes variation and group norms with open-ended questions; whereas quantitative quantifies variations and determines cause and effect with closed questions. Data within the qualitative method is verbally focused while quantitative data is numerically focused. The study designs of the two methods are quite different as well. Within quantitative research, the study design is set and does not change, whereas qualitative research allows the design to emerge and evolve based on the research findings.

The data collection models most often used in qualitative research are now described. It is important that authors reporting their work describe the data collection model used as well as the method of qualitative research. Not reporting both can discredit the rigor and validity of qualitative research.

The data collection methods for qualitative research include, but are not limited to:

♦ The interview: where persons' feelings, thoughts and experiences can be discussed with appropriate questioning by the researcher.

♦ The focus group: which usually includes a group of about 8–10 people from whom information pertinent to the research is elicited. This information is usually documented in some way and coded later. Focus groups can also be used as a way to confirm or clarify information from a questionnaire.

♦ Written narratives: these are frequently used. They require the person writing the narrative to critically reflect on the circumstances or events being studied.

♦ Observations: simple observations can also be used to gather data. The person observing a group needs to be aware of their

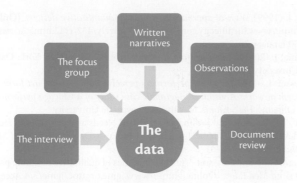

Figure 54.3 Data collection methods.

personal bias so as not to interrupt the flow of the group being observed.

◆ Document review: the review of documents, while important, does not involve the human quality found in most of the other data collection methods. Yet clearly it is needed in some instances—primarily as background information to the research.

The collection methodology is driven always driven by the research question. Sometimes, a number of different techniques are needed to gather enough data for a complete picture—see fig. 54.3 (Sullivan and Sargeant 2011).

As with any research model, qualitative research is not without its challenges. Marshall and Rossman (1995) identify at least three challenges:

◆ determining a conceptual framework that is thorough, concise and elegant

◆ developing a design that is systemic and manageable yet flexible

◆ integrating these into a coherent whole.

Within medical research there is the perception that qualitative research is cumbersome and difficult to analyse and that the analysis requires a high degree of interpretive skills (Pope and Mays 2000).The other frequent negative comment concerns the small number of participants being studied. Mays and Pope (2000) are clear that if the data analysis is done well, this is not an issue. Misunderstandings about the nature of qualitative methods and

their use in healthcare have often meant qualitative research is labeled as unscientific (Mays and Pope 2000) The most frequent criticism is the subjective nature of qualitative research. Within that statement is the assumption that subjective means biased or prejudicial. Subjectivity is part of qualitative research because the researcher is also the tool that gathers data. Many qualitative tools are used together to either guard against overly subjective research or to identify the researchers' role in the data collection (fig. 54.4).

The following criteria give insight into how to achieve rigor in qualitative research (Lingard and Kennedy 2007):

1. Adequacy and appropriateness of the sample: are the right people/activities being sampled? Is the sample size appropriate to allow sufficient insight?

2. The quality of the data collected: what is the researchers' relationship to those being researched? Are the interview and observation techniques being used in the natural setting of those being observed?

3. The clarity of the analysis process: Is there clarity in the analysis process? Can the reader determine who did the analysis, what they analysed and how they did the analysis?

Questions in medical education are becoming increasingly complex. We need all the research tools available to find answers to these questions. Both qualitative and quantitative research has a role to play in addressing the challenges we face.

Conclusions

◆ Qualitative methods can be used in medical education research to answer the questions that quantitative research is not be able to address.

◆ Qualitative research, no matter what methodology used, concerns itself with the meanings people attach to their experiences of the social world and how they make sense of that world.

◆ Qualitative research, in all methods, tries to interpret social phenomena (e.g. interactions and behaviours).

◆ The research question should determine which qualitative methodology to use as well as the data collection methods.

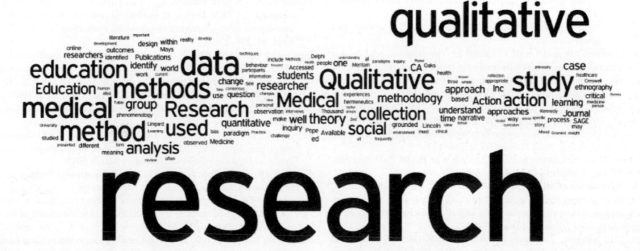

Figure 54.4 Qualitative research.

References

Bourgeois, J., Pugmire, L., Stevenson, K., Swanson, N., and Swanson, B. (2006) The Delphi method: a qualitative means to a better future. [Online]. http://www.freequality.org/documents/knowledge/Delphimethod.pdf Accessed 14 March 2013

Biklen, B. (1992) *Qualitative Research for Education; An Introduction to Theory and Methods*. 2nd edn. Needham Heights, MA: Allyn and Bacon

Creswell, J.W. (1998) *Qualitative Inquiry and Research Design: Choosing Among Five Traditions*. Thousand Oaks, CA: SAGE Publications, Inc

Creswell, J.W. (2003) *Research Design; Qualitative, Quantitative, and Mixed Methods Approaches*. 2nd edn. Thousand Oaks, CA: Sage Publications, Inc

Denzin, N.K. and Lincoln, Y.S. (eds) (2008) *Strategies of Qualitative Inquiry*. Thousand Oaks (CA): Sage Publications, Inc

Denzin, N.K. and Lincoln, Y.S. (eds) (2011) *The Sage Handbook of Qualitative Research*. Thousand Oaks, CA: Sage Publications, Inc

Devers, K.J. (1999) How will we know 'good' qualitative research when we see it? Beginning the dialogue in health services research. *Health Services Research*. 34(5/II): 1153–1188

Garrison, D., Lyness, J.M., Frank, J.B., and Epstein, R.M. (2011) Qualitative analysis of medical student impressions of a narrative exercise in the third-year psychiatry clerkship. *Acad Med.* 86(1): 85–89

Hart, E. and Bond, M. (1995) *Action research for health and social care*. Buckingham: Open University Press

Josselson, R. (2004) Hermeneutics of faith and hermeneutics of suspicion. *Narrative Inquiry.* 14(1): 1–29

Illing, J. (2007) Thinking about research: frameworks, ethics, and scholarship. In: Lingard, L. and Kennedy, T.J. (eds) *Qualitative research in Medical Education*. Edinburgh: Association for the Study of Medical Education

Jones, J. and Hunter, D. (1995) Consensus methods for medical and health services research. *BMJ.* 311: 376–380

Kuper, A., Zur Nedden, N., Etchells, F., Shadowitz, S., and Reeves, S. (2010) Teaching and learning in morbidity and mortality rounds: an ethnographic study. *Med Educ.* 44: 559–569

Lincoln, Y.S. and Guba, E.G. (1985) *Naturalistic Inquiry*. London: Sage Publications, Inc

Lingard, L. and Kennedy, T.J. (2007) *Qualitative Research in Medical Education*. Edinburgh: Association for the Study of Medical Education

Marshall, C. and Rossman, G.B. (1995) *Designing Qualitative Research*. 2nd edn. Thousand Oaks, CA: Sage Publications, Inc

Maudsley, G. (2011) Mixing it but not mixed-up: Mixed methods research in medical education (a critical narrative review). *Med Teach.* 33: 92–104

Merriam, S.B., et al. (2002) *Qualitative Research in Practice; Examples for Discussion and Analysis*. San Francisco, CA: Jossey-Bass

Meyer, J. (2000) Using qualitative methods in health related action research. *BMJ.* 320: 178–181

Mezirow, J. (1991) *Transformative Dimensions of Adult Learning*. San Francisco: Jossey-Bass Inc

Mitchell, J., Brown, J.B., and Smith, C. (2009) Interprofessional education: a nurse practitioner impacts family medicine residents' smoking cessation counselling experiences. *J Interprof Care.* 23(4): 401–409

Morrison, J. (2000). Jill Morrison. *Med Educ.* 34(6): 490–491

Pedler, M. (2005) Critical action learning. *Action Learn Res Pract.* 2(1): 1–6

Plack, M.M., Driscoll, M., Marquez, M., and Greenburg, L. (2010) Peer-facilitated virtual action learning:reflecting on critical incidents during a pediatric clerkship. *Acad Pediatr.* 10(2): 146–152

Pope, C. and Mays, N. (2000) *Qualitative Research in Health Care*. 2nd edn. London: BMJ Publishing Group

Rego, P., Peterson, R., Callaway, L., Ward, M., O'Brien, C., and Donald, K. (2009) Using a structured clinical coaching program to improve clinical skills training and assessment, as well as teachers' and students' satisfaction. *Med Teach.* 31(12): e586–595

Roberts, J.H., Sanders, T., Mann, K., and Wass, V. (2010) Institutional marginalisation and student resistance: barriers to learning about culture, race and ethnicity. *Adv Health Sci Educ.* 15(4): 559–571

Ross, J. (1999) *Ways of approaching research: quantitative designs*. [Online] http://www.fortunecity.com/greenfield/grizzly/432/rra2.htm>Accessed 30 January 2012

Saldaña, J. (2011) *Fundamentals of Qualitative Research*. New York: Oxford University Press, Inc

Schlesser, L. (2010) *How do performers perceive dance, as an art form or a form of work? A visual ethnographic case study of a Chicago performance company: The Seldoms*. MA thesis. Newcastle University.

Singh, T., Moust, J., and Wolfhagen, I. (2010) Needs and priorities of faculty development for medical teachers in India: A Delphi study, *Natl Med J India.* 23(5): 297–301

Sullivan, G.M. and Sargeant, J. (2011) Qualities of qualitative research: part 1, *J Grad Med Educ*. [Online]. http://www.jgme.org/toc/jgme/3/4 Accessed 14 March 2013

Wertz, F.J., Charmaz, K., McMullen, L.M., Josselson, R., Anderson, R., and McSpadden, E. (2011) *Five Ways of Doing Qualitative Analysis*. New York: The Guilford Press

Wong, G., Greenhalgh, T., Westhrop, G., and Pawson, R. (2012) Realist methods in medical education research: what are they and what can they contribute? *Med Educ.* 46: 89–96

Further reading

Aronoff, S.C., Evans, B., Fleece, D., Lyons, P., Kaplan, L., and Rojas, R. (2010) Integrating evidence based medicine into undergraduate medical education: combining online instruction with clinical clerkships. *Teach Learn Med.* 22(3): 219–223

Atkinson, P. and Pugsley, L. (2005) Making sense of ethnography and medical education. *Med Educ.* 39: 228–234.

Avison, D., Lau, F., Myers, M., and Nielson, P.A. (1999) Action research. *Commun ACM.* 42(1): 94–97

Babbie, E. (1995) *The Practice of Social Research*. 7th edn. Belmont, CA: Wadsworth Publishing Company

Cameron, D., Russell, D., Rivard, L., Darrah, J., and Palisano, R. (2011) Knowledge brokering in children's rehabilitation organizations: perspectives from administrators. *J Cont Educ Health Prof.* 31(1): 28–33

Coghlan, D. (2011) Action research: Exploring perspectives on a philosophy of practical knowing. *Acad Manage Ann.* 5(1): 53–87

Cook, D.A. (2010) Twelve tips for evaluating educational programs. *Med Teach.* 32: 296–301

Creswell, J.W. (2012) *Educational Research: Planning, Conducting, and Evaluating Quantitative and Qualitative Research*. 4th edn. Boston, MA: Pearson Education, Inc

Dauphinee, W.D. (2012) Educators must consider patient outcomes when assessing the impact of clinical training. *Med Educ.* 46: 13–20

Denzin, N.K. (1997) *Interpretive Ethnography; Ethnographic Practices for the 21st Century*. Thousand Oaks, CA: SAGE Publications, Inc

Driessen, E., van der Vleuten, C., Schuwirth, L., Van Tartwijk, J., and Vermunt, J. (2005) The use of qualitative research criteria for portfolio assessment as an alternative to reliability evaluation: a case study. *Med Educ.* 39: 214–220

Dyrbye, L., Cumyn, A., Day, H., and Heflin, M. (2009) A qualitative study of physicians' experiences with online learning in a masters degree program: Benefits, challenges, and proposed solutions. *Med Teach.* 31(2): e40–e46

Erlandson, D.A., Harris, E.L., Skipper, B.L., and Allen, S.D. (1993) *Doing Naturalistic Inquiry; A Guide to Methods*. Newbury Park, CA: Sage Publications, Inc

Fletcher, R.H., Aronson, M.D., and Eamranond, P. (2011) Evidence-based medicine. *UpToDate*, [Online]. http://www.uptodate.com/contents/evidence-based-medicine? Accessed 14 March 2013

Fraenkel, J.R. and Wallen, N.E. (2003) *How to Design and Evaluate Research in Education*. 5th edn. Boston, MA: McGraw Hill

Giacomini, M.K. and Cook, D. (2000) Users' guides to the medical literature: XXIII. Qualitative research in health care A. Are the results of the study valid? *JAMA.* 284(3): 357–362

Giacomini, M.K. and Cook, D. (2000) Users' guides to the medical literature: XXIII. Qualitative research in health care B. What are the results and how do they help me care for my patients? *JAMA.* 284(4): 478–482

Glaser, B.G. (2004) Naturalist inquiry and grounded theory. *Forum: Qualitative Social Research*. 5(1): Art 7

Green, J. and Britten, N. (1998) Qualitative research and evidence based medicine. *BMJ*. 316(7139): 1230–1232

Greenhalgh, T. and Taylor, R. (1997) How to read a paper: papers that go beyond numbers (qualitative research). *BMJ*. 315: 740–743

Hall, S. Qualitative Methods in Health Care Management, [Online]. http://www.ehow.com/way_5622578_qualitative-methods-health-care-management.html Accessed 14 March 2013

Hart, D. and Gregor, S. (2005) *Information Systems Foundations*. Canberra, Australia: The Australian National University

Hafferty, F.W. (1998) Beyond curriculum reform: confronting medicine's hidden curriculum. *Acad Med*. 73(4): 403–407

Hasson, F., Keeney, S., and McKenna, H. (2000) Research guidelines for the Delphi survey technique. *J Adv Nursing*. 32(4): 1008–1015

Imel, S. (1995) Race and gender in adult education. Educational Resources Information Center. [Online] http://www.calpro-online.org/eric/docgen.asp?tbl=tia&ID=92 Accessed 9 January 2012

Jaye, C. (2002) Doing qualitative research in general practice: methodological utility and engagement. *Fam Pract*. 19(5): 557–562

Keim, S. M., Howse, D., and Mendoza, K. (2008) Promoting evidence based medicine in preclinical medical students via a federated literature tool. *Med Teach*. 30(9–10): 880–884

Kuhn, J.S. and Marsick, V.J. (2005) Action learning for strategic innovation in mature organizations: key cognitive, design and contextual considerations. *Action Learn Res Pract*. 2(1): 27–48

Leddy, P.D. and Ormrod, J.E. (2010) *Practical research: Planning and design*. 9th edn. Upper Saddle River, NJ: Pearson

Lempp, H. and Seale, C. (2004) The hidden curriculum in undergraduate medical education: qualitative study of medical students' perceptions of teaching. *BMJ*. 329(7469): 770–773.

Mathison, S. (1988) Why triangulate? *Educ Res*. 17(2): 13–17

Maxwell, J.A. (1992) Understanding and validity in qualitative research. *Harvard Educ Rev*. 62(3):

McMillian, J.H. and Schumacher, S. (2010) *Research in Education. Evidence based Inquiry*. 7th edn. Upper Saddle River, NJ: Pearson Education

McNally, P. and Killion, R. (1999) *The McNally–Killion Learning Organization Model: A Case Study in Managing Change*. Chicago IL: National-Louis University.

Merriam, S.B., 1988. *Case Study Research in Education; A Qualitative Approach*. San Francisco, CA: Jossey-Bass.

Merriam, S.B. (1998) *Qualitative Research and Case Study Applications in Education*. San Francisco, CA: Jossey-Bass

Merriam, S.B. and Simpson, E.L. (1995) *A Guide to Research for Educators and Trainers of Adults*. 2nd edn. Malabar, FL: Krieger Publishing Company

Miles, M. B. Huberman, A.M. (1994) *Qualitative Data Analysis: An Expanded Sourcebook*. Thousand Oaks, CA: Sage Publications, Inc

Mills, G.E. (2003) *Introduction to Education Research*. Upper Saddle River, NJ: Merrill Prentice Hall

Monrouxe, L.V., Rees, C. E., Lewis, N.J., and Cleland J.A. (2010) Medical educators' social acts of explaining underperformance in students: a qualitative study. *Adv Health Sci Educ*. 16: 239–252

Moulton, B. and King, J.S. (2010) Aligning ethics with medical decision-making: The quest for informed patient choice. *J Law Med Ethics*. 38(1): 85–97

Moustakas, C. (1990) *Heuristic Research; Design, Methodology, and Applications*. Newbury Park, CA: Sage Publications, Inc

Moustakas, C. (1994) *Phenomenological Research Methods*. Thousand Oaks, CA: Sage Publications, Inc

Okoli, C. and Pawlowski, S.D. (2004) The Delphi method as a research tool: an example, design considerations, and applications. *Information & Management*. 42: 15–29

Parsonnet, J., Gruppuso, P.A., Katner, S.L., and Boninger, M. (2010) Required versus elective research and in-depth scholarship programs in the medical school curriculum. *Acad Med*. 85(3): 405–408

Pawson, R. (2002) Evidence-based policy: the promise of 'realist synthesis'. *Evaluation*. 8(340): 340–358

Penney, D. and Leggett, B. (2005) Connecting initial teacher education and continuing professional learning through action research and action learning. *Action Learn Res Pract*. 2(2): 153–169

Poses, R.M. and Isen, A.M. (1998) Qualitative research in medicine and health care. *J Gen Intern Med*. 13: 32–38

Presser, S., Rothgeb, J.M., Couper, M.P., et al.(eds) (2004) *Methods for Testing and Evaluating Survey Questionnaires*. Hoboken, NJ: John Wiley & Sons Inc

Pruskil, S., Burgwinkel, P., Georg, W., Keil, T., and Kiessling, C., 2009. Medical students' attitudes towards science and involvement in research activities: A comparative study with students from a reformed and a traditional curriculum. *Med Teach*. 31(6): 254–259

Ramos, K.D., Schafer, S., and Tracz, S.M. (2003) Validation of the Fresno test of competence in evidence based medicine. *BMJ*. 326: 319–321

Reason, P. and Rowan, J. (1981) *Human Inquiry; A New Sourcebook of New Paradigm Research*. Hoboken, NJ: John Wiley & Sons Inc

Rees, C. and Monrouxe, L.V. (2011) 'A morning since eight of just pure grill': a multischool qualitative study of student abuse. *Acad Med*. 86(11): 1374–1382

Ringsted, C., Hodges, B., and Scherpbier, A. (2011) 'The research compass': An introduction to research in medical education: AMEE Guide No. 56. *Medical Education Online* [e-journal]. http://informahealthcare.com/doi/abs/10.3109/0142159X.2011.595436 Accessed 14 March 2013

Roberts, T.E. (2012) To every complex problem there is a simple solution… *Med Educ*. 46: 3–12

Rosenfield, D., Oandasan, I., and Reeves, S. (2011) Perceptions versus reality: a qualitative study of students' expectations and experiences of interprofessional education. *Med Educ*. 45: 471–477

Rothwell, W.J. (1999) *The Action Learning Guidebook; A Real-Time Strategy for Problem Solving, Training Design, and Employee Development*. San Francisco, CA: Jossey-Bass Pfeiffer

Santen, S.A. and Hemphill, R.R. (2011) A window on professionalism in the Emergency Department through medical student narratives. *Ann Emerg Med*. 58(3): 288–294

Savenye, W.C., and Robinson, R.S. (2001) *The Handbook of Research for Educational Communications and Technology*. [Online]. http://www.aect.org/edtech/ed1/40/index.html Accessed 14 March 2013

Shank, G.D. (2006) *Qualitative Research: A Personal Skills Approach*. 2nd edn. Upper Saddle River, NJ: Merrill Prentice Hall

Skulmoski, G.J., Hartman, F.T., and Krahn, J. (2007) The Delphi method for graduate research. *J Inf Technol Educ*. 6: 1–21

Smith, J.K. (1983) Quantitative versus qualitative research: an attempt to clarify the issue. *Educ Res*. 12(3): 6–13

Straus, S.E., Green, M.L., Bell, D.S., et al. (2004) Evaluating the teaching of evidence based medicine: Conceptual framework. *BMJ*. 329: 1029–1032

Straus, S. E., Tetroe, J., and Graham, I. (2009) Defining knowledge translation. *Can Med Ass J*. 181(3–4): 165–168

Sterkenburg, A., Barach, P., Kalkman, C., Gielen, M., and ten Cate, O. (2010) When do supervising physicians decide to entrust residents with unsupervised tasks? *Acad Med*. 85(9): 1408–1417

Stringer, E.T. (1999) *Action Research*. 2nd edn. Thousand Oaks, CA: Sage Publications, Inc

Swanwick, T. (ed) (2010) *Understanding Medial Education; Evidence, Theory, and Practice*. Chichester: John Wiley & Sons Ltd

Tavakol, M. (2006) Training medical teachers in using qualitative research methods. *Med Educ Online* [e-journal]. http://www.med-ed-online.org/pdf/L0000010.pdf Accessed 14 March 2013

Thistlethwaite, J., Quirk, F., and Evans, R. (2010) Medical students seeking medical help: A qualitative study. *Med Teach*. 32: 164–166

Tyson, K. (1995) *New Foundations for Scientific Social and Behavioral Research; The Heuristic Paradigm*. Needham Heights, MA: Allyn and Bacon

Wear, D. (2008) On outcomes and humility. *Acad Med*. 83(7): 625–626

Wong, G., Greenhalgh, T., and Pawson, R. (2010) Internet-based medical education: a realist review of what works, for whom and in what circumstances. *BMC Med Educ*. 10(12): doi: 10.1186/1472-6920-10-12

Zuberi, R.W. (2012) Layers within layers… self-regulation in a complex learning environment. *Med Educ*. 46: 3–12

CHAPTER 55

Publishing in medical education

Steven L. Kanter, Victoria A. Groce, and Eliza Beth Littleton

I have only made this letter longer because I have not had the time to make it shorter.

Blaise Pascal, The Provincial Letters, Letter 16, 1657.

Introduction

An old aphorism states that 'you cannot write better than you can think'. In other words, the quality of your article can never be better than the quality of your reasoning about a topic. No matter how effectively and attractively you may arrange words and sentences on a page, or how authoritatively they may ring, a careful reader will discern the upper limits of the quality of the reasoning used to generate the text. This aphorism, of course, has relevance for writing about educational studies, projects, and innovations. The quality of the article about an experimental study, a curriculum project, or an educational innovation will be limited by the quality of the study, project, or innovation itself. A poorly conducted experiment, a faulty survey design, or an ill-conceived programme cannot be repaired with fancy writing. So, while the main focus of this chapter is on writing and publishing in medical education, it is important at all times to keep in mind that high-quality design and execution of educational studies and projects (covered in other chapters of this text) are critical prerequisites to good writing and successful publishing.

Given an excellent experiment or innovation, writing for a critical audience still requires careful planning and reasoning. At the very earliest stages, the scholar in medical education must consider how to conceive and undertake a topic, must follow guidelines in publication ethics, and must write with the intended audience in mind. This is not just because it is better to think ahead than to discover a significant error after submitting a manuscript to a journal but rather because planning ahead *is* the thinking that concludes with a substantive contribution to the field.

A good manuscript should have both intellectual and moral integrity. Intellectual integrity includes, but is not limited to, a clear statement of the problem, aim, or hypothesis; an appropriate summary of relevant literature; a complete description of the methods used; an accurate report of results or findings; sound arguments and logical reasoning; and conclusions that reflect the results. Moral integrity includes, but is not limited to, citation of others' works as appropriate; a clear description of the treatment of human participants in a study or project; an explicit statement of compliance with relevant ethical principles; and indication of ethical approval from an appropriate committee or other entity, as applicable.

Intellectual integrity of a manuscript

Medical education journals publish a range of articles, including reports of scientific research, scholarly articles that provide evidence and sound arguments for a perspective, reports about innovations, 'how to' articles, commentaries, editorials, point–counterpoint essays, letters to the editor, and a variety of special features (e.g. features that focus on the interface between the arts and medicine). This chapter focuses primarily on the first three types of articles, but the principles and guidelines are applicable to all writing in medical education.

Bordage (2001 p. 892) listed a set of qualities often reported by reviewers as they consider the quality of manuscripts.

- relevance: 'important, timely, relevant, critical, prevalent problem'

- problem statement: 'problem well stated, formulated'

- context: 'thoughtful, up-to-date, focused review of the literature'

- design: 'well-designed study (appropriate, rigorous, comprehensive design)'

- power: 'sample size sufficiently large'

- creativity: 'novel, unique approach to data analysis'

- realism: 'interpretation took into account the limitations of the study'

- applicability: 'practical, useful implications'

- style: 'well-written manuscript (clear, straightforward, easy to follow, logical)'.

These qualities also provide a valuable framework for planning and writing your own manuscript and for ensuring the intellectual integrity of your own paper. Let us examine some of these areas in more detail.

Problem statement and relevance

At the beginning of a manuscript, as the topic is introduced, it is critical to state explicitly the purpose or aim of the article and to give a clear statement of relevance. The purpose can be stated as a problem, hypothesis, or research question. Regardless of the format of your purpose or aim, the important point is that you communicate clearly to readers why you are writing the paper. This statement of purpose is, in a sense, a promise to the reader, and the rest of the paper should deliver on that promise. It is equally important to explain the relevance of the issue at hand.

A common reason for an editor to reject a manuscript without review is that the editor cannot discern a clear purpose (Bordage 2001). If there is a clear purpose, but it is not stated explicitly, the manuscript generally will not be judged favourably by reviewers.

Critics of medical education research have called for the community to explore education problems in expanded and more sophisticated ways. For example, Regehr (2004 pp. 939–942) pointed out that, over the last several decades, medical education research tended to focus on four major classes of problems: applied curriculum and teaching issues; skills and attitudes; learner characteristics; and evaluation of learners. Regehr went on to note that the nature of medical education reveals many more exciting opportunities for discovery.

As Turnbull (2011 pp. 1–2) notes:

> some education research starts with questions that are well structured and well scaffolded by existing research, and some starts with a program to be tested, but some…studies should start with a problem experienced by practitioners. By documenting occurrences of a problem, analysing them, bringing existing theory to bear, and systematically probing the surrounding circumstances, researchers bring disciplined inquiry to the search for root causes.

Context

A thorough summary and analysis of other researchers' perspectives is a way of helping readers understand your topic and the specific problem you wish to address. On one level, a literature review is a list of citations that back up a claim and demonstrate that other investigators have addressed similar problems or related issues. On a deeper level, a literature review can be a thoughtful and penetrating summary of each scholar's position on an issue or problem. It is not just a summary of each article an individual wrote; rather, it is a summary of that individual's work in a given area. It includes not only a scholar's claims, but also why or how the scholar believes those claims. It is a trace of each scholar's reasoning and provides a 'point of departure' for addressing your topic or problem.

To write a thoughtful literature review that also helps you defend and develop your problem statement, a good approach is to first summarize the approaches of each scholar in the 'conversation' and then compare and contrast them (Kaufer et al. 1989). As you compare and contrast, look for ways to group the summaries so that camps or schools of thought on the issue emerge. As in any group discussion, the scholars you have summarized will appear to agree or disagree with one another. In particular, they will vary in what they think is important or what is at stake.

As you articulate the substantive agreements and disagreements, you will discern both what matters to your topic or position and what matters to different groups of scholars. You will see how your problem statement shares elements of others' and also has its own unique features that may be important. Summarizing, analysing, and synthesizing others' research takes time and deep reading, but is invariably fruitful.

Design and power

Depending on the nature of the problem you plan to address, the design of a study can take different forms. For example, an observational study design may be valuable when you suspect that there is more to the problem than is currently known or when the problem requires clearer definition. Experimental study designs enable you to examine variables or ideas that you already know to be important. It should not be a surprise that, in the case of scientific reports, sound study design is one of the most important factors determining whether a study will be accepted or rejected. Among rejected manuscripts, the methods section is often the weakest and is also the section most likely to lead to a rejection in and of itself (Byrne 2000; Johnson 2008; Quinn and Rush 2009). A survey of *JAMA* reviewers revealed that the largest factor influencing reviewers toward recommending rejection of a manuscript was poor study design (Beckman and Cook 2007; Byrne 2000; Johnson 2008).

Some scholars have noted that many individuals who aspire to do research in medical education lack specific training in appropriate research methods (Albert et al. 2006; Gruppen 2007). This issue is gradually being addressed as more medical faculties offer such training (Carline 2004; Gruppen 2007). In addition, there are a growing number of certificate and degree programmes in medical education offered by medical schools throughout the world.

Implications, limitations, and conclusions

One way to ensure that your article contributes useful knowledge, and thus has a good chance of publication in a peer-reviewed journal, is to ask the reader to reconsider your original problem in light of how your findings advance thinking and/or practice. This is a critical point. If your work contributes new information that influences a field of inquiry, reviewers will likely rate it more favorably and an editor is more likely to select it for publication.

When discussing the potential implications of your findings, it is crucial not to overstate what can be gleaned from the data. In a discussion of results, the writer must transition from statements of fact to useful interpretations of those facts. Declaring conclusions that go beyond the study's findings communicates potential bias, irritates reviewers, and diminishes a reader's confidence in the overall integrity of the paper.

In a research report, you should discuss both the strengths and limitations of your methods as well as the potential value of and threats to the validity of your results. In a perspective type article, you should discuss the strengths and limitations of your arguments as well as the potential value of and threats to the validity of your line of reasoning. It is important to examine biases, confounding variables, and other limitations that may affect the interpretation of results or that may compromise the generalizability of findings (Bordage 2001; Bordage and Dawson 2003). You may wish to examine potential rival hypotheses and ideas.

Writing style

Poor writing is a common reason for manuscripts to be rejected, and studies have shown that executive and academic professionals—the kind of individuals who will be reviewing your paper—react negatively to errors in grammar and usage, particularly sentence fragments and run-on sentences (Beason 2001; Hairston 1981; Leonard and Gilsdorf 1990). Their negative reactions go beyond simply being annoyed by the errors themselves or by how the errors may interfere with ease of understanding the text. Rather, reviewers who encounter poor writing may assume that the writer who committed the errors does not value accuracy and/or is not a critical thinker. Once they have detected an error, reviewers begin to question other areas of the manuscript and wonder whether the writer has made other, non-writing mistakes in their observations or computations. As you can imagine, based on these observations, poor writing can lead to a disproportionately negative review.

The quality of writing is especially important for authors to consider if they hope to publish in a journal written in a language that is not their first language. If you are writing in a second language, or if you are not especially confident about your writing skills, consider getting external writing help from a mentor, an institution's research office, or a private tutor (Chipperfield et al. 2010).

Other flaws that put off reviewers include verbosity, use of jargon, and lack of clarity. These characteristics are common and can compromise reviewers' and editors' opinions of even a well-performed study (Bordage et al. 2001, p. 948; Quinn and Rush 2009). Readers need clear descriptions of how your intervention or innovation worked and how you tested it or what you learned from it in order to replicate your methods or determine how a novel programme might work at their own institution (Cook et al. 2007b).

Be alert to all aspects of your writing, from the overall organization of the paper to individual word choice. A first draft written without careful attention to matters of style and technique may be useful in getting your main ideas down and figuring out a basic structure (Quinn and Rush 2009). A standard format such as 'IMRaD' (introduction, methods, results, and discussion) does not in and of itself guarantee a clear paper, but for experimental research it is an obvious starting point and reflects the stages of the scientific method in action (Bordage et al. 2001, p. 948; International Committee of Medical Journal Editors 2010). Most papers are overly long in first draft and will benefit from judicious pruning (Dant 2011; Johnson 2008).

Wordiness is unappealing to reviewers, editors, and your general audience. Unnecessary verbosity may be taken by the reader as a sign of 'the researcher's own confusion about the elements of his or her study' (Bordage et al. 2001, p. 948; Quinn and Rush 2009). Clearly define unusual terms or acronyms in your paper at their first use, and as much as possible use a natural conversational style (Cantillon et al. 2009; Dant 2011; Johnson 2008).

Each journal has its own 'instructions for authors' (IFA). IFAs usually specify the types and categories of articles that a given journal will publish as well as its word limits, ethical guidelines, authorship criteria, and other requirements. It is important to comply with a journal's guidelines. Violating submission requirements may make it less likely that your manuscript will be considered for publication by a given journal.

Some professional writers put their writing aside for a period of time before revising it, and you may wish to consider such a tactic. After a brief lapse—perhaps a couple of days—the most glaring stylistic issues and redundancies often become more apparent (Dant 2011). The first author need not do all of the revising; one useful technique is to assign different sections of the paper to different authors, or to have different authors revise with an eye towards different aspects of the paper (e.g. redundancy, clarity, style, or consistency) (Quinn and Rush 2009). It can be useful to have colleagues, including those who are neither authors nor involved in the underlying study, read your paper before you submit. Two useful types of readers are a colleague who is as close as possible to your intended audience, and an intelligent, perceptive reader who has no connection to your field (Dant 2011; Johnson 2008; Quinn and Rush 2009). Quinn and Rush (2009 p. 638) suggest that you use your lay reader to make sure your paper's results and conclusions are clear: 'Ask them to proofread the paper. Then ask them to tell you in their own words what you found. That way you will know whether they got the message'. When all authors are satisfied that the paper is as good as it can be, it is time to submit the manuscript.

Moral integrity of a manuscript

Publication ethics has become increasingly prevalent as a topic of discussion at medical education meetings and has been addressed in several editorials and articles (Eva 2009; Kanter 2009). The need for ethical approval, when it is appropriate to obtain such approval, is important for ensuring the moral integrity of a manuscript and has become a requirement to get published in some medical education journals (although it is implemented in different ways).

While there have been few major ethical scandals in medical education research, the field has lagged behind clinical research in terms of describing and demanding human subjects' protection for experimental research (Roberts et al. 2001). Increasingly, however, editors are requiring authors to certify that their studies, surveys, and projects—if they involve human subjects—were overseen by appropriate ethical bodies and that there is a statement to such effect in the body of the manuscript. *Academic Medicine* requires a statement that a study received ethical approval, and requires that a manuscript about research not under the purview of an ethical approval body include a discussion of how risks and benefits were determined, how subjects' data were kept confidential, and other ways in which study authors and investigators treated human participants (Kanter 2009). *Medical Education* has a similar requirement for external oversight and requires that research not overseen by an external body explicitly demonstrate its compliance with the Declaration of Helsinki (a document stipulating human subjects' protection in research) (Eva 2009).

Almost all journals in which medical education is published forbid simultaneous submission of a manuscript to more than one journal. In addition to over-representing findings, there is the potential for copyright dispute and the potential waste of journal resources (Bordage et al. 2001, p. 950; Brice and Bligh 2004; Council of Science Editors 2009; International Committee of Medical Journal Editors 2010; Johnson 2008).

It is not uncommon for medical education research findings to be presented at a conference or symposium and subsequently for a full manuscript based on those findings to be submitted to a journal. This is permitted by some journals, but not others. The IFAs of the journal to which you plan to submit will likely include information about the circumstances under which they will consider publication of previously published data. Occasionally, some journals allow publication of previously published material when research findings are being presented to an entirely different, non-overlapping audience (e.g. in another language) (Brice et al. 2008; International Committee of Medical Journal Editors 2010). Other journals forbid publication of previously published material of any sort even with notice and full disclosure (Bordage et al. 2001, p. 950; Chipperfield et al. 2010).

Some journals require cover letters, others consider it optional. Some journals may offer a place for authors to enter comments or notes during the submission process (in place of a cover letter). In any case, the cover letter or 'comment box' is the appropriate place to alert the editor to previous publication of any part of your research in any venue. A call to the editorial office may be a useful preliminary step to clarify the journal's policies.

'Salami slicing'—i.e. 'dividing up a piece of research as thinly as possible to get the maximum number of papers out of it'—is a special case of results manipulation that is generally considered unethical. This type of publication can imply to readers that the evidence base for a conclusion is broader than is warranted by the results (by dint of a large number of publications). It can lend itself to problems of self-plagiarism, and can lead to 'subsequent papers, possibly with the most interesting results, [being] rejected' (Brice et al. 2008). Of course, sometimes researchers may conduct longitudinal research or conduct new analyses on previously reported data that leads to new knowledge, and therefore, new publications. This is not a breach of integrity, but researchers should be transparent to editors (usually through the cover letter) and readers (through clear explanation in the article itself) about previous publications relating to the same research project (Brice et al. 2008; Chipperfield et al. 2010). It is pertinent to note that there may be large studies and surveys conducted by multidisciplinary groups of individuals from several institutions. These studies often result in multiple publications as the data set and work of writing are divided among investigators—this may not be a case of 'salami slicing'.

Biomedical journals commonly use the International Committee of Medical Journal Editors (ICMJE) criteria to determine whether a contributor on a research project should be credited as an author (International Committee of Medical Journal Editors 2010). These criteria include:

(1) substantial contributions to conception and design, or acquisition of data, or analysis and interpretation of data; (2) drafting the article or revising it critically for important intellectual content; and (3) final approval of the version to be published. Authors should meet conditions 1, 2, and 3.

Council of Science Editors 2009; International Committee of Medical Journal Editors 2010.

In general, publication in a peer-reviewed journal will require authors to certify that they understand the criteria and that all individuals—and only those individuals—who meet authorship criteria have been listed as coauthors (Brice and Bligh 2004).

Proper attribution is a matter of intellectual and moral integrity in the course of reporting a study. Two major threats to integrity in authorship are *gift authorship* (in which someone who has not met one or more ICMJE criteria is given authorship credit) and *ghost authorship* (in which someone who has met all ICMJE criteria is not listed as an author) (Albert and Wager 2003; Brice et al. 2008; Council of Science Editors 2009; International Committee of Medical Journal Editors 2010; Sly 1997). In the case of contributions

that do not rise to the level of ICMJE criteria for authorship, such as secretarial assistance or general mentoring, formal acknowledgement at the end of the paper is an appropriate way to recognize these contributions without running afoul of ethical guidelines (Albert and Wager 2003).

The order in which authors are listed on a manuscript is an internal matter for the writing team and not generally a matter of journal policy (Council of Science Editors 2009). However, there are some widely accepted conventions (although there is variance among disciplines). The first author is 'generally held to have made the greatest contribution to the research', and first authorship usually is given the greatest weight in promotion and tenure decisions (Albert and Wager 2003; American Educational Research Association 1992 (rev. 1996, 2000, 2011); Dant 2011; Johnson 2008).

It is common for the last author to be the most senior member of the team. According to the International Committee of Medical Journal Editors (2010) 'this can be consistent with ICMJE criteria if this person was involved in study design, the interpretation of data, and critically reviewed the publication'. 'Last authorship' should not be an honorific. There are several approaches to arranging authors other than first and last: descending order of contributions and alphabetical order are two common ones (Albert and Wager 2003; Johnson 2008).

One author needs to be listed as the corresponding author for your paper. This is best decided early in the publication process (Albert and Wager 2003; Chipperfield et al. 2010). It is useful for the corresponding author to be someone who has access to all study data, who can answer questions about the study, and who can readily and rapidly communicate with other authors (Albert and Wager 2003).

It is good practice to discuss the order of authorship early in the study process (well before writing begins). As writing begins and different individuals make various contributions, the order may change—with the consensus of the group. If there is a change in the order of authorship after a manuscript is submitted to a journal, the editor may require written consent of all authors on the paper.

The classic triad of research misconduct includes plagiarism, falsification of data, and fabrication of data. It is beyond the scope of this chapter to address these issues in detail, but there is ample information on the websites of most medical schools and/or their parent universities about definitions, policies, procedures, and processes of inquiry and investigation should there be a breach of research conduct.

Plagiarism is, perhaps, the most common and familiar form of research misconduct. Most researchers are aware that verbatim copying of another's published work is plagiarism and a serious form of academic dishonesty (although there are cultural variations in the interpretation of the notion of plagiarism). Other forms of plagiarism, though, are less obvious. Self-plagiarism is potentially problematic despite the fact that it does not entail a researcher claiming another's work or ideas as their own, but because authors typically assign copyright to a publisher or professional association (Brice et al. 2008; Johnson 2008).

The notion of 'fair use'—a doctrine of United States copyright law—or 'fair dealing'—a doctrine of Canadian copyright law—is not an appropriate justification for plagiarizing even small portions of others' writings (Sly 1997). It is true that guidelines are not always clear as to exactly how much of an unacknowledged quotation is considered an infringement, nor exactly how and under what conditions to cite ideas that may have been inspired by another's work. Nonetheless, 'the appropriation of ideas, data, or methods from others without adequate permission or acknowledgement' is plagiarism, and it is vital to acknowledge all works from which you have taken ideas for your study (Council of Science Editors 2009).

Submitting a manuscript to a journal

There are several factors to consider when deciding to which journal to submit your manuscript, including: the focus areas of the journal; whether your desired audience reads the journal; how your paper will be distributed (free or paid access); whether your paper will be published online only or in print only or available in both media; and the urgency of your research findings or message (e.g. a perspective article about health policy related to pending legislation may not be relevant after the legislation is passed or rejected) (Chipperfield et al. 2010; Quinn and Rush 2009).

Ideally, you would like your article to appear in the most prestigious and competitive journal that your intended audience reads. It may be worthwhile to first send your article to a journal that is 'a bit of a long-shot', but if you do so, have a backup in mind in case your paper is rejected (Quinn and Rush 2009). Some experienced authors say that if your manuscripts are being accepted for publication by the first journals to which you submit, then you are not 'aiming high enough'—i.e. you cannot know if your paper would be accepted by a more competitive journal, unless you submit to that journal and take on the risk of rejection (Quinn and Rush 2009).

It is imperative to be familiar with each journal to which you are considering submitting a manuscript. Read a few issues of the journal that were published in the past year or so to gain a first-hand, in-depth understanding of that journal's article types, the nature of articles that are published, and how those articles are structured. Compare the articles that have been published with your manuscript to determine if the journal in question is a good fit. Also, familiarize yourself with the journal's submission requirements. Different journals have different submission requirements that may affect how you prepare your manuscript, including the structure and organization of the article, the word count, the format of references, the communication of ethical approval, and the disclosure of conflicts (Quinn and Rush 2009).

Each journal has its own 'personality' and editorial priorities can vary over time. Ask 'fellow authors, trusted peers, academic mentors, and librarians/information specialists' (Chipperfield et al. 2010), and read editorials and instructions for authors to help get a sense of the current focus of a particular journal. If studies similar to yours have been published in a journal, then it may be receptive to your manuscript—if your paper advances what has already been published (Chipperfield et al. 2010). In selecting a journal, you may wish to consider one that has published articles in your manuscript's bibliography.

There are three major options for publishing scholarly work in medical education (see fig. 55.1):

1. Publishing in one of the major journals that devote most or all content to medical education (e.g. *Academic Medicine*, *Medical Education*, *Medical Teacher*, *Advances in Health Sciences Education*, *Teaching and Learning in Medicine*).

2. Publishing in a journal dedicated to a particular specialty and that devotes most or all content to medical education (e.g. *Academic Radiology*, *Academic Psychiatry*, and many others).

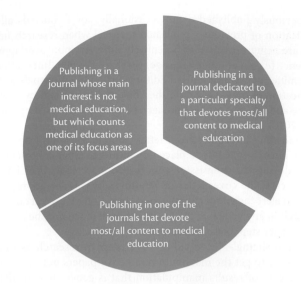

Figure 55.1 Options for publishing scholarly work in medical education.

3. Publishing in a journal whose main interest is not medical education, but which counts medical education as part of its focus areas (e.g. *BMJ*, *Journal of General Internal Medicine*, and the *American Journal of Surgery* publish some medical education content, and *JAMA* publishes an annual issue devoted to medical education). Medical education articles with interdisciplinary approaches are occasionally published in law, general education, bioethics, and general science journals.

Journals dedicated to medical education publish almost half of the scholarly articles in the field. About one-third are published in specialty journals, such as *Annals of Internal Medicine*; approximately one-tenth are published in other types of journals, including basic science journals; and a small percentage are published in general medical journals, such as *JAMA* and *BMJ* (Baernstein et al. 2007). Most medical education articles are published in English, although medical education research takes place worldwide. The bulk of studies to date have been conducted in North America and Europe, but an increasing number of submissions to medical education journals are coming from Asia and Australia (Baernstein et al. 2007; Rotgans 2012).

A variety of types of articles are found in medical education journals (Academic Medicine 2008; Advances in Health Sciences Education 2012; Medical Education 2012; Medical Teacher 2012). Figure 55.2 shows the most common types.

Journals provide guidance for prospective authors about article types, ethical guidelines, word limits, and formatting requirements. Often this can be found on the journal's website under a title like 'Instructions for Authors' or 'Author Guidelines'. If guidelines are not readily apparent when you examine the journal's website, contact the editorial office and request a copy. It is vital to carefully read and follow the guidelines for the journal to which you are submitting a manuscript.

An editor-in-chief usually has 'responsibility, authority, and accountability for the editorial content of the journal, an arrangement that is usually referred to as "editorial independence"' (Council of Science Editors 2009). Editorial independence implies that an editor-in-chief is free to make publication decisions based on the strength of scholarship and other editorial considerations,

1. Original medical education research: reports of experimental, quasiexperimental, and non-experimental (longitudinal, observational, or epidemiological) studies

2. Systematic, critical, and thematic reviews

3. Letters to the editor responding to previously published content

4. In-depth, scholarly commentary pieces, often with significant, but not extensive citations to the literature; these may be author-initiated or they may be by invitation only

5. Scholarly perspective articles that examine important issues and controversies in medical education; some may propose new theories or hypotheses

6. Book reviews

7. Special, recurring features: e.g. *Academic Medicine* publishes Point-Counterpoint essays, a Medicine & the Arts column, and a Teaching & Learning Moments feature. *Medical Education* publishes a Really Good Stuff supplement. *Medical Teacher* publishes How We…, Twelve Tips, And Finally…, and Around the World. *Advances in Health Sciences Education* publishes Methodologist's Corner and If I Had Known Then. Read guidelines carefully if you are interested in submitting for a special section, as journals often have strict requirements for structure, focus, and word count.

Figure 55.2 Types of articles in medical education journals.

and that those decisions are not influenced by the financial, political, social, or advocacy concerns of the journal's owner. It is the editor-in-chief, sometimes in consultation with associate and assistant editors and a managing editor, who ultimately determines which articles are accepted, how to organize and structure the journal, when and whether to publish supplements, and when accepted articles should appear (Council of Science Editors 2009; International Committee of Medical Journal Editors 2010). Editors have a responsibility to refrain from exhibiting bias and should avoid conflicts of interest (Council of Science Editors 2009).

Virtually all journals now require electronic submissions. Author guidelines will indicate if your paper needs to be in a specific file format. Different publications have different requirements for the content required on a title page and the formats preferred for figures and artwork. If guidelines on a topic are vague or absent, an email to the editorial office may save time and prevent reformatting at a later stage (Chipperfield et al. 2010). Many journals also require that copyright documentation and certification of authorship be submitted.

After your manuscript is submitted, the journal will respond with notification that your submission has been accepted. Most medical education journals use a web-based submission management system that allows authors to log in and check the status of manuscripts.

Different journals vary as to whether all submissions are sent to experts for peer review or whether some manuscripts are rejected without review (i.e. based only on screening by the editor and/or editorial staff). In some cases, the editorial office will check submissions to make sure they fit the scope of the journal and meet baseline standards before they are sent to peer reviewers. In other cases, all manuscripts may be sent for peer review (Council of Science Editors 2009; Hojat et al. 2003). Journals also differ on the degree to which editorial board members play a role in the review process.

Initial screening, for those journals that use it, usually takes between 1 and 4 weeks. Peer review, of course, will require

additional time. Two to four weeks is a reasonable period for turnaround, but several factors can lengthen the process: editors and editorial staff may require additional time to identify a reviewer with appropriate expertise who is available (to get a particular expert to review a manuscript, especially one who is highly sought on a specific topic, an editor may need to offer that expert additional time to do the review); the initial reviewers may disagree, and the editor may choose to send the manuscript to another reviewer to 'break the tie'; or personal circumstances may cause a reviewer to take an unusually long time to review a manuscript (Hojat et al. 2003). Sometimes additional or special reviews of a manuscript are required to examine in more detail issues of experimental design, choice of statistical tests, or appropriateness of special methods.

After review, you will receive a letter with an editorial decision. If your manuscript is rejected with an invitation to resubmit, you may choose to edit the manuscript and resend it, at which time your revised submission will generally go through some form of review again, either internally by the editor (who may or may not consult associate editors, assistant editors, a managing editor, editorial staff, or editorial board members), or external peer review. If an article is accepted, the journal will prepare it for publication. It will be copyedited and typeset, and the authors will have an opportunity to respond to the copyeditor's changes. Some journals, such as *Academic Medicine*, engage in substantive editing, in which case a professional staff editor will work with the author to improve the organization of content, strengthen arguments, and tighten prose.

The time between acceptance of a manuscript and publication of the article is changing. With traditional print journals, editing and publishing schedules required editorial staff to work 3 or 4 months ahead—i.e. in January, the staff works on the April issue. However, with online publication of articles, the lag between acceptance and publication can be much shorter. More and more journals, even those with print versions, are publishing articles electronically ahead of print.

Many journals require that a cover letter be sent with a submission. If a cover letter is required, it need not be elaborate and can be brief. Include the title and authors of your manuscript, indicate the article type (e.g. research report), and if appropriate, specify to which section of the journal your paper is being submitted. If part of your work has been presented in another venue (e.g. a conference), it is good practice to provide relevant details in the cover letter (Chipperfield et al. 2010; International Committee of Medical Journal Editors 2010). If applicable, you should also mention regulatory and ethical clearances and information about financial and other conflicts of interest (Chipperfield et al. 2010; International Committee of Medical Journal Editors 2010). Some journals do not require a cover letter, but instead require the authors to respond to a series of questions that address the aforementioned issues. In this case, there is usually a 'comment box' where authors can provide additional information as appropriate.

The title you choose comprises the most important words in your paper. This is so because the words you select play a critical role in declaring what the paper is about, in attracting a reader's attention, and in how your article will be stored and retrieved in article indexing systems. Perhaps most importantly, the title of a paper is a promise. It is a promise to the reader of what to expect; if the article does not deliver on that promise, reviewers will not rate the paper highly and editors will be less likely to accept the paper for publication (Bordage et al. 2001, p. 945).

While you may draft your paper using a working title, you should refine and polish the title before you submit (Dant 2011). An effective title should be appealing and interesting but also clear, informative, and concise.

Many journals require a title page in a particular format indicating such information as the affiliations of the authors, contact information for the corresponding author, word count, and other data. Follow the author guidelines carefully on this point.

An abstract is a clear and concise summary of your article. It is not simply an excerpt of the introduction or background paragraphs. An abstract is required for some, but not all, types of article. For example, in some journals a commentary requires an abstract, but not in other journals. Consult a particular journal's instructions for authors to determine if an abstract is required for the article type you intend to submit and to note abstract word limits; whether the abstract should be structured or unstructured; and other pertinent guidance.

While your abstract will likely be the last part of the paper you write (since it is a summary of the entire paper), it is important to give it careful thought and attention because your abstract, along with the title, is the first impression readers will get of your paper—and, in some cases, the only impression (e.g. if an author retrieves a few hundred citations to prepare a literature review, the author may screen articles on the bases of the title and abstract) (Quinn and Rush 2009). The word count for the abstract—usually around 250 words—means that every word must be carefully chosen if you want to make your abstract as informative and useful as possible. Note that different journals have different requirements for abstracts, so you may need to revise your abstract if you resubmit your article to another journal after a rejection.

A key distinction in writing an abstract is whether to use a structured or unstructured format. Journals often specify in the instructions for authors which type of abstract to use for which article type (e.g. a structured abstract often is required for a research report and an unstructured abstract may be required for a descriptive article). Structured abstracts for experimental studies may include some or all of the following categories: objective, purpose, or aim of the study; design; setting; participants; interventions; outcome measures; results; and conclusions. Review articles often use a structured format with purpose, data identification, study selection, data extraction, results of data synthesis, and conclusions (Bordage et al. 2001, p. 946; Cook et al. 2007a).

While structured abstracts work well for experimental and review articles, descriptive articles and commentaries lend themselves to a more flexible summary format. Unstructured abstracts should emphasize the most important and unique aspects of your paper and clearly state how the arguments in your paper fit into the ongoing scholarly conversation about your topic (International Committee of Medical Journal Editors 2010). Three common pitfalls in abstracts are 'inconsistencies between abstract and text, information present in the abstract but not the text, and conclusions not justified by the information in the abstract' (Bordage et al. 2001, p. 947).

Peer review

The process of peer review provides editors and authors with valuable feedback. Editors benefit from the assessments of manuscripts by experts who comment on the importance and relevance of the problem or question, the quality of logic and reasoning, the soundness of arguments, and the strength of conclusions. If the paper is about an experiment or other type of intervention, peer reviewers may comment on the study design, the appropriateness of methods used to investigate the research question, the validity of results, and the degree to which the conclusions are supported by the results.

Reviewers' feedback helps authors improve their papers by making revisions based on reviewer concerns or by explaining to editors—and perhaps to readers of the manuscript once published—why they disagree with reviewers' concerns (Purcell et al. 1998). In general, editors select reviewers who are scholars and who 'have both knowledge and experience of the manuscript topic' (Bligh 1998). These reviewers examine the manuscript to determine how the paper fits into the intellectual context of the discipline at hand, and provide comments as to how the paper could be improved (Bligh 1998; Hojat et al. 2003). In some cases, reviewers may make recommendations as to whether a paper should be published, and reviewers' opinions are strongly correlated with a journal's decision to accept or reject a manuscript (Bligh 1998).

As mentioned previously, some journals send all submitted manuscripts to peer review, while others use an initial screening process at the editorial level to reject some articles at this stage:

> editors may sometimes reject manuscripts without external peer review to make the best use of their resources. Reasons for this practice are usually that the manuscript is outside the scope of the journal, does not meet the journal's quality standard or is of limited scientific merit, or lacks originality or novel information.
>
> Council of Science Editors 2009

A review process can be double-blinded, in which the authors do not know the reviewers' identities and the reviewers do not know the authors' identities. Alternatively, a review process can be single-blinded, in which authors do not know the reviewers' identities, but reviewers can see the identities of the authors. There are advocates for open review, in which authors' and reviewers' identities are known to one another (and to readers as well, if the reviews are published with the article). In practice, even with blinding, it may be possible for reviewers to guess authors' identities, especially in a small field of study (Council of Science Editors 2009; Hojat et al. 2003).

Reviewers submit their comments to journal editors. In some cases, reviewers rate manuscripts and/or answer questions on a standardized form. Editors often forward reviewers' complete comments to authors, but may choose to forward selected points from the reviews. Some editors will not send to authors criticism that is unnecessarily personal or vituperative (Bligh 1998; Council of Science Editors 2009; Hojat et al. 2003).

Editors strive to select reviewers with relevant expertise in the matter at hand (Council of Science Editors 2009). Editors must ensure that they solicit sufficient assessments and opinions to make an informed decision on a manuscript's scholarly merits, which is why most journals seek more than one review for each paper selected for external peer review (Bligh 1998; Council of Science Editors 2009). While editors must be mindful of the need for a reasonably quick turnaround time, they must also be careful not to overburden their most reliable reviewers by requesting too many reviews in too short a period of time (Council of Science Editors 2009).

Often when you submit a paper, the journal will offer you the opportunity to recommend potential reviewers or to indicate individuals who should not review your manuscript. Journals may ask authors for reasons to justify their choices to help editors decide whether the requests are reasonable (International Committee of Medical Journal Editors 2010). Of course, it is unethical to suggest reviewers who have inherent conflicts of interest, such as close colleagues at an author's institution; advisors or mentors of an author;

or individuals who could benefit financially or otherwise if a manuscript is published.

Even the most positive reviews usually include criticism and suggestions for changes. Some of these may be minor matters of grammar or style, while others may point to substantive concerns with a literature review, theoretical grounding, or methods. You may or may not agree with a reviewer's recommendations, but it is best to respond to them in one way or another—i.e. either revise your manuscript to address the reviewer's concern or indicate (in a cover letter to the editor or as additional explanation in the manuscript itself) what is the concern and why you do not agree with it.

If your manuscript is rejected by a journal, reviewers' comments can be helpful in revising your paper for another journal (Chipperfield et al. 2010; Hojat et al. 2003; Woolley and Barron 2009). In fact, it may be crucial to address reviewer comments because when you submit your manuscript to another journal, that journal may, by happenstance, send the manuscript to the same reviewer. This is likely to happen in relatively small disciplines or if your article deals with a specialized topic for which there are few experts. If a reviewer receives your manuscript for a second time and sees no revisions or explanations based on their original concerns, the reviewer almost assuredly will recommend that the journal reject the manuscript.

It is perfectly acceptable to disagree with a reviewer's recommendations, but your written response should be accompanied by a clear rationale and be supported by citations for substantive disputes (Chipperfield et al. 2010; Johnson 2008; Quinn and Rush 2009). The most straightforward way to organize your responses to reviewers' comments is to reply on a point-by-point basis, citing the parts of your paper where changes have been made or discussing why you chose not to change your paper (Johnson 2008; Woolley and Barron 2009). Box 55.1 shows an example of how to do this:

Box 55.1 How to respond to a peer reviewer

Cover letter:

Dear <editor-in-chief>:

Enclosed please find the revised manuscript titled <name of paper>. We have addressed the reviewers' valuable suggestions and include a list of our responses and revisions.

Sincerely, <authors>

Reviewers' comments and our responses

1. Reviewer 1: *Explain why Smith received his PhD in Germany rather than the US (p. 2)*
   Response: We added historical background about the paucity of PhDs awarded in the US around the time Smith was a student.
   Where changed in manuscript: p. 3–4, under 'Smith's Background'
   New text in manuscript: At the time Smith was a student, most American graduate students pursued their PhD degrees abroad, generally in Germany or France. In fact, in 1900, only 342 people earned PhD degrees from institutions in the United States, and this was a nearly eight-fold increase over 1876.
2. Reviewer 1: *(Reviewer 1's next comment)*
3. And so forth, addressing each comment of each reviewer.

The process of responding to reviewers' questions and concerns presents an opportunity to learn more both about your topic and how to write for a particular audience. Even if a reviewer is wrong about how they interpret something you wrote, it is valuable feedback about how at least some readers will respond to your prose. In such a case, you may improve the text by adding additional explanation or clarifying statements.

Just as all authors must agree on the content of the manuscript to be submitted, so must all authors agree on revisions. All authors should be involved in the revision process and should approve the revised manuscript prior to resubmission (Quinn and Rush 2009).

During the peer review process, you are entitled to certain ethical protections. Reviewers are not allowed to share your work with others before publication or to use ideas from your manuscript in their own work before the article is published. Also, reviewers are not allowed to retain copies of your manuscript after they review it (Council of Science Editors 2009; International Committee of Medical Journal Editors 2010). Reviewers should also not '[propose] changes that appear to merely support the reviewer's own work or hypotheses' (Council of Science Editors 2009).

A reviewer should decline to review a paper if they are aware of a conflict of interest; the same considerations that would bar you from ethically recommending someone to review your paper should also bar those same people from reviewing the paper if requested to do so by the journal (American Educational Research Association 1992 (rev. 1996, 2000, 2011); Bligh 1998; Council of Science Editors 2009; Hojat et al. 2003; International Committee of Medical Journal Editors 2010). The journal to which you have submitted your manuscript may also have policies regarding communication between an author and a reviewer while a paper is under consideration. It is good practice to become familiar with these policies and to follow them carefully (Council of Science Editors 2009).

In the event that you receive a review that you believe to be unfairly biased, you can discuss your concerns with the editor working with your submission or with the editor-in-chief of the journal (Chipperfield et al. 2010; Hojat et al. 2003).

Editorial decisions about manuscripts

After the peer review process is complete, you will receive correspondence from the editorial office with a decision about your manuscript. While editorial decisions and their wording vary among journals, most journals use some form of the following four decisions: (1) Accept; (2) Accept pending minor revisions, or Conditional accept; (3) Reconsider after major revisions, or Reject with option to revise; and (4) Reject.

Journals may use other decisions that are, in essence, variations of one of the aforementioned options. For example, a journal may issue, depending on the specific circumstances, a decision of 'reject with invitation to submit a letter to the editor' or a decision of 'reject with option to submit a new manuscript on the same topic'.

Outright acceptance of an initial submission to any journal is exceedingly rare (Bligh 1998; Chipperfield et al. 2010; Council of Science Editors 2009; Hojat et al. 2003; Quinn and Rush 2009). In virtually all cases, a decision to accept a manuscript for publication will be conditioned on incorporating the suggestions made by peer reviewers and/or by the editorial staff (i.e. if you submit a manuscript that receives excellent reviews, it still is unlikely that the journal will issue decision #1; rather, the journal will first issue decision #2 and then issue decision #1 after you have made appropriate revisions and improvements). After acceptance for publication your manuscript will be copyedited and typeset. You will have the opportunity to review your paper before publication and to sign off on any changes made by the editorial staff. If you notice small errors in the paper that have been missed in the earlier stages of review, you will generally be able to fix them before publication.

If your article is of particular public interest, journal staff may release some findings to the media around the publication date. If this happens in advance of your publication date, the materials will usually be embargoed; selected journalists may receive an advance copy of your article shortly before publication but will be requested not to write news stories about it until it is officially released. The editorial staff of the journal should let you know if they will be preparing press materials on your behalf (Council of Science Editors 2009). Generally, confidentiality policies still apply in these circumstances, and you should refrain from discussing your accepted manuscript publicly until it has been published; however, in some cases (e.g. if your work has public health implications), this prohibition may be waived (International Committee of Medical Journal Editors 2010).

Editors have an affirmative obligation to 'maintain the integrity of the literature by publishing errata or corrections identifying anything of significance, retractions, and expressions of concern as quickly as possible' (Council of Science Editors 2009). While authors can let editors know that a correction or retraction may be necessary, the editor of the journal in which the work was published is usually the final arbiter (Council of Science Editors 2009). It is a normal part of the scholarly enterprise that research findings, evidence, and other conclusions may be superseded by new findings and evidence. This situation does not require correction or retraction in a journal; the 'correction' occurs by the publication of updated scholarly work that advances knowledge about the issues in question. Actions of correction or retraction by a journal are reserved for material errors or misstatements in a published work, or when there has been a lapse of integrity in the conduct or reporting of a study. Once an editor has determined that a correction or retraction is appropriate, it should be published as quickly as is practical (Council of Science Editors 2009).

An intermediate step before retraction or correction is an 'expression of concern', in which an editor 'draw[s] attention to possible problems, but does not go so far as to retract or correct an article' (Council of Science Editors 2009). Errata are generally published in a prominent fashion and indexed in services like MEDLINE to facilitate easy retrieval (Council of Science Editors 2009).

For most journals, a reject decision is final. If your manuscript is rejected, you and your coauthors may wish to revise it based on editorial and reviewer feedback, and submit it to another journal. If the manuscript has merit, most likely you will find a journal to publish it (Chipperfield et al. 2010; Hojat et al. 2003; Weber et al. 1998; Woolley and Barron 2009).

Whether a rejected manuscript is publishable in another journal depends, in part, on whether it has fatal flaws of conception, design, or methodology. The review comments and the editorial decision letter for the rejected manuscript can provide valuable information in this regard.

Conclusions

◆ Good writing reflects good work and good work reflects good thinking.

◆ High-quality writing starts with a sound project, that is planned and executed well, and that adheres to the highest standards of intellectual and moral integrity.

◆ High-quality writing is based on sound arguments, solid evidence, and valid conclusions. There are no shortcuts to good writing; it takes time.

◆ Thinking comprehensively and deeply about a problem, executing a well-planned project, and publishing a good article in a good journal is a most stimulating and rewarding experience.

References

Academic Medicine (2008) Editorial Policy, Publication Ethics, and Complete Instructions for Authors [Online]. http://journals.lww.com/academicmedicine/Pages/InstructionsforAuthors.aspx Accessed 16 July 2012

Advances in Health Sciences Education (2012) Aims and Scope [online]. http://www.springer.com/education+%26+language?SGWID=0-40406-9-10459-print_view=aimsAndScopes Accessed 16 July 2012

Albert, T., Hodges, B., and Regehr, G. (2006) Research in Medical Education: Balancing Service and Science. *Adv Health Sci Educ.* 12(1): 103–115

Albert, T. and Wager, E. (2003) How to handle authorship disputes: a guide for new researchers [Online]. Committee on Publication Ethics (COPE). http://publicationethics.org/files/u2/2003pdf12.pdf Accessed 16 July 2012

American Educational Research Association (1992 (rev. 1996, 2000, 2011)) Ethical standards of the American Educational Research Association [Online]. http://www.aera.net/AboutAERA/AERARulesPolicies/CodeofEthics/tabid/10200/Default.aspx Accessed 16 July 2012

Baernstein, A., Liss, K., Carney, P., and Elmore, J. (2007) Trends in study methods used in undergraduate medical education research, 1969–2007. *JAMA.* 298(9): 1038–1045

Beason, L. (2001) Ethos and error: how business people react to errors. *Coll Comp Commun.* 53(1): 33–64

Beckman, T. and Cook, D. (2007) Developing Scholarly Projects in Education: A Primer for Medical Teachers. *Med Teach.* 29: 210–218

Bligh, J. (1998) What happens to manuscripts submitted to the journal? *Med Educ.* 32(6): 567–570

Bordage, G. (2001) Reasons reviewers reject and accept manuscripts: the strengths and weaknesses in medical education reports. *Acad Med.* 76(9): 889–896

Bordage, G., Caelleigh, A., Steinecke, A., et al. (2001) Review Criteria for Research Manuscripts. *Acad Med.* 76(9): 897–978

Bordage, G. and Dawson, B. (2003) Experimental study design and grant writing in eight steps and 28 questions. *Med Educ.* 37(4): 376–385

Brice, J. and Bligh J. (2004) Author misconduct: not just the editors' responsibility. *Med Educ.* 39(1): 83–89

Brice, J., Bligh, J., Bordage, G., et al. (2008) Publishing ethics in medical education journals. *Acad Med.* 84(10 Suppl.): S132–S134

Byrne, D. (2000) Common reasons for rejecting manuscripts at medical journals: a survey of editors and peer reviewers. *Sci Ed.* 23(2): 39–44

Cantillon, P., McLeod, P., Razack, S., Snell, L., and Steinert, Y. (2009) Lost in translation: the challenges of global communication in medical education publishing. *Med Educ.* 43(7): 615–620

Carline, J. (2004) Funding medical education research: opportunities and issues. *Acad Med.* 79(10): 918–924

Chipperfield, L., Citrome, L., Clark, J., et al. (2010) Authors' submission toolkit: a practical guide to getting your research published. *Curr Med Res Opin.* 26(8): 1967–1982

Cook, D., Beckman, T., and Bordage, G. (2007a) A systematic review of titles and abstracts of experimental studies in medical education: many informative elements missing. *Med Educ*. 41(11): 1074–1081

Cook, D., Beckman, T., and Bordage, G. (2007b) Quality of reporting of experimental studies in medical education: a systematic review. *Med Educ*. 41(8): 737–745

Council of Science Editors (2009) CSE's White Paper on Promoting Integrity in Scientific Journal Publications [Online] (Updated 2009) http://www.councilscienceeditors.org/files/public/entire_whitepaper.pdf Accessed 14 March 2013

Dant, C. (2011) Teaching effective writing skills at an academic cancer center: reflections of an erstwhile journal editor and writer. *J Cancer Educ*. 26(2): 208–211

Eva, K. (2009) Research ethics requirements for *Medical Education. Med Educ*. 43: 194–195

Gruppen, L. (2007) Improving medical education research. *Teach Learn Med*. 19(4): 331–335

Hairston, M. (1981) Not all errors are created equal: nonacademic readers in the professions respond to lapses in usage. *College English*. 43(8): 794–806

Hojat, M., Gonnella, J., and Caelleigh, A. (2003) Impartial judgment by the 'gatekeepers' of science: fallibility and accountability in the peer review process. *Adv Health Sci Educ*. 8(1): 75–96

International Committee of Medical Journal Editors (2010) Uniform Requirements for Manuscripts Submitted to Biomedical Journals: Writing and Editing for Biomedical Publication [Online] (Updated April 2009) http://www.icmje.org/urm_main.html Accessed 16 July 2012

Johnson, T. (2008) Tips on how to write a paper. *J Am Acad Dermatol*. 59(6): 1064–1069

Kanter, S. (2009) Ethical approval for studies involving human participants: academic medicine's new policy. *Acad Med*. 84(2): 149–150

Kaufer, D., Geisler, C., and Neuwirth, C. (1989) *Arguing from Sources: Exploring Issues through Reading and Writing*. New York: Harcourt Brace Jovanovich

Leonard, D. and Gilsdorf, J. (1990) Language in change: academics' and executives' perceptions of usage errors. *J Business Commun*. 27(2): 137–158

Medical Education (2012) Author Guidelines [Online] http://onlinelibrary.wiley.com/journal/10.1111/%28ISSN%291365–2923/homepage/ForAuthors.html Accessed 16 July 2012

Medical Teacher (2012) Information for Authors [Online] http://www.medicalteacher.org/MEDTEACH_wip/pages/authinfo.htm Accessed 16 July 2012

National Commission on Writing in America's Schools and Colleges (2003) The neglected 'R': The need for a writing revolution. College Entrance Examination Board. p. 13. http://www.host-collegeboard.com/advocacy/writing/publications.html Accessed 19 July 2012

Norman, G. (2002) Research in medical education: three decades of progress. *BMJ*. 324: 1560

Purcell, G., Donovan, S., and Davidoff, F. (1998) Changes to manuscripts during the editorial process. *JAMA*. 280(3): 227–228

Quinn, C. and Rush, A. (2009) Writing and publishing your research findings. *J Invest Med*. 57(5): 634–639

Regehr, G. (2004) Trends in medical education research. *Acad Med*. 79(10): 939–947

Roberts, L., Geppert, C., Connor, R., Nguyen, K., and Warner, T. (2001) An invitation for medical educators to focus on ethical and policy issues in research and scholarly practice. *Acad Med*. 76(9): 876–885

Rotgans, J. (2012) The themes, institutions, and people of medical education research 1988–2010: content analysis of abstracts from six journals. *Adv Health Sci Educ*.17(4): 515–527

Sly, R. (1997) Ethical science writing and responsible medical practice. *Ann Allergy Asthma Immunol*. 79(6): 489–494

Turnbull, B. (2011) Practice-engaged research and development in education (Report) Community for Advancing Discovery Research in Education (CADRE). Newton MA: Education Devlopment Center Inc.

Weber, E., Callaham, M., Wears, R., Barton, C., and Young, G. (1998) Unpublished Research from a Medical Specialty Meeting: Why Investigators Fail to Publish. *JAMA*. 280(3): 257–259

Woolley, K. and Barron, J. (2009) Handling Manuscript Rejection: Insights from Evidence and Experience. *Chest*. 135(2): 573–577

CHAPTER 56

Scholarship in medical education

Christie L. Palladino, Maryellen E. Gusic,
Ruth-Marie E. Fincher, and Janet P. Hafler

What we need, then, in higher education is a reward system
that reflects the diversity of our institutions and the breadth
of scholarship, as well. The challenge is to strike a balance
among teaching, research, and service, a position supported
by two-thirds of today's faculty who conclude that 'at my
institution, we need better ways, besides publication, to
evaluate scholarly performance of faculty.

Ernest Boyer

Reproduced from The Carnegie Foundation for the Advancement of
Teaching (1989) The Condition of the Professoriate: Attitudes and Trends.
Princeton: Carnegie Foundation for the Advancement of Teaching,
with permission from the Carnegie Foundation

Evolution of the definition of educational scholarship

A 1980 report from the Carnegie Foundation, *College: The Undergraduate Experience in America*, called for the reward of faculty who devoted professional time to students and urged an expansion of the scope of scholarship to encompass all dimensions of academic work, including teaching (Boyer 1987). Faculty data collected over decades demonstrated that the majority of faculty viewed teaching as a central focus of their role, but university reward systems remained predominately weighted to reward research (Carnegie Foundation 1989; Glassick 2000). In 1990, Ernest Boyer's *Scholarship Reconsidered*, also published by the Carnegie Foundation, explicitly delineated four dimensions of scholarship:

1. Scholarship of Discovery—inquiry contributing to human knowledge and/or the intellectual climate.

2. Scholarship of Integration—making connections across disciplines and synthesizing sources of knowledge to bring new insights.

3. Scholarship of Application—applying knowledge to engage the larger society and to address important current issues.

4. Scholarship of Teaching—not only transmitting, but also transforming and advancing knowledge through teaching activities (Boyer 1990; Glassick 2000; Maurana et al. 2001).

Boyer argued for recognition and reward of faculty in all four dimensions, including teaching (Boyer 1990; Glassick 2000; Maurana et al. 2001). This expanded scope of scholarship formed a conceptual framework in which research was one, but no longer the only, recognized form of scholarship.

Building on Boyer's work, others refined the evolving definition of scholarship (Bok 1990; Diamond and Adam 1995, 2000; Huber and Hutchings 2005; Hutchings and Shulman 1999; Kreber and Cranton 2000; Rice 1992, 1996; Shulman 1999; Trigwell et al. 2000). Yet, the scholarship of teaching remained the most difficult of the four dimensions to define, and this generated discussion about the distinction between the quality of teaching and scholarship related to teaching (Glassick 2000). Hutchings and Shulman (1999) addressed these concerns by asserting that all scholarship, including the scholarship of teaching, must be presented on a platform that is: (1) 'made public'; (2) 'available for peer review and critique'; and (3) 'able to be reproduced and built on by other scholars' (Glassick, 2000, p. 879). All three criteria must be met for a product to meet the definition of scholarship. Shulman further defined the scholarship of teaching as including the scholarship of learning, emphasizing the importance of the interaction between teacher and learner, and of scholarship around the educational process itself (Morahan and Fleetwood 2008; Shulman 1999). As a consequence, all forms of scholarship, including research, are defined by: a product presented on a platform that can be peer reviewed to assess quality, and made public for others to learn from or build upon.

Despite the reconceptualization of scholarship, few medical schools modified their reward systems to recognize faculty for excellence in teaching or scholarship related to education. The terms teaching and education were often used interchangeably, excluding other educational activities from consideration in academic reward systems. In an effort to create a framework for recognizing faculty for their contributions as educators, the Association of American Medical Colleges (AAMC) Group on Educational Affairs (GEA) initiated a longitudinal educational scholarship project to recognize and reward faculty who support and advance medical education (Simpson and Fincher 1999; Fincher et al. 2000). In two publications, the group defined educational scholarship, outlined the infrastructure needed to support it, and provided examples of scholarship related to educational activities (Simpson and Fincher 1999; Fincher et al. 2000). Educator activities can be documented and assessed in five categories: teaching, curriculum development, advising and mentoring, educational leadership and administration, and learner assessment (Simpson et al. 2004). The 2006 GEA Consensus Conference on Educational Scholarship reaffirmed these five categories of educator activities and proposed the Q^2Engage model of educational scholarship (fig. 56.1) (Simpson et al. 2007a). The Q^2Engage model outlines standards to document educational activities and the pathway to scholarship:

1. $Q^{2=}$ Quantity and Quality: Educational excellence, demonstrated by documenting quantity (i.e. frequency of activities) and quality (i.e. evidence of the effectiveness of the activity).

2. Engagement with the educational community. Engagement involves two complementary processes:

   a. Taking a scholarly approach, defined as demonstrating how one's work is informed by the field of education and

   b. Producing educational scholarship, defined by demonstrating that one's work contributes to the field of education (Simpson et al. 2007a).

Table 56.1 contains questions that are aligned with the Q^2 Engage model and that address how to document the quantity and quality of educator activities and engagement with the education community (Simpson et al. 2007a, p. 1006).

Consistent with the work of the GEA, faculty at the University of Toronto linked educational activity and scholarship by defining *creative professional activity* (CPA) as a criterion for promotion (Levinson et al. 2006). CPA includes three components:

1. *Professional innovation* includes development and/or use of an innovative product or introduction or dissemination of a novel technology, process, or concept even if the faculty member was not personally involved in development of the product.

   Example: A medical educator discovers a new teaching method from the literature, implements it, tests its effectiveness in the classroom, and writes guidelines for use of the new method for colleagues.

2. *Exemplary professional practice* means that one's practice is not only worthy of being copied but actually has been 'emulated by students and colleagues to the point that the individual has become a role model within the profession' (Levinson et al. 2006, p. 569).

   Example: A faculty member establishes a novel interprofessional simulation laboratory to teach clinical skills. Faculty members from other institutions visit the lab to learn about the innovative model and then emulate the model at their centres. The developer is invited to give presentations about the model.

3. *Contributions to the development of the discipline* are often accomplished when one is serving in a leadership role in which a person contributes significantly to the discipline by serving in the role. Simply serving in an executive position in an organization does not in itself constitute 'contribution to development of the discipline' (Levinson et al. 2006, p. 569).

   Example: As a leader of a national organization, a faculty member develops guidelines for the assessment of clinical competencies and disseminates these guidelines to form new national standards (Levinson et al. 2006).

Evolution of the assessment of educational scholarship

Scholarship of educational discovery (research) may be evaluated using the same parameters as research in other fields, typically through peer-reviewed publications. However, other products encompassed by the broadened definition of scholarship were unlikely to become accepted as legitimate forms of scholarship in academic reward systems until a framework to evaluate the quality of educational scholarship was clearly delineated. In response to this need, the Carnegie Foundation commissioned a report compiling information from granting agencies, press directors, and journal editors about their definitions of excellence in scholarship (Glassick et al. 1997). From these data, Glassick developed six standards for assessing scholarship, often referred to as the 'Glassick criteria'. Importantly, the Glassick criteria can be used to assess all forms of scholarship (including research) in all disciplines; they are not limited to the assessment of educational scholarship.

The following sections are a summary of the Glassick criteria for assessing scholarship (Glassick 2000).

Clear goals

Does the scholar state the basic purpose of his or her work clearly? Does the scholar define objectives that are realistic and achievable? Does the scholar identify important questions in the field?

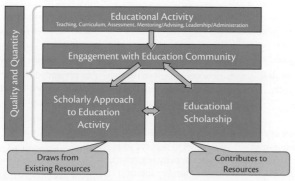

Figure 56.1 Q^2 Engage Model of Educational Scholarship (adapted from Simpson et al. 2007b, p.8) © 2007 Association of American Medical Colleges.

Table 56.1 GEA Standards for Educational Scholarship

Category and definition of educational activities	Quantity	Quality	Engagement with the educational community Draws from the field to inform own work (i.e. scholarly) and contributes to the field to inform other's work (i.e. scholarship)	
	Questions to document quantity and quality		Questions to address engagement	
Teaching: Any activity that fosters learning, including direct teaching (e.g. lecturing, tutoring, precepting) or creation of associated instructional materials.	◆ What is your teaching role? ◆ How long do you spend in teaching activities? ◆ How often do you teach? ◆ Where do you teach (e.g. course, venue)? ◆ What format do you use to teach? ◆ How many learners do you teach? ◆ What are the levels of the learners that you teach?	◆ Have you received any teaching awards? If so, what are the criteria for those awards? ◆ How do students, peers, and/or consultants rate the quality of your teaching? ◆ What is the evidence that students are learning from your teaching (e.g. self-reports, exams, standardized tests)?	◆ How is your teaching approach informed by the literature? ◆ How have discussions with colleagues impacted your subsequent practice?	◆ Have you had learning exercises accepted in peer-reviewed repositories? If so, which exercises and where? ◆ Have you been invited to present your teaching approach(es) at regional, national, and/or international conferences? If so, where?
Curriculum: A longitudinal set of systematically designed, sequenced, and evaluated education activities occurring at any training level, venue, or in any delivery format.	◆ What is your role in and contribution to the curriculum? ◆ What is the purpose of the curriculum(a) in which you are active? ◆ Who is the intended audience of the curriculum(a)? ◆ How was the curriculum(a) designed? ◆ How is the curriculum(a) evaluated?	◆ How have learners reacted to or rated the curriculum(a)? ◆ What impact has the curriculum(a) had on learning (e.g. course exams, standardized tests, observations of learners)? ◆ How has the curriculum(a) been evaluated by your peers?	◆ How are your curricular objectives informed by local, national, or international reports or standards? ◆ How does your curriculum(a) compare to other curriculum models? ◆ Have you adopted evaluation tools or models used by others in the field?	◆ Has your curriculum(a) been peer-reviewed by local, national, and/or international experts? If so, what was the result of those reviews? ◆ Have other institutions or departments adopted your curriculum(a)? ◆ Has your curriculum(a) been accepted into a peer-reviewed repository? If so, where?
Mentoring and/or advising: A developmental relationship in which an educator facilitates the accomplishment of a learner's or colleague's goals.	◆ Who are you mentoring? ◆ What is the current status of each mentoring relationship? ◆ What are the goals or purpose of the relationship? ◆ What is the duration of the relationship? ◆ What is the total time invested in mentoring?	◆ What have been the outcomes of the mentoring relationship(s)? For example, to what extent has the mentee accomplished his/her goals? Has the mentee produced products, such as awards, publications, or presentations?	◆ Have you participated in faculty development activities to enhance your effectiveness as a mentor? ◆ Have you compared your current mentoring practices with best practices? ◆ Have you obtained funding to participate in mentoring programmes?	◆ Have others adopted your mentoring practices? ◆ Have you produced publications or presentations related to your mentoring?
Education leadership and administration: Leadership activities that transform educational programmes and advance the field.	◆ With what types of leadership projects or administrative activities have you been involved? ◆ What was the rationale behind each project/ activity? ◆ What were the goals of each project/activity? ◆ What was your leadership role in each project/ activity? ◆ What was the duration of each project/activity?	◆ What have been the outcomes of each project/ activity? Have they achieved their goals? ◆ How well have faculty participated in each project/activity (formative)? ◆ How has each project/ activity impacted learner performance or faculty retention (summative)? ◆ How do peers, staff, learners, and bosses rate your leadership?	◆ Are the changes you make with projects or activities based on the literature or best practices? ◆ How does improvement under your project compare with that from other models? ◆ Have you garnered resources to support your project/activity (e.g. grants, internal funds, national funds)?	◆ Have your leadership activities been reviewed by your peers? ◆ Have you been invited to present your work locally, nationally, and/or internationally? ◆ Have other institutions adopted your work? ◆ Have you produced publications related to your leadership work?

(Continued)

Table 56.1 (*Continued*)

Category and definition of educational activities	Quantity	Quality	Engagement with the educational community
			Draws from the field to inform own work (i.e. scholarly) and contributes to the field to inform other's work (i.e. scholarship)
	Questions to document quantity and quality		Questions to address engagement
Learner assessment: All activities associated with measuring learners' knowledge, skills, and attitudes.	◆ What is your role in and contribution to learner assessment? ◆ What are the goals of the assessments you use? ◆ What types of assessments do you use (e.g. number of items)? ◆ How often do you assess learners?	◆ How reliable are the assessments you use (i.e. are they reproducible)? ◆ How valid are the assessments (i.e. how well do they measure what they are intended to measure; how accurate are they)?	◆ How do your methods of assessment reflect best practices?	◆ Have you given presentations about an innovative testing strategy? ◆ Have you published about your assessment strategy(ies)?

Adapted from D Simpson et al., 'Advancing educators and education by defining the components and evidence associated with educational scholarship', *Medical Education*, 41, 10, p. 1006, Copyright © 2007, Wiley, with permission.

Adequate preparation

Does the scholar show an understanding of existing scholarship in the field? Does the scholar bring the necessary skills to his or her work? Does the scholar bring together the resources necessary to move the project forward?

Appropriate methods

Does the scholar use methods appropriate to the goals? Does the scholar effectively apply the methods selected? Does the scholar modify procedures in response to changing circumstances?

Significant results

Does the scholar achieve the goals? Does the scholar's work add consequentially to the field? Does the scholar's work open additional areas for further exploration?

Effective presentation

Does the scholar use a suitable style and effective organization to present his or her work? Does the scholar use appropriate forums for communicating the work to its intended audiences? Does the scholar present his or her message with clarity and integrity?

Reflective critique

Does the scholar critically evaluate his or her own work? Does the scholar bring an appropriate breadth of evidence to his or her critique? Does the scholar use evaluation to improve the quality of future work?

In 1996, the AAMC's GEA scholarship project focused on operationalizing Glassick's criteria, applying the criteria to medical education and producing a list of specific sources of evidence that could be used to assess the quality of the scholarship of teaching and learning (Simpson and Fincher 1999; Fincher et al. 2000). For example, the questions in table 56.2 from the GEA project apply Glassick's criteria to evaluate teaching.

Table 56.2 Application of Glassick's criteria to teaching

Glassick criteria	Questions to apply the criterion
Clear goals	What is the evidence regarding the degree to which one's teaching objectives are clear and appropriate for the topic and level of learner?
Adequate preparation	What is the evidence that the information presented by the teacher is current and focuses on key content and issues?
Appropriate methods	What is the evidence that the teacher selects instructional methods that are appropriate for their objectives, their audiences, and their setting?
Significant results	What is the evidence that learners have achieved the teacher's objectives or of one's impact on learners?
Effective presentation	What is the evidence of how one has disseminated knowledge via graduates, advisees, curriculum reports, and/or web site data, as well as in traditional forums?
Reflective critique	What is the evidence of a sustained reflective process, including revision of instruction, changes in teaching strategies, and instituting new forms of assessment?

Adapted from Glassick CE, Huber MR, Maeroff G, *Scholarship assessed evaluation of the professoriate*, Copyright 1997, Jossey-Bass: Wiley. This material is adapted with permission from John Wiley & Sons, Inc.

Valuing educational scholarship in formal processes of recognition and reward requires documentation and evaluation using accepted frameworks and criteria

Using Glassick's criteria, faculty members can document their educational contributions and related scholarship to make their work visible and available for review by others. Traditional systems of recognition and reward require reliable judgments based on accepted and explicit standards. Work that is not documented adequately, or is not presented in a way that is easily understood by reviewers, may be misunderstood or discounted. Although an individual educator is unlikely to engage in the same level of accomplishment in each of the categories of educator activity, there should be established frameworks to document and summarize educational contributions in each domain.

Tools for documenting educational scholarship

The curriculum vitae (CV) is the accepted method for documenting most of a faculty member's activities and accomplishments. It adequately records evidence of educational discovery (research). An educator portfolio, however, also known as a teaching portfolio or a teaching dossier, is helpful to supplement a CV accurately capturing the breadth of one's educational activities and the related scholarship. It is a comprehensive record of the quantity and quality of educational activities and accomplishments and of the effectiveness of one's contributions. Summative portfolios contain at least three components (Simpson et al. 2004): a personal statement that establishes the context for reviewing the remaining components of the dossier; a summary of selected accomplishments; and evidence of excellence. Kuhn (2004) suggests the following organization for a portfolio: a narrative of one's philosophy of education, a list of teaching and scholarly activities (should incorporate created materials and data from evaluations by peers and learners), recognition of excellence (honours, awards, and thank you letters from learners), courses and study to increase one's expertise as an educator, and publications (authored educational materials). The template described by Lamki and Marchand in 2006 contains a section to summarize and provide brief narrative descriptions of one's work, an area to link activities with one's underlying philosophy, a list of professional development needs with an approach to address these needs, and appendices containing specific and objective data to support assertions in the other parts of the dossier. In this model, evidence of excellence is documented by cataloguing the dissemination of one's scholarly educational products. Despite evidence of an increasing use of portfolios in medical schools in the United States, a standardized format has not been adopted and the value assigned to the evidence in portfolios remains variable (Simpson et al. 2004). An example of a comprehensive, developmental educator portfolio is available from Gusic et al. (2007) www.mededportal.org/publication/626 (accessed 15 March 2013). Examples of a summative portfolio more appropriate for use in high-stakes assessments, such as decisions about promotion, the granting of an award, or selection into a teaching academy, are described by Simpson et al. (2007b).

Criteria for evaluating educational scholarship

Educational scholarship includes a broad array of scholarly contributions to health professional education (McGaghie and Webster 2009; Simpson et al. 2007a), including publications, peer-reviewed and invited presentations, books or chapters, educational grants, electronic publications, and other educational materials. Systems of recognition and reward for these contributions require reliable judgments based on accepted and explicit standards. Recognizing the need to further substantiate criteria that establish the impact of the work of educators, leaders of the Academic Pediatric

Association's Educational Scholars Program (APA ESP) developed a research tool for the comprehensive analysis of developmental educator portfolios (Chandran et al. 2009). The tool uses quantitative and qualitative data to measure outcomes in each of the categories of educator activity. To provide evidence of *adequate preparation* and *appropriate methods*, an educator must describe how they use systematic planning, sound conceptual models, and best practices from the literature in designing, implementing, and evaluating their work. Rigorous evaluation should be used to demonstrate *significant results*, and dissemination of one's work for review by others (*effective presentation*) allows the impact of the work to be revealed. Educators should express how they have utilized evaluation data and input from peer review to refine educational activities (*reflective critique*). This tool, with specified criteria using Glassick's framework (Glassick 1997) provides an objective approach to evaluate educational scholarship, but it may be too complex to be used in promotion and in recognition and reward decisions.

Building on this work, Baldwin et al. (2011) further refined criteria for the evaluation of educational activities, including educational scholarship, in *Guidelines for Evaluating the Educational Performance of Medical School Faculty*. Excellence in each of the five categories of educator activity is defined, evaluation items (discrete quantity and quality markers in each domain) are delineated, and examples of high-quality performance are described. Specific examples of evidence that document elements of a scholarly approach and of educational scholarship are provided. For example, a course director who uses evaluation data from learners and teachers to improve a course in addition to reviews done by the curriculum committee or an accrediting body, and national surveys, like the Association of American Medical College's (AAMC) Graduation Questionnaire, is providing evidence of use of *reflective critique*. Presenting information that demonstrates improvement in the course—i.e. improved learner performance on standardized skills examinations (an OSCE) assessing a skill that had been taught using a video during a lecture but that is now taught in a simulated clinical learning environment, documents *significant results* from changes made in the course. Although a brief, summative rating tool is provided, Baldwin et al. (2011) do not suggest a definitive rating system to go with the criteria and indicators. Institutions need to use locally accepted standards and values to develop a rating system that assigns relative weights to different measures.

In a companion resource, Educator Evaluation Guidelines (Baldwin et al. 2012), the authors add specific indicators (evidence) of quality that can be used in evaluating the impact and contribution of one's work to the community of educators. For example, an assessment tool that is developed by an educator must be designed to measure what it is intended to measure (validity of responses). Valid and reliable responses provide information for the learner, for the teacher, and for the institution in which the tool is being used. Publication of the tool and dissemination of the assessment methodology allow others to adopt this tool in their home institution. The Educator Evaluation Guidelines contain indicators for each of the five categories of educator activity contained in an educator portfolio, but application of specific criteria is not limited to the evaluation of portfolios and can be used with any tool used to document educational scholarship (Baldwin et al. 2012).

The use of explicit criteria requires infrastructure to support decision-making about educator performance. In particular, formal processes to inform departmental and institutional decision-making bodies about criteria for evaluation are required to implement a fair and rigorous process (Simpson and Fincher 1999).

In 2010, a national task force on educator evaluation was convened by the AAMC to develop a toolbox for decision makers. This resource was created to facilitate rigorous and consistent decision-making within and across institutions (Gusic et al. 2013). Input was obtained though national stakeholder discussions and from a survey of faculty affairs deans at academic health centres. The authors also used Glassick's criteria (Glassick et al. 1997) as the structure to assess quality (evidence of effectiveness through positive reviews), a scholarly approach (use of best practices from the literature and from participation in professional development activities), and scholarship (evidence of peer review, dissemination, and/or adoption by others) in each category of educator activity. An evaluator should expect to see adequate evidence of quality, a scholarly approach, and scholarship in the domain of focus for the educator, but not every indicator in the toolbox may be relevant for every educator. For example, using the indicators for educational leadership or administration, an educator with a leadership or administrative role should be expected to describe their vision for the program that they are leading. Goals for the programme must be aligned with institutional goals and with the articulated vision. Using best practice, the leader must create a timeline with milestones to meet these goals, identify and align resources, and obtain support from relevant stakeholders. Methods used to lead and manage others and the programme must be feasible, practical, and consistent with the highest standards of professionalism. There must be a plan to evaluate the programme and collect data that demonstrates that the goals of the programme were met.

The taskforce adapted Kirkpatricks' model for the evaluation of educational and training programs (Kirkpatrick and Kirkpatrick 2006) to establish criteria to measure significant results in each domain (as applicable, evidence of reaction/satisfaction, change in knowledge, skills, attitudes, and/or behaviours, observed performance in other settings, and impact within and outside of one's institution). For example, in the case of an educational leader, the reaction of the programme's stakeholders, the impact of the program on organizational processes, and the programme's contribution to advancing the mission of the institution are important results indicating the quality of the programme. Dissemination of the results of the programme evaluation in peer-reviewed publications and invitations to share the outcomes of the programme, or to peer-review similar programmes in other institutions, are evidence of *effective presentation*. Demonstrable changes made in the programme after self-analysis and review of the evaluation data show how the leader uses *reflective critique* to improve their skills as a leader and to enhance the programme.

Criteria for evaluation have multiple purposes: to inform decision makers and those who mentor educators, and to help educators develop their careers in line with expectations for performance. Knowing what is expected allows an educator to approach their work as a systematic discipline. To be an educational scholar, one does not need to create another category of work but rather, needs to learn about, and apply sound educational principles, in their work as teachers, developers of curricula, or mentors. Importantly, with the help of their own mentors, educators discover how to develop scholarship within their assigned activities. By documenting a scholarly approach and disseminating their work for peer-review, educators provide evidence of their contributions to their departments and institutions and to the community of educators. The use of accepted criteria for the evaluation of educators ensures a fair decision-making process to value the work that educators do. Institutions must ensure that educational scholarship is included in academic reward processes if education is truly valued by the organization.

In 2009, the Association for Medical Education in Europe (AMEE) published a guide that is designed to provide users with a resource for publishing research and other scholarly products and to highlight the importance of a broad range of scholarship in one's career advancement within higher education (McGaghie and Webster 2009). The AMEE guide highlights eight attributes of productive scholarly teams, based on the literature: (1) 'shared goals, common mission'; (2) 'clear leadership that may change or rotate'; (3) 'high standards'; (4) 'sustained hard work'; (5) 'physical proximity'; (6) minimal 'status differences within the team'; (7) maximum 'status of the team'; and (8) 'shared activities that breed trust' (McGaghie and Webster 2009, pp. 577–578). In addition, the guide recommends several types of skills for developing a successful career that focuses on publication and scholarship (McGaghie and Webster 2009, pp. 586–589):

Challenges for educators

Despite advances in defining, categorizing, documenting, and assessing educational scholarship, many educators do not engage in educational scholarship for various reasons, including:

1. A culture in medical education where research is still the dominant model of scholarship at many institutions (Simpson et al. 2007; Smesny et al. 2007; Irby et al. 2004; Collins and Gough 2010).

2. Increasing demands for clinical productivity for clinician educators (Smesny et al. 2007; Irby et al. 2004; Collins and Gough 2010).

3. Limited interactions with colleagues interested in educational scholarship (Goldszmidt et al. 2008; Smesny et al. 2007).

4. Limited time and support for producing scholarship (Smesny et al. 2007; Goldszmidt et al. 2008; Zibrowski et al. 2008).

5. Persistent difficulties in operationalizing the concept of educational scholarship (Purcell and Lloyd-Jones 2003).

6. Limited knowledge of how to produce educational scholarship (Goldszmidt et al. 2008; Mavis and Henry 2005).

Barriers to producing educational scholarship may be even greater in developing countries (Morahan and Fleetwood 2008). These challenges raise important questions: How might we succeed in promoting educational scholarship? How can we utilize resources and existing standards to engender support and recognition for educational scholarship?

Infrastructure to support educators and educational scholarship

For institutions to value faculty as educators and educational scholars, they must provide an infrastructure to support faculty as educators and scholars. Fincher et al. (2000) proposed Bolman and Deal's four 'frames' model as an organizational structure by which institutions can assess their capacity to support educational scholarship and target areas for improvement. The four 'frames' are: structural, human resources, political, and symbolic (Fincher et al. 2000). Institutional and organizational infrastructure at local, national, and even international level, is needed to support faculty to engage in educational scholarship. While the monetary investment necessary to support educational scholarship may be less than what is needed to support biomedical research, resources within the four frames are indispensable for enabling and recognizing faculty as educational scholars (fig. 56.2).

Simpson and colleagues (2000) at the Medical College of Wisconsin (MCW) targeted each of Bolman and Deal's four frames as part of their change strategy to recognize and reward educational scholarship. For example, they strengthened the structural frame by developing and refining promotion guidelines for a clinician–educator track and publishing the MCW Educator's Portfolio. They built human resource infrastructure through the development of faculty development programs, such as the MCW faculty mentor programme, a fellowship in medical education, a medical education seminar, and annual faculty orientation to medical education. Political support was bolstered by involving key stakeholders, such as the chair of the Rank and Tenure Committee. In addition, MCW faculty garnered further political support by establishing themselves as national leaders in medical education. The establishment of the MCW Society of Teaching Scholars and several education awards at convocations strengthened symbolic recognition for educational scholars (Simpson et al. 2000).

Initiatives that can provide support using the Bolman and Deal Four Frames Model

The teaching commons

Recent discussions in higher and medical education have highlighted the concept of the teaching commons (Huber and Hutchings 2005) as a method for creating a community for scholarship. The commons is defined as a virtual home through which educators can discuss innovative educational approaches and resources, and disseminate scholarship among peers through venues in addition

to traditional journals (Huber and Hutchings 2005; Morahan and Fleetwood 2008). As such, the commons can provide human resources and structural support by connecting educators and providing a mechanism for the dissemination of educational resource materials.

Several national and international initiatives are based on teaching commons as a conceptual foundation. The Foundation for Advancement of International Medical Education and Research (FAIMER) Institute provides a 2-year faculty development fellowship for medical educators in developing countries (Norcini et al. 2005) that includes two residential sessions in the United States and a distance learning intersession at the home institution. Fellows complete a curricular innovation project at their home institution, and co-mentor new fellows in their second year. The Mentoring-Learning Web Listserv (ML-Web), a component programme of the Institute (Norcini et al. 2005; Anshu et al. 2010), serves a function analogous to the 'teaching commons' at regional sites. ML-Web sessions are moderated by volunteer FAIMER fellows and faculty, and fellows exchange discussion emails monthly about selected topics (Norcini et al. 2005; Anshu et al. 2010). In this way, the Institute provides not only human resource infrastructure for faculty development but also structural infrastructure in the shape of the listserv to keep the dialogue active and ongoing.

For faculty who are not physically connected to a programme such as FAIMER, electronic versions of the teaching commons exist. For example, the AAMC's iCollaborative (2011) is a publically available online collective designed for the exchange of innovative educational resources, including tutorials, case studies, laboratory manuals, simulations, faculty development materials, poster presentations, and web resources. Users of iCollaborative may provide comments and feedback on resources through a system mimicking social networking (Association of American Medical Colleges 2011).

Academies of educators

Academies have emerged as organizational mechanisms for supporting the educational mission of medical schools (Irby et al. 2004). They often play a multifaceted role of symbolic support by

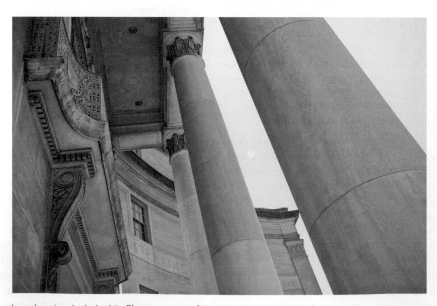

Figure 56.2 Institutions should value educational scholarship. Photo courtesy of Terry Dagradi, copyright Yale University.

recognizing faculty excellence in educational scholarship; human resource support by delivering faculty development activities; and structural support by providing a formal structure to support scholarship, often at a local or institutional level, but sometimes on a national level. In addition, academies of medical educators (see examples) are a second academic 'home' for educators, fostering a community (a commons) with other colleagues engaged in educational scholarship (Irby et al. 2004). Irby (2004) outlined four defining characteristics of academies:

1. An often broad-based mission supporting educators, curriculum development, and educational scholarship, and providing protected faculty time for education.

2. A rigorous review process to select members who are distinguished educators.

3. A formal, school-wide organizational tree with its own assigned leadership.

4. Allocation of dedicated resources to support the academy's mission.

Examples of how academies can support each of Bolman and Deal's four frames are provided in table 56.3.

On a national level, the Australian Academy of Surgical Educators, established by the Royal Australian College of Surgeons, supports activities including the design of professional development programs, development of advanced degree programmes, conduct of and collaboration on educational research, and working with hospitals and funders to establish educational fellowships (Collins and Gough 2010). In this way, the Academy supports the country's human resource and symbolic infrastructure, fostering the development and recognition of educational scholarship. In the UK, the Academy of Medical Educators (AoME) functions as an independent charitable organization (Sandars and McAreavey 2007; Academy of Medical Educators 2006). The AoME has established a set of professional standards that includes 'educational scholarship' as one of the core expectations for medical educators. Levels of membership in the UK Academy include regular *Membership*, 'for all those who are professionally involved in medical education, at any stage of their career', and *Fellowship* and *Honorary Fellowship*, granted through a peer review process of one's contributions to medical education (Academy of Medical Educators 2006, p. 'Membership'). The AoME offers masterclasses on educational development, an Annual Academic Meeting, and a series of 'Recognizing Teaching Excellence' Workshops (Sandars and McAreavey 2007; Academy of Medical Educators 2006).

Faculty development programmes

A variety of faculty development programmes provide structural and human resource support for faculty to develop skills as educators and educational scholars. For example, many institutions have developed medical education fellowships (Gruppen et al. 2006; Thompson et al. 2011). Typically, these fellowships focus on enhancing skills in teaching, curriculum design, and assessment. Most require completion of a scholarly project. One such programme, the Medical Education Scholars Program (MESP) at the University of Michigan, served the role of centralizing faculty development focused on educational scholarship (Gruppen et al. 2003). The MESP targets basic science and clinical faculty and includes content related to teaching and learning, cognition, educational assessment,

Table 56.3 Infrastructure supports for educational scholarship: examples from three academies

Bolman & Deal Model[*]	Examples[**]
Frame 1: Structural	
◆ Educational leadership positions, listed on organizational chart	◆ Dedicated academy budget and staff (UCSF; Baylor; MCW)
◆ College-wide medical education office, committee, or individual	◆ Fulbright & Jaworski L.L.P Educational Grant Fund (Baylor)
◆ Medical school library/web site	◆ Innovations funding grants for education (UCSF)
◆ Other education facilities (e.g. computer labs) and support personnel	
Frame 2: Human Resources	◆ Educational resource materials
◆ Orientation programs about medical education	◆ UCSF Teaching Scholars Program (medical education fellowship)
◆ Education handouts/web-based materials	◆ Preparing Future Faculty professional development programme (UCSF)
◆ Faculty development programmes/ workshops	◆ Medical education seminar series (Baylor)
◆ Hiring processes for education positions	◆ Annual medical education symposium (MCW)
◆ Fellowships in medical education	
Frame 3: Political	◆ Endowed chairs (UCSF)
◆ Educators in leadership positions	◆ Academies Collaborative (UCSF; Baylor)
◆ Educator coalitions for influencing decisions	◆ Educational Policy and Advocacy Working Group (UCSF)
◆ Educator roles in the selection/ election/appointment processes for key positions	◆ Sponsorship of the National Alpha Omega Alpha teaching award recipient as a visiting professor (MCW)
Frame 4: Symbolic	◆ Rigorous peer review process (UCSF; Baylor; MCW)
◆ Public documents featuring education	◆ Excellence in Teaching awards (UCSF)
◆ Rituals/traditions/ceremonies recognizing education	◆ Fulbright and Jaworski L. L. P. Faculty Excellence Award (Baylor)
◆ Public forums on education topics	◆ Baylor Academy of Distinguished Educators Showcase of Educational Scholarship
	◆ Edward J. Lennon Endowed Clinical Teaching Award and the Marvin Wagner Preceptor Award (MCW)

*Data from Fincher, R-M.E., Simpson, D.E. and Mennin, S.P. et al. (2000). Scholarship in teaching: an imperative for the 21st century. Academic Medicine, 75(9), 887–894. Data from Bolman LG, Deal TE, 'Reframing Organizations'. San Francisco, CA: Jossey-Bass, 1997.

**Data from UCSF-Haile T. Debas Academy of Medical Educators at the University of California, San Francisco (Irby et al. 2004; University of California San Francisco 2000); Baylor-Academy of Distinguished Educators at Baylor College of Medicine (Irby et al. 2004; Baylor College of Medicine 2001); MCW-The Medical College of Wisconsin Society of Teaching Scholars (Irby et al. 2004; Medical College of Wisconsin 1990).

academic leadership, and research methods. Scholars are expected to develop and implement a scholarly project during their tenure in the programme. Evaluation of the MESP has demonstrated an increase in promotions, educational grants, and new educational programmes amongst its alumni. (Gruppen et al. 2003).

Some institutions have taken a step further to establish formal degree programmes in medical education (Cohen et al. 2005; Tekian and Harris 2012). Such programmes offer a variety of delivery methods, including face-to-face, distance learning, and hybrids of the two, providing valuable opportunities even for educators who do not have such a programme at their home institution. For example, at Maastricht University in the Netherlands, participants can earn a Masters in Health Professions Education (MHPE) in a 2-year programme, largely based on distance education. In addition, the University offers an International MHPE-Brazil and a Joint Master of Health Professions Education (JMHPE) in Egypt (Cohen et al. 2005). The University of Illinois-Chicago MHPE has an educational leadership focus and offers options for on-campus or online programmes of study. Several articles have reviewed common characteristics of advanced degree programs for medical educators (Cohen et al. 2005; Tekian and Harris 2012).

Other examples

Several organizations and institutions have developed other innovative methods for supporting educational scholarship. The Medical Council of India (MCI) offers political infrastructure support in its country, increasing faculty development efforts at a national level. The Council has developed Faculty Development Programs focused on medical education at 16 regional sites throughout the country, and has developed a basic course in medical education geared for all faculty (A. Supe 2012, personal communication, 4 January). An advanced course in medical education is being initiated (A. Supe 2012, personal communication, 4 January). In addition, through the 1997 MCI Regulations on Graduate Medical Education, the Council mandated Medical Education Units (MEUs) at all medical colleges (Medical Council of India 1997). At the University of Toronto, the Research, Innovation, and Scholarship in Education (RISE) programme was established as a formally recognized programme within the Department of Psychiatry (Martimianakis et al. 2009). Activities of RISE incorporate the scholarship of teaching and include a graduate health professional education fellowship, training programmes for residents in educational research, affiliated faculty appointments with other clinical and basic science departments, and an Educational Scholars Program for faculty, among others. RISE has also enhanced support through formal affiliations with centres for education and faculty development outside of their home department of psychiatry (Martimianakis et al. 2009).

Conclusions

◆ Given that education is a core mission of medical education, there is a critical need to value faculty as educators and educational scholars. In order to do so, we must apply consistent definitions and standards of assessment to the work of educators.

◆ Medical educators participate in a variety of educational activities, which may be grouped into one of five categories: teaching, curriculum development, advising and mentoring, educational leadership and administration, and learner assessment.

◆ Within any of these five categories, educators may apply a scholarly approach (i.e. drawing from the field to inform one's work) and produce educational scholarship (i.e. making a contribution to the field through a product that is made public, available for peer review, and able to be built upon by others).

◆ Faculty should document their educational activities by reporting the quantity and quality of each activity and reporting how one has used a scholarly approach or produced scholarship from the given activity.

◆ Institutions and organizations should assess their capability to provide structural, human resource, political, and symbolic support to promote educational scholarship. Individual faculty may look to these supports and specific educational initiatives, such as teaching commons, faculty development programs, and academies for assistance in generating educational scholarship.

References

Academy of Medical Educators (AoME) (2006) Academy of Medical Educators. [Online] http://www.medicaleducators.org Accessed 20 March 2012

Anshu, S.M., Burdick, W.P., and Singh, T. (2010) Group dynamics and social interaction in a south Asian online learning forum for faculty development of medical teachers. Educ Health. 23(1): 311

Association of American Medical Colleges (2011) iCollaborative. [Online] https://www.aamc.org/icollaborative/ Accessed 20 March 2012

Baldwin, D., Chandran, L., and Gusic, M. (2011) Guidelines for evaluating the educational performance of medical school faculty: priming a national conversation. Teach Learn Med. 23(3): 285–297

Baldwin, D., Chandran, L., and Gusic, M. (2012) Educator evaluation guidelines. MedEdPORTAL, [Online] http://www.mededportal.org/publication/9072 Accessed 9 January 2012

Baylor College of Medicine (2001) Academy of Distinguished Educators. [Online] http://www.bcm.edu/fac-ed/academy/ Accessed 20 March 2012

Bok, D. (1990) Universities and the Future of America. Durham NC: Duke University Press

Boyer, E.L. (1987) College: The Undergraduate Experience in America. New York: Harper-Collins

Boyer, E.L. (1990) Scholarship Reconsidered: Priorities of the Professoriate. Princeton: Carnegie Foundation for the Advancement of Teaching

The Carnegie Foundation for the Advancement of Teaching (1989) The Condition of the Professoriate: Attitudes and Trends. Princeton: Carnegie Foundation for the Advancement of Teaching

Chandran, L., Gusic, M. and Baldwin, C., et al. (2009) Evaluating the performance of medical educators: a novel analysis tool to demonstrate the quality and impact of educational activities. Acad Med. 84(1): 58–66

Cohen, R., Murnaghan, L., Collins, J., and Pratt, D. (2005) An update on master's degrees in medical education. Med Teach. 27(8): 686–692

Collins, J.P. and Gough, I.R. (2010) An academy of surgical educators: sustaining education—enhancing innovation and scholarship. ANZ J Surg. 80: 13–17

Diamond, R.M. and Adam, B.E. (1995) The Disciplines Speak. Washington, DC: American Association of Higher Education

Diamond, R.M. and Adam, B.E. (2000) Recognizing Faculty Work: Reward Systems for the Year 2000. San Francisco: Jossey-Bass

Fincher, R-M.E., Simpson, D.E. and Mennin, S.P., et al. (2000) Scholarship in teaching: an imperative for the 21st century. Acad Med. 75(9): 887–894

Glassick, C.E., Huber, M.T., and Maeroff, G.I. (1997) Scholarship Assessed: Evaluation of the Professoriate. San Francisco: Jossey-Bass

Glassick, C.E. (2000) Boyer's expanded definitions of scholarship, the standards for assessing scholarship, and the elusiveness of the scholarship of teaching. Acad Med. 75(9): 877–880

Goldszmidt, M.A., Zibrowski, E.M., and Weston, W.W. (2008) Education scholarship: it's not just a question of 'degree'. Med Teach. 30: 34–39

Gruppen, L.D., Frohna, A.Z., Anderson, R.M., and Lowe, K.D. (2003) Faculty development for educational leadership and scholarship. Acad Med. 78(2): 137–141

Gruppen, L.D., Simpson, D., Searle, N.S., Robins, L., Irby, D.M., and Mullan, P.B. (2006) Educational fellowship programs: common themes and overarching issues. Acad Med. 81(11): 990–994

Gusic, M., Chandran, L., Balmer, D., D'Alessandro, D., and Baldwin, C. (2007) Educator Portfolio Template of the Academic Pediatric Association's Educational Scholars Program. MedEdPORTAL www.mededportal.org/publication/626 Accessed 15 March 2013

Gusic, M., Amiel, J., Baldwin, C., et al. (2013) Using the AAMC Toolbox for Evaluating Educators: You be the Judge!. MedEdPORTAL. [Online] www.mededportal.org/publication/9313 Accessed 10 May 2013

Huber, M.T. and Hutchings, P. (2005) *The Advancement of Learning: Building the Teaching Commons*. San Francisco: Jossey-Bass

Hutchings, P. and Shulman, L.S. (1999) The scholarship of teaching: new elaborations and developments. *Change*. 31(5): 11–15

Irby, D.M., Cooke, M., Lowenstein, D., and Richards, B. (2004) The academy movement: a structural approach to reinvigorating the educational mission. *Acad Med*. 79(8): 729–736

Kirkpatrick, D.L. and Kirkpatrick, J.D. (2006) *Evaluating Training Programs: The Four Levels*. 3rd edn. San Francisco: Berrett-Koehler Publishers

Kreber, C. and Cranton, P.A. (2000) Exploring the scholarship of teaching. *J Higher Educ*. 71(4): 476–495

Kuhn, G.J. (2004) Faculty development: the educator's portfolio: its preparation, uses, and value in academic medicine. *Acad Emerg Med*. 11(3): 307–311

Lamki, N. and Marchand, M. (2006) The medical educator teaching portfolio: its compilation and potential utility. *Sultan Qaboos University Med J*. 6(1): 7–12

Levinson, W., Rothman, A.I., and Phillipson, E. (2006) Creative professional activity: an additional platform for promotion of faculty. *Acad Med*. 81(6): 568–570

Martimianakis, M.T., McNaughton, N. and Tait, G.R., et al. (2009) The Research Innovation and Scholarship in Education Program: an innovative way to nurture education. *Acad Psychiatry*. 33(5): 364–369

Maurana, C.A., Woff, M., Beck, B.J., and Simpson, D.E. (2001) Working with our communities: moving from service to scholarship in the health professions. *Educ Health*. 14(2): 207–220

Mavis, B.E. and Henry, R.C. (2005) Being uninformed on informed consent: a pilot survey of medical education faculty. *BMC Med Educ*. 5(1): 12

McGaghie, W.C. and Webster, A. (2009) Scholarship, publication, and career advancement in health professions education: AMEE guide no. 43. *Med Teach*. 31: 574–590

Medical College of Wisconsin (1990) *MCW Society of Teaching Scholars*. [Online] http://www.mcw.edu/medicalschool/educationalservices/FacultyDevelopmentandResources/MCWSocietyofTeachingScholars.htm Accessed 20 March 2012

Medical Council of India (1997) Salient features of the regulations on graduate medical education. [Online] http://www.mciindia.org/RulesandRegulations/GraduateMedicalEducationRegulations1997.aspx Accessed 20 March 2012

Morahan, P. and Fleetwood, J. (2008) The double helix of activity and scholarship: building a medical education career with limited resources. *Med Educ*. 42: 34–44

Norcini, J., Burdick, W., and Morahan, P. (2005) The FAIMER Institute: creating international networks of medical educators. *Med Teach*. 27(3): 214–218

Purcell, N. and Lloyd-Jones, G. (2003) Standards for medical educators. *Med Educ*. 37: 149–154

Rice, R.E. (1992) Towards a broader conception of scholarship: the American context. In R. Whiston, and R. Geiger, (eds) *Research and Higher Education: The United Kingdom and the United States*. Buckingham: Society for Research into Higher Education and Open University Press

Rice, R.E. (1996) *Making a Place for the New American Scholar*. Washington, DC: American Association of Higher Education

Sandars, J. and McAreavey, M.J. (2007) Developing the scholarship of medical educators: a challenge in the present era of change. *Postgrad Med J*. 83: 561

Shulman, L.S. (1999) Taking learning seriously. *Change*. 31: 11–17

Simpson, D.E. and Fincher, R-M. (1999) Making a case for the teaching scholar. *Acad Med*. 74(12): 1296–1299

Simpson, D., Fincher, R-M.E., Hafler, J.P., et al. (2007a) Advancing educators and education by defining the components and evidence associated with educational scholarship. *Med Educ*. 41: 1002–1009

Simpson, D., Fincher, R-M., Hafler, J.P., et al. (2007b) *Advancing Educators and Education: Defining the Components and Evidence of Educational Scholarship*. Proceedings from the Association of American Medical Colleges Group on Educational Affairs Consensus Conference on Educational Scholarship, 9–10 February 2006, Charlotte, NC. Washington, DC: Association of American Medical Colleges

Simpson, D.E., Hafler, J., Brown, D., and Wilkerson, L. (2004) Documentation systems for educators seeking academic promotion in US medical schools. *Acad Med*. 79: 783–790

Simpson, D.E., Marcdante, K.W., Duthie, Jr., E.H., et al. (2000) Valuing educational scholarship at the Medical College of Wisconsin. *Acad Med*. 75(9): 930–934

Smesny, A.L., Williams, J.S., Brazeau, G.A., et al. (2007) Barriers to scholarship in dentistry, medicine, nursing, and pharmacy practice faculty. *Am J Pharm Educ*. 71(5): 1–9

Tekian, A. and Harris, I. (2012) Preparing health professions education leaders worldwide: a description of masters-level programs. *Med Educ*. 34(1): 52–58

Thompson, B.M., Searle, N.S., Gruppen, L.D., Hatem, C.J., and Nelson, E.A. (2011) A national survey of medical education fellowships. *Med Educ Online*. 16: 5642

Trigwell, K., Martin E., Benjamin, J., and Prosser, M. (2000) Scholarship of teaching: a model. *Higher Educ Res Devel*. 19(2): 155–168

University of California-San Francisco (2000) The Haile T. Debas Academy of Medical Educators. [Online] http://medschool.ucsf.edu/academy/ Accessed 20 March 2012

University of Illinois-Chicago Master of Health Professions Education. [Online] http://chicago.medicine.uic.edu/departments___programs/departments/meded/educational_programs/mhpe/ Accessed 20 March 2012

Zibrowski, E.M., Weston, W.W., and Goldszmidt, M.A. (2008) 'I don't have time': issues of fragmentation, prioritization and motivation for education scholarship among medical faculty. *Med Educ*. 42(9): 872–878

PART 11

Global medical education

CHAPTER 57

Medical education in developing countries

Francesca Celletti, Eric Buch, and Badara Samb

> The African continent is short of doctors and the obvious place to train doctors for Africa is in Africa. This requires medical schools. But as soon as these two simple statements are accepted, problems crowd around the scene like bees around a honeypot.
>
> Lindsay Davidson

Setting the scene

Health means people. Healthcare is about the relationship between those people who seek prevention and care services and the healthcare professionals who deliver them. All people should be able to access care when and where needed. The right to health should not be determined by the geographical, social or economical status of a country, population, or individual.

Nonetheless, we are still facing big disparities in the health conditions of the population and are falling short in meeting population health needs and expectations in many parts of the world (Evans et al. 2004; Joint Learning Initiative 2004; World Health Organization 2006).

Globally, we are facing a rapid demographic and epidemiological transition which is posing new health challenges; and health security is being undermined by new infectious and environmental threats (Institute of Medicine 2005, 2009; Commission on Social Determinants for Health 2008). However, the situation is even worse in low- and middle-income countries. Today, over a billion people worldwide lack access to quality health services and many die of common infections, maternity-related illnesses, and malnutrition (Whitehead et al. 2001). For example, an estimated 1500 women lose their lives in pregnancy and childbirth every day—lives that could be saved if a qualified health professional were available. In addition, health gains of the past 50 years have been reversed by new diseases such as, the human immunodeficiency (HIV) pandemic in sub-Saharan Africa (Buvè et al. 2002; Merson et al. 2008).

One important factor is the global health workforce crisis. Currently, the World Health Organizarion (World Health Organization 2006a) estimates that an additional 2.4 million doctors, nurses and midwives are needed worldwide; again, poor countries are more affected than others. The United States has 270 medical doctors per 100 000 people, the United Kingdom 210, and Brazil 170, while Tanzania has just 2.3, and Malawi 1.1 (World Health Organization 2006). In the 47 countries of sub-Saharan Africa, 168 medical schools produce only 9000–10 000 graduates per year (Mullan et al. 2010).

However, simply increasing the number of medical graduates will not solve the more intractable problems facing the global workforce. Solutions will need to address the poor match between current models of medical education and evolving population health needs; the insufficient alignment between the priorities of the health and education sectors; the imbalanced distribution that disadvantages rural and poor urban populations; and the challenges of keeping doctors in the communities where they are needed most (World Health Organization 2008b, 2010d).

In many cases today, educational institutions are isolated from national health systems and from health service delivery, limiting their ability to prepare graduates for the workplaces where they will practise (Dussault and Dubois 2003). Curricula may not reflect the disease burden of the areas in which doctors are most needed. Training sites are often urban tertiary centres whose practice conditions are unlike those that graduates will ultimately face. Training physicians in isolation from other professionals may prepare them poorly for team-based practice. The failure to orient medical education to the needs of the local healthcare system and the most relevant models of care may leave graduates unprepared to serve as advocates for improving the healthcare system around them.

Achieving an appropriate balance between local relevance and global excellence is a challenge and some argue that placing an emphasis on social accountability in medical education can undermine the overall technical excellence of graduates. However, a more socially accountable scale-up of medical education does not exclude investment in centres of global excellence and world-class research (Eley et al. 2008; Bianchi et al. 2008; Abdel-Rahim et al. 1992). Indeed, the need for specialist care is likely to increase with the improved provision of primary care. The approach needed is one where a greater value is assigned to the impact on population health outcomes among the criteria for measuring excellence.

While there is increasing attention paid to the need for a transformative approach to medical education (Frenk et al. 2010), there remains a paucity of published data to inform policy dialogue. Models for innovative scale-up of medical education are being implemented in a number of countries, but few outcomes have been documented—apart from some literature to suggest that the articulation of a framework of generic attributes may be an important mechanism for the development of graduate skills that transcend disciplinary content (Laidlaw et al. 2009)

It is possible, nevertheless, to identify a number of critical areas that are in need of reform if the health workforce of the future is to meet the needs of the 21st century.

The challenges of medical education

Although the challenges of medical education are many, they can be summarized into three broad categories as shown in fig. 57.1.

Quantity

In a seminal report issued by the WHO in 2006, the main issues of the global workforce crisis were outlined. The global density of doctors is 1.6/1000 population, but the country-specific ratios of physicians to population varies across the globe from a low of 0.01/1000 in Liberia to 3.7/1000 in Italy, and 2.7/1000 in the US (Joint Learning Initiative 2004; 2006). A recent study (Frenk et al. 2010) estimated a global total of about 2420 schools producing around 389 000 medical graduates every year for a world population of 7 billion people. The shortages are exacerbated by maldistribution, both between and within countries. While in India, China, Western Europe, Latin America, and the Caribbean, the number of schools is high; Central Asia, Central and Eastern Europe, and sub-Saharan Africa face severe shortages. For example, China, India, Brazil, and the USA each have more than 150 schools—which make up 35% of the world's total; while 31 countries have no medical school whatsoever (Frenk et al. 2010). Of the countries with no medical school, nine are in sub-Saharan Africa; 44 countries, including 17 in sub-Saharan Africa, have only one medical school (Frenk et al.

2010). Nearly half of countries worldwide have either one or no medical school (Frenk et al. 2010). Compounding the problem of inadequate numbers and maldistributed doctors, physicians who are trained in low-income countries often migrate to richer countries after completing their education (Bosk 1985; Fox 1993). North America, Europe, and countries in the Persian Gulf are the principal destinations of emigrating doctors who are drawn by training and financial opportunities (Bosk 1985; Fox 1993). Poor working conditions and low pay make it hard to retain qualified health professionals. In addition, some countries are unable to use all the providers they have educated since new doctors, nurses, and other health professionals cannot be deployed without sufficient budgetary resources.

One result of all this is that rural populations often have few or no physicians available to treat them. In South Africa, 46% of the population lives in rural areas, but only 12% of doctors and 19% of nurses work in such settings. Good evidence (Cooper 2002; Anand and Baernighausen 2004) indicates that higher numbers of health workers—particularly doctors, nurses, and midwives—are associated with better population health outcomes.

The successful accomplishment of the health-related millennium development goals, lifespan extension, and poverty reduction require putting in place strategies to make more doctors available where needed. The training of sufficient numbers of doctors and their even distribution is a worldwide challenge (Bosk 1985; Fox 1993; Cooper 2002; Anand and Baernighausen 2004).

Quality

No matter how many individuals are educated and deployed, medical doctors cannot improve population health unless they have the necessary competencies. Physicians need to be technically competent and efficient but they also need to be able to work in teams, to adapt to changing environments, and to initiate change where needed.

Efforts to deliver high quality education face various challenges. These include: medical teaching falling to keep up to date with the science and practice of medicine; tensions between teaching and research; the need to adjust medical education to the challenges imposed by chronic diseases; and the requirement to teach about the delivery of evidence-based and cost-effective care (World Health Organization 2010d). Historically, as the molecular revolution transformed research, teaching and research grew further apart. Consequently, the research interests of most faculty no longer relate to the subject matter taught to students. This has resulted in an institutional culture that rewards research accomplishments more than educational effectiveness.

More emphasis has to be placed on an educational culture in which trainees and physicians examine their performance and measure patient outcomes; with the ultimate aim of continually improving the quality of care they provide (Ludmerer 2003).

In low- and middle-income countries, many educational institutions have insufficient infrastructure and equipment (Mullan et al. 2010). The educational methods are static and fragmented, and shortages of teaching staff severe (Mullan et al. 2010; Frenk et al. 2010). Postgraduate education is inadequate or non-existent. Regulatory mechanisms designed to ensure the quality of education, such as accreditation, are rarely standardized and often weak and inconsistently applied—especially in the case of private sector institutions. Variability of secondary education may mean there are

There are not enough doctors globally and the crisis is most acute in low- and middle-income countries (quantity)

No matter how many individuals are educated and deployed, doctors cannot improve population health unless they have the necessary skills (quality)

Even well-educated doctors may find themselves ill-prepared to meet the challenges they face when they start practising (relevance)

Global investment in medical education is inadequate

Figure 57.1 Challenges of medical education.

not enough qualified secondary school graduates to fill university programmes.

In many settings, a variety of workplace challenges mean that even qualified health professionals do not always perform as well as they might. Poor wages and working conditions contribute to low morale, low productivity, and absenteeism. Lack of equipment and other supplies also prevent health professionals doing their jobs properly (Celletti et al. 2011).

Given these constraints, the number of graduates does not tell the whole story (Mullan et al. 2010; Frenk et al. 2010).

Relevance

Even well-educated doctors may find themselves ill-prepared to meet the challenges they face when they take up posts within a health system. The mix of skills they have acquired during their professional education is often not oriented to their workplace. The scientific content of their education may be poorly matched to the illnesses that affect the communities in which they work.

Medical schools in low- and middle-income countries tend to be isolated from the reality of health-service delivery. This limits their ability to prepare doctors to respond to evolving policies, epidemiology, and technologies relevant to their eventual workplace (Mullan et al. 2010).

Curricula may not reflect the disease burden of the areas in which doctors are most needed. Countries show wide variations in the burden of different categories of disease. In low-income countries communicable diseases, maternal and perinatal conditions, and nutritional deficiencies represent 69% of the disease burden. However, teaching tends to revolve around service delivery models with limited relevance—there is little training in public health, epidemiology, or health systems management. Clinical training sites are mostly urban tertiary centres whose practice conditions differ from secondary and primary healthcare centres. In many countries the proportion of the population receiving services in primary care centres reaches 85%, with only 1% of the population's healthcare needs being met at the tertiary level (World Health Organization 2006; Commission on Social Determinants for Health 2008; Anand and Baernighausen

2004)—and yet education often occurs in tertiary centres and graduates tend to want to stay in hospital settings. For example, less than 9% of graduates from schools in sub-Saharan Africa are practising in rural public general practice (Institute of Medicine 2001).

The failure to orient medical education to the needs of the local healthcare system and the most relevant models of care leaves graduates unprepared to serve as advocates for improving the healthcare system around them. However, there are some examples of better practice. For example, graduates from Walter Sisulu University are required to learn about the principles of social accountability, and at the same time to demonstrate high-level academic and clinical performance (World Health Organization and Global Health Workforce Alliance 2009; Dunbabin et al. 2006; Thomson et al. 2003). In any case, reformed medical education does not exclude investment in centres of excellence and world class research. What is important is to assign greater value to the impact on population health outcomes among the criteria for measuring excellence in medical education (fig. 57.2).

Other challenges relate to the suitability of the students who are recruited into the health professions. Health professionals who are not representative of the people they serve in terms of language and other social and demographic factors may find it more difficult to understand and respond to the needs of communities. Fees for professional education are high and subsidies to ensure affordability are rare, limiting the pool of potential candidates. The concentration of opportunities in urban and specialist settings also influences the types of students recruited. Potential candidates from rural or underserved areas face numerous barriers—including difficulties travelling, poor accommodation, and a lack of familiarity with an environment so far from home.

Costing and investments

Until recently there was a total absence of data on the financing of health professional education. To address this knowledge gap, the independent commission on the education of health professionals performed a study to estimate the financing of medical and nursing education worldwide (Frenk et al.2010).

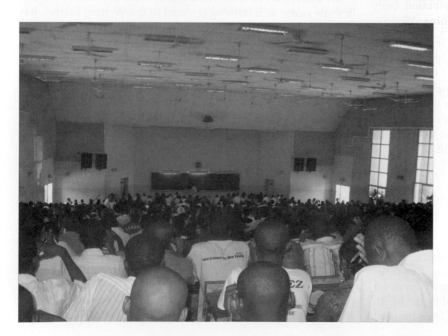

Figure 57.2 A medical class in Ghana.
Photographer: Fitzhugh Mullan, reproduced with permission.

Total yearly expenditure in health professional education has been estimated to be about $100 billion for medicine, nursing, public health, and allied health professions. The education of medical graduates alone has been estimated to cost about $47.6 billion (Frenk et al. 2010). The average unit cost per medical graduate has been calculated at around $122 000 (this is education only, not the total turnover of health education institutions). The cost can escalate if other components of medical education are included. For example, one Canadian study reported that whereas the average cost of educating a medical graduate was about Ca$286 000, the costs would escalate to Ca$787 000 if additional elements such as research and clinical services turnover were included (Erney et al. 1991). The unit cost can differ between countries: for example, the average cost of producing a medical graduate in China is estimated to be US$14 000, while in sub-Saharan Africa it is US$52 000 (Frenk et al. 2010).

Investments in professional education constitute a minimal proportion of national health investment. In the USA, for example, the highest estimate of US$55 billion for all activities by medical schools is only 2% of the national health spend—$2.5 trillion in 2009 (Valberg et al. 1994). The global picture is similar—investments in health professional education represent less than 2% of a global healthcare industry turning over an estimated $5.5 trillion yearly (Frenk et al. 2010).

Budgets of national governments and development assistance donors rarely separate out funding for health professional education (Keehan et al. 2008). Growing awareness of the implications of global health workforce shortages, including the identification of limited human resources for health as a key barrier to achieving the health-related Millennium Development Goals, has encouraged some international development partners to direct their funding towards basic health worker training (Lu et al. 2010; Institute of Medicine 2007). However, donors rarely finance medical education as part of their health development assistance. Recent exceptions include the US Medical Education Partnership Initiative (MEPI), which supports institutions in sub-Saharan African to develop or expand their models of medical education. These models are intended to strengthen medical education systems and build 'clinical and research capacity in Africa' as part of a staff retention strategy for medical schools (Collins et al. 2010, p. 1324).

At the individual level, the rising cost of medical education is a growing challenge in all countries (Josiah Macey Jr Foundation 2008; Kwong et al. 2002). Increased costs impose hardship on student families and exclude those who cannot afford them. Loan-based financing of medical education causes additional drawbacks. In the USA, the average debt of graduating students is now about $200 000 (Kwong et al. 2002). As a result, the burden of repayment can draw graduates away from socially important but less lucrative careers (United States Government Accountability Office 2009).

What is needed

A wide range of reforms are needed (fig. 57.3).

Curricula oriented towards local relevance

The 1910 Flexner Report prompted a transformation of medical education in the US and beyond, not only by highlighting inadequacies in quality and facilities, but also by making a convincing case for an approach to education that was informed by the health needs of society (Flexner 1910). One hundred years later, the need

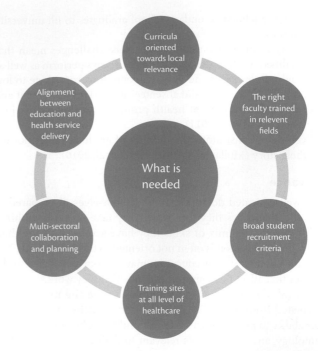

Figure 57.3 Reform of medical education.

for medical education to keep pace with evolving epidemiology, patient demographics, and health systems remains pertinent everywhere and even more so in low and middle income countries (Laidlaw et al. 2009). Academic excellence must be associated with the delivery of improvements in population health outcomes. Medical universities must teach to the local disease burden, as well as educate students to practise within the care delivery models that are likely to best serve the local population's health needs. Medical schools need to be integrated with the relevant local, regional, and national health authorities to ensure an effective alignment between medical education, research, health service delivery, and population health needs.

The current association of excellence with specialist skills, and in some cases, with training oriented to the Western market, has meant that family and community-oriented medicine and public health, usually better matched to overall epidemiological burden and needs, are often afforded 'low status' and are relatively poorly paid (Hauer et al. 2008, p. 1153). What is needed are curricula that equip graduates to address the specific epidemiology of the communities where they are deployed. This includes the incorporation of community medicine and public health into curricula as compulsory rotations, with a focus on prevention. In addition, institutional and national funding bodies should promote research directed towards national health needs and health systems.

Many schools, both in high- and low-income countries, provide examples of programmes that allow students and residents to identify and address the specific health needs of the local community. The East Carolina University created a 1-year postgraduate fellowship for primary care doctors to become specialized in diabetes care (Peterson and Burton 2007; Tanenberg et al. 2009). The family studies programme at the Arabian Gulf University has students visit local families to deliver health promotion messages (Grant et al. 2009). The Rural Track Family Practice Residency Program at SUNY-Buffalo (USA) trains residents in low-risk obstetrics at an affiliated hospital. About 75% of deliveries in the area are attended by residents and the Caesarean section rate has decreased from 24% to 19% (Anderson et al. 2007).

In Pakistan, the Aga Khan University Medical Center has a community-oriented curriculum that includes urban health projects; these have effected a drop in the infant mortality rate from 126/1000 to 64/1000 and a drop in the under five mortality rate from 177/1000 to 83/1000 between 1985–1988 and 1991 (Davidson 2002). Interns at the University College of Medical Sciences, Shahdara (Delhi, India), who underwent a community medicine posting showed a significant improvement in immunization knowledge following their posting (Pandit et al. 1991). At Bharati Vidyapeeth University Medical College, India, students work on community-based projects in secondary schools, rural areas, and urban slums (Vaidya and Gothankar 2009). Nearly all of the surveyed students felt the experience should be routine, 78% rated their experience as good or excellent, and 70% rated their community exposure as good or excellent.

At the University of Transkei, South Africa, the curriculum has gradually shifted from a traditional to a problem-based curriculum. From 1990 to 2004, 24% of students graduated from the traditional curriculum and 76% from the problem-based curriculum (Kwizera et al. 2005). Makerere University, Uganda also transitioned from a traditional curriculum to a more community-oriented, problem-based curriculum (that includes community placements) (Kaye et al. 2010). The community placements were found to have a great impact on graduates' preference and competency for rural practice.

Other studies comparing practice outcomes of graduates of community-oriented curricula with graduates of traditional curricula showed that community-oriented curricula improve: screening rates; continuity of care; and relationships with patients and the community (Tamblyn et al. 2005).

There is increasing evidence that team-based practice with partial transfer of tasks ('task-shifting') to non-physician providers may be the most effective means of care delivery, in a variety of settings (Al-Dabbagh and Al-Taee 2005; World Health Organization 2008b,c). The form and content of medical curricula need to prepare doctors to practise within this model, and will likely require the incorporation of progressive educational strategies, such as interdisciplinary and interprofessional training (World Health Organization 2008a, World Health Organization 2010b). In this regard, a systematic review of the effectiveness of interprofessional education (Samb et al. 2007), although non-conclusive, suggested a positive impact on clinical practice.

The right faculty trained in relevant fields

A challenge to medical schools in most parts of the world is hiring and retaining adequate faculty. Strategies that develop faculty; that provide adequate compensation; that promote research opportunities; and that enable continuing education and skills acquisition, are essential to faculty building.

A number of complex issues need to be addressed. Medical schools must strike a balance between faculty teaching, service, research, and management duties to ensure that course content is relevant, that clinical skills are maintained, and that career development opportunities are available. At the same time, institutions should develop incentives to ensure that teaching achievements are afforded comparable status to those of research and clinical work (Celletti et al. 2011). A devaluation of teaching has been observed

in the last few decades (World Health Organization 2010d). This has resulted in an institutional culture that rewards research accomplishments far more than educational effectiveness. Teaching, when done well, is time consuming and labour intensive, requiring close personal contact with students. In addition, it requires a generalist and synthetic orientation that in an era of increasing specialization takes greater effort to maintain.

Some progressive medical schools in the US, South Africa, and Australia have used creative approaches to faculty strengthening and expansion, incorporating doctors and nurses working in district hospitals or health clinics into the faculty body, or establishing joint appointments and affiliate positions with other institutions (Celletti et al. 2011). The Faculty Development Center of the Department of Family Practice at Cook County Hospital in Chicago teaches faculty to educate their students about practising in underserved areas (Beck et al. 2008). Of those that have completed the programme, 60% went on to practice or teach in underserved settings. The University of California-San Diego offers a 3-week faculty development programme entitled 'Addressing the Health Needs of the Underserved' and they also offer a 1-year fellowship in underserved medicine (Norman et al. 1999, p. 86). Developing clinical preceptor programmes can also be an effective means of expanding a mentoring pool, and can serve to bring community practitioners' understanding of local health needs into the university (Beck et al. 2008; Norman et al. 1999). A number of institutions have also explored the potential of international and public–private partnerships to increase pedagogical capacity and provide opportunities for students and faculty at all partner sites (Celletti et al. 2011).

Broad student recruitment criteria

Medical doctors need to direct their education, research, and service activities towards the health concerns of their communities. As such, it is essential that the students recruited represent the broad spectrum of society and are able to service a wide range of needs. These needs include: primary care including community and home based care; public health; secondary care; and tertiary care.

Educating a health workforce that is representative of the entire country's population and that meets its needs and expectations is important both in terms of equity of opportunity, effectiveness of services, and advancement of education and research.

However, substantial disparities in access to medical education exist in all countries. These disparities are determined by many issues, including gender, geographic location of secondary schools, and socioeconomic status. In addition, most medical institutions around the world tend to favour the recruitment of students with an appropriate background for, and desire to work in, tertiary care. Specialized biomedical research tends to receive more attention from funding institutions and scientific journals and offers better career opportunities than public health research and health systems research. Medical schools are a public good and have a social mission. As such they need to comply with the local needs of health systems.

Selecting students who speak local languages, communicate well with minority groups, and serve as role models for young people from disparate backgrounds, is an important transformative function of medical education in the 21st century. Many factors help to promote diversity, including: schools' recruitment and admissions policies; schools' physical locations; faculty diversity and role models; special preparatory courses; and in-school tutoring of students who may be struggling. Moreover, selecting students from underserved populations tends to produce graduates who will advocate the needs of these populations.

Evidence suggests that students recruited from marginalized communities are more likely to serve those communities for an extended period once they are qualified doctors and that community involvement in the selection of candidates may also increase engagement and retention (Freeman et al. 2009; World Health Organization 2010a). Such recruitment strategies can help identify prospective students who may be better adjusted for a lifestyle in underserved areas, more able to provide culturally sensitive and appropriate care, and more in tune with the social and economic determinants of health in the communities they serve (Laven and Wilkinson 2003). A systematic review of the effect of rural background on doctors choice of practice area found that doctors from rural areas are 2 to 2.5 times more likely to practise in rural areas (Briggs and Mantini-Briggs 2009). Graduates of the Memorial University of Newfoundland, Canada were more likely to practise in rural Canada if they had a rural background; did their residency at the local university; and were family doctors rather than specialists (Grobler et al. 2009). An evaluation of the Jefferson Medical College Physician Shortage Area Program in the USA, which recruits students from rural areas, revealed that 55% of the graduates were practising in family medicine, 67% were practising in-state, 39% were practising in rural areas, and 33% were practising in physician shortage areas (Smucny et al. 2005). In Walter Sisulu University, a total of 835 doctors have graduated, 70% of whom still practise in the underserved rural communities of the immediate area. Other graduates have found success abroad or as specialists, confounding sceptics who argued that the quality of the education of these progressive schools might prove inferior to that of more traditional schools (Celletti et al. 2011). Another study from the Congo compared graduates of an urban and a rural medical school and established that of the rural school graduates, 98% worked in the province in which they were trained and 81% worked in a rural area, in contrast to 43% and 61%, respectively, of the urban school graduates (Longombe 2009).

Training sites at all level of healthcare

Medical graduates play a key role in addressing the health needs of their country. The presence of an adequate supply of doctors is essential for building and maintaining health systems. The distribution (rural as well as urban, peripheral and central, wealthy areas, and poor ones) of the graduates of these schools is essential to the effectiveness of a country's health system.

Graduates, however, do not always choose to practise in patterns that meet local and regional health needs (sometimes they do not have the opportunity to do so). In some instances, they remain clustered in urban areas around training institutions or major hospitals. In most medical schools, hospital-centred training is the norm, and both educational institutions and teaching hospitals are found predominantly in urban areas (Institute of Medicine 2001). Such a concentration of opportunities in urban and specialist settings influences the type of students that are recruited and adversely affects the distribution of graduates when they enter clinical practice (Norman et al. 1999). Strategies that prepare students for practice in underserved communities (such as preceptorships, clinical rotations, public health training, and health policy exposure) seem

to provide good results. These include programs that focus on the national burden of disease; that address community needs; and that nurture a commitment to public service among trainees (Celletti et al. 2011).

Evidence shows that physicians trained through community health centres are 3.4 times more likely to work in a health centre and 2.7 times more likely to work in an underserved setting (Rabinowitz et al. 1999). An evaluation of the University of British Columbia's rural training found that 51% of graduates were working in rural areas and that graduates reported that they were more prepared for rural medicine—particularly in the domains of family medicine, community medicine, practice management, and behavioural science (Morris et al. 1996). The Rural Medical Education Program, which provides clinical training in rural communities at the State University of New York Upstate Medical University, also affected graduates' choice of rural practice. Significantly more graduates from the programme were working in rural areas compared to other graduates, and 84% of graduates felt that this programme had been important in their choice of geographic practice location (Whiteside and Mathias 1996). A longitudinal study that measured the career preferences of two cohorts of students at Sheffield Medical School, one that underwent hospital-based training and one that took a module on community-based medicine, showed that students in the community group had a significant shift over time towards preferring a community-based career (Smucny et al. 2005; Howe 2001). The effect of training in community health centres, which comprise a network of federally funded health clinics that serve as a safety net for the indigent, has also been studied. Family medicine residents at the University of Massachusetts Medical School were offered a choice of three ambulatory clinical training sites: a community health centre; an urban practice; and a rural practice (Howe 2001). Those trained at the community health centre were significantly more likely practise in underserved areas, both immediately after graduation and in the long term. Likewise, graduates trained at rural sites were more likely to practice in rural areas. At the Jimma University Medical School in Ethiopia, combining training in community environments with an interdisciplinary approach to medical education resulted in higher-quality graduates with skills relevant to nearby populations (Celletti et al. 2011). At Gezira University in Sudan, each student is attached to a particular family for the period of their training. Student teams consult community members to identify priorities around which they develop interventions and then seek funding for implementation and evaluation (Celletti et al. 2011).

Multisectoral collaboration and planning

A medical education aimed at addressing population health needs has far-reaching implications and requires political commitment and the engagement of multiple government sectors and of communities. In most countries, high-level political commitment to medical education reform is scarce and responsibility for medical universities lies only with the Ministry of Education. Without national planning across different sectors, the potential benefits that can be produced through medical education are reduced, and investment in medical education is unlikely to produce maximum returns in health. Significant resource and logistics coordination are required from government ministries and other stakeholders. For example, medical student numbers cannot be increased without enough well-qualified students graduating from secondary education; the need for increased infrastructure for medical education will not only require better teaching facilities, but also improvements in the surrounding environment; and new doctors cannot be deployed without budgetary allocation for salaries from the ministry of finance. Providing a good medical education therefore implies strategic planning and financial investment on a long-term and multisectoral basis.

While the challenges are daunting, there is good evidence from nations as diverse as Brazil (Celletti et al. 2011; Freeman et al. 2009; Rocha and Soares 2009), Thailand (Wibulpolprasert and Pengpaibon 2003) and Venezuela (Armada et al. 2009; Borroto Cruz and Salas Perea 2008) that such multisectoral commitment to health professional education can reap significant long-term savings in terms of population health outcomes and economic development. In Brazil, for example, integration of the health and education sectors at the highest level (the national constitution establishes joint responsibility over the education of health professionals to the Ministry of Education and the National Health System) has resulted in significantly improved utilization of health services and better chronic disease management (Rocha and Soares 2009). In Thailand, multisectoral planning facilitated rural recruitment and hometown placement initiatives that substantially increased retention of doctors in underserved areas (Wibulpolprasert and Pengpaibon 2003). In Venezuela, interdisciplinary coordination for educational innovation allowed rapid scale-up of primary care services for millions of people. The Venezuelan national training programme for Comprehensive Community Physicians, a 6-year programme, which began admitting students in 2005 (Armada et al. 2009; Borroto Cruz and Salas Perea 2008), has the goal of radically improving population health—especially in underserved areas of the country. A special emphasis has been given to public service and to recruiting poor and rural students who have had little prior opportunity to access higher education. Moreover, a community-based curriculum focused on health promotion, public health, and family medicine principles has been used together with the appointment of practising physicians as professors. In Ethiopia, the government has introduced a 'flooding and retention' human resources strategy which involves ministries, professional societies, and universities in achieving the goal of rapidly increasing the number of doctors produced by Ethiopian schools and keeping them in the country (Celletti et al. 2011; Institute of Medicine 2001). In Australia, the medical education system is run by

◆ the national government, which is responsible for policy and funding of medical education

◆ the state and territory governments, which manage and fund training hospitals for medical students and

◆ private hospitals, which fund a small amount of training for postgraduate students.

Alignment between educational institutions and health service delivery

Producing new doctors without regard for overall national human resource plans can result in a mismatch of graduates to country needs or a shortage of posts for newly qualified staff. Indeed, a good match between supply and demand is essential to ensure efficient and effective delivery of health services (Macinko et al. 2007). Some countries have introduced innovative programmes to link

the production of doctors to national and regional health sector plans.

In Brazil the public health system guarantees all citizens access to preventive and health promotion services. In order to create enough of the appropriate health workers to realize this goal, the Brazilian government established the Family Health Programme in 1994. The government focused on the reorientation of 50 medical schools so that they would be more responsive to the country's health needs, and at the same time has funded family medicine residency programs. As a result of the implementation of the Family Health Programme, infant mortality has dropped from 48/1000 to 17/1000; hospital admissions due to diabetes or stroke have decreased by 25%; and the proportion of children under 5 years old who are underweight has fallen by 67% (Macinko et al. 2007). Controlling for other health determinants, a 10% increase of Family Health Programme coverage was associated with a 0.45% decrease in the infant mortality rate, a 0.6% decline in postneonatal mortality, and a 1% decline in diarrhoea mortality (Macinko et al. 2007). The programme was also associated with an increase in the adult labour supply and school enrolment, and a decrease in fertility rates (Rocha and Soares 2009).

In the US, the Council on Graduate Medical Education (Council on Graduate Medical Education 2005) estimated that the country will have a shortage of 85 000–96 000 physicians in 2020. Their recommendations included increasing the available number of residencies to 27 000 in 2015 from the 2002 level of approximately 24 000, and increasing enrolment in medical schools by 15%. The Association of American Medical Colleges (AAMC) (2003) recommended a more drastic increase of 30% in medical school enrolment for the decade starting from 2002 by increasing class sizes at existing medical schools and by establishing new schools. The American College of Physicians (2009) recommended increasing the proportion of US doctors that work in primary care by providing incentives to lessen the financial burden of graduates entering primary care. The American Academy of Family Physicians' (AAFP) (2009) 2006 AAFP Workforce Study stated that about 39 000 additional family physicians are needed by the year 2020 to supply Americans with an adequate primary care physician supply—they recommend that 50% of US physicians should work in primary care specialties. The AAFP recommends that federal funding for family medicine departments be increased under the US Public Health Service Act. Both the Council on Graduate Medical Education (COGME) (Martinez and Martineau 1998) and the AAMC (Council on Graduate Medical Education 2005) recommended decreasing or eliminating Medicare caps for funding of residencies and fellowships.

At the regional level, in low- and middle-income countries, the ASEAN (Association of Southeast Asian Nations) Mutual Recognition Arrangement on Medical Practitioners encourages all ASEAN states to adopt mechanisms for sharing of information about medical education—resulting in harmonization in accordance with international standards. Under this agreement, medical practitioners may apply for registration outside their home countries, but within ASEAN states, if they meet certain conditions. They must:

◆ be in possession of a medical qualification recognized by the host and home country

◆ have a professional registration and practising certificate recognized by the home country

◆ have been actively practising for at least 5 years in the home country

◆ be in compliance with home country regulating bodies

◆ have not violated any professional or ethical standards

◆ declare that they have no legal proceedings pending against them, and

◆ comply with other assessments or requirements as levied by the host country.

Examples of innovation in low- and middle-income countries

There is a range of examples of innovation (fig. 57.4).

The Medical Education Partnership Initiative (MEPI)

The US President's Emergency Plan for AIDS Relief (PEPFAR) has a goal to train at least 140 000 new healthcare professionals and paraprofessionals. Through MEPI, the aim is to strengthen medical systems in Africa, to expand clinical and research capacity, and to support innovative retention strategies for doctors, nurses, midwives, and teaching staff in African countries.

MEPI will invest up to US$130 million over 5 years in grants to African institutions in a dozen sub-Saharan countries. Key to this initiative is the formation of a network of about 30 regional partners, health and education ministries, and more than 20 collaborators from the USA.

A coordinating centre will link the African sites and their US partners, leverage shared resources, and provide technical expertise. An online platform will allow all partners to share data and outcomes. MEPI will enable participating institutions to strengthen their information technology, support distance education and data sharing, and encourage the establishment of clinical registries to inform research and healthcare decision making.

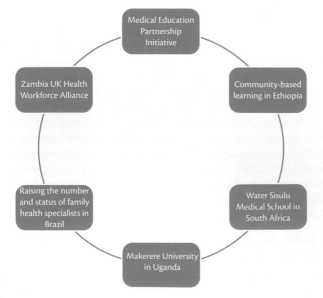

Figure 57.4 Examples of innovation.

Community-based learning in Ethiopia

Jimma Medical School in Ethiopia is a pioneer of community-based undergraduate and postgraduate education. From their first year through to graduation, medical, nursing, and allied healthcare professional students are deployed to pursue a specific educational objective through research in the community. In the final year this approach is extended to team-based learning, whereby teams of students from a range of disciplines are posted to regional, district, or community health centres. During their 8-week deployment the students learn to apply the skills they have acquired in a wide range of real-life situations. They also learn to work together with colleagues, using a joint problem-solving approach, to address the multifaceted health challenges that are common in local communities.

By using the community as a learning environment, and placing an emphasis on interdisciplinary work, the medical and nursing education programmes at Jimma Medical School have achieved a high degree of relevance. This has been shown to benefit the students—Jimma is becoming widely recognized for the high quality of its graduates—while also contributing to improving the health of the communities that participate in the programme (World Health Organization 2009).

A local solution to recruitment, education, and retention in South Africa

Walter Sisulu Medical School was founded in 1985 with a clear objective: to produce doctors with the right skills to practise in the underserved rural communities of South Africa.

The challenge was twofold. Not only did the region of Transkei need more doctors with the appropriate skills, it also needed more doctors who were motivated and willing to serve in deprived rural areas. To meet this challenge, the school needed to equip students with the right kind of scientific and professional knowledge to deal with the healthcare problems of Transkei. It also needed to recruit students with a sense of vocation, and to nurture a commitment to public service. A total of 835 doctors have now graduated from the school and as many as 70% of these are still working in the immediate area of KwaZulu-Natal and the Eastern Cape where they have made a significant contribution to alleviating healthcare problems.

What have been the key elements that have ensured this success? Students are recruited largely from the local communities. This has involved particular challenges, as the secondary educational opportunities available in the area are poor. The curricula and style of teaching have used problem-based methods to enhance learning skills, in addition to providing knowledge. The education, research, and service programmes of the school are guided by the specific health and social needs of the surrounding population. Partnership with the local health system actors has helped to develop locally relevant competencies. The curriculum integrates basic and clinical sciences with population health and social sciences. Much of the learning takes place within the community, rather than in the university or tertiary hospitals, and is located within the broad healthcare delivery system. In these ways, early clinical contact increases the relevance of theoretical teaching, and the programmes encourage a commitment to public service. The medical school's approach to faculty development has also emphasized the importance of teachers and mentors having relevant experience of practice in community medicine (World Health Organization 2009).

Flexible approaches to faculty development in Uganda

Makerere University is finding ways to better meet the country's needs and to improve health outcomes in Uganda. Like many teaching institutions in resource-constrained countries, the university is working with severe constraints. Makerere has an acute shortage of teaching staff—with around 75% of faculty posts currently vacant. To ease this situation, the university has made extensive use of modern communication technologies and partnerships that allow the programmes to call upon teaching resources and opportunities elsewhere. A mentoring programme allows staff to benefit from world-class instruction and to establish career pathways while remaining in Makerere. Fellowships and faculty exchange programmes are designed to encourage those who leave temporarily to return home. Good use is made of opportunities for teleconferencing with other universities for case conferences, and the main lecture hall is currently being rewired to allow for improved video and audio conferencing. An electronic library broadens opportunities for learning in a resource-constrained environment by allowing full access to relevant articles on a daily basis.

Makerere has also adopted other innovative educational methodologies, such as community-based learning and problem-based learning, which encourages students to seek out information and solve problems—skills they will need when practising in the rural areas of Uganda (World Health Organization 2009).

Raising the number and status of family health specialists in Brazil

Brazil has made a long-term and sustained investment in its health system over the past 20 years. Fifty percent of the population is now covered by a total of 30 000 family health teams. However, only 4% of the workforce has specialist training. One of the objectives of the current health development plan is to increase the numbers of specialist doctors with a particular emphasis on family health, in line with the principles of primary healthcare around which Brazil's health system has been built.

The traditional training institutions of Brazil lack the capacity to meet this need and tend to adopt a traditional approach that fails to promote family health. Brazil is now using an 'open university' model to offer postgraduate specialization for 52 000 family health professionals and to provide training for 110 000 health managers. The programme aims to draw on the strengths of different institutions to upgrade both the quantity and quality of graduates by creating a more robust platform for shared distance learning. Currently 12 universities are involved, with eight of these rated among the top 10 in the country. The teaching tools can range from the distribution of CDs for short-term, on-demand knowledge transfer, through to long-term diploma courses. The programme expects to increase the percentage of family health specialists in the country from the current figure of 3.5% to over 56%.

The power of academic partnerships

There are many examples of alliances between academic institutions in resource-constrained countries and high-income countries. Although some concerns have been raised around lack of coordination and the potential for undue influence on country planning, there are many examples of success—particularly in the areas of faculty development, leadership training, and curriculum development. The Fogarty International Center funds training in the USA for medical students from all over the world. The programme aims to ensure that study abroad does not contribute to brain drain. It does this through careful selection of appropriate candidates; strong interinstitutional collaborations and mentoring; and by focusing on the production of future leaders in global health. A high proportion of graduates do return home to practise medicine, and many choose a career in primary care and elect to work with disadvantaged groups. The University of Nigeria has forged a partnership with the University of Maryland, which aims to build the intrinsic capacity of in-country medical institutions with the long-term objective of building overall medical capacity in Nigeria. The programme adopts a phased approach to human resource development, starting with opportunities for faculty to travel to the US for training. This first phase involves faculty in 6–10 month placements for advanced clinical teaching. The second phase sends highly trained faculty from the US to Nigeria to teach there. In phase three, highly motivated students are recruited from Nigeria for training in the US, but with the expectation that they will return to Nigeria at the end of the 7-year programme. The partners are now working to build greater residency training in country and to transfer leadership to indigenous experts. Phase four is a strategic alliance with leading universities and teaching hospitals or medical schools to develop technical experts at all levels.

The recently launched Zambia UK Health Workforce Alliance will support the implementation of the Zambian human resources plan by providing educational faculty and other support to scale up medical training by 50% and nursing and midwifery training by 75% (World Health Organization 2009).

A medical education to meet population needs and expectations

Twenty-first century medical education should aim to put population health needs and expectations at its centre and should use population health outcomes as crucial measures in assessing the success of the educational process. Isolated improvements in individual educational institutions or narrowly defined health sector reforms are not enough. While the expansion of medical schools may serve to increase the quantity of doctors, expansion alone will not meet the equally important objectives of improving their quality. Nor will sole expansion of numbers ensure that new doctors have the competencies to provide care that their patients need. The efforts of education and health ministries will only be effective with simultaneous engagement of educational institutions, private sector providers, professional associations, civil society and communities (World Health Organization 2008c, 2009, 2010d).

The guiding principles

If medical education is to evolve to meet the changing needs of society, a number of principles must inform its transformation. These are outlined in fig. 57.5.

A practical way forward

New medical education must entail a series of interventions in the following domains: governance, education and training, research, regulation, financing, planning, implementation, and monitoring and evaluation in order to achieve the outcome of improving the quality, quantity and relevance of doctors around the world.

Medical education should:

- Be country led, context specific, and embedded in the broader socio-economic and development characteristics of communities and populations

- Respond to population health needs and expectations, whereby population health needs encompass local epidemiology, burden of disease, and broader health needs in terms of promotion, prevention, education and rehabilitation; and whereby population expectations include health equity, the delivery of people-centred services, responsiveness, and inclusion

- Prepare students to perform biomedical and technical research that can contribute to improving the wellbeing of the population

- Contribute to universal coverage of health services

- Be designed and implemented through multi-sectoral coordination of all relevant stakeholders in both public and private sectors

- Align with national health strategies and plans

- Involve all relevant institutions and constituencies, including policy makers at all levels in health, education, labour and finance; education and training institutions and associations; professional associations and regulatory bodies; health services administrators; communities and civil society; national and international research institutions; and development agencies and partners

- Address a combination of context-specific interventions, applicable in both the public and private sectors, in broad areas such as governance, education, and regulation

- Produce doctors who are globally competent, locally relevant, able to serve their local communities and national population, and advance biomedical research

- Ensure that an increase in the production of doctors is accompanied by an increase in the absorptive capacity of the labour market in academia, research, and service delivery

- Be supported by significant financial investment, long-term and effective leadership and management, good information systems, and government commitment

- Measure success based on the quantity, quality, and relevance of doctors who are practising within the health system and research institutions, and not simply on the numbers of new graduates.

Figure 57.5 Guiding principles in medical education.

Governance

1. Political commitment and leadership in the form of collaboration and shared accountability between the Ministry of Health, the Ministry of Education, and other related ministries (e.g. finance, labour, public service), at national and/or subnational level are crucial to plan and deliver medical education that is responsive to population needs.

2. The governance of medical schools should include the active participation of representatives from key stakeholder groups such as policy makers, education and training institutions, professional associations, regulatory bodies, the private sector, health services, communities and civil society, and students.

Medical schools

1. Students from underserved, underrepresented, or rural populations should be actively recruited, admitted, and retained in medical schools.

2. A system of recognition and reward that values teaching ability should be put in place for both undergraduate and postgraduate programmes.

3. Faculty should be expanded to include researchers, health service providers, service users, community members, and private sector personnel as adjunct faculty and/or teaching staff.

4. Curricula should include core competencies to address local population health needs and expectations; effective delivery of health services; education and training; and research.

5. Interprofessional learning should be expanded.

6. The educational activities of medical students should expose them to a wide range of health services, reflecting service delivery needs.

7. Postgraduate training programmes should be made available in underserved areas.

8. Partnerships between accredited medical schools that promote the exchange of students, faculty, technology and facilities, and strengthen capacities to develop and deliver core curricula should be promoted.

Regulatory frameworks

1. Accreditation and periodic reaccreditation of all medical schools and their associated clinical practice placement sites should be undertaken.

2. Universal certification and licensure (including periodic recertification) of all medical doctors should be adopted.

3. Continuous professional development (CPD) and in-service training of medical doctors (and the engagement and active participation of education institutions in their design and execution) should be introduced.

4. Compulsory service requirements after graduation in underserved geographical areas and/or populations should become common practice.

Financing

1. Increased allocation of resources targeted to medical education should be made available from both the public and private sector through taxes, grants, loans, and other mechanisms.

2. Results-based financing for medical schools should be introduced.

3. Financial assistance to students, either through subsidized education in return for compulsory service in underserved or rural areas, or as direct financial assistance to students in forms of loans, grants, and fellowships, should be provided.

Planning, implementation, and monitoring and evaluation

1. National medical education plans should be developed in consultation with all stakeholders. The plans should be informed by the needs and absorptive capacity of the labour market and aligned with national health plans.

2. The creation or strengthening of national or subnational institutions, capacities, or mechanisms to support medical education (such as legislation, policies, and procedures) should be considered.

Conclusions

◆ Low- and middle-income countries need more doctors, but not simply more of the same.

◆ Insufficient collaboration between the health and education sectors creates a crippling mismatch between medical education and the realities of health service delivery.

◆ The challenge of medical education in low- and middle-income countries relates to the quantity of doctors graduating from medical schools: the quality of medical education; and its relevance to population health needs and expectations.

◆ A transformative scale-up of medical education is needed to increase the capacity of health systems to respond to population needs and will require a broad process of multisectoral reform.

Acknowledgement

The authors are grateful to Ms Anna Wright (London School of Hygiene and Tropical Medicine) for her valuable input throughout the development of this chapter.

References

Abdel-Rahim, I., Mustafa, A., and Ahmed, B. (1992) Performance evaluation of graduates from a community-based curriculum: the housemanship period at Gezira. *Med Educ.* 26: 233–240

Al-Dabbagh, S.A. and Al-Taee, W.G. (2005) Evaluation of a task-based community oriented teaching model in family medicine for undergraduate medical students in Iraq. *BMC Med Educ.* 5: 31

American Academy of Family Physicians (2009) *Family Physician Workforce Reform: Recommendations of the American Academy of Family Physicians* (AAFP Reprint No. 305b). Leawood, KS: AAFP

American Association Medical Colleges (2003) Trends Among Foreign-Graduate Faculty at US Medical Schools, 1981-2000. *Analysis in Brief.* 3: 15–16

American College of Physicians (2009) *Recommendations for Health Care Workforce Policy to the Senate Health, Education, Labor, and Pensions Committee Staff.* http://www.acponline.org/advocacy/where_we_stand/workforce/hc_may09.pdf Accessed 15 March 2013

Anand, S. and Baernighausen, T. (2004) *Human Resources and Health Outcomes.* Oxford: Global Equity Initiative, USA, and Oxford University

Anderson, F.W.J., Mutchnick, I., Kwawukume, E.Y., et al. Who will be there when women deliver? Assuring retention of obstetric providers. (2007) *Obstet Gynecol.* 110(5): 102–116

Armada, F., Muntaner, C., Chung, H., Williams-Brennan, L., and Benach, J. (2009) Barrio Adentro and the reduction of health inequalities in Venezuela: an appraisal of the first years. *Int J Health Serv.* 39: 161–187

Art, B., De Roo, L., Willems, S., and De Maeseneer, J. (2008) An interdisciplinary community diagnosis experience in an undergraduate medical curriculum: development at Ghent University. *Acad Med.* 83(7): 675–683

Beck, E., Wingard, D.L., Zuniga, M.L., Heifetz, R., and Gilbreath, S. (2008) Addressing the health needs of the underserved: a national faculty development program. *Acad Med.* 83(11): 1094–1102

Bianchi, F., Stobbe, K., and Eva, K. (2008) Comparing academic performance of medical students in distributed learning sites: the McMaster experience. *Med Teach.* 30: 67–71

Bosk, C.L. (1985) Social controls and physicians: the oscillation of cynicism and idealism in sociological theory. In J. Swazey and S.R. Scher (eds) *Social Controls and the Medical Profession* (pp. 31–52). Boston, MA: Genn, Oelgeschlager, Gunn and Hahn

Borroto Cruz, E.R. and Salas Perea, R.S. (2008) National Training Program for comprehensive community physicians, Venezuela. *MEDICC Review.* 10(4): 35–42

Briggs, C. and Mantini-Briggs, C. (2009) Confronting health disparities: Latin American social medicine in Venezuela. *Am J Public Health.* 99: 549

Buvé, A., Bishikwabo-Nsarhaza, K., and Mutangadura, G. (2002) The spread and effect of HIV-1 infection in sub-Saharan Africa. *Lancet.* 359: 2011–2017

Celletti, F., Reynolds, T.A., Wright, A., et al. (2011) Educating a new generation of doctors to improve the health of populations in low- and middle-income countries. *PLoS Med.* 10e: 1001–1008

Collins, F.S., Glass, R.I., Whitescarver, J., et al. (2010) Public health. Developing health workforce capacity in Africa. *Science.* 330: 1324–1325

Commission on Social Determinants of Health (2008) *Closing the gap in a generation: health equity through action on the social determinants of health.* Geneva: World Health Organization

Cooper, R. (2002) Economic and demographic trends signal an impending physician shortage. *Health Affairs.* 21(1): 140–154

Council on Graduate Medical Education (2005) *Physician Workforce Policy Guidelines for the U.S. for 2000–2020.* Rockville, MD: US Department of Health and Human Services

Davidson, L. (1965) The setting up of a new medical school. *Postgrad Med J.* 41: 61–66

Davidson, R.A. (2002) Community-based education and problem solving: the Community Health Scholars Program at the University of Florida. *Teach Learn Med.* 14(3): 178–181

Dunbabin, J.S., McEwin, K., and Cameron, I. (2006) Postgraduate medical placements in rural areas: their impact on the rural medical workforce. *Rural Remote Health.* 6(2): 481

Dussault, G. and Dubois, C. (2003) Human resources for health policies: a critical component in health policies. *Human Resources for Health.* 1: 1

Eley, D., Young, L., Baker, P., and Wilkinson, D. (2008) Developing a rural workforce through medical education: lessons from down under. *Teach Learn Med.* 20: 53–61

Erney, S.L., Allen, D.L., and Siska, K.F. (1991) Effect of a year-long primary care clerkship on graduates' selection of family practice residencies. *Acad Med.* 66(4): 234–236

Evans, T., Whitehead, M., Diderichsen, F., Bhuiya, A., and Wirth, M. (2001) *Challenging Inequities in Health: From Ethics to Action.* New York: Oxford University Press

Flexner, A. (1910) *Medical Education in the United States and Canada: a report to the Carnegie Foundation for the Advancement of Teaching.* New York: The Carnegie Foundation for the Advancement of Teaching

Fox, R.C. (1993) Training in caring competence. In H.C. Hendrie and C. Lloyd (eds) *Educating Competent and Human Physicians* (pp. 199–216). Bloomington, IN: Indiana University Press

Freeman, J., Kelly, P., Levites, M.R., and Blasco, P.G. (2009) *Attitudes about family medicine among Brazilian medical students.* 42nd STFM Annual Spring Conference, Denver

Frenk, J., Chen, L., Bhutta, Z.A., et al. (2010) Health professionals for a new century: transforming education to strengthen health systems in an interdependent world. *Lancet.* 376: 1923–1958

Grant N., Gibbs, T., Naseeb, T.A., and Al-Garf, A. (2009) Medical students as family-health advocates: Arabian Gulf University experience. *Med Teach.* 29(5): e117–e121

Grobler, L., Marais, B., Mabunda, S., Marindi, P., and Reuter, H. (2009) Interventions for increasing the proportion of health professionals practising in rural and other underserved areas. *Cochrane Database Systematic Reviews*, CD005314

Hauer, K.E., Durning, S.J., Kernan, W.N., et al. (2008) Factors associated with medical students' career choices regarding internal medicine. *JAMA.* 300: 1154–1164

Howe, A. (2001) Patient-centred medicine through student-centred teaching: a student perspective on the key impacts of community- based learning in undergraduate medical education. *Med Educ.* 35(7): 666–672

Institute of Medicine (2001) *Crossing the Quality Chasm: A new health system for the 21st century.* Washington DC: Institute of Medicine

Institute of Medicine, Smolinski, M.S., Hamburg, M.A., Lederberg, J. (2005) *Microbial Threats to Health: emergence, detection, and response.* Washington DC: National Academy Press

Institute of Medicine (2007) In: Sepulveda, J., Carpenter, C., Curran, J., et al. (eds) *PEPFAR Implementation: Progress and Promise.* Washington DC: National Academy Press

Institute of Medicine (2009) *Global Issues in Water, Sanitation, and Health. Workshop summary.* Washington DC: National Academy Press

Joint Learning Initiative (2004) *Human Resources for Health: Overcoming the Crisis.* Cambridge MA: Harvard University Press

Josiah Macy Jr Foundation (2008) *Revisiting the Medical School Educational Mission at a Time of Expansion.* Charleston: Josiah Macy Jr Foundation

Kaye, D.K., Mwanika, A., and Sewankambo, N. (2010) Influence of the training experience of Makerere University medical and nursing graduates on willingness and competence to work in rural health facilities. *Rural Remote Health.* 10: 1372

Keehan, S., Sisko, A., Truffer, C., et al. (2008) Health spending projections through 2017: the baby-boom generation is coming to Medicare. *Health Affairs.* 27: w145–w155

Kwizera, E.N., Igumbor, E.U., and Mazwai, L.E. (2005) Twenty years of medical education in rural South Africa—experiences of the University of Transkei Medical School and lessons for the future. *S Afr Med J.* 95(12): 920–922

Kwong, J.C., Dhalla, I.A., Streiner, D.L., et al. (2002) Effects of rising tuition fees on medical school class composition and financial outlook. *Can Med Ass J.* 166: 1023–1028

Laidlaw, A., Guild, S., and Struthers, J. (2009) Graduate attributes in the disciplines of medicine, dentistry and veterinary medicine: a survey of expert opinions. *BMC Med Educ.* 9: 28

Laven, G. and Wilkinson, L. (2003) Rural doctors and rural backgrounds: how strong is the evidence? A systematic review. *Aust J Rural Health.* 11: 277–284

Longombe, A.O. (2009) Medical schools in rural areas—necessity or aberration? *Rural Remote Health.* 9: 1131

Lu, C., Schneider, M.T., Gubbins, P., et al. (2010) Public financing of health in developing countries: a cross-national systematic analysis. *Lancet.* 375: 1375–1387

Ludmerer, K.M. (2003) The internal challenges to medical education. *Trans Am Clin Climatol Ass.* 114: 241–253

Macinko, J., Marinho de Souza, M.F., Guanais, F.C., and da Silva Simões, C.C. (2007) Going to scale with community-based primary care: An analysis of the family health program and infant mortality in Brazil. *Soc Sci Med.* 65(10): 2070–2080

Martínez, J. and Martineau, T. (1998) Rethinking human resources: an agenda for the millennium. *Health Policy Plan.* 13: 345–358

Merson, M.H., O'Malley, J., Serwadda, D., and Apisuk, C. (2008) The history and challenge of HIV prevention. *Lancet.* 372: 475–488

Morris, C., Johnson, B., Kim, S., and Chen, F. (2008) Training family physicians in community health centers: a health workforce solution. *Fam Med.* 40: 271

Mullan, F., Frehywot, S., Omaswa, F., Buch, E., and Chen, C. (2010) Medical schools in sub-Saharan Africa. *Lancet.* 377: 1113–1121

Norman, G., Joseph, A., Theodore, A., and Maruthamuthu, M. (1999) Community-based teaching of tropical diseases: an experience with filariasis. *Trop Doct.* 29: 86

Pandit, K., Kumar, S., and Aggarwal., O.P. (1991) Knowledge of fresh medical graduates about immunization: impact of posting in community medicine. *Ind J Pediatr.* 58(3): 345–348

Peterson, C. and Burton, R. (2007) *Congressional Research Service report: U.S. health care spending: comparison with other OECD countries.* Washington DC. Congressional Research Service

Rabinowitz, H.K., Diamond, J.J., Markham, F.W., and Hazelwood, C.E. (1999) A program to increase the number of family physicians in rural and underserved areas: impact after 22 years. *JAMA.* 281: 255–260

Rocha, R. and Soares, R.R. (2009) *Evaluating the Impact of Community-Based Health Interventions: Evidence from Brazil's Family Health Program.* IZA, Discussion paper 4119. Bonn, Germany

Samb, B., Celletti, F., Holloway, J., et al. (2007) Sounding board: rapid expansion of the health workforce in response to the HIV epidemic. *N Engl J Med.* 24: 2510–2514

Smucny, J., Beatty, P., Grant, W., Dennison, T., and Wolff, L.T. (2005) An evaluation of the Rural Medical Education Program of the State University of New York Upstate Medical University, 1990–2003. *Acad Med.* 80: 733–738

Tanenberg, R.J., Cummings, D.M., Dreyfus, K.S., et al. (2009) Primary care fellowship in diabetes: an innovative program in postgraduate diabetes education. *Teach Learn Med.* 21(4): 334–343

Tamblyn, R., Abrahamowicz, M., Dauphinee, D., et al. (2005) Effect of a community oriented problem based learning curriculum on quality of primary care delivered by graduates: historical cohort comparison study. *BMJ.* 331(7523): 1002–1009

Thomson, W.A., Ferry, P.G., King, J.E., Martinez-Wedig, C., and Michael, L.H. (2003) Increasing access to medical education for students from medically underserved communities: one program's success. *Acad Med.* 78: 454–459

United States Government Accountability Office (2009) *Graduate Medical Education: trends in training and student debt.* Washington DC: United States Government Accountability Office

Vaidya, V.M and Gothankar, J.S. (2009) Community based project work as a teaching tool: students' perception. *Ind J Community Med.* 34(1): 59–61

Valberg, L.S., Gonyea, M.A., Sinclair, D.G., and Wade, J. (1994) Planning the future academic medical centre. *Can Med Ass J.* 151: 1581–1587

Whitehead, M., Dahlgren, G., and Evans, T. (2001) Equity and health sector reforms: can low-income countries escape the medical poverty trap? *Lancet.* 358: 833–836

Whiteside C. and Mathias, R. (1996) Training for rural practice. *Can Fam Physician.* 42: 1113–1121

Wibulpolprasert, S. and Pengpaibon, P. (2003) Integrated strategies to tackle the inequitable distribution of doctors in Thailand: four decades of experience. *Human Resources for Health.* 1: 12

World Health Organization (2006) *The World Health Report: working together for health.* Geneva: World Health Organization

World Health Organization (2008a) *Scaling Up, Saving Lives. Task Force for scaling up education and training for health workers.* Geneva: World Health Organization.

World Health Organization (2008b) *Task Shifting: global recommendations and guidelines.* Geneva: World Health Organization

World Health Organization (2008c) *The World Health Report 2008—primary health care (now more than ever)* Geneva: World Health Organization

World Health Organization and Global Health Workforce Alliance (2009) *What Countries Can Do Now: Twenty-Nine Actions to Scale Up and Improve the Health Workforce.* World Health Organization, Geneva Switzerland. http://www.who.int/workforcealliance/knowledge/publications/taskforces/actionpaper.pdf Accessed 1 May 2012

World Health Organization (2009) *Report on the WHO/PEPFAR planning meeting on scaling up nursing and medical education.* Geneva: World Health Organization

World Health Organization (2010a) *Global Policy Recommendations: increasing access to health workers in remote and rural areas through improved retention.* Geneva: World Health Organization

World Health Organization (2010b) *Framework for Action on Interprofessional Education and Collaborative Practice.* Geneva: World Health Organization,.

World Health Organization (2010c) *World Health Statistics.* Geneva: World Health Organization

World Health Organization (2010d) *Report on the WHO/PEPFAR First technical reference group meeting: medical education experts.* Geneva: World Health Organization

CHAPTER 58

Medical education in the emerging market economies

Manisha Nair and Premila Webster

At present it might seem that the teaching of medicine
is a by-product of the school and not the main objective,
for teaching is carried out by those who happen to find
themselves there, who have not been trained in education
nor benefited by informed criticism of their teaching
methods.

A.G. Oettlé

Introduction

The World Bank defines emerging market economies as 'economies
with relatively high levels of economic potential and international
engagement, broader than the traditional classifications [based on
the Gross National Income per capita]' (The World Bank 2011).
The countries labelled emerging market economies (EMEs) have
increased from 28 in 2006 to 61 in 2011 (The World Bank 2011),
constituting 32% of the independent nations worldwide.

Six countries of the EMEs (China, India, Indonesia, Brazil,
Pakistan, and Russia) are among the 10 most populous in the
world, comprising of 48% of the world's population with China and
India constituting 36.5% of the global population (United Nations
Department of Economic and Social Affairs Population Division
2010). According to the demographic transition theory most EMEs
are in the third stage of transition when there is a decline in death
rates with a slower decline in birth rates leading to a slower population growth and an ageing population ((Davis 1945; Thompson
1929). This appears to be accompanied by an exponential increase
in the rate of urbanization (fig. 58.1). Seven of the 10 largest conur-
bations are in five EMEs (United Nations Department of Economic
and Social Affairs Population Division 2010). These socioeconomic
and demographic changes have accelerated the pace of epidemiological transition in the EMEs, rapidly moving them from the 'age
of receding pandemics' to the 'age of degenerative and man-made
diseases' (Omran 2001, pp. 168–169). The health of the population
in most of these countries is threatened by the double burden of
lifestyle-associated diseases and new and existing infectious diseases (Brito and García 2010).

Since the cost of treating chronic diseases and disability is high,
the role of prevention becomes important, especially with the
increasing knowledge of modifiable risk factors. While retaining
the curative model of healthcare, multidimensional preventive
models will have to be developed for early detection of risk factors and timely prevention of disease (Charalambous and Rousou
2010). There is a growing awareness among policy makers of the
need for reforms in health systems and a change from an acute care
model to a patient-centred public health model (Pruitt and Epping-
Jordan 2005). The health systems and healthcare workforce in these
countries are evolving to handle these changes (Pruitt and Epping-
Jordan 2005). Consequently, the EMEs are in different phases
of health system reforms, underpinned by the common objectives of bridging the gap between population and patient-centred
approaches and shift from secondary to primary care (Pruitt and
Epping-Jordan 2005). Examples of this are shown in fig. 58.2.

Medical education in these countries will need to be tailored
to meet the challenges related to the epidemiological transition,
the growing social change that economic growth brings and the
creation of an equitable health service. This will require an understanding of the history of the evolution of medical education in
the EMEs, their relation to the health needs of population and the
impact of globalization and technical advancement on the provision of healthcare.

The evolution of medical education in EMEs

While the scientific foundation of medical knowledge in Europe
dates back to the work of Hippocrates (440 BCE) and Galen (160
CE), medical education developed in the Middle Ages, mainly in
Western Europe (Spain and Italy) as a blend of Greek, Roman,
and Arabic medicine, and 'Western medicine' evolved towards the
end of the 14th century (Jamieson 1946). The other four ancient

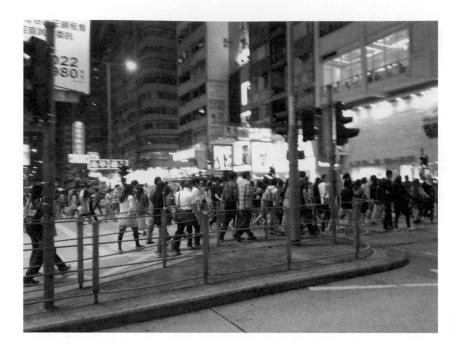

Figure 58.1 Mong Kok, an area in Hong Kong with the highest population density in the world (Mong Kok means busy corner).

1. Countries of Eastern and Central Europe, including Russia and Poland are in the process of replacing the Soviet model of clinic based specialist care by a system of integrated general practice (Szmatloch 2000; Rese et al. 2005; Farmer et al. 2003)

2. Countries in Latin America (Brazil, Chile, Argentina, Peru, and Colombia) are in the process of strengthening their primary healthcare system as part of their social and health system reforms for equity of access to quality care (Román et al. 2007; Pulido et al. 2006; Fleury 2007)

3. A few countries in South Asia (India, China, Sri Lanka, and Pakistan), while striving for universal health coverage by remodelling primary care delivery and public health systems, are struggling to maintain primary healthcare delivery in rural areas due to migration of healthcare workers both to urban areas and overseas. This is coupled with a growing and lucrative market in medical tourism (Sood 2008; Schwarz et al. 2004)

Figure 58.2 EMEs in different phases of health system reforms.

systems of medicine all have their origins in four EMEs namely, India, China, Egypt, and 'Arabia', and can be traced back to a period in history when the seeds of European medicine were not yet sown (Croizier 1970). While the Arabic system merged with the Greek and Roman ones to form the European system, the Indian, Egyptian, and Chinese systems grew independently of the European system with their roots firmly embedded in traditions and sophisticated theoretical underpinnings (Croizier 1970).

Western medicine (European medicine) was introduced in many of the EMEs during colonization between the 17th and the 19th centuries. Medical colleges were set up in British, French, German, and American colonies to train local people in Western medicine, using the curriculum and teaching methods of the 'rulers' while the traditional systems of medicine were derecognized (Bowers 1974). Some historians are of the view that the colonists established medical schools in the colonies as a means of influencing the country's systems to meet the needs of Western countries (Brown 1979).

Major reforms in medical education in most of the EMEs began in the mid-19th century, coinciding with their political, social, and economic transitions. Two distinct phases are seen in the evolution of medical education in the EMEs—the establishment phase and the development phase (see fig. 58.3).

The establishment phase is the period during which many of the EMEs were identifying and defining their medical education systems and was mainly driven by sociopolitical contexts. The phase of development can be attributed to transitions in health systems, population demography, and epidemiology, which were brought about by the rapid transitions in the economy. Considering the historical diversity of the sociopolitical contexts in the 61 EMEs, it is difficult to precisely identify a cut-off in the time period where the phase of establishment ended and development began. However, trends suggest that the phase of establishment spanned from the latter half of the 18th century to the mid-20th century.

The establishment phase

While the evolution of medical education in Europe and America can be seen as a continuous phase from its origin in 440 BCE to the present time, the evolution in the EMEs was interrupted by a period of the search for the identity of their own medical system amongst the turmoil of social, cultural and political reforms. While the medical education systems of many of the EMEs were undergoing 'Westernization', the medical education system in Russia underwent 'Sovietization', incorporating communist principles and was governed by a Central Soviet Committee in Moscow (Gantt 1924, p. 1056). The reforms were based on political philosophies rather than scientific evidence. For example, student uptake from the working classes increased, irrespective of their level of literacy. The only modification made to the prerevolution medical curriculum was inclusion of compulsory education on 'social hygiene', 'history of materialism', and 'the political organization of the Russian Socialistic Federation of Soviet Republics' (Gantt 1924, p. 1057).

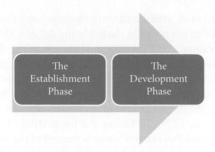

Figure 58.3 Evolution of medical education.

However, the evolution of medical education in African countries differs both in the construct of the phases as well as the time-period. The establishment phase for Africa has a different construct because it was a struggle for equal opportunities for medical education for Africans. The first medical school in South Africa was established in Cape Town in 1912 (Ncayiyana 1999) and medical education in the country followed the British model (De Villiers and De Villiers 1999), but was characterized by the absence of non-European students until the 1950s (Ncayiyana 1999). The medical education system in South Africa became a part of apartheid (Tobias 1980). Between 1968 and 1977, only 3% of the medical graduates in South Africa were of African origin, although they constituted 70.4% of the population (Tobias 1980). Even towards the end of the 20th century the situation had only marginally improved, as only 15% of the students in the eight South African medical schools were of African origin (De Villiers and De Villiers 1999). Clearly, the problems of racial imbalance in medical school entrants still persists in Africa, hence, instead of a demarcation by time period between the 'establishment phase' and 'development phase', an overlap is observed.

However, the search for an identity in medicine and medical education in the EMEs diminished by the 1960s paving the way for the 'development phase', largely due to emerging health system challenges related to the demographic and epidemiological transitions (Charalambous and Rousou 2010).

The development phase

Medical education during the development phase was influenced by demography and epidemiology rather than political and sociocultural contexts. At the outset it is important to highlight the evolving challenges to medical education in the EMEs during the period of the development phase. During the 1950s, in most of the EMEs, the health system challenges were to prevent and contain epidemics of infectious diseases through health education promoting hygiene and sanitation, maternal child health, and nutrition. In addition, there was an increased demand for paediatricians (as one-third of the population were children) and physicians for the rural population (which constituted more than 60–80% of the population).

During the 1940s and 1950s when medical schools were being established in many of these newly independent nations, fellowships were provided by both government and private foundations (such as Rockefeller) to train medical students in Britain and the United States so returning doctors could contribute to the development of medical education in these countries (Junqueira 1959; Monteiro 1959; Sheth 1959). However, in the 1960s and 1970s it was recognized that besides the prestige associated with overseas training there were no real benefits, as the doctors trained abroad were

unable to adapt their knowledge of diseases and health systems of the West to address the disease burden and/or improve health system performance in their countries (Rosa 1964). Another disadvantage was the reluctance of these doctors to work in rural areas, resulting in their congregating in the urban areas of their country, or migration to the West (Rosa 1964; Crane 1969; Beighton 1978). During this period medical educators in many EMEs highlighted the merits of the following: training in local medical schools, needs-based education, problem-solving ability, and training in rural communities (Rosa 1964).

The development phase heralded the dawn of the era of 'needs-based medical education'—the needs of the population, the needs to address disease burden and promote health, and the needs of the growing healthcare delivery system. While the generic nature of the needs have been retained, the specific features have changed over the past 60 years. For example, until the latter part of the 20th century, the population pyramid in most of these countries was broad at the base, demanding a curriculum that provided adequate training in infant and child health, but with an ageing population, the focus has shifted towards problems of ageing.

The establishment phase of medical education in the EMEs dealt mainly with two debates: the sociocultural versus scientific basis of the medical education curriculum; and the equal opportunities of education for all classes and races versus merit-based selection of students. The subjects of these debates extended into the development phase, but the nature of the debates altered. The curriculum reforms in the development phase were faced with the challenges of volume due to the growth in knowledge of diseases, treatments and diagnostics and the need for standardization of both curriculum and student selection processes. In addition, ethics, research, methods of teaching, and teacher training were also important areas of discussion. Two other factors that had an impact on medical education in EMEs at this time were the unprecedented increase in the number of medical schools and the increasing number of doctors training to be specialists.

Challenges for medical education in the EMEs

Curriculum development

As early as the 1950s it was realized that instead of loading the curriculum with knowledge acquired through rote learning, the medical education system should facilitate reasoning among students, and that this could be best achieved through integration (Oettlé 1952). One of the earlier considerations in curriculum development was the integration of basic sciences with clinical medicine. Educators in some of the EMEs including Brazil, South Africa, and India advocated vertical coordination between the subjects taught in each year (Junqueira 1959; Kaur 1960). However, from the perspective of the students who were required to pass examinations on a certain group of subjects unrelated to the preliminary years, the curriculum appeared horizontal (Oettlé 1952). Among the EMEs, Russia was probably the only country that went from an integrated medical curriculum delivered through self-directed group learning in the 1930s (where an illness was not merely discussed from a clinical or pathological perspective, but from all its complexities, including social and economic) to a theory-based system in the 1950s (Fox 1954).

During this period there was also widespread discussions, on the introduction of preventive medicine in the medical curriculum—mainly to prevent, eliminate and eradicate the infectious diseases prevalent in the EMEs (Paul 1959). While some countries such as Brazil, Colombia, Chile, Singapore, and China made concerted efforts to introduce preventative medicine in their curriculum (Paul 1959; Müller 1980; Chew 1991), others like India, Thailand, and South Africa were engaged in discussions about whether to incorporate preventive medicine in the curriculum and give it equal status with other clinical subjects (Kaur 1960; De Villiers and De Villiers 1999; Piyaratn 1982). The development phase brought about changes in the concept of public health from a subject that dealt with environmental sanitation and hygiene to one that should deal with the community level factors that result in ill health; this led to the introduction of the concept of 'clinical epidemiology' (Paul 1959). However, not everyone was in favour of public health research and training. Public health was described by a Brazilian doctor as 'a heavy routine hindering research, and training' (Junqueira 1959, p. 988). Yet others were of the opinion that public health was the business of auxiliaries and not qualified doctors.

Similar to the case of students who trained abroad but had little impact on developing the medical education and healthcare delivery systems in their native countries, there was limited usefulness of the 'imported curriculum', unless it was modified to suit the population, sociocultural, economic and health system needs of the country (Blizard 1991; Foster 1966). This gave birth to the concept of the needs-based curriculum for the EMEs in the late 1960s. Latin American countries, such as Colombia, used a more evidence-based approach, instead of importing medical education. They endeavoured to set up a medical education system by studying the needs of the local community through both local and international collaboration (Jimeñez-Arango 1966). The seven medical schools in Colombia (in 1965) joined to form the Association of Colombian Medical Schools, which monitored the standards of medical education and undertook research initiatives to shape the medical education system according to the needs of the country (Jimeñez-Arango 1966).

Another step towards needs-based education was the establishment of the community-oriented primary care model (COPC) of teaching in the 1980s in several Latin American countries such as Costa Rico, Mexico, Chile, Brazil, Cuba, and Nicaragua (Fernando 1983). In this model, the medical students were taught an integrated curriculum of medicine, and social and behavioural sciences in community settings (Fernando 1983). However, the development of the COPC model in Latin America and other methods of introducing community-based training in undergraduate curricula (which spanned the length of the 'development phase') were fraught with financial crisis, political unrest, lack of student interest, and criticism of medical educators (Fernando 1983; Mash and De Villiers 1999).

Conferences were held worldwide to discuss the structure of medical education systems for the EMEs in order to enable them to strengthen the healthcare workforce, and contribute towards their socioeconomic development (Hill 1962; Hyde 1965). Medical educators in Colombia were considered visionaries as they incorporated medical education into the National Health Plan as early as the 1960s (Jimeñez-Arango 1966). Similar national processes for curricular reforms were also described in Indonesia during the 1970s (Blizard et al. 1980) and were proposed in other South and South-East Asian countries in the following decades (Blizard 1991).

A unique example of curriculum planning in the development phase was Saudi Arabia, where equal priority was given to religious and cultural norms along with science. A female student was not allowed to study certain anatomical parts of the human body, which segregated the medical responsibilities of males and females (Basalamah et al. 1979). In China, the integration of Chinese and Western medicine that started towards the end of the establishment phase was further developed during this phase (Jain 1972), but this was not the case in India where the schools set up to teach an integrated curriculum gradually shifted to teaching either Ayurvedic or allopathic medicine (allopathic medicine is a term used for Western medicine in India) (Jeffery 1977).

Further, two characteristic features of the curriculum in the socialist countries (Russia and China) which separated them from the rest of the world were political indoctrination of the curriculum and the absence of written examinations in the student evaluation system (Fox 1954; Jain 1972).

Student selection

Another crucial element of medical education is the selection of students, which during the 'establishment phase' appeared to be influenced by political ideologies in countries such as Russia and China. During the 'development phase' when there was a drive to increase the number of medical professionals, the process of selection changed into a merit-based system, where students were mainly selected based on their academic records and scores in common entrance tests, regardless of their aptitude to work as health professionals. While this process of selecting students continues in most EMEs, research exploring students' motivation and career interests began in several countries towards the end of 20th century. A study among final-year medical students in Saudi Arabia showed that the majority of students were inclined to specialize, with few wanting to study family medicine (al-Faris et al. 1997). Their decisions were motivated by 'prestige', higher earnings, and working in speciality hospitals in the cities (al-Faris et al. 1997).

Teaching medical ethics

The concept of doctors being more 'human' and ethical in their practice was discussed widely in the development phase and a body of research in this area was undertaken. Oettlé 1952, a medical educator at the South African Institute of Medical Research while outlining the aims and tasks of undergraduate medical education laid special emphasis on 'developing the student's mind and character, and bringing out the best in him' (Oettlé 1952, p. 240), which he suggests can be done only though rigorous training in ethics. In Thailand, the medical curriculum was revised to include the four pillars of Buddhism; 'veracity, non-injury to life, justice and compassion' as the ethical basis for medical practitioners (Ratanakul 1988, pp. 302–312). This was done as the perception was that while the American system of medical education in Thailand was almost entirely centred around the 'science' of medicine and was able to increase life-expectancy in Thailand, it lacked the values of traditional Thai medicine, which was balanced by bioethics based on the principles of Buddhism (Ratanakul 1988). Similarly in Poland, philosophy of medicine was integrated into the curriculum, which taught not only the 'art of healing', but also formed the basis of medical ethics (Pedziwiatr 1999). China based their ethics curriculum on the principles of patients' rights and professional conduct (Li 2000). In South Africa, teaching of ethics and human rights to undergraduate medical students was initiated by the South African Medical Association (SAMA) in 1999 as an aftermath of the apartheid period (Williams 2000). The teaching of bioethics was included in the curriculum in most EMEs during the development phase, but the degree of incorporation varied. Although bioethics is now taught in most medical schools in the EMEs, the quality is questionable and time devoted to this subject is limited. Even with the increasing number of research projects on human subjects in many EMEs, the subject of bioethics is not seen as a priority (Drane and Fuenzalida 1991; Du 2000).

Research and the medical school

Doctors were undertaking research to learn about the diseases and their aetiology during the 19th century. The first research institute in South Africa, the South African Institute for Medical Research was set up in 1912 to investigate occupational diseases (silicosis and pneumonia), though the research was driven by economic gains rather than humanitarian ideals (Brock 1960). The medical community gradually realized that the role of a medical school was not just to educate health professionals, but also to advance medical knowledge, without which there was a risk that the institutes themselves would become redundant (Brock 1960; Oettlé 1952). Research became an important part of medical education in many of the EMEs after the World War II. However, medical schools in some South American countries were ill-equipped (due to the lack of scientific expertise and human resources), but were pushed into research to obtain grants and technical aids from US agencies (Paul 1959). In Russia it was compulsory for all postgraduate students to be involved in research; in 1954 there were 279 institutes for medical research in Russia (Fox 1954). Focus on research in medical schools continued to grow throughout the 20th century and into the 21st century, with increasing international collaborative research. However, increased medical research has not been accompanied by increased training and participation of medical students in research programmes in many EMEs (Oliveira et al. 2011).

Teaching and learning

Teaching during the development phase in the EMEs was through lectures and rote learning. There was a shortage of diagnostic equipment and teaching aids and students often did not have access to medical journals. The development of teaching methods during the 1950s and 1960s was mainly focused on improving lectures and practical demonstrations through tutorials for undergraduate students (Oettlé 1952). This propensity of students and teachers towards acquiring theoretical knowledge through rote learning without reasoning was recognized as a problem in the 1950s (Junqueira 1959; Fox 1954), but is still prevalent in many of the medical schools in the EMEs. In the 1970s, attempts were made to abolish the lecture-based, teacher-centric, didactic systems, and replace them with 'active-learning' and student-led discussions, used in the several medical schools in the United Kingdom and North America. However, this change was introduced suddenly and without appropriate preparation or training offered to the faculty. A Sri Lankan medical educator commented (Senewiratne et al. 1975, p. 28) 'a sudden exposure of students who have been taught to unquestioningly listen to a teacher throughout their school life to these new methods will result in chaos and confusion'. Medical

educators from many EMEs in Latin America and Asia suggested that this form of teaching should be introduced to the country's entire education system, rather than medical education alone (Lobo and Jouval Jr 1973; Senewiratne et al. 1975). Some countries (China for example) initiated collaborations with US universities to review the methods of teaching and student evaluation and obtained support from them to develop a uniform and comprehensive course for teaching and assessment in medical education (Stillman and Sawyer 1992).

Teacher training

In many EMEs before the mid-20th century the focus was not so much on the teachers and their level of training as on the academic ability of students. The responsibility of learning was with the students. As commented by (Oettlé 1952, p. 244):

'at present it might seem that the teaching of medicine is a by-product of the school and not the main objective, for teaching is carried out by those who happen to find themselves there, who have not been trained in education nor benefited by informed criticism of their teaching methods.

The development phase brought in a concerted effort by the World Health Organization (WHO) to emphasize the need to train teachers on learning processes, methods of teaching and student evaluation (World Health Organization 1966). However, in practice the reforms undertaken in many of the countries served merely to make the teachers proficient in lecturing (Oettlé 1952; Rao 1966). Another problem was a shortage of teachers in the growing number of medical schools. New graduates were not willing to give up a lucrative medical practice to become full-time teachers. While most preclinical teachers worked full-time, the clinical teachers gave time for teaching at their own convenience (Sheth 1959). Though discussions to set up a full-time teaching system for clinical education in EMEs started in 1958 (Paul 1959; Junqueira 1959; Sheth 1959), it made only limited progress. Besides time, the quality of teaching and the role of teachers in educating health professionals was only properly recognized in the 1970s and 1980s when several EMEs adopted programmes to 'teach the teachers to teach' and introduced 'computer-simulation', multimedia, videos, and films as additional teaching aids (Lobo and Jouval Jr 1973).

Growth of medical schools—quantity versus quality

The EMEs were economically underdeveloped during the development phase of medical education, many of them still recovering from the ravages of World War II. Some having recently gained independence had just embarked on the task of sociopolitical construction of a new nation. Hence, the priority to invest in medical education came only after provision of food, clothing and shelter to citizens. With economic growth and liberalization came a steady growth in the number of medical schools (especially in the last decade or two of the 20th century), which enrolled a great number of students—producing thousands of physicians annually. Privatization has played a key role in the economic growth of these countries, which is reflected in its growing influence in health education (Ng et al. 2005). The proliferation of private medical schools increased after many of these countries adopted the 'structural adjustment policies' of the World Bank and changed from a socialist to a free-market economy (Ladinsky et al. 2000; Bhat 1999). Private medical and nursing schools grew at an accelerated rate in

Latin America (Senf et al. 2003), Eastern and Central Europe, as well as in East and South-East Asia (Ng et al. 2005).

While the private market has grown, it is mostly unregulated, as a result of which most private universities and teaching hospitals do not provide standard quality education. In Chile there is one medical school for 675 000 inhabitants compared to one for 2.4 million in the US and 3 million in Canada (World Federation for Medical Education 1998). The Chilean healthcare teaching universities have about 60 648 students, leading to a collection of US$250 million tuition fees, but only 9.8% of these teaching programmes are accredited (Senf et al. 2003; The Lancet 2004).

Another example is India, where the number of medical schools has almost doubled in last 25 years producing the largest number of doctors (about 30 408 per year) in the world (Sood 2008). At present there are 315 medical schools recognized by the Medical Council of India (MCI) (The Lancet 2011), with inequity in distribution between the states (Sood 2008). The private schools are growing at an increased pace (Ng et al. 2005) leading to lack of adequate supervision, which impacts on the quality of education (Sood 2008; Goic G 2002). Another challenge is the shortage of educators for the increasing number of students, which has further led to a compromise in quality (Sood 2008). While research shows the existence of explicit accreditation systems in Argentina, India, Malaysia, Pakistan, Philippines, and South Africa for quality assurance of undergraduate programmes (Sánchez et al. 2008) the implementation of accreditation is variable (Sood 2008; Ajay and Manoj 2006; Medina L and Kaempffer R 2007).

Specialists versus generalists

The development phase in the EMEs saw the growth of the specialist and decline of the generalist (Hull 1948). Specialist training was a norm set by Western medical education, and in most of the EMEs the medical education curriculum was designed to promote specialization (Arechiga et al. 1985; Fox 1954; De Villiers and De Villiers 1999; Kaur 1960; Junqueira 1959). Specialization was encouraged by policy makers to address the shortage of specialists in the newly established schools in many of the EMEs. Specialists were also needed in hospitals; for example in Russia, as a third of the population in the latter half of the 20th century were children and a third of the doctors graduating were trained in paediatrics (Forrest 1948). A specialist was perceived to have prestige, social status, and better financial opportunities (Sood 2008; Ennigrou et al. 2002; Abyad et al. 2007; Hull 1948). Despite being specialist-oriented, the literature during the development phase in South-East Asia criticized their medical education systems for not being able to train adequate number of doctors in paediatrics (Robinson 1961) and family planning (Rice 1969, 1970).

However, towards the last quarter of the 20th century the political and social transitions in some countries such as South Africa (Benatar 1997) and Russia (Chernichovsky and Potapchik 1999), and economic transitions in others such as Vietnam (Ladinsky et al. 2000), India (Sood 2008), China (Schwarz et al. 2004), Thailand (Jaturapatporn and Dellow 2007), Korea (Lee 1999), and the Latin American countries (Pulido M et al. 2006; Fleury 2007) resulted in the healthcare systems becoming more decentralized and focused on population needs. This in turn created an awareness about the disconnect between the needs of the rural communities and specialist-oriented medical education in many of these countries, leading to the introduction of family medicine and training of general

practitioners. The Alma Ata Declaration in 1978 further strengthened efforts and brought in political commitment from the EMEs. Poland adopted a 3-year training programme to train general practitioners in primary healthcare, based on the British and the Norwegian models, which was found to be highly effective (Wasyluk et al. 1990). Similarly, medical schools in Mexico and Brazil introduced 2-year residency programmes in family medicine delivered by teaching clinical medicine, social and behavioural sciences, and public health in the first year, and practical training in community health centres in the second year (Abath 1985; Arechiga et al. 1985). These programmes were intended to train doctors who wished to develop a career in family medicine on local health problems and to help them understand the social and economic determinants of diseases (Arechiga et al. 1985). A postgraduate programme for training physicians in family practice was also introduced in Sri Lanka (Fernando 1983), Jordan (Abbadi et al. 1997), and Lebanon (Abyad and Sibai 1992) in the 1980s, and some medical schools in South Africa introduced rotations in family medicine and primary care during the final year of the undergraduate curriculum (Mash and De Villiers 1999). The curriculum in a newly established Saudi Arabian medical school in 1975 had an innovative approach based on population growth. It has planned two different approaches: a specialist-based curriculum for present population health demands and a preventive community based curriculum to be introduced in the next 10 years to cater to the needs of the projected population (Basalamah et al. 1979).

Despite these innovative initiatives the literature suggests that training in family medicine and primary care were kept separate from the standard medical education curriculum with only a few attempts to integrate this with the undergraduate and postgraduate curriculum—e.g. family medicine was fully integrated into the curriculum of a South African University, the University of Pretoria in 1977 and was delivered by a faculty of general practitioners (Reitz 1980). Nevertheless, the development phase in the 1970s saw a further push for generalists to work in preventive medicine. This was both due to saturation of specialists in curative medicine (Beighton 1978) and the shifting paradigm in health services from the individual to the population (Roux 1977; Ghei 1979). It was also during this period that medical educators, particularly in South Africa, envisioned that medical curricula in the next few decades would have to incorporate training in mental health and geriatrics—embedded within community medicine (Minde 1977; Wicht 1977).

The present state of medical education in the EMEs

The literature on medical education in the EMEs published in the past 12 years (2001–2012), points to four main areas of mismatch between health needs of the population and medical education. These are outlined in fig. 58.4.

Initiatives in setting up systems for education in family medicine and the training of general physicians seen in the various EMEs during the development phase have not materialized into national reforms (Senf et al. 2003; Rese et al. 2005; Román A 2008; Román AO et al. 2007). Qualitative studies conducted in two universities in Malaysia showed that there is poor understanding of the discipline of general practice among students, and most of them are unable to relate their training to actual practice in the community (Ng et al. 2005). A study conducted in Jordan found

It appears that the integration of clinical care, research, and teaching is difficult to achieve in the modern service-based healthcare system (Stern et al. 2005; Maaroos 2004)

Educational curricula are out-dated in terms of the learning and teaching methods (Supe and Burdick 2006; Maaroos 2004)

Medical education concentrates on specialization in advanced technology and disease sciences, ignoring the common health problems at the population level (Supe and Burdick 2006)

The proliferation of medical schools in EMEs appears to compromise the quality of medical education and thereby compromise the ability of health professionals to meet the health needs of the population (Hans 2008)

Figure 58.4 Mismatch between medical education and population needs.

that community-oriented training, large programmes in primary care, and faculty role models positively influence medical students to select family medicine as a career (Senf et al. 2003).

Proposals to update the medical curriculum and train medical educators to effectively implement teaching and learning methods such as problem-based learning (PBL) and community-oriented education (COE) were put forward in a few EMEs. An example is the participatory curriculum development initiative of the School of Medicine Tec de Monterrey in Mexico. To overcome the resistance to reforms from the faculty and to increase the ownership of clinical and basic scientists, teachers, and students, a curriculum committee with seven subcommittees comprising these stakeholders was created (Elizondo-Montemayor et al. 2008). These committees adopted the approach of outcome-based education (OBE), performed needs assessments of the health system, and identified gaps in existing programmes, course syllabi, and timetables (Elizondo-Montemayor et al. 2008). A follow-up of the implementation of the updated curriculum in the same school provides evidence of a gradual transition from the existing to the new curriculum (Elizondo-Montemayor et al. 2008). Similarly, a gradual replacement of the lecture-based, teacher-centric learning with PBL was found to be successful in the medical schools of Malaysia (Barman et al. 2007; Achike and Nain 2005), the United Arab Emirates (UAE) (Mpofu et al. 1997), and in the Nelson R. Mandela School of Medicine in South Africa (McLean 2004). Evaluation showed that students taught using these teaching methods were able to perform better than those who chose to continue with the traditional curriculum and acquire a more humanistic and holistic approach to the practice of medicine (McLean 2004). However, the technique needs further refining in terms of the problems presented, discussions organized, and facilitation for students to identify the relevant learning issues (Mpofu et al. 1997; Connolly and Seneque 1999). In many countries, teaching methods in medical education have increasingly become more technology driven with the use of the internet (Chen et al. 1998).

The updating of curricula and teaching methods have to be complemented with educating the educators. Several initiatives to train medical educators were undertaken in many of these EMEs through cross-cultural exchange programmes aimed at developing teaching skills, leadership, and professional bonding among medical educators worldwide (Norcini et al. 2005). Examples include the US Stanford Faculty Development Program piloted in the Kazan State Medical University (Russia), which showed that despite the differences in culture, medical curriculum, and philosophy of

teaching between the two countries, the project was successfully adapted in the Russian university and improved the technical skills of the medical faculty and contributed to their professional and personal growth (Wong and Agisheva 2007). A different method was adopted by the Medical Education Department in the Faculty of Medicine, Suez Canal University, in Egypt (Talaat and Salem 2009). It developed a distance learning diploma for health professionals, covering all domains, supported by the Egyptian National Quality Assurance and Accreditation Agency, and the Eastern Mediterranean Regional Office of the World Health Organization. Besides building professional and technical ability of the physicians, it was cost effective as it reduced the cost of training and travel expenses related to sending health professionals to other countries for training (Talaat and Salem 2009).

In spite of these various initiatives, medical education in EMEs is continuously being criticized for being unable to meet health system requirements. However, the pace required to keep medical education up to date in the face of rapid changes in demography and epidemiology, and subsequent changing health system demands is underestimated by the critics. Examples of good practice can be found in some of the EMEs—China, Sri Lanka, Cuba, and other Latin American countries which, informed by the projected demography and health needs of the population, brought in reforms in the medical education curriculum (preventive and family medicine, mental health, and palliative care) at least two decades in advance of the projected changes. Another lesson that can be learned from these pioneering countries is that reforms take time and often encounter challenges, which include the ability and training of teachers, unwillingness to adapt or change to a new system, and the educational culture of higher education in the country. The majority of them are struggling to align the initiation and implementation of reforms with the global pedagogic and local health system shifts. Clearly, all countries labelled EMEs cannot be grouped together in their degrees of alignment of medical education systems with scientific, population, and health system needs, but some common threads can be drawn.

While the population and health system needs kept changing, there were limited and patchy reforms in medical education. Some needs-based reforms undertaken in the 1950s and 1960s to meet population health needs such as setting up of medical schools and training of specialists continued even when they were no longer required. Others initiated in response to needs such as integrated curricula, PBL, and OBE were not scaled up—resulting in medical education in the EMEs lagging behind the demographic, epidemiological transitions, and health system changes.

The decrease in infectious diseases and improvement in neonatal and infant survival contributed largely to the socioeconomic changes in these countries rather than a better alignment of medical education to health system needs. While over the past 50 years medical schools kept producing ever more doctors, the shortage of physicians to cater to the rural population was not resolved and the gap between urban and rural healthcare delivery has actually widened. To quote Prywes and Freidman (1991, p. 209):

the growing gap between the two [medical education and healthcare] has been enhanced as both have become institutionalised: medical education in its academic 'ivory tower' and the healthcare delivery system in its socio-political and professional settings.

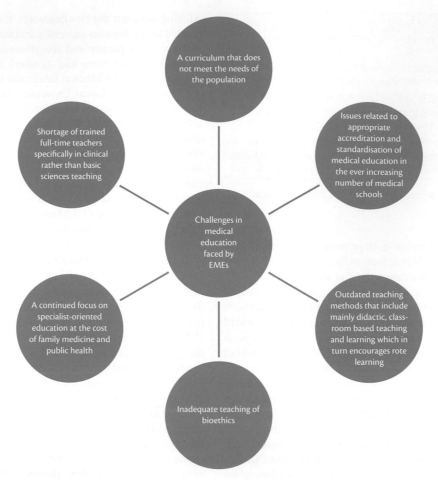

Figure 58.5 Challenges in medical education faced by EMEs.

Many EMEs still face key challenges in the medical education—see fig. 58.5.

These challenges remained to a greater or lesser extent in the EMEs depending on the pace of reforms in medical education adopted by the countries. However, medical education systems have undergone reforms in many of the EMEs and during this process several innovations such as cross-national collaborations for curricula development and standardization, community-oriented primary care models for teaching and learning, North–South collaboration for sharing teaching aids and training educators, and evaluation of the medical education systems, were introduced.

Future of medical education in the EMEs

The initiatives undertaken to reform medical education in the EMEs are appropriate but the pace is slow. OBE, PBL, community-based teaching, and the updating of curricula to reflect need appears to be the way forward. OBE can help to resolve several of the challenges facing medical education in the EMEs as it appears to have advantages such as relevance of curriculum to the health needs of the people, and an integrated approach to learning, teaching methods and assessment (Harden 1999). Clarity and self-directed learning inherent in the system make it more acceptable to teachers and students, and assessment criteria are consistent with performance-based assessment (Harden 1999). It also makes any

gaps in the curriculum explicit, thus ensuring accountability and quality (Harden 1999). The client-centred approach in healthcare, which has made the community 'the central institutional goal' (Margolis 2000) means that educational institutions will need to address community-oriented primary care and primary prevention at population level (Margolis 2000) through a balanced training in 'family medicine' (Amanda 2004). Lessons learnt from the Latin American countries (Fernando 1983) can be adapted to develop country-specific successful models. The first step would be to bring the classroom into the community (Margolis 2000; Tse et al. 2006), followed by community-based projects for students with good mentorship (Margolis 2000). Adopting models of curriculum planning that focus on outcome-based, community-oriented, PBL approaches, integrated curriculum structure and teaching, and an explicit mode of evaluation (Elizondo-Montemayor et al. 2008) will enable transformation of the 'teacher-centred' systems to 'student-led' teaching and learning (Nair and Webster 2010; Elizondo-Montemayor et al. 2008).

Another important area to be considered is information technology, which will play a key role in shaping the future of medical education in the EMEs. Studies conducted among the 'Net Generation' or 'Generation Y' (Sandars and Morrison 2007) of medical students in countries including the UK, Denmark, Vienna, Tanzania, Colombia, and Malaysia show that information technology (IT) has potential as an educational tool in enhancing teaching and learning in medical schools (Sandars and Morrison 2007; Link and Marz 2006; Sandars and Schroter 2007). The literature provides examples for utilizing IT in several areas of medical education, such as: PBL using patient simulation models (Smørdal et al. 2002; Harden 2006); training students in advanced medical technology in rural institutions (Lau and Bates 2004; Sargeant 2005); and sharing practice experiences among clinicians worldwide (Parboosingh 2002). There is consensus among the teaching and the learning communities that IT could be the way forward, especially in standardizing medical education across countries—provided appropriate training is incorporated (Valcke and De Wever 2006; Sandars and Schroter 2007). However, inertia on the part of the educators in shifting from traditional teaching methods to new ones may be a challenge (Sandars and Morrison 2007; Wise 2005); these could be overcome by a gradual shift through a 'blended approach' (Broadbent 2002).

In addition, it is essential to identify leadership potential in future doctors and train them on doctor–patient communication skills. A leadership programme in medical education was proposed under the auspices of the Pan-American Federation of Associations of Medical Schools for Latin American students to develop their leadership role in the much required areas of management, communication, planning, and motivation (Pulido 1989). Evaluation of the impact of such programmes can provide lessons to other EMEs. Although communication is an integral part of leadership programmes, more relevant to medical education is the teaching of doctor-patient communication skills. Compared to medical education in the West, where the emphasis on training medical students is to develop such communication skills, this is limited in EMEs (Claramita et al. 2011). Despite the realization that a partnership style of communication is the most appropriate in doctor–patient communications, the prevalent style in many of the EMEs is the paternalistic style. Studies in South Asia have attributed this not only to lack of training, but also to the culture, education, hierarchical, and over-burdened healthcare systems (Claramita et al. 2011).

Perhaps the task of reforming medical education in the EMEs appears daunting for an individual country, but may be possible through collaborative efforts. Such collaborations among EMEs regionally and globally are already found in countries with shared population healthcare needs and similar socioeconomic environments. These collaborations provide platforms to build political will and commitment for needs-based revision of curricula and teaching methods, improving quality, and ensuring comparable standards of medical education across the EMEs. The roots of such collaborative efforts can be traced back to the development phase of medical education in the EMEs. In 1962, a group of leading medical educators founded the Panamerican Federation of Association of Medical Schools (PAFAMS) at Viña del Mar, Chile constituting of 343 medical schools from Latin America, USA and Canada to address the prevailing problems in medical education in Latin America (Pulido 1989).

One of the issues that medical education in the EMEs will need to address is getting the balance between science (advancing medical technology) and humanities (demand for care). Perhaps lessons could be learnt by reflecting on the loss of cultural and human identity in medical education when pursuing scientific and technical advancement during the 'establishment phase'. One reason for the introduction of bioethics in the medical curriculum in many of the EMEs was dissatisfaction with Western medical training, which was considered to produce 'businessmen' rather than ethical and morally sound healers (Ratanakul 1988, p. 303). Similarly growing dissatisfaction with a highly mechanized, technocratic medical system may encourage medical educators to incorporate arts, music, religion, and culture to enhance learning and teaching of medical students. Philosophy in medicine which is taught in the University of Kraków (Zalewski 2000) may be adopted by other EMEs to enrich medical education. Since 1993, religion and spirituality in medicine is taught in undergraduate and postgraduate medicine in more than 100 medical schools in the USA and is presently included in the medical curricula of some universities in Canada, England, Germany, and Cuba (Lucchetti et al. 2012). Based on research evidence WHO, the Association of American Medical Colleges (AAMC), and the Joint Commission on Accreditation of Healthcare Organisations (JCAHO) recommend introducing spirituality in medical education and patient care (Anandarajah and Mitchell 2007).

Conclusions

◆ Medical education in the EMEs has evolved in the past 200 years, initially driven by sociopolitical and cultural factors and then by population health needs, health system requirements, and scientific progress.

◆ At present, the rapid and ongoing socioeconomic transitions, globalization, changes in population structure and related disease epidemiology, and the demands of an increasingly educated and informed population are imposing changes in healthcare systems.

◆ Medical education in many of the EMEs has not been able to keep pace with these transitions, not only lagging behind in curriculum development, and teaching and learning methods but also struggling to train doctors to provide appropriate healthcare to meet the needs of their population.

◆ Concerted efforts are being made to reform medical education to meet the needs of populations.

◆ Several innovative initiatives have been introduced but the implementation of a sustainable, fit for purpose medical education system to meet the needs of EMEs, has been patchy.

◆ As well as commitment from medical educators ready to embrace change there needs to be social and political will and regional and global collaboration to ensure that tomorrow's doctors in EMEs are fit for purpose to provide appropriate and humane care to their populations.

References

Abath, G.M. (1985) [Family medicine in Brazil]. *Educ Med Salud.* 19: 48–73

Abbadi, S., Abdallah, A.K., and Holliman, C.J. (1997) Emergency medicine in Jordan. *Ann Emerg Med.* 30: 319–321

Abyad, A., Al-Baho, A.K., Unluoglu, I., Tarawneh, M., and Al Hilfy, T.K.Y. (2007) Development of family medicine in the Middle East. *Fam Med.* 39: 736–741

Abyad, A. and Sibai, A.M. (1992) The general practitioner in Lebanon: is he a potential family physician? *Fam Pract.* 9: 437–440

Achike, F.I. and Nain, N. (2005) Promoting problem-based learning (PBL) in nursing education: A Malaysian experience. *Nurse Educ Pract.* 5: 302–311

Ajay, M. and Manoj, M. (2006) Growth of private medical education in India. *Med Educ.* 40: 1009–1011

Al-Faris, E., Kalantan, K., Al-Rowais, N., et al. (1997) Career choices among Saudi medical students. *Acad Med.* 72: 65–67

Amanda, H. (2004) Education in family medicine—gains and dangers. *Croat Med J.* 45: 533–536

Anandarajah, G. and Mitchell, M. (2007) A spirituality and medicine elective for senior medical students: 4 years' experience, evaluation, and expansion to the family medicine residency. *Fam Med.* 39: 313–315

Arechiga, A.F., Heras, H.R. and Cantu, I. Q. (1985) Family medicine: a medical care alternative for Latin America. *Soc Sci Med.* 21: 87–92

Barman, A., Jaafar, R. and Rahim, A.F.A. (2007) Perception of tutors about the problem-based learning sessions conducted for medical and dental schools' students of Universiti Sains Malaysia. *Int Med J.* 14: 261–264

Basalamah, A., Rosinski, E. and Schumacher, H. (1979) Developing the medical curriculum at King Abdulaziz University. *J Med Educ.* 54: 96–100

Beighton, P. (1978) The present state and future of the medical sciences in South Africa. *S Afr Med J.* 53: 19–21

Benatar, S.R. (1997) Health care reform in the new South Africa. *N Engl J Med.* 336: 891–896

Bhat, R. (1999) Characteristics of private medical practice in India: a provider perspective. *Health Policy Planning.* 14: 26–37

Blizard, P. J. (1991) International standards in medical education or national standards/primary health care—which direction? *Soc Sci Med.* 33: 1163–1170

Blizard, P.J., Blunt, M.J., Alibazah, P. and Husin, M. (1980) The long term effectiveness of workshops in curriculum planning and design for teaching staff in Indonesian medical schools. *Med Educ.* 14: 154–163

Bowers, J.Z. (1974) Imperialism and medical education in China. *Bull Hist Med.* 48: 449–464

Brito, A.E. and García, P.O.O. (2010) Integration of public health specialists, epidemiologists and clinicians for the care of patients suffering chronic diseases. *Revista Cubana de Salud Pública.* 36: 262–266

Broadbent, B. (2002) *ABCs of e-Learning: Reaping the Benefits and Avoiding the Pitfalls.* San Francisco: Jossey-Bass/Pfeiffer

Brock, J.F. (1960) The evolution of medical research in South Africa. *S Afr Med J.* 34: 420–421

Brown, E.R. (1979) Exporting medical education: Professionalism, modernization and imperialism. *Soc Sci Med.* 13 A: 585–595

Charalambous, A. and Rousou, E. (2010) The factors contributing to 'epidemiological transition' and its consequences in the organization of health care services and the development of health policy *Arch Hellen Med.* 27: 976–983

Chen, H.-S., Guo, F.-R., Liu, C.-T., et al. (1998) Integrated medical informatics with small group teaching in medical education. *Int J Med Informatics.* 50: 59–68

Chernichovsky, D. and Potapchik, E. (1999) Genuine federalism in the Russian health care system: changing roles of government. *J Health Polit Policy Law.* 24: 115–144

Chew, C.H. (1991) Medical education, training, and health care services in the Republic of Singapore. *West J Med.* 155: 186–188

Claramita, M., Utarini, A., Soebono, H., Dalen, J.V., and van der Vleuten, C. (2011) Doctor–patient communication in a Southeast Asian setting: the conflict between ideal and reality. *Adv Health Sci Educ.* 16: 69–80

Connolly, C. and Seneque, M. (1999) Evaluating problem-based learning in a multilingual student population. *Med Educ.* 33: 738–744

Crane, P.S. (1969) An unresolved problem for developing countries. Korea as exhibit A. *JAMA.* 209: 2039 2041

Croizier, R. C. (1970) Medicine, modernization, and cultural crisis in China and India. *Comp Studies Soc History.* 12: 275–291

Davis, K. (1945) The world demographic transition. *Ann Am Acad Polit Soc Sci.* 237: 1–11

De Villiers, P.J.T. and De Villiers, M.R. (1999) The current status and future needs of education and training in family medicine and primary care in South Africa. *Med Educ.* 33: 716–721

Drane, J.F. and Fuenzalida, H.L. (1991) Medical ethics in Latin America: a new interest and commitment. *Kennedy Inst Ethics J.* 1: 325–338

Du, Z. (2000) On the development of teachers of medical ethics in China. *Hastings Cent Rep.* 30: S37–S40

Elizondo-Montemayor, L., Hernňdez-Escobar, C., Ayala-Aguirre, F. and Aguilar, G. M. (2008) Building a sense of ownership to facilitate change: the new curriculum. *Int J Leadership Educ Theory Pract.* 11: 83–102

Ennigrou, S., Ayari, H., Skhiri, H., and Zouari, B. (2002) The general medicine and the physician general practitioner. The opinion of the teachers of the faculty of medicine of Tunis. *Tunisie Medicale.* 80: 605–615

Farmer, R.G., Sirotkin, A.Y., Ziganshina, L.E., and Greenberg, H.M. (2003) The Russian health care system today: Can American-Russian CME programs help? *Cleveland Clin J Med.* 70: 937–944

Fernando, J. (1983) Training doctors for family practice in primary health care work in Sri Lanka. *Soc Sci Med.* 17: 1457–1461

Fleury, R.N. (2007) Medical education and the needs of the health system in Brazil. *Hansenologia Internationalis.* 32: 153–154

Forrest, W.P. (1948) Medical education in the Ukraine. *Lancet.* 252: 579–582

Foster, G.M. (1966) Environmental factors bearing on medical education in the developing countries. C. Cross-cultural medical education: Some social and cultural factors. *Journal of. Med Educ.* 41(Suppl): 166–174

Fox, T.F. (1954) Russia revisited: impressions of Soviet medicine. *Lancet.* 267: 803–807

Gantt, W.H. (1924) A review of medical education in Soviet Russia. *BMJ.* 1: 1055–1058

Ghei, P.N. (1979) Reorientation of medical education to improve health care staffing. *World Hospitals.* 15: 266–268

Goic G,A. (2002) Proliferation of medical schools in Latin America. *Causes and Consequences.* 130: 917–924

Hans, K. (2008) International recognition of basic medical education programmes. *Med Educ.* 42: 12–17

Harden, R.M. (1999) AMEE Guide No. 14: Outcome-based education: Part 1- An introduction to outcome-based education. *Med Teach.* 21: 7–14

Harden, R.M. (2006) Trends and the future of postgraduate medical education. *BMJ.* 23: 798

Hill, K.R. (1962) Some reflections on medical education and teaching in the developing countries. *BMJ.* 2: 585–587

Hull, E. (1948) Impacts of general ethical and social trends upon medical care and upon medical education. *South Med J.* 41: 1103–1105

Hyde, H.V.Z. (1965) Medical education in developing countries. *J Med Educ.* 40: 298–299

Jain, K.K. (1972) Glimpses of Chinese medicine, 1971: (changes after the cultural revolution) *Can Med Ass J.* 106: 46–50

Jamieson, H.C. (1946) Medical education in the 14th century. *Can Med Ass J.* 54: 610–615

Jaturapatporn, D. and Dellow, A. (2007) Does family medicine training in Thailand affect patient satisfaction with primary care doctors? *BMC Fam Pract.* 8: 14–19

Jeffery, R. (1977) Allopathic medicine in India: A case of deprofessionalization? *Soc Sci Med.* 11: 561–573

Jimeñez-Arango, A. (1966) Medical education and medical care in developing countries. *Am J Public Health Nation's Health.* 56: 2126–2132

Junqueira, L.C. (1959) Developments in medical education in Brazil. *J Med Educ.* 34: 986–988

Kaur, R.A. (1960) Medical education in India. *Postgrad Med J.* 36: 592–597

Ladinsky, J.L., Nguyen, H.T., and Volk, N.D. (2000) Changes in the Health Care System of Vietnam in Response to the Emerging Market Economy. *J Public Health Policy.* 21: 82–98

Lau, F. and Bates, J. (2004) A review of e-learning practices for undergraduate medical education. *J Med Systems.* 28: 71–87

Lee, J.C. (1999) [Korea's health care policy of the twentieth century]. *Uisahak.* 8: 137–145

Li, B. (2000) Ethics teaching in medical schools. *Hastings Cent Rep.* 30: S30–S32

Link, T.M. and Marz, R. (2006) Computer literacy and attitudes towards e-learning among first year medical students. *BMC. Med Educ.* 6: 34–41

Lobo, L.C.G. and Jouval Jr, H.E. (1973) The use of new educational technology in the development of health manpower in Latin America: Its implications in the teaching of epidemiology. *Int J Epidemiol.* 2: 359–366

Lucchetti, G., Lucchetti, A., and Puchalski, C. (2012) Spirituality in medical education: global reality? *J Relig Health.* 51: 3–19

Maaroos, H.-I. (2004) Family medicine as a model of transition from academic medicine to academic health care: Estonia's experience. *Croat Med J.* 45: 563–566

Margolis, C.Z. (2000) Community-based medical education. *Med Teach.* 22: 482–484

Mash, B. and De Villiers, M. (1999) Community-based training in Family Medicine—a different paradigm. *Med Educ.* 33: 725–729

Mclean, M. (2004) A comparison of students who chose a traditional or a problem-based learning curriculum after failing year 2 in the traditional curriculum: a unique case study at the Nelson R. Mandela School of Medicine. *Teach Learn Med.* 16: 301–303

Medina L.E. and Kaempffer R.A.M. (2007) *Medicina y otras Carreras de la Salud en Chile. Un análisis preliminar.* 135: 1346–1354

Minde, M. (1977) History of mental health services in South Africa. Part XV. The future of mental health services. *S Afr Med J.* 51: 549–553

Monteiro, E.S. (1959) International cooperation in postgraduate medical education in Malaya. *BMJ.* 2: 330–332

Mpofu, D.J.S., Das, M., Murdoch, J.C., and Lanphear, J.H. (1997) Effectiveness of problems used in problem-based learning. *Med Educ.* 31: 330–334

Müller, H. K. (1980) Zur Entwicklung der medizinischen Wissenschaften in China. *Naturwissenschaften.* 67, 55–60.

Nair, M. and Webster, P. (2010) medical education in review: Education for health professionals in the emerging market economies: a literature review. *Med Educ.* 44: 856–863

Ncayiyana, D. (1999) Medical education challenges in South Africa. *Med Educ.* 33: 713–715

Ng, C.J., Leong, K.C., and Teng, C.L. (2005) What do medical students think about primary care in Malaysia? A qualitative study. *Educ Prim Care.* 16: 575–580

Norcini, J., Burdick, W., and Morahan, P. (2005) The FAIMER Institute: creating international networks of medical educators. *Med Teach.* 27: 214–218

Oettlé, A. G. (1952) The aims and tasks of undergraduate medical education in South Africa. *S Afr Med J.* 26: 240–241

Oliveira, N.A.D., Luz, M.C.R., Saraiva, R.M., and Alves, L.A. (2011) Student views of research training programmes in medical schools. *Med Educ.* 45: 748–755

Omran, A.R. (2001) The epidemiologic transition. A theory of the Epidemiology of population change. 1971. *Bull World Health Org.* 79: 161–170

Parboosingh, J.T. (2002) Physician communities of practice: where learning and practice are inseparable. *J Cont Educ Health Prof.* 22: 230–236

Paul, J.R. (1959) Commentaries on medical education and medical research in Latin America 1958. *Yale J Biol Med.* 31: 284–293

Pedziwiatr, M.J. (1999) Role of history and philosophy of medicine in the professional formation of a physician: writings of Polish school of philosophy of medicine. *Croat Med J.* 40: 14–19

Piyaratn, P. (1982) Doctors' roles in primary health care. *Trop Doct.* 12: 196–202

Pruitt, S.D. and Epping-Jordan, J.E. (2005) Preparing the 21st century global healthcare workforce. *BMJ.* 330: 637–639

Prywes, M. and Friedman, M. (1991) Education for leadership in health development. *Acad Med.* 66: 209–210

Pulido M.P.A., Cravioto, A., Pereda, A., Rondo N.R., and Pereira, G. (2006) Changes, trends and challenges of medical education in Latin America. *Med Teach.* 28: 24–29

Pulido, P.A. (1989) Strategies for developing innovative programs in international medical education. A viewpoint from Latin America. *Acad Med.* 64: S17–S22

Rao, K.N. (1966) Educational adaptation to the factors bearing on medical education in the developing countries. A. Medical education in developing societies. *J. Med Educ.* 41(Suppl): 175–179

Ratanakul, P. (1988) Bioethics in Thailand: the struggle for Buddhist solutions. *JMed Philos.* 13: 301–312

Reitz, C.J. (1980) Family practice as a part of undergraduate medical training in South Africa. *S Afr Med J.* 57: 461–463

Rese, A., Balabanova, D., Danishevski, K., Mckee, M. and Sheaff, R. (2005) Implementing general practice in Russia: Getting beyond the first steps. *BMJ.* 331: 204–207

Rice, D.T. (1969) Medical education and family planning—II. Implementation of administrative recommendations for the Third Conference of Deans and Principals. *Ind J Med Educ.* 8: 257–261

Rice, D.T. (1970) Medical education and family planning—III. What departments of preventive and social medicine are doing in India. *Ind J Med Educ.* 9: 1–7

Robinson, P. (1961) Undergraduate paediatric education in South-East Asia. *Acta Paed.* 50: 329–338

Román, A.O. (2008) Incorporation of specialists to primary health care to increase its efficiency. *Rev Med Chil.* 136: 1073–1077

Román, A.O, Pineda, R.S., and Señoret, S.M. (2007) [The profile and number of primary care physicians required in Chile]. *Rev Med Chil.* 135: 1209–1215

Rosa, F. (1964) A doctor for newly developing countries: principles for adapting medical education and services to meet problems. *J Med Educ.* 39: 918–924

Roux, J.P. (1977) The social revolution in health services. *S Afr Med J.* 52, 686–688.

Sánchez, I., Riquelme, A., Moreno, R., et al. (2008) Revitalising medical education: The School of Medicine at the Pontificia Universidad Cato´lica de Chile. *Clin Teach.* 5: 57–61

Sandars, J. and Morrison, C. (2007) What is the Net Generation? The challenge for future medical education. *Med Teach.* 29: 85–88

Sandars, J. and Schroter, S. (2007) Web 2.0 technologies for undergraduate and postgraduate medical education: an online survey. *BMJ.* 83: 759–762

Sargeant, J.M. (2005) Medical education for rural areas: Opportunities and challenges for information and communications technologies. *J Postgrad Med.* 51: 301–307

Schwarz, M.R., Wojtczak, A., and Zhou, T. (2004) Medical education in China's leading medical schools. *Med Teach.* 26: 215–222

Senewiratne, B., Benjamin, V.A., Gunawardena, D.A., and Kanagarajah, M. (1975) Should undergraduate medical training in a developing country be different? *BMJ.* 4: 27–29

Senf, J.H., Campos-Outcalt, D., and Kutob, R. (2003) Factors related to the choice of family medicine: A reassessment and literature review. *J Am Board Fam Pract.* 16: 502–512

Sheth, U.K. (1959) International cooperation in postgraduate medical education with regard to India. *BMJ.* 2: 328–330

Smordal, O., Gregory, J., and Langseth, K.J. (2002) PDAs in medical education and practice. In: *Proceedings of IEEE International Workshop on Wireless and Mobile Technologies in Education* (pp. 140–146). Piscataway NJ: IEEE

Sood, R. (2008) Medical education in India. *Med Teach.* 30: 585–591

Stern, D.T., Ben-David, M.F., De Champlain, A., et al. (2005) Ensuring global standards for medical graduates: a pilot study of international standard-setting. *Med Teach.* 27: 207–213

Stillman, P.L. and Sawyer, W.D. (1992) A new program to enhance the teaching and assessment of clinical skills in the People's Republic of China. *Acad Med.* 67: 495–499

Supe, A. and Burdick, W.P. (2006) Challenges and issues in medical education in India. *Acad Med.* 81: 1076–1080

Szmatloch, E. (2000) Internal medicine in Poland. *Eur J Intern Med.* 11: 355–356

Talaat, W. and Salem, H. (2009) A new opportunity for Egyptian health professions educators. *Med Educ.* 43: 498–499

The Lancet (2004) National strategies wanted to plug the brain drain. *The Lancet.* 364: 556

The Lancet (2011) Rational reform to medical education in India. *Lancet.* 377: 1212

The World Bank (2011) *Multipolarity: The New Global Economy. Global Development Horizons 2011.* Washington DC: The World Bank

Thompson, W.S. (1929) Population. *Am. J. Sociol.* 34: 959–975

Tobias, P.V. (1980) Apartheid and medical education: the training of black doctors in South Africa. *J Natl Med Ass.* 72: 395–410

Tse, A.M., Iwaishi, L.K., King, C.A., and Harrigan, R.C. (2006) A collaborative approach to developing a validated competence-based curriculum for health professions students. *Educ Health.* 19: 331–344

United Nations Department of Economic and Social Affairs Population Division (2010) *World urbanisation prospects: the 2009 revision population database* [Online] (updated 2010) www.un.org/esa/population/ Accessed 13 March 2012

Valcke, M. and De Wever, B. (2006) Information and communication technologies in higher education: evidence-based practices in medical education. *Med Teach.* 28: 40–48

Wasyluk, J.S., Wegrzyn, Z. and Woznica, I. (1990) A three-year training programme for primary health care physicians in Poland. *Scand J Prim Health Care.* 8: 127–129

Wicht, C.L. (1977) Future geriatric needs in South Africa. Hospital and teaching aspects. *S Afr Med J.* 51: 440–442

Williams, J.R. (2000) Ethics and human rights in South African medicine. *CMAJ.* 162: 1167–1170

Wise, L. (2005) Blogs versus discussion forums in postgraduate online continuing medical education, 1–6 http://incsub.org/blogtalk/images/lwise_blogtalk2005.pdf Accessed 15 March 2013

Wong, J.G. and Agisheva, K. (2007) Developing teaching skills for medical educators in Russia: A cross-cultural faculty development project. *Med Educ.* 41: 318–324

World Federation for Medical Education (1998) International standards in medical education: assessment and accreditation of medical schools' educational programmes. [A WFME position paper]. *Med Educ.* 32: 549–558

World Health Organization (1966) The training and preparation of teachers for medical schools with special regard to the needs of developing countries. *World Health Organization—Technical Report Series.* 337: 5–26

Zalewski, Z. (2000) What philosophy should be taught to the future medical professionals? *Med Health Care Philos.* 3: 161–167

PART 12

The future

CHAPTER 59

The future of health professional education

Julio Frenk, Lincoln Chen, and Catherine Michaud

The history of education is not a straight line of progress. Like any discipline, it is marked by periods of extraordinary advance, more or less intelligent reflection, and stultifying stagnation. The history of education among the health professions is no exception. After a century of rapid progress (initiated in the western medical tradition by the 1910 Flexner Report), consolidation, but more recent ossification, health professionals' education is poised again to enter a new epoch of transformation.

Richard Horton

Reprinted from *The Lancet*, 376, 9756, R Horton, 'A new epoch for health professionals' education', pp. 1875–1877, Copyright 2010, with permission from Elsevier

A century of progress

Knowledge-based health advances

Health is about people. Beyond the glittering surface of modern technology, the core space of every health system is occupied by the unique encounter based on trust between one set of people who need services and another who have been entrusted to deliver them. This trust is earned through a special blend of technical competence and service orientation, steered by ethical commitment and social accountability, which forms the core of professional work. Developing such a blend requires a prolonged period of education and a substantial investment on the part of both student and society. Through a chain of events flowing from effective learning to high-quality services to improved health, professional education at its best makes an essential contribution to the well-being of individuals, families, and communities.

Yet, the context, content, and conditions of social effort to educate competent, caring, and committed health professionals are rapidly changing across time and space. Looking backwards, our great grandparents would never have dreamed that life expectancy of their descendents would nearly double over the course of the 20th century. Unprecedented in human history, this progress was due both to improving living standards and to advances in knowledge (Frenk 2009b). There is abundant evidence that good health is at least in part knowledge-based and socially driven (Chen and Berlinguer 2001; Pablos-Mendez et al. 2005). Scientific knowledge not only produces new technologies but also empowers citizens to adopt healthy

lifestyles, improve care-seeking behaviour, and become proactive citizens conscious of their rights. In addition, knowledge translated into evidence can guide practice as well as policy. Health systems are socially driven differentiated institutions whose primary intent is to improve health, complementing the importance of social determinants and social movements in health.

In these endeavours, professionals play a critical mediating role of applying knowledge to improving health—as *knowledge producers* in research and discovery, as *knowledge reproducers* as faculty and teachers of the next generation, as *knowledge-based decision-makers* to craft and navigate health systems, and as *knowledge brokers* who link people to technology, information, and knowledge systems. There is strong evidence that health professional density and coverage have a direct impact on health outcomes (Anand and Barnighausen 2004). Health professionals are also care-givers, communicators and educators, team members, managers, and leaders. As 'knowledge-based workers', health workers are the human faces of the health system.

Flexner and scientific reforms

Dramatic reforms in the education of health professionals helped to catalyse the last century's health gains. Educating health professionals has deep historical roots in diverse societies. Coming on the heels of the discovery of the germ theory in Europe, the opening of the 20th century witnessed widespread reforms in professional education around the world. In the United States, such reports as by Flexner (1910), Welch-Rose (1915), and Goldmark (Committee for the Study of Nursing Education 1923) paved the way for major reforms in the education of health professionals (Flexner 1910; The Committee for the Study of Nursing Education 1923; Welch and Rose 1915) (fig. 59.1). These efforts imbedded a scientific foundation into the education of health professionals launching modern health sciences into classrooms and laboratories in medicine, public health, nursing, dentistry, and allied professions (Gies and Pritchett 1926;). The reforms—usually sequencing education in the biomedical sciences followed by training in clinical and public health practice—were joined by similar efforts in other world regions. Curricular reform was also linked to institutional transformation—university bases, academic hospitals linked to universities, closure of low-quality proprietary schools, and the bringing together of research and education. The goals were to advance scientifically based professionalism with high technical and ethical standards.

American philanthropy, led by the Rockefeller Foundation, the Carnegie Foundation for the Advancement of Teaching, and other like-minded organizations, promoted these educational reforms by financing the establishment of dozens of new schools of medicine and public health in the United States and around the world (Fosdick 1952).Two years after the publication of his original report, which focused on the United States and Canada, Flexner extended his study of medical education to the German Empire, Austria, France, England, and Scotland (Flexner 1912)—but the influence went beyond Western nations. The Flexner model was translated into action through the establishment of new medical schools in other countries, the earliest and most prominent being the Peking Union Medical College by the Rockefeller Foundation and executed by its China Medical Board in 1917 (Bullock 1980).

In public health, the earlier experiences at the London School of Tropical Medicine, Tulane University (Wellman 1912), and the Harvard-MIT School for Health Officers were impacted by the Welch-Rose report paving the way for a major growth in new schools starting with the Johns Hopkins School of Hygiene and Public Health (1916), the Harvard School of Public Health (1922), the School of Public Health of Mexico (1922), a renewed London School of Hygiene and Tropical Medicine (1924), and the University of Toronto School of Public Health (1927). The Welch-Rose model was also exported through Rockefeller's funding of 35 new schools of public health overseas.

This mass-scale export and adoption was a mixed blessing, with useful results in some countries but also misfits in others. Throughout the century, a recurring debate has been the appropriateness of these models of Western scientific medicine in diverse societies, many which had health problems that could be dealt with by more basic workers and did not have the resources to absorb the costs of highly trained professionals. In 1987, the pioneering Mexican school underwent major reform when it merged with the Center for Public Health Research and the Center for Infectious Disease Research to form the National Institute of Public Health—one of leading institutions of its kind in the developing world (Frenk et al. 2003). There are many other innovative examples, including several in the Arab world and south Asia, which demonstrate the capacity of public health academic institutions to respond to diverse and rapidly changing local requirements.

In parallel with the increasing engagement of national governments in health affairs, a second generation of reforms began after World War II both in industrialized and in developing nations, many of the latter having just gained independence from colonialism (Rosenberg 2007). School and university development was accompanied by expansion of tertiary hospitals and academic health centres that trained health professionals, conducted research, and provided care, thereby integrating these three spheres of activity. Pioneered in the 1950s was the concept of graduate medical education as postgraduate apprenticeship-like training through residency programmes in hospital-based academic centres (Whitcomb 2009).

The major instructional breakthroughs from the second generation of reforms were problem-based learning and disciplinarily integrated curricula. In the 1960s, McMaster University in Canada pioneered student-centred learning based on small groups as an alternative to didactic lecture-style teaching (Neville 2009). In parallel, an integrated rather than discipline-bound curriculum was experimentally developed by Newcastle University in the United Kingdom and Case Western Reserve University in the United States (Papa and Harasym 1999; Pickering 1978). Other curricular innovations included standardized patients to evaluate students on practice (Harden 1988), strengthening doctor–patient relationships through facilitated group discussions (Luban-Plozza 1995), and broadening the continuum from classroom to clinical training

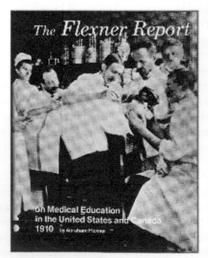 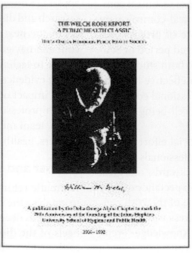 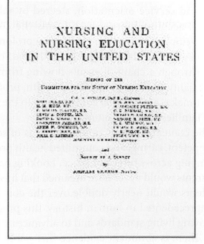

Figure 59.1 The Flexner, Welch-Rose, and Goldmark reports.
Reprinted from The Lancet, 376, Frenk et al., 'Health professionals for a new century: transforming education to strengthen health systems in an interdependent world', pp. 1923–1958, Copyright 2010, with permission from Elsevier.

through earlier student exposure to patients and an expansion of training sites beyond hospitals into communities (Chen and Bunge 1989; Kark 1981; Seipp and eds 1963; Wyon and Gordon 1971). In public health, disciplines expanded along with interdisciplinary work, and in nursing there was accelerated integration of schools into universities with more advanced graduate programmes at the masters and doctoral levels.

Recent history of reforms

Culminating in 2010 around the centennial of the Flexner Report has been a series of recent initiatives that have once again heightened national and global attention on the future of health professional education. Summarized here are four sets of major reports that focus on educating the global health workforce, nursing education, public health education, and medical education. Recommendations in these reports are increasingly coalescing into a third generation of reforms that emphasize patient and population centredness, competency-based curricula, interprofessional and team-based education, IT-empowered learning, and policy and management leadership skills. These provide a strong base for innovation and reform into the 21st century.

Global workforce education

Global workforce education has witnessed a major resurgence of policy attention, driven in part by imperatives to achieve national and global health objectives as set out by the Millennium Development Goals (MDGs). Three major reports are noteworthy in terms of education and training of the workforce: Task Force on Scaling-Up and Saving Lives (2008) (Global Health Workforce Alliance 2008), World Health Report (2006) (WHO 2006), and the Joint Learning Initiative (2004) (Joint Learning Initiative 2004). These reports all underscore the centrality of the workforce in well performing health systems for achieving health goals. All of the reports highlight the global crisis of workforce shortages estimated worldwide at 2.4 million doctors and nurses in 57 crisis countries. The crisis is severest in the world's poorest nations struggling to achieve the MDGs, particularly in sub-Saharan Africa. The shortages also highlight associated issues including imbalances of skill mix, negative work environment, and maldistribution. The reports also cite imbalanced labour market dynamics that are failing to ensure adequate rural coverage while generating unemployed professionals in capital cities and the international migration of professionals from poorer to richer countries.

These reports recommend ramping up investment in education and training. They concentrate on basic workers because of the importance of primary healthcare and the relatively longer time lag and higher costs of post-secondary education. Consequently, health professionals, although acknowledged, do not receive much attention. These reports, however, are sparking growing interest in 'task shifting' and 'task sharing', a process of delegating practical tasks from numerically limited professionals to basic health workers. All reports propose greater investment, sharing of resources, and partnerships within and across countries.

Nursing education

Nursing education was the focus of three major reports in 2010: Radical Transformation, by the Carnegie Foundation (Benner et al. 2010); Frontline Care, a UK Prime Minister commission (The Prime Minister's Commission on the Future of Nursing and Midwifery in England 2010) and the Robert Wood Johnson Foundation Initiative on the Future of Nursing, at the US Institute of Medicine (Institute of Medicine 2010). The Carnegie report concluded that while nursing has been effective in promoting professional identity and ethical comportment, there remains the challenge of anticipating changing demands of practice through strengthening of scientific education and integrating classroom and clinical teaching. The UK Commission identifies the requisite core competencies, skills, and support systems for nursing. For the National Health Service it recommends mainstreaming nursing into national service planning, development, and delivery. Pioneering work in nursing education is also being pursued in other world regions, for example in China and the Middle East.

Public health education

Public health education is the subject of two major reports by the US Institute of Medicine in 2002 and 2003, both focusing on the future of public health in the 21st century (Institute of Medicine 2002; Institute of Medicine quoted in Gebbie et al. 2003). The reports recommend that the core curricula adopt transdisciplinary and multischool approaches and instil a culture of life-long learning. They also urge that public health skills and concepts be better integrated into medicine, nursing, and other allied health fields, become more engaged with local communities and policy-makers, and be disseminated to other practitioners, researchers, educators, and leaders. Importantly, the reports argue in favour of expanding federal funding for public health development.

Medical education

Medical education has commanded comparatively greater attention as illustrated by a series of selected reports: Future of Medical Education, by the Associations of Faculties of Medicine of Canada (2010) (The Association of Faculties of Medicine of Canada 2010); Tomorrow's Doctors, by the General Medical Council of the UK (UK General Medical Council 2009); Reform in Educating Physicians, by the Carnegie Foundation (2010) (Cooke et al. 2010); and Revisiting Medical Education at a Time of Expansion, by the Macy Foundation (2008) (Josiah Macy Jr. Foundation 2008). An additional report was recently issued by the Association of American Medical Colleges: 'A snapshot of medical student education in the United States and Canada' (Association of American Medical Colleges 2010; Fagin 1997). All reports concur that health professionals in the United States, the United Kingdom, and Canada are not being adequately prepared in undergraduate, postgraduate, or continuing education to address challenges ushered in by ageing, changing patient populations, cultural diversity, chronic diseases, care-seeking behaviour, and heightened public expectations.

The focus of these reports is on core competencies beyond the command of knowledge and facts. Rather, the competencies to be developed include patient-centred care, interdisciplinary teams, evidence-based practice, continuous quality improvement, use of new informatics, and integration of public health. Research skills are valued, as are competencies in policy, law, management, and leadership. Undergraduate education should prepare graduates for life-long learning. Curriculum reforms include outcome-based programmes tracked by assessment; capacity to integrate knowledge and experiences; flexible individualization of the learning process to include student-selected components; and development of a culture of critical inquiry—all for equipping physicians with a renewed sense of socially responsible professionalism.

It is necessary to recognize the different perspectives of these major initiatives between richer and poorer countries and amongst the professions. These differences reflect the huge diversity of conditions between countries at various stages of educational and health development and the core competencies of various professions. At the same time, they also underscore the opportunities for mutual learning across diverse countries (Crisp 2010) Taken together, they form a base of convergence around a third generation of reforms that promise to address gaps and opportunities in a globalizing world.

Emerging challenges

Despite a century of progress and recent reforms, not all is well in world health. In the opening decade of the 21st century, glaring gaps and striking inequities in health persist both among and within countries (Evans et al. 2001). A large proportion of the people who inhabit our planet are still trapped in health conditions of a century earlier. The poor in developing countries continue to suffer from the unfinished agenda of common infections, malnutrition, and maternity-related health risks (Whitehead et al. 2001). Many countries are entering a new agenda of the non-communicable diseases—such as diabetes and other chronic conditions. At the same time, the health security of all is being challenged by new infectious, environmental, and behavioural threats superimposed upon rapid demographic and epidemiologic transitions (Commission on Social Determinants of Health 2008; Institute of Medicine quoted in Smolinski et al. 2005; Institute of Medicine 2009). Health systems are struggling to keep up and becoming more complex and costly, placing fresh demands on health workers. In many countries, professionals are encountering more socially diverse patients with chronic conditions who are more proactive in their health-seeking behaviour (Anderson et al. 2003; Horton 2005; Strong et al. 2005; Yach et al. 2005). Patient management requires coordinated care across time and space, demanding unprecedented team work. Professionals must integrate the explosive growth of knowledge and technologies while grappling with expanding functions—super-specialization, prevention, and complex care management in multiple sites, including different types of facilities alongside home- and community-based care (Benner et al. 2010; Cooke et al. 2010; Josiah Macy and Jr. Foundation 2008; The Association of Faculties of Medicine of Canada 2010; The Prime Minister's Commission on the Future of Nursing and Midwifery in England 2010; UK General Medical Council 2009).

Consequently, there is a slow-burning crisis in the mismatch of professional competencies to patient and population priorities due to fragmentary, outdated, and static curricula producing ill-equipped graduates from under-financed institutions. In virtually all countries, the education of health professionals has contributed to dysfunctional and inequitable health systems due to curricular rigidities, professional silos, static pedagogy, insufficient adaptation to local contexts, and commercialism of the professions. Breakdown is especially noteworthy at the primary care level, in both poorer and richer countries. The failings are systemic—for example professionals unable to keep pace—becoming mere technology managers or a continuing reluctance to serve marginalized rural communities (WHO 2010). Professionals are falling short on appropriate competencies for effective team work, and they are failing to exercise effective leadership for transforming health systems.

The renaissance of a 'new professionalism'—patient-centred and team-based—has been much discussed (ABIM Foundation et al. 2003; Cohen et al. 2007; Levinson et al. 2010; Royal College of Physicians 2005; Siantz and Meleis 2007; Swick 2000), but it has lacked the leadership, incentives, and power to deliver on its promise. Some attempts to redefine the future roles and responsibilities of health professionals have floundered amid the rigid tribalism that afflicts them. There has been strong advocacy for specific practitioner groups, but without an overall strategy for the broader health professional community to work together to meet individual and population health needs. Several well-meaning recent efforts have attempted to address these fractures, but have usually fallen short.

The Lancet Commission

Marking the centennial of the Flexner Report in 1910, the Commission on Education of Health Professionals for the 21st Century was launched in January 2010 to address these emerging challenges. This independent initiative, led by a group of 20 Commissioners from around the world, adopted a global perspective seeking to advance health by recommending instructional and institutional innovations to nurture a new generation of health professionals who would be better equipped to address future health challenges. Over the course of 2010, the Commission articulated a fresh vision with practical recommendations of specific actions that can catalyse steps towards the transformation of health professional education in all countries, rich and poor alike.

The Commission began by defining its object of study, *health professional education*. It purposefully did not confine itself to a single profession. The current division of labour among the various health professions is a social construction resulting from complex historical processes around scientific progress, technological development, economic relationships, political interests, and cultural values and beliefs. The dynamic character of professional boundaries is underscored by the continuous struggles among different professional groups to delimit their respective spheres of practice. The division of labour at any given point in time and in any given society is much more the result of those social forces than of any inherent attribute of health-related work.

Recognizing these dynamics, the Commission articulated a framework aimed at understanding the complex interactions between two core systems: education and health. Contrary to other frameworks, where the population is exogenous to the health or education systems, the provision of educational services generates the *supply* of an educated workforce to meet the *demand* for professionals to work in the health system. People are not only recipients of services but actual coproducers of their own education and health. In this systemic approach, balance between the two systems is critical for efficiency, effectiveness, and equity. Clearly, every country has its own unique history, and legacies of the past shape both the present as well as the trajectory into the future. There are two critical junctures in the framework: the first is the labour market, which governs the fit or misfit between the supply and demand of health professionals; the second is the weak capacity of many populations, especially the poor, to translate their health and educational needs into effective demand for the respective services.

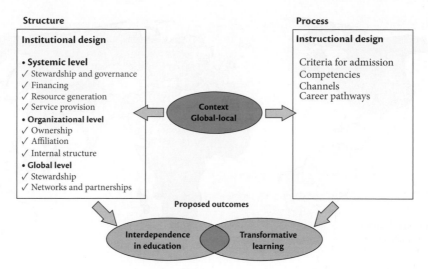

Figure 59.2 Key components of the educational system.
Reprinted from The Lancet, 376, Frenk et al., 'Health professionals for a new century: transforming education to strengthen health systems in an interdependent world', pp. 1923–1958, Copyright 2010, with permission from Elsevier.

Having specified the linkages between the health and educational spheres, our framework proceeds to identify three key dimensions of education, as shown in fig. 59.2: *institutional design* (which specifies the structure and functions of the education system), *instructional design* (which focuses on processes), and *educational outcomes* (which deal with the desired results).

Adapting a framework that was originally formulated to understand health system performance (Murray and Frenk 2000), we can think of four crucial institutional functions that apply to educational systems as well: (1) stewardship and governance; (2) financing; (3) resource generation, and (4) service provision. To have a positive impact on the functioning of health systems and ultimately on health outcomes of patients and populations, instruction must be designed consisting of four C's: (1) criteria for admission; (2) competencies and curriculum; (3) channels of instruction; and (4) career pathways.

In the case of the Commission, two outcomes were proposed for the health professional education system. *Transformative learning* is the proposed outcome of improvements in instructional design; *interdependence in education* should result from institutional reforms. All aspects of the educational system are deeply influenced by both local and global contexts. While many commonalities may be shared globally, there is local distinctiveness and richness. Such diversity offers opportunities for shared learning across all countries.

Major findings of the Lancet Commission

The Commission's major findings are presented in three subsections: institutional design, instructional design, and global–local dynamics. The institutional analysis relies mostly on quantitative data to present for the first time a global landscape of institutions, graduates, and financing—followed by such key stewardship functions as accreditation and academic systems. The examination of instructional design focuses on the purpose, content, method, and outcomes of the learning process—categorized according to the four C's: criteria for admission, competencies, channels, and career pathways. The final subsection cuts across institutions and instruction by examining the challenges of local adaptability in an interdependent globalizing world.

Institutional design

In this section, we focus on institutions of post-secondary education that offer professional degrees in medicine, public health or nursing. Such educational institutions may be independent or linked to government, part of a university or free-standing, fully accredited or even informally established. Their facilities may range from rudimentary field training sites to sophisticated campuses. And each country, of course, has its own unique legacy because institution building is a long-term, path-dependent development process.

Global landscape

Not surprisingly, enormous global diversity is observed in medical institutions. Scarcity is associated with low national income, especially impacting sub-Saharan Africa, but abundance is not concentrated solely in wealthy countries. The Commission estimates 2420 medical schools producing around 389 000 medical graduates annually for a world population of 7 billion people. It also estimates 467 schools or departments of public health and about 541 000 nursing graduates annually. The counts of both public health and nursing schools and graduates are hampered by variability in definition and data limitations.

Figure 59.3 shows the density of medical schools by major world regions. The better endowed regions are Western Europe, North Africa and the Middle-East, and Latin America and the Caribbean, while lower density is found in sub-Saharan Africa and parts of Southeast Asia. Distribution of medical institutions is skewed among nations. India, China, Brazil, and the United States—each having more than 150 schools—comprise 35% of world's total. Thirty-one countries have no medical school whatsoever, and 9 of these are in sub-Saharan Africa. Forty-four countries have only one medical school, and of these 17 are in sub-Saharan Africa. Nearly half of the countries in the world have either one or no medical school.

Financing

Due to limited data, the Commission undertook a special study on the financing of health professional education, generating the first ever estimate of the financial size of the health professional education industry. Total annual expenditures in health professional

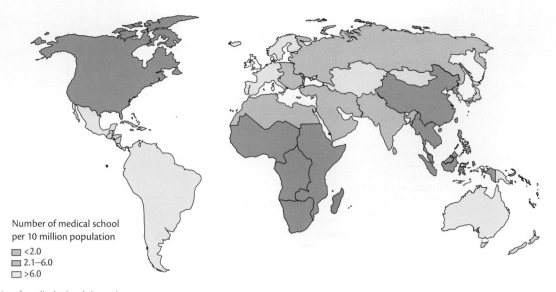

Figure 59.3 Density of medical schools by region.
Reprinted from The Lancet, 376, Frenk et al., 'Health professionals for a new century: transforming education to strengthen health systems in an interdependent world', pp. 1923–1958, Copyright 2010, with permission from Elsevier.

education is estimated at about US$100 billion for medicine, nursing, public health, and allied health professions. Educating medical graduates is estimated at US$47.6 billion and nursing graduates at US$27.2 billion, with the remaining amount estimated for public health and other related professions. Altogether, the Commission estimates a unit cost of US$122 000 per medical graduate, and a unit cost of US$50 000 per nursing graduate. Unit costs per graduate in North America are estimated at $497 000 with much lower costs estimated for China ($14 000), India ($35 000), and sub-Saharan Africa ($52 000).

Private investments in professional education may be increasing, infusing welcome funding but also generating concerns over quality and social purpose (Amin et al. 2010). Trend lines of new medical schools in India and Brazil reveal a spurt of new private establishments. The growth of private commercial medical schools raises concerns about quality, transparency, and the urban bias of their geographic location. Driven by global workforce shortages and growing market demand for health services, the explosive increase in unplanned and unregulated medical schools could generate the same type of low-quality proprietary schools that Flexner criticized.

Accreditation

Accreditation is the formal legitimization of an institution to grant degrees that enables its graduates to achieve licensing and certification for professional practice. Accreditation is usually based on external, peer, or self review, wherein an institution is assessed for its compliance with predetermined standards of structure, process, and achievement. The aim is to ensure an acceptable quality of graduates to meet the health needs of patients and populations.

Accreditation practices demonstrate great global diversity. In most countries, government performs the function, although in many nations accreditation is conducted by professional councils or associations (Woollard 2010). Two major issues of accreditation refer to the ultimate purposes and incentives driving accreditation processes and harmonizing global principles versus local adaptability. WHO has defined 'social accountability' of accreditation as 'directing education, research and service activities towards

addressing the priority health concerns of the community, region, and/or nation they have the mandate to service' (WHO and Division of Development of Human Resources for Health 1995). The imposition of greater 'social accountability' into accreditation could be instrumental in producing a professional workforce that is better aligned with societal health goals, including equity, quality, and efficiency. Another challenge is harmonizing global standards with local adaptability to diverse contexts. Global principles with local adaptability would bring consistency, transparency, and open accountability to the accreditation process, while facilitating the emergence of like-minded communities of knowledge and practice.

Academic systems

This includes aspects such as academic hospitals and training sites, primary care, institutional collaboration, and faculty development. Over the past half century, academic centres based in tertiary hospitals grew rapidly due to income from clinical services and research. The power and influence of these centres integrating the continuum of discovery–care–education correspondingly increased as did the proliferation of subspecialties of practice (Wartman et al. 2009). Efforts have been made to expand the educational options beyond tertiary hospitals to community health centres, sometimes situated amongst disadvantaged communities. Some have proposed systems that would include not just tertiary hospital centres but also networks of secondary and primary health units, including community-based programmes.

A clear danger is that tertiary academic centres can relegate or diminish the attractiveness of primary care which should be seamlessly integrated into training for health systems. Professional education must reinforce the primary function of assuring access to all of high-quality services for a defined population through proactive strategies, favoring continuity of care, guaranteeing an explicit set of entitlements, and assuring universal social protection in health (Frenk 2009a).

Collaboration, a potential power tool of academic systems, describes the opportunities for enhancing educational quality and productivity through sharing of information, academic exchange, pursuit of joint work, and synergies among institutions with different assets (Horton 2000). The purposes of education, research, and service may be advanced through sharing of curricula, exchange of faculty and students, collaborative research, and other activities. Many organizational arrangements have been employed to facilitate these synergies: networks, consortia, alliances, and partnerships. Especially noteworthy is capacity building through twinning arrangements for mutual institutional strengthening.

Faculty members, the ultimate resource of all educational institutions, are the teachers, stewards, agents of knowledge transmission, and the most important role models for students—reproducing the profession by training the next generation of professionals. Faculty challenges in most countries include heavy teaching loads, a shortage of teachers, competing demands for research and consultancy services, and the hazards of mid-career burn-out (Cooke et al. 2006; Corbett and Marsico 1981; Shanafelt et al. 2009; Shirey 2006). In some institutions, there is the dominance of research over teaching, not just in academic and clinical career paths, but in power, money, and privileges. In many institutions, teaching is not accorded the status or priority of research. Knowledge generation trumps knowledge sharing and knowledge translation. There may also be reluctance of outstanding professionals to accept full-time teaching roles due to more financially lucrative and socially rewarding opportunities in assuming senior positions in practice rather than in education (Blades et al. 2000).

Instructional design

The Commission's literature review located 11 054 articles in medical, nursing, and public health education. The papers on education in medicine (73%) are more abundant than on nursing (25%), or public health (2%). Over half of the articles (53%) focus on professional education in North America, one quarter (26%) in Europe, and the remainder (21%) in other world regions. It is noteworthy that we found little solid research evidence documenting the impact or effectiveness of educational innovations. While there is movement towards greater analytical rigor in educational research, most studies were descriptive, highlighting the importance of strengthening evidence building in the field (Harden and Grant 1999).

Challenges to instructional design can be examined systematically by considering the learning process of students from admission to graduation via the four Cs: criteria for admission, competencies, channels, and career pathways.

Criteria for admission

In many countries, the social competency of graduates may not be aligned with the social, linguistic, and ethnic diversity of patients. Health professional students may be disproportionately admitted from the higher social classes and dominant ethnic groups (Josiah Macy and Jr. Foundation 2008; The Association of Faculties of Medicine of Canada 2010). Gender stereotypes, skewed gender composition, and 'feminization' of the workforce can be problematic. Yet, the composition of entering students constitutes an important determinant of how well graduates will be able to meet the health needs of patients and populations.

Many remedies have been proposed to achieve balanced admissions, but few have turned the tide—balancing social, linguistic, and ethnic diversity, affirmative action, preferential admission for those from disadvantaged backgrounds, dispersal of training institutions into provinces and rural areas, building rural experiences into the curriculum, and payments or incentives for serving the underprivileged. Ultimately, the criteria for admission are linked to and reflect institutional purpose. A purely competitive merit-based admissions policy may recruit the best and brightest; alternatively proactive recruitment to obtain balanced rural, ethnic, and sociocultural composition may express the institutional purpose of advancing health equity. These admission goals are not mutually incompatible, and many institutions attempt to harmonize allied purposes into a coherent admissions policy (Josiah Macy Jr. Foundation 2008).

Competencies

There is a strong movement to align the curriculum as an instrument of learning to achieve requisite competencies as the educational goal. Curricula often become anchored to historical legacy that codifies the traditions, priorities, and values of the faculty. A competency-based approach realigns the 'horse-and-cart'. It is a disciplined approach to specify the health problems to be addressed, identify the requisite competencies required of graduates, tailor the curriculum to achieve competencies, and assess achievements and shortfalls. Competency-based education allows for an individualized learning process rather than the traditional, lock-step, one-size-fits-all curriculum (Gruppen et all 2010). By focusing on educational outcomes, the approach is more transparent and therefore accountable to learners, policy-makers, and stakeholders.

A growing demand in competency is team work. Team work is essential in all health systems, especially in an era of non-communicable diseases where patient care becomes a series of transitions from home to hospital to rehabilitation facilities back to home again, necessarily engaging a host of interdisciplinary professionals—social workers, nurses, therapists, doctors, and counsellors—who must work together to provide a seamless web of services (Calabretta 2002). *Interprofessional education* and *team-based learning* are instructional approaches aimed at preparing students for effective, collaborative work. So too in many settings, *trans-professional education* is assuming importance because all health professionals must learn to work beyond the medical professions with non-medical professionals—community health workers, administrators, logistics managers, office staff, and policy-makers.

Channels

Good professional education programmes mobilize all learning channels to their full potential: didactic faculty lectures, small student learning groups, team-based education, early patient or population exposure, different worksite training bases, longitudinal relationship with patients and communities, and the use of IT. Among these, the impact of e-learning is likely to be revolutionary. E-learning has traditionally included computer-assisted instruction to facilitate the delivery of stand-alone multimedia packages and distance learning for delivering instruction to remote locations (Ruiz et al. 2006). Explosive growth of the internet has brought power, speed, and versatility to both approaches (OECD 2005). The range of options available today encompass web-supplemented courses that may include online lectures, use of email, and linkages to online resources; web-dependent courses that require students to use the internet; and full online courses with little classroom or direct human interaction.

As with all technologies, the drivers of constructive change are not the hardware or software by themselves, but rather the institutional transformation, including what has been called 'humanware'. IT-empowered learning is already a reality for the younger generation in most parts of the world, and in many cases, the uptake of new digital technologies has been faster and more widespread in poorer countries. Educational institutions must now be re-engineered to ride this wave of transformation, or else they risk becoming obsolete. Put simply, the 21st century education of health professionals must focus less on memorizing and transmitting facts and more on promoting the reasoning and communication skills that will enable the professional to be an effective partner, facilitator, adviser, and advocate.

Career pathways

Graduation signifies the passage from student status to member of one of the health professions. By joining, the novice professional should understand the duties and obligations of membership as well as undertake the commitment to the professional code of conduct. As the archetype of professional work, medicine has been the subject of intense study in an effort to understand the essential attributes that distinguish professions from other occupations— and the forces that are transforming those attributes (Hafferty and McKinlay 1993). In his classical work, Freidson explained the two meanings of the word profession: as 'a special kind of occupation' and as 'an avowal or promise' (Freidson 1970).

To fulfil such a promise, professionalism 'signifies a set of values, behaviours, and relationships that underpin the trust' of the public (Royal College of Physicians 2005). Professional education, therefore, must inculcate responsible professionalism, not only by acquiring explicit knowledge and skills, but also by promoting an identity, as well as the adoption of values, commitments, and disposition of the profession (Cooke et al. 2010). Developing the fundamental attributes of professional behaviour, identity, and values is facilitated by appropriate role models, team interactions, coaching, instruction, assessment, and feedback. Included in this process is aligning the hidden curriculum so that the learning environment is made consistent with professional rhetoric and stated values.

Global-local health

While in his 1910 report Flexner concentrated on one region, he recognized the worldwide implications of his study in the '. . . advancement of medical science throughout the world'. Today's world is markedly different to that of a century ago, however. The richness of diversity is not entirely new, but the pace, scale, and intensity of global interdependence have ushered in new risks and opened new opportunities. Consider the extent of global inequality. In national income, the world's richest and poorest countries show a 100-fold difference, but in per capita healthcare expenditures there is 1000-fold gap between the richest and poorest nations. Differences of such magnitude profoundly influence the educational and health systems. How could one professional standard encompass such diversity? Every country has its unique institutional legacies in professional education. Every country's health system must develop an appropriate skill-mix of workers with requisite competencies for local effectiveness. The challenge for professional education is to adapt locally while harnessing the power of global flows of knowledge and resources.

Making the most of limited resources has led many developing countries to undertake expansion of their workforce through the training of ancillary health workers. There is ample evidence that

such workers can offer a wide range of primary health services (Bhutta et al. 2010). Yet, the effectiveness and long-term sustainability of such basic workers depend critically upon collaborative linkages with professional cadres (Buchan and Dal Poz 2002). Many community health worker programmes, indeed, have failed because they did not successfully incorporate professionals into the workforce mix (Bhutta et al. 2010); Crisp 2010; Global Health Workforce Alliance 2010). Professionals invariably are the leaders, planners, and policy-makers. They are also an invaluable resource for the training of community workers. Post-secondary educated professionals can perform complex reasoning, deal with uncertainty, anticipate and plan impending changes, and conduct many other functions essential for health systems performance. Virtually all top leaders of the health sector are professionals with post-secondary education. Complementary requisite skills for these professionals should include such key health system functions as planning, policy, and management.

After decades of stagnation, the number of medical schools in the United States and some other richer countries is again growing to meet increasing demand. Like most other wealthy countries, the US has chronic shortages of physicians, suffers from imbalances in expertise (especially a shortage of primary physicians), and also has professional maldistribution for coverage of disadvantaged populations. Medical school expansion opens an opportunity to revitalize professional education as many curricular innovations can be tested and disseminated (Josiah Macy Jr. Foundation 2008).

Among recent innovations is the integration of global perspectives into revitalized curricula. Educating professionals in intercultural sensitivities is important for increasingly diverse patient populations. The transnational flow of diseases, risks, technologies, and career opportunities also demands new competencies of professionals working in a shrinking planet. These professional competencies should be advanced through curricular inclusion of global health, including crosscultural and crossnational experiential exposure. Some see global health as an added dimension to their respective professions. Others see it as equivalent to public health studied and practiced from a perspective encompassing the entire world (Fried et al. 2010). There is growing consensus over its key tenets—universalism, global perspectives in discovery and translation, inclusion of broad determinants of health, interdisciplinary approaches, and a comprehensive framework. While having distinctive courses and training sessions in global health is important, it is even more valuable to ensure the integration of a global perspective into all courses and exercises.

Professional education is increasingly experiencing global connectedness and flows. In richer countries, a priority is interprofessional education to breakdown silos for team work, while in poorer countries, transprofessional education is even more important because of numerically larger cadres of basic and other workers. We are recognizing increasingly that we have one global pool of health professionals, with a global labour market where professionals are on the move, crossing national borders, and creating global communities of expertise. The current pattern has richer countries sending funds, models, and technical assistance to poorer countries which in return loose migrating health professionals to richer countries. Yet, more balanced flows can be established where many innovations in poorer countries can be appreciated and such models used in richer countries. Rather than exporting inappropriate models, richer countries can send teachers to educate and build indigenous health professionals in under-staffed educational institutions abroad.

The future of innovation and reform

Three generations of reform

To understand the baseline for the future of health professional education, it is important to capture the historical developments of the past century, which the Commission defines as a typology of three generations of reforms (fig. 59.4). Like all classification schemes, this one simplifies realities, but is informed by historical analyses and has heuristic value. The word generation conveys the notion that this is not a linear succession of clear-cut reforms. Instead, elements of each generation persist in the following ones, in a complex and dynamic pattern of change. The first generation, launched at the beginning of the 20th century, inculcated a science-based curriculum. Around mid-century, the second generation introduced problem-based instructional innovations. The Commission argues that now is the time for a third generation of reforms that should be systems-based.

Most countries and professional institutions possess mixed patterns of these reforms. In some countries, most schools are entirely confined to the first generation, locked into traditional and stagnant curricula and teaching methods with an inability, or even resistance, to change. Many countries are incorporating second-generation reforms, and a few countries are moving into the third generation (Azizi 1997; Kent and de Villiers 2007; Kurdak et al. 2008; Lam and Lam 2009). No country has all schools in the third generation.

Vision and recommendations

Based on these three generations of reforms, the Commission offers a vision and recommendations for health professional education reform. Fundamental is the recognition that all peoples and countries are tied together in an increasingly interdependent global health space. While each country must address local problems through building its own professional workforce for its health system, many health workers participate in a common global pool of talent—with great porosity across national borders. That common pool reflects growing interdependence in all health matters, including expanding transfers of risks and knowledge, trans-national movement of workers and patients, and growing trade in health services and products.

Of course, the common global pool of professionals and other health workers is divided by political borders and professional certification within nations. Yet cross-border flow of professional workers, patients, and health services is already significant and will grow to impact on educational content, channels, and competencies in all countries. Each profession may have distinctive and complementary skills that may be considered the core of its special niche. But there is an imperative for bringing such expertise together into teams for effective patient-centred and population-based health work. Moreover, like porous borders, the walls between task competencies of different professions are not airtight but assume various shades of grey where task-shifting and task-sharing are crafted to produce practical health outputs that would not be possible with sealed competencies.

In this global pool, professionals with post-secondary education are especially privileged because their training commanded significant time, effort, and investment by the professional, their family, and society, usually calling upon significant public financing. Professionals, therefore, have special obligations and responsibilities to acquire competencies and to perform functions beyond purely technical tasks—such as team work, ethical conduct, critical analysis, coping with uncertainty, scientific inquiry, anticipating and planning for the future, and most importantly leadership of effective health systems.

The Commission's vision calls for a new era of professional education that advances transformative learning and harnesses the power of interdependence in education. Just as reforms in the early 20th century rode on the wave of the germ theory and the establishment of the modern medical sciences, so too the Commission argues that the future will be shaped by adaptation of competencies to specific contexts drawing upon the power of global flows of information and knowledge. The Commission aspires to spark a second century of reforms in all countries and all professions facing new contexts and fresh challenges. Its vision is global not parochial, interprofessional not confined to a single group, committed to building sound evidence, encompassing of both individual and population-based approaches, and focused on instructional and institutional innovations.

In this vision, all health professionals in all countries are educated to mobilize knowledge, as well as to engage in critical reasoning and ethical conduct, so they are competent to participate in patient- and population-centred health systems as members of locally responsive and globally connected teams. The ultimate purpose is to assure universal coverage of high-quality comprehensive services essential to advancing opportunity for health equity within and among countries. The aspiration of good health commonly shared resonates with young professionals who seek value and meaning in their work.

Carrying out this vision requires a series of instructional and institutional reforms that are aimed at the two outcomes suggested earlier: transformative learning and interdependence in education.

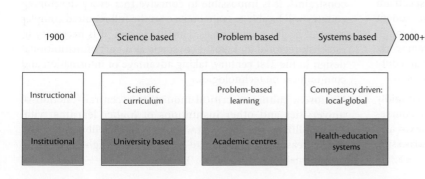

Figure 59.4 Three generations of reform.
Reprinted from The Lancet, 376, Frenk et al., 'Health professionals for a new century: transforming education to strengthen health systems in an interdependent world', pp. 1923–1958, Copyright 2010, with permission from Elsevier.

Table 59.1 Transformative learning

Level	Objective	Outcome
Informative	◆ Information ◆ Skills	Experts
Formative	◆ Socialization ◆ Values	Professionals
Transformative	◆ Leadership attributes	Change agents

The notion of transformative learning derives from the work of several educational theorists, notably Freire and Mezirow (Freire 1970; Mezirow 2000). While it has been used with different meanings (Markos and McWhinney 2003), the Commission views it as the highest of three successive levels, moving from informative to formative to transformative learning (table 59.1). Informative learning is about acquiring knowledge and skills; its purpose is to produce experts. Formative learning is about socializing students around values; its purpose is to produce professionals. Transformative learning is about developing leadership attributes; its purpose is to produce enlightened change agents. Effective education builds each level on the previous one. As a valued outcome, transformative learning involves three fundamental shifts:

◆ from fact memorization to critical reasoning that can guide the capacity to search, analyse, assess, and synthesize information for decision-making

◆ from seeking professional credentials to achieving core competencies for effective team work in health systems

◆ from non-critical adoption of educational models to creative adaptation of global resources to address local priorities.

Interdependence is a key element in a systemic approach as it underscores the ways in which various components interact with each other, without presupposing that they are equal. As a desirable outcome, interdependence in education also involves three shifts:

◆ from isolated to harmonized education and health systems

◆ from stand-alone institutions to worldwide networks, alliances, and consortia

◆ from self-generated and self-controlled institutional assets to harnessing global flows of educational content, pedagogical resources, and innovations.

Transformative learning and interdependence in education are the proposed outcomes of instructional and institutional reforms, which are described next:

Instructional reforms should encompass the entire spectrum from admission to graduation so as to generate a diverse student body experiencing a competency-based curriculum that, through the creative use of IT, prepares them for the realities of team work, in order to develop flexible career paths based on the spirit and duty of a new professionalism. Health professional education should:

◆ Adopt competency-based curricula that are responsive to rapidly changing needs rather than being dominated by static coursework. Competencies must be adapted to local contexts and should be determined by national stakeholders, while harnessing global knowledge and experiences.

◆ Promote inter- and transprofessional education that breaks down professional silos while enhancing collaborative and non-hierarchical relationships for effective team work.

◆ Exploit the power of IT for learning through development of evidence, capacity for data collection and analysis, simulation and testing, distance learning, collaborative connectivity, and management of the explosion in knowledge.

◆ Adapt locally, but harness resources globally, in a way that confers capacity to flexibly address local problems while tapping global knowledge, experience, and shared resources, including faculty, curriculum, didactic materials, and students linked internationally through exchange programmes.

◆ Strengthen educational resources, since faculty, syllabi, didactic materials, and infrastructure are necessary instruments to achieve competencies. Faculty development requires special attention through increased investments in 'education of educators', stable and rewarding career paths, and constructive evaluation linked to incentives for good performance.

◆ Promote a 'new professionalism' that uses competencies as the objective criterion for the classification of health professionals, transforming current conventional silos, and developing a set of common attitudes, values, and behaviours as accountable change agents.

Institutional reforms should align national efforts through joint planning especially in the education and health sectors, engage all stakeholders in the reform process, extend academic learning sites into communities, develop global collaborative networks for mutual strengthening, and lead in promoting the culture of critical inquiry and public reasoning. Institutions should:

◆ Establish joint planning mechanisms in every country to engage key stakeholders, especially ministries of education and health, professional associations, and the academic community, to overcome fragmentation by assessing national conditions, setting priorities, shaping policies, tracking change, and harmonizing the supply of and demand for health professionals to meet the health needs of the population.

◆ Expand from academic centres to academic systems, extending the traditional discovery–care–education continuum in schools and hospitals into primary care settings and communities, strengthened through external collaboration domestically and internationally as part of more agile and dynamic professional education systems.

◆ Link together through networks, alliances and consortia among educational institutions from around the globe and across to allied actors, such as governments, civil society organizations, business, and media. Given faculty shortages and other resource constraints, it is impossible to conceive that every developing country will be able to train on its own the full required complement of health professionals. For this reason, it is necessary to establish regional and global consortia as a part of institutional design in the 21st century, taking advantage of information and communication technologies.

◆ Nurture a culture of critical inquiry as a central function of universities and other institutions of higher learning, vital for mobilizing scientific knowledge, ethical deliberation, and public reasoning and debate to generate enlightened social transformation.

Future of health professional education

The Commission offers its recommendations recognizing that in our complex and interdependent world professional education is at a crossroads. Opportunities are opening for a fresh round of reforms to craft professional education, spurred by mutual learning due to health interdependence, changes in educational pedagogy, the public salience of health, and the growing recognition of the imperative for change.

Paradoxically, despite glaring disparities, interdependence in health is growing and the opportunities for mutual learning and shared progress have greatly expanded. Global movements of people, pathogens, products, information, lifestyles, and technologies underlie the international transfer of health risks and opportunities (Garcia et al. 2009). We are increasingly interdependent in terms of key health resources, especially skilled workers.

Alongside the rapid pace of change in health, there is a parallel revolution in education. The explosive increase not only in total volume of information, but also in ease of access to it, makes it necessary to rethink the role of universities and other educational institutions. Learning, of course, has always been experienced outside formal instruction through all kinds of interactions, but the informational content and learning potential that flows today through the airwaves and cyberspace are without precedent. In this rapidly evolving context, universities and educational institutions are broadening their traditional role as places where people go to obtain information (e. g. by consulting books in libraries or listening to experts) to incorporate novel forms of learning that transcend the confines of the classroom. The next generation of learners requires the capacity to discriminate vast amounts of information and extract and synthesize knowledge necessary for clinical and population-based decision-making. These developments point toward fresh opportunities around the modes, means, and meaning of education.

Like never before, the public salience of health in general and global health in particular has generated an environment more propitious for change. Health is assuming centre stage amongst the most pressing global issues of our time: socioeconomic development, national and human security, and the global movement for human rights. There is growing consensus that good health is not only a consequence of but also a condition for development, security, and rights. At the same time, access to high-quality healthcare with financial protection for all has become one of the major domestic political priorities around the world.

Driving forces

Since publication of the Commission Report in December 2010, follow-up activities have revealed widespread interest in reforming health professional education so that it responds better to the requirements of the 21st century. Regional networks or consortia are beginning to form to landscape diverse national situations, to engage key stakeholders, and to chart innovation and reforms. Most encouragingly, regional networks have made starts in the Middle East, Africa, Latin America, and Asia.

How these activities will eventually generate innovation and reform in health professional education will be dependent upon five key forces. These macroforces will shape both the context of health professional education as well as impose demands upon the educational process. The five forces are: demographic and epidemiologic transition; the knowledge explosion; markets; public policies; and professional leadership.

Epidemiologic–demographic transitions

Professional education will be powerfully shaped by profound demographic and epidemiologic shifts now underway in most countries, rich and poor. World population size has reached 7 billion and will increase several more billions due to growth in high fertility countries. What characterizes the demographic transition, however, is the rapid ageing of populations, the pace of urbanization, and increasing mobility of people. Along with these demographic shifts are epidemiologic transitions in which the burden of disease is shifting from common infections and childhood malnutrition to the non-communicable diseases (NCDs). Along with the emergence of chronic diseases are new threats due to environmental risks, new infectious agents, and socio-behavioral pathologies such as drugs, tobacco use, and alcoholism.

Health systems will have to be revamped to address these transitions. Prevention of NCDs will have to move beyond simple technological solutions to multidisciplinary and multi-sectoral engagement that targets lifestyle, behaviour, and regulates industry. Primary care will remain of paramount importance, but its linkages to secondary and tertiary care will have to be strengthened through integrated networks as patients with chronic conditions move up and down these tiers, including home- and facility-based care. Interprofessional and transprofessional education to strengthen workforce teams will grow in importance to properly manage these new health system demands. Educational systems will also be impacted by demographic and epidemiologic transitions. The next generation of faculty will need to be developed in light of smaller cohorts of young entrants into the profession. Feminization of the profession is likely to expand, and given greater mobility of people, cultural diversity of patients will demand greater cultural competencies of health professionals.

Explosion of knowledge

All of the knowledge roles of health professionals will be profoundly affected by the explosion of knowledge—scientists and researchers as knowledge producers, faculty and teachers as knowledge reproducers, policymakers as knowledge-based decision-makers, and professional practitioners as knowledge brokers to ensure patients and populations access knowledge for health improvements. The explosion of knowledge will translate into more and stronger technologies for prevention, therapeutics, and diagnostics, which in turn could generate more subspecialties of practice, even as primary care is also challenged. The digital revolution will undoubtedly transform both the content and the pedagogy of education. Archiving data, retrieval of information, and simulation exercises all hold promise in the future of education. Distance learning, too, could ensure lower cost and wider access. The expansion of knowledge will fundamentally challenge existing systems of education that relies on mastering a set of core facts or information, as knowledge expansion pushes beyond traditional boundaries. Higher premium will be attached to the discrimination, synthesis, and analysis of information for decision-making in clinical and population-based practice.

Market forces

Market forces will be important first through the economic effects of wealth generation and income distribution. Whether the economy grows and generates jobs and whether income is skewed or mal-distributed will profoundly affect patients and populations. Market forces, will also influence the health and educational systems. Private medical organizations are growing, backed by market-driven health insurance, pharmaceutical companies, and the vast construction and equipment industry. These private corporations will create many of the jobs needed to be supplied by educational institutions. Market forces are also attracting private investments in health professional education. While such private investment will help to expand institutional capacities, there are concerns over quality of education and imbalances in the production of professionals. Commercial investments are biased towards more lucrative professions like clinical medicine and nursing, rather than other less lucrative professions like public health and social work. Channelling private investments, ensuring quality, and balancing impact of commercial investments are important for securing a positive impact of market forces on education.

Public policy

Public policies are undertaken to further the wellbeing of society and political leadership is no less important in health professional education than in other fields. One reason is that most educational institutions in this field require public subsidies. In addition, public policies regarding the size and composition of the health system determine the demand for professional workforces. Financial investments in health professional education must be substantially increased. For a knowledge-driven system, investing less than 2% of total turnover in the development of its most skilled members is not only insufficient but unwise, putting the remaining 98% of expenditure at risk. Public policy also reflects societal values with regard to the esteem and support health professionals receive in society.

Professional leadership

Undoubtedly, the most important force driving the future of higher education in health is academic and professional leadership. For reforms to succeed, they must ultimately be accepted by academia and the organized professions. As an intergenerator of knowledge transmission, educational systems tend to resist change. It is professional leadership that can pioneer and disseminate innovations, as well as promote their adoption in standard practice. Leadership is required to progressively move to align accreditation, licensing, and certification with health goals through engaging relevant stakeholders in setting objectives, criteria, assessment, and tracking of accreditation processes. Professional leadership is also essential to the development of a stronger evidence base for educational reforms through shared learning, about what works, why, and how.

Reform, ultimately, must begin with a change in the mindset that acknowledges problems and seeks to solve them. Educational reform is a long and difficult process that cries out for leadership and requires changing perspectives, work styles, and relationships among all actors. The Commission therefore calls on the most important constituencies to embrace the imperative for reform through dialogue, open exchange, discussion, and debate over these recommendations. Professional educators are key players since change will not be possible without their leadership and ownership. So too are students and young professionals, who have a stake in their own education and careers. Other major stakeholders include professional bodies, universities, non-governmental organizations, international agencies, and donors and foundations.

Most importantly, implementation of these recommendations can be propelled by a global social movement engaging all stakeholders as part of a concerted effort to strengthen health systems. The result would be an enlightened new professionalism that can lead to better services and consequent improvements in the health of patients and populations. In this way, professional education would become a crucial component in the shared effort to address the daunting health challenges of our times, and the world would move closer to new era of passionate and participatory action to achieve the universal aspiration for equitable progress in health.

Conclusions

♦ Health professional education has not kept pace with emerging challenges of the 21st century and needs further reform to better align professional competencies to patient and population priorities.

♦ Current health and education systems face a number of major challenges—mismatch of professional competencies to needs; weak team work; gender stratification; hospital dominance over primary care; labour market imbalances; and weak leadership for health systems performance.

♦ Reforms in health professional education have evolved through successive generations, from a science-based curriculum, to problem-based instructional innovations and now require a third generation of reforms that should be systems based.

♦ Key recommendations for the future include instructional reforms (competency-driven, interprofessional and transprofessional education; IT-empowered, local-global educational resources; and a new professionalism), and institutional reforms (joint planning; global networks; and a culture of critical inquiry).

Acknowledgements

This chapter is adapted from The Lancet, 376, Frenk et al., 'Health professionals for a new century: transforming education to strengthen health systems in an interdependent world', pp. 1923–1958, Copyright 2010, with permission from Elsevier.

References

ABIM Foundation, American Board of Internal Medicine, ACP-ASIM Foundation, American College of Physicians-American Society of Internal Medicine, and Medicine, European federation of Internal (2003) Medical professionalism in the new millenium: a physician charter, *J Am Coll Surg*. 196(1): 115–118

Amin, Z., Burdick, W.P., Supe, A., and Singh, T. (2010) Relevance of the Flexner Report to contemporary medical education in South Asia. *Acad Med*. 85(2): 333–339

Anand, S. and Barnighausen, T. (2004) Human resources and health outcomes: cross-country econometric study. *Lancet*. 364(9445): 1603–1609

Anderson, L.M., Scrimshaw, S.C., Fullilove, M.T., Fielding, J E., and Normand, J. (2003) Culturally competent healthcare systems. A systematic review. *Am J Prev Med.* 24(3Suppl): 68–79

Association of American Medical Colleges (2010) A snapshot of medical student education in the United States and Canada, *Acad Med.* 85 (9): S1–S648

Azizi, F. (1997) The reform of medical education in Iran, *Med Educ.* 31(3): 159–162

Benner, P., Sutphen, M., Leonard, V., and Day, L. (2010) *Educating Nurses: a call for radical transformation*. Stanford CA: The Carnegie Foundation for the Advancement of Teaching

Bhutta, Z.A., Lassi, Z.S., Pariyo, G., and Huicho, L. (2010), Global experience of community health workers for delivery of health related Millennium Development Goals: a systematic review, country case studies, and recommendations for integration into national health systems. Geneva: Global Health Workforce Alliance

Blades, D.S., Ferguson, G., Richardson, H.C., and Redfern, N. (2000) A study of junior doctors to investigate the factors that influence career decisions. *Br J Gen Pract.* 50(455): 483–485

Buchan, J. and Dal Poz, M.R. (2002) Skill mix in the health care workforce: reviewing the evidence. *Bull World Health Org.* 80(7): 575–580

Bullock, M.B. (1980) *An American Transplant: the Rockefeller Foundation and the Peking Union Medical College*. Berkeley CA: University of California Press

Calabretta, N. (2002) Consumer-driven, patient-centered health care in the age of electronic information. *J Med Libr Assoc.* 90(1): 32–37

Chen, L and Berlinguer, G (2001) Health equity in a globalizing world. In: T. Evans, et al. (eds) *Challenging Inequities in Health: from Ethics to Action* (pp. 35–44). New York: Oxford University Press

Chen, C.C. and Bunge, F.M. (1989) *Medicine in Rural China*. Berkeley CA: University of California Press

Cohen, J.J., Cruess, S., and Davidson, C. (2007) Alliance between society and medicine: the public's stake in medical professionalism. *JAMA.* 298(6): 670–673

Commission on Social Determinants of Health (2008) *Closing the Gap in a Generation: health equity through action on the social determinants of health*. Geneva: World Health Organization

Committee for the Study of Nursing Education (1923) *Nursing and Nursing Education in the United States*. New York: The Rockefeller Foundation

Cooke, M., Irby, D.M., Sullivan, W., and Ludmerer, K.M. (2006) American medical education 100 years after the Flexner report. *N Engl J Med.* 355(13): 1339–1344

Cooke, M, Irby, D.M., O'Brien, Bridget C., and Shulman, L.S. (2010) *Educating Physicians: a call for reform of medical school and residency*. Stanford CA: The Carnegie Foundation for the Advancement of Teaching

Corbett, M.A. and Marsico, T. (1981) Faculty burn-out in nurse-midwifery education. *J Nurse Midwifery.* 26(5): 33–36

Crisp, N. (2010) *Turning the World Upside Down: the search for global health in the 21st century*. New York: Oxford University Press

Evans, T., Whitehead, M., Diderichsen, F., Bhuiya, A., and Wirth, M. (2001) *Challenging Inequities in Health: from Ethics to Action*, New York: Oxford University Press

Fagin, C. (1997) How Nursing Should Respond to the Third Report of the New Health Professions Commission. *Online Journal of Issues in Nursing.* 2(4) www.nursingworld.org/MainMenuCategories/ ANAMarketplace/ANAPeriodicals/OJIN/TableofContents/Vol21997/ No4Dec97/ThirdReportofthePewHealthProfessions.aspx Accessed 18 March 2013

Flexner, A. (1910) *Medical Education in the United States and Canada: a report to the Carnegie Foundation for the Advancement of Teaching*. New York: The Carnegie Foundation for the Advancement of Teaching, xvii, p. 346

Flexner, A. (1912) *Medical Education in Europe: a report to the Carnegie Foundation for the Advancement of Teaching*. New York: Carnegie Foundation for the Advancement of Teaching

Fosdick, R. (1952) *The story of the Rockefeller Foundation*. New York: Harper & Bros

Freidson, E. (1970) *Profession of Medicine: a study of the sociology of applied knowledge*. New York: Dodd & Mead

Freire, P. (1970) *Pedagogy of the Oppressed*. New York: Seabury Press

Frenk, J. (2009a) Reinventing primary health care: the need for systems integration. *Lancet.* 374(9684): 170–173

Frenk, J. (2009b) Globalization and health: the role of knowledge in an interdependent world. David E. Barmes Global Health Lecture. Bethesda, MD: National Institutes of Health

Frenk, J., Sepúlveda, J., Gómez-Dantés, O., and Knaul, F. (2003) Evidence-based health policy: three generations of reform in Mexico. *Lancet.* 362(9396): 1667–1671

Frenk, J., Chen, L., Bhutta, Z.A., et al. (2010) Health professionals for a new century: transforming education to strengthen health systems in an interdependent world. *Lancet.* 376(9756): 1923–1958

Fried, L.P., Bentley, M.E., Buekens, P., et al. (2010) Global health is public health. *Lancet.* 375(9714): 535–537

Garcia, P.J., Curioso, W.H., Lazo-Escalante, M., Gilman, R.H., and Gotuzzo, E. (2009) Global health training is not only a developed-country duty. *J Public Health Policy.* 30(2): 250–252

Gies, W.J. and Pritchett, H.S. (1926) *Dental education in the United States and Canada: a report to the Carnegie Foundation for the Advancement of Teaching*. New York: The Carnegie Foundation for the Advancement of Teaching

Global Health Workforce Alliance (2008) *Scaling Up. Saving Lives*. Geneva: World Health Organization

Global Health Workforce Alliance (2010) *Community Health Workers: Key Messages. Global consultation on community health workers*. Montreux, Switzerland

Gruppen, L.D., Mangrulkar, R. S., and Kolars, J. C. (2010) Competency-based education in the health professions: implications for improving global health. Working Paper. Cambridge MA: Commission on Education of Health Professionals for the 21st Century

Hafferty, F.W. and McKinlay, J.B. (1993) Introduction. In: F.W. Hafferty and J.B. McKinlay (eds) *The Changing Medical Profession: An International Perspective* (pp. 25–42). New York: Oxford University Press

Harden, R.M. (1988) What is an OSCE? *Med Teach.* 10(1): 19–22

Harden, R.M. and Grant, J. (1999) BEME Guide No.1: Best Evidence Medical Education. *Med Teach.* 21: 553

Horton, R. (2000) North and South: bridging the information gap. *Lancet.* 355 (9222): 2231–2236

Horton, R. (2005) The neglected epidemic of chronic disease. *Lancet.* 366(9496): 1514

Institute of Medicine (2002) *The Future of the Public's Health in the 21st Century*. Washington DC: National Academy Press

Institute of Medicine (2003) Summary. In: K. Gebbie, L. Rosenstock, and L.M. Hernandez, (eds), *Who Will Keep the Public Healthy: educating public health professionals for the 21st century* (pp. 3–26). Washington DC: National Academy Press.

Institute of Medicine (2005) Introduction. In: M.S. Smolinski, M.A. Hamburg, and J. Lederberg (eds) *Microbial Threats to Health: Emergence. Detection. and Response* (pp. 19–22). Washington DC: National Academy Press

Institute of Medicine (2009), *Global Issues in Water, Sanitation, and Health. Workshop summary*. Washington DC: National Academy Press

Institute of Medicine (2010) The future of nursing: leading change, advancing health. http://www.iom.edu/Reports/2010/The-Future-of-Nursing-Leading-Change-Advancing-Health.aspx Accessed 18 March 2013

Joint Learning Initiative (2004) *Human Resources for Health: Overcoming the Crisis*. Cambridge MA: Harvard University Press

Josiah Macy Jr. Foundation (2008) *Revisiting the Medical School Educational Mission at a Time of Expansion*. Charleston: Josiah Macy, Jr. Foundation

Kark, S.L. (1981) *The Practice of Community Oriented Primary Health Care*. New York: Appleton-Century-Crofts

Kent, A. and de Villiers, M.R. (2007) Medical education in South Africa—exciting times. *Med Teach.* 29(9): 906–909

Kurdak, H., Altintas, D., and Doran, F. (2008) Medical education in Turkey: past to future. *Med Teach.* 30(8): 768–773

Lam, T.P. and Lam, Y.Y. (2009) Medical education reform: the Asian experience. *Acad Med.* 84 (9): 1313–1317

Levinson, W., Lesser, C.S., and Epstein, R.M. (2010) Developing physician communication skills for patient-centered care. *Health Aff (Millwood).* 29(7): 1310–1318

Luban-Plozza, B. (1995) Empowerment techniques: from doctor-centered (Balint approach) to patient-centred discussion groups. *Patient Educ Couns.* 26 (1–3): 257–263

Markos, L. and McWhinney, W. (2003) Editors' perspectives: auspice. *J Transformative Educ.* 1(1): 3–15

Menand, L. (2010). *The Marketplace of Ideas: reform and resistance in the American university.* New York: W. W. Norton & Company, p. 102

Mezirow, J. (2000) *Learning as Transformation: critical perspectives on a theory in progress.* San Francisco: Jossey Bass

Murray, C.J.L. and Frenk, J. (2000) A framework for assessing the performance of health systems. *Bull World Health Org.* 78: 717–731

Neville, A.J. (2009) Problem-based learning and medical education forty years on. A review of its effects on knowledge and clinical performance. *Med Princ Pract.* 18(1): 1–9

OECD (2005) *Policy brief: E-learning in tertiary education.* Paris: OECD

Pablos-Mendez, A., Chunharas, S., Lansang, M.A., Shademani, R., and Tugwell, P. (2005) Knowledge translation in global health. *Bull World Health Org.* 83(10): 723

Papa, F.Jand Harasym, P.H(1999) Medical curriculum reform in North America, 1765 to the present: a cognitive science perspective. *Acad Med.* 74(2): 154–164

Pickering, G.W. (1978) *Quest for Excellence in Medical Education: A Personal Survey.* Oxford: Oxford University Press

Rosenberg, C.E. (2007) *Our Present Complaint: American Medicine. Then and Now.* Baltimore MD: Johns Hopkins University Press, vi, p. 214

Royal College of Physicians (2005) *Doctors in Society: medical professionalism in a changing world.* London: Royal College of Physicians

Ruiz, J.G., Mintzer, M.J., and Leipzig, R.M. (2006) The impact of E-learning in medical education. *Acad Med.* 81(3): 207–212

Seipp, C. and eds (1963) *Health Care for the Community.* Selected Papers of Dr John B. Grant. Baltimore MD: Johns Hopkins University Press

Shanafelt, T.D., West, C.P., Slaon, J.A., et al. (2009) Career fit and burnout among academic faculty. *Arch Intern Med.* 169(10): 990–995

Shirey, M.R. (2006) Stress and burnout in nursing faculty. *Nurse Educ.* 31(3) 95–97

Siantz, M.L. and Meleis, A.I. (2007) Integrating cultural competence into nursing education and practice: 21st century action steps. *J Transcult Nurs.* 18(1 Suppl): 86S–90S

Strong, K., Mathers, C., Leeder, S., and Beaglehole, R. (2005) Preventing chronic diseases: how many lives can we save? *Lancet.* 366(9496): 1578–1582

Swick, H.M. (2000) Toward a normative definition of medical professionalism. *Acad Med.* 75(6): 612–616

The Association of Faculties of Medicine of Canada (2010) *The future of medical education in Canada(FMEC): a collective vision for MD education.* Ottawa: The Association of Faculties of Medicine of Canada

The Committee for the Study of Nursing Education (1923) *Nursing and Nursing Education in the United States.* New York: The Rockefeller Foundation

The Prime Minister's Commission on the Future of Nursing and Midwifery in England (2010) *Front Line Care: the future of nursing and midwifery in England.* London: The Prime Minister's Commission on the Future of Nursing and Midwifery in England

UK General Medical Council (2009) *Tomorrow's Doctors: outcomes and standards for undergraduate medical education.* London: General Medical Council

Wartman, S.A., Hillhouse, E.W., Gunning-Schepers, L., and Wong, J.E. (2009) An international association of academic health centres. *Lancet.* 374(9699): 1402–1403

Welch, W.H. and Rose, W. (1915) *Institute of Hygiene: a report to the General Education Board of Rockefeller Foundation.* New York: The Rockefeller Foundation

Wellman, C. (1912) The New Orleans School of Tropical Medicine and Hygiene. *New Orleans Med Surg J.* 64: 893–915

Whitcomb, M.E. (2009) Commentary: Flexner Redux 2010: graduate medical education in the United States. *Acad Med.* 84(11): 1476–1478

Whitehead, M., Dahlgren, G., and Evans, T. (2001) Equity and health sector reforms: can low-income countries escape the medical poverty trap? *Lancet.* 358(9284): 833–836

WHO (2006) *The World Health Report: working together for health.* Geneva: World Health Organization

WHO (2010) *Increasing Access to Health Workers in Remote and Rural Areas Through Improved Retention.* Geneva: World Health Organization

WHO and Division of Development of Human Resources for Health (1995) *Defining and Measuring the Social Accountability of Medical Schools.* Geneva: World Health Organization

Woollard, R.F. (2010) Social accountability and accreditation in the future of medical education. Working Paper. Cambridge MA: Commission on Education of Health Professionals for the 21st Century.

Wyon, J.B. and Gordon, J.E. (1971) *The Khanna Study: population problems in the rural Punjab.* Cambridge MA: Harvard University Press

Yach, D., Leeder, S. R., Bell, J., and Kistnasamy, B. (2005) Global chronic diseases. *Science.* 307(5708): 317

CHAPTER 60

Faculty development for teaching improvement: from individual to organizational change

Yvonne Steinert

"The quality of teaching is not likely to become optimal until the instructors themselves are schooled in the science of imparting knowledge."

Malcolm Bateson

Reproduced from *British Medical Journal*, MC Bateson, 'Teaching the Teachers', 4, p. 59, copyright 1968, with permission from BMJ Publishing Group Ltd.

Introduction

Clinical teachers develop their knowledge, skills and teaching prowess in a number of ways. For some, this trajectory includes participation in formal workshops or courses; for others, their learning occurs in a number of informal ways, often through role modelling and practical experience in the workplace. The goal of this chapter is to describe core definitions and underlying principles of faculty development for clinical teachers, common approaches to professional development in this area, a proposed curriculum for teaching improvement, and a brief review of the available evidence. The chapter will conclude with a discussion of how faculty development can influence organizational change and how clinical teachers can pursue their own professional development.

Although this chapter focuses on clinical teachers in medicine, the general principles and strategies also apply to the professional development of other healthcare professionals. Similarly, although the chapter addresses clinicians involved in teaching and learning at all levels of the educational continuum, it is hoped that medical educators and faculty developers can refer to this chapter in the design and delivery of their faculty development programmes and activities.

Core definitions and underlying principles

What is faculty development?

Faculty development, or staff development as it is often called, refers to that broad range of activities that institutions use to *renew* or *assist* faculty in their multiple roles (Centra 1978). Moreover, although

faculty development has traditionally been defined as a planned programme designed to *prepare* institutions and faculty members for their various roles (Bland et al. 1990) and *improve* an individual's knowledge and skills in the areas of teaching, research and administration (Sheets and Schwenk 1990), clinicians engage in both formal and informal faculty development to enhance their knowledge and skills. For the purpose of this discussion, faculty development will refer to *all* activities teachers pursue to improve their teaching, in both individual and group settings (Steinert 2010d).

It has been said that the goal of faculty development is 'to teach faculty members the skills relevant to their institutional and faculty position, and to sustain their vitality, both now and in the future' (Steinert 2009, p. 391). With this objective in mind, faculty development can provide individuals with knowledge and skills about teaching and learning, curriculum design and delivery, learner assessment and programme evaluation, leadership and administration, and research and scholarship. It can also reinforce or alter attitudes or beliefs about teaching and learning, provide a conceptual framework for what is often performed on an intuitive basis, and introduce clinical teachers to a community of medical educators interested in medical education and the enhancement of teaching and learning for students, residents, and peers (Steinert 2009). In its broadest sense, faculty development should target all faculty members' roles including those of teacher, educator, researcher (and scholar) and leader (and administrator). However, for the purpose of this discussion, we will focus on the clinician's role as *teacher*.

It is also important to note that faculty development can serve as a useful instrument in the promotion of organizational change

(Steinert 2000; Steinert et al. 2007). That is, by building consensus, generating support, transmitting core content, and promoting skill acquisition, faculty development can help to implement curricular change. It can also strive to influence the institutional culture by altering the formal, informal, and hidden curriculum (Hafferty 1998), setting policy, or enhancing organizational capacities (Bligh 2005). As Swanwick (2008, p. 339) has said, faculty development should be 'an institution-wide pursuit with the intent of professionalising the educational activities of teachers, enhancing educational infrastructure, and building educational capacity for the future'.

Why faculty development?

Many institutions and organizations now offer a broad range of faculty development opportunities (McLean et al. 2008; Skeff et al. 2007). This increase in activity is due, in part, to the realization that clinicians are often not prepared for their teaching roles. It is also linked to a growing sense of public accountability, the changing nature of healthcare delivery, an ongoing pursuit of excellence, and the professionalization of teaching and medical education (Gruppen et al. 2006; Swanwick 2008). An emphasis on quality assurance in healthcare, and a desire to offer quality training programmes for students and residents (Schofield et al. 2010), are further drivers for change, as are many emerging educational priorities (e.g. the teaching and learning of professionalism, cultural awareness and humility, and interprofessional education and practice). Not surprisingly, however, despite the importance of new priorities, many faculty members feel ill-equipped to teach students and residents about these important content areas, and faculty development has a critical role to play in both individual and organizational (e.g. curricular) change.

Who are the faculty?

Although use of the term 'faculty development' is widespread, a common concern relates to the meaning of 'faculty'. For the purpose of this discussion, faculty refers to all individuals who are involved in the teaching and supervision of learners at all levels of the educational continuum (e.g. undergraduate, postgraduate, continuing professional development), in a wide range of contexts (e.g. in the classroom, at the bedside, in the outpatient clinic) and settings (e.g. the university, the hospital, and the community). As an example, Schofield et al. (2010) have reported that students in the UK are taught by university-employed clinical and non-clinical academics as well as National Health Service (NHS)-employed medical staff. In this chapter, all of these individuals are included in our definition of faculty.

Common approaches to faculty development

In reviewing the educational literature, Webster-Wright (2009, p. 702) noted that 'many professional development practices focus on delivering content rather than enhancing learning', and in so doing, she argues for a reconceptualization of professional development that moves away from learning that occurs in 'discrete, finite episodes' to a focus on continuous and authentic professional learning. Webster-Wright (2009, p. 705) also observed that 'professionals learn in a way that shapes their practice, from a diverse range of professional development activities' that include formal programmes, interactions with colleagues, and learning on

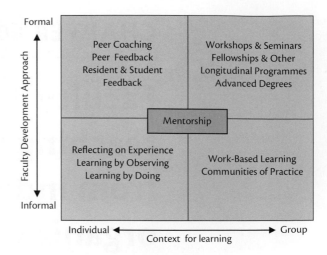

Figure 60.1 How clinicians learn about teaching.
This figure was originally prepared for a chapter on 'Becoming a Better Teacher: From Intuition to Intent' (Steinert 2010a) and is published with permission by the American College of Physicians, © 2010.

the job, and she suggests that we move towards the notion of *promoting learning* that occurs in authentic contexts rather than the *development* of our colleagues. In her opinion, the latter implies a deficit model, reinforces the notion that we 'do something to' our colleagues, and ignores a critical venue for learning. In many ways, Webster-Wright's view (2009), that we should move away from delivering and evaluating professional development programmes towards understanding and supporting learning, is also consistent with a number of recent reports (Steinert 2010a, c) that suggest that we broaden our view of how clinical teachers develop.

Figure 60.1 illustrates a number of ways in which clinicians can learn about teaching. Although we usually think about workshops, seminars, fellowships, and longitudinal programmes as the most common approach (or strategy) for faculty development, faculty members do, in fact, develop in a number of ways. As demonstrated here, clinicians can learn through both individual (independent) and group (collective) experiences while benefiting from both informal and formal approaches to teaching and learning. We will briefly examine what takes place in each quadrant, concluding with mentorship, as any strategy for self-improvement can benefit from 'the support and challenge that an effective mentor can provide' (Steinert 2010a, p.78).

Learning from experience

Clinical teachers often become adept at what they do by 'the nature of their job responsibilities' and 'learning on the job' (Steinert 2010b). Although this form of learning is not often viewed as faculty development, it is vital to self-improvement and renewal. Learning from experience can be further divided into learning by *doing*, learning by *observing* (through role modelling), and learning by *reflecting* on experience (Steinert 2010a). In fact, reflection can enhance both learning by doing and learning by observing, and it is a critical component of faculty development. The challenge for clinicians and faculty developers alike is to find ways to promote reflection in a busy clinical environment and to demonstrate that learning has, indeed, occurred. Some have suggested the benefit of using written logs of teaching encounters; others have recommended the value of personal narratives and teaching portfolios. At a practical level, Graffam et al. (2008) suggest that teachers can benefit from the use of guiding questions that tap their ability to converse and engage with the learner, model appropriate behaviours, measure performance, and structure the learning experience.

The discussion of critical incidents can be another way to promote reflection. Rademacher et al. (2010) described the use of critical incidents as a faculty development strategy to explore faculty members' professionalism. More specifically, they used teachers' personal experiences to identify challenges, discuss potential solutions, and highlight areas for further development. Although this approach is not commonly used, the analysis of critical incidents can be an innovative way in which to enhance experiential learning and reflective practice, key components in becoming a teacher.

Learning from peers, residents and students

Learning from experience can be augmented by peer feedback and learner evaluations (Steinert 2010a). Although clinical teachers are often reluctant to seek feedback from peers, it can be beneficial to discuss an educational 'problem' (or critical incident) with a colleague or ask them to observe and provide feedback after a teaching encounter. Peer coaching, which is sometimes called co-teaching, has particular appeal for clinical teachers because it occurs in the practice setting, enables individualized learning, and fosters collaboration (Steinert 2009). It also models aspects of clinical practice: the identification of individual learning goals (e.g. improving specific teaching skills); focused observation of teaching by colleagues; and the provision of feedback, analysis, and support (Flynn et al. 1994). Lochner and Gijselaers (2011) have described the components of a successful 'pedagogical consultation' that includes tailoring the consultation to individual needs, using repetition to reinforce key points, forming a 'student committee' to support the consultation, and focusing on strengths to enhance success. Irrespective of the methodology used, peer coaching (and consultation), which can promote mutually beneficial exploration and discovery, should be viewed as an important faculty development strategy (McLeod and Steinert 2009). Soliciting feedback from learners can be equally helpful, despite the fact that most clinicians do not actively seek out students' or residents' perspectives. In fact, 'taking the initiative to solicit [students'] observations and suggestions can be an integral part of the process of becoming a better teacher' (Steinert 2010a, p. 79), as an appreciative inquiry of learner evaluations can help to uncover personal strengths and areas for improvement.

Learning from structured activities

Formal (structured) activities are the most common approaches to faculty development (Steinert et al. 2006) and include workshops, seminars and short courses, fellowships and other longitudinal programmes, and certificate or degree programmes.

Workshops, seminars, and short courses are one of the most popular approaches because of their inherent flexibility and because they enable promotion of active learning through a variety of teaching methods: interactive lectures, small group discussions and exercises, role-plays and simulations, and experiential learning (Steinert 2009). Workshops and short courses are commonly used to promote skill acquisition, prepare for new curricula, or help faculty to adapt to new teaching environments.

Fellowships, of varying duration, form another structured approach to faculty development, although their focus usually extends beyond teaching improvement to include educational leadership or scholarship. More recently, integrated, longitudinal programmes (typified by teaching scholars programmes) have been developed as an alternative to fellowship programmes, as they allow clinicians to maintain most of their clinical, research, and administrative responsibilities while furthering their own professional development. Longitudinal programme components often consist of a variety of methods, including university courses, monthly seminars, and independent research projects, and they appeal to clinicians as they can continue to practice and teach while improving their educational knowledge and skills (Gruppen et al. 2006; Steinert and McLeod 2006).

Certificate or degree programmes are becoming increasingly popular in some settings, due to the 'professionalization' of medical education and an increasing desire to develop pedagogical standards at a global level (Eitel et al. 2000; Purcell and Lloyd-Jones 2003). Tekian and Harris (2012) recently described 76 masters-level programmes. As the authors suggest, an advanced degree can offer essential grounding in educational theory and practice while providing the foundation for educational research and scholarship. These programmes can also 'prepare leaders in the health professions who can manage change within their institutions, overcome organisational barriers, and effectively direct the future of healthcare delivery systems' (Tekian and Harris 2012, p. 56). Although advanced training programmes inevitably extend beyond teaching improvement, they are becoming an increasingly common approach to faculty development.

Work-based learning and communities of practice

As previously mentioned, Webster-Wright (2009) highlighted the role of work-based learning as a key component in professional development. In fact, it is in the everyday workplace, where teachers conduct their clinical, teaching, and research activities, that learning most often takes place. It is surprising that we do not currently view work-based learning as a common venue for faculty development, for by working together in a clinical or classroom setting, and discovering opportunities for learning, teachers can acquire new knowledge and refine their approaches to teaching and learning. Interestingly, faculty development activities have traditionally been conducted away from teachers' workplaces, requiring participants to take their lessons learned back to their own contexts. It is time to reverse this trend and think about how we can enhance the learning that takes place in the work environment. Learning at work is clearly a key component of the development of clinical teachers, and there is value in rendering this learning as visible (or explicit) as possible so that it can be valued as an important component of faculty development.

The notion of a community of practice is closely tied to that of work-based learning. Barab et al. (2002, p. 495) have defined a community of practice as a 'persistent, sustaining, social network of individuals who share and develop an overlapping knowledge base, set of beliefs, values, history and experiences focused on a common practice and/or mutual enterprise'. In many ways, becoming a member of a teaching community should be viewed as an approach to faculty development and we should collectively explore new ways to make this community—and the learning that it offers—more accessible to clinical teachers. We should also find ways of creating new opportunities for exchange and support, documenting the learning that takes place in the workplace, and learning to value the community of which we are a part.

Mentorship

Mentoring, a recognized component of a successful academic career (Farrell et al. 2004), is often used to promote the socialization and development of clinical faculty (Bland et al. 2009; Bligh 1999). It is therefore surprising that mentorship is not more frequently described as a faculty development strategy (Morzinski et al. 1996), for mentors can provide guidance, direction, support or expertise to faculty members on a range of topics, in a variety of settings. Mentors can also help teachers to understand the organizational culture in which they are working and introduce them to invaluable professional networks (Schor et al. 2011; Walker et al. 2002). Teachers often report that finding a mentor—and being mentored—is one of the most critical components to their becoming a better teacher (Steinert 2010b). It behoves us to recognize the value of this important strategy and to help colleagues to identify their needs and actively seek a mentor, knowing that, at times, multiple mentors for diverse purposes can be beneficial. In fact, mentorship can fall into each of the quadrants in fig. 60.1, while simultaneously serving as a compass to identify approaches to personal growth and development.

A proposed curriculum for teaching improvement

Most faculty development programmes address the clinician's role as teacher (Steinert et al. 2006). Common topics include large group lecturing and small group facilitation, clinical supervision (in both hospital and ambulatory settings), feedback, and learner assessment. Some programmes also focus on curriculum design and delivery, educational research and scholarship, or leadership in the educational context. Few programmes focus on personal effectiveness or career development.

The following section outlines a proposed faculty development curriculum for teaching improvement, which can be viewed as a road map for clinical teachers, as they pursue their own development, or by medical educators or faculty developers responsible for offering professional development opportunities. Whenever possible, however, faculty development should be aligned with a competency framework for teachers. Such an alignment can facilitate self-assessment and reflection, careful monitoring of objectives and outcomes, and the development of specific programmes (or activities).

The relevant literature currently offers a number of frameworks that can guide teaching improvement. For example, Srinivasan et al. (2011) describe a competency framework for teaching, based on the Accreditation Council for Graduate Medical Education (ACGME) competencies (Swing 2007), that includes: medical (or content) knowledge; learner-centredness; interpersonal and communication skills; professionalism and role modelling; practice-based reflection and improvement; and systems-based learning. Molenaar et al. (2009) also present a valuable framework of teaching competencies that encompasses three dimensions: six domains of teaching (e.g. development, organization, execution, coaching, assessment, and evaluation); three levels in the organization at which teachers perform (e.g. teaching, coordinating, and educational leadership); and specific competencies that consist of knowledge, attitudes, and skills (e.g. developing an effective teaching module; initiating policies to develop curricular units).

By presenting this three-dimensional framework, and describing specific core teaching competencies using concrete examples, these authors map out a course for teacher development and reflection. In a similar vein, Hesketh et al. (2001) outline a framework for excellence as a clinical educator by defining competence in terms of 12 learning outcomes that include performance of tasks (e.g. teaching large and small groups; assessing learners), approach to tasks (e.g. with an understanding of educational principles and appropriate attitudes), and professionalism as it relates to teaching (e.g. the role of the clinical educator in the organization; personal development). This framework was inspired by Harden and Crosby's (2000) description of teacher roles that include the following: information provider, role model, facilitator, assessor, and planner. Not surprisingly, each framework offers different strengths and limitations as well as a particular lens on teaching. It is, therefore, important to choose a framework that is congruent with individual and institutional values and beliefs and that will help to facilitate personal and organizational growth and development. In another study designed to define competencies for all faculty roles (including that of teacher), Milner et al. (2011) suggest a number of ways to adapt available frameworks to local contexts. In particular, they recommend that medical educators: conduct a broad exploration of the literature, with input from multiple stakeholders; ensure that faculty competencies are congruent with those defined for students and residents, reflecting a developmental approach over time; and aim for measureable competencies.

Irrespective of the model (or framework) chosen, however, the following content areas (outlined in box 60.1) can form the foundation of a faculty development curriculum for clinical teachers that can be pursued in both formal and informal settings. Moreover, although the list of suggested topics is not exhaustive and will need to be tailored to local contexts and needs, it is hoped that it will help clinicians and educators to identify areas for personal and professional development.

Teaching and learning

The broad domain of teaching and learning can be divided into four main areas: educational principles and frameworks; specific core content; methods of teaching and learning; and assessment strategies.

Educational principles and frameworks buttress the work that we do with students and residents and include: competency-based education; work-based learning; situated learning and apprenticeship as a model for teaching and learning; principles of adult learning; and lifelong learning. To the extent that is possible, teachers should understand these key concepts and find an opportunity to reflect upon their application in medical education. The role of the teacher, as described by Harden and Crosby (2000), and teachers' conceptions of teaching (Eley 2006: Peeraer et al. 2011), could also be included in this curricular component. Although teachers' core teaching beliefs undoubtedly determine their behaviour (Masunaga and Hitchcock 2011; Williams and Klamen 2006), medical educators tend to ignore the centrality of these notions in faculty development.

Depending on local contexts and priorities, specific core content should also form part of a faculty development curriculum. For example, if a core competency framework, such as the ACGME competencies (Swing 2007) or the CanMEDS framework (Frank and Danoff 2007), underpins the educational programme for

Box 60.1 A proposed curriculum for teaching improvement

Teaching and Learning
Educational principles and frameworks
For example:

◆ Competency-based education

◆ Work-based learning

◆ Situated learning and apprenticeship

◆ Principles of adult learning and lifelong learning

◆ Teachers' roles and conceptions of teaching

Specific core content
For example:

◆ Core competency frameworks and 'intrinsic competencies'

◆ Interprofessional education and practice

◆ Social responsibility and accountability

◆ Cultural diversity and humility

◆ Patient safety

◆ Hidden curricula

◆ Identity formation

◆ Physician wellbeing and health

Methods of teaching and learning
For example:

◆ Small group learning

◆ Role modelling

◆ Mentorship and coaching

◆ Experiential learning and reflective practice

◆ Work-based learning

◆ Online learning and simulation

Assessment strategies
For example:

◆ Principles of assessment

◆ Methods of assessment

◆ Strategies for effective feedback

◆ Ensuring due process

◆ Overcoming organizational and administrative barriers

Curriculum Design and Implementation
Educational Leadership
Research and Scholarship
Career Developmen

students or residents, teachers will need to be able to define these competencies, relay their importance in the clinical or classroom setting, and teach them in an effective manner (based on best practices reported in the literature). Certain roles or 'intrinsic competencies' (Sherbino et al. 2011), including health advocacy and professionalism, are known to be more challenging for clinicians and may require focused attention. In addition, emerging priorities

in undergraduate and postgraduate education (e.g. interprofessional education and practice; social responsibility and accountability; cultural diversity and humility; patient safety) should be addressed as well. Not only do clinical teachers need to role model effectively, they must also transmit core content and facilitate skill acquisition in a multitude of areas. In addition, they need to address what is often called the hidden curriculum and facilitate identity formation (Monrouxe 2010; Trede 2009) whilst promoting physician wellbeing and health. In fact, focusing on these content areas for individual teachers is a powerful example of how faculty development can promote organizational change through curricular renewal.

Methods of teaching and learning (e.g. small group learning) are commonly addressed in faculty development programmes and will continue to be an important focus. However, the following pedagogical methods, which are often utilized but not explicitly addressed, also need to be emphasized: role modelling; mentorship and coaching; experiential learning and reflective practice; and work-based learning. In addition, the effective use of educational technologies (e.g. online learning and simulation) needs to be incorporated into professional development opportunities.

To elaborate, role modelling is one of the most commonly used—and powerful—methods of teaching and learning. However, teachers usually take this important strategy for granted and rarely take the time to make the implicit learning explicit. Faculty development in this area can help teachers to become aware of the importance of role modelling, to dissect the components of this important teaching and learning strategy, to analyse facilitators and barriers to effectiveness, and to examine how the institutional culture can help to promote role modelling (Cruess et al. 2008). Similarly, although mentorship can clearly influence teaching and learning (Bland et al. 2009; Bligh 1999), clinicians are often ill-equipped to mentor effectively. Faculty development on mentoring can focus on: the role and value of mentoring in career development; the skills and strategies needed to promote mentorship; and the variables that affect this important relationship (e.g. culture, gender, discipline). Daloz's (1986) model, with its emphasis on 'support, challenge, and a vision of the individual's future career', could also be a helpful framework for promoting mentorship. Coaching, another important teaching and learning strategy, is closely related to mentorship though it does not presuppose an ongoing relationship with the learner and is often more limited to the acquisition of specific knowledge or skills. As a result, clinicians can benefit from learning specific coaching techniques that include: support, encouragement and challenge; reframing, reflection and facilitation; effective questioning; and the mindful exploration of values and beliefs (Claridge and Lewis 2005).

Although the role of experiential learning and reflective practice is frequently acknowledged by clinical teachers, they are often not aware of how to promote these essential ingredients of learning. Kolb and Fry (1975) offer a description of the learning cycle that includes four distinct phases: the ability to experience diverse situations (in both the classroom and the clinical setting); the opportunity to observe and reflect on what is being learned (which may occur individually or with peers); the development of one's own theory and understanding of the world; and the need to experiment with new ways of being in order for learning to occur. Teachers' understanding of this cycle can facilitate teaching *and* learning and help to ensure that different learning styles are respected and nurtured. Learning to promote reflective practice can also include an understanding of what we mean by reflection (Lachman and Pawlina 2006; Schön 1983), finding ways to trigger self-assessment and critical analysis, and making an implicit process more explicit.

Experiential learning and reflective practice are also closely tied to work-based learning, which has been defined as learning *for* work, learning *at* work, and learning *from* work (Swanwick 2008). It is therefore important for teachers to view everyday experiences as learning experiences, to reflect with students and residents on learning that has occurred in the work environment (Boud and Middleton 2003), and to make the 'invisible' more visible.

Assessment strategies form another essential component of a faculty development curriculum for clinical teachers. It has often been said that assessment drives learning. Assessment is also a critical step in ensuring the competence of students and residents as they prepare to enter practice. Teachers often lament that they are ill-prepared to assess students and residents in a fair, reliable, and valid manner. At the same time, learners often observe that feedback is lacking and that end-of-rotation assessments are a surprise. Faculty development in this area can include a focus on underlying principles of assessment, common (and novel) methods of assessment, strategies for giving effective feedback (formative assessment), and ways of ensuring due process. Irrespective of the context in which they are working, teachers must be able to identify, document, communicate, and remediate learners' weaknesses. Importantly, faculty development must also address the organizational and administrative barriers that can impede effective assessment, and all learners must be actively engaged in the process. A more recent trend towards competency-based assessment (Holmboe et al. 2010; 2011) also foreshadows the need for innovative faculty development programming in this area.

The content areas previously described can form the basis of a faculty development curriculum for teaching improvement. However, many clinical teachers also become involved in educational pursuits that include curriculum design and implementation, educational leadership, and research and scholarship. These content areas, as well as personal and career development, should (whenever possible) be included in a faculty development initiative for clinical teachers.

Curriculum design and implementation

Although many clinicians are involved primarily in the teaching of students and residents, some faculty members design and deliver educational courses or curricula. For this group of clinicians, a focus on principles of curriculum design and implementation would be pertinent and could highlight: the instructional design cycle, which includes a description of learning outcomes; the matching of objectives to educational content and pedagogical methods; the assessment of learners; and the evaluation of educational programmes. This component can also aim to enhance teachers' abilities to: perform literature reviews and environmental scans; facilitate stakeholder engagement; incorporate theories of innovation (Greenhalgh et al. 2004; Rogers 1995); and understand principles of programme evaluation (Musick 2006; Wholey et al. 2004). Whenever possible, we should try to empower our teachers to become agents of educational change (Hatem et al. 2011), prepared to lead curricular innovation and renewal in their own departments and specialties.

Educational leadership

Given the need for curricular change and the complexity of educational programmes in medicine, leadership training should be a key component of faculty development initiatives for clinical teachers. Although little has been written about the role of clinical leaders in the educational context, a survey designed to identify the educational and leadership skills required of programme directors with major educational and leadership responsibilities (Bordage et al. 2000) indicated the importance of nine key skill areas: oral communication; interpersonal abilities; clinical competence; educational goal-definition; educational design; problem-solving and decision-making; team building; written communication; and budgeting and financial management. Spencer and Jordan (2001) also highlighted the fact that educational change requires leadership and that we need to equip our colleagues to implement change. Possible topic areas could include personal and interpersonal effectiveness; leadership and change management; negotiation and conflict management; team building; and organizational change and development. Leadership training would also help clinical teachers to respond to the complexity and shifting priorities of healthcare systems, and in this way, achieve multiple objectives. Irrespective of the context, we need to develop leaders who will identify opportunities for change, respond effectively to emerging needs, and be prepared to take action.

Research and scholarship

Although research capacity building has long been an essential component of faculty development in its broadest sense (Bland and Ruffin 1992; Henry 1997), the need to include research and scholarship in a faculty development curriculum for teaching improvement is becoming increasingly important as clinical teachers and medical educators need to produce an evidence base for what they do. A growing awareness of the notion of scholarship as defined by Boyer (1990), which includes the scholarship of discovery, integration, application, and teaching, has also prompted the need for professional development in this area. As the field evolves, faculty development should focus on definitions of scholarship, ways of promoting scholarship among colleagues and peers, methods of disseminating scholarly work, and 'moving from innovation to scholarship' (Steinert 2011). A more traditional focus on research methods, grantsmanship and writing for publication would also be beneficial (Morzinski and Simpson 2003; Pololi et al. 2004).

Career development

A recent study on faculty members' participation in faculty development (Steinert et al. 2009) indicated that study participants believed that faculty development referred to their general development as faculty members. That is, they saw faculty development as the *development* of themselves as faculty members, including personal and career development, and not merely the enhancement of specific competencies related to teaching, research, or administration. Interestingly, however, the literature does not report many faculty development programmes focusing on career development, despite the fact that faculty members welcome the opportunity to identify career goals and values, develop collaborative relationships, and acquire skills to further their career (Miedzinski et al. 2001; Pololi et al. 2002). Given that faculty members are our most important asset (Whitcomb 2003), an investment in career development through faculty development would represent a critical step forward. Programmes in this area could focus on academic identity formation, career planning (including an overview of different career paths), and the value of mentorship (Steinert 2012). In fact, mentorship can enhance recruitment, promote retention, and create an environment that enriches the academic role (Thorndyke et al. 2006; Wingard et al. 2004), and as such, it should be viewed as a strategy to develop faculty. Time management, prevention of burnout, and promotion of wellbeing should also be considered as vital areas for professional development (Steinert 2011).

A theoretical framework for faculty development

Despite an emphasis on educational know-how and practice, theory is noticeably absent from the faculty development literature (Graffam et al. 2008; Steinert 2010b). However, a number of educational theories could be applied to faculty development and the development of clinical teachers (Bandura 1977; Bandura 1997; Steffe and Gale 1995). In our experience, situated learning (Brown et al. 1989) appears to be one of the most useful overarching frameworks for faculty development, although principles of adult learning (Knowles 1980) and experiential learning (Kolb and Fry 1975) are also pertinent, especially in the design and delivery of instructional programmes. Models of identity formation (Côté and Levine 2002) are also relevant. Although few studies have explored clinicians' lived experiences (Higgs and McAllister 2007) and the development of their identities as teachers (Starr et al. 2003), the process of becoming a teacher is a critical aspect of faculty development.

Situated learning is based upon the notion that knowledge is contextually situated and fundamentally influenced by the activity, context, and culture in which it is used (Brown et al. 1989). This view of knowledge, as situated in authentic contexts, provides a useful framework by which to understand how clinical teachers develop. This is because it brings together the cognitive base and experiential learning that is needed to facilitate the acquisition of new behaviours. Its component parts, including cognitive apprenticeship (which consists of modelling, scaffolding, fading, and coaching), collaborative learning, reflection and practice (McLellan 1996), also reinforce the value of embedding learning in authentic activities.

Closely tied to the notion of situated learning is the concept of legitimate peripheral participation (Lave and Wenger 1991). This social practice combines experiential learning and apprenticeship into a single theoretical perspective and describes the process by which a novice becomes an expert. From this perspective, teachers build new knowledge and understanding through gradual participation in the community of which they are becoming a part. As learners, they begin at the edge—or periphery—of the community, where, because of their status as learners, they have what is called 'legitimate peripheral participation'. With time, they become more involved with their colleagues, and as they participate more in the community's work, they move from the periphery to the centre. They also take on increasing responsibility for the work of the community, be it patient care, teaching, or research. According to Wenger (1998), social participation within the community is the key to informal learning and helps to create identity and meaning. Social participation within the community also complements, and can substitute for, formal learning.

An evidence-based approach to faculty development

In 2006, as part of the BEME (Best Evidence in Medical Education) Collaboration, an international group of medical educators systematically reviewed the faculty development literature to ascertain the impact of formal initiatives on teaching improvement (Steinert et al. 2006). This review was based on 53 reports that targeted practising clinicians and included workshops, seminar series, short courses, longitudinal programmes, and other interventions such as peer coaching, augmented feedback, and site visits. The results of this review indicated overall satisfaction with faculty development programmes, changes in attitudes towards teaching and faculty development, gains in knowledge and skills, and limited changes in organizational practice and student learning.

To elaborate, participants found diverse programmes to be useful, acceptable, and relevant to their objectives. Teachers also reported positive changes in attitudes toward faculty development *and* teaching as a result of their involvement in these activities, and they cited an increased awareness of personal strengths and limitations, motivation and enthusiasm for teaching and learning, self-confidence as a teacher, and a sense of belonging to a community (of like-minded individuals). In addition, they noted a greater knowledge of educational principles and strategies as well as gains in teaching skills and an appreciation of the benefits of professional development.

The BEME review also highlighted specific features that contribute to the effectiveness of formal faculty development activities. These key features included: the role of experiential learning and the importance of applying what had been learned; the provision of feedback; effective peer relationships, which included the value of role modelling, exchange of information, and collegial support; well-designed interventions that followed principles of teaching and learning; and the use of multiple instructional methods to achieve intended objectives. Awareness of these components can help teachers (to choose effective programmes) and medical educators and faculty developers (in the design and delivery of their programmes).

Despite these findings, however, there continues to be a paucity of research demonstrating the effectiveness of many faculty development activities (Hueppchen et al. 2011), and we must continue to examine the benefits of both formal and informal faculty development programmes on the individual and the organization. Comprehensive faculty development programmes are resource intensive, especially as they often require time away from clinical work, financial support, and a variety of educational tools and methodologies. As a result, we should strive to tease apart the ingredients that work (e.g. experiential learning; interaction with colleagues; feedback) and initiate more process-oriented studies that compare different faculty development strategies and the maintenance of change over time. Stes et al. (2010) suggest that the duration and nature of instructional development in higher education can positively influence behavioural outcomes. Moving forward, we should carefully consider studies outside of the field of medicine that can inform the development of clinical teachers. For example, Bell and Gilbert (1994, p. 493) analysed the learning process of science teachers and found that 'teacher development can be viewed as teacher *learning*, rather than as others getting teachers to change'. This is clearly an important lesson for all faculty members (Webster-Wright 2009). Bell and Gilbert (1994) also highlighted the iterative nature of faculty learning which they found could be divided into three domains: personal, social, and professional development. To date, medicine has primarily focused on the latter.

Faculty development and organizational change

Although medical educators agree that faculty development should focus on both the individual *and* the organization (Wilkerson and Irby, 1998), most reports focus on programmes targeting individual change and development. However, as stated previously, faculty development can serve as a useful instrument in the promotion of organizational change. For example, at the organizational level, faculty development initiatives can help to: reward and recognize clinical teachers for their contributions to the educational mission; encourage mentorship and coaching for all teachers; value and promote educational innovation and scholarship (including the scholarship of teaching); and recognize teaching excellence and educational scholarship in promotion criteria.

Changes in healthcare delivery and education have, in many ways, increased the expectations of clinical teachers. We must therefore find ways to ensure that the expectations of clinical teachers are realistic and that the rewards are appropriate and sufficient. Many clinical teachers will agree that much of their work arises from a spirit of volunteerism and wanting to contribute to the development of future generations of healthcare professionals (Steinert 2011). We need to ensure that this spirit of volunteerism can be sustained. Faculty developers should also work in tandem with other educational units to help clarify expectations of clinical teachers, protect time for teaching, develop institutional policies that promote the academic mission, and provide appropriate support for innovation and excellence. The latter might include administrative assistance, the timely provision of information (e.g. online educational resources), or new professional development opportunities. Clinical teachers face a number of environmental and systemic pressures (e.g. competing priorities and the challenge of teaching effectively in a fast-paced environment); addressing these issues in a thoughtful manner highlights the role that faculty development can play in promoting change at an organizational level. Faculty development initiatives can also help to facilitate the formative and summative evaluation of clinical teachers and the development of remedial programmes for clinical teachers who need to improve their professional and teaching behaviours. As medical educators we often tend to focus on the individual teacher and overlook the importance of organizational support and development (Steinert et al. 2007). Both foci are important.

Developing as a teacher

As described in this chapter, both formal *and* informal approaches can facilitate the clinical teacher's development (fig. 60.2). Irrespective of the approach chosen, however, it is important to identify personal needs, to determine preferred method(s) of learning, and to choose a programme (or activity) that incorporates effective teaching and learning strategies and aligns with personal goals and objectives. Finding a mentor and a community of teachers that supports the teacher's vision and goals can also be helpful.

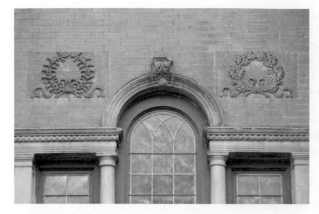

Figure 60.2 Windows of opportunity—Lady Meredith House, which houses the Centre for Medical Education and the Faculty Development Office at McGill University.
Reproduced with permission from Owen Egan.

As stated earlier, the literature describes a number of frameworks for teaching attributes and competencies (Molenaar et al. 2009; Srinivasan et al. 2011). Whenever feasible, clinical teachers should assess their strengths and possible weaknesses and consider different modalities to improve their teaching abilities. An assessment of preferred methods of learning is also indicated. Some of us prefer to learn on our own; others prefer to learn with colleagues, in a formal or informal setting. Choosing a strategy for learning is as important as selecting the topic for discussion. When participating in a more formal (or structured) programme (or activity), we should ensure that it is relevant to personally identified needs, endorses principles of adult learning, and incorporates experiential learning and reflective practice. Faculty development should also facilitate interacting with colleagues and networking (Starr et al. 2003). Identifying a mentor can be equally helpful. Clinical teachers value their mentors' support, ability to challenge personal assumptions, and assistance in framing a vision for the future (Steinert 2010b). When possible, we should consider the value of finding someone who can help to fulfill this role as we try to improve as teachers. Finding a community of teachers can also help us to refine our vision, develop our skills, and find ways to develop further. It has often been said that teaching is a 'team sport'. Achieving educational excellence cannot be accomplished in a social vacuum, and we should try to find—and value—a community of like-minded colleagues and peers (Steinert 2010d).

Two recent studies tried to examine the reasons why faculty members do—and do not—participate in formal (structured) faculty development activities (Steinert et al. 2009; 2010). Teachers' reasons for participating in organized faculty development activities included the observations that: faculty development was seen as enabling personal and professional growth; learning and self-improvement were valued at a personal level; workshop topics were viewed as relevant to the teachers' needs; and networking with colleagues was greatly appreciated. It was also reported that initial positive experiences promote ongoing development and that teachers' expectations of how the experience will be of benefit is a critical determinant. Barriers to participation included: the clinical reality and workload (which usually does not permit protected time for teaching improvement); a perceived lack of direction from, and connection to, the school of medicine; a perceived lack of recognition and financial reward for teaching; and the central location of faculty development and other logistical issues. Awareness of these motivators and perceived barriers can help to identify pathways for personal and organizational development.

This chapter has described core definitions and guiding principles, common approaches, and a possible curriculum for faculty development for teaching improvement (grounded in a theoretical framework for professional development); it has also outlined what is known about effectiveness. In so doing, we have noted the value of faculty development in promoting academic excellence and institutional vitality, the need to broaden our perspective from *formal* professional development offerings to the promotion of *informal* learning in authentic contexts, and the role of experiential learning and reflective practice in individual and group settings. We have also observed that becoming an effective teacher is a developmental process that requires individual and institutional commitment and that individuals can benefit from being part of a vibrant community of practice. What is more difficult to describe is the role of faculty development in cultivating passion and compassion in teaching and learning and nurturing the more elusive attributes of curiosity, creativity, and commitment (in ourselves and in our colleagues). One suggested avenue for future inquiry is the exploration of identity formation among clinical teachers; another is the creation and preservation of communities of practice in promoting professional growth and development. Interestingly, these two avenues of future study might also help to inform how we can encourage and support curiosity, creativity, and commitment. Graffam et al. (2008, pp. 768–74) suggest that effective teaching leads to the empowerment of the learner. In a similar vein, deliberate and strategic faculty development can empower clinical teachers to excel at what they do; and as we know, the desire to excel is a fundamental incentive for clinicians and the institutions in which they work.

Conclusions

◆ Becoming an effective teacher is a developmental process that requires individual and institutional commitment and can benefit from a vibrant community of practice.

◆ Faculty development is critical in promoting academic excellence and institutional vitality.

◆ We need to broaden our perspective of faculty development to include both *formal* professional development activities as well as *informal* learning in authentic contexts that build on the role of experiential learning and reflective practice in individual and group settings.

◆ Deliberate and strategic faculty development can enable clinicians to excel in their roles as teachers.

References

Bandura, A. (1977) *Social Learning Theory.* New Jersey: Prentice Hall

Bandura, A. (1997) *Self-Efficacy: The Exercise of Control.* New York: W.H. Freeman

Barab, S.A., Barnett, M., and Squire, K. (2002) Developing an empirical account of a community of practice: characterizing the essential tensions. *J Learning Sci.* 11: 489–542

Bell, B. and Gilbert, J. (1994) Teacher development as professional, personal, and social development. *Teach Teach Educ.* 10: 483–497

Bland, C.J., Schmitz, C.C., Stritter, F.T, Henry, R.C, and Aluise, J.J. (1990) *Successful Faculty in Academic Medicine: Essential Skills and How to Acquire Them.* New York: Springer Publishing

Bland, C., Taylor, A.L., Shollen, S.L., Weber-Main, A.M., and Mulcahy, P.A. (2009) *Faculty Success Through Mentoring.* New York: Rowman and Littlefield Publishers

Bland, C.J. and Ruffin, M.T. (1992) Characteristics of a productive research environment: literature review. *Acad Med.* 67: 385–397

Bligh, J. (1999) Mentoring: an invisible support network. *Acad Med.* 33: 2–3

Bligh, J. (2005) Faculty development. *Med Educ.* 39: 120–121

Bordage, G., Foley, R., and Goldyn, S. (2000) Skills and attributes of directors of educational programmes. *Med Educ.* 34: 206–210

Boud, D. and Middleton, H. (2003) Learning from others at work: communities of practice and informal learning. *J Workplace Learn.* 15: 194–202

Boyer, E.L. (1990) *Scholarship Reconsidered: Priorities of the Professoriate.* Princeton: Princeton University Press

Brown, J.S., Collins, A., and Duguid, S. (1989) Situated cognition and the culture of learning. *Educ Res.* 18: 32–42

Centra, J. (1978) Types of faculty development programs. *J Higher Educ.* 49: 151–162

Claridge, M.T. and Lewis, T. (2005) *Coaching for Effective Learning.* Abingdon: Radcliffe Publishing

Côté, J.E. and Levine, C.G. (2002) *Identity Formation, Agency, and Culture.* London: Psychology Press

Cruess, S.R., Cruess, R.L., and Steinert, Y. (2008) Role modelling—making the most of a powerful teaching strategy. *BMJ.* 336: 718–721

Daloz, L.A. (1986) *Effective Teaching and Mentoring.* San Francisco: Jossey-Bass

Eitel, F., Kanz, K.G., and Tesche, A. (2000) Training and certification of teachers and trainers: the professionalization of medical education. *Med Teach.* 22: 517–526

Eley, M.G. (2006) Teachers' conceptions of teaching, and the making of specific decisions in planning to teach. *Higher Educ.* 51: 191–214

Farrell, S.E., Digioia, N.M., Broderick, K.B., and Coates, W.C. (2004) Mentoring for clinician-educators. *Acad Emerg Med.* 11: 1346–1350

Flynn, S.P., Bedinghaus, J., Snyder, C., and Hekelman, F. (1994) Peer coaching in clinical teaching: a case report. *Fam Med.* 26: 569–570

Frank, J.R. and Danoff, D. (2007) The CanMEDS initiative: implementing an outcomes-based framework of physician competencies. *Med Teach.* 29: 642–647

Graffam, B., Bowers, L., and Keene, K.N. (2008) Using observations of clinicians' teaching practices to build a model of clinical instruction. *Acad Med.* 83: 768–774

Greenhalgh, T., Robert, G., MacFarlane, F., Bate, P., and Kyriakidou, O. (2004) Diffusion of innovations in service organizations: systematic review and recommendations. *The Milbank Q.* 82: 581–629

Gruppen, L.D, Simpson, D., Searle, N.S, Robins, L., Irby, D.M., and Mullan, P.B. (2006) Educational fellowship programs: common themes and overarching issues. *Acad Med.* 81: 990–994

Hafferty, F.W. (1998) Beyond curriculum reform: confronting medicine's hidden curriculum. *Acad Med.* 73: 403–407

Harden, R.M. and Crosby, J. (2000) AMEE Education Guide No. 20: The good teacher is more than a lecturer: the twelve roles of the teacher. *Med Teach.* 22: 334–347

Hatem, C.J., Searle, N.S., Gunderman, R., Krane, N.K., Perkowski, L., Schutze G.E., and Steinert, Y. (2011) The educational attributes and responsibilities of effective medical educators. *Acad Med.* 86: 474–480

Henry, R. (1997) Developing research skills for medical school faculty. *Fam Med.* 29: 258–261

Hesketh, E.A., Bagnall, G., Buckley, E.G.Friedman, M., Goodall, E., Harden, R.M., et al. (2001) A framework for developing excellence as a clinical educator. *Med Educ.* 35: 555–564

Higgs, J. and McAllister, L. (2007) Educating clinical educators: using a model of the experience of being a clinical educator. *Med Teach.* 29: e51–e57

Holmboe, E.S., Sherbino, J., Long, D.M., Swing, S.R., and Frank, J.R. (2010) The role of assessment in competency-based medical education. *Med Teach.* 32: 676–682

Holmboe, E.S., Ward, D.S., Reznick, R.K., Katsufrakis, P.J., Leslie, K.M., Patel, V.L., et al. (2011) Faculty development in assessment: the missing link in competency-based medical education. *Acad Med.* 86: 460–467

Hueppchen, N., Dalrymple, J.L., Hammoud, M.M., et al. (2011) To the point: Medical education reviews—ongoing call for faculty development. *Am J Obstet Gynecol.* 205: 171–176

Knowles, M.S. (1980) *The Modern Practice of Adult Education: From Pedagogy to Andragogy.* New York: Cambridge Books

Kolb, D. and Fry, R. (1975) Towards an applied theory of experiential learning. In C.L. Cooper (ed.) *Theories of Group Processes* (pp. 33–57). Chichester: John Wiley & Sons Ltd,

Lachman, N. and Pawlina, W. (2006) Integrating professionalism in early medical education: the theory and application of reflective practice in the anatomy curriculum. *Clin Anat.* 19: 456–460

Lave, J. and Wenger, E. (1991) *Situated Learning: Legitimate Peripheral Participation.* New York: Cambridge University Press

Lochner, L. and Gijselaers, W.H. (2011) Improving lecture skills: a time-efficient 10-step pedagogical consultation method for medical teachers in healthcare professions. *Med Teach.* 33: 131–136

Masunaga, H. and Hitchcock, M.A. (2011) Aligning teaching practices with an understanding of quality teaching: a faculty development agenda. *Med Teach.* 33: 124–130

McLean, M., Cilliers, F., and Van Wyk, J.M. (2008) Faculty development: yesterday, today and tomorrow. *Med Teach.* 30: 555–584

McLellan, H. (1996) *Situated Learning Perspectives.* New Jersey: Educational Technology Publications

McLeod, P.J. and Steinert, Y. (2009) Peer coaching as an approach to faculty development. *Med Teach.* 31: 1043–1044

Milner, R.J., Gusic, M.E., and Thorndyke, L.E. (2011) Perspective: toward a competency framework for faculty. *Acad Med.* 86: 1204–1210

Miedzinski, L.J., Davis, P., Al-Shurafa, H., and Morrison, J.C. (2001) A Canadian faculty of medicine and dentistry's survey of career development needs. *Med Educ.* 35: 890–900

Molenaar, W.M., Zanting, A., van Beukelen, P., de Grave, W., Baane, J.A., Bustraan, J.A., et al. (2009) A framework of teaching competencies across the medical education continuum. *Med Teach.* 31: 390–396

Monrouxe, L.V. (2010) Identity, identification, and medical education: why should we care? *Med Educ.* 44: 40–49

Morzinski, J.A., Diehr, S., Bower, D.J., and Simpson, D.E. (1996) A descriptive, cross-sectional study of formal mentoring for faculty. *Fam Med.* 28: 434–438

Morzinski, J.A. and Simpson, D.E. (2003) Outcomes of a comprehensive faculty development program for local, full-time faculty. *Fam Med.* 35: 434–439

Musick, D.W. (2006) A conceptual model for program evaluation in graduate medical education. *Acad Med.* 81: 759–765

Peeraer, G., Donche, V., De Winter B.Y., Muijtjens, A.M., Remmen, R., Van Petegam, P., et al. (2011) Teaching conceptions and approaches to teaching of medical school faculty: the difference between how medical school teachers think about teaching and how they say that they do teach. *Med Teach.* 33: e382–e387

Pololi, L.H., Knight, S.M., Dennis, K., and Frankel, R.M. (2002) Helping medical school faculty realize their dreams: an innovative, collaborative mentoring program. *Acad Med.* 77: 377–384

Pololi, L., Knight, S., and Dunn, K. (2004) Facilitating scholarly writing in academic medicine. *J Gen Intern Med.* 19: 64–68

Purcell, N. and Lloyd-Jones, G. (2003) Standards for medical educators. *Med Educ.* 37: 149–154

Rademacher, R., Simpson, D., and Marcdante, K. (2010) Critical incidents as a technique for teaching professionalism. *Med Teach.* 32: 244–249

Rogers, E.M. (1995) *Diffusion of Innovations.* New York: Simon and Schuster

Schofield, S.J., Bradley, S., Macrae, C., Nathwani, D., and Dent, J. (2010) How we encourage faculty development. *Med Teach.* 32: 883–886

Schön, D. (1983) *The Reflective Practitioner: How Professionals Think in Action.* New York: Basic Books

Schor, N.F., Guillet, R., and McAnarney, E.R. (2011) Anticipatory guidance as a principle of faculty development: managing transition and change. *Acad Med.* 86: 1235–1240

Sheets, K.J. and Schwenk, T.L. (1990) Faculty development for family medicine educators: an agenda for future activities. *Teach Learn Med.* 2: 141–148

Sherbino, J., Frank, J.R., Flynn, L., and Snell, L. (2011) 'Intrinsic Roles' rather than 'armour': renaming the 'non-medical expert roles' of the CanMEDS framework to match their intent. *Adv Health Sci Educ.* 16: 695–697

Skeff, K.M., Stratos, G.A., and Mount, J.F.S. (2007) Faculty development in medicine: a field in evolution. *Teach Teach Educ.* 23: 280–285

Spencer, J. and Jordan, R. (2001) Educational outcome and leadership to meet the needs of modern health care. *Qual Health Care.* 10: ii38–ii45

Srinivasan, M., Li, S.T., Meyers, F.J. Pratt, D.D., Collins, J.B., Braddock, C., et al. (2011) 'Teaching as a competency': competencies for medical educators. *Acad Med.* 86: 1211–1220

Starr, S., Ferguson, W.J., Haley, H.L., and Quirk, M. (2003) Community preceptors' views of their identities as teachers. *Acad Med.* 78: 820–825

Steffe, L. and Gale, J. (eds) (1995) *Constructivism in Education.* New Jersey: Lawrence Erlbaum

Steinert, Y. (2000) Faculty development in the new millennium: key challenges and future directions. *Med Teach.* 22: 44–50

Steinert, Y. (2009) Staff development. In J. Dent and R. Harden (eds) (2009) *A Practical Guide for Medical Teachers* (pp. 391–397). Edinburgh: Elsevier Churchill Livingstone

Steinert, Y. (2010a) Becoming a better teacher: from intuition to intent. In J. Ende (ed.) *Theory and Practice of Teaching Medicine* (pp. 73–93). Philadelphia: American College of Physicians

Steinert, Y. (2010b) Developing medical educators: a journey not a destination. In T. Swanwick (ed.) *Understanding Medical Education: Evidence, Theory and Practice* (pp. 403–418). Edinburgh: Association for the Study of Medical Education

Steinert, Y. (2010c) Faculty development: from workshops to communities of practice. *Med Teach.* 32: 425–428

Steinert, Y. (2010d) Making it all happen: faculty development for busy teachers. In P. Cantillon and D. Wood (eds) *ABC of Learning and Teaching in Medicine* (pp. 73–77). London: BMJ Publishing Group

Steinert, Y. (2011) Commentary: Faculty development: the road less traveled. *Acad Med.* 86: 409–411

Steinert, Y. (2012) Perspectives on faculty development: Aiming for 6/6 by 2020. *Perspectives on Med Educ.* [Online] 10 Feb.

Steinert, Y., Cruess, R.L., Cruess, S.R., Boudreau, J.D., and Fuks, A. (2007) Faculty development as an instrument of change: a case study on teaching professionalism. *Acad Med.* 82: 1057–1064

Steinert, Y., Macdonald, M., Boillat, M., Elizov, M., Meterissian, S., Razack, S., et al. (2010) Faculty development: if you build it, they will come. *Med Educ.* 44: 900–907

Steinert, Y. and McLeod P. (2006) From novice to informed educator: the Teaching Scholars Program for Educators in the Health Sciences. *Acad Med.* 81: 969–974

Steinert, Y., McLeod, P.J., Boillat, M., Meterissian, S., Elizov, M., and Macdonald, M.E. (2009) Faculty development: a 'Field of Dreams'? *Med Educ.* 43: 42–49

Steinert, Y., Mann, K., Centeno, A., Dolmans, D., Spencer, J., Gelula, M., and Prideaux, D. (2006) A systematic review of faculty development initiatives designed to improve teaching effectiveness in medical education: BEME Guide No. 8. *Med Teach.* 28: 497–526

Stes, A., Min-Leliveld, M., Gijbels, D., and Van Petegam, P. (2010) The impact of instructional development in higher education: the state-of-the-art of the research. *Educ Res Rev.* 5: 25–49

Swanwick, T. (2008) See one, do one, then what? Faculty development in postgraduate medical education. *Postgrad Med J.* 84: 339–343

Swing, S.R. (2007) The ACGME outcome project: retrospective and prospective. *Med Teach.* 29: 648–654

Tekian, A. and Harris, I. (2012) Preparing health professions education leaders worldwide: a description of masters-level programs. *Med Teach.* 34: 52–58

Trede, F.(2009) Becoming professional in the 21st century. *J Emerg Prim Health Care.* 7: 1–5

Thorndyke, L.E., Gusic, M.E., George, J.H., Quillen, D.A., and Milner, R.J. (2006) Empowering junior faculty: Penn State's faculty development and mentoring program. *Acad Med.* 81: 668–673

Walker, W.O., Kelly, P.C., and Hume, R.F. (2002) Mentoring for the new millennium. *Medical Education Online* [Online] 7, 15. http://www.med-ed-online.org Accessed 18 March 2013

Webster-Wright, A. (2009) Reframing professional development through understanding authentic professional learning. *Rev Educ Res.* 79: 702–739

Wenger, E. (1998) *Communities of Practice: Learning, Meaning and Identity.* New York: Cambridge University Press

Whitcomb, M.E.(2003) The medical school's faculty is its most important asset. *Acad Med.* 78: 117–118

Wholey, J.S., Hatry, H.P., and Newcomer, K.E. (2004) *Handbook of Practical Program Evaluation.* New York: John Wiley & Sons Inc

Wilkerson, L. and Irby, D.M. (1998) Strategies for improving teaching practices: a comprehensive approach to faculty development. *Acad Med.* 73: 387–396

Williams, R.G. and Klamen, D.L. (2006) See one, do one, teach one—exploring the core teaching beliefs of medical school faculty. *Med Teach.* 28: 418–424

Wingard, D.L., Garman, K.A., and Reznik V. (2004) Facilitating faculty success: outcomes and cost benefit of the UCSD National Center of Leadership in Academic Medicine. *Acad Med.* 79: S9–S11

CHAPTER 61

Educational leadership

Judy McKimm, Phil Cotton,
Anne Garden, and Gillian Needham

A medical school is a vibrant place. Such a powerhouse
of intellect and achievement needs a firm hand inside the
supple glove of deanship if ideas are to be converted into
opportunities and students are to become the doctors the
country needs.

Brian Livesley

Introduction

Medical education leaders and managers operate in a wide range of
contexts and cultures, taking on roles at varying levels of responsibility and accountability and working across and between professions and organizations. When we think of leadership, it is often at
the level of the Senior Manager, Dean, Director, Principal, or Vice
Chancellor, whereas in reality, leadership is found at all levels of
an organization. Leadership is widely dispersed, and power is diffused or shared. The range of educational leadership activities is
vast, including: leading a project, team or group to achieve a task;
programme management; curriculum development; departmental or organizational management; leading a research or publication group. And for many medical education leaders, leading and
managing the classroom (learners, activities, assessments) is a large
part of their work, often carried out as an activity that does not
involve peers. Bush (2003) terms this type of leadership 'instructional leadership'. Bolden's (2011) and others' research into distributed (or shared) leadership suggests that this is a dominant form
of leadership in public sector organizations, notably education and
healthcare sectors, the value of which lies in dispersed leadership
in which power and responsibility are shared (Kouzes and Posner
2002). Research has shifted from a scrutiny of 'who' is leading
(where power is invested in individuals who possess certain skills
or personal qualities), to 'how' they lead—the process of leadership within a social system. Uhl-Bien (2006, p. 688) for example,
describes leadership as 'a social influence process through which
emergent coordination (i.e. evolving social order) and change (i.e.
new values, attitudes, approaches, behaviours, ideologies, etc.) are
constructed and produced'.

To focus on only the most senior leaders in institutions provides a limited view of the organization and process of change.

Leadership qualities achieve nothing without a task, social interaction and engagement. A tension exists between the trait and
competency approaches to leadership, which gives rise to a one-
size-fits-all style of leadership development and the situational and
contingency approaches which require reactivity to individuals and
groups in the organization, respectively. We will now explore these
approaches.

Leading and managing change

Medical and healthcare education is a rapidly changing and complex environment, in which education leaders and managers are
required to respond to demands from multiple stakeholders and
organizations (McKimm and Swanwick 2010). As Fullan (2005,
2007) suggests, one of the main tasks of a leader is to manage
change, whether this is in response to external demands (such as a
new e-learning policy directive or reduced student numbers) or to
internal shifts (such as a member of staff leaving the organization).
Change has traditionally been conceptualized along linear models,
as in Lewin's (1951) 'freeze–unfreeze–refreeze' model in which the
leader's task is to move from the existing state to a desired state.
In the force field model Lewin (1951) suggests that while we often
look at how to drive change we should not forget to consider
removing resisting factors. He argues that removal of resisting factors is easier than adding further driving factors in effective change.
Other models such as Kotter's (1995) suggest that leaders need to
pay attention to eight interlinked steps if change is to be successful.
Thus leaders must

◆ establish a sense of urgency

◆ form a powerful guiding coalition

◆ create a vision

- communicate the vision
- empower others to act on the vision
- plan for and create short-term wins
- consolidate improvements and produce still more change
- institutionalize (embed) new approaches in the organizational culture.

It has been argued that effective change management involves identifying colleagues who are in a position to enable that change (Baulcomb 2003; Beerel 2009), but it is equally as important to ensure that leaders have a firm knowledge base in the area they are leading—to maintain credibility (Ledlow and Coppola 2011). People resist change for many reasons, such as parochial self-interest; misunderstanding; low tolerance of change; and different assessments of the situation (Kotter and Schlesinger 2008). It is therefore essential that change leaders maintain the integrity of their vision which may be more important than heroism (Iles 2011) or trying to reach compromise between competing factions.

Often people feel powerless within organizations. The transformational leader motivates others by empowering them to take forward change. Power arises from different sources—the wise leader understands this and is comfortable with the power that others bestow on them. French and Raven (1959) define the main sources of power as

- coercive power (the belief of followers that leaders can impose sanctions or punishment)
- reward power (the leader can give valued reward on compliance with instructions)
- legitimate power (the leader has the formal authority to control and give instructions)
- expert power (the leader has superior knowledge) and
- referent power (the leader is a desirable role model, with whom followers will identify and want to follow).

In contemporary society, leaders need to be comfortable with managing change and be confident to work within complex systems (Fraser and Greenhalgh 2001), using complex adaptive leadership approaches (Heifetz and Linsky 2004). In these models, the leader's task is to enable emergent change, ensuring that the organization or activity is sufficiently stimulated towards change without slipping into chaos. From this postmodern perspective, change cannot be managed and planned for, as change seems to be the only constant (Carr et al. 1996) and the leader will not know exactly what will emerge, only that something will, and change will happen (Fullan 2005).

Different writers have suggested that the multiple perspectives on change and the focus on complexity reflect post-modernity (Harvey 1988), the network society (Castells 1990), and late capitalism (Jameson 1991). Without doubt, however we frame the world in which educational leaders operate, the most effective leaders are those who can deftly juggle multiple tasks at different levels and who have an understanding of the prevailing international, national, organizational, and professional policies and strategies that impact on their work. They also need an understanding of how teams function, how to manage a project, and how to manage themselves appropriately in difficult situations. This multilevel understanding is summed up by Bolman and Gallos (2011, p. 11)

when they describe successful, academic leaders who 'establish campus arrangements and reporting relationships that offer clarity and facilitate work. Such leaders create 'caring and productive campus environments that channel talent and encourage cooperation' Bolman and Gallos (2011, p. 11). They 'respect differences, manage them productively, and respond ethically and responsibly to the needs of multiple constituencies' Bolman and Gallos (2011, p. 11).

Before we go on to discuss this in more depth, it is important to distinguish between what is meant by the terms 'leadership' and 'management'.

Leadership and management

In their study of medical school deans, Rich et al. (2008) describe the qualities needed under the broad headings of management skills, leadership skills, knowledge, and attitudes. Early leadership theories often made a distinction between leadership, management, and administration (Zaleznick 2004). Leadership was seen as: strategic, articulating a vision, and setting direction, promoting change and movement, aligning people, motivating, and inspiring (Kotter 1998; Northouse 2007) creating new paradigms and challenging systems (Covey et al 1994). Management was seen as operational, promoting order, stability, and structure (Kotter 1998), concerned with planning, budgeting, setting rules and procedures, problem-solving (Northouse 2007), and working within existing paradigms (Covey et al 1994). Administration was seen as part of the bureaucracy that made things happen for academics, similar to management. According to Bennis and Nanus (1985, p. 21) 'managers are people who do things right, leaders are people who do the right thing', picking up the notion that leadership incorporates morals or values.

This artificial distinction gave rise to a number of problems and tensions between managers and leaders. For example, take an understaffed emergency department with a 4-hour waiting time target, where, if targets are not met, financial penalties will be imposed, but whose clientele comprises many elderly people with complex conditions. Tensions are played out where 'management' (who clinicians feel do not understand the complexities of clinical practice) comes into conflict with 'clinical leaders' (who managers feel do not understand that the underlying purpose is to improve service quality). In education we see similar tensions between academics or clinicians (who just want to get on and teach) and administrators who are perceived as imposing more and more quality assurance processes. The educational leadership job in the real world is to make it all happen. The management task is to: enable the organization to remain high quality and financially viable (otherwise there will be no organization); operate within legal and regulatory constraints; and meet multiple stakeholders' demands. However, the leader also wants to promote innovation through change, motivation of people, communication, and enactment of a vision for the future that will mark out the organization as delivering leading-edge education. This can lead to instability as the organization moves from one state to another—this needs to be actively managed and planned.

It is now accepted that leadership and management are inseparable (fig. 61.1), although one difference between them is their orientation to organizational change. Fulop and Day (2010) describe this as 'hybridity' where both individual and collective, or distributed, leadership exists, and the hybrid professional manager has a crucial role. Universities and healthcare organizations are structured hierarchically,

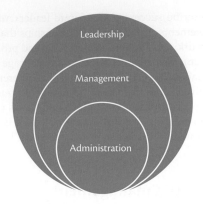

Figure 61.1 Leadership and management.

even though some flattening of organizations has occurred via matrix management structures, which are designed around functional units (e.g. marketing, admissions, or operating theatres). What makes leading and managing in these contexts challenging is that much of the workforce comprises professionals who value and demand relative autonomy and power to make professional decisions. Mintzberg (1992), suggests that professional organizations are managed by a small 'strategic apex' (e.g. senior management team), assisted by a 'supporting technostructure (systems, procedures, processes) and staff (support, administrative staff)' through a small middle line (directors, programme managers, heads of department) who themselves manage a large operating core of professionals. Effective leaders understand the purpose and methods of management (including budgeting, managing people, quality management, and programme delivery) and either learn these skills themselves or ensure that their team equips itself with these skills. When planning over the short or long term (e.g. planning a curricular change or introducing a new programme), the following tools can be useful

◆ SWOT (where the organization's internal *s*trengths and *w*eaknesses are mapped against the external *o*pportunities and *t*hreats)

◆ PESTLE (a tool used to consider external factors from *p*olitical, *e*conomic, *s*ociodemographic, *t*echnological, *l*egal, and *e*nvironmental perspectives)—also known as PEST or PESTELI

◆ options appraisals

◆ risk analyses or

◆ project management approaches.

As leaders need to be managers too, or at least understand management concepts, a management tool such as the McKinsey's 7S model can help a leader focus on the interrelated elements within an organizational system that need to be attended to when implementing the strategy (Waterman et al. 1980). The 7S model categorizes elements as either hard or soft; all elements relate to one another—change in any one of them will influence the other elements directly or indirectly.

Hard elements are easier to identify and managers can directly influence them. They include

◆ organizational structures (hierarchies or management structures, the organizational tree)

◆ strategies (at various levels in the organization) and

◆ systems (finance, IT and human resources).

Soft elements are more difficult to describe—they are less tangible and more influenced by culture, but are as important as the hard elements for organizational success. The soft elements are

◆ style (both the organization's style of working as well as the style of teams, individuals and groups)

◆ staff (the people who work for or use the organization, their behaviours, morale, and motivation)

◆ skills (capabilities and mindsets) and

◆ superordinate goals or shared values: the guiding concepts, values and aspirations that underpin an organization and that are typically enshrined in a leader's vision, mission and strategy.

Leaders and organizations

Any educational leader works in a formal organization, be it a university, college, hospital, or family practice (fig. 61.2). Increasingly, public services are becoming more integrated to facilitate easier access to services for users and more efficient care pathways. Organizations intersect with one another and so education leaders must be comfortable working across boundaries (what Bradshaw (1999) calls 'boundary spanners') and in the spaces between

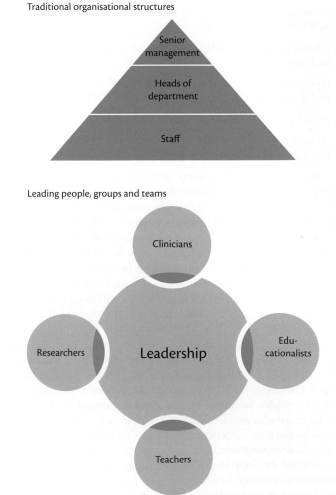

Figure 61.2 Leadership and organizations.

organizations, professions, and subcultures, requiring skills in brokering, negotiation, mediating, decision-making, conflict management, communication, and translation of concepts from one setting to another (Hartle et al 2008; Tennyson and Wilde 2000). Meyerson (2004) describes these new forms of workers as 'tempered radicals'—they are willing to work on different, external agendas and take risks. In addition to being able to work in the crowded stage of contemporary medical education (and returning to the idea of leaders being able to think on many levels) central to Bolman and Gallos' concept of a leader is the idea that leaders can embrace and utilize 'multi-frame thinking' (Bolman and Gallos 2011, p. 11): being able to consider issues, challenges and opportunities from different perspectives.

In some ways, we might see this from a sociological perspective, what Mills (1959) called the 'sociological imagination': being able to step back and look into an organization, event or system from an alternative point of view to that of the dominant culture or way of working. Many writers have taken a sociological perspective on organizations—this has been developed further by those writing on leadership to offer strategies that leaders might adopt to manage complex social systems. In his influential book, *Images of Organisations* (1997), Morgan describes organizations in terms of metaphors: these metaphors can enable deeper understanding of the perspectives of all stakeholders in an organization. The metaphors are:

* machines (systems or processes)

* organisms (complex systems in which the relationship with external environment is important)

* brains (learning and self-organization)

* cultures (the 'way we do things round here', rites, rituals, and symbols)

* political systems (with notions of power, interests, and conflict)

* psychic prisons (being trapped at work, perhaps through low pay and unsatisfactory conditions) and

* instruments of domination (organizations use these to promulgate dominant ideologies).

The way in which leaders (and those who work or study in the organization) perceive the organization can greatly influence the way that stakeholders behave and respond to situations. Conversely, the effective leader can tap into the power of metaphor to communicate ideas and vision: the notion that one of the roles of a leader is to 'manage meaning' can be seen throughout history, from Winston Churchill's 'Iron Curtain' to Martin Luther King's 'I have a dream' speeches. All are powerful images conveyed through rhetoric that served to shape and change the reality of different societies and those who lived within them.

Coming back to education, Bolman and Deal's (1991) original conceptualization of an organization was described in terms of four frames. The frames are four different ways of looking at educational organizations (or the departments or activities within them) from the perspective (or metaphor) of the machine, family, jungle, and theatre.

From the frame of the 'machine', the leader needs to focus on ensuring that rational systems and processes are in place (rules, roles, and policies), which themselves align with organizational and professional goals and purposes.

In the 'family frame', relationships are important, talents are recognized and developed, and people feel motivated and proud to belong to the organization. The leader's challenge is to find 'fit' between individuals' and organizational needs.

From the 'jungle' perspective, the organization demonstrates a diversity of views, beliefs and values, with competition for scarce resources. Becher and Trowler (2001) describes these as academic tribes and territories. In medical education, such academic tribes (healthcare scientists, psychologists, and clinical researchers) who control laboratories, classrooms, curricula, and assessments, intersect with professional tribes (doctors, nurses, and allied health professionals) who occupy different territories (clinics, wards, and operating theatres) and who work within clinical protocols, procedures, and cultures. This raises challenges for medical educators, as curricula and educational programmes are moving towards integrated, competency-based models (Hodges 2010; Whitehead 2010). Understanding the perspectives of different tribes is vital if leaders are to enact strategies and effect meaningful change. Barrow et al.'s (2011) research in New Zealand explored newly graduated doctors' and nurses' perceptions of leadership, followership, power, and authority and found striking differences in beliefs as to how teams worked, where the locus of power and control was invested and who should lead multidisciplinary teams. This has implications for how we teach, who we teach and what we teach, and leaders need to engage with this emerging evidence.

Bolman and Gallos point out that there are opportunities too within the 'jungle', as a diversity of views and approaches can act as 'a wellspring of creativity and innovation' (Bolman and Gallos 2011, p. 12). Trying to use diversity within teams or organizations can be a challenge for educational leaders.

Bolman and Gallos' (2011) image of the 'theatre' considers the educational organization as an ongoing drama, where culture and meaning is created and cocreated as the actors play out their roles. Here, the leader needs to pay attention to the management of meaning—how symbols, rites, and rituals (such as logos, graduation ceremonies, and daily routines) reinforce the 'reality' and keep learners and teachers engaged. This idea also reflects dominant educational thinking, drawing from theories of the social construction of meaning and reality, which map onto constructivist concepts. Just as the teacher's task is to integrate multiple realities in the learning environment, so must the leader orchestrate players into a unified team who know their parts and work towards common outcomes.

This highlights the importance leaders need to place on the culture of the organization. Culture can be defined as 'the way we do things round here' (Deal and Kennedy 1982, p. 4) and as 'values, beliefs and taken for granted routines' (Schein 1985, p. 1). In medical education, these can be deeply held beliefs (for example about the moral purpose of medicine) or grounded in routine and practice, such as carrying out selection in a certain way, or delivering a programme using teaching and assessment methods that have been used for many years. As we discuss elsewhere, quite often competing cultures and subcultures exist, and the leader's role is therefore to question and challenge these taken for granted ideas, models of practice, and professional identities. This can be difficult when a leader is immersed in a culture. Sometimes a 'credible outsider' can manage this sensitively, through appropriate questioning, enabling an articulation of needs and values, working with mutual respect and motivating people to improve the current situation collaboratively.

Leading people, groups, and teams

Lieff and Albert (2010) studied the nature and practices of medical school deans and described how medical education leaders employed all four of Bolman and Deal's frames for understanding their work. Lieff introduces a fifth domain of 'interpersonal and work style' ('knowing how to socially situate people in an organization so that they work in their areas of strength'). Leadership is thus relational and contextual. Souba (2010) describes a new model of leadership performance in healthcare in which conversational domains become contextual. This perspective echoes work on dialogic leadership, which uses skills and techniques such as appreciative inquiry (Isaacs 1999), 'World café', storytelling or taking multiple perspectives to solve 'wicked problems'. Argyris and Schön (1978) distinguish between 'inquiry' and 'advocacy'. Inquiry requires bystanding and following; advocacy requires a balance between moving and opposing. An effective leader will work to find a balance between inquiry and advocacy in conversations.

As Davies and Davies (2012) suggest, educational leaders need to pay attention to emotion as well as reason. Later in this chapter we explore how leaders need to develop self-insight but here we want to highlight two relevant concepts

- emotional intelligence (EI) and
- affective leadership.

Goleman's (2000) work on EI has been influential on leadership development, although the underpinning research does not provide robust empirical evidence for the theory. Salovey and Mayer (1990, p. 31) describe EI as 'the ability to perceive emotion, integrate emotion to facilitate thought, understand emotions and to regulate emotions to promote personal growth'. Goleman (2000) suggests that the competencies required for emotional intelligence are:

- self awareness
- self management
- social awareness
- relationship management.

In terms of leadership, Goleman et al. (2002) suggest that effective leaders are able to draw on a range of styles to suit to the situation, primarily to motivate others, and to regulate their own (and others') disruptive emotions. Although personality traits and EI are important, these are only part of the range of attributes of a leader. Where EI might be more relevant to medical leadership is where it intersects with 'emotional labour', the work that healthcare professionals and teachers do on a day-to-day basis because they work primarily with people. Medical education leadership is primarily 'people work', and because students, teachers, trainers, and clinicians work daily with people with pressing needs and high emotions, they need to understand how emotions affect their behaviours, responses, and performance (Howe 2008). Humphrey et al. (2008) suggest that effective transformational leaders are those who perform emotional labour through 'deep acting'—they are empathic and use genuine emotional expressions: in other words they are authentic. They use trust and transparency and they care about their followers (Avolio and Gardner 2005). Leaders who break trust lose their followers' commitment and respect.

Leaders who have high EI and can use emotion safely and appropriately in the workplace can be seen to employ 'affective leadership' (Newman et al 2009). This artistry is the 'dance of leadership' (Denhardt and Denhardt 2006): 'a metaphor for the artful use of affect (expressed emotion) in leadership…through carefully moderated emotional display that shows situational awareness, contextual sensitivity and recognition of an individual's needs' (Held and McKimm, 2012, p. 60). As long as participants follow the 'dance steps', using rapid cognition, emotion, and rational thought, leaders and followers can use emotion to work collaboratively. Moss (2009) suggests that leaders also need to pay attention to spiritual intelligence, ensuring that ethics, values, and vision are used to support individuals in their emotional labour and people work. This helps people derive meaning from their work—it can be inspiring and motivating; it facilitates creativity and innovation; and it ensures people stay connected.

Knowing your team, both how they perform as individuals and how they work together is an essential skill for a leader. Again there are many tools available—the personality tools already mentioned help leaders to identify how individuals may complement each other and where there are areas of potential conflict. Specific tools such as the Aston Team Performance Inventory or the still widely used Belbin Team role inventory can also help identify the strengths and potential weaknesses of a team. For the developing leader, there is a further reason to know their team well. It is rare for one individual to have all the capabilities required for leadership. No one individual can be a complete leader and a good leader is one who is aware of their limitations and is strategic in selecting others who will offset these limitations (Ancona et al 2007). The concept of the 'ontological leader' (Erhard et al. 2011; Souba 2011, 2010), who pays attention to being as well as doing, who is aware of process, who has a strong sense of self and is aware of their impact on others fits well with the approaches to leadership discussed earlier. Fullan (2005) suggests that the new work of educational leaders working in complex adaptive systems is to find adaptive (rather than technical) solutions. Heifetz and Linsky (2004) suggest that an adaptive challenge consists of a gap between aspiration and reality, demanding a response outside our current repertoire; adaptive work is needed to narrow the gap—this is difficult learning; the people with the problem are both the problem and the solution; and adaptive work generates disequilibrium and avoidance. So hard conversations are needed, people need to be given space, time and security to explore solutions and make changes, whilst avoiding 'groupthink' or getting stuck (Fullan 2005).

Leadership theories and concepts

A range of leadership theories and concepts have been described in the literature—it is not possible to do them all justice in this chapter. Here, we discuss some of the more dominant and influential theories and explore how these might have meaning for medical education leaders. Although there is a loose chronology of leadership theories, and at certain times or in certain cultures, some forms of leadership seem more acceptable than others (Storey 2004), today, an existing or aspiring leader can select from a huge menu of styles, approaches, ways of working, and behaviours. The most important factor, however, is that leadership is always relational (Binney et al 2004)—it is about how you behave and interact with others. As a result, developing self-insight and 'emotional intelligence' is vital (Goleman 2000).

At the start of the last century, descriptions of leaders gave rise to the dominant 'great man' or trait theory: aspiring leaders would emulate these 'great men'. From the 1940s, dominant theories tended to focus on leadership styles, supported by the underpinning concept that leaders could change and develop (Jago 1982). Leaders were distinct from managers and administrators, not only in the tasks that they did but also in terms of skills. In the 1950s and 1960s behavioural and relational theories began to articulate how individuals perform better when their needs are met, with the result that the organization does better. Thus, leaders and organizations began to involve workers (sometimes termed followers) in improving organizational performance and achieving goals, and so motivation theorists emerged.

In the 1960s and 1970s there was an interest in situational (Hersey and Blanchard 1993) and contingent leadership theory, in which the leader is not only an orator and vision-maker but reacts to the business, organizational, and social contexts in which they and their organization operate. Selznick (1957) regards leadership as managing the human side of organizations, infusing purpose and values. Contingency theories suggest that leaders need a variety of skills and approaches, and must be able to select from a repertoire to deal with different situations effectively. The leadership style chosen is therefore contingent on the situation. Whilst it is true that education leaders need to behave somewhat differently in different situations (such as chairing a meeting or relaxing with your close team), this view denies the value of leaders displaying authenticity and openness which is more prevalent in later conceptions of leadership (McKimm and Leiff in press).

Following the high-profile falls in the 1970s and 1980s of some political and business leaders, the charismatic leader (who as Maccoby (2007) suggests can sometimes be narcissistic to the extent that they fail to realize the impact of their behaviours and lose sight of organizational goals) started to fall out of favour as the dominant leadership form. These 'heroic individual' theories based on individuals' characteristics gave way to post-heroic theories including distributed and shared leadership theories and theories of followership. There is much overlap and recycling of theories through the literature. Leadership theory neither emerged from nor was tested in medical education. However, several dominant theories (sometimes called 'new paradigm' (Bryman 1996) models of leadership)—transactional, transformational, and servant leadership theories—possibly have greatest resonance with the still emerging language of leadership in healthcare education.

The focus of transactional leadership is improving the performance of the organization, and the leader exchanges reward for compliance with objectives and rules. This form of engagement is sometimes termed reciprocity (Heifetz et al 2004). Transformational leadership is an expansion of the transactional model, in which everyone is involved through collaborative decision making to drive organizational improvement (Bass and Avolio 1994). Transformational leaders create value congruency and trust, and are committed to change being achieved.

Servant leadership first emerged from the beliefs and values in the Roman Catholic Church and is about service to followers, with the leader valuing the people who are in the organization (Greenleaf 2002). Servant leaders gain influence from serving and Greenleaf (2002) suggests that an individual serves first and then, through conscious choice and a wish to make a difference, aspires to lead. The concept of servant leadership is relevant to healthcare and education, particularly in the public sector, enshrining ideas such as stewardship (caring for something for the next generation), community decision-making, listening, empowering others, persuasion, and commitment to the growth of people. Fullan (2007) describes this as education's moral purpose—bringing the idea of 'value-led leadership' firmly to the fore. Fullan (2001) suggests that effective change leaders are those who can work with members of a community using five skills: coherence making; defining the moral purpose; understanding the change (and its impact); building relationships; and knowledge creation and sharing. The skilled leader who has good self-insight does all this with energy, enthusiasm, compassion, and hope. Unfortunately, we see many examples of leaders who fail to engage others in a change process because they lack one of more of these personal qualities. More recently, a focus on different forms of leadership that acknowledge collaboration, community engagement, network forms of knowledge, and environmental and organizational sustainability have emerged (Cardona 2000; Scott, 2004; van Zwanenberg 2003; McKimm and Swanwick 2009, p18; Fullan 2005). Western (2012, p. 18) also discussed the concept of ecoleadership as an emerging leadership discourse within the post-heroic paradigms, describing it as : 'about connectivity, inter-dependence and sustainability, underpinned by an ethical, socially responsible stance . . . it is fuelled by the human spirit, for some this is underpinned by spirituality, for others not'.

Framing leadership in these terms is relevant to medical and healthcare educators and echoes other refrains in the education literature around social responsibility and accountability (Boelen and Woollard 2011), promoting global health and cultural diversity (McKimm and McLean 2011), student, trainee, patient and carer empowerment, and community engagement (Fullan 2005). The notion of collaborative or shared leadership (Lambert 2002) also underpins interprofessional education and collaborative health practice. The World Health Organization (2007, 2009) suggests that collaborative practice leads to improved health outcomes:

- improved patient care

- improved access to and coordination of health outcomes

- more appropriate use of resources

- improved patient safety, reduced clinical errors

- decrease in complications, hospital stays, cost of care

- funding often geared to collaboration for innovation.

Northouse (2007) describes leadership as a process, involving influence in a group context with goal attainment. This brings us back to the earlier notions that leadership is relational and cannot be properly understood without reference to followers. Leaders and followers are not exclusive groups, and many followers will lead and many leaders will follow. There are several typologies of followership that Kellerman (2008) asserts are different and of a particular time, culture, and order. However, they are more similar than different; they all involve dominance and deference. Kellerman identifies isolates, bystanders, participants, activists, and diehards, and Kelley (1988) identifies alienated, passive, conformist, pragmatic, and exemplary followers. Kelley's exemplary followers act with intelligence, independence, courage, and a strong sense of ethics. In addition, the typologies involve a spectrum of engagement from passive to active.

Followers transcend their own needs for the success of the organization and it is the task of the leader to make this happen, what Bass and Avolio (1996) describe as 'idealised influence'. According to Alimo-Metcalfe (1998), leaders transform followers by pulling them to a future state. Rost (1991) makes it clear that leaders and followers work in relationships based on influence to bring about changes for their mutual purposes. Leadership is thus what leaders and followers do together. As organizations become flatter, Rost (1993) challenges theorists and activists to set aside the concept of followership. However, the literature on followership continues to increase. Grint and Holt (2011) provide a typology of followership based on authority, and certainty and uncertainty, and the relative complexity of problems ('wicked' and 'tame' problems) that organizations face. They describe individual and collective responsibility of people working in the health service. In many ways the approach to problems, some more fixable than others, is captured in the theory of adaptive leadership (Heifetz and Linsky 2004). Central to the understanding of leaders and followers is power, which is a relationship and not a possession; the result is that followers are never powerless. Kelley (1988) suggests four roles are involved in the leader–follower relationship: passive followership (looks to the leader to make decisions, passive engagement, sometimes negative energy), active followership (independent critical thinkers, supportive of the organization and leader's goals and vision), little 'l' leadership (leading tasks, teams, and groups), and big 'L' leadership (leading big initiatives or holding senior positions).

Grint (2005) describes four views of leadership: leadership as the person (who requires interaction with others to effect change); leadership as the results (or outcomes, some of which are more measurable than others); leadership as the process (through different behaviours of leaders and followers); and leadership as the position (whether rank or status determines the leadership). Each successive description of a leader, a change, or an organization yields another theory or style. The lack of agreed definitions of leaders and leadership in the literature makes the straightforward application of theory to medicine and medical education problematic (Turnbull James 2011).

Institutional variability also confounds our understanding of what is successful leadership in medical education (Rich et al 2008). Mennin (2010) describes the nature of medical schools as complex adaptive systems. Clinical academics continuously move between the clinical environment and the university context. In clinical settings, leadership is often related to position or profession and in medical schools professional practice is valued by both leaders and followers. Mintzberg (2009) asserts that important criteria in healthcare are the style of problem solving, the context and the sum total of decision-making. However, Turnbull James (2011) shifts away from individuals and their profiles; named leaders are invariably part of a network of colleagues. The King's Fund, informing the Commission on Leadership and Management in the NHS, states that staff need both transformational leadership to lead change and transactional leadership (management) to hold stability (King's Fund 2011).

Contemporary leadership involves creating vision, strategy, communication, and dealing with conflicts. Leaders undoubtedly require management skills for enhancing services and patient care; for supporting teamwork; and to realize patient engagement. This is leadership for a purpose and there is recognition of how structures, processes, demands, and language shape leaders (Souba 2011).

Leadership in healthcare has both context and purpose which involve the achievement of quality patient care, and satisfaction through the management of teams (Firth-Cozens and Mowbray 2001). In the 1980s, transactional methods were increasingly employed to measure and monitor healthcare excellence, effectiveness, and quality. These became political devices as well as methods to develop and enhance leadership in healthcare—and in holistic systems such as the UK National Health Service, they continue to prevail. Any assessment of leadership has to go beyond performance monitoring and to look at effects on staff and the organization through which healthcare is delivered.

Many leadership approaches emphasize a framework whereby the skills, attitudes, or competencies of leadership can be learned. Kotter (1990) defines leadership skills and practices, and establishes methodologies for developing leaders. In the UK, all clinicians can reference their leadership development to the widely endorsed Medical Leadership Competency Framework (MLCF) (NHS Institute for Innovation and Improvement 2010). In healthcare, the normative model of professional leadership is of heroic leaders. Although the MLCF emphasizes shared leadership, it is also underpinned by the belief that problems of leadership can be addressed by developing individuals rather than systems. Leadership programmes that focus on developing individuals need to be relevant to day to day practice. In clinical working lives, leadership requires individual resilience and robust personal skills. Kelley's (1998) view sees leadership as a solution-oriented practice, getting things done operationally rather than strategizing.

Leadership development programmes must be situated in the practice of those developing what should be both their leadership and their management skills (Fulop 2010). Programmes should focus on building trust and collective leadership (Grint 2005). The essential people management skills that include creating a meaningful vision and implementing change require a high degree of emotional intelligence (Goleman 2000). Furthermore, the post-heroic theories have moved from individual leader development to leadership development that focuses on continuing organizational development (Turnbull James 2011). A distributed and shared leadership approach which facilitates open and diffuse boundaries needs to develop the 'social capital' of the organization (the ability of the organization to develop systems in alignment with its goals and mission) instead of focussing on developing 'individual capital', which focuses on developing the individual's leadership skills (Bolden et al. 2011).

Developing leaders at all levels

During the first decade of the 21st century, UK health strategy has focused on health improvement and leadership development. In 2008 an expert group wrote that:

> formal leadership training is presently seen as limited and there is a need to include this in professional training as an essential precursor for senior posts in hospital medicine, general practice and public health… The role of educational leaders is also viewed as crucial for future excellence and professionalism
>
> Scottish Medical and Scientific Advisory Committee (2009.

In medical education it is understood that career pathways are necessary to guide the novice. Some students enter medical school sure of their final career goal; others have no formed idea or even understanding of where their educational journey will lead. These career tracks define the path to a doctor's main identity. En route a proportion of doctors choose to follow a parallel track as an academic. Awareness of this possibility often develops from student years where university-based educators are also researchers. There is an inevitability that students will encounter clinical researchers—they are also required to be research aware (General Medical Council 2009). The concept of moving through a clinical academic continuum of research awareness to engagement to activity is well described (The Academy of Medical Sciences 2012). At the time of writing, a similar continuum cannot be clearly articulated for clinical educators and leaders.

Many professional guidance frameworks define leadership, management, teaching and assessing as important to good patient care (CanMEDS 2010; General Medical Council 2011). And it is required that those involved in teaching 'are responsible for developing the skills and practices of a competent teacher' (General Medical Council 2011, p. 8), although not necessarily the skills of an educational leader. To develop educational leaders at every level it is necessary to define the stages of a career and construct a coherent approach that ensures that every doctor is educationally aware and every role filled by a doctor is clear in its educational requirements and responsibilities. A few doctors will pursue an educational career track to a role with a major educational component (e.g. director of medical education). Those currently in post will have followed many different tracks to their educational role; not all will have a primary medical degree. Some will have recognized qualifications in education or leadership. Others will have gained expertise through experience. For students and doctors it is still not straightforward to describe a career track in medical education that connects with other curricular competencies. This poses problems in developing educational leaders—different countries have addressed this in different ways.

The UK MLCF was first published in 2008 and was updated in 2011 (Academy of Medical Colleges and NHS Institute for Innovation and Improvement 2008). It was designed to help address a perceived deficit in medical leadership and sets out the leadership competencies that doctors need to become more engaged and involved in planning, delivering and transforming health services. Although not specifically focusing on educational leadership, many of the competencies and curriculum activities are relevant to educational leadership as well as clinical leadership. The Academy of Medical Educators has produced professional standards that help to direct current and future educational leaders (AoME 2012). However, these competency frameworks only provide the starting point and it is how they are interpreted at policy, organizational and individual levels that will determine whether they help to develop educational and clinical leadership capacity (General Medical Council 2012b).

Educational leadership awareness for medical students

The journey from novice to expert is long. Factors determining progress include an individual's learning style and commitment; an institution's philosophy of teaching; specific curricula; and available educational environments. Every interaction for the student is formative and at this stage improving a student's conscious recognition of the educational processes can be key. That transition from school pupil to adult learner can be enriched by the student gaining an active

understanding of educational theory as well as medical knowledge. Some students will enter medical school with an awareness of education. All UK students are now required to acquire skills in education as well as clinical leadership. *Tomorrow's Doctors* (General Medical Council 2009) requires students to 'function effectively as a mentor and teacher including contributing to the appraisal, assessment and review of colleagues, giving effective feedback, and taking advantage of opportunities to develop these skills' (General Medical Council 2009 p. 27) and to 'demonstrate ability to build team capacity and positive working relationships and undertake various team roles including leadership and the ability to accept leadership by others' (General Medical Council 2009 p. 28). Many schools now teach and assess skills in facilitating learning, giving presentations, educational research and leadership. A few schools offer an intercalated option in medical education or clinical leadership. The provision of a theoretical basis for education and leadership coupled with role modelling and guided opportunities for engagement in teaching and little 'l' leadership helps to ensure a deep and enduring awareness of the possibilities ahead in medical education.

The MLCF guides the student into gaining an understanding of their personal qualities:

◆ acting with integrity

◆ self development

◆ self management

◆ self awareness

and working with others:

◆ working within teams

◆ encouraging contribution

◆ building and maintaining relationships

◆ developing networks.

These domains are the cornerstones of leadership development, fostering emotional intelligence and humanity—shared requirements for leaders of whatever kind (Jordan et al. 2008). The challenge for undergraduate education is identifying and negotiating sufficient curriculum time for in-depth self-development.

Educational leadership engagement for early years doctors in training

The early years' curriculum is usually generic, a common path that all must follow. It focuses on supporting and developing new graduate doctors through the transition from student to doctor. It offers opportunity to build on further MLCF domains of managing services:

◆ managing performance

◆ managing people

◆ managing resources

◆ planning

and improving services:

◆ facilitating transformation

◆ encouraging innovation

◆ critically evaluating

◆ ensuring patient safety.

These domains should stretch the new doctor in the increasingly familiar educational environment that is their workplace, ensuring they engage with and understand the context in which they work and learn. Relevant to enhancing educational leadership, the domains enable opportunities for exposure to a wide range of educational activities on which the leadership lens can be focused. Workplace learning and its plethora of assessment tools, some assessments of learning and others assessments for learning could offer opportunity to develop and assess leadership skills (General Medical Council 2012a). Evidence of progression is demonstrated through maintaining a portfolio of practice that incorporates logs of reflection, achievement, and skills completed. Skills such as team working and communication are assessed formally and informally (although they are not defined explicitly in leadership terms). Again, although educational leadership is not specifically addressed, for the educationally curious these early years are a time of immersion in educational methods and a time of choice for the potential educational leader. The possibility of embarking on a postgraduate qualification in medical education (often including an educational leadership module) arises at this stage. Some institutions offer academic track programmes including options in medical education. These programmes are competitive and offer protected time for academic endeavour, often coming with built-in mentorship. As a foundation for a future educational leadership career they are worth considering.

Educational leadership activities for doctors in training

All curricula for UK doctors include a mandatory component of recognizable education and leadership development, (e.g. The UK Foundation Programme Office 2011). The qualification route is achievable, with a number of part-time and distance learning products available in both medical education and leadership. Success requires commitment, both intellectual and financial, but evidence of such commitment is becoming a prerequisite for recognition and promotion to educational leadership roles. The last decade has also seen a rise in the number of fellowships in education and clinical leadership.

Supporting and developing trainers for future educational leaders

Most healthcare systems have recognized that many of their current medical and educational leaders have experience but have not followed a conventional or even explicit career track. The last decade has seen the rise of healthcare leadership strategies such as the Scottish Government's Delivering Quality through Leadership: NHS Scotland Leadership Development Strategy. Such approaches are enabling leadership development at all levels.

Table 61.1 Possible career track for medical education leaders

Level: Educational track	Relevant to: Career track	(UK) educational qualification	(UK) resource source
I Educationally aware	All medical students	None—embedded curricular requirement	Undergraduate medical curricula
II Educationally engaged	All doctors in training	None—embedded curricular requirement	Foundation & Specialty Training Curricula
III Educationally active	Some doctors in training e.g. Academic Foundation trainee; Clinical Teaching Fellow All teachers, trainers, and supervisors	Postgraduate Certificate/Diploma/Masters in (Clinical/Medical) Education; MPhil; PhD Recognized trainer training/faculty development Membership of: the Academy of Medical Educators (or equivalent) or Higher Education Academy	Higher education institutes Medical schools, deaneries & Specialty Colleges Academy of Medical Educators Higher Education Academy
IV Educational leader (usually a sessional role)	E.g. Phase/Year Coordinator; Educational Supervisor; Associate Adviser/Associate Dean/Assistant GP Director	Recognized trainer training/faculty development—enhanced & tailored to role Leadership training—including Postgraduate qualifications (PG Cert/Dip/Masters in Business Administration)	Medical schools, deaneries & Specialty Colleges. ASME Higher education institutes
V Educational leader (usually a substantial time commitment)	Director of Medical Education/PG Dean/GP Director Dean/Head/Principal of School	As above Fellowship of the Academy of Medical Educators (or equivalent) or Higher Education Academy Member of the Faculty of Medical Leadership and Management (or equivalent)	Academy of Medical Educators Higher Education Academy Faculty of Medical Leadership and Management

Is educational leadership in need of specialty status?

Developing a career track in educational leadership takes commitment and achievement. In many healthcare systems, senior recognition is from a doctor's base specialty and it is that specialty that may define their registration, licensure and scope of practice. Only when medical education is recognized as a legitimate career track will it be possible to fully integrate curricular requirements, rather than the alongside approach currently necessitated by the predominance of the clinical specialty curriculum. Table 61.1 sets out an approach to a career track. There is also a need to support a 'catch up cohort' of current doctors with educational responsibilities who have not had the benefit of following some of the curricula just described.

As education is at the heart of health improvement, educational leadership needs to flourish and so must be organized in a way that is recognizable, navigable, and accessible. This requires that whatever the current health system's approach to organizing career progression, a linked and integrated arrangement for educational leadership progression is in place. The recently established Faculty of Medical Leadership and Management provides medical leaders (and others who have leadership roles in medical management and education) with a home organization that acts as both a reference point and a community of practice (McKimm et al 2009).

Developing and understanding self as a leader

While the previously mentioned frameworks set out the qualities and competencies required for leadership, attaining these requires application and practice (NHS Leadership Centre 2003; Academy of Medical Royal Colleges and NHS Institute for Innovation and Improvement 2008).

There is a huge knowledge base for leadership and a wealth of resources available for aspiring leaders to acquire knowledge. Numerous books, articles, and journals are available and courses abound. The first step in leadership development, therefore, is to identify the way in which this information will be best assimilated. Individuals may prefer role play, study, action learning sets, or discussion groups, depending on their learning style (Honey and Mumford 1982).

However, while it is a tantalizing thought that somewhere there might be a book to be read or a learning activity to be undertaken which would transform the individual into an outstanding leader, the reality is quite different. Being a leader is not something taught but is learned from experience and practice (Adair 1997). Books and articles can provide background principles and knowledge but it is only by putting these into practice and experimenting and reflecting on the outcome that an individual can develop as a leader.

Beginning as a leader

Leadership does not occur in a vacuum; being a leader is a social construct, dependent on the situation—in particular the team being led and the circumstances and culture in which it operates. Adair, in his description of functional leadership, describes a leader as: 'one who, by virtue of his personality, knowledge and training, is able to provide the functions necessary to enable the group to achieve its task and to hold it together as a working team' and

Box 61.1 Factors to be considered in leadership development

- An understanding of self
- An ability to put learning into practice
- An understanding of the team

leadership as 'an interaction among leader, group members, and situation' (Adair 1968). Leadership development is therefore multifactorial (box 61.1).

An understanding of self

'Personality predicts leadership and affects the performance of the team—who we are is how we lead' (Hogan and Kaiser 2005). An understanding of self is essential to develop as a leader. Knowing how others perceive us can provide a more accurate insight into leadership behaviour and may aid personal development (Alimo-Metcalfe, 1998). Specifically, it leads to:

- An understanding of strengths and weaknesses and the effect these may have on the team.
- An understanding of behaviour under stress and the pressure points that trigger stress.
- An appreciation of which leadership styles come easily and which will require some practice to develop.
- An ability to maximize the effectiveness of the team.

Several tools are available to help identify strengths and weaknesses. Objective assessment of personality can be carried out using tools such as the Myers-Briggs Personality Type Indicator (MBPI) and the five factor NEO Personality Inventory (NEO-PI). While there is little objective evidence that such knowledge improves leadership, studies such as that of Judge et al. (2002) or Siebert and Kraimer (2001) identify those personality traits most often recognized in leaders, providing insight into areas requiring development.

Multisource feedback may also be useful in this context but requires careful application and skilled feedback from an experienced facilitator otherwise its effectiveness may be hampered by unintended consequences (Sargeant et al. 2007). However, there is some evidence that when used with appropriate support, it may aid leadership development (Thach 2002)—particularly when used to identify specific areas for improvement (Bass and Avolio 1996).

As well as knowing what one's strengths are as a potential leader, it is crucial that an individual knows the stresses that might derail them. Frequently, those personal attributes which make an individual a good leader are those which, under stress, will cause problems for them and their team. Hogan and Hogan (2001) have identified 11 such derailers. Under stressful conditions, an individual whose strength lies in their enthusiasm for the role may become volatile and unpredictable; one who is cautious may become overcautious and risk-averse; one who is shrewd may become mistrustful and vindictive; one who is independent may become detached and withdrawn; one who is focused may become passive–aggressive and stubborn; one who is confident may become arrogant and opinionated; one who is charming may become manipulative; one who is vivacious may become dramatic and histrionic; one who is imaginative may become eccentric; one who is diligent may become a perfectionist and over-controlling; and one who is dutiful may become dependent or indecisive. Knowing this allows the potential leader to recognize the situation early and take preventative action.

There are many leadership styles. Goleman (2000) describes the following styles, all of which may be appropriate in different situations: coercive (demanding immediate compliance); authoritative (mobilizing people toward a vision; affiliative (creating harmony and building emotional bonds); democratic (obtaining consensus through participation); pace-setting (setting and expecting high standards of performance); and coaching (developing people for the future). However, the coercive and pace-setting styles tend to have a deleterious effect on the climate of the organization, especially if used inappropriately and too frequently. Bush (2003), in considering leadership in the educational setting, discusses formal, political, ambiguity, subjective, collegial, and cultural models—there are many others. The important issue about considering the different styles is to appreciate that there is no one 'right' model. Different styles are appropriate for different occasions and good leaders are aware that their preferred style will not work for all occasions. By reflecting on the leadership style that comes most easily to their personality, and using appropriate situations to try different styles, a developing leader can build a repertoire of approaches that will enhance their effectiveness in different situations.

An ability to put learning into practice

As has already been mentioned, leadership is learned from experience and practice (Adair 1997). The most practical advice therefore that can be given to someone who wishes to develop as a leader is: 'Just do it'. All the actions of leadership, setting vision; setting direction; motivation; coping with change, are all things that have to be done so without the action you cannot be a leader. Leadership involves taking risks, a leader who does not take risks will not progress their organization. However, safeguards and supports are required to enable the leader to develop while doing. Nonaka and Takeuchi (2011) suggest that leaders also need to display and develop practical wisdom.

New educational leaders may be offered a coach or mentor. Much has been written about the role of coaching, but at its centre is the emphasis on developing the talents and resources of the potential leader within the context of their work. Coaching and mentoring have been described as learning relationships which help people to take charge of their own development, to release their potential and to achieve results which they value (Connor and Pakora 2007). One of the most widely used methods is that of Whitmore (2002) which uses the GROW model:

Goals   What do you want?

Reality   What is happening now?

Options   What could you do?

Will   What will you do?

Another process which has been identified as helping leaders develop is the use of reflective practice. Bennis (1994) encourages all executives to practise the 'three Rs: retreat, renewal, and return' as a means of bringing about renewal and change in an organization. Reflective practice has been described as 'the capacity to reflect on

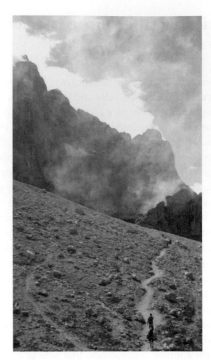

Figure 61.3 Leadership—the road ahead.

action so as to engage in a process of continuous learning' (Schon 1983). At its simplest, reflective practice involves thinking about an action or decision and its consequences, critically reviewing what happened and generating alternate solutions. This can be done in a variety of ways but usually involves taking time out to do it, either alone or with a colleague.

Action learning sets (Revans 1998), having a role model or structured observation and discovery are all means by which a new leader can develop while doing the job. Developing and understanding yourself as a leader, therefore, is an experiential process, underpinned by awareness of self and your team, during which the learning of the knowledge and skills of leadership is practised. Like all experiential learning, it is a lifelong journey and you can only make progress by focussing on the road ahead (fig. 61.3).

Conclusions

◆ Effective and imaginative medical education leadership and management are essential to ensure that quality education is delivered.

◆ Whilst it is now commonly accepted that educational knowledge and skills need to be both taught and assessed, it is less well recognized that medical educational leadership needs to be learned and developed, not just 'on the job' but through more formal and planned ways.

◆ Leadership development is crucial to develop existing and future educational leaders and managers who can weave deftly through the multifaceted, complex, and rapidly changing health service and education environments in which medical education is played out.

◆ Leaders need to be credible and visible, and able to lead and manage change, and collaborate and work with many groups of (often competing) stakeholders.

References

Academy of Medical Educators (2012) *Professional Standards*. [Online] http://www.medicaleducators.org/index.cfm/profession/profstandards/ Accessed 9 April 2013

Academy of Royal Colleges and NHS Institute for Innovation and Improvement (2008) Medical Leadership Qualities Framework. London: AoMRC

Adair, J. (1968) *Training for leadership*. London: MacDonald and Co

Adair, J. (1997) *Leadership Skills*. London: Chartered Institute of Personnel and Development

Alimo-Metcalfe, J. (1998) 360 degree feedback and leadership development. *Int J Select Assess*. 6: 35–44

Alimo-Metcalfe, B. (1998) *Effective leadership*. London: Local Government Management Board

Ancona D., Malone T.W., Orlikowski, W.J., and Senge, P.M. (2007) In praise of the incomplete leader. *Harvard Business Review*. 85: 92–100

Argyris, C., and Schön, D. (1978) *Organizational learning: A theory of action perspective*, Reading, MA: Addison Wesley

Avolio B.J. and Gardner W.L. (2005) Authentic leadership development: Getting to the root of positive forms of leadership. *The Leadership Quarterly*. 16: 315–338

Barrow, M., McKimm, J., and Gasquoine, S. (2011) The policy and the practice: early career doctors and nurses as leaders and followers in the delivery of health care. *Adv Health Sci Educ*. 16(1): 17–29

Bass, B.M. and Avolio, B.J. (1994) *Improving Organizational Effectiveness Through Transformational Leadership*. Thousand Oaks, CA: Sage

Bass, B.M. and Avolio, B.J. (1996) 'Postscript'. In *Improving Organisational Effectiveness Through Transformational Leadership*. London: Sage

Baulcomb, J.S. (2003) Management of change through force field analysis. *J Nurs Manag*. 11(4): 275–280

Becher, T. and Trowler, P. (2001) *Academic Tribes and Territories: Intellectual enquiry and the cultures of disciplines*. Milton Keynes: Open University Press

Beerel, A. (2009) *Leadership and Change management*. London: Sage Publications.

Bennis, W. (1994) *On Becoming a Leader*. Reading, MA: Addison-Wesley

Bennis, W. and Nanus, N. (1985) *Leaders: the strategies for taking charge*. New York: Harper and Row

Binney, G., Wilke, G., and Williams, C. (2004) *Living Leadership: a practical guide for ordinary heroes*. London: Pearson Books

Boelen, C. and Woollard, R. (2011) Social accountability: the extra leap to excellence for educational institutions. *Med Teach*. 33(8): 614–619

Bolden, R., Hawkins, B., Gosling, J., and Taylor, S. (2011) *Exploring Leadership: Individual, Organisational and Societal Perspectives*. Oxford: Oxford University Press

Bolden, R., Petrov, G., and Gosling, J. (2009) Distributed leadership in Higher Education: Rhetoric and reality. *Educ Manag Admin Leadership*. 37(2): 257–277

Bolden, R. (2011) Distributed leadership in organisations: a review of theory and research. *Int J Manag Rev*. 13(3): 251–269

Bolman, L. and Deal, T. (1991) *Reframing organisations: Artistry, Choice and Leadership*. San Francisco, CA: Jossey Bass

Bolman, L.G. and Gallos, J.V. (2011) *Reframing Academic Leadership*. San Francisco, CA: Jossey Bass

Bradshaw, L. (1999) Principals as boundary spanners: working collaboratively to solve problems. *NASSP Bull*. 83: 38

Bryman, A. (1996) Leadership in organisations. In S.R.Clegg, C. Harvey, and W.R. Nord (eds) *Handbook of Organisational Studies*. London: Sage

Bush, T. (2003) *Theories of Educational Management and Leadership*. London: Sage

CANMEDS Physician Competency Framework (2010) [Online] http://rcpsc.medical.org/canmeds/index.php Accessed 23 May 2012

Cardona, P. (2000) Transcendental leadership. *The Leadership and Organisation Development Journal*. 21(4): 201–206

Carr, D.K., Hard, K. J., and Trahant, W.J. (1996) *Managing the Change Process: a field book for change agents, consultants, team leaders and reengineering managers*. New York: McGraw Hill

Castells, M. (1990) *The Rise of the Network Society*. Oxford: Blackwell

Connor, M.P., and Pakora, J.B. (2007) *Coaching and Mentoring at Work: Developing Effective Practice*. Maidenhead McGraw Hill

Covey, S., Merrill, A.R., and Merrill, R.R. (1994) *First Things First*. New York: Simon and Schuster

Davies, B. and Davies, B.J. (2012) The nature and dimensions of strategic leadership. In M. Preedy, N. Bennett, and C. Wise (eds) *Educational Leadership: context, strategy and collaboration* (pp. 83–95). Milton Keynes: Open University Press

Deal, T. and Kennedy, A.E. (1982) *Corporate Cultures*. Reading, MA: Addison-Wesley

Denhardt, B. and Denhardt, V. (2006) *The Dance of Leadership: the art of leading in business, government and society*. Armonk NY: M.E. Sharpe

Department of Health (2011) *Service Increment for Teaching in England*. [Online] http://webarchive.nationalarchives.gov.uk/+/www.dh.gov.uk/en/Publicationsandstatistics/Publications/PublicationsPolicyAndGuidance/Browsable/DH_5651084 Accessed 9 April 2013

Erhard, W.H., Jensen, M.C., and Granger, K.L. (2011) Creating leaders: an ontological model. *Harvard Business School Negotiation, Organisations and Markets Research Papers*. Number 11–037

Firth-Cozens, J. and Mowbray, D. (2001) Leadership and the quality of care. *Qual Health Care*. 10(Suppl II): ii3–ii7

Fraser, S. and Greenhalgh, T. (2001) Coping with complexity: educating for capability. *BMJ*. 323:799–803

French, J.R.P. and Raven, B. (1959) The bases of social power. In D. Cartwright and A. Zander (eds) *Group Dynamics* (pp. 150–167). New York: Harper & Row

Fullan, M. (2001). *Leading in a Culture of Change*. San Francisco, CA: Jossey-Bass.

Fullan, M. (2005) *Leadership and Sustainability: Systems Thinkers in Action*. Thousand Oaks, CA: Corwin Press

Fullan, M. (2007) *The New Meaning of Educational Change*. 4th edn. London: Teachers College Press

Fulop, L. (undated) Exemplary leadership, the clinician manager, and a thing called 'hybridity'. [Online] www.download.bham.ac.uk/hsmc/liz-fulop.pdf. Accessed 10 March 2012

Fulop, L. and Day, G. E. (2010) From leader to leadership: clinician managers and where to next? *Aust Health Rev*. 34(3): 344–351

General Medical Council (2009) *Tomorrow's Doctors: Outcomes and standards for undergraduate medical education*. [Online] http://www.gmc-uk.org/education/undergraduate/tomorrows_doctors.asp Accessed 17 June 2012

General Medical Council (2011) *Good Medical Practice: Teaching and training, appraising and assessing*. [Online] http://www.gmc-uk.org/guidance/good_medical_practice/teaching_training.asp Accessed 17 June 2012

General Medical Council (2012a) *Workplace Based Assessments: a guide for implementation*. [Online] http://www.gmc-uk.org/Workplace_based_assessment_31381027.pdf Accessed 21 December 2011

General Medical Council. (2012b) *Recognition and Approval of Trainers: a consultation*. [Online] http://www.gmc-uk.org/education/10264.asp (accessed 17 June 2012)

Goleman, D. (2000) Leadership that gets results. *Harvard Business Review*. March/April: 78–90

Goleman, D., Boyatzis, R., and McKee, A. (2002) *Primal Leadership*. Boston: Harvard Business School Press

Greenleaf, R.K. (2002) *Servant Leadership: A Journey Into the Nature of Legitimate Power and Greatness*. New York: Paulist Press

Grint, K. (2005) *Leadership: Limits and Possibilities*. Basingstoke: Palgrave MacMillan

Grint, K. and Holt, C. (2011) Followership in the NHS. In: *The Future of Leadership and Management in the NHS. No more heroes*. Report from The King's Fund Commission on Leadership and Management in the NHS. London: The Kings Fund

Hartle, F., Snook, P., Apsey, H., and Brownton, R. (2008) *The training and development of middle managers in the children's workforce*. Report by the

Hay Group to the Children's Workforce Development Council (CWDC). [Online] www.cwdcouncil.org.uk Accessed 5 June 2012

Harvey, D. (1988) *The Condition of Post-modernity*. Cambridge MA: Polity Press

Heifetz R.A. and Linsky M. (2004) When leadership spells danger. *Educ Leadership*. 61(7): 33–37

Heifetz, R.A., Kania, J.V., and Kramer, M.R. (2004) *Leading Boldly*. Stanford CA: Stanford Social Innovation

Held, S. and McKimm, J. (2012) Emotional intelligence, emotional labour and affective leadership. In M. Preedy, N. Bennett, and C. Wise (eds) *Educational Leadership: context, strategy and collaboration* (pp. 52–64). Milton Keynes: Open University Press

Hersey, P. and Blanchard K. (1993) *Management of Organizational Behavior: Utilizing human resources*. 6th edn. Englewood Cliffs, NJ: Prentice Hall, Inc.

Hodges, B. (2010) A tea-steeping or i-doc model for medical education? *Acad Med*. 85: s34–s44

Hogan, R. and Hogan, J. (2001) Assessing leadership: A view from the dark side. *Int J Select Assess*. 9: 40–51

Hogan, R. and Kaiser, R.B. (2005) What we know about leadership. *Rev Gen Psychol*. 9: 169–180

Honey, P. and Mumford, A. (1982) *The Manual of Learning Styles*. Maidenhead: Peter Honey Publications

Howe, D. (2008) *The Emotionally Intelligent Social Worker*. Basingstoke: Palgrave McMillan

Humphrey, RH, Pollack, J.M., and Hawver, T. (2008) Leading with emotional labour. *J Manag Psychol*. 23(2): 151–168

Iles, V. (2011) Leading and managing change. In T. Swanwick and J. McKimm (eds) *The ABC of Clinical Leadership* (pp. 19–23). Oxford: Blackwell Publishing

Isaacs, I. (1999) Dialogic leadership. *The Systems Thinker*. 10(1): 1–5

Jago, A.G. (1982) Leadership: perspectives in theory and research. *Manag Sci*. 28(3): 315–336

Jameson, F. (1991) *Postmodernism, or, the Cultural Logic of Late Capitalism*. London: Verso

Jordan, P.J., Ashkanasy, N.M., and Daus, C.S. (2008) Emotional intelligence: rhetoric or reality? In S. Cartwright and C.L. Cooper (eds) *The Oxford Handbook of Personnel Psychology* (pp. 37–58). Oxford: Oxford University Press

Judge, T.A., Bono, J.E., Ilies, R., and Gerhardt, M.W. (2002) Personality and leadership: A qualitative and quantitative review. *J Appl Psychol*. 87: 765–780

Kellerman, B. (2008) *Followership: How Followers Are Creating Change and Changing Leaders*. Boston MA: Harvard Business Press

Kelley, R.E. (1988) In praise of followers. *Harvard Business Review*. 66: 142–148

Kelley, R.E. (1998) Followership in a leadership world. In L.C. Spears (ed.) *Insights on Leadership: service, stewardship, spirit, and servant leadership* (pp. 170–184). New York: John Wiley & Sons Inc.

The King's Fund (2011) The Future of Leadership and Management in the NHS. No more heroes. Report from The King's Fund Commission on Leadership and Management in the NHS. London: The Kings Fund

Kotter, J.P. (1990) *A Force for Change: How leadership differs from management*. New York: Free Press

Kotter, J. (1995) Leading change: why transformation efforts fail. *Harvard Business Review*. March–April: 1–20

Kotter, J.P. (1998) What leaders really do. In: *Harvard Business Review on Leadership* (pp. 37–60). Boston: Harvard Business School Press

Kotter, J.P. and Schlesinger, L.A. (2008) *Choosing strategies for change*, Harvard Business Review. July, 2008.

Kouzes, J. M. and Posner, B. Z. (2002) *The Leadership Challenge*, San Francisco: Jossey Bass

Lambert, L. (2002) *Educational leadership*. [Online] johnwgardnertestsite.pbworks.com Accessed 9 April 2013

Ledlow, G.R. and Coppola, N. (2011) *Leadership for Health Professionals: Theory, Skills, and Applications*. London: Jones & Bartlett Learning International

Lewin, K. (1951) *Field Theory in Social Science; selected theoretical papers*. New York: Harper & Row

Lieff, S, and Albert, M. (2010) The mindsets of medical education leaders; how do they conceive of their work? *Acad Med*. 85(1): 57–62

Livesley, B. (1989) Book review medicine and books. *BMJ*. 299: 1172

Maccoby, M. (2007) *The Leaders we Need and What Makes us Follow*. Boston: Harvard Business School Press

McKimm, J and Leiff, S. (in press) Medical education leadership. In J.A. Dent and R.M. Harden (eds) *A Practical Guide for Medical Teachers*. 4th edn. London: Elsevier Churchill Livingstone

McKimm, J. and McLean, M (2011) Developing a global health practitioner: time to act? *Med Teach*. 33(8): 626–631

McKimm, J., Rankin, D., Poole, P., Swanwick, T., and Barrow, M. (2009) Developing medical leadership: a comparative review of approaches in the UK and New Zealand, *Int J Publ Serv Leadership*. 5(3): 12–26

McKimm, J. and Swanwick, T. (2010) Educational Leadership. In T. Swanwick (ed.) *Understanding Medical Education* (pp. 419–437). Oxford: Wiley Blackwell and Association for the Study of Medical Education

McKimm, J. and Swanwick, T. (2009) *Educational Leadership*. Edinburgh: Association for the Study of Medical Education

Mennin, S. (2010) Self-organisation, integration and curriculum in the complex world of medical education. *Med Educ*. 44: 20–30

Meyerson, D. (2004) The tempered radicals. *Stanford Social Innovation Review*. 2(2): 14–23

Mills, C. Wright (1959) *The Sociological Imagination*. Oxford: Oxford University Press

Mintzberg, H. (1992) *Structure in Fives; Designing Effective Organisations*. Harlow: Prentice Hall

Mintzberg, H. (2009) *Managing*. USA: Berrett Koehler

Morgan, G. (1997) *Images of Organization* Thousand Oaks, CA: Sage

Moss, B. (2009) Ethics, vision and values: the challenge of spirituality. In J. McKimm and K. Phillips (eds) *Leadership and Management in Integrated Services* (pp. 93–105). Exeter: Learning Matters

Newman, M.A., Guy, M.E., and Mastracci, S.H. (2009) Beyond cognition: affective leadership and emotional labour. *Public Admin Rev*. 69: 6–20

NHS Institute for Innovation and Improvement (2010) *Enhancing Engagement in Medical Leadership: Medical Leadership Competency Framework*. 3rd edn. [Online] http://www.institute.nhs.uk/images/documents/Medical%20Leadership%20Competency%20Framework%203rd%20ed.pdf Accessed 16 June 2012

NHS Leadership Centre (2003) *NHS Leadership Qualities Framework*. London: NHS Leadership Centre

NHS Medical Careers. [Online] http://www.medicalcareers.nhs.uk Accessed 16 June 2012

Nonaka, I. and Takeuchi, H. (2011) The wise leader. *Harvard Business Review*. May: 59–67

Northouse, P.G. (2007) *Leadership: Theory and Practice*. 4th edn. Thousand Oaks, CA: Sage

Revans R.W. (1998) *ABC of Action Learning*. London: Lemos and Crane

Rich, E.C., Magrane, D., and Kirch, D.G. (2008) Qualities of the medical school dean: insights from the literature. *Acad Med*. 83: 483–487

Rost, J.C. (1991) *Leadership for the 21st Century*. New York: Praeger

Rost, J.C. (1993) *Leadership for the 21st Century*. Westport, CA: Praeger Publishers

Salovey, P., and Mayer, J. (1990) *Emotional Intelligence*. Amityville, NY: Baywood Publishing

Sargeant J, Mann, K., Sinclair, D., van der Vleuten, C., Metsemakers, J. (2007) Challenges in multisource feedback: intended and unintended outcomes. *Med Educ*. 41: 583–591

Schein, E.H. (1985) *Organizational Culture and Leadership*. San Francisco: Jossey-Bass

Schön, D. (1983) *The Reflective Practitioner, How Professionals Think In Action*. New York: Basic Books

Scott, S. (2004) *Fierce conversations: Achieving Success at Work and in Life One Conversation at a Time*. New York: The Berkley Publishing Group

Scottish Medical and Scientific Advisory Committee (2009) *Promoting Professionalism and Excellence in Scottish Medicine: a report from the Scottish Medical and Scientific Advisory Committee. SMJ.* 54(supplement 2): 17

Selznick, P. (1957) *Leadership in Administration A Sociological Interpretation.* New York: Harper & Row

Siebert, S.E. and Kraimer, M.L. (2001) The five-factor model of personality and career success. *J Vocat Behav.* 158(1): 1–21

Souba, C. (2010) Perspective: the language of leadership. *Acad Med.* 85: 1609–1618

Souba, W. (2011) Perspective: a new model of leadership performance in health care. *Acad Med.* 86(10): 1241–1252

Storey, J. (2004) Changing theories of leadership and leadership development. In J. Storey (2004) (ed.) *Leadership in Organisations: Current Issues and Key Trends* (pp. 11–37). Abingdon: Routledge

Tennyson, R. and Wilde, I. (2000) *The guiding hand: Brokering partnerships for sustainable development. Report to UN Department of Public Information theory, proxy to practice.* Paper for the Pan-Canadian Education Research Forum

Thach, E.C. (2002) The impact of executive coaching and 360 feedback on leadership effectiveness. *Leadership & Organization Development Journal.* 23: 205–214

The Academy of Medical Sciences. *Careers in Academic Medicine.* [Online] http://www.academicmedicine.ac.uk/careersacademicmedicine.aspx Accessed 16 June 2012

The Scottish Government. *Delivering Quality Through Leadership: NHS Scotland Leadership Development Strategy.* [Online] http://www.scotland.gov.uk/Publications/2009/10/29131424/0 Accessed 16 June 2012

The UK Foundation Programme Office (2011) *The Foundation Programme.* [Online] http://www.foundationprogramme.nhs.uk/pages/home/training-and-assessment Accessed 16 June 2012

Turnbull James, K. (2011) Leadership in context. Lessons from new leadership theory and current leadership development practice. In: *The Future of Leadership and Management in the NHS. No more heroes.* Report from The King's Fund Commission on Leadership and Management in the NHS. London: The Kings Fund

Uhl-Bien, M. (2006) Relational leadership theory: Exploring the social processes of leadership and organising. *The Leadership Quarterly.* 17: 654–676

Van Zwanenberg, Z. (2003) *Modern Leadership for Modern Services.* Alloa: Scottish Leadership Foundation

Waterman, R.H., Peters, T.J., and Philips, J.R. (1980) Structure is not organisation. *Business Horizons.* June: 14–26.

Western, S. (2012) An overview of leadership discourses. In M. Preedy, N. Bennett, and C. Wise (eds) *Educational Leadership: Context, Strategy and Collaboration* (pp. 11–24). Milton Keynes: The Open University

Whitehead, C. (2010) Recipes for medical education reform: Will different ingredients create better doctors? *Soc Sci Med.* 70: 1672–1676

Whitmore, J. (2002) *Coaching for Performance.* 3rd edn. London: Nicholas Brealey

World Health Organization (2007) *Everybody's Business: Strengthening health systems to improve health outcomes. WHO's Framework for Action.* Geneva: WHO

World Health Organization (2009) *Framework for action on interprofessional education and collaborative practice.* Geneva: WHO

Zaleznick, A. (2004) Managers and leaders: Are they different? *Harvard Business Review.* 82(1): 74–81

Index

A

abductive reasoning 622
abuse issues 277
academic partnerships between low-
    and high-income countries 679
academic records 390
academic systems 702–3
academies of educators 664–5
accountability 514
    social accountability 672
accreditation 346–7
    continuing professional development 357
    Lancet Commission findings 702
action research 643
    in e-learning development 177
    participatory (PAR) 621–2
administration 723
admission
    criteria 703
    dropout relationships 400–5
    open admission versus selection 401–2
    see also selection
adult learning 101–2, 351
affective leadership 726
affordance 168
ageing population 326, 707
ambulatory care 5, 221–2
    assessment 229
    learning enhancement 225–8
    learning opportunities 222
    teachers in 228–9
    teaching evaluation 229–30
    teaching venues 222–5
    when to teach in 228
ambulatory care teaching centres (ACTC) 224,
    226, 230
analytic judgement standard-setting
    method 427
andragogy 101, 241
Angoff standard-setting procedure 416–17,
    424–5
application forms 390–1
appraisal system 269
appreciative inquiry (AI) 40
apprenticeship 211, 303
    cognitive 261

Approaches to Teaching Inventory 303
aptitude tests 390, 501
artefacts 282, 566
    feedback relationship 571
arthritis educator programme 315–16
assessment 6–7, 409–18, 432, 606
    advanced clinical assessments 34
    in ambulatory care setting 229
    classroom assessment techniques
        (CATs) 458
    clinical ability 436–9
    cognitive ability 433–7
    concept map use 96–7
    constructive alignment 69
    continuing professional development 358
    cost and value 606–9
    effectiveness 607
    e-learning 182
    examination preparation 252
    facilitator assessments 34
    faculty development 716
    formative 191, 411, 457, 478–86
        see also formative assessment
    impact on learning 479–81
    instrument selection 432–3, 440
    integrated assessment 69–70
        clinical assessments 70
        written assessments 69–70
    knowledge application 504–5
    learners' needs see learners' needs assessment
    learning environment 105–7
    medical humanities 241
    mentoring and 269
    methods 411–13
    Miller's Pyramid 504
    peer assessments 33, 541
    performance 491–2, 496–7, 515–16
    postgraduate medical education 345–6, 347
    problem-based learning 32–4
    professionalism 6–7, 500–10
        difficulties 503
        pitfalls 509–10
        reasons for 502
    progress testing 69–70
    psychometrics 413–16
    purpose of 409–11, 421

rating scales 437
reliability 414–16, 544
for relicensure 513, 516–21
scholarship 659–62
for selection 385
self-assessment 34, 57, 250, 459
simulated patient use 203–4
    in situ assessment 203–4
simulations 33
stakes 421
standard setting 416–17, 421–30, 608–9
student-selected components (SSCs) 57–8
student teaching abilities 307
summative 191, 411, 457–8, 478
technology application 490–8
    benefits 491–3
    history 490–1
triple jump exercise 33
undergraduate medical education 330
validity 413–14, 492, 528–9, 543, 607
workplace-based 458–9, 508–9, 515, 537–46,
    608
    see also specific types of assessment; test-
        enhanced learning
assignments 251–2
assimilation theory 86–8
assumptions 282
attitudes
    formation of 153
    performance relationship 364
attribution research 472
audiovisual technologies 169
authentic learning 64

B

Beck Depression Inventory (BDI) 127
behaviourist perspectives 17, 127, 455, 565
Best Evidence Medical Education (BEME)
    systematic review 156–7
blogs 178
blueprinting 550
borderline group standard-setting method
    426–7, 528
borderline regression standard-setting method
    427, 528
boundaries, professional 43

Bourdieu, P. 141–2
Brazil, open university model 679
breakout model 225
buzz groups 157

C
California Personality Inventory (CPI) 129
career development 716–17
career pathways 704
case-based discussion (CBD) 540–1
case-based learning 40
   integration in 65
   see also problem-based learning (PBL)
causal-comparative research designs 628–30
cause and effect 617
central tendency error 437
change management 722–3
checklists
   objective structured clinical exams 526–7
   workplace-based assessment 537–8
classroom assessment techniques (CATs) 458
climate 364
   performance relationship 364–5
clinical attachments 54
   integrated learning 66–7
clinical competence 330
clinical evaluation exercise (CEX) 539
   mini-CEX 539–40, 543
clinical investigations suite 225–6
clinical placements 67–8, 215–16
CmapTools 95–6
coaching 367
   remediation 367
cognitive apprenticeship 261
cognitive architecture 75–6, 77
   see also information processing
cognitive-behaviour therapy (CBT) 127
cognitive load theory 74, 77
   cognitive load effects 79–82
      expertise reversal effect 80–1
      guidance fading effect 81, 83
      imagination effect 81, 83
      intrinsic element interactivity effect 81, 83
      isolated elements effect 81, 83
      modality effect 80, 84
      problem completion effect 79, 83
      redundancy effects 80, 83
      split-attention effect 79–80, 84
      transient information effect 80, 84
      variability effect 81–2
      worked example effect 79, 83
   curriculum and course design implications 82–4
   see also instructional design
   extraneous cognitive load 79
   germane cognitive load 79
   intrinsic cognitive load 78–9
   see also information processing
cognitive theories of learning 17
   small group work 152
collaborative competencies 44–5
   see also interprofessional education (IPE)
collaborative inquiry 41
collaborative learning 94–5, 152
   e-learning 179
   see also small group learning
collaborative practice 358–9
communities of practice (CoP) 120, 151, 213
   continuing professional development 352
   faculty development 713

community-based medical education 328–9
   Ethiopia 678
community service 328
competence 343–4
   clinical 330
   digital 179
competency 343–4
competency-based education (CBE) 330, 343–4, 703
complex adaptive system (CAS) 26
complexity theory 352–3
computer adaptive testing (CAT) 491
computer-assisted learning (CAL) 245–6
   see also e-learning
concept learning 86, 87, 446
concept maps 86, 87–8, 249
   directedness 88
   learning assessment 96–7
   software 95–6
   teaching students to use 88–94
   techniques 89–94
   use with groups 94–6
concurrent validity 128
conflict theory 137–8
Consortium of Longitudinal Integrated Clerkships (CLIC) 67
constructivist perspectives 17, 63–4, 87, 136, 455–6, 565, 619–20, 624
   transitions and 377
construct validity 128, 413, 628
consultation skill development 201
   video recording 228
content recontextualization 214, 216
content validity 628
Context, Inputs, Processes and Products (CIPP) model 26
contextual learning 26
continuing medical education (CME) 350
   e-learning and 180
continuing professional development (CPD) 5, 341, 350–9
   accreditation 357
      maintenance of certification 357–8
   activities 355
   assessment 358
   design 353–4
   domains influencing behaviour change 353
   effectiveness 355
   evaluation of educational outcomes 356
   external influences 356–7
   implementation 353–4
   interprofessional education influence 358–9
   patient safety influence 358
   performance relationship 364
   theoretical foundations 350–1
      adult learning theory 351
      complexity theory 352–3
      learning in communities of practice 352
      reflective practice 351–2
      self-directed and lifelong learning 351
      work-based learning 217–18, 352
   theories informing practice change 353
continuous quality improvement (CQI) 41, 515, 589–98
   see also quality
contrasting groups standard-setting method 426
control theory 26
conversation analysis (CA) 119
cooperative learning (CL) 26, 152
copyright issues 169

correlation research designs 628
cost issues 56, 601–10
   assessment cost and value 606–9
      work-based assessment 544
      written assessments 562
   e-learning cost and value 603–6
   escalating healthcare costs 244
   evaluation activities 583–4
   Lancet Commission findings 701–2
   medical education in developing countries 673–4
   objective structured clinical exams 531–2
   simulation cost and value 602–3
   technology 493
Council of Elders 316
counterbalanced study design 634–5
creative thinking skills 249
   development 251
criterion validity 413, 628
critical discursive psychology 120
critical theory 152–3, 247, 281, 620–1, 624
cueing effect 412
cultural–historical activity theory (CHAT) 566
culture 282
   feedback support 5, 566–7, 570–1
   performance relationship 364–5
   quality culture 594–5
      quality management relationship 596–8
curriculum 3–4, 5
   context 13, 19–22
   contradictions 15
   curriculum creep 32
   definition 13, 14
   design 18–19, 22
      with formative assessment 483
      see also instructional design
   developing countries 674–5
   diversity 13
      case for 19
      localizing content 19
   emerging market economies 685–6
   hidden curriculum 100–1, 143, 283, 289, 328
   ideology 15
   implementation 334–5
   influences on 16–18
      paradigms of learning 16
      political influences 16
      professional and social theories 16–18
   integration 64–6, 328, 498
      horizontal integration 65
      vertical integration 65–6
   knowledge base and 15–16
   learning to teach inclusion 307
   limits of 14, 64
   local relevance 674–5
   models 18
   omissions 14–15
   organ-based 31
   postgraduate medical education 344–5
   practice and 15
   professionalism integration 278–9
   resident as teacher programmes 291, 293
   spiral 65, 333
   student-selected components (SSCs) 50–9
      assessment 57–8
      cost issues 56
      curriculum issues 53–4
      definition 50–1
      global perspective 52
      implementation 51–2

learning outcomes and competencies 52–3
  models 52
  practical aspects 56–7
  staff engagement 57
  types of 54–6
for teaching improvement 714–17
theory 13
undergraduate medical education 332–5
  alignment of values and outcomes 332–3
  planning with implementation in mind 333–4
curriculum vitae (CV) 389–90, 662

D

day surgery unit (DSU) 223, 226
deductive theory 616
deep profiling 115
delivery 4–5
Delphi technique 644
demographic changes 326, 707
dependent variables 627
determinism 616, 624
developing countries 8, 671–81
  academic partnerships 679
  challenges 672–4
    costing and investments 673–4
    quality 672–3
    quantity 672
    relevance 673
  innovation examples 678–9
  meeting population needs 679
  requirements 674–8
    broad student recruitment criteria 675–6
    education alignment with health service delivery 677
    faculty training 675
    local relevance of curricula 674–5
    multisectoral collaboration and planning 676–7
    training sites at all levels of healthcare 676
diagnostic and treatment centres (DTC) 224–5
didactic teaching 41
digital competences 179
direct observation of procedural skills (DOPS) 229, 413, 540
disciplinary action 502–3
  see also remediation
discourse
  analysis (DA) 120, 139–41
  large group teaching as 166–8
discrimination 277
discussion boards 179
discussion groups 157
distance learning 245
distributive justice 388
divergent validity 128
dramaturgy theory 119
DREEM (Dundee Ready Educational Environment Measure) 105–6
dropout 6, 398–405
  estimation of 398–9
  failure time analysis techniques 404–5
  predictor variables 399–400
    sociodemographic variables 403–4
  reasons for 399
  selection relationships 400–5
    active selection versus lottery 402–3
    selection method effects 403
    selection versus open admission 401–2
due process 520

E

Ebel's standard-setting method 425–6
educational ecologies 170
educational leadership see leadership
educational supervision 367
  see also supervision
elaboration 152
e-learning 4, 174–83, 331
  case studies 177–8
  collaborative learning 179
  context 177
  continuing medical education (CME) 180–1
  cost and value 603–6
  effectiveness 604
  evaluation 177–8
  framework 174–8
  future developments 181–3
    assessment 182
    cost-effectiveness 182–3
    immersive learning environments 181–2
    research 183
    sharing online resources 182
    ubiquitous learning 181
    understanding effective e-learning processes 182
  informal learning 178–9
  instructional design 176
  interprofessional education 41–2
  sharing online resources 606
  tutor importance 180
  usability testing 179–80
  see also technology
elective study 55–6, 246
emerging adulthood 114–15
emerging market economies 683
  challenges 685–8
    curriculum development 685–6
    growth of medical schools 687–8
    medical ethics teaching 686–7
    research 687
    specialists versus generalists 688
    student selection 686
    teacher training 687
    teaching and learning 687
  medical education evolution 683–5
e-moderation 179
emotional intelligence (EI) 131, 726
  measurement 131–2
epidemiologic changes 326, 707
epigenetic system 77, 78
epistemological assumptions 616
EPITOMISE logbook 227
e-portfolios 181, 229, 496, 571
espoused values 282
essay questions 33, 433, 560–1
  modified (MEQ) 33, 433, 560–1
    technology application 493–6
ethics
  of evaluation 586–7
  publication 650
  teaching in emerging market economies 686–7
Ethiopia, community-based learning 678
ethnography 640
evaluation 7, 460, 577–87
  approaches 582
  budgeting 583–4
  data analysis 583
  data collection 582
  dimensions of 581

e-learning 177–8
  ethics of 586–7
  evaluator role definition 580–1
  history of 577–8
  initiation/commissioning 580
  learners' needs assessment 460
  mentoring implementation 273
  meta-evaluation 584–5
  planning 581–2
  problem-based learning 32
  realistic 623
  reporting the findings 585–6
  resident as teacher programmes 292–5
  scholarship 659–62
    criteria 662–3
  standard setting 429–30
  theories 578–9
  utility 586
evidence-based practice 41
examination preparation 252
examinations see assessment
experiential learning 40
  continuing professional development 351–2
  faculty development 712–13, 715–16
  mentor role 269–71
  professionalism 281
  remediation and 366
experimental research design 630, 631–5
  counterbalanced design 634–5
  meta-analysis research designs 635–6
  non-equivalent comparison group design 634
  one-group, pretest, and post-test design 634
  one-shot case study design 634
  post-test only, control group design 635
  pre-experimental research 631–4
  pretest and post-test, control group design 635
  quasiexperimental research 634–5
  Solomon four group design 635
  static group comparison design 634
  time series design 634
expertise reversal effect 80–1
extended matching question format (EMQs) 435–6, 558
Eysenck Personality Questionnaire (EPQ) 127

F

facilitators
  ambulatory care 228–9
  e-learning 180
  interprofessional education 42
  online discussions 179
  preparing teachers as 42
  problem-based learning 28–9, 34
  small group learning 153
  student assessment 34
factor analysis 127–9
facts, learning of 446
faculty development 454, 498, 665–6, 675, 711–19
  approaches 712–14
    communities of practice 713
    learning from experience 212–13
    learning from peers, residents and students 713
    learning from structured activities 713
    mentorship 714
    work-based learning 713
  career development 716–17
  challenges 703

faculty development (*cont'd*)
  curriculum for teaching improvement
      714–17
  definition 711–12
  developing countries 675, 679
  developing as a teacher 718–19
  educational leadership 716
  evidence-based approach 717–18
  organizational change and 718
  research and scholarship 716
  theoretical framework 717
failure time analysis 404–5
falsification principle 618
feedback 7, 57, 251, 252, 479, 564–72
  concept map use and 95
  in context 566–7
  continuum 571–2
  cultural aspects 570–1
feedback (*Cont.*)
  effective feedback 481
  faculty development 713
  feedback activity 567–8
  feedback givers 568
  feedback receivers 568
  in formative assessment 481
  mentors 273
  peer feedback 57
  peer review 654–5
  postgraduate medical education 346
  practical models 569–70
  professionalism 280, 508
  reconceptualization 571–2
  responding to 57
  simulated patient use 204
  in simulation-based education 193
  support 570–1
  technology application 491, 492, 493
  test-enhanced learning 450
  theoretical perspective 565–6
  timing 569
  types of 569
fellowships 713
feminist perspectives 620
Flexner Report 341, 373, 697–8
focused discussion 228
formative assessment 191, 411, 457, 478–86
  curriculum design with 483
  definition 479–80
  for educational institutions 483–4
  feedback 481
  impact on learning 479–81
  in medical education 484–5
  objective structured clinical exams 524–5
  professionalism 504
  student perspectives 482–3
  teacher perspectives 482
  workplace-based assessment 545
Foucault, M. 139–41
Foundation for Advancement of International
    Medical Education and Research (FAIMER)
    664
functionalism 137

G
generalizability theory 415
general mental ability (GMA) tests 390
global workforce education 699
  see also developing countries; emerging
      market economies
goal setting, in self-regulated learning 471–2

Goffman, E. 138–9
goldfish bowling 158
governance 680
grade point average (GPA) 390, 403
gradual release 216, 217
grandstand model 225
grand theories 616
grounded theory 622–3, 640–1
guidance fading effect 81, 83

H
Hacking, Ian 143
halo effect 437
Harding, Sandra 143
Hawthorne effect 618
health
  knowledge-based advances 697
  performance relationship 363–4
healthcare trends 244
health psychology 127
hermeneutics 642
hidden curriculum 100–1, 143, 283, 289, 328
higher specialist training 341
Hogan Development Survey (HDS) 126
hubris syndrome 365
humanist approaches 17, 565
  see also medical humanities

I
ice breaking 40
identity 4
  acquiring additional identities 43
  cues 115
  development in emerging adulthood 114–15
  dramaturgy theory 119
  ethnomethodology 119–20
  future directions 121
  individual perspectives 113–14
  moral identity 115–16
  narrative approaches 117–18
      autobiographical past and imagined future
          117–18
      positioning theories 118
      structural theories 117
  possible identities 116
  professional boundaries and 43
  self-verification theory 115
  social or contextual perspectives 116–17
  sociocultural perspectives 120–1
  theoretical perspectives 113
identity status 114–15
imagination effect 81, 83
immersive learning environments 181–2
independent variables 627
inductive theory 616
information processing 75–6, 466
  borrowing and reorganizing principle 76
  environmental organizing and linking
      principle 78
  information store principle 76
  narrow limits of change principle 77
  in problem-based learning 26
  randomness as genesis principle 76–7
  see also cognitive load theory
information retrieval 247
information storage 247
information technology (IT)
  in emerging market economies 690–1
  feedback support 571
  use in assessment 497–8

see also e-learning; technology
inpatient to outpatient shift 328–9
institutional ethnography (IE) 142–3
institutionalized bias 503
instructional design 74–84
  e-learning 176
  four-component model (4C/ID-model) 82–4
      learning tasks 82–3
      part-task practice 84
      procedural information 83–4
      supportive information 83
  knowledge categories 74–5
  simulation-based education 190–1, 194–5
instrumentation 627–8
  reliability 627
  validity 628
integrated learning 63–70, 249
  clinical experience and 66–9
      clinical attachments 66–7
      community-based longitudinal placements
          67–8
  curriculum and 64–6, 328
  integrated assessment 69–70
      clinical assessments 70
      written assessments 69–70
  outcomes 67
  patient-centred 68–9
integrated panels 157–8
Integrated Systems Model (ISM) 26–7
  see also integrated learning; problem-based
      learning (PBL)
intellectual property issues 169
intercalated degrees 56
interdisciplinary teaching 328
  see also interprofessional education (IPE)
interprofessional education (IPE) 38–47,
    329–30
  acquiring additional identities 43
  boundaries and identities 43
  building on experience 42–3
  case study 39, 43
  continuing professional development and
      358–9
  IPE process 39–40
  learning methods 40–1
      e-enhanced learning 41–2
      mixing and matching 42
      practice-based learning 42
  outcomes 44–5
      supporting evidence 45–7
  patient involvement 43–4
  simulated patient use 201
interviews 388–9
intimate examination skills 315
intrinsic element interactivity effect 81, 83
isolated elements effect 81, 83
item total score correlation (ITC) 529
IT resources, problem-based learning 31

J
Jimma Medical School, Ethiopia 678
job analysis 386
journal clubs 355

K
Kirkpatrick's Model of Learning 292, 294
knowing-in-action 351
knowledge
  application assessment 504–5
  categories 74–5

biologically primary knowledge 74–5
biologically secondary knowledge 75
growth of 244, 343, 707
types of knowing 623–4
working 504
knowledge-to-action (KTA) cycle 356
knowledge translation (KT) 356

L
Lancet Commission 700–1
major findings 701–5
academic systems 702–3
accreditation 702
admission criteria 703
career pathways 704
channels 703–4
competencies 703
financing 701–2
global landscape 701
global–local health 704–5
large group learning 163–71
cognition and 164–5
continuing professional development 355
as discourse 166–8
in educational ecologies 170
follow up 166
literature review 164
preparation 165
presentation 165–6
technology use 168–9
variations 166
Latour, Bruno 143
leadership 9, 566, 708, 722–32
affective 726
change leadership 722–3
contingent 727
development 728–9, 731, 732
educational leadership 731
activities 730
awareness 729
engagement 729–30
faculty development 716
leading people, groups, and teams 726
management and 723–4
organizations and 724–5
performance relationship 365
servant 727
situational 727
theories and concepts 726–8
trainers for future educational leaders 730
transactional 566, 727
transformational 566, 723, 727
learner-centred approach 228
individualized learning plans 455
simulation-based education 188–9
learner-centric ecological approach 178
learner/employee recontextualization 215
learners' needs assessment 453–9
assessing 457–9
evaluation 460
learning 455–7
planning 455
struggling learners 459–60
learning
adults 101–2, 351
in ambulatory care 222
approaches to 245–6, 455–6
authentic 64
case-based 40
channels 703–4

collaborative 94–5, 152
computer-assisted (CAL) 245–6
see also e-learning
concept 86, 87, 446
contextual 26
cooperative 26, 152
deep learning skills 250–1
distance 245
facts 446
individualized learning plans 455
Kirkpatrick's model 292, 294
learning by doing 188
mastery learning 191–2
meaningful 86–8
observation-based 40
outcomes 52–3, 455, 505
paradigms 16, 17
practice-based 42
propositional 86, 87
representational 86
resources 456
rote 86
self-directed 182, 189, 245, 251
situated 64, 200, 717
styles 456
task-based 227
team-based 329
to teach *see* students learning to teach
transformative 64, 153, 705–6
see also e-learning; experiential learning;
    integrated learning; large group
    learning; problem-based learning (PBL);
    small group learning; test-enhanced
    learning; work-based learning
learning contracts 227
learning environment 3–4, 100–7
adult learning and 101–2
assessment of 105
qualitative analysis 106
quantitative analysis 105–6
SWOT analysis 106
emotional aspects 103
environment–person reciprocal exchange
    472–3
immersive 181–2
importance of 105
improvement of 107
managed (MLE) 176–7
needs assessment 457
opportunities 104
organizational aspects 103
people 104
personal perceptions 103–4
professionalism and 283–4
resources 104
small group learning 154–5
social aspects 103
teaching or learning activities 104
virtual (VLEs) 56, 104–5, 176–7
Learning Environment Inventory 105
learning portfolios 57, 249, 346, 543
e-portfolios 181, 229, 496, 571
professionalism assessment 509
workplace-based assessment 542–3
learning resources
identification of 247
problem-based learning 31
sharing online resources 182
lectures 4, 163–4
cognition and 164–5

as discourse 166–8
follow up 166
methods and systems 168
preparation 165
presentation 165–6
see also large group learning
lecture theatres 168–9
legitimate peripheral participation (LPP) 120,
    213, 279
faculty development 717
leniency error 437
libraries 31
licensure 514
see also relicensure
logbooks 227, 229
workplace-based assessment 542–3
logical error 437
logic model 515–16
long case assessment 439
longitudinal integrated attachments 66–7

M
McKinsey's 7S model 724
Makerere University, Uganda 679
managed learning environments (MLEs) 176–7
management 723–4
manuscripts *see* publication
market forces 708
Marxist perspectives 620–1
mastery learning 191–2
Mayer–Salovey–Caruso Emotional
    Intelligence Test (MSCEIT) 131
meaningful learning 86–8
means–end analysis 79
MedEdPORTAL 27
media sharing 178
medical compentencies 124–5
emotional intelligence and 131
medical education
changing approaches 211–12
cost 7
developing countries 8, 671–81
challenges 672–4
innovation examples 678–9
requirements 674–8
developments 245–6
emerging challenges 700
emerging market economies
    683–91
challenges 685–8
evolution 683–5
future 690–1
present situation 688–90
evaluation 7, 460
formative assessment in 484–5
future directions 9, 144–5, 707
globalization 144
guiding principles 679–80
history 137–8
planning 455
reforms 697–700, 705
driving forces 707–8
global workforce education 699
nursing education 699
public health education 699
recommendations 705–6
research 7–8
socialization 138–9
transitions 372–9
future research 378–9

medical education (*cont'd*)
    interventions 377–8
    medical student to junior doctor/
        postgraduate 374–5
    perspectives 375–7
    preclinical to clinical medical
        training 373–4
    specialty trainee to consultant 375
    see also postgraduate medical education
        (PME); undergraduate medical
        education (UGME)
Medical Education Partnership Initiative
    (MEPI) 678
medical humanities 233–41
    assessment 241
    educational drivers 233–4
    educational objectives 233, 241
    knowing the body 236
    listening 237–9
    medical gaze 236–7
    medical models of normality 239–40
    metaphor 234–6
    patient narratives 237–8
    reflective practitioner 240
    teaching methods 240–1
medicalization of society 136–7
Medical Leadership Competency Framework
    (MLCF) 728, 729
medical textbooks 141
membership categorization analysis (MCA)
    119–20
mental health education, patient involvement
    316–17
mentoring 5, 265–73, 367, 454
    appraisal system 269
    barriers to 267–8
        identification of 272
    benefits of 266–7
        to mentee 266
        to mentor 266–7
        to organization 267
    confidential advisors 273
    faculty development 714
    formative assessment systems 269
    implementation 272–3
        evaluation 273
    mentee roles 271–2
    mentors 272–3
        incentives 273
        peer feedback 273
        roles of 269–71
        training 272
    models 268–9
    remediation 367
meta-analysis research designs 635–6
metacognition 470
meta-evaluation 584–5
metaphor 234–6
Meyer, John W. 143
middle-range theories 616
mini-CEX 538–40, 544
    validity 543
Minnesota Multiphasic Personality Inventory
    (MMPI) 126, 129
mistreatment 277
modality effect 80, 84
modified essay questions (MEQ) 33, 433,
    560–1
    technology application 493–6
MOOCs (massively open online courses) 170

moral identity 115–16
motivation 152
    improvement 471
    resident teachers 289
    self-regulated learning 466, 471–2
multimedia learning 176
multiple-choice questions (MCQs) 411–12,
    434–5, 458, 553–8
    extended matching question format (EMQs)
        435–6, 558
    integrated learning assessment 69
    problem-based learning assessment 32–3
    question flaws 554–7
        convergence strategy 554–5
        elimination of 557–8
        grammatical clues 55, 554
        incongruous options 554
        irrelevant difficulty 556–7
        long correct answer 555
        use of absolute and vague terms 556
    technology application 493, 494
    true/false format 434, 551–3
multiple mini-interview (MMI) 389
musculoskeletal examination skills 315–16
music 237–9, 240
Myers–Briggs Type Indicator (MBTI) 126

N

narrative 117
    coherence 117
    identity approaches 117–18
    patient narratives 237–8
narrative research 642–3
Nedelsky's standard-setting method 423–4
needs assessment *see* learners'
    needs assessment
NEO Personality Inventory 126
    Revised (NEO-PI-R) 129
net generation 175–6
nine events of instruction 176
nominal group technique 644
non-equivalent comparison group study design
    634
note taking skills 253
nursing education 699

O

objective setting 271
objective structured clinical examinations
    (OSCEs) 33, 140, 330, 412, 437–9, 459,
    524–34
    administration 534
    appeals 534
    formative 524–5
    integrated learning assessment 70
    mark sheet processing 534
    practical considerations 529–32
    raters 527, 533
    reporting results 534
    scoring instruments 526–7, 532
    setting standards 527–8
    simulated patient use 203
    standardized patients 525
    station writing 532–3
    subjectivity 412
    summative 524–5
    test security 529
    validity 528–9
objective structured teaching examination
    (OSTE) 292, 294, 307

objectivism 617
observational research design 628–30
    causal-comparative research designs 628–30
    correlation research designs 628
    experimental research designs 630
    survey research designs 628
observation-based learning 40
obsessive–compulsive disorder 127
one-group, pretest, and post-test study design
    634
one-shot case study design 634
online learning *see* e-learning
ontological assumptions 615
oral/viva voce examinations 436
organizational change
    faculty development and 718
    management and leadership 722–3
organizational culture *see* culture
organizational justice 388
organizational socialization 376–7
organizational values 594–6
    competing values framework 594
organizations 724–5
outpatient clinics 222
    learning enhancement 225
    simulated patient use 223
    see also ambulatory care

P

paradigms 638–9
parallel consulting 68–9
Parallel Rural Community Curriculum (PRCC),
    Flinders University, Australia 67–8
parents as teacher programmes 317
participatory action research (PAR) 621–2
patient-centred care 300, 304
patient-centred learning 68–9
patient education 300, 304
patient involvement 5, 311–21
    active involvement 311
    classification 312–13
        Cambridge Framework 312–13
    future directions 320–1
    interprofessional education 43–4
    learners' perspectives 318
    mental health 316–17
    outcomes 317
    parents as teacher programmes 317
    Patient Instructor (PI) programmes 315
    patients' perspectives 318
    practical considerations 318–20
        preparation and training 319
        recruitment 319
        remuneration 320
        representativeness 319
        retention and sustainability 320
    professionals' perspectives 318
    rationale 313–14
        government and professional policy
            313–14
        patients as experts 314–15
        social accountability 314
    senior mentor programmes (SMPs) 316
    as teachers of clinical skills 315–16
    teaching in ambulatory care 228, 229
    terminology 312
    theoretical perspectives 314–15
patient journey record book 228
patient surveys 541–2
pedagogic recontextualization 214, 216

pedagogy 241, 377
  remediation 365–6
  transitions and 377
peer assessments 33
  workplace-based 541
peer-assisted learning (PAL) 228, 305–6
  planning and implementation 306
  potential disadvantages 306
  reported benefits 306
peer feedback 57
  faculty development 713
  mentors 273
peer review 654–5
peer teaching 250
performance 363–9
  assessment 491–2, 515–16
    technology application 496–7
  determinants of 363
    climate and culture 364–5
    health 363–4
    medical education 364
    personality 129–30, 364
    team working and leadership 365
    workload and sleep 365
  reassessment 368
  underperformance identification 362–3
  see also assessment
personality 4
  Five Factor Model 364
  inventories 390–1
  leadership and 731
  performance relationship 129–30
  professionalism relationship 124
  stress relationship 130–1
  theoretical approaches 125–8
    behaviour theories 127
    biological theories 127
    cognitive-social-learning theories 127
    cognitive theories 127
    humanistic theories 126–7
    psychodynamic theories 125–6
    trait theories 127–8, 129
Personal Qualities Assessment
  (PQA) 131–2, 391
phenomenography 366
phenomenology 641–2
physical examination skills 202, 315–16
placebo effect 618
plagiarism 57–8
  detection software 491
  publication 651–2
political validity 392–3
portfolio see learning portfolios; teaching
  portfolio
positioning theories 118
positivism 615, 616–18, 638–9
postgraduate medical education (PME) 216–17,
  340–7
  changes and trends 342–3
  competency-based training 343–4
  definition 341
  development and implementation
    344–7
    accreditation 346–7
    assessment 345–6
    challenges 347
    curriculum 344–5
    feedback 346
    teaching skills 245
  historical perspective 340–1

supervision 257–9
  versus higher specialist training 341
postpositivism 618–19, 624, 639
post-test only, control group study design 635
post-traumatic stress disorder (PTSD) 19
power 140
power distance 365
practice-based learning, interprofessional
  education 42
PRECEDE (Predisposing, Reinforcing and
  Enabling Causes in Educational Diagnosis
  and Evaluation) model 353
predictive validity 128
prepositivism 638
President's Emergency Plan for AIDS Relief
  (PEPFAR) 678
pretest and post-test, control group design 635
PRISMS model 64
problem-based learning (PBL) 3, 25–6, 246, 331
  assessment 32–4
    advanced clinical assessments 34
    concept map use 97
    essay questions 33
    facilitator assessments 34
    multiple choice exams 32–3
    objective structured clinical exams
      (OSCEs) 33
    peer assessments 33
    self-assessment 34
    simulations 33
    triple jump exercise 33
  effectiveness 34–5
  evaluation of 32
  facilitators 28–9
    number of 29
    selection of 28–9
    training of 29
  grading systems 32
  groups 29–31
    optimal group composition 30
    optimal group size 29–30
    resources 31
    role assignments 30
    time management 30–1
  integration in 65
    Integrated Systems Model (ISM) 26–7
  interprofessional education 41
  methods 25
  modules (PBLMs) 27
  problems (cases) 27–8
    characteristics of 27
    selection issues 27–8
    sources of 27
  small groups 158
  underlying theories 26
problem completion effect 79, 83
problem-solving 79, 249
procedural justice 388
professionalism 124, 144, 275–84, 500–1
  as an educational issue 277
  assessment 6–7, 500–10
    difficulties 503
    methods 508–9
    pitfalls 509–10
    reasons for 502
    steps 505–8
  contemporary issues 502
  development of 501
  educational environment and 283–4
  integration into curricula 278–9

content 279
educational outcomes 279
mistreatment and abuse 277
professional conflict situations 278
  assessment of observed behaviour 278
  learning benefit resulting in patient harm
    278
selecting for 501
teaching and learning methods 282–3
theoretical considerations 279–84
  experiential learning 281
  reflective practice 280–1
  role modelling 279–80
  self-directed learning 281–2
  situated learning theory 279
  socialization theory 282
professional theories 16–18
programme theory 578–9
progress testing
  integrated learning 69–70
  problem-based learning 33
projective tests 126
propositional learning 86, 87
proximity error 437
psychoanalysis 125–6
publication 8, 648–56
  intellectual integrity of a manuscript 648–50
    conclusions 649
    context 649
    design and power 649
    problem statement and relevance 649
    writing style 650
  manuscript submission 652–4
    choice of journal 652
    cover letter 651, 653
    editorial decisions 655–6
    electronic submission 653
    title 653–4
  moral integrity of a manuscript 650–2
    authorship issues 651
    plagiarism 651–2
  peer review 654–5
public awareness 244
public health education 699
public policy 708

Q
qualitative research 638, 639
  action research 643
  ethnography 640
  grounded theory 640–1
  hermeneutics 642
  in medical education 639–40, 644–5
  mixed method research 644
  narrative research 642–3
  phenomenology 641–2
quality 7, 589–98
  definition 590
  in higher education 590–1
  improvement (QI) 358, 515
    continuous quality improvement (CQI) 41,
      515, 589–98
  management 335, 591–4
    effectiveness 591–4
    implications for practice 598
    organizational culture importance
      596–8
    total quality management (TQM) 591–2
  medical education in developing countries
    672–3

quality (*cont'd*)
    quality culture 594–5
    research on quality conceptions 590–1
    written assessments 561
quantitative research 626
    methods 626–36
        dependent variables 627
        independent variables 627
        instrumentation 627–8
        observational research design 628–30
        research question clarification 626–7
        threats to internal and external validity 630–1
        see also experimental research design

R

raters, objective structured clinical exams 527
    recruitment 533
rating scales 437
    objective structured clinical exams 526–7
    workplace-based assessment 538
realistic evaluation 623
recontextualization 214–15, 216
recruitment
    broad student recruitment criteria 675–6
    for patient involvement 319
    raters 533
    standardized patients 533
    see also selection
redundancy effect 80, 83
references, use in selection 389
reflection/reflective practice 57, 188–9, 248–9, 260–1, 453–4
    continuing professional development and 351–2
    faculty development 715–16
    feedback role 568
    mentor role 270
    professionalism and 280–1, 508–9
    in self-regulated learning 469
    strategic reflective thinking 472
reflective practitioners 240, 280
reform 3, 5, 697–700, 705
    driving forces 707–8
    global workforce education 699
    nursing education 699
    public health education 699
    recommendations 705–6
regulatory frameworks 680
reliability 128, 414–16
    instrumentation 627
    workplace-based assessment 544–5
    written assessments 551
relicensure 513–21
    assessment for 513
        challenges 519–20
        examinations 519
        frameworks 516–18
        measurement instruments 518–19
        risks 520–1
    bases 516
    definition 514
remediation 362–9, 458–9, 502–3
    evidence 366–7
    mentoring and coaching 367
    pedagogic theory 365–6
    remediation programmes 367–8
    supervision 367
    underperformance identification 362–3
    see also performance

replicability, test-enhanced learning 444
report back model 225
representational learning 86
research design *see* experimental research design; qualitative research; quantitative research
research projects 54–5
    assessment issues 54
residency 342
    see also postgraduate medical education (PME)
resident teachers 288–96
    attributes 289–90
    challenges 289
    motivations 289
    needs of 290
    resident as teacher programmes 291–6
        content 291, 293
        design 295
        evaluation 292–5
        implementation 295–6
        instructional methods 292, 293
    roles 288–9
retrieval practice *see* test-enhanced learning
reusable learning object (RLO) 182
ritual behaviour 155
robustness, test-enhanced learning 444
role modelling 260
    faculty development 715
    in learning to teach 305
    professionalism 279–80
role play 158
Rorschach test 126
Rosenberg Self-Esteem scale 126
rote learning 86

S

scholarship 8, 658–66
    assessment 659–62
    challenges for educators 663
    definition 658–9
    documentation tools 662
    evaluation criteria 662–3
    faculty development 716
    four frames model 663–4
    standards 660–1
    supporting infrastructure 663–4, 665
    support initiatives 664–6
        academies of educators 664–5
        faculty development programmes 665–6
        teaching commons 664
scoring
    objective structured clinical exams 526–7
    for relicensure 519
    scores versus standards 421
SCORM (Sharable Content Object Reference Model) 606
script concordance tests (SCTs) 558–9
Second Life 105
selected response questions 434–6
    extended matching question format (EMQs) 435–6, 558
    multiple choice questions (MCQs) 32–3, 69, 411–12, 434–5, 458, 553–8
    true/false format 434, 551–3
selection 6, 385
    developing countries 675–6
    dropout relationships 400–5
        active selection versus lottery 402–3
        selection method effects 403
        selection versus open admission 401–2

emerging market economies 686
    future research 393–4
    methods 388–92
        academic records 290
        CVs and application forms 389–90
        interviews 388–9
        mental ability and aptitude tests 390
        personality inventories 390–1
        references 389
        selection centres 391–2
        situational judgement tests 391
    process 385–7
    for professionalism 501
    selection system design 392–3
    validity 387
        candidate reactions 387–8
        fairness 388
    see also admission
selection centres (SCs) 391–2
self-assessment 34, 57, 250, 352, 459
    continuing professional development 358
    feedback role 568
    leadership qualities 731–2
    professionalism 508
Self-Assessment Inventory (SAI) 132
self-awareness 352
self-determination theory 26
self-directed learning (SDL) 245, 251, 470
    continuing professional development 351
    professionalism 281–2
    see also self-regulated learning (SRL)
self-efficacy beliefs 251
self-regulated learning (SRL) 182, 189, 453, 465–75
    clinical education 474
    contextualized and task-specific strategies 471
    cyclical feedback loop model 466, 467–9
        conceptual advantages 469
        forethought 468
        performance phase 468–9
        relevance of 473
        self-reflection 469
    future directions 474–5
    motivation and 466, 471–2
    multi-phase self-regulation training 470–1, 473
    preclinical education 473
    self-monitoring 467
    social-cognitive account 467
    strategic reflective thinking 472
    see also self-regulated learning (SRL); study skills
self-regulation 352
    medical education relationship 469–70
    theories of 466–7
    see also self-regulated learning (SRL)
self-verification theory 115
seminars 157, 713
senior mentor programmes (SMPs) 316
servant leadership 727
sexual harassment 277
shadowing 216
shift work, performance relationship 365
short answer questions (SAQs) 434, 559–60
short case assessment 439
simulated patients (SPs) 198–205
    hybrid simulation 202–3
    reasons for use 199–200
    required characteristics 204–5
        ability 204

credibility 205
  suitability 204
simulated outpatient clinic 223–4
theoretical underpinnings 200
use in assessment 203–4
  feedback 204
  objective structured clinical exams
      (OSCEs) 203
  in situ assessment 203–4
use in teaching 201–3
  consultation skill development 201
  interprofessional education 201
  physical examination skills 202
  procedural skills development 202–3
simulation 602
  cost and value 602–3
  see also simulation-based assessment;
      simulation-based education (SBE)
simulation-based assessment 492
  performance assessment 496–7
simulation-based education (SBE) 4–5, 186–7,
    330–1
  as a bridge to clinical practice 189
  case studies 193–5
  challenges 192–3
  cost and value 602
  drivers for 187
  evidence for effectiveness 189–90
    programme design level 190
    simulation encounter level 190
    simulation environment level 190
  feedback 193
  implementation 195
  instruction design 190–1, 194–5
  in interprofessional education 41
  learner-centred simulation 188–9
  learning and 187–8
    learning by doing 188
  mastery learning 192
  programme design 190–3
  range of simulation modalities 187
  simulation as social learning 193
  simulation use in assessment 33
  test-enhanced learning 447
  see also simulated patients (SPs)
Simulation-based Training for Enhancement of
    Procedural Skills (STEPS) 193–4
single best answer (SBA) multiple-choice
    questions see multiple-choice questions
    (MCQs)
situated learning 64, 200
  faculty development 717
  professionalism 279
situational judgement tests (SJTs) 391, 559–60
Sixteen Personality Factor questionnaire (16PF)
    129
skill development 153
  consultation skills 201
  physical examination skills 202, 315–16
  procedural skills 202–3
  simulated patient use 201–3
  simulation-based training 193–4
  test-enhanced learning 447
  see also study skills
sleep deprivation, performance relationship 365
small group learning 4, 151–9, 329
  active learning 155–6
  cognitive theory 152
  continuing professional development 355
  engagement in learning 155

evaluation 159
  group interaction 156
  influencing factors 152–5
    activity 155
    learners 154
    learning environment 154–5, 158–9
    learning outcomes expected 152–3
    tutor 153–4
  preparation 155, 156–7
    learners 155, 156
    staff 156–7
  social theory 151–2
  techniques 157–8
Smith, D. 142–3
snowballing 157
social accountability 672
social bookmarking 178
social cohesion 152
socialization 282, 376–7
social loafing 155–6
social networks 103, 178–9
social software 178–9
social theories 16–18, 565
  of self-regulated learning 467
  of small group work 151–2
  social learning theory 17
Solomon four group study design 635
SPICES model 64
spiral curriculum 65, 333
split-attention 79–80, 84
staff development see faculty development
Stages of Change Theory 353
standardized learners 292
standardized patients 31, 330, 525
  recruitment 533
  in test-enhanced learning 447–8
  training 532, 533
standards 421
  supporting evidence 423
  types of 422
  versus scores 421
standard setting 416–17, 421–30, 608–9
  choice of method 422–3
  compromise methods 428–9
  evaluation 429–30
  examinee-centred approaches 426–8
    analytic judgement method 427
    borderline group method 426–7, 528
    borderline regression method 427, 528
    contrasting groups method 426
    generalized examinee-centred method 427
  implementation 429
  objective structured clinical exams 527–8
  responsibility for 422
  test-centred approaches 423
    Angoff's method 416–17, 424–5
    Ebel's method 425–6
    Nedelsky's method 423–4
static group comparison study design 634
station clinics 224
stress
  personality relationship 130–1
  simulated patients 205
structured interviews 388–9
structured logbook 227
student advice, student-selected component
    opportunities 56
student assistantships 216
student-selected components (SSCs) see
  curriculum

students learning to teach 300–7
  aligning with intended outcomes 304
  appreciating the purpose of teaching 303–4
  assessment 307
  gaining practical experience 305
  identifying with a teaching role 302–3
  inclusion in the curriculum 307
  learning to teach patients 304
  reasons for 300–1
  role models 305
  specific teaching techniques 304
  specific training in teaching 305
student support, student-selected component
    opportunities 56
study guide 227
study skills 244
  application and problem-solving 249
  creative thinking skills 249
  integration of learning 249
  learning with understanding 247–8
  reflection 248–9
  self-assessment 250
  study plan development 246–7
  study skills courses 252–3
  teacher's roles 250–3
  teaching peers 250
study strategies 456
summative assessment 191, 411, 457–8, 478
supervision 5, 257–62, 367
  in ambulatory care 225
  by residents 288
    see also resident teachers
  feedback provision 568
    see also feedback
  functions 257–8
  levels of 258–9
  models 261–2
  patient safety and 259–60
  remediation 367
  of resident teachers 296
  theoretical perspectives 260–1
survey research designs 628
survival analysis 404–5
SWOT analysis, learning environment 106
symbolic interactionism 138–9

T
task-based learning (TBL) 227
task classes 83
teaching
  colleagues 300–1
  curriculum for teaching improvement
      714–17
  expectancy 152
  patients 300, 304
  peers 250
  perspectives on good teaching 303
  skills 345
  see also facilitators; students learning to teach
teaching clinics 223
teaching commons 664
teaching instinct 221
Teaching Perspectives Inventory (TPI) 303–4
teaching portfolio 662
team-based learning (TBL) 329
team-working 703
  performance relationship 365
  small group learning relationship 153
technology 174, 176–7, 489–90
  definition 490

technology (cont'd
  in large group teaching 174
  use in assessment 490–8
    benefits 491–3
    e-portfolio 496, 571
    history 490–1
    information technology (IT) 497–8
    performance assessment 496–7
    validity 492
    virtual patients 496
    written assessments 493–6
  see also e-learning
tempered radicals 725
test-enhanced learning 443–50
  generalizability 444–5
  implementation 445
    aligning retrieval practice with educational
      objectives 446–7
    feedback 450
    repetition 448–9
    spacing 449–50
    type of test 447–8
  robustness and replicability 444
  testing effect research 444
  theoretical mechanisms 445
tests see assessment
Thematic Apperception Test (TAT) 126
theoretical perspectives 615–25
  constructivism 17, 63–4, 87, 136, 377, 455–6,
    565, 619–20, 624
  critical theory 152–3, 247, 281, 620–1, 624
  deductive theory 616
theoretical perspectives 615–25 (Cont.)
  grand theories 616
  grounded theory 622–3, 640–1
  inductive theory 616
  middle-range theories 616
  participatory action research (PAR) 621–2
  positivism 615, 616–18, 638–9
  postpositivism 618–19, 624, 639
  realistic evaluation 623
  social reality 615–16
    epistemological assumptions 616
    ontological assumptions 615
  types of knowing 623–4
Theory of Planned Behaviour 353
time series study design 634
transactional leadership 566, 727
transfer-appropriate processing 445
transformational leadership 566, 723, 727
transformative learning 64, 153, 705–6
transient information effect 80, 84
transitions 372
  definition 372
  future research 378–9
  history of 372–3
  interventions 377–8
  medical student to junior doctor/
    postgraduate 374–5
  perspectives 375–7
    constructivist pedagogy 377
    interruption of medical education
      continuum 376

key characteristics of human development
  376
    organizational context 376–7
  preclinical to clinical medical training 373–7
  specialty trainee to consultant 375
tribalism 43
triple jump exercise 33
true/false questions 434, 551–3
  problems with 552–3
tutorials 157
tutors see facilitators

U
Uganda, Makerere University 679
UK Clinical Aptitude Test (UKCAT) 393
undergraduate medical education (UGME) 325–35
  changes since 1970 326–31
    assessment 330
    demographics and epidemiology 326
    healthcare delivery 328–9
    healthcare roles 329–30
    medical knowledge and technology 328
    science and technology of learning 331
    societal and consumer expectations 330–1
  context 325
  curriculum planning 332–4
  implementation 334–5
  performance relationship 364
  prior to 1970 325–6
underperformance identification 362–3
  see also performance; remediation
unprofessional behaviour 124
  mistreatment and abuse 277
  see also professionalism

V
validity 128, 423
  assessments 413–14, 492, 607
    objective structured clinical exams 528–9
    workplace-based assessment 543, 544–5
  external 630
    threats to 630–1
  incremental 387
  instrumentation 628
  internal 630
    threats to 630–1
  political 392–3
  selection procedures 387
value 601
  e-learning cost and value 603–6
  simulation cost and value 602–3
  see also organizational values
variability effect 81–2
video recording, student–patient consultation 228
virtual learning environments (VLEs) 56,
  104–5, 176–7
virtual patients 228, 496
viva voce examinations 436
voluntarism 616, 624

W
waiting time analysis 404
Walter Sisulu Medical School, South Africa 678

Web 2.0 178, 603
  see also e-learning; technology
Wikis 178
work-based learning 5, 209–18
  conceptualization 212–14
    sociocognitive theories 212–13
    sociocultural accounts 213–14
  continuing professional development 217–18,
    352
  faculty development 713, 716
  initial professional formation 215–16
  knowledge transfer 214–15
  literature review 210–11
  postgraduate training 216–17
worked example effect 79, 83
working knowledge 504
working memory 77, 78, 79
  see also cognitive load theory
workload, performance relationship 365
workplace-based assessment (WBA) 458–9,
  515, 537–46, 608
  acceptability 544
  checklists 537–8
  cost-effectiveness 544
  educational impact 544
    enhancement 545–6
  educational rationale 537
  instruments 538–43
    CBD 540–1
    DOPS 540
    logbooks 542–3
    mini-CEX 538–40
    patient surveys 541–2
    peer assessment 541
    portfolios 542–3
    single versus multiple observations 542
  practicability 544
  professionalism 508–9
  rating scales 538
  reliability 544–5
  summative versus formative assessment
    545
  validity 543, 544–5
workplace recontextualization 214–15, 217
workshops 713
writing style 650
written assessment 69–70, 549–62
  assessment criteria 550–1
  blueprinting 550
  cost and feasibility 562
  learning outcomes 550
  marking schemes 550–1
  purpose of 549
  quality assurance (QA) 561
  reliability 551
  technology use 493–6
  types of 551–61
    see also specific types

Z
zone of proximal development (ZPD)
  481